COMPLETE GUIDE TO

SYMPTOMS, ILLNESS & SURGERY

Revised Sixth Edition

By H. Winter Griffith, M.D.

Revised and updated by
Stephen Moore, M.D.
and
Kenneth Yoder, M.D.

Surgical Illustrations by
Mark Pederson

Editor
Jo A. Griffith

A Perigee Book

A PERIGEE BOOK
Published by the Penguin Group
Penguin Group (USA) Inc.
375 Hudson Street, New York, New York 10014, USA

Penguin Group (Canada), 90 Eglinton Avenue East, Suite 700, Toronto, Ontario M4P 2Y3, Canada
(a division of Pearson Penguin Canada Inc.) • Penguin Books Ltd., 80 Strand, London WC2R 0RL, England
Penguin Group Ireland, 25 St. Stephen's Green, Dublin 2, Ireland (a division of Penguin Books Ltd.)
Penguin Group (Australia), 250 Camberwell Road, Camberwell, Victoria 3124, Australia (a division of Pearson
Australia Group Pty. Ltd.) • Penguin Books India Pvt. Ltd., 11 Community Centre, Panchsheel Park, New
Delhi—110 017, India • Penguin Group (NZ), 67 Apollo Drive, Rosedale, Auckland 0632, New Zealand
(a division of Pearson New Zealand Ltd.) • Penguin Books (South Africa) (Pty.) Ltd., 24 Sturdee Avenue,
Rosebank, Johannesburg 2196, South Africa

Penguin Books Ltd., Registered Offices: 80 Strand, London WC2R 0RL, England

While the author has made every effort to provide accurate telephone numbers, Internet addresses, and other
contact information at the time of publication, neither the publisher nor the author assumes any responsibility
for errors, or for changes that occur after publication. Further, the publisher does not have any control over and
does not assume any responsibility for author or third-party websites or their content.

PUBLISHING HISTORY
First Perigee edition / July 1995
Fifth Perigee edition / March 2006
Sixth Perigee edition / December 2012

Sixth Perigee edition ISBN: 978-0-399-16151-3

The Library of Congress has cataloged the fourth Perigee hardcover edition as follows:

Griffith, H. Winter (Henry Winter), 1926–1993
Complete guide to symptoms illness & surgery / H. Winter Griffith ;
surgical illustrations by Mark Pederson.— 4th ed.
p.
Includes index.
ISBN 0-399-52609-9
1. Medicine, Popular—Handbooks, manuals, etc. 2. Symptoms—Handbooks, manuals, etc.
3. Surgery—Handbooks, manuals, etc. I. Title.
RC81.G834 2000
616—dc21   00-036049

PRINTED IN THE UNITED STATES OF AMERICA

10 9 8 7 6 5 4 3 2

PUBLISHER'S NOTE: Neither the publisher nor the author is engaged in rendering professional advice or
services to the individual reader. The ideas, procedures, and suggestions contained in this book are not
intended as a substitute for consulting with your physician. All matters regarding your health require medical
supervision. Neither the author nor the publisher shall be liable or responsible for any loss or damage allegedly
arising from any information or suggestion in this book.

Most Perigee books are available at special quantity discounts for bulk purchases for sales promotions,
premiums, fund-raising, or educational use. Special books, or book excerpts, can also be created to fit specific
needs. For details, write: Special Markets, Penguin Group (USA) Inc., 375 Hudson Street, New York,
New York 10014.

ALWAYS LEARNING   PEARSON

Contents

About the Author

H. Winter Griffith, M.D., authored many medical books, including the best-selling *Complete Guide to Prescription & Nonprescription Drugs, Complete Guide to Symptoms, Illness & Surgery for People Over 50, Complete Guide to Sports Injuries*, and *Complete Guide to Pediatric Symptoms, Illness & Medications*, all from Perigee Books. Others include *Instructions for Patients, Drug Information for Pediatric Patients, Vitamins, Minerals and Supplements* and *Medical Tests— Doctor-Ordered and Do-It-Yourself.*

Dr. Griffith received his medical degree from Emory University in 1953. After 20 years in private practice, he established a basic medical-science program at Florida State University. He subsequently became an Associate Professor of Family and Community Medicine at the University of Arizona College of Medicine. Until his death in 1993, Dr. Griffith lived in Tucson, Arizona.

Editors

Stephen Moore, M.D.
Family Physician, Tucson, Arizona.

Kenneth Yoder, M.D.
Surgeon, Tucson, Arizona.

Preface

Continuing with the work of H. Winter Griffith, M.D., this sixth edition of Complete Guide to Symptoms, Illness & Surgery revises and updates the topics from the fifth edition and adds a select number of important new illness and surgery topics. The information provided on the charts in this book can be of great help to patients and their families. It is presented in an understandable and easy-to-read format. As a practicing family physician, I place a tremendous amount of importance on my patients' understanding of their particular ailments. I cannot stress enough how important it is to the healing process for patients to fully comprehend all aspects of their condition. Your best chance to achieve and maintain optimal health is to participate fully in taking care of yourself. This book provides a tool to help you reach that goal. However, this book does not replace the services of your own health care provider. Be sure to follow his or her instructions and advice. If they differ from what you read in these pages, talk to your doctor or health care provider. They are the best source if you have questions or concerns.

Stephen Moore, M.D.

Take Care of Yourself

YOUR ROLE

As a patient, you can and should share responsibility with your health care provider for your medical care. Knowing the "what," "why," and "how" of a medical problem enables you to get maximum benefit from your medical treatment.

Many thoughtful and assertive patients wish to be more involved with their medical care. They don't want to be passive and powerless in matters that affect their own bodies. They don't want instructions or advice that is incomplete or lacking in credibility. They seek—and sometimes demand—enough information so they can think for themselves and participate in important medical decisions affecting them.

Patients who are well educated about their illnesses or a recommended surgical procedure are more likely to have a greater satisfaction with their medical care. The educated patient will have a better understanding and fewer surprises about the treatment steps, the expected outcome, and possible complications.

THE INFORMATION GAP

Somehow, and sometimes for justifiable reasons, a health care provider's medical information does not get explained, translated or transmitted into usable form for the most important member of the health-care team—the patient.

Even when information *is* competently conveyed to the patient by a doctor, nurse or other health professional, the patient has no follow-up written checklist to remind and reinforce what he or she has learned. This book is intended to provide patients and their families with the missing checklist and to supplement information you have received from your health care provider.

SIMPLE, CONCISE INFORMATION

Condensing the available mass of medical and surgical knowledge into one volume has required much simplification. We have tried not to omit major facts and concepts, but, of necessity, many details have been left out.

It is impossible to include all the factors and circumstances that affect each individual's health. Thus, your health care provider may take into account other factors not included here when he or she makes a precise diagnosis and recommends treatment for you.

The information in this book barely scratches the surface of all the information available about various medical subjects. It is supplemental to the knowledge doctors and other medical professionals have acquired. In addition to a medical education, most doctors have extensive clinical experience—and ideally, a great deal of wisdom and compassion.

WHAT YOU CAN FIND IN THIS BOOK

This book contains three major sections: Symptoms, Illnesses and Disorders, and Surgeries. Information for each is organized in chart form. The three chart formats vary somewhat, and each format is explained in detail in the following pages.

The book contains an appendix section to supplement information in the charts. The appendix entries cover a variety of topics that do not fit into the chart format used in the other sections. The topics include: a number of special diets; suggestions to reduce stress; instructions for breast, skin, and testicle self-exams; guidelines for safe drug use; information about condom usage as well as other subjects.

Also in the Appendix is a list of resources for additional information. If you want more, in-depth information about symptoms, illnesses, surgeries or other medical problems discussed in this book, the list provides a starting place to find that type of information. The resource list contains names, addresses, telephone numbers, and websites of organizations and government health agencies devoted to specific disorders.

A glossary section of medical-related terms is also included. This includes definitions of medical tests and medical terms that are used throughout the book. In addition, it will give a brief description of some rare illnesses and disorders that are not covered in the other sections due to lack of space.

WHAT YOU CAN'T FIND IN THIS BOOK

This book will not help you diagnose or treat your own illnesses in most cases. It can be a valuable starting point. Printed words cannot replace the knowledge and expertise that your health care provider provides.

This book does not replace the services of doctors and other health care providers. It is not a substitute for communication between you and your health care provider. Only he or she knows your medical history and special circumstances about your health. Only you know the intensity and exact quality of your symptoms. The printed page cannot capture or convey the *feelings* that accompany illness.

HOW YOU WILL BENEFIT

Yet, armed with introductory knowledge about symptoms, illness, and surgical procedures discussed in this book, you benefit in the following ways:
• You can better understand the nature of your illness.

• You can more easily recognize circumstances when medical help is necessary.
• You can learn useful facts about how to prevent disease and injury.
• You can confirm, refresh your memory and help your family learn and understand the facts regarding your illness.
• You can review a checklist of ways to make yourself better if you are ill.
• You can ask questions if treatment steps mentioned in the book differ greatly from what your health care provider advises. Recognize that medical professionals may have differing opinions, ideas, or practices on the course of treatment for a particular illness. Plus, newer and improved methods of treatment continue to be developed.

You should feel free to ask questions and discuss your concerns about treatment options with your health care provider. He or she should welcome and answer your questions. If not, you may want to consult another health care provider.

Your best chance to achieve and maintain optimal health is to participate fully in taking care of yourself. This book provides a tool to help you reach that goal.

Guide to Symptoms Charts

The symptoms charts are designed to suggest one or more illnesses and disorders that a specific symptom might indicate. Each chart focuses on one common symptom as shown on the list at the beginning of the section. The chart for *SWEATING, EXCESSIVE* appears on the facing page.

These charts do not include every possible *sign* or *symptom* the human body can exhibit, but they represent the most familiar and easily recognizable ones. *Signs* are observed. *Symptoms* are felt or experienced. A sign may be observed by the patient or by someone else. Symptoms are feelings only the patient can describe.

The charts provide a guide for how serious symptoms are. They give you clues as to what symptoms can mean. They refer you to other sections of the book for further information. *However, they are not intended as self-diagnosis charts*. No book should replace a competent doctor's diagnosis! The charts are only to help you decide how to proceed when you or someone else develops symptoms.

Refer to the numbers on the sample chart for an explanation of each heading described below.

1—SYMPTOM NAME

Charts are titled and arranged alphabetically by the name that is most common or that best describes the symptom (**SWEATING, EXCESSIVE**).

In cases where the symptom name is ambiguous, or the symptom can apply to several parts of the body, the body part is part of the title. For example,

SWELLING (a symptom) appears as separate charts titled: **ABDOMINAL SWELLING; ANKLES, SWOLLEN; SWELLING OR LUMP;** and **TESTICLES OR PENIS, PAINFUL OR SWOLLEN**. One chart is alphabetized by the symptom name, **SWELLING OR LUMP**. The rest are alphabetized by the body part the swelling affects.

If you can't find your symptom under its own name, refer to the list at the start of the section and check alphabetically for the main part of the body it affects.

2—SYMPTOMS & FACTORS

The main symptom is grouped in the first column with other symptoms or factors that frequently accompany it. Each group represents one or more separate illnesses or disorders that the symptom can indicate.

For instance, excessive sweating can mean many things, depending on what other symptoms appear with it. When accompanied by chest pain, excessive sweating can be a sign of heart attack. When accompanied instead by weight loss, coughing with blood, fever and fatigue, it can be a strong indication of serious lung disorders. Another entry relating to a disorder of the thyroid gland presents yet another possibility.

Often, none of the symptom groups will match your present problem. Your doctor knows your medical history and can perform a physical examination and use laboratory tests to diagnose your condition.

SWEATING, EXCESSIVE

SYMPTOMS & FACTORS	POSSIBLE PROBLEM	WHAT TO DO*
• Excessive sweating. • Anxiety or excitement.	Normal occurrence with stress.	• See Anxiety Disorder, Generalized. • See Stress.
• Excessive sweating. • Overweight.	Effect of excess weight.	See Obesity & Overweight.
• Excessive sweating in woman older than 38. • Irregular menstrual periods.	Hormone changes, end of menstrual cycles approaching.	• See Menopause. • See Perimenopause.
• Excessive sweating in woman during menstrual period. OR • Excessive sweating due to tension or apprehension. OR • Excessive sweating following coffee consumption.	No underlying disorder.	Nothing.
Excessive sweating in teenager.	Normal occurrence during adolescence.	Nothing.
• Sweating. • Palpitations, tremors, flushing. • Symptoms of anxiety when exposed to, or thinking of, a particular stimulus.	Fears.	See Phobias.
• Excess sweating. • Unpleasant body odor.	Several disorders.	See Hyperhidrosis.
• Skin is cool and moist. • Prolonged exposure to hot temperature.	Excessive fluid loss.	See Heatstroke or Heat Exhaustion.
• Excessive sweating. • Chest pain.	Heart attack.	• Call doctor now! • See Heart Attack.
• Excessive sweating at night. • Weight loss. • Persistent cough with blood in sputum. • Fever. • Fatigue.	Infection or cancer.	• See Hodgkin's Disease. • See Tuberculosis.
• Excessive sweating, plus 2 or more of following: • Weight loss. • Increased appetite. • Anxiety. • Sleeping problems.	Overactive thyroid gland.	See Hyperthyroidism.
• Excessive sweating. • Use of prescription, nonprescription or illegal drug.	Adverse reaction or side effect of drug.	• Consult doctor about prescription drug. • Discontinue use of non-prescription or illegal drug.
• Excessive sweating. • Fever.	Normal occurrence with fever.	See Fever charts (in this Symptoms section).

*All references are to Illness section unless noted otherwise.

3—POSSIBLE PROBLEM

The center column provides a short description of what a symptom group can indicate and may briefly define the illness or disorder to which you are referred in the third column.

In some cases, a group of symptoms can indicate more than one illness—sometimes they are totally unrelated. In that event, each description is listed next to an editor's bullet. For instance, one group of symptoms that we have discussed can indicate lung inflammation or infection, *or* cancer.

No attempt has been made to include every possible illness or disorder signaled by a symptom group. The identifications are based on illnesses that are *more obvious, most common, or most serious*. For similar reasons, some rare illnesses described on illness charts in this book may not be referred to on symptom charts.

4—WHAT TO DO

The more serious medical problems that require immediate help are usually preceded by directions to call your doctor *now*. Below that, you will often be directed to the illness chart in this book that explains the problem. For instance, one entry has the instructions:

• Call doctor now.
• See Heart Attack.
• See Coronary Artery Disease.

All "See ..." instructions refer to illness charts. Exceptions to this rule will be noted on the symptom chart.

If the chart says "Call doctor now," don't waste precious time looking up the illness in this book. Wait to read more about it when the crisis has passed. Call your doctor immediately!

If anyone develops dramatic symptoms that you think represent life-threatening danger, call for *emergency help*. Dial 911 and report your address or location (with directions if needed).

In extreme situations, render what first aid you can, such as giving cardiopulmonary resuscitation (CPR). Yell for help from anyone within range.

Additional emergency information appears on the pages just before the index.

Guide to Illness & Disorders Charts

The information about illness and disorders is organized in 578 condensed, easy-to-read charts. They cover the majority of illnesses (diseases or disorders) and some injuries that can affect humans.

Each topic is described in a one-page format as shown in the sample chart for *HYPERTHYROIDISM*.

Major sections of the chart format are numbered and explained in the next few pages.

Most of the charts in this section refer to an illness. In some cases, however, charts refer to disorders, injuries or problems that are not really illnesses. The chart, *TEETHING*, is not about a disease—or even a disorder. It deals with a normal process that all people experience. It would be a disorder only if it did *not* occur.

But teething can be a medical problem. It often affects an infant's sense of well-being, and it may require treatment. Because teething is so common, and because some treatments for it are appropriate and others are not, it is included with illness charts.

1—CHART NAME

Charts are arranged alphabetically by the most-common name for the illness, disorder or medical problem. Other names or terms for these appear in parentheses below the main heading. Hyperthyroidism may also be referred to as thyrotoxicosis, toxic goiter, or Graves' disease.

The chart names in this book, and most of the alternate names, are listed in the index. To find information about a medical problem, check the index.

2—GENERAL INFORMATION

This section includes seven topics: *Definition; Body Parts Involved; Sex or Age Most Affected; Signs & Symptoms; Causes; Risk Increases With;* and *How to Prevent.* Each is discussed separately.

3—DEFINITION

A short definition of the problem or disease is provided. Sometimes the definition must include information from other categories, such as causes, body parts involved, and others. The definition may also include information of general interest, such as how common a disease is, or whether it is contagious, cancerous, or inherited.

4—BODY PARTS INVOLVED

This is usually a list of specific body parts or organs, such as bones, skin, or liver. Sometimes general body systems, such as central nervous system, genitourinary system, or gastrointestinal system, will be listed. The list usually includes body parts affected at the beginning of the disease, as many diseases spread to other body parts as they progress.

Of course, some illnesses involve all body cells—even from the beginning. Then the words "Total body" appear.

5—SEX OR AGE MOST AFFECTED

Some medical problems affect specific population groups only. Others affect all ages and both sexes indiscriminately. This section explains whether the medical problem occurs more often in males or females, or whether the incidence is about equal in either sex. It also lists the age group usually affected. These are generalizations, and variations can occur with specific individuals.

Sometimes labels, such as "newborns" or "adolescents," are used to describe age ranges. These labels are arbitrary names for specific ages, but they are commonly used in medical texts. Following are the age classifications:

- Newborns (0 to 2 weeks)
- Infants (2 weeks to 1 year)
- Young children (1 to 5 years)
- Older children (5 to 12 years)
- Adolescents (12 to 20 years)
- Young adults (20 to 40 years)
- Middle-aged adults (40 to 60 years)
- Older adults (over 60 years)

6—SIGNS AND SYMPTOMS

Signs are observed. *Symptoms* are felt or experienced.

A sign may be observed by the patient or by someone else, or it may represent physical findings determined by laboratory tests, x-rays, and other diagnostic measures. Symptoms are feelings only the patient can describe.

Refer to the chart. The first item under this heading—hyperactivity—is a sign. It can be observed by the patient and others around him or her. The next three items—feeling warm or hot all the time, tremors and sweating—are signs *and* symptoms. They can be observed by others and they can be felt by the patient. The fifth—itching skin—is a symptom that only the patient can feel and describe.

Signs and symptoms are listed together in this book; no attempt is made to separate the two. On most charts, a wide range of possible signs and symptoms are listed. *It is unlikely that any patient will have all, or even most, of the possible signs and symptoms.* The presence or absence of signs and symptoms may vary according to:

- The age and sex of the patient.
- Extent of the illness.
- The stage of the illness.
- Medical and family history.
- Current state of health.

7—CAUSES

Many times the cause of a disorder is unknown. Causes for most medical problems include the following:
- Inherited or congenital defects.
- Infections from bacteria, viruses, parasites, yeasts, or fungi. All of these are sometimes referred to as "germs," but most people associate "germs" with bacteria only.
- Physical injury.
- Toxins (poisons) from a wide range of sources, such as contaminated food, environmental pollution, and bites from poisonous snakes or insects.
- Allergies.
- Tumors. These may be benign or malignant. Benign tumors do not spread to adjacent or distant organs and threaten life. Malignant (cancerous) tumors can.
- Endocrine disorders. This means too many or too few hormones are produced from the pituitary gland, thyroid gland, parathyroid gland, pancreas, adrenal glands, ovaries, testicles, or thymus gland.
- Mental or emotional disorders, such as anxiety, depression, or schizophrenia.
- Diseases caused by defects in the body's immune system. These include disorders of hypersensitivity, such as rheumatic fever, rheumatoid arthritis, systemic lupus erythematosus, and many others.

HYPERTHYROIDISM
(Graves' Disease)

 GENERAL INFORMATION

DEFINITION—Hyperthyroidism means the thyroid gland is overactive and produces too much thyroid hormone. The most common form of hyperthyroidism is called Graves' disease. The thyroid hormone is used by the body to regulate metabolism (producing energy).

BODY PARTS INVOLVED—Thyroid gland and most other body organs, especially the endocrine system.

SEX OR AGE MOST AFFECTED—Both sexes (mostly women); adults ages 20 to 50.

SIGNS & SYMPTOMS
* Anxiety, nervousness, and restlessness.
* Feeling warm or hot all the time; sweating; itchy skin.
* Heart palpitations.
* Weight loss, even though appetite increases.
* Sleeplessness, fatigue, and weakness.
* Frequent bowel movements.
* Women may have less menstrual flow.
* Eyes appear to bulge out, there is swelling around the eyes, and may have vision changes.
* Goiter (visibly enlarged thyroid) may occur.
* Hair loss.
* Tremor of the hands.
* High blood pressure.

CAUSES—Graves' disease is an autoimmune disorder. In these disorders, the immune system by mistake attacks the body itself in different ways. In Graves' disease, abnormal antibodies from the immune system cause the thyroid to produce more hormone. Other causes of hyperthyroidism may be due to thyroid disorders.

RISK INCREASES WITH
* Thyroid nodules or tumors.
* Thyroiditis (inflammation of thyroid gland).
* Personal or family history of thyroid or autoimmune diseases.
* Radiation treatment.
* Females more than males.
* Excess iodine intake.
* Stress may be a contributing factor.

HOW TO PREVENT—No known way to prevent.

 WHAT TO EXPECT

DIAGNOSTIC MEASURES
* Your health care provider will do a physical exam.
* Medical tests include blood studies for thyroid levels. Radioactive iodine studies may be done.

APPROPRIATE HEALTH CARE
* Treatment usually involves drugs to reduce thyroid hormone levels. Permanent treatment involves use of radioactive iodine or surgery. With these two treatments, thyroid hormone production is decreased. Sometimes, hypothyroidism (too little thyroid hormone) occurs, which will need to be treated.
* Radioactive iodine treatment is usually done as an outpatient. The iodine (taken by mouth) causes the thyroid gland to shrink over a period of months.
* Surgery to remove part of the thyroid (called a thyroidectomy) may be advised in some cases.
* For eye symptoms, an exam and follow-up care by an eye specialist (ophthalmologist) is often prescribed.

POSSIBLE COMPLICATIONS
* Thyroid eye disease (e.g., visual loss or double vision).
* Heart problems.
* Bone mineral loss (osteoporosis).
* Dermopathy (a skin disorder).
* Hypothyroidism (low thyroid hormone levels).
* Thyroid crisis (rare and possibly fatal complication).

PROBABLE OUTCOME—Treatment is effective in controlling the disorder. It may take 6 months for thyroid levels to return to normal.

 HOW TO TREAT

GENERAL MEASURES—Follow medical advice.

MEDICATION
* Antithyroid drugs to depress thyroid activity are usually prescribed. Follow-up blood tests are done to adjust the dosage until thyroid hormone levels are normal.
* Beta blockers to treat the heart and nervous system symptoms may be prescribed.
* Thyroid replacement drugs may be prescribed if the thyroid gland becomes underactive due to treatment.
* Avoid drugs or supplements that contain iodide. It may interfere with drugs used in treatment.

ACTIVITY—Usually no limits in otherwise healthy persons. In older persons or those with heart problems, decrease activity until thyroid levels are normal.

DIET—No special diet.

 CALL YOUR DOCTOR IF

* You or a family member has symptoms of hyperthyroidism.
* Symptoms worsen or new symptoms occur.

8—RISK INCREASES WITH

Many disorders have known risk factors that can trigger the problem, make it more likely to occur, or increase its duration and intensity. The most common risk factors include:
- Age, especially older persons or newborns and infants.
- Stress—either physical or emotional.
- Anxiety, depression and other mental or emotional problems.
- Fatigue or overwork.
- Poor nutrition due to improper diet or disease.
- Obesity.
- Recent or chronic illness that can lower resistance to other diseases.
- Recent surgery or injury.
- Genetic factors, such as family or ethnic tendency toward a disease.
- Use of drugs, such as alcohol, tobacco, caffeine, narcotics, psychedelics, hallucinogens, marijuana, sedatives, hypnotics or cocaine.
- Use of medications, whether prescription or nonprescription. Even necessary drugs cause adverse reactions and side effects that can complicate treatment and outcome of medical problems.
- Exposure to allergens, environmental pollutants, or poisons.
- Geographic areas.
- Crowded or unsanitary living conditions.
- Socioeconomic factors (e.g., income, poverty, social class, and education).

9—HOW TO PREVENT

Prevention can be of two types— prevention of the initial disease or prevention of a relapse or recurrence after recovery.

Prevention of any medical problem is the *best treatment*. Researchers continue to discover ways to prevent, delay or diminish some illness, pain, disability, and untimely deaths. These are included whenever available.

The causes and risk factors for a disease often provide the best clues for prevention. Many diseases, however, cannot be prevented at present.

10—WHAT TO EXPECT

This section includes four topics: *Diagnostic Measures; Appropriate Health Care; Possible Complications;* and *Probable Outcome*. Each is discussed separately below.

11—DIAGNOSTIC MEASURES

Your own observation of symptoms is usually the first—and often, most important—diagnostic measure. It is the first step toward medical treatment. For that reason, it is listed under this heading on almost all illness charts. Exceptions are made for a few medical problems, such as those that are signaled by unconsciousness, in which case self-observation is impossible.

A medical history and physical exam by a health care provider are also almost universal requirements before treatment for any disorder can begin. Even if a medical problem is usually treated at home, a history and exam will be necessary if complications develop that require medical treatment.

Additional diagnostic measures include laboratory studies and other medical tests. The most-common include:
- Studies of body fluids, such as blood, serum, plasma, or spinal fluid.
- Microscopic and chemical examination of excreted material, such as urine or stools.
- CT (computerized tomography) scans or x-rays of the affected body part.
- ECG (electrocardiogram), EEG (electroencephalogram), and EMG (electromyogram).

• Therapeutic trial of medication. This is used sometimes for a critically ill patient without a specific diagnosis while awaiting laboratory results.

You may not undergo every diagnostic test listed on the chart, and conversely, you may undergo tests not listed. Some tests are performed only if previous tests have not provided enough information. Others are performed only when complications develop. Most medical diagnostic tests mentioned in this book are defined in the Glossary.

12—APPROPRIATE HEALTH CARE

Self-care or home care is sometimes listed as the first form of appropriate health care. It is an important part of care for many disorders. Sometimes total self-care suffices if you have previous experience with a medical problem and a source to review important points in treatment.

Usually, however, a medical problem should be diagnosed by a doctor before you attempt self-care. Once your doctor diagnoses an illness and outlines a treatment program, self-care or home care is often important. Treatment measures outlined in this book are designed to guide you, whether you are caring for yourself or taking care of someone else.

Effective self-care includes maintaining a positive attitude about yourself and being determined to improve or heal. During illness, a sense of humor and a positive outlook are helpful in addition to the medication or other treatments.

Medical care is often necessary, not only to diagnose and prescribe treatment for a medical problem, but to supervise self-care (or hospitalization, when necessary) and to provide additional medical treatment such as surgery.

In addition, even the simplest medical problems sometimes develop complications and require a doctor's care. In those cases, a doctor's treatment can be appropriate even though it applies to a small fraction of cases.

Find a personal physician who communicates well with you and with whom you can establish a good rapport and mutual respect.

Psychotherapy, counseling, or biofeedback training may be the only useful health care for a medical problem caused mainly by stress or emotional problems.

Counseling and therapy are also helpful in providing personal and family support, especially with illnesses that are terminal or represent major lifestyle adjustments.

Rehabilitation is often helpful for illnesses or injuries that cause temporary or permanent disability. Rehabilitation may be provided by trained physical therapists or physiatrists (medical doctors who specialize in physical therapy). If rehabilitation is mentioned as appropriate health care, ask your doctor for information specific to your disability.

13—POSSIBLE COMPLICATIONS

Complications are additional medical problems triggered by or as a result of the original illness. Complications sometimes occur, despite accurate diagnosis and competent treatment. Some are preventable, a few are inevitable—but most are rare.

14—PROBABLE OUTCOME

Outcome (or prognosis) is a very important concern of the patient (and the family) in any illness. "What is going to happen to me? Is there a cure? How will this disease or injury affect my life?"

No one can completely predict the outcome of an illness or accident. The predicted or expected outcome information in this section is based on averages.

Patients and doctors work toward optimal results, but medicine is an inexact science. Response to treatment depends on many variables, and there are many unanswered questions about health and disease.

Some illnesses are considered incurable at present. The term "incurable" is a general one that includes everything from insignificant conditions that are mere annoyances to fatal diseases that bring certain death in a short time. For that reason, additional information about life expectancy is sometimes included for incurable illnesses. Again, individual variations are common, but the predictions are an attempt to answer a patient's most important questions. They help you adopt optimistic but realistic expectations.

In almost all cases—no matter how serious the illness—symptoms can be relieved or controlled to minimize pain and discomfort.

15—HOW TO TREAT

This section provides the checklist mentioned earlier that reminds you of instructions your doctor has given you. The information should not replace your doctor's instructions, because treatments vary a great deal between individuals.

If the instructions don't seem to fit your problem, ask your doctor or nurse for answers that apply uniquely to you.

The four major headings include: *General Measures; Medication; Activity;* and *Diet.*

16—GENERAL MEASURES

The instructions under this heading apply to home treatment. They cover common matters, such as soaks for skin problems, use of crutches, appropriate clothing, bandages, or bathing.

They are not complete and may not apply to everybody, but they provide a good review of general measures helpful for most patients.

17—MEDICATION

Information under this heading is generally of two types—drugs your doctor may prescribe, and nonprescription drugs you can take safely.

Prescription drugs are named by generic name or drug class. A brief description of a drug's purpose and effect is usually given. The Glossary contains entries for some generic drugs and drug classes mentioned in this book.

Additionally, you may refer to the book *Complete Guide to Prescription & Nonprescription Drugs.*

For general instructions about safe use of medicine, see the Appendix section.

18—ACTIVITY

Patients are often confused about whether they must stay in bed during an illness. They are often concerned with returning to work or school, and whether activity will be restricted after recovery. General answers to these questions are found under this heading.

In some topics, guidelines are given for resuming sexual relations—an important area that patients are sometimes reluctant to mention. If the illness has been life-threatening, as with a heart attack, or if it involves abdominal or genital organs, this is particularly pertinent information.

Exercise references are often included, and when not specified otherwise, references to regular physical exercise mean an *aerobic* exercise such as walking.

19—DIET

Diet information can vary from "no special diet" to references to special diets. Some of these special diets are included in the Appendix section.

For additional specialized diets, consult your doctor or a dietitian.

20—CALL YOUR DOCTOR IF

For most medical problems, a phone call or visit to your doctor is recommended to establish a diagnosis.

After diagnosis, when the course of an illness differs from what is expected, your doctor wants to know. Many developing complications can be averted with prompt medical treatment. Specific symptoms are often listed that indicate complications.

Of course, if any other symptoms begin that you believe are related to your illness or the drugs you take, call your doctor about them, too.

Guide to Surgeries Charts

The information about common surgeries, procedures, or medical tests is organized in two-page charts (first page has written information and second page has illustrations). See sample chart on *THYROID GLAND REMOVAL* on facing page (its illustration page is not shown).

Generally, the surgery topics in this section are those commonly performed as treatment for a disorder, such as thyroid-gland removal, or as a diagnostic procedure, such as dilatation and curettage. The topics may be about a minor procedure such as a toenail removal, or a major lifesaving procedure such as a heart transplant.

Sometimes a surgery is mentioned on an illness chart as part of treatment for that disorder. For instance, thyroid-gland removal is mentioned on the chart for hyperthyroidism (the previous sample chart) as a possible treatment.

Each major heading on the surgery information page is numbered in the sample chart, and the numbered sections are explained in the next few pages.

1—NAME OF SURGERY
Charts are arranged alphabetically by the name that most simply describes the surgical procedure. In some cases, medical professionals refer to the surgery by a more technical name. The technical name may appear in parentheses below the main title.

Thyroid-gland removal is clearly understood by everyone, but your surgeon may refer to it as *thyroidectomy*. Both names are included on the chart, and the surgery appears in the index under both names.

2—GENERAL INFORMATION
This section contains four topics: *Definition; Body Parts Involved; Reasons for Surgery;* and *Surgical Risk Increases With*. Each topic is discussed separately.

3—DEFINITION
A short definition of the surgery may include information about how common the procedure is and whether or not the medical problem requiring surgery is caused by congenital defects or is the result of disease or injury.

4—BODY PARTS INVOLVED
Body parts can refer to specific organs, such as the brain, or to body systems, such as the central nervous system.

Body parts are often defined in the text, if space permits. If you are not familiar with the body parts listed, and the parts are not defined in the text, check the Glossary for information.

5—REASONS FOR SURGERY
This section lists the most common reasons for a surgical procedure. (Of course, it cannot include *all* possible reasons.)

If the medical problems listed are unfamiliar to you, refer to the index. Some have separate illness charts, and the rest may be explained in the Glossary.

6—SURGICAL RISK INCREASES WITH
Risk factors make a surgery more complicated or delay healing. Following are common risk factors for most surgeries:

THYROID GLAND REMOVAL
(Thyroidectomy)

 GENERAL INFORMATION

DEFINITION—Removal of part or all of the thyroid gland.

BODY PARTS INVOLVED—Thyroid gland, the organ in the neck below the Adam's apple that controls the body's metabolism; lymph nodes in the neck.

REASONS FOR SURGERY
- Hyperthyroidism.
- Benign or cancerous tumors of the thyroid.
- Goiter (see Glossary).

SURGICAL RISK INCREASES WITH
- Adults over 60.
- Obesity; poor nutrition.
- Smoking.
- Untreated hyperthyroidism (see Glossary).
- Diabetes.
- Use of some prescription and nonprescription drugs. Inform your doctor of any drugs, medications, or vitamin and herb supplements you are using or have used in the last month.

 WHAT TO EXPECT

WHO OPERATES—General surgeon.

WHERE PERFORMED—Hospital.

DIAGNOSTIC TESTS
- Before surgery: Blood studies; ultrasound; CT scan; needle biopsy; radioactive-iodine uptake and scan (see Glossary for all).
- After surgery: Blood studies.

ANESTHESIA—General anesthesia by injection and inhalation with an airway tube placed in the windpipe.

DESCRIPTION OF OPERATION
- An incision is made in the neck following natural skin lines.
- Neck muscles are cut or retracted.
- Blood supply to the thyroid gland is clamped.
- The thyroid gland is cut free and removed, and a drain is left in place. In certain cases, some normal thyroid gland tissue is left intact.
- If cancer is present, some lymph nodes may be removed around the thyroid.
- The muscles are closed and the skin is closed with sutures or clips, which can usually be removed in 2 to 10 days after surgery.

POSSIBLE COMPLICATIONS
- Hoarseness or loss of voice, if vocal-cord nerves are damaged during surgery.
- Hypothyroidism (see Glossary).
- Hypoparathyroidism (see Glossary).
- Excessive bleeding.
- Surgical-wound infection.

AVERAGE HOSPITAL STAY—0 to 3 days.

PROBABLE OUTCOME—Underlying problem cured in most patients. Cancer that is present but has not spread may require radiation treatment. Allow about 6 weeks for recovery from surgery.

 POSTOPERATIVE CARE

GENERAL MEASURES
- A hard ridge should form along the incision. As it heals, the ridge will gradually recede.
- Shower as usual. You may wash the incision gently with mild, unscented soap. After showering, replace any wet dressings with clean, dry ones.

MEDICATION
- Your doctor may prescribe:
  - Pain relievers. Don't take prescription pain medication longer than 4 to 7 days. Use only as much as you need.
  - Thyroid hormones
  - Antibiotics to fight or prevent infection.
- You may use nonprescription drugs, such as acetaminophen, for minor pain. Avoid aspirin.

ACTIVITY
- Return to daily activities and work as soon as possible to promote healing.
- Resume driving 2 weeks after you return home.
- Resume sexual relations when able.

DIET—No special diet.

 CALL YOUR DOCTOR IF

- Pain, swelling, redness, drainage, or bleeding increases in the surgical area.
- You develop symptoms of infection including headache, muscle aches, dizziness, fever, or a general ill feeling.
- You develop symptoms of hypothyroidism, including excessive weakness, fatigue, intolerance to cold, menstrual irregularities, constipation, or dry and coarse skin and hair.
- You develop symptoms of hypoparathyroidism (see Glossary) including dry hair, brittle fingernails, dry or scaly skin, or irregular heartbeat.
- New, unexplained symptoms develop.

- Poor nutrition from any cause.
- Chronic illness.
- Recent illness, surgery, or injury.
- Genetic factors.
- Obesity.
- Smoking.
- Alcoholism.
- Age, especially newborns and infants or older adults.
- Stress, anxiety, depression, or other emotional problems.
- Use of drugs of abuse, such as narcotics, psychedelics, hallucinogens, marijuana, sedatives, hypnotics, or cocaine.
- Use of some drugs or medications, whether prescription or nonprescription. Medicines most likely to increase surgical risk include antihypertensives, muscle relaxants, tranquilizers, sleep inducers, insulin, sedatives, cortisone, beta-adrenergic blockers, calcium-channel blockers, and antibiotics.

These same drugs, of course, are lifesaving for some serious illnesses, but they can complicate treatment and outcome of other medical or surgical problems.

7—WHAT TO EXPECT

This section includes eight topics: *Who Operates; Where Performed; Diagnostic Tests; Anesthesia; Description of Operation; Possible Complications; Average Hospital Stay;* and *Probable Outcome.* Each topic is discussed separately.

8—WHO OPERATES

A routine surgery is often performed by a general surgeon or by a doctor who specializes in the body system involved. For instance, either a general surgeon or an obstetrician-gynecologist might remove an ovarian cyst.

Highly complicated surgeries, such as a heart transplant, are usually done by surgeons with additional specialized training.

We have included the type of surgeon most likely to perform the procedure, but variations can occur. In many communities general surgeons perform operations that are customarily performed elsewhere by a surgical specialist.

Your surgeon should not be uneasy about discussing with you before surgery his or her previous experience and education. Most competent surgeons welcome and sometimes recommend a second opinion when the surgery to be performed is elective rather than an emergency.

9—WHERE PERFORMED

A surgical procedure may be performed in any of the following places:
- A doctor's or medical office.
- An independent, outpatient surgical facility.
- A hospital outpatient surgical facility.
- The operating room of a hospital.
- An emergency room.

10—DIAGNOSTIC TESTS

Diagnostic tests related to surgery can occur before, during, or after the surgical procedure.

Laboratory studies are helpful in diagnosis and in providing necessary anatomical information prior to surgery. Many tests are the same as those discussed earlier in diagnosis of illnesses.

Some tests are especially useful in surgery. Examples include:
- Special x-ray studies of the gastrointestinal tract (upper GI series or lower GI series).
- Intravenous studies of the kidney and urinary tract (intravenous pyelogram and retrograde pyelogram).
- Coronary angiography (x-ray studies of the coronary arteries performed during a cardiac catheterization procedure).

• Biopsy (microscopic study of tissue) before surgery to establish a diagnosis prior to extensive surgery (usually for cancer) and biopsy afterward of tissue removed during the surgical procedure.

11—ANESTHESIA

Anesthesia makes surgery possible without pain. Prior to giving anesthesia, most surgeons prescribe preoperative medications. These generally consist of:
• Tranquilizers or sedatives to help reduce apprehension.
• Pain relievers (frequently a narcotic drug such as morphine). This medication also reduces apprehension and decreases the amount of anesthesia needed.
• An anticholinergic drug, such as scopolamine or atropine, to decrease secretions from the nose, throat, and lungs during the operation.

The type of anesthesia used depends on the surgical problem, the age, and general condition of the patient, and sometimes on the availability of personnel to administer the anesthesia.

If an operation can be performed with any of several types of anesthesia, you have a right to know the advantages and disadvantages of each. If you wish, you have the right to participate in the selection. Don't hesitate to ask questions.

Before you have any anesthesia, tell your doctor or dentist about any allergic responses you have had to anesthesia in the past. Also inform him or her about any prescription or nonprescription drugs you take, and about any cardiovascular disease, heartbeat irregularities, or peripheral vascular disease you have.

If a chart lists several anesthesia options for a surgery, you will have one of them, but not all.

The various types of anesthesia include:

Local Anesthesia—This is usually an injectable form of a drug ending in "caine," such as novocaine or lidocaine.

Local anesthesia is frequently injected into an injury site, such as a fracture, and bleeding from the injury disperses the anesthetic to all pain-sensitive parts of the injury. Local anesthesia may also be used to block a specific nerve bundle, allowing a pain-free procedure such as a tooth extraction.

Regional Anesthesia—This is used when it is desirable for the patient to remain conscious during the operation. Regional anesthesia works only on the part of the body upon which surgery is performed. Types of regional anesthesia include spinal or epidural anesthesia.

Spinal anesthesia involves an injection of local anesthetic into the spinal canal, above the level of the surgery site. It relieves pain satisfactorily for many procedures below the waist, such as surgery of the rectum, genitourinary tract or lower extremities.

A special type of low-spinal anesthesia is called caudal anesthesia or "saddle block" (it affects the body area that comes into contact with a horse saddle).

Epidural anesthesia involves an injection of local anesthetic into the extradural (epidural) space in the lower back. It is used to block pain for the abdominal region.

General Anesthesia—This form of anesthesia is usually administered by inhalation or injection, or a combination of the two.

A short-acting hypnotic or sedative is injected into a vein, followed by a muscle relaxer. This quickly produces light sleep and allows placement of an airway tube (endotracheal tube) without discomfort. The tube is connected to hoses that lead to gas machines.

The anesthesiologist controls the flow

of anesthesia gases and monitors many body functions, such as blood pressure, breathing rate, pulse, and ECG, while the patient sleeps.

When you awaken, the endotracheal tube may still be in place or may have been removed. Unless your respiration needs continued machine support, the endotracheal tube is usually removed in the recovery room.

The tube will make your throat sore for about 24 hours. This is normal and requires no treatment.

12—DESCRIPTION OF OPERATION

The surgical procedure is described in brief, nontechnical terms. Individual surgeons may use slightly varying techniques, but the basic steps are included and only details vary.

If you want additional information, your surgeon can give more details. An Internet search can also help you find resource materials with fuller descriptions and explanations. Be sure the website is a reliable one (such as those provided by the government, a university, or hospital).

During some surgeries of the gastrointestinal tract, a hollow tube is passed through your nose into your stomach after you are asleep. The tube will probably be in place when you awaken in the recovery room. The purpose of the tube is to keep the stomach empty to prevent vomiting or aspiration of material while you are asleep. It also keeps the stomach decompressed until normal muscular movement of the gastrointestinal tract can resume after surgery. An empty stomach is more comfortable and helps prevent complications that may arise if the stomach becomes distended with air or gas.

The average time in surgery and in the recovery room are left out because

variations are too great. Factors that affect the time limits depend upon:
• The exact techniques chosen.
• The experience and preference of the surgeon.
• The availability and experience of assistants and operating room personnel.
• The presence or absence of complications during surgery.
• The age and condition of the patient prior to surgery.

Don't hesitate to ask your surgeon to estimate the time your operation will require.

13—POSSIBLE COMPLICATIONS

Complications are additional medical problems related to the surgery that occur during or after the procedure. They sometimes happen despite accurate diagnosis, skillful surgery, competent assistance and well-equipped operating rooms. Some complications are preventable, and a few occur frequently— but most are rare.

14—AVERAGE HOSPITAL STAY

This estimate is based on an average. It varies according to how healing and recuperation progress and whether complications develop before, during, or after surgery. It is also influenced by the amount insurance companies will allow as reimbursement of specific procedures.

15—PROBABLE OUTCOME

This heading relates to the surgery's effect on the underlying disorder and the average length of time required to recover from surgery. Estimates are based on the assumption that complications do not occur and healing proceeds normally. Complications can alter the course of healing dramatically. A positive outlook following surgery is an important factor in good outcome and rapid healing.

16—POSTOPERATIVE CARE

This section generally provides instructions for self-care during recuperation after hospitalization. It should serve as a reminder for instructions given you by your surgeon. It does not replace your doctor's instructions.

The section has four major topics: *General Measures; Medication; Activity; and Diet.*

17—GENERAL MEASURES

Some questions are almost universal following surgery. Most patients are unsure how to care for a surgical wound. They have questions about pain, bathing, stitches, clothing, and other matters. These questions are answered in this section.

18—MEDICATION

Drugs usually prescribed after surgery are described, along with brief instructions for their use.

See Safe Use of Medicine (in Appendix) for general instructions.

19—ACTIVITY

Resumption of activity is a strong area of concern for postsurgical patients. Guidelines may be provided for when to return to school or work, when to resume driving, when to resume sexual relations, and what types of exercise are appropriate. Again, it should serve as a reminder for instructions given you by your surgeon; it should not replace specific medical instructions.

20—DIET

During surgery with general anesthesia, the gastrointestinal tract is kept empty. After the patient awakens, clear liquids are usually provided until the gastrointestinal tract begins to function again. When appropriate, this information is included in the surgery charts. Additional diet instructions often refer to special diets in the Appendix section.

21—CALL YOUR DOCTOR IF

Call your doctor if healing and recuperation after surgery don't follow the usual course of events. Excessive bleeding and general or surgical-wound infection are common dangers after most surgical procedures, and these are always mentioned on surgery charts when appropriate.

Other reasons listed can serve as reminders of possible complications. If you develop symptoms you believe are related to your surgery—even if they don't appear on the chart—call your doctor about them.

Symptoms

Symptoms Charts

Find your main symptom on this list and then look at that chart for additional symptoms you may have. Remember, anytime you have symptoms that cause concern, consult a health care provider.

Abdominal Pain, Recurrent Attacks
Abdominal Pain, Sudden Attack
Abdominal Swelling
Ankle Pain
Ankles, Swollen
Anxiety & Nervousness
Appetite Loss
Arm or Hand Pain
Backache or Back Pain
Behavioral or Emotional Changes
Bleeding, Rectal
Bowel, Lack of Control
Breast Pain or Lumps
Breath, Bad
Breathing Difficulty
Bruising or Blood Spots Under the Skin,
    Unexplained
Burping or Gas
Chest Pain
Confusion (Person Over Age 65)
Confusion (Person Under Age 65)
Constipation
Convulsions (Seizures)
Cough
Cough With Blood
Coughing In Children
Depression
Diarrhea (Infant 0 To 6 Months)
Diarrhea (Person Over 6 Months)
Dizziness
Ear, Ringing or Buzzing Sounds
Earache
Eye Pain, Swelling, Dryness, Itching,
    Tearing
Face Pain
Facial Skin Problems
Faintness or Fainting
Fatigue or Tiredness
Fever (Child 0 To 2 Years)
Fever (Child Over 2 Years)
Fever (Person Over Age 12)
Foot Problems
Genital Sores, Blisters, Warts or Boils
Hair Growth In Women, Excessive
Hair Loss
Headache
Hearing Loss
Heartbeat Irregularity

Hip Pain
Impotence, Male Sexual
Itching
Joint Aches or Pain
Knee Pain
Leg Pain
Memory Problems
Menstrual Periods, Late or Absent
Menstrual Periods, Painful or Heavy
Mouth, Sore, Tingling, Dry
Muscle Pain, Ache, Cramp, Weakness
Neck Pain
Nose, Stuffy or Runny
Numbness, Tingling or Prickling
Sexual Intercourse, Painful For Man
Sexual Intercourse, Painful For Woman
Shoulder Pain
Skin, Bumps on
Skin Problems (Child Under Age 2)
Skin Problems (Person Over Age 2)
Skin Rash With Fever
Skin Rash Without Fever
Sleeping Problems
Speaking Difficulty
Stool, Abnormal Appearance
Swallowing Difficulty
Sweating, Excessive
Swelling or Lump
Testicles or Penis, Painful or Swollen
Throat, Sore
Tongue, Sore
Toothache
Trembling or Twitching
Urination, Change in Frequency
Urination, Lack of Control
Urination, Painful
Urine, Abnormal Color
Vaginal Bleeding, Unexpected
Vaginal Discharge, Abnormal
Vaginal Itching
Vision Disturbance or Loss
Voice Loss or Hoarseness
Vomiting (Infant 0 To 6 Months)
Vomiting, Recurrent Attacks
Vomiting, Sudden Attack
Weight Gain
Weight Loss
Wheezing

ABDOMINAL PAIN, RECURRENT ATTACKS

SYMPTOMS & FACTORS	POSSIBLE PROBLEM	WHAT TO DO*
• Recurrent pain in upper right abdomen that may spread to chest, back, or shoulders. • No fever.	Gallbladder disorder.	See Gallstones.
• Recurrent pain in lower abdomen. • Nausea. • Diarrhea (may be bloody). • General ill feeling. • Fever during attacks.	Inflammatory disease of small or large intestine.	• See Colitis, Ulcerative. • See Crohn's Disease.
• Pain or cramping in the upper abdomen. • Appetite loss. • Weight loss.	• Inflammation. • Ulcer. • Digestive problem.	• See Celiac Disease. • See Gastritis. • See Ulcer, Peptic.
• Cramping pain in lower left abdomen (male). • Constant urge to have a bowel movement.	Rectum inflammation.	See Proctitis.
• Recurrent pain in upper abdomen. • Poor appetite. • Unexplained weight loss.	• Cancer. • Disorder of pancreas.	• See Kidney Cancer. • See Pancreatitis. • See Pancreatic Cancer. • See Stomach Cancer.
• Recurrent pain in lower abdomen. • No fever. • Recurrent diarrhea, usually without blood.	• Inflammation of large intestine. • Tumor.	• See Colon Cancer. • See Diverticular Disease.
• Recurrent cramps or pain or discomfort in abdomen. • Passing gas; belching. • Abdomen pressure.	• Gastrointestinal problem. • Ovarian problem.	• See Gas & Gas Pain. • See Gastroesophageal Reflux Disease. • See Indigestion. • See Ovarian Cancer • See Ovarian Cyst or Tumor, Benign.
• Recurrent pain in upper right abdomen. • Vomiting. • Fever during attacks.	Gallbladder inflammation.	See Cholecystitis or Cholangitis.
• Recurrent pain in lower abdomen. • Alternating diarrhea and constipation; feeling bloated.	Disorder of muscle contractions in colon.	See Irritable Bowel Syndrome.
Pain or discomfort in abdomen with swelling, lump, or bulge.	Intestinal protrusion.	See Hernia.
• Pain in lower abdomen. • Nausea, constipation.	Inflammation.	See Appendicitis.
• Pain in abdomen (pelvic area). • Urgent need to urinate.	Bladder problem.	See Interstitial Cystitis.
Pain in the pelvic, lower stomach, and back areas.	• Chronic pain. • Uterine lining problem.	• See Chronic Pelvic Pain. • See Endometriosis.

*All references are to Illness section unless noted otherwise.

ABDOMINAL PAIN, SUDDEN ATTACK
(continued on next page)

SYMPTOMS & FACTORS	POSSIBLE PROBLEM	WHAT TO DO*
Abdominal pain following excessive consumption of alcohol or food.	Stomach inflammation.	• See Gastritis • See Indigestion.
• Abdominal pain. • Diarrhea. • Vomiting.	• Infections of digestive tract. • Food poisoning.	• See Food Poisoning. • See Gastroenteritis. • See Salmonella Infections.
• Abdominal pain. • Diarrhea. • Flatulence and bloating.	Reaction to swallowed substance.	See Food Allergy.
• Abdominal pain that may spread to back and genital area. • Low fever. • Frequent, painful, possibly bloody urination.	Infection in urinary tract.	• See Bladder Infection, Female. • See Bladder Infection, Male. • See Kidney Infection, Acute.
• Mild pain in lower abdomen. • Constipation or gas. • Recent diet change, such as adding more fiber.	Intestinal disturbance caused by diet change.	Consult doctor if discomfort persists.
• Severe abdominal pain, plus any of following: • Temperature of 100°F (37.8°C) or higher. • Constipation. • Abdominal swelling. • Vomiting.	Serious abdominal disorder.	• Call doctor now. • See Intestinal Obstruction. • See Aneurysm. • See Appendicitis. • See Peritonitis.
• Lower abdomen pain or cramps. • Menstrual period late (4 or more weeks). • Vaginal bleeding or spotting.	Early stage of pregnancy developing outside uterus.	See Ectopic Pregnancy.
• Off and on abdominal pain that began in small of back, spreading to genital area. • No fever at onset of pain. • Cloudy or dark or bloody urine.	Kidney problem.	See Kidney Stones.
• Pain in lower abdomen in woman. • Bad-smelling vaginal discharge. • Painful intercourse. • Pain when urinating.	Infection of reproductive organs.	See Pelvic Inflammatory Disease.
• Burning pain of abdominal skin with tenderness along pain route. • Skin blisters.	Virus infection.	See Herpes Zoster.
• Sharp or extreme pain in abdomen. • Bloating. • Nausea or vomiting.	• Gallbladder disorder. • Pancreas problem.	• See Gallstones. • See Pancreatitis

*All references are to Illness section unless noted otherwise.

ABDOMINAL PAIN, SUDDEN ATTACK
(continued from previous page)

SYMPTOMS & FACTORS	POSSIBLE PROBLEM	WHAT TO DO*
• Pain in lower abdomen in females. • Unexplained vaginal bleeding.	Several disorders.	See Vaginal Bleeding, Unexpected (in this Symptoms section).
Recurrent abdominal pain for 1 week or more.	Several disorders.	See Abdominal Pain, Recurrent (in this Symptoms section).
• Sense of fullness in abdomen or rectal area. • Mucous discharge, sometimes tinged with blood. • Firm mass that can be felt.	Rectal tissue disorder.	See Rectal Prolapse.
• Abdominal cramps. • Intermittent diarrhea. • Gas and abdominal bloating.	Parasitic infection.	See Amebiasis.

*All references are to Illness section unless noted otherwise.

ABDOMINAL SWELLING

SYMPTOMS & FACTORS	POSSIBLE PROBLEM	WHAT TO DO*
• Lower abdominal swelling that is slowly increasing. • No signs of pregnancy. • Persistent constipation.	• Intestinal disorder. • Ovarian problem.	• See Constipation. • See Ovarian Cancer. • See Ovarian Cyst or Tumor, Benign.
Abdominal swelling in woman 1 to 5 days before or during menstrual period.	Fluid retention caused by hormone changes.	• See Premenstrual Syndrome. • See Premenstrual Dysphoric Disorder.
• Abdominal swelling, bloated and full feeling. • Gas or belching. • Abdominal pain or discomfort.	• Heartburn. • Stones in gallbladder.	• See Gallstones. • See Indigestion.
• Abdominal swelling in last 24 hours. • Severe abdominal pain. • Fever. • Diarrhea or constipation. • Vomiting.	Serious abdominal disorder.	• Call doctor now. • See Intestinal Obstruction.
• Abdominal swelling. • Swollen ankles. • Breathing difficulty, especially at night.	Fluid in abdomen and other body parts caused by heart condition.	• Consult doctor. • See Heart Failure.
• Abdominal swelling. • Puffy ankles that hold a dent when pressed with finger. • Decreased urination.	Kidney disorder.	• Consult doctor. • See Glomerulonephritis. • See Wilms' Tumor (children only).
• Abdominal swelling. • Yellow skin and eyes.	Liver disorder.	• Consult doctor. • See Cirrhosis of the Liver.
• Abdominal swelling. • Overweight.	Effect of excess weight.	See Obesity & Overweight.
• Abdominal swelling in woman of childbearing age. • Tender, enlarged breasts. • Morning nausea. • No menstrual period for 2 months or longer.	Pregnancy.	Consult doctor to confirm pregnancy.
• Swollen abdomen in an infant. • Weight loss or slow weight gain. • Loose, pale, bad-smelling stools.	Gluten intolerance.	See Celiac Disease.

*All references are to Illness section unless noted otherwise.

ANKLE PAIN

SYMPTOMS & FACTORS	POSSIBLE PROBLEM	WHAT TO DO*
• Severe pain in ankle following injury. • Ankle can't move or bear weight. • Ankle swells rapidly and may turn bluish color.	Injury.	• See Bone Fracture. • See Sprains & Strains.
• Pain in ankles or other joints, such as knees or fingers. • Affected joints red, warm, swollen. • No fever.	• Joint inflammation. • Degenerative condition of joints.	• See Arthritis, Rheumatoid. • See Arthritis, Juvenile Idiopathic (children only). • See Gout. • See Osteoarthritis.
• Moderate pain in ankle following injury. • Ankle can move and bear weight.	Mild ligament injury.	See Sprains & Strains.
• Pain in ankle. • Ankle swollen, red, and hot. • Fever. • Recent infection, such as gonorrhea.	Joint infection.	See Arthritis, Infectious.
• Pain in ankles or other joints. • Affected joints red, warm, swollen. • Fever. • General ill feeling. • Recent illness, such as sore throat or skin infection.	Complication of prior streptococcal infection.	• Consult doctor. • See Rheumatic Fever.
• Acute attack of swelling and pain in one or more joints. • Attacks may last for 2 or more days.	Joint disorder.	See Pseudogout.

*All references are to Illness section unless noted otherwise.

ANKLES, SWOLLEN

SYMPTOMS & FACTORS	POSSIBLE PROBLEM	WHAT TO DO*
• Swollen ankle. • Injury to ankle in last 4 months.	Normal swelling following injury.	If ankle becomes painful, consult doctor.
• Swollen ankles. • Recent confinement for several hours, such as car, bus, train, airplane. • No pain.	Normal occurrence.	• Elevate legs. When possible, avoid prolonged sitting or standing—move around frequently. • If swelling persists more than 48 hours, consult doctor.
Swollen, painful ankle.	Several disorders.	See Ankle Pain (in this Symptoms section).
• Swollen ankles. • Use of prescription or nonprescription drug.	Adverse reaction or side effect of drug.	• Consult doctor about prescription drug. • Discontinue use of nonprescription drug.
• Swollen ankles. • Menstrual period due in a few days.	Fluid retention caused by hormone changes or excess salt intake.	See Premenstrual Syndrome.
Swollen or distended veins in ankles.	Dilated, twisted, or blocked veins.	• See Thrombophlebitis, Superficial. • See Varicose Veins.
• Swollen ankles. • Pregnancy.	Common occurrence during pregnancy, but may be sign of high blood pressure.	See Preeclampsia & Eclampsia.
• Swollen ankle. • Calf of swollen leg is tender. • Pain when flexing ankle.	Blood clot in deep vein.	• Call doctor now. • See Thrombosis, Deep-Vein.
• Swollen ankles. • Chronic breathing difficulty that is worsening. • Cough that is worse when lying down.	Fluid in lungs and other body parts caused by heart condition.	See Heart Failure.
• Swollen ankles. • Use of oral contraceptives, cortisone drugs, or nonsteroidal anti-inflammatory drugs.	• Adverse reaction or side effect of drug. • Blood clot in deep vein.	• Consult doctor. • See Thrombosis, Deep-Vein.

*All references are to Illness section unless noted otherwise.

ANXIETY & NERVOUSNESS
(continued on next page)

SYMPTOMS & FACTORS	POSSIBLE PROBLEM	WHAT TO DO*
• Anxiety, plus any of following: • Inability to listen attentively and remember. • Clinging dependency. • Cold or hot flashes. • Cool, sweaty hands. • Abdominal cramps. • Diarrhea or constipation. • Dizziness. • Dry mouth. • Lack of concentration. • Faintness. • Rapid heartbeat. • Impotence in men. • Low frustration level. • Muscle tension and pain (backache, neck ache, headache). • Painful menstruation. • Painful sexual intercourse. • Pale or flushed skin. • Restlessness. • Tightness in chest. • Frequent urination.	Effect of anxiety or stress.	• See Anxiety Disorder, Generalized. • See Stress.
Anxiety about any of following: enclosed spaces, airplanes, crowds, heights, "going crazy," infection, or other situations.	Psychological disorder.	See Phobias.
• Anxiety, plus 2 or more of following: • Weight loss. • Bulging eyes. • Excessive sweating. • Fatigue. • Rapid or irregular heartbeat.	Overactive thyroid gland.	See Hyperthyroidism.
• Anxiety. • Dizziness or lightheadedness. • Rapid breathing. • Frequent sighing.	Decreased carbon dioxide in blood.	See Panic Disorder.
• Anxiety. • Use of prescription or nonprescription drug.	Adverse reaction or side effect of drug.	• Consult doctor about prescription drug. • Discontinue use of nonprescription drug if symptoms persist.
• Nervousness or anxiety. • Weakness, hunger, headache.	Low blood sugar.	• See Diabetes Hypoglycemia. • See Hypoglycemia. Reactive.
• Nervousness and irritability in a female. • Menstrual period is due.	Hormone fluctuation.	• See Premenstrual Syndrome. • See Premenstrual Dysphoric Disorder.

*All references are to Illness section unless noted otherwise.

ANXIETY & NERVOUSNESS
(continued from previous page)

SYMPTOMS & FACTORS	POSSIBLE PROBLEM	WHAT TO DO*
• Anxiety. • Recent withdrawal from tobacco, alcohol, or drug, such as sleeping pills.	Withdrawal symptom.	• Consult doctor about drug withdrawal. • See Alcoholism. • See Smoking Addiction. • See Substance Abuse.
• Anxiety behavior in a child. • Restlessness, inability to be still. • Unable to pay attention to directions.	Behavioral syndrome.	See Attention Deficit Hyperactivity Disorder in Children.
• Anxiety involving recurrent, intrusive and distressing recollection of an event. • Reliving of an event.	Psychological disorder.	See Post-Traumatic Stress Disorder.

*All references are to Illness section unless noted otherwise.

APPETITE LOSS
(continued on next page)

SYMPTOMS & FACTORS	POSSIBLE PROBLEM	WHAT TO DO*
• Appetite loss. • Nausea and vomiting. • Fever.	Irritation or infection of digestive tract.	See Gastroenteritis.
• Appetite loss. • Use of vitamins or prescription or nonprescription drug, especially: anticancer drugs, digitalis, aminophylline, narcotics, antihistamines, ephedrine, methylphenidate, diphenyl-hydantoin, or amphetamines.	Adverse reaction or side effect of drug.	• Consult doctor about prescription drug. • Discontinue use of nonprescription drugs.
• Appetite loss, plus 2 or more of following: • Fever. • Sore throat. • Headache. • Painful swelling in neck, armpit or groin. • Fatigue. • Jaundice (yellow skin and eyes). • Pain in upper right abdomen.	Virus infection.	See Mononucleosis, Infectious.
• Appetite loss. • Depression or anxiety.	Effect of stress.	• See Anxiety Disorder, Generalized. • See Anorexia Nervosa. • See Depression. • See Stress.
• Decrease in appetite (especially in a child). • Low-grade fever. • Runny nose and cough.	Virus infection.	See Respiratory Syncytial Virus.
• Appetite loss. • Emotional upset such as grief.	Temporary emotional situation.	• Appetite will return in time. Drink plenty of fluids. • See Grief.
• Appetite loss (sudden). • Headache. • Nausea or vomiting. • Bloody, decreased urine. • Puffy face.	Kidney disorder.	See Glomerulonephritis.
• Appetite loss. • Nausea at sight of food, plus 2 or more of following: • Jaundice (yellow skin and eyes). • Vomiting. • Tenderness over liver area. • Fever. • Weakness and fatigue.	Liver disorder.	• See Cirrhosis of the Liver. • See Hepatitis, Viral.
• Appetite loss. • Weight loss. • Vague feeling of illness or fatigue.	Early signs of cancer or other disorder.	Consult doctor.

*All references are to Illness section unless noted otherwise.

APPETITE LOSS
(continued from previous page)

SYMPTOMS & FACTORS	POSSIBLE PROBLEM	WHAT TO DO*
• Appetite loss with weight gain. • Loss of energy, fatigue. • Decreased sex drive. • Dry skin and hair. • Constipation.	Underactive thyroid gland.	See Hypothyroidism.
• Appetite loss. • Excessive alcohol consumption.	Vitamin deficiency caused by alcohol.	See Alcoholism.
• Appetite loss. • Weight loss, plus 2 or more of following: • Paleness. • Sore, red, smooth, burning tongue. • Yellowish skin.	Vitamin B-12 and/or folic-acid deficiency.	• See Anemia, Pernicious. • See Folic Acid Deficiency.
• Gradual appetite loss in woman 45 or older. • Fatigue. • Menstrual changes.	Normal occurrence with the decreasing estrogen level of menopause.	• See Menopause. • See Perimenopause.
• Appetite loss. • Fluid retention. • Reduced urine production.	Kidney disease.	See Nephrotic Syndrome.
• Appetite loss in child. • Irritability. • Paleness.	Disorder of red-blood cells.	See Anemia, Iron-Deficiency.
• Appetite loss. • Nausea. • Pregnancy or possible pregnancy.	Effect of hormone change during pregnancy.	Eat small, frequent meals.
Appetite loss in child around age 2.	Normal occurrence caused by slowed growth rate.	Appetite will return when growth accelerates.
• Poor appetite. • Sleeping problems. • Lack of energy. • Feelings of hopelessness, self-pity.	Chronic mild depression.	See Dysthymia.
• Appetite loss and weight loss. • Tender mass in upper right abdomen. • Pain in upper right abdomen.	Cancer.	See Hepatocellular Carcinoma.

*All references are to Illness section unless noted otherwise.

ARM OR HAND PAIN

SYMPTOMS & FACTORS	POSSIBLE PROBLEM	WHAT TO DO*
• Pain in elbow, wrist, or finger joint when bending arm or hand. • No redness or swelling.	Tendon inflammation.	• See Tendinitis. • See Tennis Elbow.
• Pain in arm or hand. • Numbness or tingling in arm or hand. • Weakness in arm or hand.	Pressure on nerves in wrist.	• See Carpal Tunnel Syndrome. • See Thoracic-Outlet Syndrome.
• Severe pain in arm after injury. • Arm not misshapen.	Muscle or ligament injury.	See Sprains & Strains.
• Severe pain in arm after injury. • Arm misshapen.	Broken bone.	• Call doctor now. • See Bone Fracture.
• Pain in arm during exercise. • Feeling of pressure in chest.	Temporary lack of oxygen to heart.	• Call doctor if pain lasts longer than 5 minutes. • See Angina Pectoris. • See Coronary Artery Disease.
• Pain in elbow, wrist, or finger joint. • Affected joint red and swollen. • Fever and general ill feeling.	Bone or joint infection.	• Consult doctor. • See Arthritis, Infectious. • See Osteomyelitis.
• Pain in elbow, wrist, or finger joints. • Joints are red, warm, swollen. • Fever. • Recent illness, such as sore throat, gonorrhea, or skin infection.	Complication of prior streptococcal infection.	See Rheumatic Fever.
• Discomfort in fingers. • Fingers turn pale, then bluish, then red, when exposed to cold.	Circulation disorder.	See Raynaud Disease & Phenomenon.
• Pain in elbow, wrist, or finger joint. • Affected joint is red, warm, swollen.	Joint inflammation.	• See Arthritis, Juvenile Idiopathic (children only). • See Arthritis, Rheumatoid. • See Bursitis. • See Gout. • See Osteoarthritis. • See Psoriatic Arthritis.
• Pain in arm or hand. • Numbness or tingling in arm or hand. • Stiff neck and cracking sound with neck movement.	Pressure on nerves in neck.	See Cervical Spondylosis.
Pain around fingernails.	Tissue inflammation.	See Paronychia.
• Arm or leg pain (may be burning or aching) and swelling. • Changes in skin color.	Unknown.	See Regional Pain Syndrome, Complex.

*All references are to Illness section unless noted otherwise.

BACKACHE OR BACK PAIN
(continued on next page)

SYMPTOMS & FACTORS	POSSIBLE PROBLEM	WHAT TO DO*
• Sudden backache. • Recent fall or injury to back. • Pain only at injury site.	Muscle injury or muscle spasm.	• See Back Pain, Low. • See Disc, Herniated. • See Sprains & Strains.
• Sudden sharp pain down back of leg. • Recent heavy lifting or strenuous exercise.	Pressure on large nerve in leg.	See Back Pain, Low.
• Sudden backache in person over age 60. • Sharp pain in one place over the spine. OR • Recent confinement to bed or wheelchair.	Bone damage caused by softening of bones.	• Consult doctor. • See Osteoporosis.
• Backache. • Fever. • Painful urination.	Kidney infection.	See Kidney Infection, Acute.
• Backache in person older than 60. • Pain in other joints.	Degenerative condition.	See Osteoarthritis.
• Backache. • Overweight • Recent heavy lifting or new or strenuous exercise.	Strain of back muscle or ligament.	• See Back Pain, Low. • See Obesity & Overweight.
• Chronic back pain. • Numbness in extremities that is worsening.	Pressure on spinal cord.	• See Spinal-Cord Tumor. • See Spinal Stenosis.
• Sudden backache. • Recent fall or injury to back, plus any of following: • Difficulty moving arm or leg. • Loss of bladder or bowel control. • Numbness or tingling in extremities.	Damaged spinal cord.	• Call doctor now. • Don't move injured person.
• Backache in female. • Wearing high heels.	Poor weight distribution.	Wear lower heels.
• Chronic backache. • Repetitive work such as computer use.	Poor posture, incorrect chair or desk height.	• Correct problem with posture or equipment. • See Back Pain, Low.
Backache that is worse in morning.	• Lack of adequate back support during sleep. • Chronic inflammation.	• Sleep on back or side. • Use mattress that is not too firm or too soft. • See Spondylitis, Ankylosing.

*All references are to Illness section unless noted otherwise.

BACKACHE OR BACK PAIN
(continued from previous page)

SYMPTOMS & FACTORS	POSSIBLE PROBLEM	WHAT TO DO*
• Backache that worsens with lifting. • Lump in back or front of the vagina or projecting outside of it.	Fallen uterus.	See Uterine Prolapse.
• Pain in bones in back. • Weight loss. • Symptoms of anemia.	Cancer.	See Multiple Myeloma.
• Back pain in female. • Pain with sexual intercourse. • Blood in the urine.	Disorder of the uterus.	See Endometriosis.
• Chronic back pain. • Pain may affect other body parts. • Follows an injury or illness.	Persistent pain.	See Chronic Pain Syndrome.
• Back pain. • Visible curving of the upper body.	Curvature of the spine.	See Scoliosis.

*All references are to Illness section unless noted otherwise.

BEHAVIORAL OR EMOTIONAL CHANGES
(continued on next page)

SYMPTOMS & FACTORS	POSSIBLE PROBLEM	WHAT TO DO*
• Behavior that involves thoughts of failure, inadequacy, and negativity. • Lack of energy. • Sleeping problems. • Poor appetite.	Mild or clinical depression.	• See Depression. • See Dysthymia.
• Behavioral changes. • Use of a prescription or nonprescription drug.	Adverse reaction or side effect of drug.	• Consult doctor about prescription drug. • Discontinue nonprescription drug.
Obsessions and/or compulsive behaviors that consume more than an hour a day.	Psychological disorder.	See Obsessive Compulsive Disorder.
Anxiety symptoms when exposed to, or thinking of, a particular stimulus.	Psychological disorder.	See Phobias.
• Recurrent, intrusive and distressing recollection of an event. • Reliving of an event.	Psychological disorder.	See Post-Traumatic Stress Disorder.
• Start of winter season. • Depression. • Irritability. • Tiredness.	Lack of light.	See Seasonal Affective Disorder.
• Fear of going crazy. • Fear of dying. • Sense of terror or doom. • Palpitations. • Rapid heartbeat.	Severe anxiety.	See Panic Disorder.
• Behavioral changes in a female. • Week to 14 days before OR • Beginning of menopause.	Hormone fluctuations.	• See Menopause. • See Perimenopause. • See Premenstrual Dysphoric Disorder. • See Premenstrual Syndrome.
• Trouble concentrating. • Easily distracted. • May be restless. • Doesn't complete tasks.	Behavioral syndrome.	• See Attention Deficit Hyperactivity Disorder. in Children. • See Attention Deficit Hyperactivity Disorder. in Adults.
• Irritability. • Paleness, fatigue, lethargy. • Abdominal discomfort. • Headache. • Tremor.	Inhalation or ingestion of lead.	See Lead Poisoning.
Behavioral changes in an elderly person.	Mental deterioration.	• See Alzheimer's Disease. • See Dementia.

*All references are to Illness section unless noted otherwise.

BEHAVIORAL OR EMOTIONAL CHANGES
(continued from previous page)

SYMPTOMS & FACTORS	POSSIBLE PROBLEM	WHAT TO DO*
• Behavioral changes. • Recent withdrawal from tobacco, alcohol, or drug, such as sleeping pills.	Withdrawal symptom.	• Consult doctor about drug withdrawal. • See Alcoholism. • See Smoking Addiction. • See Substance Abuse.
• Behavioral or personality changes. • Stiff neck. • General ill feeling. • Headache, vomiting, fever.	Brain inflammation.	See Encephalitis, Viral.
• Confusion. • Restlessness and anxiety. • Weakness. • Muscle cramps.	Electrolyte disorder.	See Sodium Imbalance.
Episodes of mania (excited) and episodes of depression (feeling down and sad).	Mental disorder.	See Bipolar Disorder.
In infant: Restlessness, poor sleep habits, profuse sweating, delayed motor skills.	Vitamin deficiency.	See Vitamin Deficiencies.
• Behavior changes. • Stressful life event (sometimes called a stressor).	Reaction to an event.	See Adjustment Disorders.
Child is not behaving, talking, playing, or learning new skills as expected for their age group.	Developmental problem.	See Autism.
Child's behavior changes (avoiding family or friends, sleeping problems, school problems, emotional upsets).	Possible child abuse.	See Child Abuse.
• Behavior includes: delusions (fixed false, unreal beliefs) and hallucinations (hearing voices or seeing things that are not there). • Becomes more withdrawn.	Mental disorder.	See Schizophrenic Disorders.

*All references are to Illness section unless noted otherwise.

BLEEDING, RECTAL

SYMPTOMS & FACTORS	POSSIBLE PROBLEM	WHAT TO DO*
• Bright red bleeding. • Rectal pain and itching.	Dilated rectal and anal veins.	See Hemorrhoids.
• Rectal bleeding. • Pain with bowel movements. • Discomfort when cleaning after bowel movements.	Tear in the skin or sphincter muscle or abnormal passage.	• See Anal Fissure. • See Anal Fistula.
Bright red rectal bleeding following injury, insertion of foreign object in the rectum, or anal sex.	Traumatic tear in the skin or sphincter muscle surrounding the rectum.	Consult doctor immediately.
Rectal bleeding in a child with severe abdominal pain.	Telescoping of intestine into itself.	See Intussusception.
Rectal bleeding plus unexplained bleeding from other body orifices.	Bleeding disorder.	• See Anemia, Aplastic. • See Leukemia, Acute.
• Bloody diarrhea with mucus. • Abdominal pain.	Inflammation of bowel.	See Colitis, Ulcerative.
• Blood, mucus, or pus in stool. • Diarrhea and abdominal cramps. • Fever.	Bacteria infection.	See Dysentery, Bacillary.
Blood in stool that is mixed with feces and appears black or dark red.	Bleeding from an abnormality in the stomach, duodenum, or colon.	• Consult doctor. • See Colon Cancer. • See Colon Polyps. • See Crohn's Disease. • See Diverticular Disease. • See Stomach Cancer. • See Ulcer, Peptic.
• In male, rectal bleeding. • Constant urge to have a bowel movement when little or no stool present. • Rectal or abdominal pain.	Rectum inflammation.	See Proctitis.
• Mucous discharge, sometimes tinged with blood. • Sense of fullness in abdomen or rectal area. • Firm mass that can be felt.	Rectal tissue disorder.	See Rectal Prolapse.

*All references are to Illness section unless noted otherwise.

BOWEL, LACK OF CONTROL

SYMPTOMS & FACTORS	POSSIBLE PROBLEM	WHAT TO DO*
• Lack of bowel control, plus any of following: • Recent childbirth with episiotomy. • Recent surgery of vagina. • History of rectal surgery. • Anal fissure or fistula. • Hemorrhoids.	Rectal or anal abnormalities caused by any of several factors.	• Consult doctor. • See Anal Fissure. • See Anal Fistula. • See Constipation. • See Hemorrhoids.
• Lack of bowel control. • Cramping, bloating, constipation, or diarrhea.	Incontinence.	See Incontinence, Fecal.
• Lack of bowel control. • Convulsions or unconsciousness.	Brain abnormality, such as tumor or stroke.	Call doctor now.
• Lack of bowel control, plus any of following: • Slurred speech. • Weakness or paralysis of any part of body. • Unconsciousness. • Blurred vision.	• Decreased blood supply to brain. • Pressure on spinal cord.	• Call doctor now. • See Spinal-Cord Tumor. • See Stroke.
• Lack of bowel control. • Acute diarrhea.	Unable to control bowel function	See Diarrhea, Acute.
• Lack of bowel control. • Laxative use.	Excess use of laxatives.	See Laxative Abuse.
• Frequent leakage of small amounts of stool. • Chronic constipation, especially in child or person over 65.	Irregular bowel function.	See Fecal Impaction.
Lack of bowel control in a young child who once was toilet-trained.	• Regressive behavior. • Emotional disturbance.	See Encopresis.

*All references are to Illness section unless noted otherwise.

BREAST PAIN OR LUMPS

SYMPTOMS & FACTORS	POSSIBLE PROBLEM	WHAT TO DO*
• Breast lump that can be felt. • May have mild breast discomfort or feel some pain.	• Cyst. • Tumor.	• Consult doctor. • See Breast Cancer. • See Fibrocystic Breast Changes.
• Pain or tenderness in breasts before menstrual periods. • Irregular periods. • Woman over age 38.	Thickening of gland tissue in breasts caused by hormonal changes.	• See Menopause. • See Perimenopause.
• Throbbing pain in breast of new mother. • Hard, tender, red lump on breast, or inflamed nipple. • Fever.	Breast infection.	See Mastitis.
• Breast pain. • Use of estrogen medications.	Adverse reaction or side effect of drug.	Consult doctor.
• Pain or tenderness in breasts. • Possible pregnancy.	Common sensitivity during pregnancy.	Wear a support bra as breasts enlarge.
Swollen, tender, hard breasts within 4 days of delivering baby.	Engorgement of breast tissue with milk.	Consult doctor.
• Sore nipples in woman who is breast-feeding. OR • Sharp pain in nipple of nursing mother when breast-feeding baby. • No fever. • No other symptoms related to breast.	Cracked or sore nipples. Common occurrence during first weeks of breast-feeding.	• Wash nipples and apply lanolin cream after breast-feeding. • Consult doctor if fever develops.
• Pain or tenderness in breasts. • Menstrual period due in a few days.	Discomfort caused by hormone changes.	• See Premenstrual Syndrome. • See Premenstrual Dysphoric Disorder.
• Breast pain or discomfort in woman with large breasts. • May also have pain in back neck, or shoulders.	Size of breasts.	Consult doctor.
• Breast pain. • Breast is tender, red, or hard. • Fever and chills. • Tenderness in the area under the arm.	Bacterial infection.	See Breast Abscess.

*All references are to Illness section unless noted otherwise.

BREATH, BAD

SYMPTOMS & FACTORS	POSSIBLE PROBLEM	WHAT TO DO*
• Bad breath. • Bleeding gums. OR • Aching teeth and gums when eating hot, cold, or sweet foods.	Gum inflammation or infection.	• See Gingivitis. • See Periodontitis. • See Trench Mouth.
• Bad breath. • Dentures.	Food particles trapped in dentures.	Consult dentist if home-cleaning techniques fail.
• Bad breath. • No visit to dentist in last 6 months or poor dental hygiene.	Tooth decay or plaque deposits.	• Consult dentist. • See Gingivitis. • See Tooth Decay.
• Bad breath. • Recent consumption of garlic, onions, or alcohol.	Metabolism of these substances.	Nothing. Breath will return to normal.
• Bad breath. • Cold or sore throat.	Symptom of infection.	Nothing. Breath will return to normal.
• Bad breath caused by dry mouth. • Use of drugs causing dry mouth, such as: diuretics, antihistamines, some drugs for high-blood pressure, cancer, and angina.	Effects of dry mouth on odor control.	• Drink plenty of water or citrus juices. Chew sugarless gum or suck on hard candies. • Consult doctor if problem is causing concern.
• Bad breath. • Persistent cough with bad-smelling sputum.	Chronic lung infection.	• See Bronchiectasis. • See Lung Abscess.
• Bad breath. • Fever.	Common occurrence with fever and illness.	See Fever charts (in this Symptoms section).
• Bad breath. • Pain when swallowing.	Swallowing problem or infection.	• See Dysphagia. • See Tonsillitis..
• Bad breath. • Chest pain, shallow breathing.	Infection.	See Empyema.
• Bad breath. • Sore mouth or tongue.	Infection or sores in mouth or tongue.	See Sore Mouth (in this Symptoms section).

*All references are to Illness section unless noted otherwise.

BREATHING DIFFICULTY
(continued on next page)

SYMPTOMS & FACTORS	POSSIBLE PROBLEM	WHAT TO DO*
• Sudden breathing difficulty. • Severe chest pain spreading to jaw, neck, or arms.	Possible heart attack	• Call doctor now. • See Heart Attack.
• Mild breathing difficulty that may be increasing such as when exercising. • May have heart palpitations.	Heart problem.	• See Coronary Artery Disease. • See Heart Rhythm Irregularity. • See Heartbeat, Rapid. • See Hypertrophic Cardiomyopathy.
• Breathing difficulty. • Fever. • Cough with green-yellow or brownish sputum.	Infection of breathing passages.	• See Bronchitis, Acute. • See Pneumonia (all charts).
• Difficult breathing. • Tingling or numbness. • Sneezing, wheezing, or itching. • Exposure to allergens.	Allergic reaction.	• Call doctor now. • See Anaphylaxis.
• Breathing difficulty. • Lightheadedness. • Numbness or tingling in hands and feet. • Stress, fear, or anxiety.	Decreased carbon dioxide in blood.	• See Anxiety Disorder Generalized. • See Panic Disorder.
• Difficult breathing. • Chest tightness. • Wheezing.	Airway inflammation.	See Asthma.
• Mild breathing difficulty. • Noisy breathing.	Spasm of bronchial tubes.	See Wheezing (in this Symptoms section).
• Chronic breathing difficulty that is worsening. • Persistent cough with sputum. • Dusty working conditions.	Lung inflammation.	• See Asbestosis. • See Pneumoconiosis. • See Silicosis.
• Chronic breathing difficulty that is worsening. • No dusty working conditions. • Persistent cough with sputum.	Chronic inflammation or infection of breathing passages.	• See Bronchitis, Chronic. • See Bronchiectasis. • See Chronic Obstructive Pulmonary Disease. • See Emphysema.
• Shortness of breath. • Chest pain. • Shock.	Lung collapse.	See Atelectasis.
• Shortness of breath. • Ascent to high altitude. • Headache, nausea.	Lack of oxygen.	See Altitude Illness.
• Trouble breathing. • Dizziness. • Headache. • Nausea and vomiting.	Gas inhalation.	See Carbon Monoxide Poisoning.

*All references are to Illness section unless noted otherwise.

BREATHING DIFFICULTY
(continued from previous page)

SYMPTOMS & FACTORS	POSSIBLE PROBLEM	WHAT TO DO*
• Difficult breathing in child under 6. • Barking cough. OR • Wheezing with rapid, shallow breathing.	Inflammation or infection.	• See Bronchiolitis. • See Croup.
• Shortness of breath. • Tiredness and weakness. • Paleness.	Lack of red blood cells.	See Anemia (all charts).
• Shortness of breath. • Fatigue. • Irregular heartbeat.	Heart inflammation.	See Myocarditis.
• Rapid breathing. • Dull or sharp pain in front of chest. • Cough, fever, chills.	Heart inflammation.	See Pericarditis.
• Sudden breathing difficulty. • Sharp chest pain that worsens with inhalation.	• Blood clot in lung. • Collapsed lung.	• Call doctor now. • See Pneumothorax. • See Pulmonary Embolism.
• Chronic breathing difficulty that is worsening. • Swollen legs or ankles.	Fluid in lungs and other body parts caused by heart condition.	See Heart Failure.
• Extreme shortness of breath. • Heart failure.	Lack of oxygen in blood.	• Call doctor now. • See Pulmonary Edema.
• Shortness of breath with activity. • Feeling weak and tired. • Chest pain. • Fainting or near fainting.	Heart disease.	See Cor Pulmonale.
• Rapid, shallow breathing. • Chest pain. • Chills and fever.	Lung infection.	See Empyema.

*All references are to Illness section unless noted otherwise.

BRUISING OR BLOOD SPOTS UNDER THE SKIN, UNEXPLAINED

SYMPTOMS & FACTORS	POSSIBLE PROBLEM	WHAT TO DO*
• Unexplained blood spots under skin. • Fever. • Pain in affected area. • Headache. • Weakness. • General ill feeling.	Bacterial, viral, or parasitic, infection.	Consult doctor.
• Unexplained bruising or blood spots under skin. • Use of prescription or nonprescription drug, such as: anticoagulants, aspirin, sulfa drugs, Digitoxin, quinine, quinidine, antihistamines, phenothiazines, antidepressants, local anesthetics, penicillin, mercury, bismuth, cortisone drugs, or anticonvulsants.	Adverse reaction or side effect of drug.	Consult doctor.
Unexplained bruising in healthy child.	Possible child abuse.	See Child Abuse.
• Unexplained bruising or blood spots under skin. • Swollen gums that bleed occasionally.	Poor nutrition.	• Consult doctor. • See Vitamin Deficiencies.
Unexplained blood spots under skin following violent coughing, vomiting, or choking.	Raised pressure in blood vessels of head and neck.	Consult doctor.
• Unexplained bruising in newborn. • Jaundice (yellow skin and eyes).	Blood disorder.	See Rh Incompatibility.
• Unexplained bruising or blood spots under skin. • Recent virus infection.	Blood disorder.	• Call doctor now. • See Thrombocytopenia.
• Unexplained bruising on lower extremities. • Abdominal pain. • Red, swollen, and tender joints.	Allergic disorder.	See Purpura, Henoch Schönlein.
• Frequent bruises. • Painful, swollen joints. • Excessive bleeding from minor cuts.	Blood disorder.	See Hemophilia.
• Unexplained bruising or blood spots under skin. • Kidney or liver disorder.	Kidney problem.	See Renal Failure, Chronic.
• Easy bruising and spontaneous bleeding. • Fever, tiredness, paleness. • General ill feeling.	Cancer.	See Leukemia, Acute.

*All references are to Illness section unless noted otherwise.

BURPING OR GAS

SYMPTOMS & FACTORS	POSSIBLE PROBLEM	WHAT TO DO*
• Burping. • Discomfort and fullness after eating.	Air swallowed while eating.	• See Heartburn. • See Indigestion.
• Burping that worsens after eating fatty foods. • Pain in upper right abdomen that may spread to back.	Gallbladder disorder.	See Gallstones.
• Gas or bloating. • Consumption of cow's milk or other dairy product.	Inability to digest lactose.	See Lactose Intolerance.
• Gas. • Pale, bad-smelling stool. • Unexplained weight loss.	Poor digestion.	See Malabsorption.
Burping that worsens when bending or lying down.	Stomach acid in esophagus.	See Gastroesophageal Reflux Disease.
• Passing gas frequently. • Recurrent cramps or pain in lower abdomen.	Intestinal gas.	See Gas & Gas Pain.
Burping excessively plus any of the following: drinking carbonated beverages, eating too quickly, not chewing food properly, chewing gum, or sucking hard candies.	Swallowed air.	Change eating habits. Avoid causative agent.
• Gas. • Alternating constipation and diarrhea. • Lower abdominal pain that is relieved by passing gas or bowel movements.	Disorder of muscle contractions in colon.	See Irritable Bowel Syndrome.
• Burping. • Discomfort and fullness after eating. • Nausea, poor appetite.	Tumor.	See Stomach Cancer.
• Gas. • High-fiber diet or consumption of gas-causing foods.	Effect of diet.	Nothing. Improves eventually.
• Indigestion symptoms (burping). • Pain in upper abdomen. • Pain comes and goes.	Ulcer.	See Ulcer, Peptic.
• Gas and abdominal bloating. • Abdominal cramps. • Intermittent diarrhea.	Parasitic infection.	See Amebiasis.

*All references are to Illness section unless noted otherwise.

CHEST PAIN
(continued on next page)

SYMPTOMS & FACTORS	POSSIBLE PROBLEM	WHAT TO DO*
• Severe chest pain spreading to jaw, neck, or arms. • Sudden breathing difficulty.	Possible heart attack	• Call doctor now. • See Heart Attack.
• Mild chest pain or heart palpitations. • Mild breathing difficulty that may be increasing such as when exercising.	Heart problem.	• See Coronary Artery Disease. • See Heart Rhythm Irregularity. • See Heartbeat, Rapid. • See Hypertrophic Cardiomyopathy.
• Chest pain. • Sudden breathing difficulty. • May have had recent surgery or illness.	• Collapsed lung. • Blood clot.	• Call doctor now. • See Atelectasis. • See Pulmonary Embolism.
• Chest pain or discomfort that may feel like indigestion. • Symptoms occur while exercising, after a big meal, or with strong emotions.	Temporary lack of oxygen to heart.	See Angina Pectoris.
• Sharp chest pain that worsens with inhalation. • Sudden breathing difficulty. • No other factors.	Collapsed lung.	• Call doctor now. • See Pneumothorax.
• Chest pain. • Shortness of breath. • Cough. • Fever in some cases.	• Lung infection. • Inflammation of membranes around lungs. • Fungal infection.	• See Blastomycosis. • See Empyema. • See Pleural Effusion. • See Pleurisy. • See Pneumonia (all charts).
• Chest pain on one side. • Burning feeling at pain site. • Skin rash at pain site.	Virus infection of sensory nerves.	See Herpes Zoster.
• Burning feeling in chest. • Cough, wheezing, low fever.	Infection of bronchial tubes.	See Bronchitis, Acute.
• Chest pain on one side. • Recent chest injury, chest surgery, or severe cough.	Pulled muscle or broken rib.	• See Bone Fracture. • See Sprains & Strains.
• Pain in the chest or upper abdomen. • Heartburn or burping.	Digestive disorder.	• See Gastroesophageal Reflux Disease. • See Heartburn. • See Hiatal Hernia. • See Indigestion.

*All references are to Illness section unless noted otherwise.

CHEST PAIN
(continued from previous page)

SYMPTOMS & FACTORS	POSSIBLE PROBLEM	WHAT TO DO*
• Chest pain (sharp, dull, or pressing). • Fatigue, shortness of breath. • Dizziness, anxiety.	Heart valve disorder.	• See Mitral Valve Prolapse. • See Valvular Heart Disease.
Chest pain that worsens when swallowing.	Several disorders.	See Swallowing Difficulty (in this Symptoms section).
• Pain in chest wall. • Affected area sensitive to touch.	Cartilage inflammation.	See Costochondritis.
• Chest pain, palpitations. • Rapid heartbeat. • Shortness of breath. • Numbness or tingling around mouth, hands, or feet. • Emotional changes.	Severe anxiety.	See Panic Disorder.
• Dull or sharp pain in front of chest. • Rapid breathing. • Cough, fever, chills.	Heart inflammation.	See Pericarditis.
• Burning pain in the center of the chest and upper abdomen. • Pregnant.	Pregnancy symptom.	See Heartburn During Pregnancy.
Chest pain without symptoms or factors listed on this chart.	Many disorders, including stress and anxiety.	Consult doctor. Chest pain should never be ignored.

*All references are to Illness section unless noted otherwise.

CONFUSION (PERSON OVER AGE 65)

SYMPTOMS & FACTORS	POSSIBLE PROBLEM	WHAT TO DO*
• Confusion. • Use of drugs, including: antihistamines, appetite suppressants, muscle relaxants, pain killers, sedatives, tranquilizers, or mind-altering drugs, such as marijuana, cocaine, LSD, and heroin.	• Adverse reaction or side effect of drug. • Drug interaction.	Consult doctor.
• Confusion. • Slurred speech. • Weakness in extremities.	Decreased blood supply to brain.	• Call doctor now. • See Stroke. • See Transient Ischemic Attack.
• Sudden confusion. • Unusually long time since eating. OR • Use of insulin or oral hypoglycemic drug.	Low blood sugar.	Drink sweet drink or eat sweet snack. If confusion lasts longer than 10 minutes, call doctor.
• Confusion sudden or appearing overtime. • Fall or head injury in last 2 months.	Effect of injury.	• Call doctor now. • See Head Injury. • See Subdural Hemorrhage & Hematoma.
• Sudden confusion. • Signs of physical illness, such as fever, cough, or loss of bladder control.	Effect of illness.	Call doctor now.
• Sudden confusion. • Exposure to cold conditions. • Cold hands and feet.	Drop in body temperature.	See Hypothermia.
• Confusion appearing over several weeks, plus 2 or more of following: • Inability to remember recent events. • Decline in attention to personal appearance or cleanliness. • Personality change.	• Poor nutrition. • Mental deterioration.	• See Alzheimer's Disease. • See Dementia. • See Vitamin Deficiencies.
• Confusion. • Dehydrated. • Poor diet, lack of fluid intake.	Electrolyte imbalance.	• See Dehydration. • See Fluid & Electrolyte Disorder.

*All references are to Illness section unless noted otherwise.

CONFUSION (PERSON UNDER AGE 65)

SYMPTOMS & FACTORS	POSSIBLE PROBLEM	WHAT TO DO*
• Confusion. • Use of drugs, including: antihistamines, appetite suppressants, muscle relaxants, pain killers, sedatives, tranquilizers, or mind-altering drugs, such as marijuana, cocaine, LSD, and heroin.	• Adverse reaction or side effect of drug. • Drug interaction.	Consult doctor.
• Confusion, plus any of following: • Blurred vision. • Dizziness. • Numbness or tingling in any part of body. • Speaking difficulty. • Weakness in extremities.	Decreased blood supply to brain.	• Call doctor now. • See Stroke. • See Transient Ischemic Attack.
• Confusion in a child. • Lethargy, weakness, paralysis in an arm or leg. • Personality changes.	Brain and liver infection.	See Reye's Syndrome.
• Confusion. • Alcohol consumption either alone or with drug.	• Adverse reaction or side effect of alcohol. • Drug interaction.	• Consult doctor. • Stop drinking alcohol.
• Confusion. • Excessive dieting.	Vitamin deficiency.	Consult doctor for proper method of weight control.
• Confusion in a woman of childbearing age. • Sudden fever of 101°F (38.3°C) or higher. • Vomiting. • Skin rash.	Infection.	• Call doctor now. • See Toxic Shock Syndrome.
• Confusion, plus any of following: • Heart disease. • Lung disease. • Diabetes.	Complication of underlying disorder.	Call doctor now.
• Confusion, plus any of following: • Agitation. • Delirium. • Disorientation. • Inability to recognize others. • Hallucinations.	• Mental illness. • Low blood sugar. • Bleeding inside skull. • Tumor.	• Call doctor now. • See Brain Tumor. • See Diabetes Hypoglycemia. • See Subdural Hemorrhage & Hematoma.
• Confusion. • Dehydrated. • Poor diet, lack of fluid intake.	Electrolyte imbalance.	• See Dehydration. • See Fluid & Electrolyte Disorder.

*All references are to Illness section unless noted otherwise.

CONSTIPATION

SYMPTOMS & FACTORS	POSSIBLE PROBLEM	WHAT TO DO*
• Constipation. • Pain with bowel movements. • Occasional blood in stool.	• Varicose veins in anus. • Split in skin around anus.	• See Constipation. • See Hemorrhoids.
• Constipation. • Use of prescription or nonprescription drug.	Adverse reaction or side effect of drug.	• Consult doctor about prescription drug. • Discontinue use of nonprescription drug.
• Constipation. • Pain in lower abdomen within last week.	Inflammation of large intestine.	• See Colon Cancer. • See Diverticular Disease. • See Intestinal Obstruction.
• Chronic constipation. • Recurrent pain in lower abdomen.	Disorder of muscle contractions in colon.	See Irritable Bowel Syndrome.
• Constipation, plus 2 or more of following: • Fatigue. • Unexplained weight gain. • Dry skin or hair. • Decreased tolerance to cold.	Underactive thyroid gland.	See Hypothyroidism.
• Chronic tendency toward constipation. • Frequent suppression of urge for bowel movement. OR • Regular laxative use.	Poor bowel reflexes.	See Constipation.
• Lack of normal bowel movements. • Sense of fullness, but unable to pass stool. • Pain or cramps in stomach.	Irregular bowel function.	See Fecal Impaction.
Constipation while dieting.	Lack of adequate water or fiber in diet.	Include more fiber in your diet.
• Chronic tendency toward constipation. • No other symptoms.	Lack of adequate water or fiber in diet.	See Constipation.
• In male, constant urge to have a bowel movement when little or no stool present. • Rectal or abdominal pain.	Rectum inflammation.	See Proctitis.
• Chronic constipation or chronic diarrhea. • Gas and bloating. • Laxative use.	Excess laxative use.	See Laxative Abuse.

*All references are to Illness section unless noted otherwise.

CONVULSIONS (SEIZURES)

SYMPTOMS & FACTORS	POSSIBLE PROBLEM	WHAT TO DO*
First time seizure (convulsion).	Several disorders.	Call doctor right away.
• Seizures (convulsions). • Headache, nausea, vomiting. • Confusion.	• Infection or tumor. • Breathing poisonous gas.	• See Brain or Epidural Abscess. • See Brain Tumor. • See Carbon Monoxide Poisoning.
• Seizures (convulsions). • Irregular heartbeat. • Lethargy. • Poor appetite.	Electrolyte problem.	See Calcium Imbalance.
• Seizures. • Fainting and unconsciousness.	Heart problem.	See Cardiac Arrest.
Seizures (convulsions).	Brain disorder.	See Epilepsy.
• Seizure (convulsion). • Fever. • Infant or young child.	Unknown cause.	See Febrile Seizure.
• Seizure (convulsion). • Pregnant woman.	High blood pressure.	See Preeclampsia & Eclampsia.
• Seizures (convulsions). • Recurrent headaches. • Weakness, vision changes, slurred speech.	Bleeding in the brain.	See Subdural Hemorrhage & Hematoma.
• Seizure (convulsion). • Reduced urine output. • Swelling in legs, ankles, or feet.	Kidney disorder.	See Renal Failure, Acute.
• Seizure (convulsion). • Diabetes.	Extreme low blood sugar.	See Diabetes Hypoglycemia.

*All references are to Illness section unless noted otherwise.

COUGH
(continued on next page)

SYMPTOMS & FACTORS	POSSIBLE PROBLEM	WHAT TO DO*
• Recent cough. • Stuffy or runny nose. • Sore throat.	Virus infection.	See Cold, Common.
• Recent cough. • Fever.	Inflammation or infection of breathing passages.	• See Bronchitis, Acute. • See Influenza. • See Influenza, H1N1.
• Persistent cough following cold or flu. • History of persistent cough during previous cold or flu seasons.	Chronic inflammation or infection.	• See Bronchitis, Chronic. • See Sinusitis.
• Persistent cough with sputum. • Chronic breathing difficulty that is worsening. • No dusty working conditions.	Chronic inflammation or infection of breathing passages.	• See Chronic Obstructive Pulmonary Disease. • See Emphysema.
• Chronic cough. • Smokers in the home.	Effect of second-hand smoke.	• Encourage smoker to quit or stop smoking inside the house. • See Smoking Addiction.
• Recent cough with green-yellow or rusty sputum. • Fever. • Breathing difficulty.	Lung infection.	• See Coccidioidomycosis. • See Histoplasmosis. • See Pneumonia (all charts).
• Persistent cough with sputum that is worsening. • Fever. • Unexplained weight loss. • Fatigue. • Excessive sweating at night.	Lung infection or inflammation.	• See Bronchiectasis. • See Lung Abscess. • See Tuberculosis.
• Sudden cough without sputum. • Inhalation of irritating substance or fumes such as smog.	Irritation of breathing passages.	Avoid exposure to chemicals, dust and cigarettes.
• Recent cough without sputum. • Hoarseness or voice loss.	Inflammation of vocal cords.	See Voice Loss or Hoarseness (in this Symptoms section).
• Cough. • Chest pain. • Chills, fever, sweats. • Shortness of breath.	Fungal infection.	See Blastomycosis.
• Cough. • Chills, fever, loss of appetite. • Contact with birds.	Infection transmitted by birds.	See Psittacosis.
• Sudden violent cough. • Inhalation of foreign object.	Normal coughing to expel object from lungs.	Consult doctor if cough lasts longer than 1 hour.
Persistent cough without sputum.	• Spasm of bronchial tubes. • Tumor.	• See Asthma. • See Lung Cancer.

*All references are to Illness section unless noted otherwise.

COUGH
(continued from previous page)

SYMPTOMS & FACTORS	POSSIBLE PROBLEM	WHAT TO DO*
• Cough. • Shortness of breath.	Several disorders.	See Breathing Difficulty (in this Symptoms section).
• Slow onset of dry, nonproductive cough. • Fever. • Shortness of breath. • Immune disorder such as HIV or AIDS.	Protozoan infection.	See *Pneumocystis Jiroveci* Pneumonia.
• Cough, sore throat, increased saliva. • Fatigue, slight fever. • Recent animal bite.	Virus infection.	See Rabies.
• Cough, sometimes with mucus. • General ill feeling. • Have or have had had dusty working conditions.	Lung inflammation.	• See Pneumoconiosis. • See Silicosis.
• Cough, sometimes with mucus. • Fever. • Headache, sometimes severe.	Fungal infection.	See Cryptococcosis.
• Coughing, sneezing, and postnasal drip. • Runny or stuffy nose. • Watery and itchy eyes. • Possible exposure to mold.	Mold allergy.	See Mold Allergy.

*All references are to Illness section unless noted otherwise.

COUGH WITH BLOOD

SYMPTOMS & FACTORS	POSSIBLE PROBLEM	WHAT TO DO*
• Cough with blood. • Recent surgery. OR • Recent bed confinement because of illness or injury.	Blood clot in lung.	• Call doctor now. • See Pulmonary Embolism.
• Cough with blood. • Persistent cough following recent cold or flu.	Bleeding in breathing passages.	Call doctor now.
• Persistent cough with blood for several weeks. • Fever of 100°F (37.8°C) or higher. • Unexplained weight loss. • Fatigue. • Excessive sweating at night.	• Bacterial inflammation or infection of lung. • Tumor.	• Call doctor now. • See Lung Abscess. • See Lung Cancer. • See Tuberculosis.
• Cough with blood or frothy pink or brownish sputum. • Breathing difficulty. • History of high blood pressure or heart disorder.	Fluid in lungs.	• Consult doctor. • See Pulmonary Edema.
• Cough with blood or brownish sputum. • Fever. • May have chest pain, breathing difficulty, headache, or fatigue.	Lung infection.	• Call doctor now. • See Pneumonia (all charts).

*All references are to Illness section unless noted otherwise.

COUGHING IN CHILDREN

SYMPTOMS & FACTORS	POSSIBLE PROBLEM	WHAT TO DO*
• Cough. • Fever.	Virus infection.	• See Cold, Common. • See Influenza. • See Influenza, H1N1.
• Cough, sometimes with wheezing. • Runny nose. • Low grade fever. • Being tired. • Infant or child may refuse to eat. • Ear ache.	Virus infection.	See Respiratory Syncytial Virus.
• Cough. • Severe breathing difficulty. • Wheezing. OR • Bluish face or fingertips.	• Spasm of bronchial tubes. • Swelling in vocal cords.	• Call doctor now. • See Asthma. • See Croup.
• Cough. • Use of prescription or nonprescription drug.	Adverse reaction or side effect of drug.	• Consult doctor about prescription drug. • Discontinue use of non prescription drug.
• Cough. • Fever. • Rapid or difficult breathing.	Infection of breathing passages.	• Call doctor now. • See Bronchitis, Acute. • See Bronchiolitis. • See Pneumonia (all charts).
• Severe uncontrollable cough. • Noisy "whooping" gasps for air following cough.	Bacterial lung infection.	See Whooping Cough.
• Cough. • Noisy breathing with wheezing. • Possible inhalation of small foreign object, such as peanut.	Coughing to expel object from lung.	Call doctor now or seek emergency help.
• Cough. • Sore throat.	Several disorders.	See Throat, Sore (in this Symptoms section).
• Persistent cough in an infant. • Abdominal swelling. • Frequent, bad-smelling stools.	Inherited disorder.	See Cystic Fibrosis.
• Cough. • Chronic runny or stuffy nose.	Enlarged adenoids.	Consult doctor.
• Cough. • Adult smokers in house or child may have smoked.	Irritation caused by tobacco smoke.	• Adult smokers should smoke outside. • Talk to child about hazards of smoking.

*All references are to Illness section unless noted otherwise.

DEPRESSION

SYMPTOMS & FACTORS	POSSIBLE PROBLEM	WHAT TO DO*
• Depression. • May or may not have other symptoms such as stress.	Emotional reaction	• See Depression. • See Stress.
• Depression. • Illness or health problems such as: rheumatoid arthritis, multiple sclerosis, heart or lung disease, cancer, pain, sexual problems, hormonal changes in women.	Any illness, severe or mild, can cause significant depression.	• Consult doctor. • See Depression. • See chart in Illness section for a particular disorder or condition.
• Depression. • Use of prescription or nonprescription drug. OR • Excessive alcohol consumption.	Adverse reaction or side effect of drug or alcohol.	• Consult doctor. • See Alcoholism.
• Depression. • Recent virus infection with fever such as: flu, infectious mononucleosis, or hepatitis.	Common occurrence following infection.	Consult doctor if depression worsens or lasts longer than 2 weeks.
Depression following traumatic or sad event, such as death in family.	Normal occurrence for 3 to 6 months following such experiences.	• Feelings are a normal part of mourning and will gradually improve over time. Seek medical help if depression worsens. • See Grief.
Periods of depression at times and then periods of manic (excited) behavior,	Mood/mental disorder.	See Bipolar Disorder.
Depression experienced at the start of winter season.	Lack of light.	See Seasonal Affective Disorder.
Chronic depressive mood.	Mild depression.	See Dysthymia.
Depression in a woman following childbirth.	Common occurrence for several weeks after delivery.	See Postpartum Mood Disorders.
• Depression. • Other changes in behavior in an older person.	Dementia.	• See Alzheimer's Disease. • See Dementia.
• Depression. • Lack of sleep.	Sleep problem.	• See Insomnia. • See Sleep Disorders, Temporary.
• Depression. • Persistent fatigue over the last 6 months.	Unknown cause.	See Chronic Fatigue Syndrome.

*All references are to Illness section unless noted otherwise.

DIARRHEA (INFANT 0 TO 6 MONTHS)

SYMPTOMS & FACTORS	POSSIBLE PROBLEM	WHAT TO DO*
• Diarrhea. • Fever. • Vomiting.	Infection of digestive tract.	• See Dehydration. • See Diarrhea, Acute. • See Gastroenteritis.
• Diarrhea. • Baby content, alert, and feeding well. • Baby taking nonprescription drug.	Adverse reaction or side effect of drug.	• Consult doctor. • Discontinue use of drug unless recommended by doctor.
• Diarrhea. • Baby taking prescription drug for some other disorder.	Adverse reaction or side effect of drug.	Consult doctor. Dose may need adjustment, substitution, or discontinuation.
• Diarrhea. • Itching at night. OR • Worms in stool.	Parasites.	• See Pinworms. • See Roundworms.
• Diarrhea. • Recent addition of solids to diet.	Baby too young to digest solid food.	• Consult doctor. • Wait until age 4 months before trying solids.
• Diarrhea. • Pulling at the ear.	Ear infection.	See Ear Infection, Middle.
• Diarrhea. • Baby seems content, alert, and feeds well on bottle feedings. • Sugar added to any formula or water. OR • Less than recommended amount of water added to baby's orange juice. OR • Fruit juice sweetened with sugar.	Upset digestion due to excess sugar.	• Consult doctor. • Don't add sugar to baby's food. • Use recommended amounts of water to dilute juice.
• Diarrhea. • Abdominal pain. • Flatulence and bloating.	Reaction to a swallowed substance.	• See Food Allergy. • See Lactose Intolerance.
• Diarrhea. • Vomiting.	Several disorders.	See Vomiting (Infant 0 to 6 months) (in this Symptoms section).
• Loose, pale, bad-smelling stools. • Weight loss or slow weight gain. • Swollen abdomen, abdominal pain.	Gluten intolerance.	See Celiac Disease.

*All references are to Illness section unless noted otherwise.

DIARRHEA (PERSON OVER 6 MONTHS)

SYMPTOMS & FACTORS	POSSIBLE PROBLEM	WHAT TO DO*
• Diarrhea. • Nausea or vomiting.	Viral, bacterial, or parasitic infection of digestive tract.	• See Diarrhea, Acute. • See Dysentery, Bacillary. • See Gastroenteritis. • See Pseudo-membranous Colitis.
• Diarrhea for 24 hours or longer. • Consumption of spoiled food or contaminated food or water.	Effect of toxins in food.	• See Food Poisoning. • See Listeriosis. • See Salmonella Infections.
• Recurrent attacks of diarrhea. • Pain in lower abdomen.	• Intestinal parasites. • Inflammation. • Several disorders.	• See Amebiasis. • See Crohn's Disease. • See Giardiasis. • See Recurrent Abdominal Pain (in this Symptoms section).
• Diarrhea. • Use of prescription or nonprescription drug.	Adverse reaction or side effect of drug.	• Consult doctor about prescription drug. • Discontinue use of nonprescription drug.
• Diarrhea. • Abdominal cramping and bloating. • Mucus in stools.	Bowel problem.	• See Colitis, Ulcerative. • See Irritable Bowel Syndrome.
Recurrent attacks of diarrhea during periods of stress.	Effect of stress.	• See Anxiety Disorder, Generalized. • See Irritable Bowel Syndrome. • See Stress.
• Diarrhea. • Use of sorbitol, a common sweetener found in many diet products.	The sugar is not absorbed by the small intestine.	Discontinue use of the product with sorbitol.
• Diarrhea. • Abdominal pain. • Hives, rash (called eczema), itching, redness, and swelling.	Reaction to a swallowed substance.	See Food Allergy.
Chronic, frequent, loose stools in young child.	Intestinal problem.	See Diarrhea, Chronic, Non-Specific of Childhood.
• Explosive diarrhea. • Weakness and faintness. • Recent stomach surgery.	Intestinal disorder.	See Dumping Syndrome.
• Diarrhea, bad-smelling stools. • Weight loss, gas. • Weakness.	Nutritional disorder.	See Malabsorption.
• Chronic diarrhea or chronic constipation. • Gas and bloating. • Laxative use.	Excess laxative use.	See Laxative Abuse.

*All references are to Illness section unless noted otherwise.

DIZZINESS

SYMPTOMS & FACTORS	POSSIBLE PROBLEM	WHAT TO DO*
• Dizziness. • Use of prescription or nonprescription drug.	Adverse reaction or side effect of drug.	• Consult doctor about prescription drug. • Discontinue use of nonprescription drug.
• Dizziness. • Decreased hearing. • Noises in ear. OR • Earache.	Infection or disorder of inner ear.	• See Labyrinthitis. • See Ménière's Disease.
Dizziness when turning head in person over age 50.	Pressure on nerves in neck.	See Cervical Spondylosis.
Dizziness when standing suddenly.	• Temporary drop in blood pressure. • Red blood cell disorder. • Inner ear problem.	• Avoid rising suddenly. • See Anemia, Iron-Deficiency. • See Benign Paroxysmal Positional Vertigo.
• Dizziness. • Stress or anxiety.	Hyperventilation.	• See Anxiety Disorder, Generalized. • See Panic Disorder. • See Phobias. • See Stress.
Dizziness (spinning sensation).	• Travel by air, sea, or motor vehicle. • Inner ear problem.	• See Benign Paroxysmal Positional Vertigo. • See Motion Sickness.
• Dizziness. • Headache. • Faintness. • Nausea, vomiting.	Toxic gas inhalation.	See Carbon Monoxide Poisoning.
• Dizziness. • Excess sun or heat exposure.	Body overheated.	See Heatstroke or Heat Exhaustion.
• Dizziness, plus any of following: • Speaking difficulty. • Blurred vision. • Numbness or tingling in any part of body. • Weakness or paralysis in extremities.	Decreased blood supply to brain.	• Call doctor now. • See Stroke. • See Transient Ischemic Attack.
• Dizziness. • Headache, vague symptoms.	High blood pressure.	See Hypertension.
• Dizziness. • Recurrent morning headache. • Nausea or vomiting.	• Bleeding inside skull. • Tumor.	• Call doctor now. • See Brain Tumor. • See Subdural Hemorrhage & Hematoma.
• Dizziness. • Irregular heartbeat.	Heart rhythm disorder.	• See Atrial Fibrillation. • See Heart Block. • See Heart Rhythm Irregularity.

*All references are to Illness section unless noted otherwise.

EAR, RINGING OR BUZZING SOUNDS

SYMPTOMS & FACTORS	POSSIBLE PROBLEM	WHAT TO DO*
• Ear noises. • Use of prescription or nonprescription drug.	Adverse reaction or side effect of drug.	• Consult doctor about prescription drug. • Discontinue use of nonprescription drug.
• Ear noises. • Hearing loss.	Damaged auditory nerve.	See Hearing Impairment or Loss.
• Noises in the ear. • Dizziness.	Fluid in the ear.	See Ménière's Disease.
• Strange, loud ear noises. • Severe, uncomfortable tickling in ear.	Insect in outer-ear canal.	Consult doctor.
Ear noises after airplane flight.	Middle-ear problem caused by change in air pressure.	See Barotitis Media.
Noise in ear (ringing, buzzing, roaring, whistling, or hissing).	Damaged auditory nerve.	See Tinnitus.
• Ringing in ear. • Slow, progressive hearing loss.	Abnormal bone growth in middle ear.	See Otosclerosis.

*All references are to Illness section unless noted otherwise.

EARACHE

SYMPTOMS & FACTORS	POSSIBLE PROBLEM	WHAT TO DO*
• Earache. • Sticky, green-yellow discharge from ear canal or middle ear.	Ear infection.	• See Ear Infection, Middle. • See Ear Infection, Outer. • See Eardrum, Ruptured.
• Earache. • Fever.	Infection of middle ear.	See Ear Infection, Middle.
• Earache or ear feels plugged up. • Stuffy nose.	Common occurrence with cold or allergy.	• See Cold, Common. • See Hay Fever.
Earache that worsens when earlobe is pulled.	Infection of outer-ear canal.	See Ear Infection, Outer.
• Earache. • Pain in tooth or jaw.	• Tooth or gum infection. • Inflammation of joint in jaw.	• Consult dentist. • See Tooth Abscess. • See Temporomandibular Joint Disorder.
• Earache. • Blocked feeling in ear that cannot be cleared by swallowing. • Diminished hearing.	Wax in ear canal.	See Earwax Blockage.
• Earache that began during airplane flight. • Blocked feeling in ear that cannot be cleared by swallowing.	Middle-ear damage caused by change in air pressure.	See Barotitis Media.

*All references are to Illness section unless noted otherwise.

EYE PAIN, SWELLING, DRYNESS, ITCHING, TEARING

(continued on next page)

SYMPTOMS & FACTORS	POSSIBLE PROBLEM	WHAT TO DO*
• Eye pain. • Eye injury without visible damage.	Minor injury.	See Eye Contusion or Laceration.
• Pain behind eye. • Area of tenderness over nose or cheekbones. • Pain that worsens when bending forward. • Recent cold or nasal allergies.	Sinus infection.	See Sinusitis.
• Itching, watery eyes. • Frequent sneezing, stuffy nose, with clear discharge.	Allergy.	See Hay Fever.
• Eye pain. • Watery, red eye.	Foreign object in eye.	See Eye, Foreign Body in.
• Eye pain. • Red, swollen bump on eyelid. • Red eye.	Infection of hair follicle on eyelid.	See Stye.
• Eye pain. • Red eye. • Gritty feeling in eye. • Stickiness around eye.	Infection of eye membrane.	See Conjunctivitis.
• Eye pain. • Red eye. • Gritty feeling in eye.	Inadequate tear production.	Use nonprescription artificial tears. Consult doctor if discomfort lasts longer than 2 days.
• Eye pain. • Eyelid curls inward. • Red eyelid and eye.	Disorder of eyelid.	See Ectropion & Entropion.
Swelling on eyelid.	Eye infection.	See Chalazion.
• Redness and greasy scales on the eyelid edges. • Eyelashes that fall out.	Infection.	See Blepharitis.
• Pain around eye. • Sudden onset of headache. • Headache appears at same time on consecutive days.	Chronic headache disorder.	See Headache, Cluster.
• Eye pain. • Sensitivity to light. • Tearing.	Inflammation of the cornea.	See Keratitis.
• Eye pain. • Purple-red inflamed area in one or more areas of the white of the eye.	Inflammation.	Consult doctor.

*All references are to Illness section unless noted otherwise.

EYE PAIN, SWELLING, DRYNESS, ITCHING, TEARING

(continued from previous page)

SYMPTOMS & FACTORS	POSSIBLE PROBLEM	WHAT TO DO*
• Dryness of eyes. • Foreign body sensation. • Dryness of mouth. • Parotid gland enlargement (chipmunk look).	Autoimmune disorder.	See Sjögren's Syndrome.
Sudden appearance of blood in the white of the eye.	Spontaneous bleeding.	See Subconjunctival Hemorrhage.
• Persistent tearing of one or both eyes. • Drainage of mucous and pus from tear duct.	Obstructed tear duct.	See Tear Duct Infection or Blockage.
• Eye itching, burning, stinging, or redness. • Eye irritation, discomfort, pain, or excess tearing.	Eye dryness.	See Dry Eye Syndrome.
• Severe eye pain. • Recent eye injury with visible damage. • Loss of vision.	Serious injury.	Call doctor now.
• Pain behind eye. • Tenderness in temple on affected side.	Inflammation of arteries in temples.	• Call doctor now. • See Polymyalgia Rheumatica & Giant Cell Arteritis.
• Pain behind eye, plus any of following: • Eyes sensitive to light. • Lethargy. • Confusion. • Pain that worsens when bending head forward. • Severe headache.	• Inflammation of membranes around brain. • Bleeding in membrane around brain.	• Call doctor now. • See Meningitis, Aseptic. • See Meningitis, Bacterial. • See Subarachnoid Hemorrhage.
• Eye pain. • Blurred vision.	• Eye injury. • Inflammation in eye. • Excess pressure in eye.	• See Corneal Abrasion & Ulcer. • See Glaucoma, Angle-Closure.
• Eye pain. • Sensitivity to light. • Eye redness. • Tears, blurred vision.	Inflammation.	See Iritis.

*All references are to Illness section unless noted otherwise.

FACE PAIN

SYMPTOMS & FACTORS	POSSIBLE PROBLEM	WHAT TO DO*
• Pain on one side of face or all over head. • Tight feeling around head.	Headache.	• See Headache, Migraine. • See Headache, Tension.
• Pain or tenderness around eyes and cheekbones that worsens when bending head forward. • Recent cold or nasal allergies.	Sinus infection.	See Sinusitis.
Throbbing pain on one side of face that worsens at night, when eating or when touching a particular tooth.	Infection around tooth.	Consult doctor or dentist.
• Aching pain over or around jaw joint. • Jaw that sometimes clicks when opening. • Frequent headaches.	Inflammation of joint in jaw.	See Temporomandibular Joint Disorder.
• Pain around ear. • Sudden paralysis on one side of face.	Facial paralysis.	See Bell's Palsy.
• Parotid gland enlargement (chipmunk look). • Dryness of eyes and mouth.	Autoimmune disorder.	See Sjögren's Syndrome.
• Face pain. • Recent rash at site of pain.	Virus infection of sensory nerves.	See Herpes Zoster.
• Frequent contractions of muscles on the side of the face. • Tooth-grinding noises at night.	Tooth problem.	See Tooth Grinding.
• Severe pain on one side of face over eye. • Redness of white of eye. • Blurred vision.	Excess pressure in eye.	See Glaucoma, Angle-Closure.
Sharp pain on one side of face when face is touched or when chewing.	Damaged nerve.	See Trigeminal Neuralgia.
• Face pain, plus any of following: • Chest pain. • Neck pain. • Shoulder pain. • Arm pain.	Heart attack.	• Call doctor now. • See Heart Attack.
• Pain and swelling in tongue area or behind the ear. • Dry mouth. • May be hard to open mouth wide.	Gland infection.	See Salivary Gland Infection.

*All references are to Illness section unless noted otherwise.

FACIAL SKIN PROBLEMS

FAINTNESS O
(continued o

SYMPTOMS & FACTORS	POSSIBLE PROBLEM	
• Pimples. • Painful, red bumps • Bumps with white or yellow centers. • Blackheads.	Skin disorder beginning after puberty.	
• Flushed face that may last minutes or hours to several days. • Facial tenderness.	Disorder of tiny blood vessels.	
Blister or red, rough, or painful area around mouth.	Virus infection.	See Herpes Simplex.
Sore on face or lip that doesn't heal in 3 weeks.	Skin cancer.	• See Carcinoma, Basal Cell. • See Carcinoma, Squamous Cell.
• Blister-like rash on one side of face. • Painful, burning sensation at site 1 or 2 days before rash appears.	Virus infection of sensory nerves.	See Herpes Zoster.
Blisters that burst and become crusty.	Skin infection.	See Impetigo.
Red, itching, scaling rash on face.	Allergic reaction.	See Eczema, Dyshidrotic.
• Rash (usually on the cheeks). • Fatigue. • Fever. • Joint pain.	Autoimmune disorder.	See Lupus Erythematosus, Systemic.
Red bumps on cheeks, on either side of nose and on scalp (sometimes).	Autoimmune disorder.	See Lupus Erythematosus, Discold.
• Rough, red patch on cheek, nose or forehead. • Person over age 35.	Skin damage caused by sun exposure.	• See Sunburn. • See Keratosis, Actinic.
Patch of skin on face that is lighter or darker than surrounding skin.	Disorder of skin pigment.	See Vitiligo.
• Rash (especially in children) starting on cheeks, then spreading to other body parts. • Slight tiredness or fatigue.	Virus infection.	See Erythema Infectiosum.
• Change in face mole's size, color or sensitivity. OR • A new mole or lump on face.	Skin cancer.	See Melanoma.

*All references are to Illness section unless noted otherwise.

...CTORS	POSSIBLE PROBLEM	WHAT TO DO*
	No underlying disorder.	See Fainting.
...ss when standing ...ly.	Temporary drop in blood pressure.	Avoid rising suddenly.
...aintness following bed confinement.		
• Faintness. • Breathing deeply, rapidly or sighing before faintness.	Effect of stress. No underlying disorder.	• See Anxiety Disorder, Generalized. • See Panic Disorder. • Consult doctor if happens repeatedly.
• Faintness. • Use of drug for high blood pressure.	Adverse reaction or side effect of drug.	Consult doctor.
• Faintness. • Dizziness.	Several disorders.	See Dizziness (in this Symptoms section).
• Faintness or fainting. • Feeling that heart speeds or slows before faintness. • Known heart disease.	Heart rhythm disorder.	• Call doctor now. • See Atrial Fibrillation. • See Cardiac Arrest. • See Heart Block. • See Heart Rhythm Irregularity.
• Faintness, plus any of following: • Blurred vision. • Speaking difficulty. • Confusion. • Numbness or tingling in any part of body. • Weakness or paralysis in extremities.	Decreased blood supply to brain.	• Call doctor now. • See Stroke. • See Transient Ischemic Attack.
• Fainting. • Seizure disorder.	Minor seizure.	See Epilepsy.
Faintness after several hours in strong sunshine or hot environment.	Excess heat exposure.	• Call doctor now. • See Heatstroke or Heat Exhaustion.
• Faintness. • Diabetes.	Low blood sugar.	• Drink sweetened juice or beverage or eat something sugary or starchy. • See Diabetes Hypoglycemia.
• Faintness. • Fatigue. • Shortness of breath. • Person older than 50.	• Disorder of red blood cells. • Heart disease.	• See Anemia, Pernicious. • See Heart Failure.
Faintness when turning head (in person older than 50).	Pressure on nerves in neck.	See Cervical Spondylosis.

*All references are to Illness section unless noted otherwise.

FAINTNESS OR FAINTING
(continued from previous page)

SYMPTOMS & FACTORS	POSSIBLE PROBLEM	WHAT TO DO*
• Fainting. • Shortness of breath before faintness. • Recent strenuous exercise.	Temporary change in blood chemistry.	Consult doctor if happens repeatedly.
• Fainting and weakness. • Sweating, irregular heartbeat. • Recent stomach surgery. • Diarrhea.	Intestinal disorder.	See Dumping Syndrome.
• Faintness. • Headache, dizziness, nausea, and vomiting.	Toxic gas inhalation.	See Carbon Monoxide Poisoning.
• Fainting and weakness. • Sweating, headache, confusion. • Excessive hunger.	Low blood sugar.	See Hypoglycemia, Reactive.

*All references are to Illness section unless noted otherwise.

FATIGUE OR TIREDNESS
(continued on next page)

SYMPTOMS & FACTORS	POSSIBLE PROBLEM	WHAT TO DO*
• Fatigue. • Appetite loss. • Weight loss.	• Disorder of red blood cells. • Folic deficiency.	• See Anemia (all charts). • See Folic Acid Deficiency.
• Fatigue, plus 2 or more of following: • Appetite loss. • Fever. • Headache. • Painful swelling in neck, armpit or groin. • Jaundice (yellow skin and eyes). • Sore throat.	Virus infection.	See Mononucleosis, Infectious.
• Fatigue. • Use of prescription or nonprescription drug.	Adverse reaction or side effect of drug.	• Consult doctor about prescription drug. • Discontinue use of nonprescription drug.
• Fatigue. • Coarse skin and hair. • Low voice. • Loss of sex drive. • Puffy face.	Underactive thyroid gland.	See Hypothyroidism.
• Fatigue, fever, headache. • Sore throat. • Diarrhea or constipation. • Stomach pains.	Bacterial infection.	See Typhoid Fever.
• Fatigue in woman at menopause. • Appetite loss.	Normal occurrence with decreasing estrogen level of menopause.	• See Menopause. • See Perimenopause.
• Fatigue. • Pregnancy. • Shortness of breath.	Dietary deficiency of pregnancy, particularly of protein, calcium, vitamins or iron.	• Consult doctor. • Eat extra protein foods. • Take supplements if prescribed.
• Fatigue. • Depression or anxiety.	Effect of stress.	• See Anxiety Disorder, Generalized. • See Depression. • See Stress.
• Loss of appetite, tiredness. • Swelling of lymph nodes. • Fever, night sweats, weight loss.	Cancer.	See Lymphoma, Non-Hodgkin's.
• Ongoing fatigue for several months. • Numerous other symptoms.	Unknown infection or problem.	See Chronic Fatigue Syndrome.

*All references are to Illness section unless noted otherwise.

FATIGUE OR TIREDNESS
(continued on next page)

SYMPTOMS & FACTORS	POSSIBLE PROBLEM	WHAT TO DO*
• Fatigue. • Chest discomfort with exertion that is relieved by rest.	Narrowing of coronary arteries.	• Consult doctor. • See Atherosclerosis. • See Coronary Artery Disease. • See Valvular Heart Disease.
• Fatigue. • Increased hunger and thirst. • Weight loss. • Frequent urination, especially at night.	Blood sugar problem.	• See Diabetes Type 1. • See Diabetes Type 2.
• Tiredness. • Depression. • Increased appetite. • Beginning of winter.	Lack of light.	See Seasonal Affective Disorder.
• Fatigue and weakness. • Intermittent fever, chills, sweating. • Weight loss.	• Heart valve or heart lining infection. • Viral infection.	• See Endocarditis. • See HIV & AIDS.
• Fatigue. • Fever, rash (usually on the cheeks). • Joint pain.	Autoimmune disorder.	See Lupus Erythematosus, Systemic
• Fatigue. • Appetite loss. • Weight loss. • Hair loss. • Skin that darkens.	Inadequate cortisone hormone.	See Addison's Disease.
• Fatigue. • Cough. • Fever. • Weight loss. • Shortness of breath.	• Lung infection. • Tumor.	• See Bronchiectasis. • See Influenza. • See Influenza, H1N1. • See Lung Cancer. • See Pneumonia (all charts). • See Tuberculosis.
• Fatigue. • Headache and nausea. • Recent trip to foreign country.	Parasite infection.	See Malaria.
• Fatigue. • Shortness of breath. • Irregular heartbeat.	Heart inflammation.	See Myocarditis.
• Fatigue, slight fever. • Cough, sore throat, increased saliva. • Animal bite.	Virus infection.	See Rabies.
• Fatigue. • Chills, fever, sweating. • Tenderness along spine.	Bacterial infection.	See Brucellosis.

*All references are to Illness section unless noted otherwise.

FATIGUE OR TIREDNESS
(continued from previous page)

SYMPTOMS & FACTORS	POSSIBLE PROBLEM	WHAT TO DO*
• Fatigue and lethargy. • Paleness. • Behavioral changes. • Abdominal discomfort.	Inhalation or ingestion of lead.	See Lead Poisoning.
• Tiredness. • Fever. • Swollen lymph glands.	Protozoan infection.	See Toxoplasmosis.
• Fatigue and sleep problems. • Muscle aches and pains. • Areas of the body are tender to the touch.	Chronic pain disorder.	See Fibromyalgia.
• Fatigue and weakness. • Tingling sensation in arms, hands, legs, and feet. • Urinary frequency.	Endocrine disorder.	See Hyperaldosteronism.
• Lethargy, weakness, paralysis in an arm or leg (in a child). • Confusion. • Personality changes.	Brain and liver infection.	See Reye's Syndrome.
• Fatigue. • Appetite loss. • Nausea, plus some of following: • Jaundice (yellow skin and eyes). • Vomiting. • Tenderness over liver. • Fever. • Weakness.	Liver disorder.	• See Cirrhosis of the Liver. • See Hepatitis, Viral.
• Fatigue. • Sleep disturbances, malaise. • Loss of concentration. • Travel.	Disturbance in the body's physiological processes.	See Jet Lag.
• Fatigue. • Problems with walking. • Bowel and bladder problems.	Autoimmune disorder.	See Multiple Sclerosis.
• Tiredness and weakness. • Pale skin, eyes, and fingernails. • General ill feeling.	• Anemia. • Cancer.	• See Anemia Hemolytic. • See Leukemia, Acute. • See Leukemia, Chronic.
Tiredness and weakness in pregnant woman.	Anemia.	See Anemia During Pregnancy.

*All references are to Illness section unless noted otherwise.

FEVER (CHILD 0 TO 2 YEARS)

SYMPTOMS & FACTORS	POSSIBLE PROBLEM	WHAT TO DO*
• Fever. • Runny nose. • Recent exposure to contagious disease, such as measles, mumps, or chickenpox.	Early stage of contagious illness.	Consult doctor.
• Fever. • Diarrhea.	Infection of digestive tract.	• Consult doctor. • See Gastroenteritis.
• Fever. • Runny nose.	Virus infection.	• See Cold, Common. • See Respiratory Syncytial Virus. • Consult doctor if temperature rises.
• Fever. • Infant overdressed. • Hot weather or environment.	Overheating.	• Remove some of infant's clothing. • Offer water to drink. • Give cool sponge bath.
• Fever. • Crying as if in pain. • Pulling at ear.	Infection of middle ear.	• Consult doctor. • See Ear Infection, Middle.
• Fever. • Convulsions.	Effect of high fever.	• Call doctor now. • See Febrile Seizure.
• Fever. • Infant of 3 months or younger.	Many possibilities. Signs of illness at this age require prompt medical evaluation.	Consult doctor.
• Fever. • Rash.	Several disorders.	See Rash With Fever (in this Symptoms section).
Fever on several occasions over a 3-week period.	Uncertain problem.	See Fever of Unknown Origin.
• Fever. • Noisy breathing.	Swelling in vocal cords.	• Consult doctor. • See Croup.
• Fever. • Rapid or difficult breathing.	Infection of breathing passages.	• Call doctor now. • See Bronchitis, Acute. • See Bronchiolitis. • See Pneumonia (all charts).

*All references are to Illness section unless noted otherwise.

FEVER (CHILD OVER 2 YEARS)

SYMPTOMS & FACTORS	POSSIBLE PROBLEM	WHAT TO DO*
• Fever. • Diarrhea.	Infection of digestive tract.	See Gastroenteritis.
• Fever. • Earache. • Child pulls at ear.	Infection of middle ear.	See Ear Infection, Middle.
• Fever. • Cough. • Runny nose.	Virus infection.	• See Cold, Common. • See Influenza. • See Influenza, H1N1. • See Respiratory Syncytial Virus.
• Fever. • Rash.	Several disorders.	• See Chickenpox. • See Erythema Infectiosum. • See Measles. • See Rubella. • See Scarlet Fever.
• Fever. • Convulsions.	Several disorders.	• Call doctor now. • See Febrile Seizure.
• Fever in child age under age 5. • Rash. • Irritability.	Childhood disorder.	See Roseola Infantum.
• Fever of 102°F (38.9°C) or higher. • No other symptoms.	Infection.	Consult doctor.
• Fever. • Cough. • Rapid or difficult breathing.	Infection of breathing passages.	See Pneumonia (all charts).
• Fever. • Rash.	Several disorders.	See Rash With Fever (in this Symptoms section).
• Fever. • Abdominal pain.	Several disorders.	See Abdominal Pain, Sudden Attack (in this Symptoms section).
• Fever. • Swelling between ear and jaw.	Virus infection.	See Mumps.
• Fever. • Sore throat or hoarseness.	Infection of upper respiratory tract.	• See Herpangina. • See Laryngitis. • See Pharyngitis. • See Tonsillitis.
• Fever. • Runny nose. • Recent exposure to contagious disease, such as measles, mumps, or chickenpox.	Early stage of contagious illness.	Consult doctor.
• Fever. • Child seems very ill. • Headache, stiff neck.	Infection of membranes around brain.	• Call doctor now. • See Meningitis, Aseptic.

*All references are to Illness section unless noted otherwise.

FEVER (PERSON OVER AGE 12)
(continued on next page)

SYMPTOMS & FACTORS	POSSIBLE PROBLEM	WHAT TO DO*
• Fever. • Cough. • Headache. • Aches in bones or joints. • Stuffy or runny nose.	Virus infection.	• See Cold, Common. • See Influenza. • See Influenza, H1N1.
• Fever for 24 hours without other symptoms. OR • Recurrent fever with normal temperature between fevers.	Several disorders.	• Consult doctor. • See Fever of Unknown Origin.
• Fever. • Nausea or vomiting. • Diarrhea.	Infection of digestive tract.	• See Gastroenteritis. • See Listeriosis.
• Fever. • Pain in back below last rib.	Infection of urinary tract.	See Kidney Infection, Acute.
Fever after several hours in strong sunshine or hot environment.	Excess heat exposure.	• See Heatstroke or Heat Exhaustion. • See Sunburn.
• Fever. • Cough. • Shortness of breath, even when resting.	Lung infection.	See Pneumonia (all charts).
• Fever. • Cough with gray-yellow sputum. OR • Wheezing.	Infection of bronchial tubes.	See Bronchitis, Acute.
• Fever. • Use of prescription or nonprescription drug.	Adverse reaction or side effect of drug.	• Consult doctor about prescription drug. • Discontinue use of nonprescription drug.
• Fever. • Painful urination. • Frequent urination.	Urinary-tract infection.	• See Bladder Infection, Female. • See Bladder Infection, Male. • See Kidney Infection, Acute.
• Fever. • Sore throat.	Infection.	• See Pharyngitis. • See Tonsillitis.
• Fever. • Rash. • Aching, weakness.	Problem of blood cells.	See Agranulocytosis.
• Fever. • Rash.	Several disorders.	See Rash With Fever (in this Symptoms section).
• Sudden high fever. • Vomiting and watery diarrhea. • Rash resembling sunburn.	Blood poisoning.	See Toxic Shock Syndrome.

*All references are to Illness section unless noted otherwise.

FEVER (PERSON OVER AGE 12)
(continued from previous page)

SYMPTOMS & FACTORS	POSSIBLE PROBLEM	WHAT TO DO*
• Fever. • Other symptoms similar to cold (cough, tiredness, chills).	Fungal infection or tick caused disorder.	• See Blastomycosis. • See Coccidioidomycosis. • See Histoplasmosis. • See Lyme Disease. • See Rocky Mountain Spotted Fever.
• Fever. • Headache, plus any of following: • Pain bending forward. • Lethargy. • Confusion. • Nausea or vomiting.	Infection of membranes around brain.	• Call doctor now. • See Meningitis, Aseptic.
• Intermittent fever and chills. • Fatigue and weakness. • Weight loss. • Vague aches and pains.	Heart valve or lining infection.	See Endocarditis.
• Fever and sometimes, chills. • General ill feeling. • Headache. • Muscle ache.	Bacterial or viral infection.	• See Encephalitis, Viral. • See Legionnaire's Disease. • See West Nile Virus.
• Low-grade fever. • Weight loss. • Recurrent respiratory and skin infections.	Virus infection.	See HIV & AIDS.
• Intermittent fever. • Chills. • Marked fatigue. • Enlarged lymph glands.	Bacterial infection.	See Brucellosis.
• Fever. • Chills, muscle aches, cough. • Exposure to field mice or other rodents.	Virus infection.	See Hantavirus.
• Fever. • Tiredness. • Swollen lymph glands.	Protozoan infection.	See Toxoplasmosis.
• Fever. • Tiredness and weakness. • Pale skin, eyes, and fingernails. • General ill feeling.	Cancer.	• See Leukemia, Acute. • See Leukemia, Chronic.
• Fever. • Headache, overall feeling of discomfort, and body aches. • Foreign travel.	• Protozoan infection. • Viral infection.	• See Malaria. • See Severe Acute Respiratory Syndrome.

*All references are to Illness section unless noted otherwise.

FOOT PROBLEMS
(continued on next page)

SYMPTOMS & FACTORS	POSSIBLE PROBLEM	WHAT TO DO*
Excessively sweaty feet.	No underlying disorder.	• Wash and dry feet twice a day. Apply antiperspirant and a foot powder. • Wear cotton socks.
• Foot pain. • Big toe turned inward.	Bony protrusion.	See Bunion.
Small blisters on toes or soles.	Skin condition.	See Eczema, Dyshidrotic.
Pain in foot following injury.	• Broken bone. • Ligament injury.	• See Bone Fracture. • See Sprains & Strains.
• Pain and tenderness in the sole of the foot under the heel. • Pain often occurs after resting or after rising in the morning.	Tissue inflammation.	• See Heel Pain. • See Plantar Fasciitis.
• Pain in foot joint, especially big toe. • Affected joint red, warm, swollen.	Joint inflammation.	See Gout.
• Pain on bottom of foot. • Small growth or area on sole that hurts when walking.	Skin growth caused by virus.	See Warts.
• Itching foot. • Skin between toes red, soft, and peeling.	Fungus infection.	See Athlete's Foot.
Pain in foot after walking or running.	Blood circulation problem.	See Buerger's Disease.
• Pain on bottom of foot. • Red, swollen area on sole.	Infection caused by a penetrating wound or splinter.	Consult doctor. You may need tetanus protection.
• Pain in toe joints. • Affected joints red, warm, swollen.	Inflammatory disease of joints.	See Arthritis, Rheumatoid.
Pain, dull ache, or burning feeling in the ball of one or both feet.	Foot pain problem.	See Metatarsalgia.
• Aching feet. • Significantly overweight.	Effect of excess weight.	See Obesity & Overweight.
• Pain in toe joints, ankles, knees, or hips. • Person over age 50.	Degenerative condition of joints.	See Osteoarthritis.

*All references are to Illness section unless noted otherwise.

FOOT PROBLEMS
(continued from previous page)

SYMPTOMS & FACTORS	POSSIBLE PROBLEM	WHAT TO DO*
Numbness, hardness or paleness in skin exposed to subfreezing temperatures.	Tissue injury.	See Frostbite.
• Tingling and numbness in feet or hands. • Shooting pain that may worsen at night.	Nerve disorder.	See Peripheral Neuropathy.
Pain, burning, tingling, or numbness in the ball of the foot.	Foot nerve problem.	See Morton's Neuroma.
• New sores or ulcers on the foot that take a long time to heal. • Diabetes.	Foot infection.	See Diabetes Feet & Skin Problems.
• Pain in toe joints. • Affected joints red, warm, swollen. • Fever. • Recent illness, such as sore throat or skin infection.	Complication of prior streptococcal infection.	See Rheumatic Fever.

*All references are to Illness section unless noted otherwise.

GENITAL SORES, BLISTERS, WARTS OR BOILS

SYMPTOMS & FACTORS	POSSIBLE PROBLEM	WHAT TO DO*
• Scaling patches on the skin of the groin, thighs, buttocks, or groin. • Patches have well-defined edges.	Fungal infection.	See Tinea Cruris.
Painless blister on genitals.	Sexually transmitted disease.	See Granuloma Inguinale.
• Painless red sore on genitals. • Enlarged lymph glands in neck, armpit, or groin. • Headache. • Rash on skin.	Sexually transmitted disease.	See Syphilis.
Skin problem on penis.	• Inflammation • Cancer.	• See Balanitis. • See Penile Cancer.
• Small flesh colored bumps or tiny cauliflower like bumps. • Warts may produce no symptoms, or cause itching, burning, tenderness or pain.	Sexually transmitted disease.	See Warts, Genital.
• Skin problems on genitals (blisters, sores, warts, rash, redness, irritation). • Sexually active person.	Sexually transmitted disease.	• See Chlamydia • See Gonorrhea. • See Herpes, Genital. • See HIV & AIDS. • See Molluscum Contagiosum. • See Pelvic Inflammatory Disease. • See Sexually Transmitted Diseases. • See Syphilis. • See Trichomoniasis. • See Vaginosis, Bacterial. • See Warts, Genital.
Genital sores on a child.	Possible child abuse.	See Child Abuse.

*All references are to Illness section unless noted otherwise.

HAIR GROWTH IN WOMEN, EXCESSIVE

SYMPTOMS & FACTORS	POSSIBLE PROBLEM	WHAT TO DO*
• Excessive hair growth over 4 or 5 months. • Unexplained weight gain. • Menstrual changes or absent periods. • Deep voice.	Disorder or tumor of ovaries or adrenal gland.	• See Cushing's Syndrome. • See Ovarian Cancer. • See Ovarian Cyst or Tumor, Benign. • See Polycystic Ovary Syndrome.
• Excessive hair growth over 2 months or less. • Use of prescription drug, such as hormones, cortisone drugs or anticonvulsants.	Adverse reaction or side effect of drug.	Consult doctor.
• Excessive hair on face or body that developed before age 20. • Similar hairiness in other female family members.	Genetic causes, no underlying disorder.	Research methods for removal of unwanted hair.
Excessive hair growth, especially on face, in woman who has had ovaries removed or is over age 40.	Normal occurrence with decreasing estrogen level of menopause.	• Consult doctor. • Research methods for for removal of unwanted hair.
Excessive hair growth during pregnancy.	Hormone changes of pregnancy.	Nothing. Hair growth decreases after delivery.
• Excessive hair growth on the face and body. • May have irregular or no menstruation and acne.	Several possible causes.	See Hirsutism.

*All references are to Illness section unless noted otherwise.

HAIR LOSS

SYMPTOMS & FACTORS	POSSIBLE PROBLEM	WHAT TO DO*
• Hair loss. • Use of prescription drug or radiation therapy, especially for cancer or circulatory disorders.	Adverse reaction or side effect of drug or radiation.	Consult doctor.
Sudden hair loss in patches on head.	Skin disorder.	• See Alopecia Areata. • See Lichen Planus. • See Ringworm. • See Telogen Effluvium.
Hair thinning in a woman within 2 to 3 months following childbirth.	Effect of hormonal changes.	Nothing. Hair growth will return to normal.
Gradual hair loss in women, especially thinning of hair on top of head.	Normal occurrence with aging.	See Baldness, Pattern.
Receding front hairline or thinning of hair on top of head in men.	Hereditary baldness occurring in men at any age.	See Baldness, Pattern.
• Hair loss. • Frequent use of any of following hair-care products or styles: permanent waves, dyes, bleaches, curling irons or hot rollers, straighteners, tight braids, ponytails, or cornrows.	Hair damage.	• Change hair style, avoid damaging products or styles. • Consult doctor if hair loss persists.
Hair loss in 2 to 3 months following serious illness.	Temporary effect of illness and high fever.	Nothing. Hair should return to normal within few months.
Pulling out of hair.	Psychological disorder called trichotillomania.	Consult doctor.

*All references are to Illness section unless noted otherwise.

HEADACHE
(continued on next page)

SYMPTOMS & FACTORS	POSSIBLE PROBLEM	WHAT TO DO*
• Headache. • Use of prescription or nonprescription drug.	Adverse reaction or side effect of drug.	• Consult doctor about prescription drug. • Discontinue use of nonprescription drug.
• Severe headache. • Fever.	Common occurrence with infection.	See Fever charts (in this Symptoms section).
• Headache. • Recent head injury. • No other symptoms.	Common occurrence after head injury.	See Head Injury.
• Headache. • Vision disturbance before headache. • Nausea or vomiting.	Migraine.	See Headache, Migraine.
• Headache in forehead or back of head. • Tense, stressed feeling. • Sleeping difficulty.	Effect of stress.	• See Anxiety Disorder, Generalized. • See Depression. • See Headache, Tension. • See Stress.
• Sudden onset of headache. • Pain around eyes. • Headache occurs at same time every day.	Chronic headache disorder.	See Headache, Cluster.
• Pain or tenderness around eyes and cheekbones that worsens when bending head forward. • Recent cold or nasal allergies.	Sinus infection.	See Sinusitis.
• Headache and may have pain around eyes and cheekbones. • Runny or stuffy nose.	Virus infection.	See Cold, Common.
• Headache. • Decreased consumption of caffeine-containing beverages (coffee, colas, cocoa, tea).	Caffeine withdrawal.	• Reduce consumption of caffeine gradually. • Use a nonprescription pain reliever, such as acetaminophen.
• Headache, plus any of following: • Unusually long time since eating. • Excessive alcohol consumption. • Stuffy, smoky, or noisy room. • Exposure to strong sunlight.	Circumstantial headache. No underlying disorder.	Use a nonprescription pain reliever, such as acetaminophen.
• Headache after excessive alcohol consumption. • Nausea or vomiting.	"Hangover."	Use a nonprescription pain reliever, such as acetaminophen.

*All references are to Illness section unless noted otherwise.

HEADACHE
(continued from previous page)

SYMPTOMS & FACTORS	POSSIBLE PROBLEM	WHAT TO DO*
• Severe headache that worsens when bending head forward. • Eyes sensitive to light. • Lethargy. • Confusion. • No recent head injury.	Bleeding in membrane around brain.	• Call doctor now. • See Subarachnoid Hemorrhage. • See Brain or Epidural Abscess.
• Headache that worsens when bending head forward. • Fever. • Eyes sensitive to light.	Infection of membranes around brain.	• Call doctor now. • See Meningitis, Aseptic. • See Meningitis, Bacterial.
• Headache. • Eye pain. • Blurred vision. • Nausea or vomiting. • No injury to eye.	Excess pressure in eye.	• Call doctor now. • See Glaucoma, Angle-Closure.
• Ongoing headaches. • Other symptoms that are vague and may develop over time.	• High blood pressure. • Tumor.	• See Hypertension. • See Brain Tumor. • See Pituitary Tumor.
Headache after reading or straining to see.	Strain on neck muscles (not strain on eyes).	See Headache, Tension.
• Headache, nausea, vomiting. • Ascent to higher altitude.	Lack of oxygen.	See Altitude Illness.
• Headache. • Dizziness. • Nausea, vomiting. • Faintness.	Gas inhalation.	See Carbon Monoxide Poisoning.
• Headache. • Stiff neck. • Fever.	Fungal infection.	See Cryptococcosis.
• Headache. • General ill feeling. • Chills and fever. • Muscle aches.	Bacterial infection.	See Legionnaire's Disease.
• Headache. • Fatigue and nausea. • Travel to foreign country.	Parasite infection.	See Malaria.
• Headache, fainting, weakness. • Sweating, confusion. • Excessive hunger.	Low blood sugar.	See Hypoglycemia, Reactive.
• Headache, fever, fatigue. • Sore throat. • Diarrhea or constipation. • Stomach pains.	Bacterial infection.	See Typhoid Fever.
• Headache. • General ill feeling. • Fever and sometimes, chills. • Muscle ache.	Bacterial or viral infection.	• See Encephalitis, Viral. • See Legionnaire's Disease. • See West Nile Virus.

*All references are to Illness section unless noted otherwise.

HEARING LOSS

SYMPTOMS & FACTORS	POSSIBLE PROBLEM	WHAT TO DO*
• Hearing loss. • Use of prescription or nonprescription drug.	Adverse reaction or side effect of drug.	• Consult doctor about prescription drug. • Discontinue use of nonprescription drug.
• Hearing loss. • Sticky, green-yellow discharge from ear.	• Infection of middle-ear canal or outer ear. • Injury to eardrum.	• See Ear Infection, Middle. • See Ear Infection, Outer. • See Eardrum, Ruptured.
• Hearing loss. • Dizziness.	Disorder or infection of inner ear.	• See Labyrinthitis. • See Ménière's Disease.
• Hearing loss, especially of high-pitched sounds. • Exposure to excessive noise, such as a jackhammer.	Damage caused by exposure to harmful noise levels.	See Hearing Impairment or Loss.
• Hearing loss. • Earache.	Infection or blockage.	See Earache (in this Symptoms section).
Gradual hearing loss in person over age 60.	Common occurrence with aging.	Consult doctor.
• Gradual hearing loss over several weeks or months. • History of similar hearing loss in other family members.	Poor function of middle-ear bones.	See Otosclerosis.
• Hearing loss. • Recent cold or sore throat.	Blockage of canal between middle ear and back of throat (eustachian tube).	• See Cold, Common. • Consult doctor if hearing loss lasts longer than 3 days.
Gradual hearing loss over several weeks or months without other symptoms.	Earwax problem.	See Earwax Blockage.
• Some degree of hearing loss. • Noise in ear (ringing, buzzing, roaring, whistling or hissing).	Acoustic nerve disorder.	See Tinnitus.
• Hearing loss. • Plugged feeling in ear. • Change in air pressure (flying, diving).	Ear damage.	See Barotitis Media.

*All references are to Illness section unless noted otherwise.

HEARTBEAT IRREGULARITY

SYMPTOMS & FACTORS	POSSIBLE PROBLEM	WHAT TO DO*
• Irregular heartbeat. • General ill feeling. • History of heart disease.	Disorder of heart rate or rhythm.	• Call doctor now. • See Aneurysm. • See Atrial Fibrillation. • See Calcium Imbalance. • See Heart Block. • See Heart Rhythm Irregularity. • See Heartbeat, Rapid. • See Hypertrophic Cardiomyopathy. • See Potassium Imbalance. • See Valvular Heart Disease.
• Irregular heartbeat. • Use of prescription or nonprescription drugs, such as: thyroid medication, digitalis preparations, diuretics, diet pills, stimulants, caffeine, decongestants, cold remedies, including nasal sprays, illegal drugs, including marijuana, cocaine, psychedelics, amphetamines.	Adverse reaction or side effect of drug.	• Consult doctor about prescription drug. • Discontinue use of nonprescription or illegal drug.
• Irregular heartbeat. • Unexplained weight loss. • Anxiety. • Excessive sweating. • Fatigue.	Overactive thyroid gland.	See Hyperthyroidism.
• Rapid or irregular heartbeat. • Recent tension or worry.	Effect of stress.	• See Anxiety Disorder, Generalized. • See Panic Disorder. • See Phobias. • See Stress.
• Irregular heartbeat. • Excessive smoking. OR • Excessive consumption of caffeine-containing beverages such as coffee, cola, tea, or cocoa.	Effect of nicotine or caffeine.	Decrease nicotine or caffeine use.
• Rapid or irregular heartbeat. • Fever.	Infection.	See Fever charts (in this Symptoms section).
• Heartbeat irregularity. • Shortness of breath. • Fatigue.	Heart inflammation.	See Myocarditis.
• Rapid heartbeat following exercise, emotional upset or exposure to cold. • Tremors and nervousness. • Feelings of doom.	Adrenal tumor.	See Pheochromocytoma.

*All references are to Illness section unless noted otherwise.

HIP PAIN

SYMPTOMS & FACTORS	POSSIBLE PROBLEM	WHAT TO DO*
• Hip pain. • Chills and fever.	Joint infection.	See Arthritis, Infectious.
• Hip pain. • Limited hip joint movement.	• Bursa inflammation. • Joint injury.	• See Bursitis. • See Dislocation or Subluxation.
• Chronic hip pain. • Pain may affect other body parts. • Follows an injury or illness.	Persistent pain.	See Chronic Pain Syndrome.
• Hip pain or ache. • Fatigue. • Tender areas of the body.	Chronic disorder.	See Fibromyalgia.
• Severe hip pain. • Swelling, tenderness in hip. • Recent fall or injury.	Bone fracture.	See Hip Fracture.
• Hip pain in a child. • Limping.	Hip disorder.	• See Legg-Calvé Perthes disease. • See Transient Synovitis of the Hip.

*All references are to Illness section unless noted otherwise.

IMPOTENCE, MALE SEXUAL
(Erectile Dysfunction)

SYMPTOMS & FACTORS	POSSIBLE PROBLEM	W...
• Sexual impotence. • Use of prescription or nonprescription or mood-altering drugs, such as: antihypertensives, narcotics, cocaine, antidepressants, antihistamines, antiulcer drugs, diuretics, hormones, beta-adrenergic blockers, tranquilizers, reserpine, marijuana, digitalis, skeletal-muscle relaxants, sedatives, hypnotics, or phenothiazines.	Adverse reaction or side effect of drug.	nonpr... or mood-altering drug.
• Sexual impotence. • Chronic illness.	• Low level of testosterone (male sex hormone). • Diminished blood circulation to genitals.	• Consult doctor. • See Atherosclerosis. • See Diabetes Type 1. • See Diabetes Type 2. • See Cirrhosis of the Liver. • See Hypothyroidism. • See Multiple Sclerosis. • See Pituitary Gland, Underactive. • See Prostatic Hypertrophy, Benign.
• Sexual impotence. • Excessive alcohol consumption.	Effect of alcohol.	See Alcoholism.
• Sexual impotence. • Anxiety or depression.	Effect of stress.	• See Anxiety Disorder, Generalized. • See Depression. • See Stress.
• Sexual impotence. • History of sexually transmitted disease.	Scarring or other effect of infection.	• See Gonorrhea. • See HIV & AIDS. • See Herpes, Genital. • See Sexually Transmitted Diseases. • See Syphilis. • See Urethritis. • See Warts, Genital.
• Sexual impotence. • History of premature ejaculation or other sexual dysfunction.	Psychosexual problem.	• See Erectile Dysfunction. • See Premature Ejaculation.
• Sexual impotence. • Acute illness with fever.	Temporary effect of illness.	Nothing. Sexual function will return when illness subsides.

*All references are to Illness section unless noted otherwise.

FACTORS	POSSIBLE PROBLEM	WHAT TO DO*
...ids. ...re frequently wet or ...d to chemicals.	Effect of chemicals or moisture.	See Dermatitis, Contact.
...ching on head or between toes. Small bald patches on scalp.	Fungus infection.	• See Athlete's Foot. • See Ringworm.
• Itching on head. • Tiny white spots on hair that won't come off.	Parasites.	See Lice.
• Itching. • Insect bite or sting.	Reaction.	See Insect Bites & Stings.
• Itching or bleeding around anus. • Painful bowel movements.	• Varicose veins in anus. • Split in skin around anus.	• See Anal Fissure. • See Hemorrhoids.
Itching around anus following severe diarrhea.	Normal response to irritation.	Apply ointment containing zinc oxide.
• Itching. • Diarrhea. • Abdominal pain. • Flatulence and bloating. • Rash.	Reaction to a swallowed substance.	See Food Allergy.
• Intense itching and burning. • Bright red skin rash. • Contact with poisonous plant.	Allergic reaction to plant.	See Poison Ivy, Oak, Sumac.
• Itching. • Yellow skin and eyes.	• Liver disorder. • Blood disorder.	Call doctor now.
• Itching. • General ill feeling.	• Blood disorder. • Overactive thyroid gland. • Adverse reaction or side effect of drug. • Cancer.	• Consult doctor. • See Drug Allergy. • See Hodgkin's Disease. • See Hyperthyroidism. • See Polycythemia.
• Itching. • Rash. section).	Several skin disorders.	See Rash Without Fever (in this Symptoms
Itching in genital area in females.	Irritation or infection.	See Vaginal Itching (in this Symptoms section).
Itching around anus, especially at night.	• Parasites. • Several causes.	• See Pinworms. • See Pruritus Ani.
• Itching. • Wheezing, coughing, sneezing. • Swelling around face and hands. • Difficult breathing.	Allergic reaction.	• Call doctor now. • See Anaphylaxis.

*All references are to Illness section unless noted otherwise.

JOINT ACHES OR PAIN

SYMPTOMS & FACTORS	POSSIBLE PROBLEM	WHAT TO DO*
• Joint redness, swelling, tenderness, and pain. • Chills, fever.	Bacterial infection.	See Arthritis, Infectious.
• Joint swelling, warmth, pain. • Stiffness occurs in the morning. • Child may have rash.	• Autoimmune disorder. • Pain condition.	• See Arthritis, Juvenile Idiopathic (if young child). • See Arthritis, Rheumatoid. • See Fibromyalgia.
• Joint pain, swelling, tenderness. • Pain may spread to other areas. • Limited movement of joint.	Inflammation.	See Bursitis.
• Multi-joint pain (no swelling or redness). • Chronic fatigue for months.	Chronic disorder.	See Chronic Fatigue Syndrome.
• Sudden joint pain, swelling. • Limited movement.	Joint injury.	See Dislocation or Subluxation.
• Joint aches or pain, with redness, and swelling. • Fever and fatigue. • Skin rash.	Autoimmune disorder.	See Lupus Erythematosus, Systemic.
• Joint pain or stiffness. • Bone pain (especially at night). • Skin over the bones is warm.	Bone disorder.	See Paget's Disease of Bone.
• Joint pain and swelling. • Headache, fever, loss of appetite. • Itching, red skin rash.	Inflammation.	See Purpura, Henoch Schönlein.
• Sudden onset of joint pain. • Usually in big toe, but may be in other joints. • Joint is hot, swollen, and tender.	Excess of uric acid in the blood.	See Gout.
• Joint aches. • Weight loss, fever, fatigue, general ill feeling. • High blood pressure.	Autoimmune disorder.	See Polyarteritis Nodosa.

*All references are to Illness section unless noted otherwise.

KNEE PAIN

SYMPTOMS & FACTORS	POSSIBLE PROBLEM	WHAT TO DO*
• Pain in knee. • Feeling that knee "catches" or won't bear weight.	Muscle or cartilage problem.	• See Patellofemoral Pain Syndrome. • See Sprains & Strains.
• Pain in knee following injury. • Knee won't bear weight. • Knee misshapen.	Broken bone or dislocation.	• Call doctor now. • See Bone Fracture. • See Dislocation or Subluxation.
• Pain in knee. • Knee red, warm, swollen. • Fever. • General ill feeling.	Bone or joint infection.	See Osteomyelitis.
• Pain in knee and other joints. • Affected joints red, warm, swollen. • Fever. • Recent illness such as sore throat, gonorrhea, or skin infection.	Complication of prior infection.	• See Arthritis, Infectious. • See Rheumatic Fever.
• Pain in knee or other joints. • Affected joints red, warm, swollen. • No fever.	Joint inflammation.	• See Bursitis. • See Arthritis, Juvenile Idiopathic (children only). • See Arthritis, Rheumatoid. • See Gout. • See Osgood-Schlatter Disease (older children and adolescents only). • See Psoriatic Arthritis.
• Chronic pain in knee. • Knee sometimes "catches" or won't support weight. OR • Persistent discomfort in knee, fingers or other joints without other symptoms.	Degenerative joint disease.	See Osteoarthritis.
• Pain in knee in child under 12. • Hip pain. • Limp.	• Degenerative condition of hip joint in children. • Inflammation.	• See Legg-Calvé Perthes Disease. • See Transient Synovitis of the Hip.
• Acute attack of swelling and pain in the knee. • Attack lasts for 2 or more days.	Joint disorder.	See Pseudogout.

*All references are to Illness section unless noted otherwise.

LEG PAIN

SYMPTOMS & FACTORS	POSSIBLE PROBLEM	WHA
• Leg pain. • Back pain.	Muscle strain or sciatica.	See Bac...
• Leg pain following strenuous exercise or following injury. • Leg can bear weight.	Muscle, tendon, ligament, or bone problem.	• See Shin Sp... • See Sprains & .
• Leg pain. • Restricted movement, swelling and tenderness around a tendon.	Tendon inflammation.	See Tendinitis.
• Leg pain following injury. • Leg won't bear weight.	Broken bone.	• Call doctor now. • See Bone Fracture.
Sharp pain down back of leg, especially when coughing, sneezing, or laughing hard.	Pressure on large nerve in leg.	• See Disc, Herniated. • See Backache & Back Pain (in this Symptoms Section).
• Leg cramping or pain. • Tired sensation in leg. • Symptoms start while walking.	Blood vessel problem.	See Peripheral Vascular Disease.
• Leg ache after standing for time. • Large veins in legs.	Disorder of veins.	See Varicose Veins.
• Shooting pain in leg. • Tingling and numbness that begins in hands or feet. • Gradual muscle weakness.	Nerve disorder.	See Peripheral Neuropathy.
• Pain in calf. • One vein red, hot, and firm.	Blood clot in superficial vein.	See Thrombophlebitis, Superficial.
• Pain in calf when flexing ankle. • Swollen, tender calf.	Blood clot in deep vein.	• Call doctor now. • See Thrombosis, Deep-Vein.
• Persistent pain in part of leg. • Fever, general ill feeling.	Bone infection or cancer.	• See Multiple Myeloma. • See Osteomyelitis.
• Pain in calf after walking. • Pain disappears with rest.	Circulatory disorder.	• See Atherosclerosis. • See Buerger's Disease. • See Claudication.
• Leg pain. • Painful or stiff hip on same side.	• Degenerative condition of joints (in adult). • Inflammation (in child).	• See Legg-Calvé Perthes Disease. • See Osteomyelitis. • See Transient Synovitis of the Hip.
• Leg pain along sciatic nerve. • Recurrent low backache. • Stiffness.	Joint disease.	See Spondylitis, Ankylosing.
• Leg or arm pain (may be burning or aching) and swelling. • Changes in skin color.	Pain syndrome.	See Regional Pain Syndrome, Complex.
• Leg sensations (may be painful) • Sensations occur while resting.	Movement disorder.	See Restless Legs Syndrome.

All references are to Illness section unless noted otherwise.

	POSSIBLE PROBLEM	WHAT TO DO*
	Common occurrence with aging, no underlying disorder.	• Consult doctor at next appointment. • Write lists to help your memory. This is not the beginning of serious mental decline.
...location of keys, ...glasses, or forgetting items on shopping list. • Depression or tension.	Effect of stress.	• See Anxiety Disorder, Generalized. • See Depression. • See Stress.
• Inability to remember a period of time. • Use of prescription or nonprescription drug, especially for sleeping difficulty.	Adverse reaction or side effect of drug.	Consult doctor.
Total memory loss.	Psychological disorder.	Consult doctor.
• Inability to remember a period of time. • Recent head injury.	Brain injury.	• Call doctor now. • See Head Injury.
Inability to remember episodes of excessive-alcohol consumption.	Effect of alcohol.	• Consult doctor. • See Alcoholism.
• Inability to remember recent events while remembering long-ago events, plus 2 or more of following: • Poor attention span in conversations or with instructions. • Decline in attention to personal appearance or cleanliness. • Personality change. • Decline in ability to cope with everyday matters.	Mental deterioration.	• See Alzheimer's Disease. • See Dementia. • See Vitamin Deficiencies.
• Inability to remember a period of time, plus events surrounding any of the following: • Epileptic seizure. • Diabetic coma. • Period before and after surgery. • Severe, feverish, illness such as meningitis or pneumonia.	Common occurrence following these situations.	Nothing.
• Memory problems and confusion. • Inability to speak or move part of body. OR • Low body temperature.	Decrease in blood supply to brain or exposure to cold extremes.	• Call doctor now. • See Hypothermia. • See Stroke.
• Memory loss. • Headaches, vomiting. • Vision changes.	Tumor.	• Call doctor now. • See Brain Tumor.
• Memory problems. • Recent surgical procedure with general anesthetic.	Often occurs.	Memory should return to normal.

*All references are to Illness section unless noted otherwise.

MENSTRUAL PERIODS, LATE OR ABSENT

SYMPTOMS & FACTORS	POSSIBLE PROBLEM	WHAT TO DO*
• Menstrual periods absent, plus one or more of following: • Stress, tension, or worry. • Strenuous exercise or activity. • Chronic illness. • Change in lifestyle such as new job or new home.	• Hormone changes. • Effect of stress. • Chronic illness. • Result of surgery. • Endocrine problem. • Disordered eating.	• See Amenorrhea, Secondary. • See Anorexia Nervosa. • See Female Athlete Triad. • See name of your chronic illness in Illness Section.
Menstrual periods have never started.	Hormone changes of puberty have not occurred.	• Consult doctor if older than 16. • See Amenorrhea, Primary.
• Menstrual period late by 2 or more weeks. • Sexual intercourse within last month.	Pregnancy.	• Consult doctor to confirm pregnancy. • Take a home pregnancy test.
• Menstrual periods absent. • Use of prescription drug.	Adverse reaction or side effect of drug.	• Consult doctor. • See Amenorrhea, Secondary.
Menstrual periods absent in woman over age 38.	• Normal menstrual irregularities at this age. • Endometrial overgrowth.	• See Endometrial Hyperplasia. • See Menopause. • See Perimenopause.
• Menstrual periods absent. • Overweight.	Hormone problem.	Consult doctor.
Menstrual periods absent since delivery of baby.	Normal occurrence caused by hormone changes following childbirth.	• If bottle-feeding, consult doctor if periods do not resume within 8 weeks after delivery. • If breast-feeding, consult doctor if periods do not resume within 4 weeks after weaning.
• Menstrual periods absent. • Round face, puffy eyes. • Abnormal hair growth.	Hormone imbalance.	See Cushing's Syndrome.
• Irregular menstrual flow (light or heavy at times). • Excess hair growth on body. • Overweight.	Endocrine problem.	See Polycystic Ovary Syndrome.
• Irregular menstrual periods. • Discomfort or pain in lower abdomen. • Pain or bleeding with intercourse.	Cancer.	• See Ovarian Cancer. • See Uterine Malignancy.

*All references are to Illness section unless noted otherwise.

MENSTRUAL PERIODS, PAINFUL OR HEAVY

SYMPTOMS & FACTORS	POSSIBLE PROBLEM	WHAT TO DO*
• Excessive menstrual flow. • Menstrual period lasts more than 7 days.	Menstrual irregularity.	See Menorrhagia.
Menstrual period more painful or heavier than usual, especially during last days of period.	Disorder of lining of pelvic organs.	• See Dysmenorrhea. • See Endometriosis.
• Current menstrual period more painful or heavier than usual. • Period arrived one week or more late.	Early pregnancy, miscarriage, or pregnancy outside uterus.	• Consult doctor. • See Ectopic Pregnancy. • See Miscarriage.
Menstrual periods more painful or heavier since receiving intrauterine contraceptive device (IUD).	Common side effect of using IUD.	Consult doctor.
• Menstrual periods more painful or heavier than usual. • No other pelvic or genital symptoms.	Benign growth in uterus.	See Uterine Fibroids.
Menstrual periods painful or heavy since discontinuing use of oral contraceptives.	Hormone changes caused by discontinuing pill.	Consult doctor.
• Menstrual periods painful. • Periods began within last 3 years. • Healthy otherwise.	No disease.	See Dysmenorrhea.
Menstrual period heavy in woman who has recently. delivered a baby.	Normal occurrence during first 2 menstrual periods following childbirth.	Consult doctor if heavy periods persist.
Menstrual flow always heavy.	No underlying disorder.	Consult doctor for blood test for anemia.
• Heavy menstrual flow. • Bleeding between normal menstrual periods.	Excessive estrogen.	See Endometrial Hyperplasia.
Painful, prolonged or irregular bleeding through the vagina.	Several causes.	See Uterine Bleeding, Dysfunctional.
• Heavy menstrual flow or light menstrual flow alternating. • Excess hair growth on body. • Overweight.	Endocrine problem.	See Polycystic Ovary Syndrome.
• Menstrual periods more painful or heavier than usual. • Bad-smelling vaginal discharge. • Fever.	Infection of reproductive organs.	• Call doctor now. • See Pelvic Inflammatory Disease.

*All references are to Illness section unless noted otherwise.

MOUTH, SORE, TINGLING, DRY
(continued on next page)

SYMPTOMS & FACTORS	POSSIBLE PROBLEM	WHAT TO DO*
• Sore mouth. • Blisters or red, rough or painful areas on lips or in mouth.	Virus infection.	• See Hand, Foot & Mouth Disease. • See Herpes Simplex. • See Stomatitis, Herpetic.
• Sore mouth. • Creamy-white patches in mouth or tongue.	Fungus infection.	See Thrush.
Mouth sores that are shallow, usually red, and may have a white coating over them.	Inflammation.	See Canker Sores.
• Dry mouth. • Use of prescription or nonprescription medication.	Adverse reaction or side effect of medication.	• Consult doctor about prescription drug. • Discontinue nonprescription drug if dry mouth is causing problems.
• Sore mouth. • Fever. • Sores in mouth. • Use of prescription or nonprescription drugs.	Adverse reaction or side effect of drug.	Call doctor now.
• Sore mouth. • Red, painful gums that bleed easily. • Bad breath.	Bacterial infection.	See Trench Mouth.
• Sore mouth. • Use of new cosmetics.	Allergic reaction caused by chemical.	Discontinue use of new cosmetic.
• Dry mouth. • Stress or apprehension.	Normal occurrence.	Dry mouth will disappear when stress is diminished.
Small white patch in the mouth that feels firm, rough, and stiff.	Tobacco use or or unknown problem.	See Leukoplakia, Oral.
• Dry mouth. • Decreased urination. • Severe thirst.	Electrolyte disorder.	• See Dehydration. • See Fluid & Electrolyte Disorder.
• Sore mouth. • Rough or split corners of mouth.	Vitamin or mineral deficiency.	• See Anemia, Aplastic. • See Folic Acid Deficiency. • See Vitamin Deficiencies.
• Bleeding from the gums. • Easy bruising. • Tiredness, low fever, anemia.	Cancer.	See Leukemia, Acute.

*All references are to Illness section unless noted otherwise.

MOUTH, SORE, TINGLING, DRY
(continued from previous page)

SYMPTOMS & FACTORS	POSSIBLE PROBLEM	WHAT TO DO*
• Pale, painless lump in mouth. • Lump may enlarge, ulcerate, and bleed.	Cancer.	See Oral Cancer.
• Mouth tingling. • Sneezing, coughing, wheezing. • Watery eyes. • Difficult breathing.	Allergic reaction.	• Call doctor now. • See Anaphylaxis.
• Dryness of mouth. • Dryness of eyes. • Parotid gland enlargement (chipmunk face).	Autoimmune disorder.	See Sjögren's Syndrome.
• Numbness and tingling around the mouth. • Palpitations, rapid heartbeat. • Shortness of breath. • Emotional fears.	Severe anxiety.	See Panic Disorder.
• Soft or firm mass in the in the floor of the mouth or jaw. • There may be pain or swelling.	Tumor.	See Salivary Gland Tumor.

*All references are to Illness section unless noted otherwise.

SYMPTOMS & FACTORS	POSSIBLE PROBLEM	WHAT TO DO*
• Muscle cramp while relaxed or resting in bed. OR • Muscle cramp in arm or leg during or after exercise. OR • Muscle cramp after sitting in awkward position.	Common occurrence, usually no underlying disorder.	• Massage muscle and use heat to relieve pain. • See Sprains & Strains. • See Tendinitis.
Recurrent leg cramps when walking.	Circulatory disorder.	• See Atherosclerosis. • See Buerger's Disease. • See Claudication.
Muscle cramp following exposure to heat.	Heat exhaustion.	See Heatstroke or Heat Exhaustion.
Pain, tenderness, and limited movement in muscle.	Inflammation.	See Bursitis.
• Recurrent muscle cramps. • Tender nodules on skin. • Stiffness and weakness.	Inflammation of connective tissue.	See Fibromyalgia.
• Muscle cramp. • Use of diuretic drug for high blood pressure or heart disorder.	Adverse reaction or side effect of drug.	Consult doctor.
• Muscle cramp. • Numbness, tingling in arms or legs. • Irregular heartbeat.	Electrolyte disorder.	• See Calcium Imbalance. • See Fluid & Electrolyte Disorder.
• Muscle aches. • Chills, fever, cough. • Exposure to field mice or other rodents.	Virus infection.	See Hantavirus.
• Muscle aches. • Fever, tiredness. • Exposure to cats, cat litter, or dirt soiled by cats.	Protozoan disorder.	See Toxoplasmosis.
• Muscle weakness in hands, feet, and arms. • Weakness spreads within 72 hours. • Shock.	Inflammatory nerve condition.	See Guillain-Barré Syndrome.
• Weakness. • Ducklike gait. • Falling, difficulty in getting up after falling.	Muscle deterioration.	See Muscular Dystrophy.
• Weakness in the pelvic or shoulder muscles. • Skin rash on the face, shoulders, arms, and over joints.	Connective tissue disorder.	See Polymyositis.

*All references are to Illness section unless noted otherwise.

MUSCLE PAIN, ACHE, CRAMP, WEAKNESS
(continued from previous page)

SYMPTOMS & FACTORS	POSSIBLE PROBLEM	WHAT TO DO*
• Muscle cramps (usually in the legs). • Confusion, restlessness, or anxious. • Weakness.	Electrolyte disorder.	• See Fluid & Electrolyte Disorder. • Sodium Imbalance.
• Weakness of arm and leg muscles. • Weakness of facial muscles.	Autoimmune disorder.	See Myasthenia Gravis.
• Muscle pain, aches, soreness, stiffness, and/or swelling. • New or changed exercise or activity.	Excess exercise or activity.	See Delayed Onset Muscle Soreness.
Muscle weakness, twitching, stiffness, and cramping.	Nerve disorder.	• See Amyotrophic Lateral Sclerosis. • See Parkinson's Disease.
• Muscle weakness over time. • Older persons.	Muscle loss with aging.	See Sarcopenia.
• Muscle ache. • General ill feeling. • Headache. • Fever and sometimes, chills.	• Bacterial or viral infection. • Inflammatory disorder.	• See Encephalitis, Viral. • See Legionnaire's Disease. • See Polymyalgia Rheumatica & Giant Cell Arteritis. • See West Nile Virus.

*All references are to Illness section unless noted otherwise.

NECK PAIN

SYMPTOMS & FACTORS	POSSIBLE PROBLEM	WHAT TO DO*
• Stiffness or severe neck pain on waking. • No pain before going to bed.	Uncomfortable sleeping position.	Consult doctor if pain lasts longer than 24 hours.
• Sudden, severe neck pain. • Injury to neck.	Muscle injury.	See Sprains & Strains.
• Neck pain. • Stressful situation.	Muscle tension.	Take a hot shower or have someone massage your neck muscles to relieve tension.
• Severe neck pain. • Sharp pain in shoulders or arms when moving head.	• Slipped disc in neck. • Neck-muscle injury.	• See Disc, Herniated. • See Torticollis. • See Whiplash.
• Neck and shoulder pain. • Working at computer or other repetitive task for many hours.	Muscle spasm.	• Have computer screen at proper eye level and chair at correct height. • Take a break every hour.
• Sudden neck pain, especially when bending head forward, plus any of following: • Lethargy. • Confusion. • Eyes sensitive to light. • Nausea or vomiting. • Severe headache.	Infection or bleeding in membrane around brain.	• Call doctor now. • See Meningitis, Aseptic. • See Subarachnoid Hemorrhage.
• Sudden, severe neck pain. • Recent strong jolt. • Difficulty controlling arms or legs. • Loss of bowel or bladder control.	Damaged spinal cord.	Call doctor now.
• Stiff neck. • Behavioral or personality changes. • General ill feeling. • Headache, vomiting, fever.	Brain inflammation.	See Encephalitis, Viral.
Swelling or lump in neck.	Several disorders.	See Swelling or Lump (in this Symptoms section).
• Chronic neck pain that is worsening. • Numbness or tingling in arm or hand. • Person over age 40.	Pressure on nerves in neck.	See Cervical Spondylosis.

*All references are to Illness section unless noted otherwise.

NOSE, STUFFY OR RUNNY

SYMPTOMS & FACTORS	POSSIBLE PROBLEM	WHAT TO DO*
• Stuffy or runny nose (clear, watery discharge) plus any of following: • Fever. • Cough. • Headache. • Aches in bones or joints. • Sore throat.	Virus infection.	• See Cold, Common. • See Influenza. • See Influenza, H1N1.
• Stuffy or runny nose (clear, watery discharge). • Itching eyes. • Sneezing.	Nasal allergy.	See Hay Fever.
• Runny nose. • Cough, lethargy. • Appetite loss (some cases). • Low-grade fever.	• Virus infection. • Bacterial infection.	• See Respiratory Syncytial Virus. • See Whooping Cough.
• Stuffy or runny nose (thick, cloudy, yellow-green discharge). • Pain or tenderness around eyes and cheekbones that worsens when bending head forward.	Sinus infection.	See Sinusitis.
• Chronic "stuffy nose" feeling. • Impaired sense of smell. • Feeling of fullness in the face.	Growth in nasal cavity.	See Nasal Polyps.
• Obstruction of air through the nostrils. • Nasal discharge.	Septum problem.	See Nasal Septum, Deviated.
• Chronic "stuffy nose" feeling. • Use of nasal decongestants for more than 3 days.	Decongestant is suddenly withdrawn after extended use or they are overused.	Consult doctor.
• Runny or stuffy nose. • Coughing, sneezing, and postnasal drip. • Watery and itchy eyes.	Mold allergy.	See Mold Allergy.

*All references are to Illness section unless noted otherwise.

NUMBNESS, TINGLING, OR PRICKLING
(continued on next page)

SYMPTOMS & FACTORS	POSSIBLE PROBLEM	WHAT TO DO*
• Numbness or tingling in feet or hands after sitting in one position a long time or waking from deep sleep. • No underlying disorder.	• Stretching of, or pressure on, a nerve. • Temporary decrease in blood supply to a nerve.	Nothing. Feeling returns in a few minutes.
• Numbness or tingling in any part of body. • Use of prescription drug.	Adverse reaction or side effect of drug.	Consult doctor.
• Numbness or tingling in hands and fingers, especially at night. • Sharp pain in hand or arm, especially at night. • Weak grip.	Pressure on nerves in wrist.	See Carpal-Tunnel Syndrome.
• Numbness and tingling in injured area of the skin. • Formation of scar tissue.	Normal occurrence.	Nothing.
• Numbness or tingling on one side of body, plus any of following: • Weakness in extremities. • Dizziness. • Confusion. • Blurred vision. • Speaking difficulty.	Decreased blood supply to brain.	• Call doctor now. • See Stroke. • See Transient Ischemic Attack.
• Numbness or tingling in an arm or leg. • Weakness in the affected side. • Recent heavy lifting or strenuous exercise.	Pressure on nerves.	See Disc, Herniated.
• Numbness or tingling in fingers or toes. • Blue fingers or toes in cold weather. • Redness and pain when numbness subsides and feeling returns.	Disorder of blood circulation in fingers and toes.	See Raynaud Disease & Phenomenon.
• Numbness or tingling in hands, arms, neck, or shoulder. • There may be pain or stiffness.	Pressure on nerves.	• See Cervical Spondylosis. • See Thoracic-Outlet-Syndrome.
• Numbness or tingling in hands and face, especially around lips. • Dizziness.	Decreased carbon dioxide in blood.	See Panic Disorder.
• Numbness, tingling in arms or legs. • Muscle cramps. • Irregular heartbeat.	Electrolyte disorder.	• See Calcium Imbalance. • See Fluid & Electrolyte Disorder.

*All references are to Illness section unless noted otherwise.

NUMBNESS, TINGLING, OR PRICKLING
(continued from previous page)

SYMPTOMS & FACTORS	POSSIBLE PROBLEM	WHAT TO DO*
• Numbness and tingling that begins in hands and feet. • Shooting pain that may worsen at night.	Nerve disorder.	See Peripheral Neuropathy.
• Numbness in fingers, toes, cheeks, nose, ears hands, legs, or feet. • Frequent urination.	Endocrine disorder.	See Hyperaldosteronism.
• Tingling sensation in arms, hands, legs, and feet. • Tight skin. • Swallowing difficulty.	Autoimmune disorder.	See Scleroderma.
• Numbness and tingling. • Fatigue. • Lack of coordination.	Autoimmune disorder.	See Multiple Sclerosis.
• Prickling or tingling of skin. • Itching and rash. • Thin tracks on skin.	Hookworm infestation.	See Larva Migrans, Cutaneous.
• Tremors and nervousness. • Rapid heartbeat following exercise, emotional upset, or exposure to cold. • Feelings of doom.	Adrenal tumor.	See Pheochromocytoma.

*All references are to Illness section unless noted otherwise.

SEXUAL INTERCOURSE, PAINFUL FOR MAN

SYMPTOMS & FACTORS	POSSIBLE PROBLEM	WHAT TO DO*
• Pain during ejaculation. • Burning when urinating. • Discharge from penis.	Infection of urethra or prostate gland.	• See Gonorrhea. • See Prostatitis. • See Urethritis.
• Pain in penis during intercourse. • Red, swollen, tender bumps, or sores on skin or tip of penis.	Skin inflammation or infection.	• See Balanitis. • See Herpes, Genital.
• Pain in penis during intercourse. • Partner tense, difficult to arouse or uncomfortable during intercourse.	Lack of lubrication in partner's vagina.	• See Dyspareunia. • See Vaginismus.
• Pain in tip of penis after intercourse. • Use of latex condom. OR • Partner uses contraceptive cream or douching solution.	Skin reaction to cream, solution, or condom.	• Consult doctor. • See Dermatitis, Contact. • See Latex Allergy.
• Pain in penis before, during or after intercourse. • Usually no other symptoms or factors.	Psychosexual problem.	• See Dyspareunia. • See Erectile Dysfunction.
A prolonged, painful, tender erection unaccompanied by sexual arousal.	Penis disorder.	• Call doctor now or seek emergency care. • See Priapism.

*All references are to Illness section unless noted otherwise.

SEXUAL INTERCOURSE, PAINFUL FOR WOMAN

SYMPTOMS & FACTORS	POSSIBLE PROBLEM	WHAT TO DO*
• Painful intercourse only when partner penetrates vagina deeply. • Heavy, painful periods.	Disorder of lining of pelvic organs.	See Endometriosis.
• Painful intercourse. • Abnormal vaginal discharge.	Several disorders.	• See Abnormal Vaginal Discharge (in this Symptoms section). • See Cervical Cancer. • See Vaginitis.
• Painful intercourse. • Tenderness over bladder. • Frequent, painful urination.	Bladder inflammation.	See Bladder Infection, Female.
Painful intercourse in woman past menopause or over age 45.	Normal occurrence caused by decreased vaginal secretions.	• See Menopause. • See Perimenopause.
• Painful intercourse. • Recent childbirth.	Inflammation or scarring caused by a stretched or torn vagina or episiotomy repair.	• Wait at least 3 weeks before resuming sexual relations after childbirth. • Consult doctor if pain lasts longer than 8 weeks.
• Painful intercourse. • Vaginal itching.	Several disorders.	See Vaginal Itching (in this Symptoms section).
• Painful intercourse. • Vagina seems too tight.	Muscle spasm.	• See Dyspareunia. • See Vaginismus.
• Painful intercourse. • Abnormal vaginal bleeding. • Genital itching.	Cancer.	See Vaginal or Vulval Cancer.
• Painful intercourse. • Recent start or increase in sexual activity.	No underlying disorder.	• Wait 2 to 3 days for symptoms to disappear before resuming sex. • See Dyspareunia. • See Vaginismus.
• Dryness of vagina causing painful intercourse. • Dryness of eyes and mouth.	Autoimmune disorder.	See Sjögren's Syndrome.
• Pain with intercourse. • Bad smelling vaginal discharge. • Frequent, painful urination.	Infection.	See Pelvic Inflammatory Disease.
• Pain with intercourse. • Lump in back of the vagina or projecting outside of it. • Vague backache.	Fallen uterus.	See Uterine Prolapse.
• Pain with intercourse. • Chronic pain in the pelvic, lower stomach, and back areas.	Chronic pain.	See Chronic Pelvic Pain.
• Painful intercourse. • No other specific symptoms.	• Vaginal malformation. • Lack of experience and education.	• Consult doctor. • See Sexual Dysfunction, Female.

*All references are to Illness section unless noted otherwise.

SHOULDER PAIN

SYMPTOMS & FACTORS

- Pain in shoulder following injury.
- Shoulder misshapen.
- Bruising in affected area.
- Inability to move shoulder.

- Pain in shoulder following injury.
- Shoulder appearance normal.
- Shoulder movement uncomfortable.

- Pain in shoulder, especially when moving arm.
- No other symptoms.

- Pain in shoulder and other joints.
- Affected joints red, warm, swollen.

- Sudden pain in shoulder.
- No fever.

SKIN, BUMPS ON
(continued on next page)

POSSIB

Skin t
pre

SYMPTOMS & FACTORS

Thickened bump on toe.

Bumps on skin that are cysts, blisters, scaly patches, white patches or sores.

Rough, hard bump on hand o foot with tiny black dots in

Painful, red bump with yellow center in par with hair.

- Small rais firm, white sandpa
- Bu fol

SYMPTOMS & FACTORS	POSSIBLE CAUSES	WHAT TO DO
		• See Pseudogout.
• Shoulder and neck pain. • Working at computer for many hours.	Muscle spasm.	• Have computer screen at proper eye level and chair at correct height. • Take a break every hour.
• Sudden pain in shoulder or other joint. • Affected joint red, warm, swollen. • Fever. • Recent illness, such as sore throat or skin infection.	Complication of prior streptococcal infection.	See Rheumatic Fever.
• Pain in shoulder when moving arm. • Stiffness and severity of pain increasing.	• Inflammation. • Pressure on nerves.	• See Shoulder, Frozen. • See Thoracic-Outlet Syndrome.
• Pain between shoulder blades. • Tightness, pressure, squeezing, or mild ache in the chest. • Heart disorder.	Lack of blood to heart.	• Consult doctor. • See Angina Pectoris.

*All references are to Illness section unless noted otherwise.

	E PROBLEM	WHAT TO DO*
...nickening caused by ...ssure.		See Corn or Callus.
	Several disorders.	See Skin Problems (in this Symptoms section).
...y ...ump.	Skin growth caused by virus.	See Warts.
...white or ...t of body	Infected hair follicle.	See Boils.
...ed bumps that are ..., and have a dry ...per feel. ...mps are in clusters in hair ...cles.	Common skin disorder.	See Keratosis Pilaris.
• Bumps or rash. • Fever.	Several disorders.	See Rash With Fever (in this Symptoms section).
• Papules (small, raised bumps) that are flat-topped with well-defined borders. • Papules don't itch or hurt.	Benign skin disorder.	See Keratoses, Seborrheic.
• Nodules under the skin that are dome-shaped. • Nodules feel "doughy," smooth and are easily movable.	Benign fat-cell tumors.	See Lipomas.
Rough, small bumps on skin of anus, vagina, or penis.	Skin growth caused by virus.	See Warts, Genital.
• Light-red bumps with raised edges. • Severe itching.	Allergic reaction.	See Hives.
• Dark, slow-growing lump. OR • Change in mole size or color. • Borders of mole become irregular. • Bleeding or pain in mole.	Skin cancer or precancerous lesion.	• See Dysplastic Nevi. • See Melanoma.
Single lump that grows.	• Skin growth caused by virus. • Skin cancer, especially if center is an open sore. • Spread of cancer from other body parts.	• Consult doctor. • See Carcinoma, Basal-Cell. • See Carcinoma, Squamous Cell.
Red bumps on the cheeks, either side of nose, and scalp.	Autoimmune disorder.	See Lupus Erythematosus, Discoid.
• Skin symptoms that vary. • Use of latex product, such as rubber gloves.	Allergic reaction.	See Latex Allergy.

*All references are to Illness section unless noted otherwise.

SKIN, BUMPS ON
(continued from previous page)

SYMPTOMS & FACTORS	POSSIBLE PROBLEM	WHAT TO DO*
• Nodules in the armpit. • Nodules are firm, tender, and domed.	Blocked glands.	See Hidradenitis Suppurativa.
• Red lumps appear on the shins or about the knees or ankles. • Flu-like infection may precede the skin symptoms.	Skin inflammation.	See Erythema Nodosum.
• Small red, raised bumps (papules) on the skin of the thighs, buttocks, or armpits. • Followed by other symptoms: muscle aches, fatigue, chills, fever, stiff neck, headache, backache, nausea, and vomiting.	Tick bite.	See Lyme Disease.
• Small, raised, itchy bumps. • Color is pinkish, purplish, or reddish-purple. • Irregular white lines on the skin.	Inflammatory condition.	See Lichen Planus.
• Small, raised bumps (papules) on the skin. • Bumps are firm, smooth, domed with a central pit, and skin-colored or white.	Virus infection of the skin.	See Molluscum Contagiosum.
• Small bump(s) on the skin. • Look like a spider or insect bite. • May be red, swollen, painful, or warm to the touch.	Bacterial infection.	See Methicillin-resistant Staphylococcus Aureus.

*All references are to Illness section unless noted otherwise.

SKIN PROBLEMS (CHILD UNDER AGE 2)

SYMPTOMS & FACTORS	POSSIBLE PROBLEM	WHAT TO DO*
Rash in diaper area.	Chemical skin irritation.	See Diaper Rash.
• Rash or blotches. • Hot weather or environment.	Sweat retention.	• Remove excess clothing. • Consult doctor if rash lasts longer than 24 hours or child seems ill. • See Prickly Heat.
Greasy, scaling, crusty patches on scalp.	Cradle cap.	• See Dermatitis, Seborrheic. • Cradle cap usually disappears when hair grows.
• Rash. • Fever.	Several disorders.	See Rash With Fever (in this Symptoms section).
Rash, spots, blisters, or discoloration in infant 3 months or younger.	Several disorders.	Consult doctor.
Inflamed skin with itching, flaking, patches.	Allergic skin disorder.	See Eczema, Dyshidrotic.
Blisters on face that burst and become crusty and may itch.	Skin infection.	See Impetigo.
Patch of skin that is lighter or darker than surrounding skin.	• Disorder of skin pigment. • Benign skin growth.	• See Pityriasis Alba. • See Skin Growths, Benign.
• Small, itching blisters, usually in a thin line. • Broken blisters leave scratch marks.	Disease of the skin.	See Scabies.
• Dark red or purple spots that don't fade when skin is pressed or stretched. • Headache, fever, and loss of appetite may occur first.	Allergic disorder.	See Purpura, Henoch Schönlein.
• Small raised bumps on the skin (often on the face). • Bumps don't hurt or itch.	Virus infection.	See Molluscum Contagiosum.
Redness, pain, and itching in the genital area.	Vaginal skin problem.	See Vulvovaginitis Before Puberty.
• Small, raised itch bumps. • Bumps swell and produce pink or red lesions (wheals). • Wheals form larger areas of redness.	Allergic disorder.	See Hives.

*All references are to Illness section unless noted otherwise.

SKIN RASH WITH FEVER
(continued on next page)

SYMPTOMS & FACTORS	POSSIBLE PROBLEM	WHAT TO DO*
• Raised, red, itching bumps that become blisters on face, trunk, and genitals. • Fever.	Virus infection.	See Chickenpox.
• Red rash. • Fever and fatigue. • Swelling around neck.	Virus infection.	See Rubella.
• Rash starting on cheeks and then spreading. • Fever. • Young child.	Virus infection.	See Erythema Infectiosum.
• Rash in child age under age 5. • Fever. • Irritability.	Childhood disorder.	See Roseola Infantum.
• Red spots or blotches on face or trunk. • Fever, plus 2 or more of following: • Dry cough. • Sore, red eyes. • Runny nose. • Sore throat. • Headache.	• Virus infection. • Rickettsia infection.	• See Hand, Foot & Mouth Disease. • See Measles. • See Rocky Mountain Spotted Fever.
• Painful red, blister-like rash on body. • Fever. • General ill feeling.	Virus infection.	See Herpes Zoster.
• Purple spots, plus 2 or more of following: • Fever. • Headache. • Pain when bending head forward. • Eyes sensitive to light. • Vomiting.	Infection of membranes around brain.	• Call doctor now. • See Meningitis, Bacterial.
• Red rash. • Fever. • Rapid heartbeat. • Fatigue and weakness. • Excessive thirst.	Bacterial infection.	• Call doctor now. • See Toxic Shock Syndrome.
• Purple rash. • Fever.	Allergic disorder.	See Purpura, Henoch Schönlein.

*All references are to Illness section unless noted otherwise.

SKIN PROBLEMS (PERSON OV...
(continued on next page)

SYMPTOMS & FACTORS	POSSIBLE PROBLE...	
• Red, circular, flat, scaling lesions. • May be on the scalp, skin, nails, and bearded area of the face.	Fungal infection.	
• Rash. • Use of prescription or nonprescription drug.	Adverse react... effect of drug...	
Red skin areas covered with silvery scales.	Chronic skin disorder.	See...
Flaking, white scales over reddish patches on the skin where hair grows.	Dandruff or cradle cap.	See Dermatitis, Seborrheic.
Painful, red bump with white or yellow center in part of body with hair.	Infected hair follicle.	See Boils.
Patch of skin that is lighter or darker than surrounding skin.	• Disorder of skin pigment. • Yeast infection of skin.	• See Pityriasis Alba. • See Tinea Versicolor. • See Vitiligo.
Yellow or greenish-yellow tint to the skin (jaundice).	Numerous disorders or drugs.	Call doctor now.
• Yellow-orange tint to the skin. • Consumption of large amounts of carrots or yellow vegetables.	Excess of carotene in the system.	Stop eating offending food for 2 to 6 weeks. Resume eating it in moderation.
• A new mole or dark lump. OR • Change in a mole or skin lesion.	Skin cancer or precancerous lesion.	• See Dysplastic Nevi. • See Melanoma.
• Dome-shaped cyst. • Cyst is whitish or skin-colored.	Infected cyst.	See Epidermoid Cyst.
• Blister-like rash. • Burning sensation at site 1 or 2 days before rash appears.	Virus infection of sensory nerves.	See Herpes Zoster.
• Small groups of bumps. • Usually with a hair in the middle of each bump.	Bacterial or fungal skin infection.	See Folliculitis.
Reddish, scaly, oval patches on chest, back or abdomen without fever or other symptoms.	Inflammatory skin disorder.	See Pityriasis Rosea.
• Skin symptoms that vary. • Use of latex product, such as rubber gloves.	Allergic reaction.	See Latex Allergy.
Itching rash without fever.	Several disorders.	See Rash Without Fever (in this Symptoms section).

*All references are to Illness section unless noted otherwise.

	POSSIBLE PROBLEM	WHAT TO DO*
...d	Skin infection.	See Cellulitis.
...g.		
...(blue-red nodules) ...and trunk. ...on.	Skin cancer.	See Kaposi Sarcoma.
...s, hardness, or ...ss in skin exposed to ...ng temperatures.	Tissue injury.	See Frostbite.
• Painless blister on genitals that ulcerates and heals quickly. • Enlarged lymph glands in groin.	Lymphogranuloma venereum.	Consult doctor.
Pain, redness, and tenderness at the base of the spine.	Infected cyst.	See Pilonidal Disease.
• Small, movable, nontender nodule that appears under the skin of the finger. • The nodule enlarges and becomes pink and ulcerates.	Fungal infection.	See Sporotrichosis.
New scars on the skin that arise in an area of injury, burn or other skin problem.	Defective healing process.	See Keloids.
• Clusters of small, itching blisters. • Clusters appear on both sides of the body in the same place.	Inflammation of skin.	See Dermatitis, Herpetiformis.
• Sudden appearance of warm, painful, or tender nodules (usually start on front of leg). • Color changes from pink to red to blue to brown.	Inflammatory skin disease.	See Erythema Nodosum.
• Small, raised bumps on the skin in the shape of a ring. • Pink or violet color with a dome or slightly flat shape.	Chronic benign skin disorder.	See Granuloma Annulare.
• Small raised bumps on the skin that appear first as pinhead size, but grow rapidly. • Bumps bleed easily if injured.	Skin disorder of unknown cause.	See Granuloma, Pyogenic.
• Blackheads, red, tender bumps. • Bumps fill with pus.	Blocked skin glands.	See Hidradenitis. Suppurative.
• New sores or ulcers that take a long time to heal. • Diabetes.	Skin infection.	See Diabetes Feet & Skin Problems.

*All references are to Illness section unless noted otherwise.

SYMPTOMS & FACTORS	POSSIBLE PROBLEM	WHAT TO DO*
• Rash. • Fever.	Several disorders.	See Rash With Fever (in this Symptoms section).
Skin problems in child under 2.	Several disorders.	See Skin Problems (Person Under Age 2) (in this Symptoms section).
• Redness, swelling, spots, or lumps on the skin. • May have itching or pain or burning or tingling.	Bite or sting.	See Insect Bites & Stings.
Skin problem on feet.	Several disorders.	See Foot Problems (in this Symptoms section).
Blisters on face that burst and become crusty and may itch.	Skin infection.	See Impetigo.
Skin problem on penis.	• Inflammation. • Infection.	• See Balanitis. • See Herpes, Genital. • See Syphilis.
Skin problem on face.	Several disorders.	See Facial Skin Problems (in this Symptoms section).
Itching without change in skin appearance.	Several disorders.	See Itching (in this Symptoms section).
Bumps on skin.	Several disorders.	See Skin, Bumps on (in this Symptoms section).
• Small, itching blisters, usually in a thin line. • Broken blisters leave scratch marks.	Mite infestation.	See Scabies.
• Raised, thick, flat-top, bumps. • Dark brown or black. • May be a few to 100s. • Not painful.	Benign skin growth.	See Keratoses, Seborrheic.
• Tight skin. • Tingling sensation in arms, hands, legs, and feet. • Swallowing difficulty.	Autoimmune disorder.	See Scleroderma.
Redness, pain, and itching in the genital area in a young girl.	Vaginal skin problem.	See Vulvovaginitis Before Puberty.
• Plaques (flat areas with the following characteristics): • Bright red patches with poorly defined borders. • Severe itching.	Yeast infection of the skin.	See Candidiasis of Skin.

*All references are to Illness section unless noted otherwise.

SKIN RASH WITH FEVER
(continued from previous page)

SYMPTOMS & FACTORS	POSSIBLE PROBLEM	WHAT TO DO*
• Red rash. • Paleness around mouth. • Fever. • Bright red, sore throat. • Swollen tonsils. • Enlarged glands in neck.	Complication of preceding streptococcal infection.	• Call doctor now. • See Scarlet Fever.
• Mild skin rash on chest, back, and abdomen. • Fever, fatigue, and paleness. • Pain caused by joint inflammation.	Complication of preceding streptococcal infection.	See Rheumatic Fever.
• Rash that starts with a small red spot and then spreads. • Rash resembles a bulls-eye. • Fever or flu-like symptoms. • Recent outdoors activity.	Tick-caused disorder.	See Lyme Disease.
• Red rash or spots that begins on palms, soles, arms, and legs. • Rash develops into blisters. • Fever (sometimes).	Inflammatory disorder.	See Erythema Multiforme.

*All references are to Illness section unless noted otherwise.

SKIN RASH WITHOUT FEVER
(continued on next page)

SYMPTOMS & FACTORS	POSSIBLE PROBLEM	WHAT TO DO*
• Light-red bumps with raised edges. • Severe itching.	Allergic reaction.	See Hives.
• Itching rash. • Use of prescription or nonprescription drug.	Adverse reaction or side effect of drug.	• Call doctor now. • See Drug Allergy.
Itching, red, scaling, or moist rash under cosmetics, jewelry or new clothing.	Allergic reaction.	See Dermatitis, Contact.
Itching, red, scaling or moist rash, especially on hands.	Skin disorder aggravated by stress.	See Dermatitis, Atopic.
• Itching, red, scaling, or moist rash, plus: • Recent contact with plant, such as poison ivy, poison oak, poison sumac, primrose, or mango. OR • Recent contact with irritating detergents or other chemicals.	Allergic or irritant reaction.	• See Dermatitis, Contact. • See Poison Ivy, Oak, Sumac.
• Itching rash around genitals or anus. • No other symptoms or factors.	Vaginal infection.	See Vulvovaginitis, Candidiasis.
Red bumps in a small area without other symptoms.	Insect bites.	See Insect Bites & Stings.
• Red rash. • Rash is located in areas of heavy perspiration.	Obstruction of sweat glands.	See Prickly Heat.
• Red rash scattered over body. • Severe itching at night. • Gray lines or red, sore spots between fingers or on wrists.	Parasites.	See Scabies.
• Rash that consists of small, white blisters with pus inside. • Blisters are located in hair follicles of the skin.	Bacterial or fungal skin infection.	See Folliculitis.
Red, scaling patch that spreads into a ring.	Fungus infection.	See Ringworm.
Rash without fever in child under 2.	Several disorders.	See Skin Problems (Child Under Age 2) (in this Symptoms section).
• Red rash that begins on palms, soles, arms, and legs. • Rash develops into blisters.	Inflammatory disorder.	See Erythema Multiforme.

*All references are to Illness section unless noted otherwise.

SKIN RASH WITHOUT FEVER
(continued from previous page)

SYMPTOMS & FACTORS	POSSIBLE PROBLEM	WHAT TO DO*
• Red, raised rash or skin lesions. • Rash appears on cheeks in a "butterfly" appearance.	Autoimmune disorder.	• See Lupus Erythematosus, Discoid. • See Lupus Erythematosus, Systemic.
• Rash starting on cheeks then spreading. • Slight tiredness or fatigue. • Young child.	Virus infection.	See Erythema Infectiosum.
• Skin rash, progressing to thin, raised lines on the skin. • Contact with soil or sand.	Hookworm infestation.	See Larva Migrans, Cutaneous.
• Skin rash (that may itch) on face, shoulders, arms, and over joints. • Weakness in the pelvic or shoulder muscles.	Connective tissue disorder.	See Polymyositis.
• Red skin rash, sometimes with small blisters. • A burning reaction similar to those that follow prolonged sun exposure. • Dizziness, nausea, vomiting. • Brief sun exposure.	Sensitivity to sun.	See Photosensitivity.
• Scaling patches on the skin of the groin, thighs, and buttocks, armpit, or groin. • Patches have well-defined edges.	Fungal infection.	See Tinea Cruris.

*All references are to Illness section unless noted otherwise.

SLEEPING PROBLEMS
(continued on next page)

SYMPTOMS & FACTORS	POSSIBLE PROBLEM	WHAT TO DO*
Sleep disturbance (difficulty falling asleep, staying asleep or remaining asleep).	Many causes.	• See Insomnia. • See Sleep Problems, Temporary.
• Sleeping problems (sleepiness or insomnia). • Use of prescription or nonprescription drug, such as: appetite suppressants, decongestants, or diuretics.	Adverse reaction or side effect of drug.	Consult doctor.
Sleeping problems following late, heavy dinner or consumption of 3 or more alcoholic beverages at night.	Common occurrence.	• Eat lighter or earlier dinner. • Decrease alcohol consumption.
• Sleeping problems. • Use of caffeine-containing beverage or drug.	Stimulant effect of caffeine.	Decrease use of caffeine, especially during late afternoon or evening.
• Sleeping problems. • Sedentary lifestyle.	Common occurrence.	Begin an exercise program. Consult your doctor first if you have any chronic illness or are at risk for heart disease.
Change in sleep pattern in person over age 60.	Normal occurrence, less sleep may be needed with aging.	Nothing.
• Inability to fall asleep. • Daytime tension.	Effect of stress.	• See Anxiety Disorder, Generalized. • See Stress.
• Wakefulness during night. • Fatigue. • Loss of pleasure in usual activities. • Poor appetite or overeating.	Depression.	• See Depression. • See Dysthymia.
• Sleeping problems. • Recent withdrawal from narcotics, sleeping pills, tranquilizers or alcohol.	Withdrawal symptom.	Nothing. Normal sleep pattern should return within several weeks.
• Sleeping problems. • Use of illegal drug.	Adverse reaction or side effect of drug.	• Discontinue use of drug. • See Substance Abuse.

*All references are to Illness section unless noted otherwise.

SLEEPING PROBLEMS
(continued from previous page)

SYMPTOMS & FACTORS	POSSIBLE PROBLEM	WHAT TO DO*
• Sleepiness. • Constipation. • Decreased tolerance for hot or cold.	Underactive thyroid gland.	See Hypothyroidism.
• Sleeping problems. • Excessive sweating. • Unexplained weight loss. • Increased appetite. • Anxiety. • Rapid or irregular heartbeat.	Overactive thyroid gland.	See Hyperthyroidism.
Sleep attacks that may occur up to 10 times a day.	Sleep disorder.	See Narcolepsy.
• Fitful sleep. • Shortness of breath when awake.	Fluid in lungs caused by heart condition.	See Heart Failure.
• Long periods of not breathing when asleep. • Choking while sleeping. • Snoring.	Breathing problem.	See Sleep Apnea.
• Difficulty in remaining asleep. • Stiffness and weakness. • Sudden, painful muscular spasms.	Muscle inflammation.	See Fibromyalgia.
• Child has sleepless nights. • Child is restless during day.	Behavioral syndrome.	See Attention Deficit Hyperactivity Disorder in Children.

*All references are to Illness section unless noted otherwise.

SPEAKING DIFFICULTY

SYMPTOMS & FACTORS	POSSIBLE PROBLEM	WHAT TO DO*
• Speaking difficulty. • Use of prescription or nonprescription drug.	Adverse reaction or side effect of drug.	Consult doctor.
• Inability to complete words without repeating first consonants. OR • Inability to speak when ready to say something.	Stammering or stuttering in children and stress in adults.	Consult doctor or speech therapist.
• Expressionless speech with abnormal tone and phrasing. • Trembling that is worse at rest. • Shuffling walk.	Disorder of central nervous system.	See Parkinson's Disease.
Normal pronunciation, but confused words or ideas in person under age 45.	Psychiatric disorder.	Consult doctor.
• Normal pronunciation but confused words or ideas, plus 1 or more of following: • Poor attention span with conversations or instructions. • Decline in attention to personal appearance or cleanliness. • Personality changes.	Mental deterioration.	• See Alzheimer's Disease. • See Dementia.
Speaking difficulty because of inability to move muscles on one side of face.	Disorder of facial nerves.	See Bell's Palsy.
• Speaking difficulty. • Vague eye problems. • Weakness, difficulty in walking and balance.	Nervous system disorder.	See Multiple Sclerosis.
Speaking difficulty because of pain in mouth or tongue.	Infection or sores in mouth or tongue.	See Mouth, Sore, Tingling, Dry (in this Symptoms section).
• Speaking difficulty, plus any of following: • Blurred vision. • Numbness or tingling in any part of body. • Weakness in extremities. • Dizziness.	Decreased blood supply to brain.	• Call doctor now. • See Aneurysm. • See Stroke. • See Thrombosis Embolism, Arterial. • See Transient Ischemic Attack.
• Speaking difficulty. • Vomiting with blood. • Yellow skin or eyes.	Inherited disorder.	See Wilson Disease.

*All references are to Illness section unless noted otherwise.

STOOL, ABNORMAL APPEARANCE

SYMPTOMS & FACTORS	POSSIBLE PROBLEM	WHAT TO DO*
• Stool that is very dark, black, or contains black material, plus any of following: • Recent consumption of green, leafy vegetables, licorice, chocolate, grapes, raisins, or cranberries. • Current use of iron-supplement tablets. • Recent use of Pepto-Bismol.	No underlying disorder.	Nothing. If discoloration continues, consult doctor.
• Red-looking stools. • Recent consumption of beets, tomatoes, red-colored drinks or cereal, cherry-flavored medicines.	Stools are reddish due to something you ate or drank.	Nothing. If discoloration continues, consult doctor.
• Dark or black stool. • Use of prescription or nonprescription drug.	Adverse reaction or side effect of drug.	• Consult doctor about prescription drug. • Discontinue use of nonprescription drug.
Light colored or almost white stool.	Gluten intolerance.	See Celiac Disease.
• Blood in stool OR • Stool has a black or dark-red color.	Several disorders.	See Bleeding, Rectal (in this Symptoms section).
Worms in stool.	Parasitic infection.	• Call doctor now. • See Pinworms. • See Roundworms.
• Pale stool. • Yellow skin and eyes (jaundice).	Gallbladder or liver disorder.	• Call doctor now. • See Cholecystitis or Cholangitis. • See Hepatitis, Viral.
• Bloody or black stool. • Change in bowel habits. • Cramping in abdomen.	Cancer.	See Colon Cancer.
• Black stool. • Symptoms of indigestion. • Weight loss, poor appetite.	Cancer.	See Stomach Cancer.
• Bloody stools. • Diarrhea, vomiting, cramping. • Consumed foods or beverages that may be spoiled or contaminated.	Gastrointestinal problem.	See Food Poisoning.
• Pale, foamy, bulky, bad-smelling stool. • No jaundice.	Poor digestion.	See Malabsorption.

*All references are to Illness section unless noted otherwise.

SWALLOWING DIFFICULTY

SYMPTOMS & FACTORS	POSSIBLE PROBLEM	WHAT TO DO*
• Swallowing difficulty. • Sensation that food is stuck high in chest. • Occasional chest pain, especially when bending forward or lying down.	Discomfort in upper digestive tract.	See Gastroesophageal Reflux Disease.
• Swallowing difficulty. • Sore throat. • Fever.	Throat infection.	• See Herpangina. • See Pharyngitis. • See Mumps. • See Strep Throat. • See Tonsillitis.
Normal swallowing with sensation that food is stuck.	Effect of stress.	• Increase fluid intake when eating. • See Anxiety Disorder, Generalized.
• Swallowing difficulty. • Recent swallowing of foreign object, such as fish bone. • Sore throat.	Object stuck in throat.	Call doctor now.
• Swallowing difficulty that is chronic or worsening. • Sensation that food is stuck high in chest.	Esophagus muscle disorder.	• See Dysphagia. • See Hiatal Hernia.
• Swallowing difficulty. • Pain with swallowing. • Bloody mucus regurgitation.	Tumor or esophagus disorder.	• See Esophageal Stricture. • See Esophagus Cancer.
• Swallowing difficulty. • Drooping eyelids. • Arm and leg weakness.	Autoimmune disorder.	See Myasthenia Gravis.
• Severe swallowing difficulty. • Muscle pain and spasms. • Fever. • Difficulty in using chest muscles to breathe.	Infection in a wound or injury site.	See Tetanus.
• Swallowing difficulty. • Hardening and thickening of the skin of the fingers and face.	Connective tissue disease.	See Scleroderma.
• Swallowing difficulty. • Muscle weakness of neck, chest, and extremities. • Drooping eyelids. • Double vision. • No fever.	Toxin from contaminated food.	• Call doctor now. • See Botulism.
• Swallowing difficulty. • Weight loss. • Hoarseness.	Cancer.	• See Laryngeal Cancer. • See Thyroid Cancer.
• Swallowing difficulty. • Sore throat. • Fever. • Muffled voice or cry.	Inflammation of epiglottis.	• See Epiglottitis.

*All references are to Illness section unless noted otherwise.

SWEATING, EXCESSIVE

SYMPTOMS & FACTORS	POSSIBLE PROBLEM	WHAT TO DO*
• Excessive sweating. • Anxiety or excitement.	Normal occurrence with stress.	• See Anxiety Disorder, Generalized. • See Stress.
• Excessive sweating. • Overweight.	Effect of excess weight.	See Obesity & Overweight.
• Excessive sweating in woman older than 38. • Irregular menstrual periods.	Hormone changes, end of menstrual cycles approaching.	• See Menopause. • See Perimenopause.
• Excessive sweating in woman during menstrual period. OR • Excessive sweating due to tension or apprehension. OR • Excessive sweating following coffee consumption.	No underlying disorder.	Nothing.
Excessive sweating in teenager.	Normal occurrence during adolescence.	Nothing.
• Sweating. • Palpitations, tremors, flushing. • Symptoms of anxiety when exposed to, or thinking of, a particular stimulus.	Fears.	See Phobias.
• Excess sweating. • Unpleasant body odor.	Several disorders.	See Hyperhidrosis
• Skin is cool and moist. • Prolonged exposure to hot temperature.	Excessive fluid loss.	See Heatstroke or Heat Exhaustion.
• Excessive sweating. • Chest pain.	Heart attack.	• Call doctor now! • See Heart Attack.
• Excessive sweating at night. • Weight loss. • Persistent cough with blood in sputum. • Fever. • Fatigue.	Infection or cancer.	• See Hodgkin's Disease. • See Tuberculosis.
• Excessive sweating, plus 2 or more of following: • Weight loss. • Increased appetite. • Anxiety. • Sleeping problems.	Overactive thyroid gland.	See Hyperthyroidism.
• Excessive sweating. • Use of prescription, nonprescription or illegal drug.	Adverse reaction or side effect of drug.	• Consult doctor about prescription drug. • Discontinue use of nonprescription or illegal drug.
• Excessive sweating. • Fever.	Normal occurrence with fever.	See Fever charts (in this Symptoms section).

*All references are to Illness section unless noted otherwise.

SWELLING OR LUMP
(continued on next page)

SYMPTOMS & FACTORS	POSSIBLE PROBLEM	WHAT TO DO*
• Nodule or bump under the skin. • Nodule feels "doughy," smooth and easily movable.	Benign fat-cell tumor.	See Lipomas.
• Painful, red lump or swelling. • Recent injury to area.	Bleeding under skin.	• See Sprains & Strains. • See Tendinitis.
Lump in breast.	• Benign changes. • Cancer.	• Consult doctor. • See Breast Cancer. • See Fibrocystic Breast Changes.
Soft lump or swelling in groin or near navel that disappears when pressed or enlarges with cough.	Protruding intestinal tissue.	See Hernia.
Swelling between ear and jaw.	• Virus infection of glands. • Salivary gland problem. • Infection around tooth.	• See Mumps. • See Salivary Gland Infection. • See Tooth Abscess.
• Lump or swelling in neck, armpit, or groin. • Fever.	Virus infection.	See Mononucleosis, Infectious.
Swelling or lump in child 3 months or younger.	Several disorders.	Consult doctor.
• Swelling on both sides of neck, toward front. • Sore throat.	Bacterial or viral infection.	• See Mononucleosis, Infectious. • See Pharyngitis. • See Tonsillitis.
• Swelling at both sides of back of neck. • Pink rash. • Fever.	Virus infection.	See Rubella.
• Tender swelling in armpit, groin, elbow or base of neck. • Sore, cut, or bite on hand, arm, leg or shoulder on same side as swelling.	Infected bite or wound.	Consult doctor.
Tender or hard lump in neck just below Adam's apple.	Inflammation or tumor of thyroid.	• See Thyroid Cancer. • See Thyroid Nodule. • See Thyroiditis.
• Tender lump on elbow or in armpit. • Fever. • Exposure to cats.	Virus infection.	See Cat-Scratch Disease.
Swelling in front of neck with movement when swallowing.	Thyroid goiter.	Consult doctor.

*All references are to Illness section unless noted otherwise.

SWELLING OR LUMP
(continued from previous page)

SYMPTOMS & FACTORS	POSSIBLE PROBLEM	WHAT TO DO*
• Swelling in neck, armpit, or groin. • Recent vaccination, such as tetanus or typhoid.	Swelling caused by vaccination.	Consult doctor.
• Mass in abdomen that can be felt, especially in young child. • Cramping abdominal pain.	Intestinal obstruction.	• Call doctor now. • See Intussusception.
Lump or swelling in neck, armpit, or groin without other symptoms or factors.	• Infection. • Tumor.	• See Hodgkin's Disease. • See Lymphoma, Non-Hodgkin's.
• Lump or swelling in neck, armpit or groin. • Use of prescription drug, especially for epilepsy or thyroid disorder.	Adverse reaction or side effect of drug.	Consult doctor.
• Swollen lymph nodes. • Low-grade fever. • Weight loss. • Recurrent respiratory and skin infections.	Virus infection.	See HIV & AIDS.
• Hard mass in right, upper abdomen. • Unexplained weight loss and appetite loss. • Pain and bleeding tendency.	Liver tumor.	See Hepatocellular Carcinoma.
• Swelling in rectum. • Pain during bowel movement. • Rectal redness.	Bacterial infection.	See Anorectal Abscess.
• Lump in the vagina. • Pelvic pressure. • Backache.	Prolapse of organ.	See Uterine Prolapse.
• Swelling of part of the arm or leg or entire arm or leg, including fingers or toes. • Restricted range of motion in arm or leg.	Lymph gland disorder.	See Lymphedema.
• Fluid build-up causing swelling in legs, ankles, or feet. • Decreased urine.	Kidney condition.	See Renal Failure, Acute.
• Swelling due to fluid retention. • Puffy eyes and ankles. • Weight gain (due to fluid).	Kidney damage.	See Nephrotic Syndrome.

*All references are to Illness section unless noted otherwise.

TESTICLES OR PENIS, PAINFUL OR SWOLLEN

SYMPTOMS & FACTORS	POSSIBLE PROBLEM	WHAT TO DO*
• Pain in testicles or penis. • Forceful blow, injury, or wound in lower abdomen or genitals.	Injury to genitourinary tract.	See Genitourinary Injury.
• Sudden, painful swelling in testicle. • No injury to genital area.	Testicle infection or a twisted testicle.	• Call doctor now. • See Epididymitis. • See Testicular Torsion.
Swelling or lump on one testicle.	Cyst or tumor.	• Consult doctor. • See Testicular Cancer.
• Pain in testicles. • Swelling between ear and jaw. • Fever.	Virus infection of glands.	• Consult doctor. • See Mumps.
• Ache (and sometimes pain) in the testicle. • Feeling of heaviness or dragging in the scrotum (the pouch of skin that contains the testicles).	Varicose veins.	See Varicocele.

*All references are to Illness section unless noted otherwise.

THROAT, SORE

SYMPTOMS & FACTORS	POSSIBLE PROBLEM	WHAT TO DO*
• Sore throat. • Fever. • Swelling on both sides of neck toward front. • Red, swollen tonsils with specks of pus on surface.	Bacterial or viral infection.	• Request throat culture. • See Diphtheria. • See Mononucleosis, Infectious. • See Strep Throat. • See Tonsillitis.
• Sore throat. • Excessive smoking or alcohol consumption. OR • Smoke-filled environment.	Throat irritation or inflammation.	See Pharyngitis.
• Sore throat. • Runny nose. • Itching eyes.	Allergic reaction.	See Hay Fever.
• Sore throat. • Hoarseness or voice loss.	Several disorders.	• See Laryngitis. • See Voice Loss or Hoarseness (in this Symptoms section).
• Sore throat. • Swallowing is painful. • Feeling that food "gets stuck" as you swallow.	Several disorders.	See Dysphagia.
• Sore throat. • Fever, plus any of following: • Aches in bones or joints. • Cough. • Headache. • Stuffy or runny nose.	Virus infection.	• See Cold, Common. • See Influenza. • See Influenza, H1N1
• Sore throat. • Fever. • Swelling or tenderness between ear and jaw.	Virus infection of glands.	See Mumps.
• Sore throat. • Fever. • Muffled voice or cry.	Bacterial infection of epiglottis.	See Epiglottitis.
• Sudden sore throat with redness, inflammation, and painful swallowing. • Fever. • General ill feeling.	Virus infection.	See Herpangina.
• Sore throat. • Cough, chills, fever. • Muscle and joint aches. • Skin rash.	Fungal infection.	See Coccidioidomycosis.

*All references are to Illness section unless noted otherwise.

TONGUE, SORE

SYMPTOMS & FACTORS	POSSIBLE PROBLEM	WHAT TO DO*
• Sore tongue. • Use of prescription or nonprescription drugs.	Adverse reaction or side effect of drug.	Consult doctor.
• Sore tongue. • Discomfort confined to one spot.	Abrasion from denture or irregular tooth.	Consult dentist.
• Sore tongue. • Pain on one side of face.	Nerve inflammation or damage.	See Trigeminal Neuralgia.
• Sores on tongue. • Sores are small, very painful, and shallow.	Several causes.	See Canker Sores.
• Sore tongue. • Hard lump on tongue or in mouth.	Cancer.	See Oral Cancer.
• Sore tongue. • Discomfort involves whole tongue.	• Anemia. • Inflammation or infection.	• See Anemia, Pernicious. • See Tongue Inflammation.
• Sore tongue. • Fatigue and weakness. • Loss of appetite and weight loss.	Lack of folic acid.	See Folic Acid Deficiency.
• Sore tongue. • Cracked, fissured, red tongue. • Mouth ulcers.	Poor nutrition.	• Consult doctor. • See Vitamin Deficiencies.

*All references are to Illness section unless noted otherwise.

TOOTHACHE

SYMPTOMS & FACTORS	POSSIBLE PROBLEM	WHAT TO DO*
• Toothache, plus any of following: • Fever. • Swollen face or gums. • Continual pain that interferes with sleep.	Tooth problem.	• Call dentist now. • See Tooth Abscess. • See Tooth Decay.
• Toothache over several teeth. • Red, swollen, bleeding gums.	Gum infection.	• See Gingivitis. • See Periodontitis.
• Recurrent toothache. • No other symptoms.	Tooth decay.	• Consult dentist. • See Tooth Decay.
• Toothache when biting food. • Recent tooth filling.	• Common occurrence following a filling. • Filling not level.	Consult dentist if pain lasts longer than 1 week.
• Cheek pain that resembles a toothache. • Nasal condition. • Feeling of pressure inside the head.	Sinus infection.	See Sinusitis.
• Gnawing pain in lower teeth and neck. • Chest discomfort beneath breastbone. • Shoulder or arm pain. • Sweating.	Insufficient oxygen to heart.	• Call doctor now. • See Angina Pectoris. • See Coronary Artery Disease.

*All references are to Illness section unless noted otherwise.

TREMBLING OR TWITCHING

SYMPTOMS & FACTORS	POSSIBLE PROBLEM	WHAT TO DO*
• Trembling or twitching, especially of tongue and face muscles. • Use of prescription or nonprescription drug, especially phenothiazine.	Adverse reaction or side effect of drug.	• Consult doctor about prescription drug. • Discontinue use of nonprescription drug.
Trembling in one part of body, especially when affected part is at rest.	Movement disorder.	• See Essential Tremor. • See Parkinson's Disease.
• Trembling. • Alcohol withdrawal.	Withdrawal symptom.	See Alcoholism.
• Trembling. • Excessive consumption of coffee or tea. OR • Use of nonprescription drug containing caffeine.	Adverse effect of caffeine.	Decrease use of caffeine.
• Trembling, plus 2 or more of following: • Weight loss. • Fatigue. • Excessive sweating.	Overactive thyroid gland.	See Hyperthyroidism.
• Painful twitching on side of face. • Pain is triggered by stroking or touching the face.	Nerve disorder.	See Trigeminal Neuralgia.
Twitching in one small part of body, such as eyelid.	Fatigue or tension. Usually no underlying disorder.	• Nothing. • Consult doctor if you feel ill or if muscles seem weak.
Trembling in any part of body without other symptoms or factors.	Inherited tendency to tremble, especially from anxiety or stress.	Consult doctor to confirm diagnosis.
• Leg twitching or leg sensations (uncomfortable, to irritating, to painful). They may come and go. • Lying down and trying to relax causes the symptoms.	Movement disorder.	See Restless Legs Syndrome.
Unexpected body jerks when falling asleep.	Involuntary muscle spasms. No underlying disorder.	Nothing.

*All references are to Illness section unless noted otherwise.

URINATION, CHANGE IN FREQUENCY
(continued on next page)

SYMPTOMS & FACTORS	POSSIBLE PROBLEM	WHAT TO DO*
• Frequent urination, especially at night. • Increased urine production. • Excessive consumption of tea, coffee, caffeine drink, or alcohol.	Effect of caffeine or alcohol.	Decrease consumption of caffeine or alcohol.
• Frequent urination, especially at night. • Increased urine production. • Use of diuretic drug for heart disease or high blood pressure.	Effect of diuretic drug.	Consult doctor if you are concerned.
• Frequent urination. • Anxiety or excitement. OR • Cold weather.	Normal occurrence.	Nothing.
• Frequent urination. • Burning and stinging on urination. • Increased urge to urinate.	Infection.	• See Bladder Infection, Female. • See Bladder Infection, Male. • See Urethritis.
• Frequent urination. • Painful urination. • Blood in urine.	Stones.	See Kidney Stones.
• Frequent urination. • Possible pregnancy.	Normal occurrence during first 3 months and last 3 months of pregnancy.	Consult doctor to confirm pregnancy.
• Frequent urination. • Pain with urination.	Several disorders.	See Urination, Painful (in this Symptoms section).
• Frequent urination, especially at night. • Increased hunger and thirst. • Fatigue. • Weight loss.	Blood sugar problem.	• See Diabetes Type 1. • See Diabetes Type 2.
• Frequent urination in man older than 50, plus 2 or more of following: • Involuntary urine leak after urination. • Weak urinary stream. • Difficulty starting urination. • Increased waking at night to urinate.	Disorder of prostate gland.	• See Prostate Cancer. • See Prostatic Hypertrophy, Benign. • See Prostatitis.
• Frequent urination in a woman. • Intense urge to urinate followed quickly by uncontrollable urine leak.	Incontinence problem.	See Incontinence, Urge.
• Frequent urination. • Difficulty controlling bladder.	Several disorders.	See Urination, Lack of Control (in this Symptoms section).

*All references are to Illness section unless noted otherwise.

URINATION, CHANGE IN FREQUENCY
(continued from previous page)

SYMPTOMS & FACTORS	POSSIBLE PROBLEM	WHAT TO DO*
• Passage of large amounts of urine. • Colorless urine. • Excessive thirst.	Hormone disorder.	See Diabetes Insipidus.
• Frequent urination. • Pelvic pain and pressure. • Sensation of incomplete emptying of bladder. • Pain during intercourse. • Burning on urination.	Inflammation in area of bladder.	See Interstitial Cystitis.
• Decreased urine. • Smoky or slightly red urine.	Kidney infection.	See Glomerulonephritis.
• Decreased urine. • Fluid build-up causing swelling in legs, ankles, or feet.	Kidney condition.	See Renal Failure, Acute.

*All references are to Illness section unless noted otherwise.

URINATION, LACK OF CONTROL

SYMPTOMS & FACTORS	POSSIBLE PROBLEM	WHAT TO DO*
Small urine leak in female when coughing, sneezing, laughing, or running.	Incontinence problem.	See Incontinence, Stress.
Loss of urine right after feeling an urge to urinate.	Incontinence problem.	See Incontinence, Urge.
• Lack of urinary control. • Use of prescription drug.	Adverse reaction or side effect of drug.	Consult doctor.
• Lack of urinary control. • Cloudy, bad-smelling urine.	Infection of urinary tract.	• See Bladder Infection, Female. • See Bladder Infection, Male. • See Urethritis.
Dribbling of urine after urination in male over age 50.	• Disorder of prostate gland. • Inflammation of urethra.	• See Prostate Cancer. • See Prostatic Hypertrophy, Benign. • See Urethritis.
• Lack of urinary control. • Lack of bowel control.	Decreased blood supply to brain.	• Call doctor now • See Stroke.
• Lack of urinary control. • Constipation for longer than 1 week.	Pressure on bladder from fecal impaction.	See Fecal Impaction.
• Lack of urinary control in person over age 60. • Personality change. • Decline in attention to personal appearance or cleanliness.	• Mental deterioration. • Poor nutrition.	• See Alzhelmer's Disease. • See Dementia. • See Vitamin Deficiencies.
Lack of urinary control in child over age 3-1/2.	Several causes.	See Bed-Wetting.

*All references are to Illness section unless noted otherwise.

URINATION, PAINFUL

SYMPTOMS & FACTORS	POSSIBLE PROBLEM	WHAT TO DO*
• Painful urination. • Pain in one side of back, between waist and last rib. • Fever.	Kidney infection.	See Kidney Infection, Acute.
• Painful urination. • Frequent urination.	Bladder inflammation.	• See Bladder Infection, Female. • See Bladder Infection, Male.
• Painful urination. • Painful blisters on genitals. • Fever.	Sexually-transmitted virus infection.	• See Herpes, Genital. • See Sexually Transmitted Diseases.
• Painful urination in female. • Green-yellow or white discharge from vagina. • Itching around genitals.	Vaginal infection.	• See Trichomoniasis. • See Vulvovaginitis, Candidiasis.
• Painful urination in man. • Thick, yellow-green discharge from penis.	Sexually-transmitted infection.	• See Gonorrhea. • See Urethritis.
• Painful urination in woman. • Bad-smelling vaginal discharge. • Pain or tenderness in lower abdomen. • Fever.	Sexually-transmitted infection.	• See Gonorrhea. • See Urethritis.
• Painful urination in man. • Heavy feeling or dull pain between scrotum and anus. • Fever.	Infection of prostate gland.	See Prostatitis.
• Burning urination. • Blood in urine. • Pain in pelvic area.	Abnormal growth in bladder.	See Bladder Tumor.
• Painful urination or inability to urinate. • Forceful blow, injury or wound in lower abdomen or genitals.	Injury to genital tract.	See Genitourinary Injury.
• Discomfort on urinating. • Vaginal discharge (female). • Urethral discharge (male).	Infection.	See Chlamydia.
• Pain or discomfort with urination. • Discharge from urethra. • Small ulcers on mouth, tongue, or on tip of penis in males.	Inflammatory disease.	See Reactive Arthritis.
• Discomfort with urination (male). • Painless sore or lesion on penis.	Cancer.	See Penile Cancer.

*All references are to Illness section unless noted otherwise.

URINE, ABNORMAL COLOR

SYMPTOMS & FACTORS	POSSIBLE PROBLEM	WHAT TO DO*
• Pink, red, smoky-brown, or other color change in urine. • Use of new prescription drug in last 24 hours.	Side effect of drug.	Consult doctor if color change not expected.
• Dark yellow or orange urine. • Recent use of laxatives containing senna. OR • Recent consumption of rhubarb.	Effect of chemicals in these substances.	Nothing.
• Pink, red, or smoky-brown urine. • Recent consumption of beets, red berries, or other red food.	Effect of natural or artificial color.	Nothing.
Pink, red, or smoky-brown urine.	Disorder of urinary tract.	• Consult doctor. • See Bladder Infection, Female. • See Bladder Infection, Male. • See Bladder Tumor. • See Glomerulonephritis. • See Kidney Cancer. • See Kidney Infection (both Acute and Chronic). • See Kidney Stones. • See Prostatic Hypertrophy, Benign. • See Tuberculosis. • See Wilms' Tumor (children only).
• Clear, dark-brown urine. • Pale stool. • Yellow skin and eyes.	Liver disorder.	See Hepatitis, Viral.
• Dark yellow or orange urine. • Fever. OR • Very hot weather. OR • Decreased fluid intake.	Concentrated urine.	• See Fever charts (in this Symptoms section). • See Dehydration. • See Heatstroke or Heat Exhaustion.
• Dark yellow or orange urine. • Diarrhea. • Vomiting.	Concentrated urine.	• See Diarrhea (in Symptoms section). • See Vomiting, Recurrent Attacks (in this Symptoms section).
• Green or blue urine. • Have eaten certain foods. • Use of certain drugs.	Effect of artificial color in food or drug.	Nothing. If concerned, consult doctor.
• Colorless urine. • Excessive thirst. • Passage of large amounts of urine.	Hormone disorder.	See Diabetes Insipidus.

*All references are to Illness section unless noted otherwise.

VAGINAL BLEEDING, UNEXPECTED

SYMPTOMS & FACTORS	POSSIBLE PROBLEM	WHAT TO DO*
Vaginal bleeding during first 3 months of pregnancy.	Spontaneous abortion.	• Call doctor now. • See Miscarriage.
Vaginal bleeding during 4th to 9th month of pregnancy.	Abnormal location of placenta.	• Call doctor now. • See Abruptio Placenta. • See Placenta Previa.
• Unexpected vaginal bleeding. • Severe abdominal pain. • Pregnancy possible. OR • Current use of intrauterine contraceptive device (IUD).	Pregnancy developing outside uterus.	• Call doctor now. • See Ectopic Pregnancy.
• Unexpected vaginal bleeding in woman over age 45. • Last menstrual period more than 6 months ago.	• Hormone changes. • Tumor or cancer.	• See Cervical Cancer. • See Menopause. • See Ovarian Cancer. • See Postmenopausal Bleeding. • See Uterine Malignancy. • See Vaginal or Vulval Cancer.
• Unexpected vaginal bleeding in woman over age 45. • Use of prescription drug for hormone replacement therapy.	Breakthrough bleeding.	Consult doctor.
• Unexpected vaginal bleeding. • Vaginal discharge.	• Several disorders. • Cancer.	• See Cervical Cancer. • See Cervical Polyps. • See Uterine Malignancy. • See Vaginal or Vulval Cancer.
• Unexpected vaginal bleeding. • Pain in lower abdomen.	Uterine or ovarian problem.	• See Cervical Polyps. • See Ovarian Cancer. • See Uterine Bleeding, Dysfunctional. • See Uterine Fibroids. • See Uterine Malignancy.
• Unexpected vaginal bleeding. • Recent insertion of intrauterine contraceptive device (IUD).	Complications caused by IUD.	Consult doctor.
• Unexpected vaginal bleeding. • Use of oral contraceptives.	Breakthrough bleeding, common occurrence in women taking pill.	Consult doctor.
• Excessive menstrual flow. • Menstrual period lasts more than 7 days.	Menstrual irregularity.	See Menorrhagia.
• Changes in menstrual cycle. • Course skin. • Sleepiness.	Underactive thyroid gland.	See Hypothyroidism.
• Unexpected vaginal bleeding. • Insertion of foreign object into vagina.	Vaginal injury.	Consult doctor.

*All references are to Illness section unless noted otherwise.

VAGINAL DISCHARGE, ABNORMAL

SYMPTOMS & FACTORS	POSSIBLE PROBLEM	WHAT TO DO*
• Heavy vaginal discharge. • Vaginal pain.	Irritation or infection of cervix.	See Cervicitis.
• Foul-smelling, frothy discharge that is most apparent several days after a menstrual period. • Vaginal itching and pain. • Pain with intercourse.	Vaginal parasitic infection.	See Trichomoniasis.
Discharge has a "fishy" smell.	Vaginal bacterial infection.	See Vaginosis, Bacterial.
• Heavy vaginal discharge that is normal in color and consistency. • Vaginal itching or soreness.	Irritation or infection.	See Vaginal Itching (in this Symptoms section).
White, curd-like vaginal discharge.	Vaginal fungus infection.	See Vulvovaginitis, Candidiasis.
• Green-yellow, bad-smelling vaginal discharge. • Tampon, diaphragm, or cervical cup left in vagina.	Vaginal infection.	• Remove tampon, diaphragm or cup if you can. • If not, consult doctor.
• Heavy vaginal discharge that is normal in color and consistency. • Use of oral contraceptives. OR • Possible pregnancy.	Normal occurrence caused by hormone changes.	Consult doctor to confirm pregnancy.
Heavy vaginal discharge that is normal in color and consistency during ovulation occurring during middle days between periods.	Normal occurrence.	Nothing.
• Vaginal discharge. • Reddening of vagina.	Vaginal infection.	• See Chlamydia. • See Vaginitis.
• Vaginal discharge, which may or may not smell bad. • Redness, itching in genital area. • Young girl (before puberty).	Infection.	See Vulvovaginitis Before Puberty.
• Red or brown vaginal discharge. • Occasional spotting of blood between menstrual periods.	Several disorders.	• See Cervical Polyps. • See Vaginal Bleeding, Unexpected (in this Symptoms section).
• Green-yellow, bad-smelling vaginal discharge. • Pain in lower abdomen. • Frequent or painful urination.	Infection of reproductive organs.	• See Gonorrhea. • See Pelvic Inflammatory Disease.
• Heavy, bad-smelling vaginal discharge 2 or more days after childbirth. • Fever. • Abdominal pain.	Infection of uterus.	See Postpartum Infection.

*All references are to Illness section unless noted otherwise.

VAGINAL ITCHING

SYMPTOMS & FACTORS	POSSIBLE PROBLEM	WHAT TO DO*
• Vaginal itching. • Unusual vaginal discharge.	Several disorders.	• See Pruritus Vulvae. • See Vaginitis. • See Vulvovaginitis Before Puberty. • See Vaginal Discharge, Abnormal (in this Symptoms section).
• Vaginal itching. • Use of antibiotics.	Vaginal infection.	See Vulvovaginitis, Candidiasis.
• Vaginal itching. • Abnormal vaginal bleeding.	Cancer.	See Vaginal or Vulvar Cancer.
• Vaginal itching. • Sores in genital area.	Viral infection.	See Herpes, Genital.
• Vaginal itching. • Use of chemical spray, ointment, cream, douche, or contraceptive foam.	Irritation caused by chemical or drug.	Discontinue use of possible irritant.
Vaginal itching in woman over age 38.	Decreasing level of estrogens at menopause.	See Pruritus Vulvae.

*All references are to Illness section unless noted otherwise.

VISION DISTURBANCE OR LOSS
(continued on next page)

SYMPTOMS & FACTORS	POSSIBLE PROBLEM	WHAT TO DO*
• Sensitivity to light. • Discharge from eye. • Pain in eye.	Infection.	See Conjunctivitis.
• Blurred vision. • Difficult reading. • Poor night vision.	Clouding of eye lens.	See Cataract.
• Blurred vision in past 2 days. • Eye pain.	Inflammation.	See Iritis.
• Blurred vision or sensitivity to light. • Use of prescription drug.	Adverse reaction or side effect of drug.	Consult doctor.
• Loss of peripheral vision in small areas. • Blurred vision on one side.	Excess pressure in eye.	See Glaucoma, Open-Angle.
• Blurred or fuzzy vision. • Squinting to see objects that aren't close to you. OR • Unable to see objects that are right in front of you.	Uncorrected vision problem.	Have an eye examination.
• Flashes of light or wavy spots in vision. • Severe headache. • Nausea and vomiting.	Headache.	See Headache, Migraine.
• Sensitivity to light. • Eye pain. • Tears.	Infection.	See Keratitis.
Uncoordinated eye movements that may cause vision problems.	Eye muscle disorder.	See Strabismus.
• Double vision. • Bulging eyes.	Overactive thyroid gland.	• Consult doctor. • See Hyperthyroidism.
• Vision disturbance. • Recent head injury.	Bleeding inside skull.	• Call doctor now. • See Subdural Hemorrhage & Hematoma.
Sudden, partial or total loss of vision in one or both eyes.	• Decreased blood supply to back of eye or brain. • Disorder of central nervous system.	• Call doctor now. • See Brain Tumor. • See Multiple Sclerosis. • See Stroke. • See Transient Ischemic Attack.

*All references are to Illness section unless noted otherwise.

VISION DISTURBANCE OR LOSS
(continued from previous page)

SYMPTOMS & FACTORS	POSSIBLE PROBLEM	WHAT TO DO*
• Blurred vision in one eye. • Flashing lights. • Floating spots. • No pain.	Disorder of blood vessels and structures in back of eye.	See Retinal Detachment.
• Double vision. • Drooping eyelids. • Swallowing difficulty.	Autoimmune disorder.	See Myasthenia Gravis.
• Blurred vision. • Diabetes.	Diabetic retinopathy.	Consult doctor.
• Poor night vision. • Dry, inflamed eyes. • Rough skin. • Loss of appetite.	Lack of vitamin A.	See Vitamin Deficiencies.
• Changes in vision. • Headache, nausea, vomiting. • Seizures. • Excessive thirst.	Tumor.	See Pituitary Tumor.
• Blurred vision. • Dizziness.	Ear problem.	See Benign Paroxysmal Positional Vertigo.

*All references are to Illness section unless noted otherwise.

VOICE LOSS OR HOARSENESS

SYMPTOMS & FACTORS	POSSIBLE PROBLEM	WHAT TO DO*
Hoarseness following excessive smoking or alcohol consumption.	Inflammation of vocal cords caused by alcohol or tobacco.	• Decrease smoking or alcohol consumption. • See Laryngitis.
• Hoarseness following excessive use of voice. OR • Exposure to tobacco smoke or toxic fumes.	Inflammation of vocal cords caused by overuse or exposure.	If hoarseness doesn't disappear in a few days, consult doctor.
• Hoarseness, plus 2 or more of following: • Dry skin or hair. • Decreased tolerance for cold. • Fatigue. • Unexplained weight gain.	Underactive thyroid gland.	See Hypothyroidism.
• Voice loss or hoarseness. • Tender or hard lump in neck just below Adam's apple.	Tumor of thyroid.	See Thyroid Nodule.
Hoarseness following cold, cough, or sore throat.	Inflammation of vocal cords caused by nasal drainage.	See Laryngitis.
• Hoarseness. • Recent tension or depression.	Effect of stress.	See Anxiety Disorder, Generalized.
• Voice loss or hoarseness for longer than 1 week. OR • Recurrent attacks of hoarseness or voice loss in last 6 months.	• Inflammation of vocal cords. • Tumor.	• See Laryngeal Cancer. • See Oral Cancer. • See Vocal-Cord Nodules.

*All references are to Illness section unless noted otherwise.

VOMITING (INFANT 0 TO 6 MONTHS)

SYMPTOMS & FACTORS	POSSIBLE PROBLEM	WHAT TO DO*
• Vomiting. • Diarrhea.	Infection of digestive tract.	See Gastroenteritis.
• Vomiting. • Infant appears healthy. • No other symptoms.	• Single episode—no underlying disorder. • More than one episode—several disorders, such as food allergies or milk intolerance.	• Consult doctor if vomiting lasts longer than 6 hours. • Consult doctor for repeated vomiting. • See Food Allergy. • See Lactose Intolerance.
• Vomiting. • Recent playful bouncing. OR • Travel by airplane, boat or motor vehicle.	Disturbed equilibrium.	• Don't bounce after feedings. • See Motion Sickness.
• Vomiting. • Fever.	Infection.	See Fever (child 0 to 2 years) (in this Symptoms section).
• Vomiting. • Cough or runny nose.	Virus infection.	Consult doctor if vomiting lasts longer than 6 hours.
• Vomiting. • Use of prescription drug.	Adverse reaction or side effect of drug.	Call doctor now.
• Forceful vomiting. • Possible accidental ingestion of drug, household cleaning supply, or poison. OR • Recent head injury.	• Chemical irritation of stomach and toxic effect of chemical on brain. • Internal bleeding.	• Call doctor now or go to emergency room. • See Head Injury.
• Vomiting. • Fever of 101°F (38.3°C) rectally or higher, plus any of following: • Lethargy. • Eyes sensitive to light. • General ill appearance. • Crying with urination.	• Infection in membranes around brain. • Urinary-tract infection.	Call doctor now.
• Vomiting. • Swelling or lump in groin or testicle.	Protruding intestinal tissue.	See Hernia.
• Infant vomits forcefully after each feeding. • Infant appears healthy.	Constriction in outlet to stomach.	See Pyloric Stenosis.
• Vomiting. • Recurrent attacks of screaming or crying, as if in great pain.	Blockage in intestines.	• Call doctor now. • See Intestinal Obstruction. • See Intussusception.

*All references are to Illness section unless noted otherwise.

VOMITING, RECURRENT ATTACKS

SYMPTOMS & FACTORS	POSSIBLE PROBLEM	WHAT TO DO*
• Recurrent vomiting. • Burning sensation in chest or upper abdomen, especially when bending forward or lying down.	Stomach acid in esophagus.	See Gastroesophageal Reflux Disease.
• Recurrent vomiting. • Occasional pain or tenderness in upper right abdomen. • No fever.	Gallbladder disorder.	See Gallstones.
• Recurrent vomiting. • Occasional pain or tenderness in upper right abdomen. • Fever.	Gallbladder inflammation.	See Cholecystitis or Cholangitis.
• Recurrent vomiting. • Poor appetite. • Jaundice (yellow skin and eyes).	Gallbladder or liver disorder.	• See Gallstones. • See Hepatitis, Viral.
• Recurrent vomiting. • Use of prescription or nonprescription drug.	Adverse reaction or side effect of drug.	Consult doctor.
• Recurrent vomiting. • Pain or tenderness in center of upper abdomen. • Pain relieved by vomiting.	Peptic-ulcer disease.	See Ulcer, Peptic.
Vomiting within hours after drinking alcohol.	Stomach inflammation.	See Gastritis.
Recurrent, self-induced vomiting.	Psychological disorder.	See Bulimia.
• Vomiting. • Extreme dizziness. • Loss of balance.	Inner ear disorder.	See Labyrinthitis.
• Recurrent vomiting. • Poor appetite. • Ongoing pain in upper abdomen.	Tumor.	See Stomach Cancer.
• Recurrent vomiting without nausea. • Recurrent headaches, especially in morning.	Bleeding inside skull or tumor.	• Consult doctor. • See Brain Tumor. • See Subdural Hemorrhage & Hematoma.
• Bloody vomit. • Bleeding from several body parts.	Blood-clotting problem.	See Disseminated Intravascular Coagulation.
• Vomiting with blood. • Speaking difficulty. • Yellow skin or eyes.	Inherited disorder.	See Wilson Disease.
• Vomiting. • Extreme abdominal pain, swelling, and gas.	Disorder of the pancreas.	See Pancreatitis.
• Nausea or vomiting. • Pregnancy.	Pregnancy problem.	• See Hyperemesis Gravidarum. • See Nausea & Vomiting in Pregnancy.

*All references are to Illness section unless noted otherwise.

VOMITING, SUDDEN ATTACK
(continued on next page)

SYMPTOMS & FACTORS	POSSIBLE PROBLEM	WHAT TO DO*
• Vomiting. • Diarrhea. • Fever.	Infection of digestive tract.	• See Gastroenteritis. • See Listeriosis.
• Vomiting. • Feelings of nervousness and apprehension (such as before going on stage).	Emotional upset.	• Vomiting should stop when emotions calm down. • See Anxiety Disorder, Generalized. • See Panic Disorder.
• Vomiting. • Headache.	Headache disorder.	See Headache, Migraine.
• Vomiting. • Use of prescription or nonprescription drug.	Adverse reaction or side effect of drug.	• Consult doctor about prescription drug. • Discontinue use of nonprescription drug.
• Vomiting. • Jaundice (yellow skin or eyes).	Gallbladder or liver disorder.	• Consult doctor. • See Gallstones. • See Hepatitis, Viral.
Recent, recurrent vomiting attacks.	Several disorders.	See Vomiting, Recurrent (in this Symptoms section).
• Vomiting. • Consumption of spoiled, contaminated or improperly prepared food.	Effect of toxins in food.	• See Botulism. • See Food Poisoning. • See Salmonella Infections. • See Trichinosis.
• Vomiting. • Dizziness.	Infection or disorder of inner ear.	• See Labyrinthitis. • See Ménière's Disease.
• Vomiting. • Excessive consumption of alcohol or rich food.	Stomach inflammation.	See Gastritis.
Vomiting of blood or dark "coffee ground" material.	Bleeding in stomach.	• Call doctor now. • See Ulcer, Peptic.
• Vomiting. • Severe abdominal pain. • No pain relief from vomiting.	Several disorders.	• Call doctor now. • See Appendicitis.
• Vomiting. • Dizziness, headache, faintness.	Gas inhalation.	See Carbon Monoxide Poisoning.
• Vomiting. • Headache, plus any of following: • Eyes sensitive to light. • Drowsiness or confusion. • Pain when bending head forward.	Infection or bleeding in membranes around brain.	• Call doctor now. • See Meningitis, Aseptic. • See Meningitis, Bacterial. • See Subarachnoid Hemorrhage.
• Vomiting. • Headache. • Head injury in last 24 hours.	Brain injury.	• Call doctor now. • See Head Injury.

*All references are to Illness section unless noted otherwise.

VOMITING, SUDDEN ATTACK
(continued from previous page)

SYMPTOMS & FACTORS	POSSIBLE PROBLEM	WHAT TO DO*
• Vomiting. • Abdominal pain or swelling. • Inability to have bowel movement.	Blockage in intestines.	• Call doctor now. • See Intestinal Obstruction.
• Vomiting. • Eye pain. • Blurred vision.	Excess pressure inside eye.	• Call doctor now. • See Glaucoma, Angle-Closure.
• Vomiting and watery diarrhea. • Sudden high fever. • Rash that resembles sunburn.	Blood poisoning.	See Toxic Shock Syndrome.

*All references are to Illness section unless noted otherwise.

WEIGHT GAIN

SYMPTOMS & FACTORS	POSSIBLE PROBLEM	WHAT TO DO*
• Weight gain. • Change from active to sedentary lifestyle.	Calorie intake too high for current activity level.	Decrease food consumption and increase physical activity.
• Weight gain. • No other symptoms.	More calories consumed than burned.	• See Obesity & Overweight. • See Obesity, Childhood.
• Weight gain. • Depression.	Compensatory overeating.	See Depression.
• Weight gain. • Feeling of depression and tiredness. • Start of, or during, winter season.	Lack of light.	See Seasonal Affective Disorder.
• Weight gain. • Use of prescription or nonprescription drug that causes fluid retention, such as: steroids, cortisone drugs, oral contraceptives, or nonsteroid anti-inflammatory drugs.	Adverse reaction or side effect of drug.	Consult doctor.
• Weight gain. • Decreased tolerance for cold. • Dry skin or hair. • Fatigue. • Constipation.	Underactive thyroid gland.	See Hypothyroidism.
• Weight gain. • Recently discontinued smoking.	Normal occurrence.	Weight gain will soon stop. But be careful about what you eat. Get plenty of exercise.
• Rapid weight gain during pregnancy. • Puffiness in the face, hands, and feet that is worse in the morning.	Complication of pregnancy.	See Preeclampsia & Eclampsia.
• Weight gain. • High blood pressure or history of heart, kidney, or liver disease.	Fluid retention caused by disorder of blood vessels, heart, liver, or kidney.	• See Hypertension. • See Heart Failure. • See Nephrotic Syndrome. • See Cirrhosis of the Liver.
• Weight gain with accumulation of fat over upper back and trunk. • Round face and puffy eyes.	Endocrine disorder.	See Cushing's Syndrome.
Weight gain due to fluid retention.	Several disorders.	• See Ankles, Swollen (in this Symptoms section). • See Abdominal Swelling (in this Symptoms section).

*All references are to Illness section unless noted otherwise.

WEIGHT LOSS

SYMPTOMS & FACTORS	POSSIBLE PROBLEM	WHAT TO DO*
• Weight loss. • Increased thirst and hunger. • Fatigue. • Frequent urination.	Diabetes.	• See Diabetes Type 1. • See Diabetes Type 2.
• Weight loss. following: • Excessive sweating. • Fatigue and anxiety. • Rapid heartbeat.	Overactive thyroid gland.	See Hyperthyroidism.
• Weight loss. • Anxiety, stress, or depression.	• Effect of stress. • Psychological disorder.	• See Anorexia Nervosa. • See Anxiety Disorder Generalized. • See Bulimia. • See Depression. • See Stress.
• Weight loss. • Use of prescription drug.	Adverse reaction or side effect of drug.	Consult doctor.
• Weight loss. • Cramping or pain in stomach. • Black, tarry, or bloody stool.	Cancer.	• See Colon Cancer. • See Stomach Cancer.
• Weight loss. • Recurrent pain in upper abdomen.	Intestinal disorder.	• See Colitis, Ulcerative. • See Crohn's Disease. • See Irritable Bowel Syndrome. • See Ulcer, Peptic.
• Weight loss. • Excessive sweating at night. • Fever and fatigue. • Persistent cough with blood in sputum.	Lung inflammation or infection.	• See Bronchiectasis. • See Bronchitis, Chronic. • See Tuberculosis.
• Weight loss. • Pale, bulky, bad-smelling stool. • Recurrent diarrhea. • Recurrent respiratory and skin infections.	• Poor digestion. • Virus infection.	• See Malabsorption. • See HIV & AIDS.
• Unexplained weight and appetite loss. • Abdominal discomfort or pain. • Other vague symptoms.	Cancer.	• See Hepatocellular Carcinoma. • See Pancreatic Cancer.
• Weight loss in female. • Fatigue (sometimes). • Not having monthly periods or periods that are not regular.	Eating behavior.	See Female Athlete Triad.
• Weight loss. • Increased physical activity.	Normal occurrence.	Consult doctor if weight loss is not expected and continues longer than 2 weeks.

*All references are to Illness section unless noted otherwise.

WHEEZING

SYMPTOMS & FACTORS	POSSIBLE PROBLEM	WHAT TO DO*
• Wheezing. • Fever.	Infection of bronchial tubes.	• See Bronchiolitis (young children). • See Bronchitis, Acute.
• Wheezing. • Breathing difficulty.	Spasm of bronchial tubes.	• Call doctor now. • See Asthma.
• Wheezing with a "barking" cough in an infant or young child. • Difficulty in breathing.	Viral infection.	See Croup.
• Wheezing. • Possible inhalation of foreign object, such as peanut.	Foreign object in larynx or bronchial tubes.	Call doctor now.
• Persistent, mild wheezing. • Cough (may have gray or green-yellow sputum).	Chronic infection of breathing passages.	• See Bronchiectasis. • See Bronchitis, Chronic. • See Chronic Obstructive Pulmonary Disease. • See Emphysema.
• Wheezing. • Cough with frothy pink, brownish, or white sputum.	Fluid in lungs.	• Call doctor now. • See Pulmonary Edema.
• Wheezing. • Breathing difficulty. • Swelling in face or hands. • Itching all over, hives.	Allergic reaction.	• Call doctor now or seek emergency help. • See Anaphylaxis. • See Drug Allergy.
• Symptoms similar to asthma (wheezing). • Flushed skin on the head and neck. • Diarrhea.	Tumor.	See Carcinoid Syndrome.

*All references are to Illness section unless noted otherwise.

Illness & Disorders

ABRUPTIO PLACENTA

GENERAL INFORMATION

DEFINITION—Abruptio placenta is separation of the placenta (also called the afterbirth) from the uterine wall before the baby is born. The placenta carries all nutrients and oxygen to the fetus. A separation can cause complications for the mother and the fetus. With a small separation, there may be no or few symptoms. Larger separations usually cause symptoms.

BODY PARTS INVOLVED—Uterus.

SEX OR AGE MOST AFFECTED—Females.

SIGNS & SYMPTOMS
- Bleeding may be external (vaginal bleeding) or it may be concealed (bleeding remains in the uterus).
- Mild pain or discomfort, or there may be severe pain in the lower abdomen or back.
- Decreased fetal movement.
- Hard, tender abdomen. Uterine contractions.

CAUSES—The cause is unknown. Certain risk factors do exist.

RISK INCREASES WITH
- High blood pressure (hypertension).
- Smoking.
- Women over age 35 or younger than 20.
- Women who have had more than 4 or 5 pregnancies.
- A previous pregnancy with placental separation.
- Pregnancy with more than one fetus.
- Excess amniotic fluid (polyhydramnios).
- Chronic disorder (such as diabetes) or renal infection.
- Injury from motor vehicle accident, falls, or abuse.
- Short umbilical cord.
- Abnormal uterus or uterine tumor.
- Premature rupture of the membranes (water breaks before the onset of labor).
- Use of alcohol or drugs of abuse (such as cocaine).

HOW TO PREVENT
- There is no sure way to prevent the problem.
- Avoid risk factors such as smoking, alcohol, or cocaine use. Get treatment for high blood pressure.

WHAT TO EXPECT

DIAGNOSTIC MEASURES
- Your own observation of symptoms.
- Your obstetric provider will do a physical exam and ask questions about your symptoms.
- Medical tests will include blood studies and blood clotting tests. An ultrasound (see Glossary) may be done.

APPROPRIATE HEALTH CARE
- Treatment depends on the severity of the separation, the condition of the fetus, and the duration of the pregnancy. Hospital care is usually needed (except for mild cases) so the mother can be observed for any complications. If the placenta separation is slight, you may be able to return home for bed rest and close observation.
- In the hospital, fluids may be given through a vein (IV). A blood transfusion may be needed.
- Labor may be induced, if the pregnancy is at term or if there are signs of fetal distress.
- Surgery to deliver the unborn child by cesarean section, or vaginal delivery (sometimes).

POSSIBLE COMPLICATIONS
- Premature delivery of the child. This may lead to other complications for the newborn.
- Intrauterine growth restriction (IUGR) of the fetus.
- Shock or life-threatening bleeding in the mother.
- Blood clotting problems for the mother (disseminated intravascular coagulopathy or DIC).
- Risk of abruptio placentae in a future pregnancy.
- Uncontrolled bleeding after delivery may lead to an emergency hysterectomy.
- Death of child and/or mother.

PROBABLE OUTCOME—When the separation is less severe and with immediate medical care, the outlook for mother and fetus is good.

HOW TO TREAT

GENERAL MEASURES—Abruptio placentae requires emergency medical care, but there is usually time to obtain advice by telephone and arrange safe transportation to the hospital.

MEDICATION—A drug to induce labor may be used if immediate delivery is required.

ACTIVITY—Whether you are in the hospital or have been able to return home, follow all medical instructions about any activity limits.

DIET
- A liquid-only diet may be prescribed until it is decided if surgery will be needed.
- If you are resting at home, continue with regular diet.

CALL YOUR DOCTOR IF

- You have bleeding (anything more than slight spotting) during pregnancy. This is an emergency!
- You have any other new symptoms.

ACNE
(Acne Vulgaris)

GENERAL INFORMATION

DEFINITION—Acne is a common skin condition. It can be mild to severe and can cause distress for the person affected.

BODY PARTS INVOLVED—It usually affects the skin on the face, chest, and back.

SEX OR AGE MOST AFFECTED—Acne has affected almost all people at some point during their lives. In teenagers, it is more common in males than in females. In adults, it is more common in women than men.

SIGNS & SYMPTOMS
- Mild acne can cause blackheads (open comedones) or whiteheads (closed comedones).
- Pimples (also called zits). These are skin pores that have become pus-filled (clogged and bacteria-infected).
- Severe acne produces many pimples.
- Redness and inflammation around pimples.
- Cysts (larger, firm swellings in the skin).

CAUSES—Glands in the skin make an oily substance called sebum. Sebum usually empties onto the skin surface through a pore (small opening) and causes no problems. With acne, the sebum becomes plugged up in the pore. Sex-hormone changes during the teen years play a role. Acne is not caused by unclean skin or by foods.

RISK INCREASES WITH
- Family history of acne.
- Teenagers and young adults.
- Endocrine disorders.
- Use of some drugs, such as cortisone.

HOW TO PREVENT
- Acne cannot be prevented at present. Certain factors (triggers) can cause a flare up. Avoid them where possible.
- Flare up of acne can be caused by some make-up and lotions, certain foods, sunlight, friction (tight clothes, bicycle helmets), and hormone changes in females before their periods.

WHAT TO EXPECT

DIAGNOSTIC MEASURES
- Your own observation of symptoms.
- See your health care provider if home treatments are not helping or acne is more severe. A skin exam will be done and treatment options will be discussed.

APPROPRIATE HEALTH CARE
- Medical treatment will depend on the severity of the acne, any infection or inflammation, and if you are a female who may become pregnant.

- Treatment may include drugs (for topical use and/or taken by mouth).
- Cosmetic surgery (dermabrasion) may be recommended to remove scars after acne heals.
- Removal or drainage of a cyst may be done.

POSSIBLE COMPLICATIONS
- Poor self-image, depression, and emotional stress.
- Permanent pitting of the skin.

PROBABLE OUTCOME
- Most cases respond well to treatment. It may take several months. Acne tends to disappear after teen years.
- Despite treatment, acne can have flare ups.

HOW TO TREAT

GENERAL MEASURES
- Wash face with a mild soap once or twice a day and after exercising. Clean skin gently; don't scrub. An antibacterial soap may help. Rinse soap off completely.
- Shampoo hair daily, especially if it is oily. Don't let hair hang in the face. Use dandruff-preventing shampoo if needed.
- Avoid oil-based cosmetics. Use thinner, lotion-style, water-based products.
- Don't squeeze, scratch, pick, or rub the skin. Acne heals better without damage to the skin. Removal of comedones (blackheads) may be done by your health care provider.

MEDICATION
- Use nonprescription cream or lotion products to treat the acne. These may contain benzyl peroxide, sulfur, salicylic acid, or resorcinol.
- Antibiotic may be prescribed for bacteria infection.
- For more severe cases, topical or oral retinoids (a form of vitamin A), hormone drugs, or stronger acne drugs may be prescribed. Some drugs may increase your sensitivity to sunlight and increase the risk of sunburn.
- Caution: if you are pregnant or planning a pregnancy, tell your health care provider before using acne drugs.

ACTIVITY—No limits.

DIET—Foods don't cause acne, but some foods may make it worse. To find any food problems, stop eating foods that you think may make the acne worse. Then reintroduce them one at a time. If acne flares up 2 to 3 days after a food is eaten, leave that food out of your diet.

CALL YOUR DOCTOR IF

- You or a family member has acne and self-care is not helping.
- Acne worsens or recurs despite treatment.

ACNE ROSACEA
(Rosacea; Adult Acne)

 GENERAL INFORMATION

DEFINITION—Acne rosacea is a chronic inflammation of skin of the nose, cheeks, forehead, and chin. Rarely, the neck, chest, ears, or scalp may be affected. Extensive nose and cheek involvement, mostly in men, is called rhinophyma.

BODY PARTS INVOLVED—Face, especially the nose, and surrounding areas.

SEX OR AGE MOST AFFECTED—Acne rosacea tends to start between ages 30 and 50. It is more common in women, but more severe in men.

SIGNS & SYMPTOMS
- Symptoms vary from person to person and sometimes in the same person. They may be mild or more severe.
- Flushing or blushing.
- Persistent redness.
- Unsightly red, thickened skin on the nose and cheeks. Small blood vessels are visible on the skin surface.
- Papules (small raised bumps) and pustules (small, white blisters with pus) on affected skin.
- Burning, stinging, itching, swelling, dryness, or tightness of affected skin.
- Eyes may be red, burning, watery, or irritated.

CAUSES—Unknown. Hereditary and environmental factors appear to play a role.

RISK INCREASES WITH
- Fair skinned people.
- Family history of acne rosacea.

HOW TO PREVENT—Cannot be prevented. Flare-ups may be triggered by hot liquids, spicy foods, alcohol, emotional stress, some skin care products, sun exposure, hot and cold weather, heavy exercise, and hot baths.

 WHAT TO EXPECT

DIAGNOSTIC MEASURES
- Your own observation of symptoms.
- Your health care provider can diagnose the condition by an exam of the affected skin area. Medical tests are usually not needed.

APPROPRIATE HEALTH CARE
- Treatment will depend on each individual's needs and severity of the symptoms. Treatment may include drugs and skin treatments.
- Surgery (such as laser therapy) may be done for visible blood vessels, to reduce redness, or to remove excess tissue from the nose.
- Psychotherapy or counseling, if disfigurement causes distress.

POSSIBLE COMPLICATIONS
- Emotional problems (such as lack of self confidence and low self-esteem).
- Eye complications.
- Scarring may occur, but it is rare.
- Permanent, thickened, bulbous, red skin on the nose (usually in older men).

PROBABLE OUTCOME—There is no cure. Symptoms can be controlled with treatment and self-care. Acne rosacea is a disease of remissions and frequent flare-ups.

 HOW TO TREAT

GENERAL MEASURES
- Learn what factors cause flare-ups for you and avoid them. Keep a day-to-day diary of your activities and flare-ups to identify your trigger factors.
- Wash your face with a mild soap once or twice a day and after exercising. Clean skin gently; don't scrub. An antibacterial soap may help. Rinse soap off completely.
- Don't squeeze, scratch, pick, or rub the skin.
- Reduce stress in your life if possible. Counseling may help if the condition is adding to your stress.
- To learn more: National Rosacea Society, 106 James St., Barrington, IL 60016; (888) 662-5874; website: www.rosacea.org.

MEDICATION
- Antibiotics (for the skin or taken by mouth) may be prescribed.
- Topical or oral retinoids (a form of vitamin A) or other drugs may be prescribed depending on the symptoms. Caution—if you are pregnant or planning a pregnancy, tell your health care provider before using acne drugs.
- Don't use nonprescription cortisone creams or lotions without medical advice. They may cause the condition to worsen.

ACTIVITY—Limit time spent in sunny, windy, very hot, or cold weather. Use a sunscreen (SPF 30 or higher).

DIET—Avoid food or drink triggers. Drink plenty of water.

 CALL YOUR DOCTOR IF

You have symptoms of acne rosacea. This condition can be helped with treatment.

ADDISON'S DISEASE
(Adrenal Insufficiency)

 GENERAL INFORMATION

DEFINITION—Addison's disease is a rare disorder that leads to failure of the adrenal glands. The adrenal glands produce hormones (cortisol and aldosterone) that affect almost every body organ and tissue. These hormones help the body respond to stress, maintain blood pressure, help heart and blood vessel function, and are involved in metabolism.

BODY PARTS INVOLVED—Adrenal glands.

SEX OR AGE MOST AFFECTED—Addison's often affects people ages 30 to 50, but can occur in all age groups. It affects men and women equally.

SIGNS & SYMPTOMS
- Symptoms may develop slowly over months or years and occur when levels of hormones produced by the adrenal glands are too low.
- Weakness and fatigue.
- Nausea, vomiting, stomach pain, diarrhea, and appetite and weight loss.
- Low blood pressure (faintness and dizziness).
- Darkening of the skin. This includes: skin folds, lips and inside mouth or nose, scars, joints such as elbows or knees, creases of the palm, or nipples.
- Craving for salty foods.
- Behavior or mood changes, including irritability or depression.

CAUSES
- Primary adrenal insufficiency is usually caused by an autoimmune disorder. For unknown reasons, the body's immune system attacks the adrenal glands. Other causes are tuberculosis, AIDS, adrenal gland infection, cancer that has spread to the adrenal glands, or other disorders.
- Secondary adrenal insufficiency occurs when another condition causes the adrenal gland to not produce enough hormones. This is usually due to a pituitary gland problem. In some cases, prolonged or improper use of steroid hormones may be a cause.

RISK INCREASES WITH
- Other autoimmune diseases.
- Disorders mentioned in Causes.
- Family history of Addison's disease.

HOW TO PREVENT—No preventive measures.

 WHAT TO EXPECT

DIAGNOSTIC MEASURES
- Your own observation of symptoms.
- Your health care provider will do a physical exam and ask questions about your symptoms.
- Medical tests may include blood and urine studies, tests to measure adrenal function, and CT or MRI.

APPROPRIATE HEALTH CARE
- Treatment involves replacing the hormones the adrenal glands are not making.
- Hospitalization for an adrenal crisis (see Possible Complications).

POSSIBLE COMPLICATIONS
- Adrenal crisis caused by injury or illness. Symptoms may include pain, weakness, low blood pressure, high or low temperature, fainting.
- Increased risk of infections.

PROBABLE OUTCOME—Addison's disease can be controlled with hormone replacement. A normal lifestyle can be expected.

 HOW TO TREAT

GENERAL MEASURES
- This is a lifelong condition. Learn how to care for yourself. Attention to drug schedules is vital.
- Learn about adrenal crisis and its relationship to body stress (e.g., infection, surgery, or injury). A temporary increase in hormone therapy is usually required.
- Advise any doctor or dentist who treats you that you have Addison's disease.
- You may be taught how to give yourself cortisone injections in case of emergency.
- Wear a medical alert type bracelet or tag stating that you have Addison's disease and its emergency care.
- Stay up-to-date on vaccines, such as those for influenza and pneumonia.
- To learn more: National Adrenal Diseases Foundation, 505 Northern Blvd., Great Neck, NY 11021; (516) 487-4992 (not toll free); website: www.nadf.us.

MEDICATION—Drugs to replace the hormones cortisol and aldosterone will be prescribed as needed. Never stop taking or change your drugs without medical advice.

ACTIVITY—No limits.

DIET—Special diet may be prescribed (e.g., to maintain balance of sodium and potassium).

 CALL YOUR DOCTOR IF

- You or a family member has symptoms of Addison's disease.
- After diagnosis, infection, injury, or dehydration develops. Drugs may need a dosage change.
- Swollen ankles, weight gain, or new symptoms occur.

ADJUSTMENT DISORDERS

GENERAL INFORMATION

DEFINITION—An adjustment disorder occurs when a person's response to a stressful life event (sometimes called a stressor) is out of proportion to what would be a normal reaction. The person is unable to adjust and this causes problems in both social and work (or school) situations or other functions of daily living.

BODY PARTS INVOLVED—Nervous system.

SEX OR AGE MOST AFFECTED—Both sexes, usually in adults.

SIGNS & SYMPTOMS
- Symptoms or behavior changes occur within three months of onset of the stressor. They usually last no more than six months after the end of the stressor.
- Symptoms vary from person to person. They are often more severe in teens and the elderly.
- Changes in sleeping and eating patterns.
- Withdrawal (avoids social activities and friends).
- Fearful about the future.
- Low self-esteem and feeling emotionally numb.
- Feeling tense, anxious, and depressed.
- Feelings of fear, rage, guilt, or shame.
- Denial of the stressful event (acting as if it never occurred).

CAUSES—A disruption in the normal process of adapting to a stressful event. Everyone reacts differently to an event. It depends on its importance and the intensity of the event. It depends on the person's personality, temperament, age, and well-being.

RISK INCREASES WITH
- The degree of undesired change a stressor causes.
- Whether the stressor was sudden or expected.
- The importance of the stressor in the person's life.
- Lack of support systems (e.g., family, friends, religious, cultural, and social ties).
- How well a person responds to stressful life events.

HOW TO PREVENT—No specific preventive measures known.

WHAT TO EXPECT

DIAGNOSTIC MEASURES
- Your own or other's observation of symptoms.
- Your health care provider will do a physical exam and ask questions about your symptoms and the changes that are going on in your life.

- It is important to identify the stressor that has led to the symptoms. It can be anything that is important to you. The stressor may be only one event or a string of events. It may seem minor to some, but is important to you.

APPROPRIATE HEALTH CARE
- Treatment may include self-care, counseling, and in some cases, drug therapy. This depends on severity of symptoms and impact on your lifestyle.
- Counseling or psychotherapy may be recommended. Several therapy methods are effective and are often needed for a brief period. Family therapy (including marital counseling) may be recommended for some.

POSSIBLE COMPLICATIONS
- Difficulty maintaining relationships or jobs.
- Lingering problems in teenagers.
- Self-treatment using alcohol or drugs to overcome un-desired symptoms and feelings.
- Chronic anxiety and depression.

PROBABLE OUTCOME—It usually clears up on its own after the person adapts to the changed situation, or the stressor ends. Treatment can help in other cases. These disorders are common and are often only temporary.

HOW TO TREAT

GENERAL MEASURES
- Learn to cope with stress. Keeping a journal about your stressors and feelings, talking to a friend, or joining a support group may help.
- Take good care of your physical health (diet, exercise, and sleep).

MEDICATION—Since adjustment disorders are usually of short duration, drugs are normally not needed. A drug may be prescribed for specific symptoms depending on their severity.

ACTIVITY—No limits. A routine physical exercise program is recommended. Physical activity helps reduce anxiety and stress.

DIET—Eat a well-balanced diet to maintain good health.

CALL YOUR DOCTOR IF

- You or a family member has symptoms of an adjustment disorder.
- Symptoms continue to worsen after treatment begins.

AGRANULOCYTOSIS
(Granulocytopenia; Neutropenia)

GENERAL INFORMATION

DEFINITION—Agranulocytosis is a reduction in the normal number of circulating white blood cells in the bloodstream. These cells are the first to attack bacterial and fungal infections. It is not contagious.

BODY PARTS INVOLVED—Blood and bone marrow.

SEX OR AGE MOST AFFECTED—Both sexes; all ages.

SIGNS & SYMPTOMS
- Fever, sometimes with chills.
- Aching, weakness or discomfort.
- Sore throat.
- Ulcers (especially in the mouth and throat), which do not produce pus.
- Any sign of infection in someone who has had agranulocytosis in the past. This may signal a recurrence.

CAUSES—Increased destruction or impaired production of white blood cells (neutrophils or granulocytes) in the bone marrow. This can be caused by a variety of conditions, but in some cases no cause is found.

RISK INCREASES WITH
- Certain drugs (such as carbamazepine or clozapine).
- Chemotherapy (anticancer drugs).
- Radiation therapy.
- Autoimmune disorders.
- Disorders that damage the bone marrow.
- Some hereditary disorders.
- Exposure to certain toxic chemicals.

HOW TO PREVENT—No specific preventive measures.

WHAT TO EXPECT

DIAGNOSTIC MEASURES
- Your own observation of symptoms.
- A health care provider will do a physical exam and ask questions about your medications and family medical history.
- Medical tests may include blood and urine studies and bone marrow biopsy.
- Genetic testing may be done if a hereditary disorder is suspected.

APPROPRIATE HEALTH CARE
- Possible hospital care for intensive treatment and isolation to avoid infections.
- Stopping any medication that may be the cause. Sometimes this provides a cure.
- Other treatments may include bone marrow transplant, stem cell transplants, and treatment to stimulate the production of white blood cells.

POSSIBLE COMPLICATIONS
- Dangerous, sometimes fatal infections (bacterial, fungal, viral or others)—even with vigorous treatment.
- Chronic infections that can cause organ damage and other problems.
- Adverse effects of the treatment.

PROBABLE OUTCOME—Depending on cause, usually curable with intensive treatment.

HOW TO TREAT

GENERAL MEASURES
- The following are helpful until blood counts are normal:
  - Be extra careful about personal cleanliness.
  - Keep the mouth clean by rinsing frequently with warm salt water (1 teaspoon salt to 8 oz. water) or gargling with hydrogen peroxide.
  - Pay particular attention to oral hygiene. Brush teeth gently with a very soft brush, avoiding irritation of the gums.
  - Avoid contact with harmful materials, such as cleaning chemicals, glue, insecticide, fertilizer, and paint remover.
  - Avoid contact with large crowds or people with infections.

MEDICATION
- You may be prescribed intravenous and oral antibiotics if the white blood cell count is very low.
- Drugs to stimulate bone marrow to produce more white blood cells may be prescribed.
- Stopping use of any drug that is suspected of causing agranulocytosis.

ACTIVITY
- Rest or limit activity during the acute stage. Resume normal activities gradually after symptoms ease.
- Avoid overexercising until blood counts are normal.

DIET—No special diet.

CALL YOUR DOCTOR IF

- You or a family member has symptoms of agranulocytosis.
- The following occurs after treatment:
  - Any sign of infection, especially fever.
  - Swelling of the feet and ankles.
  - Painful urination or decreased urine output in one day.

ALCOHOLISM

 ## GENERAL INFORMATION

DEFINITION
● Alcoholism is a chronic, progressive disease that involves dependence on, or an addiction to, alcohol.
 - Craving. A strong need or urge to drink.
 - Loss of control. Not being able to stop drinking once drinking has begun.
 - Physical dependence. Withdrawal symptoms, such as upset stomach, sweating, shakiness, and anxiety after stopping drinking.
 - Tolerance. The need to drink greater amounts of alcohol to get "high."

BODY PARTS INVOLVED—Brain; central nervous system; liver; heart.

SEX OR AGE MOST AFFECTED—Both sexes, but occurs 4 times more often in men than women. The incidence of alcoholism in children is increasing.

SIGNS & SYMPTOMS
● Need for alcohol at the start of the day.
● Use of alcohol to relieve stress or forget problems.
● Insomnia and nightmares.
● Vision, hearing, perception, and alertness problems.
● Monday-morning hangovers and loss of work days.
● Makes promises to limit or stop drinking, but fails.
● Lies about drinking. Sneaks drinks at work or school.
● Anger and guilt when asked about drinking.
● Blackouts, personality and mood changes, confusion, memory loss, depression, anxiety, and fatigue.
● Tremors, violent shakes, hallucinations, or convulsions when there is no alcohol in the body.
● Poor nutrition and poor hygiene. Bad breath.
● Lack of sexual interest and loss of potency.
● Problems with money, work, or family.

CAUSES—Not fully understood. It appears to be a combination of genetic, environmental, and personality factors.

RISK INCREASES WITH
● Family history of alcoholism.
● Males more than females.
● Personal history of other substance abuse.
● A person's genetic makeup may increase risk.
● Begin drinking alcohol before age 16.
● Mental health problems. These include anxiety, depression, aggressive or impulsive behaviors, schizophrenia, low self-esteem, and others.
● Peer pressure and social acceptance of alcohol use.
● Ease of getting alcohol.
● Stress (e.g., in relationships or unemployment).

HOW TO PREVENT—Avoid or limit alcohol. Women have no more than one drink a day and men no more than two drinks a day.

 ## WHAT TO EXPECT

DIAGNOSTIC MEASURES—Your health care provider will do a physical exam and ask about your symptoms. You may be asked verbal questions or asked to fill out a written form about your alcohol use. Medical tests may include blood and urine studies.

APPROPRIATE HEALTH CARE
● Treatment depends on the severity of the alcohol problem, other illnesses (physical, emotional, or mental), and how motivated you are to change. Treatment usually involves withdrawal of alcohol and detoxification, and long-term support to help you remain sober.
● Specific treatment steps include counseling (may be all that is needed), drugs (in some cases), inpatient care at a hospital or treatment center, or referral to a health care provider who treats addiction problems.

POSSIBLE COMPLICATIONS
● Damage to the brain, liver, heart, and other organs.
● Fetal alcohol syndrome in child of alcoholic mother.
● Without treatment, alcoholism can be fatal.
● Suicide or fatal motor vehicle accidents.

PROBABLE OUTCOME—Treatment can help. It has varying success rates. Some people are able to quit on their own. Relapse is somewhat common, but many people have a full recovery.

 ## HOW TO TREAT

GENERAL MEASURES
● The first and most difficult step of treatment is admitting the problem exists.
● Reassess your lifestyle to identify and alter factors that encourage drinking.
● Join support group (e.g., Alcoholics Anonymous).
● To learn more: National Institute on Alcohol Abuse & Alcoholism, website: www.niaaa.nih.gov.

MEDICATION
● Your health care provider may prescribe:
 - Drugs that reduce the craving for alcohol.
 - Drugs that cause unpleasant physical symptoms when alcohol is consumed.
 - Drugs that reduce the pleasure of alcohol.
 - Drugs for withdrawal symptoms, as needed.

ACTIVITY—Exercise daily. It helps to maintain your physical and mental well-being.

DIET—Normal, well-balanced diet, vitamin supplements may be recommended.

 ## CALL YOUR DOCTOR IF

● You or a family member has symptoms of alcoholism. It is an illness that can be treated.
● You have a relapse after recovery.

ALOPECIA AREATA

GENERAL INFORMATION

DEFINITION—Alopecia areata is sudden hair loss in circular patches on the scalp. The hair loss does not occur with other visible evidence of scalp disease.

BODY PARTS INVOLVED—Hair; scalp; eyebrows; eyelashes; beard; genital area; underarm (sometimes).

SEX OR AGE MOST AFFECTED—Alopecia can occur at any age, from birth to older adults. Many cases start before age 20.

SIGNS & SYMPTOMS
• Sudden hair loss in sharply defined circular patches. In rare cases, body hair loss may be total (alopecia universalis).
• Pain and itching may occur in some cases.
• Nails may be affected, such as pitting, in more severe cases.

CAUSES—Unknown. It is thought to be one of a group of autoimmune disorders. In these disorders, the immune system by mistake attacks the body itself. Heredity and emotional stress or psychiatric disorders may play a role.

RISK INCREASES WITH
• Family history of alopecia areata.
• Stressful life event preceding the hair loss may be a factor.
• Certain medical disorders may occur along with alopecia, but do not appear to be a cause or risk factor.

HOW TO PREVENT—Cannot be prevented at present.

WHAT TO EXPECT

DIAGNOSTIC MEASURES
• Your own observation of symptoms.
• Your health care provider will do a physical exam of the affected scalp area. Medical tests are usually not needed unless some underlying disorder is suspected.

APPROPRIATE HEALTH CARE
• In a simple, self-limited case where the alopecia is not noticeable, no treatment may be needed. In other cases, drugs may be used for treatment depending on amount of hair loss and age of patient. No one treatment helps everyone with the disorder.
• For loss of eyebrow hair, dermatography may help. Small dots of colored pigment are injected into eyebrow area.

POSSIBLE COMPLICATIONS
• Loss of all hair.
• Slow or incomplete regrowth.
• Treatment may not be effective in extensive hair loss.
• Disorder frequently recurs.

PROBABLE OUTCOME—The outcome varies depending on the amount of hair loss. There is no permanent cure and the disorder may come and go. Most people have only a few areas of alopecia and regrowth occurs in about a year.

HOW TO TREAT

GENERAL MEASURES
• A change in hair-style may cover the affected area.
• Consider wearing a hairpiece or wig until the hair grows in again.
• Continue to bathe and shampoo as usual. The disorder is not contagious. Don't tug on normal hair close to areas of hair loss.
• Seek counseling if coping with the hair loss is causing emotional problems. Support groups are also available.
• To learn more: National Alopecia Areata Foundation, 14 Mitchell Blvd., San Rafael, CA 94903; (415) 472-3780 (not toll free); website: www.naaf.org.

MEDICATION
• Topical steroids or topical anthralin may be prescribed. Follow instructions carefully.
• Topical minoxidil (a drug used for hair growth) may help. Its effectiveness is highly variable.
• In some cases, you may have injections of steroids into affected areas.
• Oral cortisone drugs may be recommended.
• Topical immunotherapy may be recommended. This involves producing a skin reaction to help hair growth.
• Photochemotherapy with PUVA may be recommended. It combines the use of a drug that sensitizes the skin along with a controlled dose of ultraviolet light.

ACTIVITY—No limits.

DIET—No special diet.

CALL YOUR DOCTOR IF

• You or a family member has symptoms of alopecia areata.
• The following occurs during treatment:
  - Hair loss increases or hair loss doesn't improve.
  - Areas show signs of infection (redness, swelling, tenderness, warmth) after injection treatment.

ALTITUDE ILLNESS

 GENERAL INFORMATION

DEFINITION
• Altitude illness results from travel to higher than normal altitudes. It can affect anyone, no matter what their age or how healthy they are. Types include:
- Acute mountain sickness (AMS); the most common.
- High-altitude pulmonary edema (HAPE) and high-altitude cerebral edema (HACE). These are less common.

BODY PARTS INVOLVED—These illnesses affect most body systems, especially the brain, heart, lungs, gastrointestinal tract, circulatory system and electrolytes.

SEX OR AGE MOST AFFECTED—Young adults of both sexes.

SIGNS & SYMPTOMS
• Mild symptoms may begin when you climb or travel to around 7,000 to 8,000 feet.
- Headache, feeling lightheaded and weak.
- Nausea or vomiting.
- Sleeping problems.
• As you go higher, more severe symptoms may occur.
- Cough and trouble with breathing.
- Unsteady walk.
- Confusion; hallucinations (seeing things that aren't there).
- Coma (person cannot be aroused).

CAUSES—There is less oxygen in the air at higher altitudes. Symptoms start to develop when the body tries to adjust to having less oxygen than it normally has. People who live at high altitudes have adapted to these lower oxygen levels and do not get sick.

RISK INCREASES WITH
• Some people are more susceptible. It is unclear why certain people get sick while others do not. At 14,000 feet, most people will have at least mild symptoms.
• People with severe heart or lung disease or people with sickle-cell anemia.
• Going too high too quickly.

HOW TO PREVENT
• Educate yourself before your trip. Find out how high the altitude will be. Know the symptoms of altitude illness. Find out if medical help will be handy.
• Ask your health care provider for advice about high altitude travel for children, for pregnant women, and for people with chronic health problems. The travel may be considered safe, but find out for sure.
• While on the trip, slowly adjust to the change in altitude. Rest for a day or two at each 1,000 to 2,000 feet. Take it easy, don't overdo, drink fluids, but not alcohol.

 WHAT TO EXPECT

DIAGNOSTIC MEASURES—Your health care provider will ask about your symptoms, may do a physical exam, and have medical tests performed to check on your heart, lungs, and other body systems.

APPROPRIATE HEALTH CARE
• Treatment steps will depend on your symptoms. You may be advised to go to a lower altitude. This is the most important and only sure treatment step.
• For more severe symptoms, you will need to go to a lower altitude immediately. You may need pure oxygen breathed in through a mask for a period of time. A hospital stay may be necessary until you recover.

POSSIBLE COMPLICATIONS—Serious outcomes, including death, are rare. They are only likely to occur if the person is unable to go down to a lower level, or is not able to get medical help.

PROBABLE OUTCOME—Most cases are mild and do not need medical treatment. Recovery takes only one to a few days.

 HOW TO TREAT

GENERAL MEASURES
• If mild symptoms occur, rest for a day or two at that altitude. You may want to go back down (to descend) to a lower altitude. Do not travel higher (to ascend) until the symptoms resolve or get much better.
• Symptoms should improve in a few days if you rest, drink plenty of fluids, don't drink alcohol, and avoid heavy exercise.

MEDICATION
• Ask your health care provider's advice before you travel about drugs that can help prevent or treat symptoms. Drugs do have side effects, so be cautious.
• For mild symptoms, such as headache, you may use pain relievers, such as ibuprofen or naproxen.
• In severe cases, drugs will be given to treat complications and help speed recovery.

ACTIVITY—Resume daily activities gradually upon returning to your normal altitude.

DIET—Increase fluid intake, avoid alcohol, eat small meals.

📞 **CALL YOUR DOCTOR IF**

You or a family member has altitude illness symptoms, or wants to discuss symptoms that occurred on a trip.

ALZHEIMER'S DISEASE
(Presenile Dementia)

GENERAL INFORMATION

DEFINITION—Alzheimer's disease (AD) is a brain disorder that involves gradual mental deterioration. The more gradual form, with slow development of symptoms, begins around ages 65 to 70. A rapidly progressive form begins in adults around ages 36 to 45.

BODY PARTS INVOLVED—Brain.

SEX OR AGE MOST AFFECTED—Both sexes, usually beginning in middle age or older adults.

SIGNS & SYMPTOMS
- Early stages:
  - Forgetful of recent events.
  - Increasing difficulty doing mental tasks, such as usual work, balancing a checkbook, or maintaining a household.
  - Personality or mood changes, such as poor impulse control, poor judgment, fearful, depression, confusion.
- Later stages:
  - Difficulty doing simple tasks, such as choosing clothing, solving problems.
  - Failure to recognize familiar persons.
  - Loses interest in hygiene or appearance.
  - Difficulty feeding self.
  - Belligerence; denials that anything is wrong.
  - Loss of usual sexual inhibitions.
  - Wandering away, anxiety and insomnia.
- Advanced stages:
  - Complete loss of memory, speech, and muscle function. This includes bladder and bowel control.

CAUSES—Damage to or loss of brain cells for unknown reasons.

RISK INCREASES WITH
- Family history of Alzheimer's disease.
- Other genetic factors.
- Aging.
- Research shows that factors related to blood circulation may be involved (such as those causing heart disease or stroke, especially smoking cigarettes).

HOW TO PREVENT—None specific; research continues. A healthy lifestyle may help.

WHAT TO EXPECT

DIAGNOSTIC MEASURES
- Your own or other's observation of symptoms.
- Your health care provider will do a physical exam and ask questions about the symptoms. There is no specific test to diagnose Alzheimer's. Medical tests may include cognitive tests (answering questions). Blood, urine, and spinal fluid studies, heart studies, CT, MRI, PET scans, or others help rule out other disorders. Certain genetic tests help to identify inherited forms of Alzheimer's.

APPROPRIATE HEALTH CARE
- Treatment will depend on the stage of the disease. Different drugs are available that can help slow the progress of the disease.
- Drugs to treat the behavior symptoms can help make a patient more comfortable and make their care easier.

POSSIBLE COMPLICATIONS
- Infections. They are a major cause of death in Alzheimer's patients.
- Final stages of the disease will lead to death.

PROBABLE OUTCOME—There is no cure. Treatment helps slow the progress and helps relieve the symptoms. Patients may progress from onset of symptoms to end-stage disease in 8 to 10 years. This varies from person to person. Those with end-stage disease often need the care provided in an assisted living facility that handles Alzheimer's patients.

HOW TO TREAT

GENERAL MEASURES
- A diagnosis of Alzheimer's is overwhelming, both for the patient and the family. Educate yourselves as much as possible about what to expect and how to plan for it. With early diagnosis, the patient can help take part in making decisions for the future.
- Caring for a family member with Alzheimer's is a difficult task. Caregivers need to take care of themselves. Joining a support group for caregivers may be helpful.
- To learn more: Alzheimer's Association, 225 N. Michigan Ave., Flr. 17, Chicago, IL 60601; (800) 272-3900; website: www.alz.org.

MEDICATION
- Drugs that slow the progress of the disease for a limited time are usually prescribed.
- Drugs as needed to help control behavior symptoms (insomnia, agitation, wandering, depression, anxiety, and others) will be prescribed.

ACTIVITY—With time, all patient activity will require supervision.

DIET—Regular diet. Feeding help will eventually be needed.

CALL YOUR DOCTOR IF

- You or a family member has symptoms of Alzheimer's disease.
- Caregiver has questions or concerns about the patient's symptoms or treatments.

AMEBIASIS
(Amebic Dysentery; Entamebiasis)

 GENERAL INFORMATION

DEFINITION—Amebiasis is a parasitic infection of the intestines (bowels). Amebiasis is found worldwide, but occurs most often in developing countries. In the United States, the disease is fairly rare in the general population. Amebic dysentery is a rare, more severe form.

BODY PARTS INVOLVED—Intestinal tract (especially the colon and liver).

SEX OR AGE MOST AFFECTED—Both sexes; all ages.

SIGNS & SYMPTOMS
- Only about 1 in 10 persons with the infection will have symptoms. Symptoms occur when the parasites (amoebas) invade the walls of the intestine.
- Diarrhea with bad-smelling stools. Constipation may alternate with diarrhea.
- Gas and stomach bloating, cramps, and tenderness.
- Amebic dysentery may cause bloody stools, stomach pain, chills, and fever.

CAUSES—A parasite, *Entamoeba histolytica*. The infection starts when someone swallows amoeba cysts (they can't be seen) that contaminate food or water. The cysts travel to the intestines and can live there without causing symptoms. Then, for unknown reasons, the amoebas invade the intestine wall. When this happens, symptoms occur. Symptoms usually begin one to four weeks after exposure, but can take a few days or a year.

RISK INCREASES WITH
- Immigrants from developing countries.
- Travel to a foreign country. In developing countries, the drinking water may be contaminated. In addition, some places use human feces for fertilizer.
- Male homosexuals.
- Living in institutions where there are poor sanitary conditions.

HOW TO PREVENT
- No specific preventive steps. No vaccine is available.
- Wash hands often to prevent spread of any germs.
- Travelers to countries where there is a risk of infection need to take proper precautions regarding food and drink.
- Use safe sex measures to help prevent spread of infection.

 WHAT TO EXPECT

DIAGNOSTIC MEASURES
- Your own observation of symptoms.
- Your health care provider will do a physical exam and ask about your symptoms and recent travels.
- Medical tests may include blood and stool studies. If liver involvement is a concern, other tests may be done.

APPROPRIATE HEALTH CARE
- Treatment is with drugs. A stool sample may be rechecked after treatment is complete to be sure the infection is cleared up.
- In severe cases of dysentery, hospital care may be needed. Fluid replacement may be necessary to manage dehydration due to diarrhea.

POSSIBLE COMPLICATIONS—The amoebas can travel through the blood stream to other parts of the body and cause infection in different organs. This can lead to an amebic liver abscess (pus-filled area) or brain abscess.

PROBABLE OUTCOME—In most cases, amebiasis is curable in three weeks with treatment.

 HOW TO TREAT

GENERAL MEASURES—Amebiasis is contagious. Be extra careful about personal cleanliness. Bathe frequently. Wash hands with warm water and soap after each bowel movement and before handling food.

MEDICATION—Antibiotic drugs to treat amebiasis are usually prescribed. These are most often taken by mouth, but in some cases may be injected.

ACTIVITY—Get extra rest until diarrhea and other symptoms improve.

DIET—No special diet. Be sure to drink plenty of fluids to help prevent dehydration.

 CALL YOUR DOCTOR IF

- You or a family member has symptoms of amebiasis.
- The following occur during treatment:
  - Stomach cramps go on longer than 24 hours.
  - Diarrhea or blood in stool increases.
  - Vomiting begins.
  - Pain begins over liver or jaundice (yellow skin or eyes) occurs.
  - A skin rash appears.

AMENORRHEA, PRIMARY

GENERAL INFORMATION

DEFINITION—Primary amenorrhea is complete absence of menstruation in a young woman who is at least 16 years old, or at age 14 with a lack of normal growth or absence of secondary sexual development. It is a rare disorder, as over 95% of girls have their first menstrual period by age 15. Most girls begin menstruating by age 14; average age is 12 years, 8 months.

BODY PARTS INVOLVED—Endocrine system; reproductive system.

SEX OR AGE MOST AFFECTED—Young females.

SIGNS & SYMPTOMS—Lack of menstrual periods after puberty.

CAUSES—A failure of certain complex body functions that normally result in menstruation. There are a number of disorders or health problems that can lead to the failure.

RISK INCREASES WITH
- Delayed puberty.
- Congenital problems, such as the absence or abnormal formation of female organs (vagina, uterus, and ovaries).
- Intact hymen (membrane covering the vaginal opening) has no opening to allow passage of menstrual flow.
- Disorders (tumors, infections, or other problems) of the endocrine system, including the pituitary, hypothalamus, thyroid, parathyroid, adrenal, and ovarian glands.
- Chromosome disorders or chronic illness.
- Polycystic ovaries (Stein-Leventhal syndrome).
- Pregnancy.
- Severe nutritional or physical stressors such as anorexia, competitive sports, or intense training (e.g., in gymnasts, ballet dancers, or long distance runners).
- Use of drugs, including oral contraceptives, anticancer drugs, barbiturates, narcotics, cortisone drugs, chlordiazepoxide, and reserpine.
- Family tendency to start menstruation late.
- Excessive dieting or weight loss.
- Extreme obesity.
- Rarely, prior gynecological surgery.

HOW TO PREVENT—No specific preventive measures. Avoid risk factors where possible.

WHAT TO EXPECT

DIAGNOSTIC MEASURES
- Your health care provider will do a physical exam and a pelvic exam. Questions will be asked about your medical history and about your lifestyle (e.g., diet, exercise, etc.).
- Medical tests may include urine and blood studies; hormone levels; and liver, thyroid, and adrenal function. Other tests may be done to diagnose an underlying disorder.

APPROPRIATE HEALTH CARE
- Treatment may involve hormone replacement therapy. Treatment for amenorrhea not related to hormone deficiency depends on the cause.
- Counseling may help if amenorrhea is related to stress, results from an eating disorder, or for emotional concerns about sexual development.
- Surgery to correct abnormalities of the reproductive system or for cysts may rarely be needed.

POSSIBLE COMPLICATIONS
- Emotional stress about sexual development.
- May lead to infertility.
- Other complications may occur, depending on the underlying cause.

PROBABLE OUTCOME
- The absence of menstruation is not a health risk in itself, but the cause should be found.
- Amenorrhea is often curable with hormone treatment or treatment of the underlying cause. Treatment may be delayed to age 18, unless the cause can be identified and treated safely.
- Causes that sometimes cannot be corrected include chromosome disorders and abnormalities of the reproductive system.

HOW TO TREAT

GENERAL MEASURES
- Seek help in resolving emotional stress.
- Don't use mood-altering, mind-altering stimulants or sedative drugs.

MEDICATION
- Hormones may be prescribed if there is a hormone imbalance. They may correct the problem.
- Birth control pills may be prescribed for polycystic ovary syndrome.
- Bromocriptine may be prescribed for pituitary tumor.

ACTIVITY—Exercise regularly, but not to excess. Reduce exercise or athletic activities if they are too strenuous.

DIET—If you are overweight or underweight, a change in diet to correct weight problem may bring on a period.

CALL YOUR DOCTOR IF

- You or a family member is 16 years old and has never had a period.
- Periods don't begin within 6 months, despite treatment.

AMENORRHEA, SECONDARY

GENERAL INFORMATION

DEFINITION—Secondary amenorrhea is absence of menstruation in a woman who has previously menstruated.

BODY PARTS INVOLVED—Endocrine system; reproductive system.

SEX OR AGE MOST AFFECTED—Females over age 16.

SIGNS & SYMPTOMS
- No menstrual periods for at least 3 to 6 months.
- Other symptoms may include infertility, acne, excess hair growth (hirsutism) or hair loss, obesity, galactorrhea (breasts produce milk when not breast-feeding), headaches, and vaginal dryness.

CAUSES—A stopping of certain complex body functions that normally result in menstruation. There are a number of conditions or health problems that can lead to the failure. Pregnancy is one of the most common causes.

RISK INCREASES WITH
- Breast-feeding an infant.
- Discontinuing use of birth-control pills.
- Menopause (if a woman is over 35 and not pregnant).
- Emotional stress or psychological disorder.
- Surgical removal of the ovaries or uterus, or complications as a result of gynecological surgery.
- Disorder of the endocrine system, including the pituitary, hypothalamus, thyroid, parathyroid, adrenal, and ovarian glands.
- Hormone imbalance.
- Chronic illness, such as diabetes or tuberculosis.
- Obesity or eating disorders (anorexia or bulimia).
- Strenuous program of physical exercise, such as long-distance running, gymnastics, or ballet.

HOW TO PREVENT—To help avoid amenorrhea, maintain a healthy lifestyle.

WHAT TO EXPECT

DIAGNOSTIC MEASURES
- Your health care provider will do a physical exam and a pelvic exam. Questions will be asked about your medical history and your family's medical history, and about your lifestyle (e.g., diet, exercise, etc.).
- Medical tests may include a pregnancy test, studies of hormone levels, and a Pap smear.
- Surgical diagnostic procedures such as laparoscopy or hysteroscopy may be recommended. These procedures use a special instrument to see inside the body's organs.

APPROPRIATE HEALTH CARE
- Treatment will depend on the cause. It may include lifestyle changes, drugs, treatment of an underlying disorder, and rarely, surgery.
- Counseling may help if amenorrhea is related to stress or other emotional problems.

POSSIBLE COMPLICATIONS
- None likely, if there is no serious underlying cause.
- May experience estrogen deficiency symptoms, such as hot flashes and vaginal dryness. May affect fertility.
- Reduced bone density (osteoporosis).

PROBABLE OUTCOME
- Amenorrhea is not a threat to health. Whether it can be corrected varies with the underlying cause.
- If from pregnancy or breast-feeding, menstruation will resume when these conditions cease.
- If from discontinuing use of oral contraceptives, periods should begin in 2 months to 2 years.
- If from menopause, periods will become less frequent or may never resume. Hysterectomy also ends menstruation permanently.
- If from endocrine disorders, hormone replacement usually causes periods to resume.
- If from eating disorders, successful treatment of that disorder will help menstruation to resume.
- If from diabetes or tuberculosis, menstruation may never resume.
- If from strenuous exercise, periods usually resume when exercise is decreased.

HOW TO TREAT

GENERAL MEASURES—Keep a record of menstrual cycles to aid in early detection of recurrent amenorrhea.

MEDICATION
- Progesterone and/or estrogen may be prescribed. If bleeding occurs after progesterone is withdrawn, the reproduction system is functional.
- Drugs to treat an underlying disorder may be prescribed.

ACTIVITY—Exercise regularly, but not to excess. Reduce exercise or athletic activities if they are too strenuous.

DIET—If overweight or underweight, a change in diet to correct the problem may be helpful.

CALL YOUR DOCTOR IF

- You or a family member has amenorrhea.
- Periods don't resume within 6 months.

AMYOTROPHIC LATERAL SCLEROSIS
(Lou Gehrig's Disease)

GENERAL INFORMATION

DEFINITION—Amyotrophic lateral sclerosis (ALS) is a progressive breakdown of the cells of the spinal cord. This results in gradual loss of muscle function.

BODY PARTS INVOLVED—Central nervous system; muscle system, especially in the hands, forearms, legs, head and neck.

SEX OR AGE MOST AFFECTED—It usually affects people ages 40 to 60 years, and occurs more often in men than women.

SIGNS & SYMPTOMS
- Muscle twitching and weakness. It begins in the hands and spreads to the arms and legs. The weakness then begins to affect muscles that control breathing and swallowing.
- Muscle cramps.
- Stiffening and spasticity of muscle groups.
- Weight loss.
- Slurring of speech.
- Mental function is rarely affected.
- Sudden involuntary bursts of laughter or crying.

CAUSES—Unknown. Research is ongoing.

RISK INCREASES WITH
- Age over 40.
- Family history of ALS.
- Smoking.

HOW TO PREVENT—Cannot be prevented at present.

WHAT TO EXPECT

DIAGNOSTIC MEASURES
- Your own observation of symptoms.
- Your health care provider will do a physical exam and ask questions about your symptoms. No one test diagnoses ALS.
- Medical tests include nerve studies (electromyography and nerve conduction velocity). Tests may include blood and urine studies, x-rays, and others.

APPROPRIATE HEALTH CARE
- There is no specific treatment. Supportive care is provided to relieve symptoms and for complications.
- Counseling may be helpful in finding ways for both the patient and the family to cope with the diagnosis.
- Surgery for tracheostomy is usually required once breathing difficulties develop.
- In later stages of the disease, the patient will require complete nursing care.
- Patient and family may benefit from hospice care.

POSSIBLE COMPLICATIONS
- The disorder affects the patient's personal relationships, career, income, muscle coordination, sexuality, and energy.
- Progressive inability to walk and to do things involved with daily living, such as being able to feed oneself.
- Wheelchair use is needed.
- Pressure sores or skin infections due to being bedridden or in a wheelchair.
- Pneumonia due to swallowing difficulty and choking.
- The disorder is eventually fatal due to respiratory muscle weakness.

PROBABLE OUTCOME
- This condition is currently considered incurable. It is usually fatal in 2 to 5 years, but 20% of patients survive 5 years and 10% survive 10 years.
- Medical research into causes and treatment continues. There is hope for more effective treatment.

HOW TO TREAT

GENERAL MEASURES
- Aids for helping with daily living are available. These can help maintain some function and quality of life.
- Learn to do self-suction in order to handle increased amount of secretions in the lungs.
- Take special care to prevent pressure sores.
- To learn more: ALS Association, 1275 K St., Ste 1050, Washington, DC 20005; (800) 782-4747; website: www.alsa.org.

MEDICATION
- Riluzole may be prescribed. It can help delay the progress of ALS for a few months.
- Antibiotics may be prescribed for infections.
- Drugs to help reduce spasticity and to decrease excess saliva are often prescribed.

ACTIVITY
- Stay as active as possible. Weakness will gradually limit movement. A physical therapy program can help to maintain independence as long as possible.
- Obtain equipment that will aid in mobility, such as a walker or wheelchair.

DIET—If swallowing is difficult, eat soft, easy-to-swallow foods. (See Soft Diet in Appendix.)

CALL YOUR DOCTOR IF

- You or a family member has symptoms of amyotrophic lateral sclerosis.
- After diagnosis, symptoms occur that cause concern.

ANAL FISSURE

GENERAL INFORMATION

DEFINITION—Anal fissure is a laceration, tear, or crack in the anal canal.

BODY PARTS INVOLVED—Anus.

SEX OR AGE MOST AFFECTED—All ages. It is most common in infants, young children, adults over 60, and women more than men.

SIGNS & SYMPTOMS
- Sharp pain with passage of a hard or bulky stool. The pain may last up to an hour, and returns with the next bowel movement.
- Pain when sitting on a hard surface.
- Streaks of blood on the toilet paper, underwear, or diaper.
- Itching around the rectum.
- Refusal to have a bowel movement (in children).

CAUSES—The exact cause is unknown. Symptoms usually occur after the stretching of the anus from a large, hard stool.

RISK INCREASES WITH
- Constipation or prolonged diarrhea.
- Childbirth.
- Inflammatory bowel disease (e.g., Crohn's disease).
- Certain infections (e.g., HIV or tuberculosis), anal trauma, or low fiber diet may play a role.

HOW TO PREVENT
- Avoid constipation by:
  - Drinking at least 8 glasses of water daily.
  - Eating a diet high in fiber.
  - Using stool softeners, if needed.
- Don't strain when having a bowel movement.
- Avoid anal trauma.

WHAT TO EXPECT

DIAGNOSTIC MEASURES
- Your own observation of symptoms.
- Your health care provider will do a physical exam of the anus and rectum to confirm the diagnosis. Other medical tests are usually not needed.

APPROPRIATE HEALTH CARE
- Treatment usually begins with self-care. Conservative therapy is safe, has few side effects, and is usually the first step in therapy. The next steps may involve prescribed topical drugs, botulinum injection, or surgery.
- Minor surgery may be needed to remove the fissure if conservative treatment is not successful. (See Anal Fissure Treatment in Surgery section.)

POSSIBLE COMPLICATIONS—Fissure may become chronic and fail to heal.

PROBABLE OUTCOME—Most fissures heal on their own. Others can be treated successfully. Most infants and young children recover after the stool is softened.

HOW TO TREAT

GENERAL MEASURES
- Gently clean the anus with soap and water after each bowel movement.
- To relieve muscle spasms and pain around the anus, apply a warm towel to the area.
- Sitz baths also relieve pain. Use 8 inches of warm water in the bathtub, 2 or 3 times a day for 10 to 20 minutes.

MEDICATION
- For minor discomfort, use nonprescription topical anesthetics, such as lidocaine gel.
- Use stool softeners (e.g., docusate sodium or docusate calcium).
- Topical nitroglycerin may be prescribed. It can cause headache in some patients.
- Topical calcium channel blockers may be prescribed (e.g., diltiazem or nifedipine). An oral form of the drug is sometimes prescribed.
- Botulinum toxin (Botox) injections may be prescribed to help relax the sphincter muscles.

ACTIVITY—No limits. Being physically active helps reduce risk of constipation.

DIET—Eat a high-fiber diet and drink extra fluids to prevent constipation.

CALL YOUR DOCTOR IF

- You or your child has symptoms of an anal fissure.
- Pain continues despite treatment.
- Drugs used for treatment cause side effects.

ANAL FISTULA

GENERAL INFORMATION

DEFINITION—Anal fistula is a very small tube or tract that leads from the anal canal (the last part of the rectum) to the skin near the anal opening. Watery pus drains through this opening and causes irritation to the skin. Some fistulas cause no symptoms.

BODY PARTS INVOLVED—Anus.

SEX OR AGE MOST AFFECTED—Both sexes, can affect all ages.

SIGNS & SYMPTOMS
- Discharge from the anus. There may be bleeding.
- Skin irritation or itching around the anus.
- Pain when passing a bowel movement.
- Tender lump near the anus.

CAUSES
- Anal fistulas are usually caused by a prior anorectal abscess. An anorectal abscess is caused by a bacterial infection of one of the glands in the anal canal. Some patients will have both an abscess and fistula.
- Other anal fistulas may be caused by infection, injury (trauma), disease, or radiation therapy.

RISK INCREASES WITH
- Inflammatory bowel disease (e.g., Crohn's disease).
- Diverticulitis, tuberculosis, chlamydial infection, large intestine cancer, HIV infection, certain other disorders, or radiation therapy.

HOW TO PREVENT—There are no specific preventive measures. Getting medical care for an anorectal abscess may help.

WHAT TO EXPECT

DIAGNOSTIC MEASURES
- Your own observation of symptoms.
- Your health care provider will ask questions about your symptoms and medical history. A physical exam of the anal area will be done.
- Medical studies (usually under anesthesia) are needed for diagnosis. An anoscope (a flexible tube with a lighted end) is used to see inside the anus and anal canal.
- Other tests may be done for complex fistulas or to look for an underlying disorder (e.g., Crohn's). These may include blood tests, MRI, sigmoidoscopy, x-rays, ultrasound, and others.

APPROPRIATE HEALTH CARE
- Treatment depends on the results of the medical tests and exact location of the fistula. Some anal fistulas can be simple and others are more complex and difficult to treat. There are several treatment options and each has benefits and risks. They will be discussed with you.
- Treatment may involve surgery (called fistulotomy or fistulectomy) to open the fistula. Advancement flap is a surgical option. Seton procedures use a surgical thread to allow for fistula draining and healing. Fibrin glue injection and anal fistula plug are other options.

POSSIBLE COMPLICATIONS
- Treatment may lead to complications. Some degree of fecal incontinence (unable to control bowels) may develop. Pain, infection, bleeding, delayed healing, and other complications may occur.
- Rarely, a temporary colostomy (feces is diverted to an outside opening) may be required.
- Anal fistula can recur.

PROBABLE OUTCOME—Anal fistula treatment can provide satisfactory results in most cases. The goals are to heal the fistula, relieve the symptoms, avoid sphincter muscle problems and other complications, and prevent fistula recurrence. In some cases, more than one type of treatment may be needed. Healing time will vary and may take weeks to months.

HOW TO TREAT

GENERAL MEASURES
- Gently clean the anus with soap and water after each bowel movement.
- Sitz baths help relieve discomfort. Sit in a tub of warm water (not hot) for 10 to 15 minutes several times a day. Dry the area carefully and completely after bathing.

MEDICATION
- To prevent constipation, use stool softeners.
- Antibiotics may be prescribed if infection is present.
- Drugs for pain may be prescribed after treatment.

ACTIVITY—You will be advised about resuming work and normal activities depending on the specific treatment.

DIET—A high fiber diet may be recommended.

CALL YOUR DOCTOR IF

- You or a family member has anal fistula symptoms.
- Symptoms recur or new symptoms develop after treatment.

ANAPHYLAXIS
(Allergic Shock)

GENERAL INFORMATION

DEFINITION—Anaphylaxis is a life-threatening allergic response to drugs or other allergy-causing substances (allergens). Reactions that happen the fastest are often the worst.

BODY PARTS INVOLVED—Blood vessels throughout the body; heart; lungs; skin.

SEX OR AGE MOST AFFECTED—Both sexes; all ages.

SIGNS & SYMPTOMS
- Any of the following can happen within seconds or a few minutes after being exposed to something that you are very allergic to:
  - Tingling or numbness around the mouth.
  - Sneezing, coughing, or wheezing.
  - Swelling around the face or hands.
  - Feeling anxious.
  - Weak, rapid pulse; pounding heartbeat.
  - Stomach cramps, vomiting, and diarrhea.
  - Itching all over. Hives often appear.
  - Watery eyes.
  - Chest feels tight; trouble breathing.
  - Swelling or itching in the mouth or throat.
  - Faintness; loss of consciousness.

CAUSES
- Sometimes the body overreacts when it tries to rid itself of the material it is allergic to. This can be life-threatening. Allergens that most often cause reactions:
  - Drugs of all types, especially penicillin. Shots are a bigger risk than eyedrops or drugs taken by mouth.
  - Stings or bites from insects, such as bees, wasps, hornets, biting ants, and some spiders.
  - Vaccines.
  - Pollen.
  - Injected chemicals used with some types of x-rays.
  - Foods, especially peanuts, tree nuts (pecans, walnuts), eggs, milk, shellfish, and fish.

RISK INCREASES WITH
- A previous mild allergy to allergens listed in Causes.
- A history of rashes, hay fever, or asthma.

HOW TO PREVENT
- If you have an allergic history:
  - Tell your health care provider before you accept any new drugs. Before you are given a shot, ask what it is. Always remain in a medical office 15 minutes after receiving any shot. Report any symptoms right away.
  - Keep a special kit, such as EpiPen, with you at all times. Be sure your family knows how to use the kit if you need it.
  - If you are allergic to insect stings, wear clothing that covers all of your body when you are outside.
- Wear a medical alert type bracelet or necklace showing that you have allergies.
- Ask your health care provider about allergy therapy that can make you less allergic.
- People with previous severe reaction to insect stings should consider immunization (allergy shots) as a preventive measure.

WHAT TO EXPECT

DIAGNOSTIC MEASURES—Skin tests to determine sensitivities.

APPROPRIATE HEALTH CARE
- Health care provider's treatment.
- Long-term treatment may involve steps to make your body less sensitive to things to which you are allergic.

POSSIBLE COMPLICATIONS—If not treated quickly, anaphylaxis can cause shock, cardiac arrest, and/or death.

PROBABLE OUTCOME—Full recovery (if treated quickly).

HOW TO TREAT

GENERAL MEASURES
- If you see signs of anaphylaxis in someone and they stop breathing:
  - Call 911 (emergency) for medical help. If the victim is a child, perform lifesaving measures for 1 minute before calling for emergency help.
  - Begin CPR (cardiopulmonary resuscitation). Do uninterrupted chest presses—about 2 a second until help arrives.
- Be aware that a reaction may happen when taking any medicine. Be ready to respond quickly if symptoms develop. If you have had a severe allergic reaction in the past, always carry your anaphylaxis kit.

MEDICATION
- Epinephrine shots are the only immediate treatment for this condition.
- Other drugs may be given after the epinephrine that will help prevent the return of symptoms.

ACTIVITY—Return to your normal activities as soon as symptoms are better. Make sure you are not alone for 24 hours, in case symptoms come back.

DIET—Avoid foods to which you are allergic.

CALL YOUR DOCTOR IF

You or a family member has symptoms of anaphylaxis. This is an emergency!

ANEMIA, APLASTIC

GENERAL INFORMATION

DEFINITION—Aplastic anemia is a blood disorder that involves decreased bone marrow production of white and red blood cells and platelets. Bone marrow is the sponge-like tissue inside the bones.

BODY PARTS INVOLVED—Bone marrow; lymphatic system; blood.

SEX OR AGE MOST AFFECTED—Both sexes; all ages.

SIGNS & SYMPTOMS
- Paleness.
- Weakness, tiredness, faintness, and breathlessness.
- Frequent infections.
- Spontaneous bleeding from the nose, mouth, rectum, vagina, gums, or other sites.
- Red dots of bleeding under the skin.
- Unexplained bruising.
- Ulcers in the mouth, throat and rectum.

CAUSES—Bone marrow contains stem cells that develop into red blood cells, white blood cells, or platelets. These are all important in maintaining functions of the body. Stem cells can be damaged due to known or unknown factors and the cells do not develop properly. This leads to aplastic anemia.

RISK INCREASES WITH
- Exposure to certain chemicals (such as benzene and pesticides).
- Use of certain drugs, especially anticancer drugs, immunosuppressive drugs, or chloramphenicol.
- Pregnancy (rarely).
- Radiation therapy.
- Severe illness.
- Some autoimmune or blood disorders.

HOW TO PREVENT
- No specific preventive measures.
- Avoid prolonged exposure to toxic compounds, such as benzene, that are used in many industrial chemicals.
- Don't use drugs that cause aplastic anemia if substitute drugs are available.

WHAT TO EXPECT

DIAGNOSTIC MEASURES
- Your own observation of symptoms.
- Your health care provider will do a physical exam and ask questions about drugs you take and exposure to chemicals.
- Medical tests usually include blood studies and for some, a bone marrow biopsy.

APPROPRIATE HEALTH CARE
- Treatment may include drug therapy, blood transfusions, or bone marrow transplant.
- Mild cases may not need treatment. Routine follow up is done to watch for complications.
- Severe cases will need hospital care.
- Blood transfusions are often done to relieve symptoms and to control the bleeding.
- Stem cell transplant (also called bone marrow transplant) may be needed for severe cases.

POSSIBLE COMPLICATIONS—Poor response to treatment, resulting in uncontrollable infections and bleeding. Complications are fatal in 50% to 70% of those with severe aplastic anemia.

PROBABLE OUTCOME—If the cause can be identified and treated successfully, the disorder is curable. Stem cell transplant is also a cure. Anemia caused by immunosuppressive drugs usually improves once the drugs are withdrawn. Full recovery often requires 6 to 8 months.

HOW TO TREAT

GENERAL MEASURES
- The following are helpful until blood counts are normal:
  - Be extra careful about personal cleanliness.
  - Pay particular attention to oral hygiene. Brush teeth gently with a very soft brush, avoiding irritation of the gums.
  - Avoid contact with harmful materials, such as cleaning chemicals, glue, insecticide, fertilizer and paint remover.
  - Avoid contact with large crowds or people with infections.

MEDICATION
- Your health care provider may prescribe:
  - Immunosuppressive drugs to suppress the immune system.
  - Drugs to stimulate the bone marrow to produce new blood cells.
  - Antibiotics or antivirals for infections.
  - Medicated mouthwash to suppress fungus infections.

ACTIVITY
- Rest as needed during treatment. Resume normal activities gradually after symptoms ease.
- Avoid contact sports or activities that put you at risk of injury and bleeding.

DIET—No special diet. You may be prescribed iron and vitamin supplements.

CALL YOUR DOCTOR IF

- You or a family member have symptoms of aplastic anemia.
- Any sign of infection or other symptoms occur during or after treatment.

ANEMIA DURING PREGNANCY

GENERAL INFORMATION

DEFINITION—Anemia during pregnancy is a low level of red cells and hemoglobin in the blood. Hemoglobin is the protein inside red blood cells that carries oxygen. Common anemias in pregnancy include iron deficiency anemia and folate (folic acid) deficiency. Other anemias are glucose-6-phosphate dehydrogenase (G6PD) deficiency, thalassemia, and sickle cell anemia.

BODY PARTS INVOLVED—Blood cells.

SEX OR AGE MOST AFFECTED—Pregnant females.

SIGNS & SYMPTOMS
- Usually no symptoms are apparent.
- Fatigue, weakness, or fainting.
- Pale skin, gums, eyes, and nailbeds.
- Palpitations (awareness of the heartbeat).
- Shortness of breath with activity.

CAUSES
- The anemia usually results from an increased need for iron. Your body is making more blood so it needs more iron. Often the diet alone does not provide enough iron to meet the needs. Also, the growing baby takes all the iron it needs from you, no matter how much you have in your system.
- In some cases, anemia during pregnancy is due to a lack of folic acid or one of the B vitamins. It may also be caused by an inherited medical problem such as sickle cell anemia or thalassemia.

RISK INCREASES WITH
- Women who are unable to eat well because of nausea or vomiting.
- Having a multiple pregnancy (e.g., twins) where iron stores are used up more quickly.
- Having two pregnancies fairly close together.
- Diet has insufficient iron content.
- A heavy menstrual flow in the months prior to the pregnancy.

HOW TO PREVENT
- Eat foods rich in iron, such as red meat, dried beans, whole-grain breads and cereals, eggs, or dried fruit.
- Eat foods high in folic acid, such as wheat germ, beans, peanut butter, oatmeal, mushrooms, collards, broccoli, and asparagus.
- Eat foods high in vitamin C, such as citrus fruits and fresh, raw vegetables.
- Take prenatal vitamin and mineral supplements, if they are prescribed.
- Get tested for certain anemias if you are at risk. Your obstetric provider will discuss the details.

WHAT TO EXPECT

DIAGNOSTIC MEASURES
- Your own observation of symptoms.
- Your obstetric provider will do blood studies during your pregnancy. These can help diagnose anemia.

APPROPRIATE HEALTH CARE—Medical care will involve treatment for any underlying cause. Supplements are needed for most anemias.

POSSIBLE COMPLICATIONS
- There may be some risk of preterm birth and low birth weight.
- Folic acid deficiency may cause birth defects (neural tube defects).

PROBABLE OUTCOME—Mild cases of anemia should cause no problems. Anemia can be treated with iron supplements or folic acid supplements.

HOW TO TREAT

GENERAL MEASURES—Follow medical advice about treatment.

MEDICATION
- Iron, folic acid, and other supplements may be prescribed. Take iron supplements 1 hour before eating or between meals. Iron can turn bowel movements black, and often causes constipation. Iron sometimes may be taken with meals if it has caused an upset stomach.
- If you are taking a calcium supplement in addition to an iron supplement, take them at different times of day, as calcium will interfere with iron absorption.

ACTIVITY—Rest often until the anemia improves.

DIET—Eat a healthy pregnancy diet.

CALL YOUR DOCTOR IF

- You or a family member is pregnant and has symptoms of anemia.
- You have diarrhea, constipation, nausea, or abdominal pain during pregnancy.
- You have unexplained bleeding during pregnancy.

ANEMIA, HEMOLYTIC

GENERAL INFORMATION

DEFINITION—Hemolytic anemia is due to red blood cells being destroyed faster than the bone marrow can produce them. In the intrinsic type, the destruction is due to a defect in the red blood cells themselves. In the extrinsic type, healthy red blood cells are produced, but are destroyed by the body.

BODY PARTS INVOLVED—Blood; bone marrow; and the spleen.

SEX OR AGE MOST AFFECTED—Both sexes; all ages.

SIGNS & SYMPTOMS
- Sometimes there are no symptoms. The anemia may be diagnosed on a routine health exam.
- Fatigue and weakness.
- Pale skin, eyes, and fingernails.
- Shortness of breath.
- Irregular heartbeat.
- Jaundice (yellow skin and eyes, dark urine).

CAUSES—Bone marrow cannot produce red blood cells fast enough to make up for those being destroyed. This is a process known as hemolysis. More than 200 causes for hemolysis exist. Some are due to inherited disorders and some are acquired disorders. Sometimes, the cause is unknown.

RISK INCREASES WITH
- Inherited disorders. These include hereditary spherocytosis, glucose-6-phosphate dehydrogenase (G6PD) deficiency, sickle cell anemia, or thalassemia.
- Infections such as hepatitis, cytomegalovirus, Epstein-Barr virus, typhoid fever, streptococcus, or *Escherichia coli* (*E. coli*).
- Leukemia or lymphoma.
- Use of certain drugs, such as penicillin, antimalarials, sulfa, or acetaminophen.
- Various tumors.
- Family history of hemolytic anemia.

HOW TO PREVENT
- Don't take any drugs that have previously caused hemolytic anemia.
- Seek genetic counseling before having children if you have a family history of inherited hemolytic anemia.

WHAT TO EXPECT

DIAGNOSTIC MEASURES
- Your own observation of symptoms.
- Your health care provider will do a physical exam and ask questions about your symptoms.
- Medical tests include blood and urine studies. Other tests may be done to help diagnose an underlying cause for anemia.

APPROPRIATE HEALTH CARE
- Treatment depends on the specific hemolytic problem. Treatment may include drugs, blood transfusions, stopping drugs, or surgery.
- Mild cases may not need treatment.
- Surgical removal of the spleen may be recommended.

POSSIBLE COMPLICATIONS
- Varies depending on the cause of the anemia.
- It may cause existing heart or lung disease to worsen.

PROBABLE OUTCOME
- If hemolytic anemia is acquired, it can usually be cured when the cause, such as a drug, is stopped.
- If it is due to an underlying disorder, the outcome depends on the course of the primary disease.
- If hemolytic anemia is inherited, it is currently considered incurable. However, symptoms can be relieved or controlled.

HOW TO TREAT

GENERAL MEASURES—If removal of the spleen is required, see Spleen Removal in Surgery section for an explanation of surgery and postoperative care.

MEDICATION
- Drugs may be prescribed depending on the specific cause of anemia. These may include corticosteroids, immune globulin, folic acid, iron therapy, and others.
- Drugs that are causing the anemia will be stopped.

ACTIVITY—No limits, except those caused by the symptoms.

DIET—No special diet. Fava beans should be avoided in certain patients (you will be advised).

CALL YOUR DOCTOR IF

- You or a family member has symptoms of hemolytic anemia.
- Fever, cough, sore throat, swollen joints, muscle aches, or bloody urine occur during treatment.
- Signs of infection occur in any part of the body (redness, pain, swelling, fever).
- New, unexplained symptoms develop. Drugs used in treatment may produce side effects.

ANEMIA, IRON-DEFICIENCY

GENERAL INFORMATION

DEFINITION—Iron-deficiency anemia is a condition caused by inadequate amounts of iron in the body. Iron is present in all cells and has several vital functions.

BODY PARTS INVOLVED—Blood, which affects all body cells.

SEX OR AGE MOST AFFECTED—Both sexes; all ages. It is more common in women of childbearing age.

SIGNS & SYMPTOMS
- There may be no symptoms. It may be diagnosed on a routine health exam.
- Fatigue and weakness.
- Pale skin, eyes, and fingernails.
- General feeling of discomfort.
- Being more sensitive to cold.
- Shortness of breath.
- Dizziness.
- Restless leg syndrome (odd sensations in the legs).

CAUSES—Iron is involved with red blood cell production. When iron stores are low, fewer red blood cells are produced and this leads to anemia. iron deficiency may result from low iron intake in the diet, increased iron loss, or excessive iron requirements.

RISK INCREASES WITH
- Growth spurts in children and young teens.
- Women before menopause.
- Heavy menstrual bleeding.
- Pregnancy.
- Lack of iron in diet (e.g., vegan diet or fad diet).
- Celiac disease, Crohn's disease, gastric or bowel surgery, gastritis, peptic ulcer disease, or certain cancers.
- Ongoing use of nonsteroidal anti-inflammatory drugs (e.g., aspirin).
- People in lower income groups.
- Frequent blood donations.

HOW TO PREVENT
- Can't always be prevented. Get adequate iron intake with a well-balanced diet to reduce risk.
- Correct problems causing excess blood loss.

WHAT TO EXPECT

DIAGNOSTIC MEASURES
- Your own observation of symptoms.
- Your health care provider will do a physical exam and ask questions about your symptoms and diet.
- Medical tests may include blood, urine, and stool studies. Other tests may be done to diagnose disorders that could be the cause of the anemia.

APPROPRIATE HEALTH CARE
- Iron deficiency can be treated with iron supplements. Other treatment will depend on the underlying cause. The cause needs to be treated so the iron deficiency does not recur.
- Severe symptoms may require hospital care. Blood transfusions are rarely needed.

POSSIBLE COMPLICATIONS
- Complications are rare in mild anemia.
- If the anemia is more severe, heart complications can occur. Children may have developmental problems.

PROBABLE OUTCOME—Usually curable with treatment. It may take 2 months for the iron levels to return to normal. Some outcomes will also depend on the underlying cause.

HOW TO TREAT

GENERAL MEASURES
- The most important part of treatment for iron-deficiency anemia is to correct the underlying cause.
- Avoid risk of infections.

MEDICATION
- Oral iron supplements (always follow your health care provider's instructions):
  - Take iron on an empty stomach (at least 1/2 hour before meals) for best absorption. If it upsets your stomach, take it with a small amount of food (except milk).
  - If you take other drugs, wait at least 2 hours after taking iron before taking them. Antacids, tetracyclines, allopurinol, and vitamin E especially interfere with iron absorption.
  - Iron supplements may cause black bowel movements, diarrhea, or constipation.
  - Too much iron is dangerous. A bottle of iron tablets can poison a child. Keep iron supplements out of the reach of children.
- In some cases, the iron may be given by injection.

ACTIVITY—No limits. You may need to reduce activities until symptoms of fatigue are gone.

DIET
- Eat iron-rich foods, including meat, fish, poultry, beans, raisins, egg yolks, and leafy green vegetables.
- Increase dietary fiber to prevent constipation.

CALL YOUR DOCTOR IF

- You or a family member has symptoms of iron-deficiency anemia.
- Nausea, vomiting, fever, stomach pain, constipation, or severe diarrhea occur during treatment.

ANEMIA, PERNICIOUS
(B-12 Deficiency Anemia)

 GENERAL INFORMATION

DEFINITION—Pernicious anemia results from the failure of the digestive tract to absorb vitamin B-12. Vitamin B-12 (also called cobalamin) is needed for making red blood cells and keeping the nervous system functioning.

BODY PARTS INVOLVED—Blood, which affects all body cells; stomach.

SEX OR AGE MOST AFFECTED—Adults of both sexes, between ages 40 and 70.

SIGNS & SYMPTOMS
- Symptoms develop slowly. It may take time to notice.
- Weakness, especially in the arms and legs.
- Bright red, smooth, burning, or sore tongue.
- Numbness or tingling in the hands and feet.
- Difficulty maintaining proper balance and walking.
- Loss of sense of position (e.g., in a dark room).
- Nausea, appetite loss, and weight loss.
- Low-grade fever.
- Constipation or diarrhea.
- Pale or yellowish skin.
- Bleeding gums and mouth sores.
- Shortness of breath, chest pain, rapid heartbeat.
- Depression, confusion, poor memory, and dementia.

CAUSES
- Pernicious anemia is due to a lack of intrinsic factor. This is a substance made by cells in the stomach that makes it possible to absorb vitamin B-12. The reason for the lack of intrinsic factor is unknown. It may be an autoimmune reaction, a genetic factor, or both.
- Other vitamin B-12 deficiency-caused anemias may be due to a variety of factors.

RISK INCREASES WITH
- Stomach surgery, stomach cancer, or gastritis.
- Diabetes and autoimmune disorders.
- Myxedema, Graves' disease, other thyroid disorders.
- Genetic factors, such as in people of Northern European ancestry. It is rare in blacks and Asians.
- Family history of pernicious anemia.
- Strict vegetarian diet or infants breast-fed by a mother on a strict vegetarian diet.
- Lack of stomach acid in older adults.
- Parasitic infections and intestinal diseases.
- Drugs such as H2 blockers, proton pump inhibitors, colchicine, neomycin, and aminosalicylic acid.
- Poor diet, such as due to alcoholism or aging.

HOW TO PREVENT—Pernicious anemia cannot be prevented.

 WHAT TO EXPECT

DIAGNOSTIC MEASURES
- Your own observation of symptoms.
- Your health care provider will do a physical exam and ask questions about your symptoms and your diet.
- Medical tests include blood test of vitamin B-12 levels, to check for antibodies to the intrinsic factor, and to measure the body's ability to absorb vitamin B-12.

APPROPRIATE HEALTH CARE
- Treatment usually involves vitamin B-12 replacement. Lifetime treatment is needed for pernicious anemia. Some symptoms should start to clear up in a few days after treatment begins, while others may take several months.
- Any underlying disorder (such as thyroid problems) will be treated also.

POSSIBLE COMPLICATIONS
- Congestive heart failure.
- Nerve damage that cannot be reversed.
- Gastric cancer.

PROBABLE OUTCOME
- For pernicious anemia, lifelong vitamin B-12 therapy will help symptoms and prevent complications.
- For vitamin B-12 deficiency-caused anemia, vitamin B-12 therapy or diet changes can prevent deficiency.

 HOW TO TREAT

GENERAL MEASURES—Stop drinking alcohol if it is a cause of the vitamin B-12 deficiency.

MEDICATION
- Vitamin B-12 replacement will be prescribed. Some patients are given injections (they can be self-administered). For other patients (or in addition to injections), the vitamin may be taken by mouth or as a nasal gel.
- Iron supplements may be prescribed.
- Avoid taking high amounts of folic acid. It can mask the signs of vitamin B-12 deficiency.

ACTIVITY—Activity may be limited short term.

DIET
- Eat a well-balanced diet.
- People on strict vegetarian diets can change the diet or take vitamin B-12 supplement for life.

 CALL YOUR DOCTOR IF

- You or a family member has symptoms of pernicious anemia.
- Symptoms don't improve with treatment.

ANEURYSM

GENERAL INFORMATION

DEFINITION—An aneurysm is a ballooning or bulge in the wall of a blood vessel (almost always an artery). It can affect the arteries in the chest, abdomen, brain, legs, or heart wall. Aneurysms have thin, weak walls and have a tendency to rupture (burst) and cause hemorrhage (bleeding).

BODY PARTS INVOLVED—Arteries. Aneurysms occur most often in the aorta (major artery in the chest and abdomen), arteries that supply the brain or legs, or heart wall.

SEX OR AGE MOST AFFECTED—Adults of both sexes, usually over age 50.

SIGNS & SYMPTOMS
- Often, no symptoms occur unless the aneurysm ruptures. Symptoms that occur depend on affected artery.
- Thoracic (chest) aneurysm produces pain in the chest, neck, back, and abdomen. The pain may be sudden and sharp.
- Cerebral aneurysm in a brain artery produces headache (often throbbing), weakness, paralysis or numbness, pain behind the eye, vision change, partial blindness, and eye pupils of different sizes.
- Abdominal aneurysm produces back pain (sometimes severe), abdomen pain, and groin pain.
- Peripheral aneurysm in a leg artery causes poor circulation in the leg, with weakness and paleness or swelling, and bluish color.
- Ventricular aneurysm in the wall of the heart causes irregular heartbeat, shortness of breath, and chest pain.

CAUSES—Arterial walls become weak due to defect, disease, or injury. This may be due to an acquired condition or it may be congenital (present at birth).

RISK INCREASES WITH
- Adults over 55.
- Family history of aneurysms.
- Atherosclerosis (hardening of the arteries).
- High blood pressure.
- Congenital weak artery.
- Polycystic disease or connective tissue disorders.
- Complications of blood infections.
- Fibromuscular dysplasia.
- Injury (trauma).
- Cigarette smoking.
- Emphysema.

HOW TO PREVENT—No specific way to prevent aneurysms. Seek treatment for any risk factors where possible.

WHAT TO EXPECT

DIAGNOSTIC MEASURES—See Appropriate Health Care.

APPROPRIATE HEALTH CARE
- Emergency treatment is needed for persons with symptoms of a ruptured aneurysm. Once the aneurysm is diagnosed, surgery may be performed. This is done to stop any bleeding and to prevent the aneurysm from recurring. Treatments called endovascular procedures can be done to plug or clog the blood vessel.
- Unruptured aneurysms may be diagnosed when a person has no symptoms. Sometimes they are found when medical tests are done for other reasons. The decision to treat or not treat these aneurysms with surgery is difficult. Both options carry risks. Your health care provider will discuss the risks and benefits of each with you. The size of the aneurysm, its location, the patient's symptoms, age, health status, and preferences must all be considered.
- Sometimes, the aneurysm can be removed and replaced with a graft (artificial blood vessel), or wrapped with a protective sleeve to prevent rupturing. See Aneurysm Repair in Surgery Section.

POSSIBLE COMPLICATIONS—Stroke or a rupture of the aneurysm.

PROBABLE OUTCOME
- Diagnosed, unruptured aneurysms may or may not be treated. You may be followed up with regular medical exams to watch for problems.
- Outcome of a ruptured aneurysm varies. Some persons are treated and recover with little or no damage. Others die before, during, or after treatment.

HOW TO TREAT

GENERAL MEASURES—None specific.

MEDICATION
- After surgery, anticoagulants to prevent blood clots and pain relievers are usually prescribed.
- Antibiotics as needed to prevent infection.

ACTIVITY—If surgery is done, you will be advised of any limits.

DIET—No special diet.

CALL YOUR DOCTOR IF

- You or a family member has symptoms of a ruptured aneurysm. This is an emergency! Call for help; rest in bed until help arrives.
- You or a family member has minor pain or aching in the chest, abdomen, or legs. Fever or weight loss occurs for no apparent reason.

ANGINA PECTORIS

GENERAL INFORMATION

DEFINITION—Angina pectoris is chest pain or discomfort due to a decrease in the blood (and oxygen) supply to the heart muscle (myocardium). Angina may be stable (symptoms are predictable), or unstable (symptoms are unexpected and usually occur while at rest).

BODY PARTS INVOLVED—Coronary arteries.

SEX OR AGE MOST AFFECTED—Men over age 35 and postmenopausal women.

SIGNS & SYMPTOMS
* Tightness, squeezing, pressure, fullness, ache, or pain in the center of the chest. Pain may feel like indigestion.
* Discomfort or pain may also occur in the neck, jaw, shoulder, arm, or back.
* Symptoms may occur with exercise, strong emotions, heavy meals, or with temperature extremes. Some persons have angina while resting.

CAUSES—Angina occurs when the heart needs more blood and oxygen and is unable to get what it requires. This is called ischemia. Coronary artery disease (CAD) is the main cause. In CAD, one or more of the arteries supplying blood to the heart is narrowed or blocked. Angina also occurs if the blood does not carry enough oxygen.

RISK INCREASES WITH
* High blood pressure, atherosclerosis, diabetes, high cholesterol, personal or family history of heart disease.
* Obesity, inactivity, smoking, or excess alcohol use.
* Metabolic syndrome (a group of risk factors).

HOW TO PREVENT—Prevention involves preventing the coronary artery disease that leads to angina. Don't smoke. Get treatment for chronic disorders such as diabetes, high blood pressure, and obesity. Exercise regularly. Reduce high cholesterol with diet or drugs.

WHAT TO EXPECT

DIAGNOSTIC MEASURES
* Your own observation of symptoms.
* Your health care provider will do a physical exam and ask questions about your symptoms.
* A number of medical tests will be done to assess heart function and to diagnose any underlying disorder.

APPROPRIATE HEALTH CARE
* Treatment usually involves drug therapy to relieve angina symptoms, slow the progress of heart disease, and prevent complications.
* If drugs cannot control the angina, there are other treatment options. They include balloon angioplasty to open blocked coronary arteries, stenting (a tiny metal tube or coil is placed in the artery to keep it open), or surgery to bypass severely blocked coronary arteries.

POSSIBLE COMPLICATIONS—Heart attack, unstable angina, and/or death.

PROBABLE OUTCOME—Most angina symptoms can be relieved with lifestyle changes and/or drug therapy. Other treatment may be needed to correct underlying diseases.

HOW TO TREAT

GENERAL MEASURES
* Don't smoke. Find a way to quit.
* Avoid angina triggers, if possible, that increase the heart's workload, such as anger, temperature extremes, high altitude (except in commercial airline flights), or sudden bursts of activity.
* To learn more: American Heart Association, local branch listed in telephone directory, or call (800) 242-8721; website: www.americanheart.org.

MEDICATION
* Nitroglycerin relieves acute symptoms of angina or it can be used before activities. It does not affect symptoms of other disorders. It can work within seconds to relieve pain. Keep it with you for immediate use.
* Drugs to prevent blood clots will be given after procedures such as balloon angioplasty or stenting.
* Other drugs for coronary disease, such as aspirin, beta-blockers, cholesterol-lowering drugs, ACE inhibitors, or calcium channel blockers may be prescribed. If they are, it is important to follow the prescribed drug regimen.

ACTIVITY
* Learn to adjust activities to lessen angina attacks.
* Don't use angina as an excuse not to exercise. A regular moderate exercise routine (determined by your health care provider) can help to control symptoms.

DIET
* Low-fat, low-cholesterol diet is often recommended.
* A weight loss diet may help if overweight.

CALL YOUR DOCTOR IF

* You or a family member has symptoms of angina pectoris.
* Despite nitroglycerin and rest, the angina pain lasts longer than 10 to 15 minutes, is getting worse, or pain stops and then returns. This may be an emergency!
* Angina symptoms occur more often.

ANIMAL BITES

GENERAL INFORMATION

DEFINITION—Animal bites are bite wounds to humans from dogs, cats, or other animals (including humans).

BODY PARTS INVOLVED—Usually the hands, face or legs.

SEX OR AGE MOST AFFECTED—All ages and both sexes, but more often occurs in children and males.

SIGNS & SYMPTOMS
- Bite wounds can be tears, punctures, scratches, ripping, or crushing injuries.
- Dog bites usually involve the hands, face, or the legs and feet.
- Cat bites usually involve the hands, followed by legs, feet, face, and trunk.

CAUSES
- Most bite wounds are from a domestic pet known to the victim. Large dogs are the most common source.
- Human bites are often the result of one person striking another in the mouth with a clenched fist.

RISK INCREASES WITH—Exposure to domestic pets or wild animals.

HOW TO PREVENT
- Education on how to avoid animal bites, for children as well as adults.
- Avoid stray animals.
- To prevent complications from possible animal bites, keep tetanus immunizations up-to-date.

WHAT TO EXPECT

DIAGNOSTIC MEASURES
- Your own observations.
- Health care provider's examination.
- Culture of wound fluids, x-rays (if wound is near a bone or joint), exploratory surgery sometimes to determine extent of injuries.

APPROPRIATE HEALTH CARE
- Self-care for minor wounds.
- Call 911 if a person has been seriously wounded or is bleeding heavily. if the wound is severe, or the bite was from a wild animal or one behaving strangely.
- Medical care may include wound cleaning and surgical closure if needed.
- Wound will usually be left open to heal to lessen risk of infection.
- If hand is injured, it may be put in a splint.

POSSIBLE COMPLICATIONS—Infection, extensive soft tissue injuries with scarring, hemorrhage, rabies, and sometimes death.

PROBABLE OUTCOME
- Wounds should steadily improve and close over within 7 to 10 days.
- Dog bites rarely become infected. Cat bites and human bites frequently become infected.

HOW TO TREAT

GENERAL MEASURES
- For first aid:
  - Wash hands before and after caring for the wound.
  - If the wound is bleeding, apply pressure to the area with clean towel or cloth until bleeding stops. Clean wound with soap and water, dry the area, apply an antibiotic ointment, and cover it with sterile gauze or clean cloth.
  - Elevate the injured extremity to prevent swelling.
- If appropriate, contact the local health department or animal control about the bite.
- If possible, the animal that caused the bite should be checked for rabies. Call an animal control office for instructions.

MEDICATION
- Preventive antibiotic treatment may be prescribed.
- Antitetanus injection may have to be given.
- Sometimes, an antirabies vaccine or serum may have to be given.

ACTIVITY—No limits, except those caused by the injury.

DIET—No special diet.

CALL YOUR DOCTOR IF

- You or a family member suffers from an animal bite that causes concern.
- The bite does not begin to heal within 2 to 3 days or signs of infection develop.
- New or unexplained symptoms develop. Drugs used in treatment may produce side effects.

ANORECTAL ABSCESS

GENERAL INFORMATION

DEFINITION—An anorectal abscess is a collection of pus (due to infection) that develops in the anus and rectum. An abscess may occur on the edge of the anal opening or deep in the rectum.

BODY PARTS INVOLVED—Anus; rectum.

SEX OR AGE MOST AFFECTED—Both sexes; all ages. They are more common in men.

SIGNS & SYMPTOMS
- Swelling around the rectum.
- Redness around the rectum.
- Dull or throbbing pain around the rectum.
- Difficulty or pain with bowel movement.
- Unable to sit comfortably.
- Fever and chills.
- Bleeding or discharge if abscess ruptures.

CAUSES—Bacterial infection. It may occur in the glands inside the rectum that produce mucus. Bacteria in the stool can also infect a scratch or cut in the skin or in the rectum.

RISK INCREASES WITH
- Diabetes.
- Crohn's disease, ulcerative colitis, or diverticulitis.
- Engaging in anal sex.
- Weak immune system due to illness or drugs.
- Blood cell cancers such as leukemia or lymphoma.

HOW TO PREVENT—No specific preventive measures.

WHAT TO EXPECT

DIAGNOSTIC MEASURES
- Your own observation of symptoms.
- Your health care provider can diagnose the abscess with a physical exam of the affected area.
- Medical tests are usually not needed, but may include an x-ray or internal exam of the rectum with a special instrument.

APPROPRIATE HEALTH CARE
- Treatment most often involves outpatient surgery to open and drain the abscess.
- For an abscess deeper in the rectum, the patient may need hospital care.

POSSIBLE COMPLICATIONS
- An extra opening (fistula) may develop between the anus and the outside of the body.
- Abscess may recur.
- Urinary retention.

PROBABLE OUTCOME—With treatment, complete healing in 6 weeks to several months (if no complications).

HOW TO TREAT

GENERAL MEASURES
- Follow your health care provider's instructions for changing bandages and other care after surgery. Keep that area of the body clean.
- A sitz bath may provide comfort after surgery. Sit in a bathtub (or a plastic sitz bath) of warm water (not hot) for 10 to 15 minutes several times a day.
- Use warm compress as needed for pain.
- Have a bowel movement when you need to, even though you may anticipate pain.

MEDICATION—Drugs may be prescribed for pain, infection, and to help prevent constipation.

ACTIVITY—Move legs often as you recover from surgery. Return to normal activities as soon as possible after surgery.

DIET—An increase in fiber in the diet may help lower the risk of constipation. Drink plenty of fluids.

CALL YOUR DOCTOR IF

- You or a family member has symptoms of anorectal abscess.
- New or unexplained symptoms develop after surgery.

ANOREXIA NERVOSA

GENERAL INFORMATION

DEFINITION—Anorexia nervosa is a type of eating disorder. A person refuses to eat enough to maintain a normal weight for height and age. It develops over time.

BODY PARTS INVOLVED—All body cells.

SEX OR AGE MOST AFFECTED—It can occur in both sexes. It most often affects young females ages 12 to 25.

SIGNS & SYMPTOMS
- Weight loss of at least 15% of ideal body weight.
- Continues to diet when not overweight. May restrict food intake or binge on food and then purge.
- Person feels fat even when extremely thin.
- Intense fear of becoming fat.
- Obsessed with food, but denies being hungry.
- Excess exercising.
- Stopping of menstrual periods or never starting.
- Uses diuretics, laxatives, emetics, and amphetamines.
- Depressed, moody, irritable, withdrawn, ritual or odd behaviors, and insomnia.
- Hair loss, dry skin, feeling cold, brittle nails, low blood pressure, and poor blood circulation.

CAUSES—Unknown. There are many theories. It involves using food and weight to deal with emotional problems, such as issues of self-worth and control for the patient.

RISK INCREASES WITH
- Young females.
- Starting a normal weight-loss diet. The person refuses to stop dieting after a reasonable weight loss.
- Some personality traits such as perfectionism, obsessiveness, or low self-esteem.
- Family history of eating disorders.
- Family influence (overprotective or placing too much value on physical appearance).
- Society, cultural, and peer pressure to be thin.
- Emotional stress.
- Athletes, ballet dancers, cheerleaders, or models.

HOW TO PREVENT—No specific preventive measures. Early treatment may help keep it from progressing.

WHAT TO EXPECT

DIAGNOSTIC MEASURES
- Your health care provider can usually diagnose anorexia with a physical exam and by asking questions about your symptoms, eating habits, and weight concerns. There is no one test to diagnose anorexia.
- Medical tests may be done to check for possible underlying disorder, physical problems, or complications.

APPROPRIATE HEALTH CARE
- Treatment may include counseling for the patient and the family, nutrition counseling, and drug therapy if needed. Hospital care may be required if the weight is extremely low or there are life-threatening symptoms.
- A dental exam is usually recommended.
- Counseling focuses on the misconceptions that patients have of themselves (physically, mentally, emotionally). Support groups may help some patients.

POSSIBLE COMPLICATIONS—Electrolyte imbalance, irregular heartbeat, esophagitis, gastritis, lack of menstrual periods, nerve disorders, anemia and weakness, infertility, osteoporosis, or suicide.

PROBABLE OUTCOME
- Treatable if the patient recognizes the problem, wants help, and is compliant with treatment.
- Therapy may continue over several years. Relapses are common, especially when stressful situations occur.
- About 40% make a good recovery in 5 years, 40% have symptoms, but function fairly well, and 20% have severe, ongoing symptoms.

HOW TO TREAT

GENERAL MEASURES
- Denial of the severity or even the existence of a problem is common in patients. Most patients resist treatment and behavioral change at first. Some want a quick and easy solution that is not feasible.
- The goal is for the patient to establish healthy eating patterns to regain normal weight.
- To learn more: National Eating Disorders Association; 603 Stewart St., Suite 803, Seattle, WA 98101; (800) 931-2237; website: www.nationaleatingdisorders.org.

MEDICATION
- Drugs may be prescribed for specific symptoms such as depression, anxiety, or agitation.
- Vitamin/mineral supplements may be advised.

ACTIVITY—May be limits until weight is gained. Then exercise for fitness—not to lose weight.

DIET—A dietitian will help you plan healthy meals that are not rigid, but provide food choices. Calories will be slowly increased over time to reach your individual needs.

CALL YOUR DOCTOR IF

- You have symptoms of anorexia nervosa or observe them in a family member.
- Weight loss continues, despite treatment.

ANXIETY DISORDER, GENERALIZED

GENERAL INFORMATION

DEFINITION—Generalized anxiety disorder is an illness that involves constant worry even though little or nothing is wrong. A person feels tense most of the time and always expects the worst to happen. They may worry about health, money, family, work, or an unknown or unspecified threat. Symptoms may be severe and interfere with daily living. Attempts to avoid the anxiety lead to more anxiety.

BODY PARTS INVOLVED—Central nervous system; endocrine system.

SEX OR AGE MOST AFFECTED—Anxiety usually comes on slowly and can start in childhood, adolescence, or as an adult. It is more common in women.

SIGNS & SYMPTOMS
- Feeling that something undesirable or harmful is about to happen.
- Constant worry about things (big and small).
- Aches and pains for unknown reasons.
- Feeling tired.
- Unable to relax.
- Muscle tension, headaches, backache.
- Trouble falling or staying asleep.
- Dry mouth, swallowing difficulty, or hoarseness.
- Twitching or trembling.
- Unable to focus or concentrate.
- Feeling irritable or grouchy.
- Nausea, diarrhea, weight loss.
- Sweating or hot flashes.
- Easily startled.

CAUSES—It is most likely a combination of hereditary factors, environmental factors (such as childhood experiences), and chemical disturbances in the brain.

RISK INCREASES WITH
- Females.
- Stressful events or crisis in one's life.
- Family history of anxiety disorders.
- Other emotional or mental illness (depression, panic disorder, phobias, or dysthymia).
- Medical illness (e.g., chronic pain, asthma, or others).
- Alcohol or substance abuse.
- Lack of social connections.
- Certain personality factors (being shy or a worrier).
- Living in poverty, in a minority group, or immigrants.

HOW TO PREVENT—There are no specific preventive measures.

WHAT TO EXPECT

DIAGNOSTIC MEASURES
- Your own observation of symptoms.
- Your health care provider will do a physical exam and ask questions about your symptoms.
- There is no specific test to diagnose anxiety. Medical tests may be done to rule out other health disorders. A mental health test may be done.

APPROPRIATE HEALTH CARE
- Treatment may involve psychotherapy (treatment of emotional and mental problems), self-care, and drugs.
- Cognitive-behavior therapy (CBT) is often recommended. Cognitive therapy teaches how to change thoughts, behaviors, or attitudes. Behavior therapy teaches ways to reduce anxiety with deep breathing and muscle relaxation.

POSSIBLE COMPLICATIONS
- Impaired social and work functioning.
- Depression, panic disorder, or social phobia.
- Dependence on drugs or alcohol.

PROBABLE OUTCOME—Anxiety can be controlled with treatment. Overcoming anxiety often results in a richer, more satisfying life.

HOW TO TREAT

GENERAL MEASURES
- Self-care steps may include:
  - Talking to a friend or family member about your feelings. This sometimes defuses your anxiety.
  - Keeping a journal about your anxious thoughts or emotions. Consider the causes and possible solutions.
  - Joining a self-help group.
  - Learning relaxation techniques. For some people, meditation is effective.
  - Reducing stress in your life where possible.
- To learn more: National Institute of Mental Health; 6001 Executive Blvd, Bethesda, MD 20892-9663; (866) 615-6464; website: www.nimh.nih.gov.

MEDICATION
- Antianxiety drugs may be prescribed.
- Antidepressants may be prescribed.

ACTIVITY—Stay active. Physical exertion helps reduce anxiety.

DIET—No special diet. Avoid caffeine and other stimulants and alcohol.

CALL YOUR DOCTOR IF

- You or a family member has symptoms of anxiety and self-treatment has failed.
- Symptoms recur after treatment.

APPENDICITIS

GENERAL INFORMATION

DEFINITION—Appendicitis is an inflammation of the appendix. The appendix is a small tube-like pouch that is part of the large intestine. The appendix has no known function, but it can become diseased. Symptoms vary widely.

BODY PARTS INVOLVED—Appendix; cecum; peritoneum (lining of intestinal tract).

SEX OR AGE MOST AFFECTED—All ages, but rare in children under 2. The incidence peaks between ages 15 and 24.

SIGNS & SYMPTOMS
- Pain that frequently begins close to the navel and moves toward the right lower abdomen. Pain becomes persistent. It worsens with moving, breathing deeply, coughing, sneezing, walking, or being touched.
- Nausea and sometimes vomiting.
- Constipation and inability to pass gas.
- Diarrhea (occasionally).
- Low fever (begins after other symptoms).
- Abdominal swelling (late stages).

CAUSES—The exact cause is unknown. The appendix may be blocked with feces from the intestinal tract which leads to infection. When infected, the appendix becomes swollen, inflamed, and filled with pus.

RISK INCREASES WITH
- Viral or bacterial infection of the gastrointestinal tract.
- Family history of appendicitis.
- Cystic fibrosis.
- Diet that is low in fiber.

HOW TO PREVENT—No specific preventive measures.

WHAT TO EXPECT

DIAGNOSTIC MEASURES
- Your own observation of symptoms.
- Your health care provider will do a physical exam and ask questions about your symptoms.
- Medical tests may include blood and urine studies, x-ray, CT, ultrasound, or other tests to confirm the diagnosis.

APPROPRIATE HEALTH CARE
- Treatment involves surgery to remove the appendix (appendectomy). Because appendicitis can be hard to diagnose, surgery may be delayed until symptoms and signs progress enough to confirm the diagnosis.
- Surgery may be done with a laparoscope (a tube-like instrument with a light on the end). Small incisions (3 to 4) are made in the abdomen. The appendix is removed using instruments inserted into the incisions.

- Open surgery may be done. This involves one larger incision in the abdomen to remove the appendix. This type of surgery is done if the appendix has ruptured (burst).
- If an abscess has formed, surgery may be delayed until the abscess is drained and has time to heal.

POSSIBLE COMPLICATIONS
- Rupture of the appendix, abscess (pus-filled area), and peritonitis. Rupture occurs earlier in children, but is more common in older persons.
- Wound infection or other surgery complications.
- Bowel obstruction.

PROBABLE OUTCOME—After treatment, most people recover without complications. People can live a normal life without their appendix.

HOW TO TREAT

GENERAL MEASURES
- Don't take any laxatives, enemas, or drugs for pain prior to diagnosis. Laxatives may lead to rupture, and pain or fever reducers make diagnosis more difficult.
- For an explanation of surgery and postoperative care, see Appendectomy in Surgery section.

MEDICATION
- Antibiotics for infection and drugs for pain are usually prescribed after surgery.
- Stool softeners to prevent constipation may be recommended.

ACTIVITY
- Rest in a bed or chair until surgery.
- Resume normal activities gradually after surgery.

DIET
- Don't eat or drink anything until appendicitis has been diagnosed. Anesthesia for surgery is much safer if the stomach is empty. If you are very thirsty, wash your mouth out with water.
- After surgery, a liquid diet is used for a short time. A regular diet may be resumed as the intestinal tract returns to normal.

CALL YOUR DOCTOR IF

- You or a family member has symptoms of appendicitis.
- The following occur after surgery:
  - Fever of 101.5°F (38.6°C) or higher.
  - Increased redness, swelling, or pain at the incision site or if the site has drainage.
  - Vomiting or diarrhea occurs.

ARTHRITIS, INFECTIOUS
(Septic Arthritis)

 GENERAL INFORMATION

DEFINITION—Infectious arthritis is an infection in one (usually) or more joints. It is a rare, but serious, condition.

BODY PARTS INVOLVED—Any joint, but most common in larger ones, such as the hip, or those subject to trauma, such as the knee or joints in the hands.

SEX OR AGE MOST AFFECTED—Both sexes; all ages.

SIGNS & SYMPTOMS
- Redness, swelling, tenderness and pain (often throbbing) in the affected joint. Pain sometimes spreads to other joints. It worsens with movement.
- Chills and fever (sometimes high).
- Pain in the buttocks, thighs or groin (sometimes).

CAUSES
- Entry into a joint by bacteria—usually streptococci or staphylococci. Other causes are rare (e.g., gonococcal in sexually active persons, viral, or fungi). Germs gain entry from:
    - Infection elsewhere in the body.
    - Infection next to the joint.
    - Injury to the joint (e.g., puncture wounds and skin abrasions).

RISK INCREASES WITH
- Adults over 60.
- Diabetes or rheumatoid arthritis.
- Certain infections in the body.
- Weak immune system due to illness or drugs.
- Recent joint surgery, injections into joint, or joint injury.
- Excess alcohol use.
- IV drug abuse.
- Prosthetic (artificial) joint.
- Having skin disorders.

HOW TO PREVENT
- Can't always be prevented.
- Protect exposed joints, such as the knee, during activities involving injury risks.
- Get prompt medical treatment for infections.
- If you have an artificial joint, your health care provider will discuss steps to prevent infections.

 WHAT TO EXPECT

DIAGNOSTIC MEASURES
- Your own observation of symptoms.
- A health care provider will do a physical exam and ask questions about illnesses or any contact with infected persons.
- Medical tests may include blood counts, blood culture, culture of fluid from the infected joint, and x-ray or ultrasound of affected joints.

APPROPRIATE HEALTH CARE
- Treatment usually involves drug therapy and joint drainage (removing fluid from the joint).
- Hospital care is typically needed.
- The joint may require splinting for a time.
- Physical therapy is usually prescribed.

POSSIBLE COMPLICATIONS
- Decreased range of motion of the joint, chronic pain, or permanent joint damage.
- Osteomyelitis (bone infection).
- An artificial joint may need to be replaced.
- Rarely, septic shock and respiratory failure.

PROBABLE OUTCOME—Curable with early diagnosis and treatment. Recovery may take weeks or months. A number of patients will still have, or develop joint problems in the future. Delayed treatment or patients with other health problems increases risk of complications.

 HOW TO TREAT

GENERAL MEASURES
- Apply heat or cold (whichever feels better) to painful joints.
- Follow medical instructions for self-care after the infection clears up.

MEDICATION
- Antibiotics (often intravenous) or other drugs to treat the infection will be prescribed.
- Drugs may be prescribed for a short time to relieve pain.

ACTIVITY
- Rest the affected joint to help relieve pain.
- Physical therapy is usually started as soon as patient can tolerate the joint movement.
- Resume normal activities gradually as symptoms improve.

DIET—No special diet.

 CALL YOUR DOCTOR IF

- You or a family member has symptoms of joint infection. Call immediately.
- After treatment, any new or recurring symptoms cause concern.

ARTHRITIS, JUVENILE IDIOPATHIC

GENERAL INFORMATION

DEFINITION
• Juvenile idiopathic arthritis (JIA) is a chronic inflammatory disease of the joints. It affects children under age 16 and can start at any age. JIA types are based on symptoms in the first 6 months of the disease. Types:
- Systemic arthritis—affects at least 1 joint. Inflammation occurs in other parts of the body besides the joints.
- Oligoarthritis (prior name pauciarticular)— affects 1 to 4 joints.
- Polyarthritis-rheumatoid factor negative or positive (prior name polyarticular)—affects 5 or more joints.
- Others types—psoriatic arthritis, enthesitis-related arthritis, and undifferentiated arthritis.

BODY PARTS INVOLVED—Any body joint (e.g., knees, hands, and feet).

SEX OR AGE MOST AFFECTED—It often starts at 2 to 5 years and occurs more frequently in girls.

SIGNS & SYMPTOMS
• Symptoms vary for each type. Symptoms may occur often or rarely and from mild to severe.
• Joint symptoms may include swelling, warmth, pain, or aching. Children may not complain about joint pain.
• Stiffness occurs in the morning or after a nap.
• Child may limp or develop clumsiness. The child may refuse to walk without being able to explain why.
• Fevers and rashes may come and go.
• Swollen lymph nodes.
• Red eye, eye pain, or photophobia (light sensitivity).

CAUSES—Idiopathic means unknown cause. There appears to be genetic and immune system factors. Trauma (injury), infection, or emotional stress may be trigger factors.

RISK INCREASES WITH
• Family history of JIA.
• Family history of autoimmune disease (e.g., rheumatoid arthritis, multiple sclerosis, or others).

HOW TO PREVENT—Cannot be prevented.

WHAT TO EXPECT

DIAGNOSTIC MEASURES
• Your own observation of symptoms.
• Your child's health care provider will do a physical exam. Questions will be asked about the symptoms and if they have gone on for at least 6 weeks.
• No specific test is available to diagnose JIA. Medical tests may include blood and joint fluid studies, x-rays, or others.

APPROPRIATE HEALTH CARE
• Treatment involves steps to relieve symptoms, preserve joint function, prevent complications, and help the child live as normal a life as possible.
• Treatment may include drug therapy, exercise, eye and dental care, help with emotional concerns, and other medical care as needed. You and your child's health care team will decide on a program based on your child's special needs.
• Rarely, surgery is needed for joint problems.

POSSIBLE COMPLICATIONS
• Joint, bone, eye, or other body system complications.
• Behavior and school difficulties; growth retardation.
• Side effects of drugs used for therapy.

PROBABLE OUTCOME—Outcome depends on type of JIA and response to treatment. Early diagnosis and treatment helps improve outcome. Some children will have permanent remission.

HOW TO TREAT

GENERAL MEASURES
• Children should attend regular school on a daily basis. Where needed, the school system should provide extra services to accommodate the child's needs.
• Learning techniques to control pain may help.
• Help morning stiffness with a warm bath or shower, sleeping in a sleeping bag, doing range-of-motion exercises, or use a heating pad or cold pack (if it feels better).
• The child should be as independent as can be.
• To learn more: American Juvenile Arthritis Organization, PO Box 7669, Atlanta, GA 30357; (800) 283-7800; website: www.arthritis.org.

MEDICATION
• Nonsteroidal anti-inflammatory drugs to help pain and inflammation will be prescribed.
• Other drugs are usually prescribed to help alter the progress of the disease and delay/prevent joint damage.

ACTIVITY
• Occupational therapy helps with daily activities.
• Physical therapy helps keep joints mobile and muscles strong. Your child will be taught how to perform daily exercises at home.
• Splints may be used for joint support.
• In general, contact sports should be avoided. Have child try other sports and activities.

DIET—Provide a healthy diet.

CALL YOUR DOCTOR IF

• Your child has symptoms of juvenile idiopathic arthritis.
• After diagnosis, symptoms worsen or change.

ARTHRITIS, RHEUMATOID

GENERAL INFORMATION

DEFINITION—Rheumatoid arthritis is a chronic, inflammatory disease that mainly affects the joints.

BODY PARTS INVOLVED—Joints, including cartilage, synovial membranes, muscles and ligaments; blood vessels; rarely, the eyes.

SEX OR AGE MOST AFFECTED—It often begins between ages 25 and 50, and is more common in women than in men.

SIGNS & SYMPTOMS
- Joint pain, redness, warmth, and tenderness. It usually affects the same joints on both sides of the body—fingers, hands, wrists, elbows, shoulders, feet, and ankles.
- Morning stiffness.
- Muscle aches, weakness, fever, and weight loss.
- Feeling generally unwell.
- Nodules (bumps) under the skin (sometimes).

CAUSES—Unknown. It is probably caused by an autoimmune disorder in which the body's immune system attacks its own normal tissues. Infection may also be a factor.

RISK INCREASES WITH
- Family history of rheumatoid arthritis or other autoimmune disorders.
- Genetic factors.
- Women.
- Native Americans (occurs more often).

HOW TO PREVENT—No specific preventive measures.

WHAT TO EXPECT

DIAGNOSTIC MEASURES
- Your own observation of symptoms.
- Your health care provider will do a physical exam and ask questions about the symptoms.
- No specific test is available to diagnose arthritis. Medical tests may include blood and joint fluid studies. CT, MRI, and x-rays of the involved joints.

APPROPRIATE HEALTH CARE
- Treatment involves steps to relieve symptoms, to preserve joint function, to prevent complications, and to help the person live as normal a life as possible.
- Treatment steps include drug therapy, physical therapy, occupational therapy, surgery, and lifestyle changes. A treatment plan is based on your special needs.
- Occupational therapy helps with activities of daily life.
- Treatment to help symptoms such as pain include relaxation techniques, counseling, meditation, stress reduction, biofeedback, and support groups. Flare-ups may be triggered by emotional stress.

- Surgery may be recommended for one or more joints. It may involve joint replacement, tendon reconstruction, joint realignment, or removing inflamed tissue. See Knee Replacement; Hip Replacement; and Arthroplasty, Shoulder in Surgery Section.

POSSIBLE COMPLICATIONS
- 5% to 10% of patients are eventually disabled.
- Drugs used in treatment can have side effects.
- Heart, lung, blood vessel, or eye problems.
- Anemia.

PROBABLE OUTCOME—The outcome varies. The disease course may be short and limited or progressive and severe. It is presently incurable. Pain relief, prevention of disability, and an active, normal life span are often possible.

HOW TO TREAT

GENERAL MEASURES
- Help the morning stiffness with a warm bath or shower, doing range-of-motion exercises, or a heating pad or cold pack (if it feels better).
- Be sure to educate yourself about the disorder. Avoid arthritis treatment fads.
- To learn more: Arthritis Foundation, PO Box 7669, Atlanta, GA 30357; (800) 283-7800; website: www.arthritis.org.

MEDICATION
- Nonsteroidal anti-inflammatory drugs (NSAIDs), such as naproxen or ibuprofen, or others will be prescribed.
- Drugs for pain, such as acetaminophen may be used.
- Disease-modifying antirheumatic drugs (DMARDs), biologic response modifiers, or steroids are classes of drugs that are often prescribed.

ACTIVITY
- Physical therapy will help maintain strength and joint mobility. Follow instructions for home exercising.
- Exercising in a heated pool is good for joints.
- Activity options include low impact aerobics, flexibility exercises, yoga, tai chi, or hydrotherapy.
- Mobility aids and splints may be recommended.

DIET—Eat a normal, well-balanced diet. Avoid arthritis diet fads, which are common. Lose weight if you are overweight. Being overweight stresses the joints.

CALL YOUR DOCTOR IF

- You or a family member has symptoms of rheumatoid arthritis.
- Symptoms appear in different joints or other symptoms get worse during treatment.

ASBESTOSIS

GENERAL INFORMATION

DEFINITION—Asbestosis is inflammation of the lung due to breathing asbestos particles. It is a chronic disorder, but is not contagious.

BODY PARTS INVOLVED—Lungs.

SEX OR AGE MOST AFFECTED—Men over age 40 who have been exposed to asbestos.

SIGNS & SYMPTOMS
- Shortness of breath.
- Cough that produces little or no sputum.
- General ill feeling.
- Fitful sleep.
- Appetite loss and weight loss.
- Chest pain.
- Hoarseness.
- Coughing up blood.
- Bluish nails.

CAUSES—Long-term exposure to small particles of asbestos at work or from other sources. The outer part of the lung becomes irritated by the asbestos fibers. This leads to inflammation and to a thickening and scarring of the lung tissue (pulmonary fibrosis). It may take up to 20 years or more between exposure to asbestos and the symptoms of the disease. This period may be shorter after intense exposure.

RISK INCREASES WITH
- Work that involves asbestos.
- Smoking.
- Excess alcohol use.

HOW TO PREVENT
- During exposure to asbestos, wear a protective mask or external-air-supplied hood.
- Follow recommended industrial safety procedures to suppress asbestos dust.
- For workers in asbestos industries: have regularly scheduled x-rays to detect any shadow on the lungs. If a problem develops, the person should stop working with asbestos, even if there are no symptoms.
- Don't smoke.

WHAT TO EXPECT

DIAGNOSTIC MEASURES
- Your own observation of symptoms.
- Your health care provider will do a physical exam and ask about your symptoms and past exposure to asbestos.
- Medical tests usually include a CT or x-rays of the lungs and lung function tests. A bronchoscopy may be done (an instrument with a lighted tip is used to view inside the lungs and remove tissue for a biopsy).

APPROPRIATE HEALTH CARE
- There is no specific treatment for asbestosis. Treatment can help relieve the symptoms and prevent complications.
- Obtain medical care for any respiratory infection, including the common cold.
- Chest physical therapy techniques will be provided by a respiratory therapist.
- Supplemental oxygen may be required.

POSSIBLE COMPLICATIONS
- Chronic obstructive pulmonary disease (COPD).
- Heart failure due to lung disease.
- It may lead to cancer of the lungs (the risk is greatly increased in cigarette smokers).
- Tuberculosis.

PROBABLE OUTCOME—There is no cure. In a few patients, it may remain unchanged, but in most, it is slowly progressive (even without further exposure to asbestos). Symptoms can usually be relieved or controlled.

HOW TO TREAT

GENERAL MEASURES
- Avoid any further contact with asbestos.
- Stop smoking. Find a way to quit that works for you.
- Learn and practice bronchial drainage.
- Use a cool-mist humidifier (if advised) to loosen bronchial secretions so they can be coughed up easily.
- Keep flu and pneumococcal vaccines up-to-date.
- Avoid crowds and persons with infections.
- To learn more: American Lung Association, 61 Broadway, 6th Floor, New York, NY 10006; (800) 586-4872; website: www.lungusa.org.

MEDICATION
- Bronchodilators (inhaled or oral) may help open up the bronchial tubes and allow passage of air. This is supervised at first by an inhalation therapist.
- For minor discomfort, use nonprescription drugs, such as acetaminophen or aspirin.

ACTIVITY—Regular exercise in whatever forms possible is important to preserve lung capacity.

DIET—No special diet.

CALL YOUR DOCTOR IF

- You or a family member has symptoms of asbestosis.
- New symptoms develop or other symptoms get worse, despite treatment.

ASTHMA

GENERAL INFORMATION

DEFINITION—Asthma involves blockage of normal airflow into and out of the lungs. The blockage develops when certain allergens or irritants are inhaled and cause a reaction in the airways. They become swollen (inflamed), produce excess mucus, and the airway muscles tighten. This leads to the wheezing and other symptoms.

BODY PARTS INVOLVED—Lungs; bronchi; bronchioles.

SEX OR AGE MOST AFFECTED—It affects all ages but 50% of the cases are in children under age 10. Boys with asthma outnumber girls. In adult-onset asthma, women are more often affected.

SIGNS & SYMPTOMS
● Chest tightness. Wheezing upon breathing in or out.
● Coughing, especially at night, may have thick, clear or yellow sputum.
● Rapid, shallow breathing that is easier with sitting up.
● Breathing difficulty that gradually gets worse.
● Neck and chest may be sucked in with each breath.
● Severe symptoms of an asthma attack may be:
  - Cough that sounds tight and dry.
  - Rapid heartbeat and abnormal rapid rate of breathing that becomes more labored.
  - Can speak only a few words in one breath.
  - Sweating, and much anxiety and distress.

CAUSES—The exact cause remains unclear. Genetic factors, airway sensitivity, and environmental factors appear to play a role. Asthma attacks are due to triggers (e.g., smoke, polluted air, molds, dust, aspirin, cold air, lung infections, and others).

RISK INCREASES WITH
● Other allergies, such as eczema or hay fever.
● Family history of asthma or allergies.
● Exposure to air pollutants.
● Obesity.
● Smoking; exposure to second-hand smoke.
● For adults, exposure to occupational irritants (fumes, gases, latex products, metals, and others).
● Low birth weight.

HOW TO PREVENT—No specific preventive measures for original disease. Avoiding risk factors where possible may help.

WHAT TO EXPECT

DIAGNOSTIC MEASURES
● Your own observation of symptoms.
● Your health care provider will do a physical exam and ask questions about your symptoms.

● Medical tests may include x-rays, pulmonary-function tests, an exercise tolerance test, and allergy tests (usually skin testing).

APPROPRIATE HEALTH CARE
● Treatment will depend on the severity of the symptoms. It may include daily drug therapy, drug therapy for attacks, avoiding triggers, lifestyle changes, self-care, and education. A written treatment plan is usually provided. It should be followed carefully.
● Counseling may help, if asthma is stress-related.
● Treatment (allergy shots) to desensitize the immune system to specific allergens may be recommended.
● Hospital care sometimes for severe attacks.

POSSIBLE COMPLICATIONS
● Pneumonia, pneumothorax, or respiratory failure.
● Status asthmaticus (an attack that cannot be relieved).
● Poorly controlled asthma; chronic symptoms.
● Missed workdays or school absenteeism.
● Problems of stress, depression, or anxiety.

PROBABLE OUTCOME
● Symptoms can be controlled with treatment.
● Half the children will outgrow asthma.

HOW TO TREAT

GENERAL MEASURES
● Identify and avoid your triggering factors.
● A peak flow meter may be used at home. It is a small device that measures how well air flows into and out of the airways. You will be instructed on its use.
● To learn more: Asthma & Allergy Foundation of America, 1233 20th St., Suite 402, Washington, DC 20036; (800) 727-8462; website: www.aafa.org.

MEDICATION
● Asthma drugs are divided into 2 categories:
  - Quick relief. Prescribed for relief of asthma exacerbations and to prevent exercised-induced asthma (EIA) symptoms.
  - Long-term control. Prescribed for use on a daily basis to prevent symptoms.

ACTIVITY—Stay active. Avoid sudden bursts of activity. Swimming is a good exercise to try.

DIET—No special diet, but avoid foods to which you are sensitive. Drink plenty of fluids daily.

CALL YOUR DOCTOR IF

● You or a family member has symptoms of asthma.
● Symptoms don't improve, despite treatment.
● Peak flow is in a zone that worries you.

ATELECTASIS

GENERAL INFORMATION

DEFINITION—Atelectasis is the collapse of lung tissue affecting part or all of one lung. It prevents normal lung function.

BODY PARTS INVOLVED—Lungs.

SEX OR AGE MOST AFFECTED—Atelectasis can affect all ages, but is more common in children under age 10.

SIGNS & SYMPTOMS
- Sudden, major collapse:
  - Chest pain.
  - Shortness of breath; rapid breathing.
  - Shock (weakness, pale skin, rapid heartbeat).
  - Dizziness.
- Gradual collapse:
  - Cough.
  - Fever.
  - Shortness of breath.
  - Sometimes, no symptoms are noticed.

CAUSES
- Obstructive atelectasis (most common type):
  - Thick mucous plugs from infection or other disease.
  - Inhaled objects, such as small toys or peanuts.
  - Surgery of the chest (thoracic) or abdomen.
- Nonobstructive atelectasis:
  - Pleural effusion (fluid in the lungs).
  - Pneumothorax (air in space around the lung).
  - Tumors.
  - Lack of surfactant (a substance in the lungs).
  - Scarring of lung tissue (due to disease such as asthma or cystic fibrosis).
  - Trauma (injury) to the lung.
  - Enlarged lymph glands.

RISK INCREASES WITH
- Anesthesia.
- Lung diseases (e.g., emphysema, asthma, or cancer).
- Obesity.
- Smoking.
- Injury to the chest.
- Conditions that limit physical activity (e.g., bed rest).

HOW TO PREVENT
- Medical care to help prevent postsurgical problems.
- Keep small objects that might be inhaled away from young children (such as peanuts).

WHAT TO EXPECT

DIAGNOSTIC MEASURES
- Your own observation of symptoms.
- Your health care provider will do a physical exam.

- Medical tests may include blood studies to measure oxygen and carbon dioxide levels, x-rays, or CT of the chest.

APPROPRIATE HEALTH CARE
- Treatment depends on the cause. It may include drug therapy, chest physical therapy, bronchoscopy, and (rarely) surgery.
- Chest physical therapy may be done to help remove mucous from the lungs. It involves clapping, patting, and massaging the chest and back over the lungs. The lungs may be suctioned with a small plastic tube.
- Bronchoscopy may be done to remove foreign objects or a mucous plug. This involves using an instrument with a lighted tip to see inside the lungs.
- Disabling, chronic atelectasis may have to be treated with surgery to remove the affected part of the lung.
- A tumor may require surgery or radiation therapy.

POSSIBLE COMPLICATIONS—Infection and chronic lung damage.

PROBABLE OUTCOME—Outcome is generally good. It usually resolves with treatment. Complications are rare, but will depend on any underlying cause.

HOW TO TREAT

GENERAL MEASURES
- Cooperate with requests to turn, cough and breathe deeply after surgery. Hold a pillow tightly against surgical incisions during the coughing exercises.
- Stop smoking.
- To learn more: American Lung Association, 61 Broadway, 6th Floor, New York, NY 10006; (800) 586-4872; website: www.lungusa.org.

MEDICATION
- Antibiotics for infection will be prescribed.
- Bronchodilators to assist breathing may be prescribed.
- Pain relievers may be prescribed.

ACTIVITY—Resume your normal activities as soon as symptoms improve. Take frequent showers. Try to avoid low-humidity environments.

DIET—No special diet. Drink plenty of water or other fluids daily to thin lung secretions.

CALL YOUR DOCTOR IF

- You or a family member has symptoms of atelectasis.
- Symptoms return after treatment. Atelectasis can recur.

ATHEROSCLEROSIS
(Hardening of the Arteries)

 GENERAL INFORMATION

DEFINITION
- Atherosclerosis is the hardening or narrowing of the arteries. Arteries are blood vessels that carry blood and oxygen to the heart, brain, and other body parts. Atherosclerosis leads to:
  - Coronary artery disease (a risk for heart attack or heart failure).
  - Carotid artery disease (a risk for stroke).
  - Peripheral artery disease—which affects legs, arms, stomach, or kidneys—(a risk for intermittent claudication (leg cramps), poor wound healing, and infections).
  - Aneurysms (a bulge in an artery wall).
  - Kidney disease.

BODY PARTS INVOLVED—All arterial blood vessels in the body.

SEX OR AGE MOST AFFECTED—It can begin in childhood and progress slowly as people age. In some people, it progresses more rapidly. Up to age 45, it is more common in men. After menopause, women are equally affected.

SIGNS & SYMPTOMS
- Symptoms often are absent until atherosclerosis reaches advanced stages. Symptoms depend on what part of the body has a decreased blood flow and the extent of disease.
- Muscle cramps if it involves leg blood vessels.
- Angina pectoris (chest pain) or a heart attack if it involves blood vessels to the heart.
- Stroke or transient ischemic attack if it involves vessels to the neck and brain.
- Abdominal cramps or pain if blood vessels to the abdomen are involved.

CAUSES—Plaque (made up of cholesterol, muscle cells, fibrous tissue, and calcium) builds up on artery walls that have been damaged in some way. Plaque deposits can grow large enough to reduce blood flow and can also crack or break apart and form clots. Clots can block blood flow or travel to another part of the body and cause serious or fatal problems.

RISK INCREASES WITH
- High blood pressure.
- Diabetes.
- High levels of LDL (the bad cholesterol).
- Low levels of HDL (the good cholesterol).
- Obesity and/or lack of physical activity.
- Smoking.
- Family history of atherosclerosis.
- Diet high in saturated fats and trans fatty acids.

HOW TO PREVENT
- Eat a healthy, low-fat, high-fiber diet. Maintain a healthy weight. Exercise daily. Don't smoke.
- Control diabetes and high blood pressure.
- Control cholesterol levels.

 WHAT TO EXPECT

DIAGNOSTIC MEASURES
- Your own observation of any symptoms.
- Your health care provider may do a physical exam. Questions will be asked about your symptoms, smoking, alcohol use, drug use, exercise, and personal and family medical history. Blood pressure and pulse rate are checked. A stethoscope is used to listen for sounds of blood flow in the arteries.
- Blood studies are done for cholesterol, triglycerides, and blood sugar. Heart function tests (such as exercise stress tests and coronary calcium scores) and blood flow tests may be done.

APPROPRIATE HEALTH CARE
- Treatment includes drug therapy and lifestyle changes. Treatment for organ damage caused by atherosclerosis depends on organ involved.
- Lifestyle changes include diet changes, losing weight, stopping smoking, and exercising.

POSSIBLE COMPLICATIONS
- Coronary artery disease, which is the number one cause of death in men and women.
- Other disorders as listed in Definition.

PROBABLE OUTCOME—There is no cure, but atherosclerosis can be slowed or even partially reversed. If organ damage has developed due to reduced blood flow, the outcome will vary.

 HOW TO TREAT

GENERAL MEASURES—To learn more: American Heart Association, local branch listed in telephone directory, or call (800) 242-8721; website: www.americanheart.org.

MEDICATION—Drugs may be prescribed to slow or sometimes reverse the effects of atherosclerosis (e.g., for high cholesterol, blood clot prevention, or high blood pressure).

ACTIVITY—Activity may depend on state of health. Try to exercise for 30 or more minutes a day 5 to 7 days a week.

DIET—Eat a low-fat, high-fiber diet, that includes fruits and vegetables. Begin a weight-loss diet, if overweight.

 CALL YOUR DOCTOR IF

You or a family member has symptoms of, or concerns about, atherosclerosis.

ATHLETE'S FOOT
(Tinea Pedis; Ringworm of the Feet)

 GENERAL INFORMATION

DEFINITION—Athlete's foot is a common, contagious fungal (tinea) infection of the skin on the feet.

BODY PARTS INVOLVED—Feet, especially the soles and skin between toes (usually 4th and 5th toes).

SEX OR AGE MOST AFFECTED—It usually affects males more than females and teens and adults (rare in young children).

SIGNS & SYMPTOMS
- Moist, soft, gray-white or red scales on feet, especially between toes.
- Dead skin between toes.
- Itching in inflamed areas.
- Damp, musty foot odor.
- Small blisters on the feet (sometimes).

CAUSES—Infection by *Trichophyton rubrum* or other fungus. The germs can be spread by direct contact with an infected person, or by contact with the germs on shoes, socks, shower, or pool surfaces. Animals can also carry the germs and infect a human.

RISK INCREASES WITH
- Infrequent changes of shoes or socks.
- Use of locker rooms and public showers.
- Persistent moisture around the feet (e.g., wearing air-tight shoes).
- Hot, humid weather.
- People who have immune system problems due to illness or medications.
- Diabetes.
- People who are more susceptible to the infection.
- Having other fungal infection (e.g., jock itch).

HOW TO PREVENT
- Keep feet clean and dry. Bathe feet often. Dry completely between the toes. Apply talcum or antifungal powder to help maintain dryness.
- Wear rubber or wooden sandals in public showers.
- Go barefoot when possible.
- Change socks daily Wear socks made of cotton, wool, or other natural, absorbent fibers. Avoid synthetics.
- Wear shoes that are not air-tight.

 WHAT TO EXPECT

DIAGNOSTIC MEASURES
- Your own observation of symptoms.
- See your health care provider if the symptoms are severe, don't respond to self-care, or you have a chronic illness. Your health care provider can usually diagnose athlete's foot by looking at the affected skin area. Certain skin tests may be done to rule out other skin disorders.

APPROPRIATE HEALTH CARE—Your health care provider may recommend special drug therapy.

POSSIBLE COMPLICATIONS
- A bacterial infection may develop in the affected area.
- A skin rash can sometimes develop on the hands and face (rare).

PROBABLE OUTCOME—Usually curable in 3 weeks with treatment, but recurrence is common. In some cases, the infection is more severe and will take longer to control.

 HOW TO TREAT

GENERAL MEASURES
- After soaking or bathing, carefully remove scales and material between the toes daily.
- Use a hair dryer to blow warm air on the feet to make sure they are completely dry.
- Keep affected areas cool and dry. Go barefoot or wear sandals during treatment. If socks are worn, keep them dry. If they get wet, change to dry ones.

MEDICATION
- Use nonprescription antifungal powders, creams, or ointments (such as terbinafine). Follow instructions on the product.
- For severe cases, you may be prescribed oral, or stronger topical antifungal drugs.
- Antibiotics may be prescribed if a bacterial infection develops.

ACTIVITY—No limits. Avoid activities that cause feet to sweat until healing is complete.

DIET—No special diet.

 CALL YOUR DOCTOR IF

- You or a family member has symptoms of athlete's foot that persist, despite self-treatment.
- New, unexplained symptoms develop. Drugs used in treatment may produce side effects.

ATRIAL FIBRILLATION

GENERAL INFORMATION

DEFINITION—Atrial fibrillation is an abnormal heart rhythm. Fibrillation is a "quivering" of muscles. Atrial pertains to the atria, the upper chambers of the heart. An abnormal rhythm reduces the flow of blood through the heart to the brain and other body parts.

BODY PARTS INVOLVED—Heart muscles; the atrium (also called auricle), a chamber of the heart that connects to the left ventricle (main chamber); heart's electrical conduction system.

SEX OR AGE MOST AFFECTED—It usually affects older adults and men more than women.

SIGNS & SYMPTOMS
- There may be no symptoms.
- Irregular and often rapid beating of the heart.
- Weakness, dizziness, shortness of breath, chest pain, or faintness may occur.

CAUSES—The heart has an electrical system that controls the heart rate and the heart's contractions. The average heart beats at a rate of 60 to 100 times per minute. With atrial fibrillation, the electrical system does not function as it should. The atria quiver instead of contracting and the heart rate increases (may exceed 160 beats a minute). There are different risk factors that can lead to atrial fibrillation and sometimes no cause is found.

RISK INCREASES WITH
- Increased age.
- Coronary heart disease.
- High blood pressure.
- Abnormal heart muscle.
- Mitral valve disease.
- Hyperthyroidism.
- Lung disease (chronic obstructive pulmonary disease, emphysema).
- Pericarditis (heart lining inflammation).
- Pulmonary embolism.
- Congestive heart failure.
- Recent heart or lung surgery.
- Excessive alcohol use.
- Congenital (present at birth) heart defects.
- Lone atrial fibrillation in young, healthy adults.

HOW TO PREVENT—No specific preventive measures. Avoid risk factors where possible.

WHAT TO EXPECT

DIAGNOSTIC MEASURES
- Your own observation of symptoms.
- Your health care provider will do a physical exam and ask questions about your symptoms. A stethoscope (device for listening to body sounds) is used to detect heart rhythms.
- Medical tests may include blood studies, an electrocardiogram, or other heart function tests.

APPROPRIATE HEALTH CARE
- Treatment is aimed at treating the cause of the atrial fibrillation, slowing the heart rate, converting the abnormal rhythm to normal, preventing a recurrence, and preventing complications.
- Treatment steps may include drug therapy, electrocardioversion, surgery, or other procedures.
- Abnormal heart rhythm may be converted to normal rhythm with drug therapy or with electric shock (electrocardioversion). An electric shock stops the abnormal activity and allows the normal rhythm to take over.
- Recurring atrial fibrillation may be treated with a variety of procedures. These include a pacemaker or atrial defibrillator implantation, AV node ablation, Maze procedure (atrial surgery), and pulmonary vein isolation.
- Some patients may be left in atrial fibrillation long-term if the heart rate is under control.

POSSIBLE COMPLICATIONS
- Stroke.
- Arterial thrombosis or embolus (blood clots).
- Congestive heart failure.
- Other heartbeat irregularities can lead to cardiac arrest.

PROBABLE OUTCOME—It can often be controlled with treatment. Atrial fibrillation tends to become a chronic condition.

HOW TO TREAT

GENERAL MEASURES
- Don't smoke.
- Learn to check your own pulse for rate (beats per minute) and rhythm (regular or irregular).
- To learn more: American Heart Association, local branch listed in telephone directory, or call (800) 242-8721; website: www.americanheart.org.

MEDICATION—Drugs may be prescribed for the underlying risk factor, to slow the heart rate, maintain normal heart rhythm, and to prevent blood clots.

ACTIVITY—Try to exercise for 30 or more minutes a day 5 to 7 days a week. Activity may depend on your health status.

DIET—Eat a low-fat, high-fiber diet that includes fruits and vegetables. Begin a weight loss diet, if overweight.

CALL YOUR DOCTOR IF

- You or a family member has symptoms of atrial fibrillation.
- Any change in heart rate, chest pain, weakness, shortness of breath, or swollen feet and ankles occurs.

ATTENTION-DEFICIT HYPERACTIVITY DISORDER IN ADULTS

GENERAL INFORMATION

DEFINITION—Attention-deficit hyperactivity disorder (ADHD) in adults always begins in childhood. As children with ADHD or ADD (attention deficit disorder) get older, their hyperactive-impulsive qualities often decrease, while the inattentive and disorganized patterns of behavior persist. These behaviors can impact all areas of adult life. Symptoms of adult ADHD vary from person to person and may be mild to severe. Many adults with ADHD also have mood or anxiety disorders.

BODY PARTS INVOLVED—Brain.

SEX OR AGE MOST AFFECTED—Adults. Males are more often affected than females.

SIGNS & SYMPTOMS
- Trouble in focusing or concentrating.
- Restlessness.
- Difficulty in starting or completing tasks.
- Delays, postpones, or puts off doing things.
- Disorganized.
- Does not appear to hear.
- Poor time management.
- Frequently losing things.
- Unstable relationships.
- Chronic lateness and forgetfulness.

CAUSES—Unknown. Hereditary, environmental factors, and altered brain function and anatomy appear to be involved.

RISK INCREASES WITH
- Family history of ADHD.
- Males more than females.
- Certain environmental factors (e.g., mother who smoked or abused alcohol while pregnant).

HOW TO PREVENT—Cannot be prevented.

WHAT TO EXPECT

DIAGNOSTIC MEASURES
- Your own or other's observation of symptoms.
- Your health care provider may do a physical exam. Questions will be asked about your symptoms (in childhood and current) and how they affect work or school and relationships with friends and family. You may be asked to fill out a questionnaire. There is no specific test to confirm the diagnosis.

APPROPRIATE HEALTH CARE
- Treatment will depend on each individual's needs and severity of the symptoms. Treatment typically involves drugs and/or psychological counseling.
- Counseling (sometimes called life coaching) may focus on improving certain skills such as organization and time management.

- Cognitive behavioral therapy helps you control your behavior and change negative thinking patterns into positive ones.
- Family and marital counseling can help with your personal relationships.

POSSIBLE COMPLICATIONS
- Poor school performance or problems at work.
- Trouble with the law.
- Alcohol or drug abuse.
- Frequent car accidents or other accidents.
- Problems with relationships; low self-esteem.

PROBABLE OUTCOME—Treatment can help improve symptoms and allow patients to lead productive lives. ADHD in adults is a lifelong condition and may require ongoing treatment.

HOW TO TREAT

GENERAL MEASURES
- Educate yourself about ADHD.
- Find ways to keep yourself organized. Keep an appointment book or planning calendar. Make a list of tasks to be done each day. Break down larger tasks into smaller steps. Use sticky pads to write notes to yourself. Carry a notepad or electronic device with you. Set up filing systems (paper and computer).
- Follow a routine that is as consistent as possible from day to day.
- Ask for help from family members or others.
- Join an adult ADHD support group to share experiences and coping techniques.
- To learn more: Children & Adults with Attention Deficit/Hyperactivity Disorder (CHADD), 8181 Professional Pl., Suite 150, Landover, MD 20785; (800) 233-4050; website: www.chadd.org.

MEDICATION
- Stimulant drugs or other drugs approved for ADHD may be prescribed. It may take time to find the drug and dosage that works best for you. Your health care provider will discuss their benefits and risks.
- Drugs to treat other diagnosed disorders may be prescribed (e.g., for anxiety or depression).

ACTIVITY—Exercise daily. It can improve your mood, relieve stress, calm your mind, and help burn off excess energy.

DIET—Eat a healthy diet. Ask your health care provider if you need to make any specific diet changes.

CALL YOUR DOCTOR IF

- You or a family member has symptoms of adult ADHD.
- New or worsening symptoms develop.

ATTENTION-DEFICIT HYPERACTIVITY DISORDER IN CHILDREN

 GENERAL INFORMATION

DEFINITION—Attention-deficit hyperactivity disorder (ADHD) is a consistent pattern of behavior that includes inattention, hyperactivity, and impulsivity. It is called ADD (attention deficit disorder) without hyperactivity. ADHD is common in children.

BODY PARTS INVOLVED—Brain.

SEX OR AGE MOST AFFECTED—Boys are affected more than girls. The symptoms may appear at ages 4 to 7 and peak between 8 and 10. It also affects adults.

SIGNS & SYMPTOMS
- Squirms in seat; fidgets with hands or feet.
- Unable to stay seated when required to do so.
- Easily distracted.
- Blurts out answers before a question is finished.
- Difficulty waiting turn in games and lines.
- Difficulty following instructions.
- Unable to sustain attention in work or play activities.
- Shifts from one uncompleted project to another.
- Difficulty playing quietly. Talks excessively.
- Interrupts or intrudes on others.
- Doesn't appear to listen.
- Loses items needed for tasks.
- Often engages in dangerous activities without considering consequences.

CAUSES—Unknown. Genetic and environmental factors appear to play a role.

RISK INCREASES WITH
- Family history of the disorder.
- Males more than females.
- Certain environmental factors (e.g., mother smoking or abusing alcohol while pregnant).

HOW TO PREVENT—No preventive measures known.

 WHAT TO EXPECT

DIAGNOSTIC MEASURES
- The child's teacher may be the first to notice the behavior. A school psychologist, your child's doctor, or a special health care provider may diagnose the disorder.
- Several methods are used to help make the diagnosis. These include observing the child doing activities, tests (mental, social, and intelligence), parent's and teacher's evaluation, and rating scales about behaviors.

APPROPRIATE HEALTH CARE
- Treatment for children includes appropriate classroom setting, behavior therapy, drug therapy, and help for parents in managing the child's behavior. A combination of these techniques will have the best outcome.
- Counseling can help, as can behavior and cognitive therapy. These help patients focus on ways to change the undesired behavior.
- Special education classes for all or part of the day may be needed for some children.

POSSIBLE COMPLICATIONS
- Higher risk of school, work, and relationship problems; conduct disorders; antisocial behavior; car accidents.
- Other conditions may be associated with ADHD such as learning diabilities and mood or conduct disorders.

PROBABLE OUTCOME—Most children improve with treatment. Symptoms often decrease with age.

 HOW TO TREAT

GENERAL MEASURES
- Help your child at home by providing a structured environment, well-defined behavior limits, and consistent use of parenting techniques.
- Stay in close contact with the child's teacher. Arrange for extra lessons or tutoring if needed.
- Support groups or parenting skills training are helpful.
- To learn more: Children & Adults with Attention Deficit/Hyperactivity Disorder (CHADD), 8181 Professional Pl., Suite 150, Landover, MD 20785; (800) 233-4050; website: www.chadd.org.

MEDICATION—Stimulant drugs (they have a calming affect on persons with ADHD) or other drugs approved for ADHD may be prescribed. Some of these drugs have side effects, such as sleep problems, depression, headache, loss of appetite, stomach ache, and others. Drug benefits and risks will be explained to you.

ACTIVITY—Schedule routine physical activity for your child. It can help a child focus, become more calm, and burn excess energy.

DIET—Provide healthy meals for your child. Ask your child's health care provider about whether you need to make any diet changes.

 CALL YOUR DOCTOR IF

- You believe your child or a family member has symptoms of ADHD or ADD.
- New or worsening symptoms develop.

AUTISM

GENERAL INFORMATION

DEFINITION—Autism is a disorder that involves the way a child develops. Parents may notice that an infant or child is not behaving, talking, playing, or learning new skills as expected for their age group. Asperger's syndrome is like autism, but without the disabilities. It can range from mild to severe.

BODY PARTS INVOLVED—Total body.

SEX OR AGE MOST AFFECTED—It is usually discovered by the time a child is age 2 and a half, but could be later.

SIGNS & SYMPTOMS
- Does not talk or may talk using nonsense words. May use a sing-song voice and repeat what they hear. Unable to carry on a conversation.
- Does not respond to name and avoids eye contact.
- Is over active; wants to play alone; does not smile.
- Repeats the same movements over and over such as rocking and flapping or twisting hands.
- Has special routines and does not like change.
- Does not want to be touched, such as being cuddled.
- May injure self by head-banging or biting.
- Is bothered by noises.
- Overly interested in lights or moving objects.

CAUSES—Unknown. It appears to have a genetic basis, but nongenetic factors are also involved. It is known that parents do not cause autism. There is no scientific proof to link childhood vaccines to autism.

RISK INCREASES WITH—Unknown. It does affect boys more than girls.

HOW TO PREVENT—None known. Autism cannot currently be detected at birth or through any prenatal tests.

WHAT TO EXPECT

DIAGNOSTIC MEASURES
- Your own observation of symptoms.
- Diagnosis is difficult, as the signs and symptoms may appear to be caused by another disorder or problem. There is no specific test for autism.
- Your health care provider (usually a mental health professional) will perform an exam of your child and ask you about your child's behavior and other signs or symptoms you may have observed.
- Tests for speech and other skills may be done to see how your child is developing compared to normal levels for his or her age group.

APPROPRIATE HEALTH CARE
- Treatment for autism should be started as soon as a child is diagnosed. Speech and behavior therapy and social skills training will help children with autism.
- There is no cure for autism. Treatments can help with many of the symptoms. The treatment plan for each child will depend on how mild or severe their symptoms are. Some children may be able to attend regular public schools. Others may require a special classroom.
- The treatment steps take time and patience. Different treatment methods may need to be tried for a child.
- Counseling may help some parents cope with the stress involved with raising an autistic child.
- Other treatments for autism are being studied and may be recommended for your child in the future. There are certain treatments that parents or others have tried and found to work for one or a few children. These treatments may or may not work for other autistic children. Always talk to your child's health care provider before you try any new type of treatment.

POSSIBLE COMPLICATIONS
- Parents of an autistic child have an increased risk of having another child with the disorder.
- Stress for the family raising an autistic child.
- Autistic children are at a higher risk for seizures.

PROBABLE OUTCOME—The future is unknown for most autistic children. A child may be mentally retarded, have normal intelligence, or even have a genius-like ability. As they get older, their symptoms may improve, stay about the same, or worsen. Some children will need supervision for life. Some may be able to live independently.

HOW TO TREAT

GENERAL MEASURES
- Join an autism family support group.
- To learn more: Autism Society of America, 7910 Woodmount Avenue, Suite 300, Bethesda, MD 20814-3015; (800) 328-8476; website: www.autism-society.org.

MEDICATION—There are no drugs that specifically treat autism. Drugs may be prescribed for certain symptoms (e.g., self-injury behavior, aggression, hyperactivity, or others).

ACTIVITY—Help your child to stay as physically active as possible.

DIET—Provide child a healthy diet. Seek medical advice before starting any special diet.

CALL YOUR DOCTOR IF

Your child is not developing as expected for his or her age.

BACK PAIN, LOW
(Sciatica)

 GENERAL INFORMATION

DEFINITION—Low back pain is pain and stiffness that affects the lower part of the back (the area from the rib cage to the tailbone). It is usually acute (lasting a few days to a few weeks). It is a common medical problem.

BODY PARTS INVOLVED—Lower back.

SEX OR AGE MOST AFFECTED—Can affect anyone at anytime; often occurs in ages 20 to 65.

SIGNS & SYMPTOMS
- Symptoms may develop quickly or have a slow onset.
- Pain, stiffness, and soreness in the lower back. It may be ongoing, or only occur when you are in certain positions. The pain may get worse by coughing, sneezing, bending, or twisting.
- The symptoms may occur in a cycle, starting with a muscle spasm; the spasm then causes pain; the pain results in another muscle spasm.
- Sciatica (pain that runs down the leg) in some cases.

CAUSES
- It is usually caused by sprains or strains that can affect the lower back's muscles, tendons, ligaments, nerves, joints, discs, and bones. This back pain is sometimes referred to as non-specific low back pain as it is unclear just what part(s) of the lower back are causing the pain. (Even x-rays or other tests are often not helpful.)
- Specific back pain is less common. It can be caused by disorders such as spinal stenosis or arthritis.

RISK INCREASES WITH
- Ages 20 to 65.
- Family history of back pain.
- Previous back injury, back surgery, or spine problem.
- Overweight.
- Smoking.
- Poor body mechanics and poor posture.
- Work or tasks that require a lot of sitting or heavy lifting, bending or twisting, or repetitive motions.
- Bone and joint conditions of the back.
- Injury or a fracture.
- Congenital problem (being born with).
- Pregnancy.
- Certain sports or recreational activities.
- Emotional factors (e.g., stress, depression, others).

HOW TO PREVENT
- Low back pain cannot always be prevented.
- Exercise (both aerobic and strength-building).
- Lift heavy objects carefully. Use good posture. Lose weight, if overweight. Don't smoke.

 WHAT TO EXPECT

DIAGNOSTIC MEASURES
- Your own observation of symptoms.
- Your health care provider will do a physical exam and ask questions about your back pain symptoms and activities.
- Medical tests may be done in some cases. Tests may include x-rays, CT, or MRI.

APPROPRIATE HEALTH CARE
- The treatment that works best for most people is a combination of self-care and drug therapy (to help relieve symptoms).
- Counseling (e.g., for depression or stress).
- Other therapy options may help some people. These can include massage, chiropractic care, yoga, acupuncture, ultrasound, or electrical nerve stimulation. Surgery for disc damage may rarely be needed.

POSSIBLE COMPLICATIONS—Chronic or recurring low back pain.

PROBABLE OUTCOME—Most people will recover within 2 to 6 weeks.

 HOW TO TREAT

GENERAL MEASURES
- An ice pack, cold massage, heating pad, or warm compress may help to reduce pain.
- Stop smoking. Find a plan that works for you.
- To learn more: National Institute of Arthritis & Musculoskeletal & Skin Disorders, (877) 226-4267; website: www.niams.nih.gov.

MEDICATION
- Use nonprescription pain drugs such as aspirin, ibuprofen, or acetaminophen.
- Stronger pain drugs, anti-inflammatories, muscle relaxants, or antidepressants may be prescribed.

ACTIVITY
- Avoid or limit any bed rest (no more than 1 to 2 days). Resume your usual activities as soon as possible.
- As pain eases, begin an exercise program. Focus on back and abdominal strength, flexibility, and posture.
- Physical therapy may be prescribed.

DIET—No special diet. A weight-reduction diet may help if overweight is a problem.

☎ CALL YOUR DOCTOR IF

- You or a family member has low back pain that persists for 3 or 4 days after self-care.
- Back pain is severe or recurrent.

BALANITIS

GENERAL INFORMATION

DEFINITION—Balanitis is an inflammation of the glans (head) of the penis and sometimes the foreskin as well. It is a common condition in males. It occurs more often in males who have a foreskin (have not been circumcised).

BODY PARTS INVOLVED—Penis and foreskin.

SEX OR AGE MOST AFFECTED—Males of all ages.

SIGNS & SYMPTOMS
- Tenderness, redness, itching, and swelling of the head of the penis.
- Inflammation of the foreskin.
- Unable to retract foreskin (phimosis).
- Impotence.
- Discharge from the penis.
- Burning during urination (rare).

CAUSES—The inflammation is a reaction to infection (most common cause), injury, or irritation of the penis. Sometimes the cause is unknown.

RISK INCREASES WITH
- Diabetes.
- Poor hygiene.
- Allergy to chemicals in clothing, contraceptive cream, or condom latex.
- Reaction to certain drugs.
- Trauma or minor injury to the foreskin and penis.
- Presence of foreskin.
- Sexual partner affected by vaginitis (rare).
- Being very obese.

HOW TO PREVENT
- Wash daily with soap and water and wash after sexual intercourse. Clean carefully under the foreskin.
- Control diabetes or other medical conditions.
- Weight loss for obese males.
- Using a latex condom during intercourse may help to prevent some infections.

WHAT TO EXPECT

DIAGNOSTIC MEASURES
- Your own observation of symptoms.
- Your health care provider can usually diagnose the disorder by an exam of the penis.
- A culture of the discharge from the penis and tests for other medical disorders (such as diabetes) may be done. If balanitis persists, a biopsy (tissue sample is removed for an exam) may be done to rule out cancer.

APPROPRIATE HEALTH CARE
- Treatment usually involves drugs applied to the penis and practicing good hygiene.
- A foreskin that cannot be retracted may be treated with topical steroid drugs, stretching techniques (done for 2 to 3 weeks), or by a special slit made in the foreskin.
- Surgery may be recommended to circumcise the penis if balanitis recurs often or scar tissue develops.

POSSIBLE COMPLICATIONS
- Chronic inflammation can cause:
  - Scarring and narrowing of the opening of the penis (urethral stricture).
  - Phimosis (difficult to retract the foreskin).
  - Paraphimosis (unable to replace the foreskin to cover the head of the penis).
  - Urinary tract infection.

PROBABLE OUTCOME—Usually curable in 1 to 2 weeks with treatment.

HOW TO TREAT

GENERAL MEASURES—Use warm-water soaks to relieve pain or discomfort.

MEDICATION
- Antibiotics to be applied to the penis are usually prescribed. Rarely, antibiotics to be taken by mouth may be prescribed.
- Steroid skin creams may be prescribed.
- Use acetaminophen or ibuprofen to relieve minor pain.

ACTIVITY
- Avoid sexual intercourse during treatment.
- Resume your normal activities when the infection is cured.

DIET—No special diet.

CALL YOUR DOCTOR IF

- You or a family member has symptoms of balanitis.
- Symptoms don't improve in 3 days, despite treatment.

BALDNESS, PATTERN

GENERAL INFORMATION

DEFINITION—Pattern baldness is the gradual, painless hair loss that occurs in a certain pattern as a person ages. The medical term is androgenetic alopecia. The earlier the hair loss begins, the greater the eventual loss. Some persons have short periods of intense hair loss followed by long, stable periods.

BODY PARTS INVOLVED—Hair; scalp.

SEX OR AGE MOST AFFECTED—In men, hair loss appears as early as the teens; in women, it rarely appears before their 50's.

SIGNS & SYMPTOMS
- In men, hair thins on top of the head and recedes in the temple and front areas.
- In women, hair tends to thin on top of the head.
- Both sexes may have scattered hair loss.

CAUSES—It is probably due to a combination of hormonal and genetic factors. Male hormones (most often, androgens) are an important factor in balding. Estrogen (a female hormone) may be protective in women, because hair loss rarely begins before menopause. Hair loss that occurs after illness, pregnancy, or as an adverse reaction to drugs is a different form of baldness. Normal everyday stress is not a cause of pattern baldness.

RISK INCREASES WITH—Family history of pattern baldness.

HOW TO PREVENT—Some drug therapies have been shown to slow or reverse baldness to some degree in some men. Other medical treatments are undergoing study.

WHAT TO EXPECT

DIAGNOSTIC MEASURES
- Your own observation of symptoms.
- Medical history and physical exam by a health care provider, if diagnosis is in doubt.

APPROPRIATE HEALTH CARE—There is usually no need for medical care. If you do have concerns about the hair loss, see your health care provider. If it is not a typical hair loss, medical tests may be done to see if there is another cause.

POSSIBLE COMPLICATIONS
- There are no medical complications.
- Baldness can cause emotional distress, such as anxiety and a negative effect on self-image.

PROBABLE OUTCOME
- There is no cure. Balding can range from partial loss to complete baldness.
- In most cases, men let the process run its course. Use of a hairpiece or hair transplant is acceptable to some. Drug therapy may help others.

HOW TO TREAT

GENERAL MEASURES
- If you are not comfortable with the hair loss, there are options that you can consider.
  - Wear a hairpiece (toupee or a wig) or get a hair weave (synthetic hair is sewn into existing hair). Be sure to use care in keeping your scalp clean under the hairpiece.
  - Have a hair-transplantation procedure or scalp-reduction surgery. Be sure to seek information about the risks and benefits before undergoing these procedures.
  - Use drug therapy.
- Be cautious about buying and using hair products that claim to thicken or strengthen hair. They often use oils or waxes to give an effect of thickening.

MEDICATION
- A nonprescription topical drug, minoxidil, seems to help hair growth in some patients. Its effectiveness varies greatly. If it helps you, you need to continue its use indefinitely to sustain hair growth.
- Finasteride is a drug taken by mouth that can be prescribed for hair loss in men. It is not approved for use in women as it may cause birth defects.

ACTIVITY—No limits.

DIET—No special diet.

CALL YOUR DOCTOR IF

You or a family member has concerns about hair loss.

BAROTITIS MEDIA
(Barotrauma)

 GENERAL INFORMATION

DEFINITION—Barotitis media is damage to the middle ear caused by pressure changes.

BODY PARTS INVOLVED—It affects the middle ear and the eustachian tube (a tube from the ear to the back of the nose and throat).

SEX OR AGE MOST AFFECTED—Both sexes; all ages.

SIGNS & SYMPTOMS
- Hearing loss (to varying degrees).
- A plugged feeling in the ear.
- Mild to severe pain in the ears, or over the cheekbones and forehead.
- Dizziness.
- Ringing noises in the ear.
- Crying in infants or young children.

CAUSES
- Damage caused by sudden, increased pressure in the air around you. This occurs in the rapid descent of an airplane or while scuba diving. In these activities, air moves from passages in the nose into the middle ear to maintain equal pressure on both sides of the eardrum. If the tube leading from the nose to the ear doesn't function properly, pressure in the middle ear is less than the outside pressure. The negative pressure in the middle ear sucks the eardrum inward. Blood and mucus may appear later in the middle ear. This damage is more likely if you have a nose or throat infection when scuba diving or traveling by air.
- Injury to external or middle ear (boxing, water skiing, accidents, etc.).

RISK INCREASES WITH
- Recent lung, nose, or throat infection.
- Airplane flight.
- Scuba diving.
- Sky diving.
- High-altitude mountain climbers.
- High-impact sports.
- Pregnancy.

HOW TO PREVENT
- If possible, don't fly when you have a lung, nose, or throat infection. If you must fly anyway, use nonprescription decongestant tablets or sprays. Follow the package instructions.
- During air travel:
  - While taking off or landing, suck on hard candy or chew gum to cause frequent swallowing.
  - Take a moderate-size breath and hold your nose. Try to force air into the eustachian tube by gently puffing out the cheeks with the mouth closed. This is called the Valsalva maneuver.
  - Give an infant a bottle of water or juice while taking off or landing during airplane travel.

 WHAT TO EXPECT

DIAGNOSTIC MEASURES
- Your own observation of symptoms.
- See your health care provider if symptoms continue. An ear exam usually confirms the diagnosis.

APPROPRIATE HEALTH CARE
- In most cases, no treatment is necessary and symptoms disappear in hours or days.
- Rarely, surgery may be required to open the eardrum and release fluid trapped in the middle ear. A plastic tube may be placed in the eardrum to keep it open. The tube falls out on its own in 9 to 12 months.

POSSIBLE COMPLICATIONS
- Permanent hearing loss.
- Ruptured eardrum.
- Middle ear infection.
- Tinnitus (hearing noises in the ear) or vertigo.

PROBABLE OUTCOME—Most cases of barotitis media heal with self-care.

 HOW TO TREAT

GENERAL MEASURES—If fluid drains from the ear, place a small piece of cotton in the outer-ear canal to absorb it.

MEDICATION
- For minor pain, you may use nonprescription decongestants and pain relievers, such as acetaminophen.
- Your health care provider may prescribe other oral or nasal decongestants or oral antihistamine and anti-inflammatory drugs.
- Antibiotics may be prescribed if infection is present.

ACTIVITY—Resume your normal activities as soon as symptoms improve.

DIET—No special diet.

☎ CALL YOUR DOCTOR IF

- You or a family member has symptoms of barotitis media.
- The following occur during treatment: severe headache or other pain, fever, and dizziness.
- New, unexplained symptoms develop. Drugs used in treatment may produce side effects.

BED-WETTING
(Enuresis)

GENERAL INFORMATION

DEFINITION—Bed-wetting (enuresis) is the repeated urination during sleep by a child who is old enough (usually by age 5) to have urinary control. Some children have been wetting the bed all along. This is called primary nocturnal enuresis. Some children start bed-wetting after having been dry at night for at least 6 months. This is called secondary nocturnal enuresis. Most children who wet the bed are healthy.

BODY PARTS INVOLVED—Urinary tract.

SEX OR AGE MOST AFFECTED—It is more common in boys than in girls.

SIGNS & SYMPTOMS—Repeated bed-wetting at night (occasionally during the day). This is not usually a concern until a child is older than 5.

CAUSES—Genetic factors (e.g., inherited) are involved. Delays in maturing, deep sleep, small bladder capacity, polyuria (excess urine), stress, or trauma may play a role. In a few children, a medical illness or other health problem may be the cause.

RISK INCREASES WITH
- Family history of bed-wetting.
- Illness such as diabetes or urinary-tract infection.
- Stress or trauma in a child (e.g., parents divorce, new sibling, moving to new home, abuse, hospital care, and others).

HOW TO PREVENT
- No effective preventive methods are known.
- Show your child love, support, and understanding for this problem.

WHAT TO EXPECT

DIAGNOSTIC MEASURES
- Your own observation of symptoms.
- Talk to your child's health care provider about the bed-wetting problem. A physical exam will be done and questions asked about the symptoms and your child's lifestyle.
- Medical tests are sometimes done to rule out diabetes or other medical problems as causes. These can include urine studies or imaging tests.

APPROPRIATE HEALTH CARE
- Medical care is usually not needed unless there is a health problem diagnosed or parents are interested in drug therapy as a treatment option.
- Counseling may be recommended for the child and the family if there are emotional or stress problems.

POSSIBLE COMPLICATIONS
- Child feels anxious, embarrassed, and shameful. May lead to social withdrawal, loss of self-esteem, or other problems. Parents become frustrated.
- Urinary-tract infection.

PROBABLE OUTCOME—If there are no medical or emotional problems, children normally outgrow the bed-wetting problem. Treatment measures are successful in many cases.

HOW TO TREAT

GENERAL MEASURES
- Follow any medical care advice from your child's health care provider.
- Protect the mattress with a heavy plastic cover.
- Stop using diapers or plastic pants by age 4. They may make it easy for the child to keep on wetting.
- Have the child change the sheet on the bed and do the laundry, if he or she is old enough.
- Have a night light so the child can find the bathroom.
- Have the child urinate at bedtime. You can also wake the child at night to urinate, but this is hard on parents.
- Reward the child for staying dry with praise and hugs. Use gold stars or happy faces to mark dry nights on a calendar.
- Try alarms that are triggered by wetting. These may be used in undergarments, pajamas, or mattresses.
- Respond gently to accidents. Don't blame, nag, restrict, or punish the child who has wet the bed. This can cause him or her to give up or lead to other problems. Your child's bed wetting should resolve with time.

MEDICATION
- The drug vasopressin may be prescribed if other methods fail and the family favors drug therapy.
- Certain other drugs may be recommended for some.

ACTIVITY—No limits.

DIET—Encourage your child to drink as needed during the day. Limit or discontinue any fluid intake during the 2 to 3 hours before bedtime.

CALL YOUR DOCTOR IF

- You are concerned about your child's bed-wetting and your child is older than 6.
- The child has any problems when urinating.

BELL'S PALSY

GENERAL INFORMATION

DEFINITION—Bell's palsy is a paralysis or weakness on one side of the face. The onset may be sudden, or may come on over several days.

BODY PARTS INVOLVED—7th cranial nerve and the facial muscles that connect to the nerve.

SEX OR AGE MOST AFFECTED—Both sexes. It most often affects people over the age of 13 and occurs more often in young adults.

SIGNS & SYMPTOMS
- Sudden paralysis on one side of the face, including muscles to the eyelid.
- Pain in or around the ear on the affected side.
- Numbness on the side of the face.
- Flat, expressionless features on one side of the face.
- Distorted smiles and frowns; drooling.
- Changes in taste, saliva, or tear formation.

CAUSES—Unknown. It may be linked to a viral infection. The paralysis is probably caused by swelling and inflammation of the facial nerve as it passes through the temporal bone of the skull.

RISK INCREASES WITH
- Common cold, flu, other upper respiratory infection.
- Pregnancy.
- Diabetes.

HOW TO PREVENT—No preventive measures.

WHAT TO EXPECT

DIAGNOSTIC MEASURES
- Your own observation of symptoms.
- Your health care provider will do a physical exam of the affected area.
- Medical tests such as x-ray may be done to rule out other causes. A nerve study of the facial nerves may be done to determine the extent of nerve damage.

APPROPRIATE HEALTH CARE
- Treatment may include self-care measures, drug therapy if needed, and surgery.
- Surgery on the facial nerve may (rarely) be needed.
- Counseling may help for any emotional problems that develop.

POSSIBLE COMPLICATIONS
- Eye irritation or injury, because the eye does not close properly and is exposed to dust. If unprotected, the eye may develop ulcers on the cornea.
- Incomplete recovery from paralysis. Results may be slight, mild, or severe.
- Emotional and self-esteem problems.

PROBABLE OUTCOME
- The amount of paralysis determines the extent of recovery. Most patients recover completely with or without treatment.
- Recovery usually begins in 3 weeks and is gradual. Recovery time varies and may take 3 to 6 months.

HOW TO TREAT

GENERAL MEASURES
- If you have pain, apply heat to the area twice a day. Use a moist, warm towel and apply for 15 minutes. Cover or close the eye during heat treatments.
- If you cannot wink or close your eye well, you should buy a pair of wrap-around, plastic sports goggles. Wear them to protect your eye from dirt, dust, and dryness.
- At night, apply an eye patch to shut the lid so that the eye stays moist and protected. Sometimes, a patch will be necessary during the daytime.
- As muscle strength returns, use facial massage and exercises. Massage muscles of the forehead, cheek, lips and eyes using cream or oil. Exercise the weak muscles in front of a mirror. Open and close the eye; wink, smile, and bare your teeth. Perform the massage and exercises for 15 to 20 minutes several times a day.
- Brush and floss teeth regularly.

MEDICATION
- You may be prescribed eye drops for comfort and protection of the exposed eye.
- Antiviral drugs may be prescribed.
- Cortisone drugs may be prescribed to reduce swelling and inflammation of the affected nerve.

ACTIVITY—Maintain your normal activities.

DIET—A soft diet may be necessary for a period of time.

CALL YOUR DOCTOR IF

- You or a family member has symptoms of Bell's palsy.
- Eye becomes red or irritated, despite treatment.
- Drooling or pain worsens or fever occurs.
- New, unexplained symptoms develop. Drugs used in treatment may produce side effects.

BENIGN PAROXYSMAL POSITIONAL VERTIGO

GENERAL INFORMATION

DEFINITION
- Benign paroxysmal positional vertigo (BPPV) is a common, inner ear disorder that causes dizziness or vertigo with certain movements of the head.
  - Benign means "not very serious."
  - Paroxysmal means "sudden and variable in onset."
  - Positional, because it comes about with a change in head position.
  - Vertigo, causing a sense of the room spinning or whirling.

BODY PARTS INVOLVED—Inner ear and the nervous system.

SEX OR AGE MOST AFFECTED—Both sexes; all ages. It is more common in people over age 40 and in women more than men.

SIGNS & SYMPTOMS
- A sensation of dizziness or vertigo (spinning). Vertigo begins 5 to 10 seconds after the head moves and lasts less than a minute. Feeling off balance may last longer.
- Most often, only one ear is affected, so symptoms occur when the head is turned that way. Symptoms are brought on when getting out of bed, rolling over in bed, or when looking up for an object on a high shelf.
- Falling, or a feeling of falling.
- Feeling lightheaded or woozy.
- Visual blurring.
- Nausea and vomiting (sometimes).
- Faintness, changes in heart rate and blood pressure, fear, anxiety, or (less often) panic.

CAUSES—It is thought to be caused by small crystals of calcium carbonate (also called "ear rocks," otoconia or otoliths) in the inner ear. The crystals normally help tell the brain about your head position. Sometimes the crystals become dislodged from their location in the vestibule and move into a semicircular canal. This can disrupt the ear's balance centers and cause the symptoms.

RISK INCREASES WITH
- Head injury.
- Degeneration of the vestibular system of the inner ear (usually in older people).
- Ear infection or disorder.
- Surgery.
- Central nervous system disease.

HOW TO PREVENT—No preventive measures.

WHAT TO EXPECT

DIAGNOSTIC MEASURES
- Your health care provider will do an exam of the ears and ask questions about your symptoms and activities.

- When BPPV occurs, there is an involuntary movement of the eyes, which is called nystagmus. To make the diagnosis, the patient's head is put into certain positions and the eye movements are observed. Medical tests may be done to confirm the diagnosis.

APPROPRIATE HEALTH CARE
- Treatment may involve watchful waiting. No treatment is done at first to see if the problem resolves itself.
- An office procedure (e.g., Epley maneuver) may be done for treatment. It is performed by placing a patient's head in various positions. This will cause the crystals to loosen and return to normal movement. This procedure takes about 5 to 10 minutes. Frequently, only one office procedure is needed. It is painless and has few side effects if any. There may be mild vertigo for a few days afterwards.
- Rarely, if other treatment is not effective, severe symptoms may require surgery.

POSSIBLE COMPLICATIONS—BPPV symptoms may come and go, recur after treatment, or become chronic.

PROBABLE OUTCOME—The condition usually clears up on its own within several weeks. It may recur. Treatment can hasten healing. It does not cause hearing loss or ear noises (tinnitus).

HOW TO TREAT

GENERAL MEASURES
- Self-treatment may be helpful. This can be done if symptoms recur, or office procedure was not effective. Instructions will be given on proper techniques for the head maneuvers. They are then done at home several times a day, usually for 2 weeks.
- To learn more: Vestibular Disorders Assn., PO Box 4467, Portland, OR 97208-4467; (800) 837-8428; website: www.vestibular.org.

MEDICATION—Usually not needed for this disorder. Drugs may be prescribed for specific symptoms, such as nausea.

ACTIVITY—Activities may be limited for 24 to 48 hours after the procedure is done. Specific instructions will be given.

DIET—No special diet.

CALL YOUR DOCTOR IF

- You or a family member has symptoms of benign paroxysmal positional vertigo.
- Symptoms recur after treatment.

BIPOLAR DISORDER
(Manic-Depressive Disorder)

 GENERAL INFORMATION

DEFINITION—Bipolar disorder is a condition in which a person has episodes of mania (being excited and high) and of depression (being sad and down). These episodes can alternate with periods of normal behavior. Episodes may last days, weeks, or months. There are several types of bipolar disorder (ranging from mild to more severe).

BODY PARTS INVOLVED—Brain.

SEX OR AGE MOST AFFECTED—Symptoms usually appear between ages 15 to 25, but the disorder can affect all ages and both sexes.

SIGNS & SYMPTOMS
- Mania:
  - Higher than normal energy levels.
  - Getting up earlier and earlier in the morning. A person may not sleep at all for 3 to 4 days.
  - Easily distracted and restless. Excited to start new projects, but then rarely finish.
  - May go on spending sprees.
  - May become sexually promiscuous.
  - Often irritable. Often has attacks of rage.
  - Speech becomes rapid; may not make sense.
  - May have very high opinion of one's abilities.
  - May forget to eat. May lose weight. Can become exhausted.
  - May have delusions of grandeur.
- Depression:
  - Becomes more and more withdrawn. Sleep may be disturbed. Late rising becomes a habit.
  - May stay in one's room. May be afraid to face the world. Often lacks self-esteem.
  - Self-neglect.
  - Sex drive is lowered.
  - Slow speech and movement.
  - Imagined problems multiply.
  - Worries about imagined illnesses.

CAUSES—There is no single cause. Genetics plays a part. Other factors may include changes in chemicals in the brain and environmental factors, such as stress.

RISK INCREASES WITH—Family history of bipolar disorder.

HOW TO PREVENT—No preventive measures.

 WHAT TO EXPECT

DIAGNOSTIC MEASURES
- Your health care provider will usually do a physical exam and ask questions about your symptoms and activities.
- Psychological testing may be done. Other medical tests may be done to rule out infections or disorders that could cause the symptoms.

APPROPRIATE HEALTH CARE
- Treatment will depend on the specific symptoms. Follow your health care provider's instructions. Schedule regular office visits. Your health care provider will monitor the effectiveness of the treatment and watch for side effects.
- Hospital care may be required for severe symptoms. A stay at a mental health facility may be recommended.
- Electroconvulsive therapy (ECT) may be considered if other treatment steps are not successful.

POSSIBLE COMPLICATIONS
- Relapse, especially if drug therapy is stopped.
- Problems at work, school, or home.
- Failure to get better.
- Alcohol or drug abuse.
- Suicide.

PROBABLE OUTCOME—Long-term therapy can help reduce how often and how severe the episodes are.

 HOW TO TREAT

GENERAL MEASURES
- Do not stop taking your medicine when you feel better. This may cause a relapse.
- Education and counseling can help you, and your family, cope with the condition. Family members should learn to recognize signs of a coming episode.
- Seek support groups. Call a suicide prevention hotline if needed.
- To learn more: Depression and Bipolar Support Alliance, 730 N. Franklin St., Suite 501, Chicago, IL 60610; (800) 826-3632; website: www.dbsalliance.org.

MEDICATION—Drugs will be prescribed to help relieve symptoms of the depression and the manic episodes. Other drugs may be prescribed to help prevent mood swings. Changes in drugs or dosages may be needed at various times to manage the symptoms.

ACTIVITY—Maintain daily activities. Exercise on a regular basis.

DIET—Try to eat healthy meals even if you have little or no appetite.

 CALL YOUR DOCTOR IF

- You or a family member has symptoms of depression or mania.
- Symptoms don't improve with treatment.
- You feel suicidal or hopeless. Call 911.

BLADDER INFECTION, FEMALE
(Cystitis in Women)

GENERAL INFORMATION

DEFINITION—Bladder infection (cystitis) is a disorder of the urinary bladder (the organ that stores urine). Bladder infections are very common. Up to one-third of all females will have one at some point in their lives.

BODY PARTS INVOLVED—Urinary bladder.

SEX OR AGE MOST AFFECTED—Females of all ages.

SIGNS & SYMPTOMS
- Pressure, burning, or stinging during urination.
- Frequent urination, although the amount of urine may be small; increased urge to urinate.
- Sensation of incomplete bladder emptying.
- Pain in the abdomen over the bladder or lower back.
- Blood in the urine; bad-smelling urine.
- Low fever and, possibly, chills.
- Painful sexual intercourse.
- Lack of urinary control (sometimes).
- A need to urinate more often at night.

CAUSES—The infection is caused by bacteria (germs) that enter the urinary tract system. A woman's urethra opening (tube from bladder to outside) is short in length and close to the anus, which makes it easier for germs to travel from the bowel area. Germs inside the urethra can travel up into the bladder, causing infection and inflammation.

RISK INCREASES WITH
- Sexual intercourse.
- Previous urinary tract infections.
- Pregnancy.
- Aging and associated conditions (e.g., menopause).
- Diabetes or other disorder affecting immune system.
- Certain types of birth control (e.g., diaphragm, spermicidal agent, or condom).
- Urinary tract problems (tumors, calculi, or strictures).
- Insertion of an instrument into the urinary tract (e.g., catheter or cystoscope).
- Poor hygiene or incomplete bladder emptying.

HOW TO PREVENT
- Urinate within 15 minutes after intercourse.
- Drink plenty of water every day.
- Get medical care for urinary tract infections.
- Don't douche, use feminine hygiene sprays, or deodorants. Avoid bubble baths.
- Clean the anal area after bowel movements. Wipe from the front to the rear, rather than rear to front.
- Wear underwear that has a cotton crotch.
- Avoid postponing urination. Be sure to completely empty the bladder with urination.

- In women with frequent recurrence of infection, antibiotics may be prescribed for use before or after sexual intercourse or on a regular basis.
- Drinking cranberry juice or using cranberry products (e.g., dried or supplement) may help.

WHAT TO EXPECT

DIAGNOSTIC MEASURES
- Your health care provider may do a physical exam.
- Medical tests will include a urine test.

APPROPRIATE HEALTH CARE—Treatment is usually with antibiotic drugs.

POSSIBLE COMPLICATIONS—Inadequate treatment can lead to chronic bladder infections, kidney infection, and (rarely) kidney failure.

PROBABLE OUTCOME
- Curable in a few days to 2 weeks with treatment.
- Recurrence is common.

HOW TO TREAT

GENERAL MEASURES
- Warm baths or using a heating pad on the abdomen may help relieve discomfort.
- Pour a cup of warm water over genital area while urinating to help ease burning and stinging.
- To learn more: National Kidney Foundation, 30 E. 33rd St., New York, NY 10016; (800) 622-9010; website: www.kidney.org.

MEDICATION
- Antibiotics for bacterial infection will be prescribed. Antibiotics may reduce the effectiveness of some birth control pills. If you are using birth control pills, discuss this with your health care provider.
- Urinary analgesics may be prescribed for pain. If phenazopyridine (Pyridium) is taken, it will turn the urine color to bright orange.

ACTIVITY—Avoid sexual intercourse until you have been free of symptoms for 2 weeks to allow inflammation to heal.

DIET—Drink plenty of fluids daily.

CALL YOUR DOCTOR IF

- You or a family member has symptoms of a bladder infection.
- Blood appears in the urine.
- Discomfort and other symptoms don't improve after you have taken the antibiotics for 48 hours or symptoms recur after treatment.

BLADDER INFECTION, MALE
(Cystitis in Men)

 GENERAL INFORMATION

DEFINITION—Bladder infection (cystitis) is an infection of the urinary bladder (the organ that stores urine).

BODY PARTS INVOLVED—Urinary bladder.

SEX OR AGE MOST AFFECTED—It can occur in males of any age. After age 50, men are affected more often (due to prostate problems).

SIGNS & SYMPTOMS
- Burning and stinging when you urinate.
- Urinating more often. The amount of urine may be small.
- Feeling like you need to go even when your bladder is empty.
- Pain in the pubic area or low back pain.
- Discharge from the penis.
- Blood in the urine.
- Low-grade fever.
- Urine that smells bad.
- Not being able to control urination.

CAUSES—The most common cause is bacteria (or germs) from the skin near the rectum and genitals. The germs spread into the urethra (tube that goes from the bladder to the outside). The germs then travel to the bladder and cause irritation and inflammation. Prostate problems in older men add to the cause.

RISK INCREASES WITH
- Blockage in the urinary tract. This may be due to kidney stones or tumor.
- Enlarged prostate gland.
- Poor hygiene.
- Uncircumcised penis.
- Aging and its associated conditions.
- Use of a catheter to empty the bladder.
- Failure to completely empty the bladder.
- Defects in the urinary tract.
- Anal intercourse or intercourse with an infected woman.
- Diabetes or weak immune system.

HOW TO PREVENT
- Drink plenty of fluids daily.
- Use a latex condom during sex. This can help prevent the spread of any infection.
- Avoid the use of catheters, if possible.
- Urinate when you feel the urge, empty the bladder completely, and keep genital area clean.
- Get medical care for any prostate infection.

 WHAT TO EXPECT

DIAGNOSTIC MEASURES
- Your health care provider will usually do a physical exam and ask questions about your symptoms.
- Medical tests include urine studies. Additional tests may be done to rule out other disorders.

APPROPRIATE HEALTH CARE—Treatment is usually with drugs, or sometimes surgery if a physical defect is the cause.

POSSIBLE COMPLICATIONS
- Recurrent or chronic bladder infections.
- Kidney infection.

PROBABLE OUTCOME
- Usually curable with treatment.
- Complicated infections in males are sometimes more difficult to treat.

 HOW TO TREAT

GENERAL MEASURES
- Warm baths may provide relief from symptoms.
- To learn more: National Kidney Foundation, 30 E. 33rd St., Suite 1100, New York, NY 10016; (800) 622-9010; website: www.kidney.org.

MEDICATION
- Drugs for bacterial infection are usually prescribed. To be sure of a cure, finish the entire prescribed dose even if symptoms improve. If infection is recurrent, drug therapy for 6 months to 2 years may be recommended.
- Drugs to relieve painful urination symptoms may be prescribed.

ACTIVITY
- Reduce activities as needed until symptoms improve.
- Avoid sexual intercourse until you have been free of symptoms for 2 weeks.

DIET
- Drink plenty of fluids daily.
- Drink cranberry juice if recommended by your health care provider.

 CALL YOUR DOCTOR IF

- You or a family member has symptoms of a bladder infection.
- Fever develops.
- Blood appears in the urine.
- Symptoms don't improve in one week.
- New, unexplained symptoms develop. Drugs used in treatment may produce side effects.
- Symptoms return after treatment.

BLADDER TUMOR

GENERAL INFORMATION

DEFINITION—A bladder tumor is an abnormal tissue growth in the bladder. It may be cancerous or noncancerous (benign). If the tumor is cancerous, it may spread to lymph nodes, bones, liver, and/or lungs.

BODY PARTS INVOLVED—Urinary bladder.

SEX OR AGE MOST AFFECTED—The tumors are most common in people over age 50 and occur more often in men than women.

SIGNS & SYMPTOMS
- There are often no symptoms in the early stages.
- Blood in the urine.
- Pain or burning when urinating.
- Needing to urinate more frequently. There may be only small amounts of urine passed.
- Fever.
- Unexplained weight loss.

CAUSES—Unknown in some cases. Exposure to cancer-causing substances in the environment may be the cause in some cases.

RISK INCREASES WITH
- Smoking.
- Family history of bladder tumors.
- Prior radiation or chemotherapy or having a catheter.
- Exposure to certain industrial dyes, chemicals, paints, solvents, ink, and others.

HOW TO PREVENT
- Avoid exposure to chemical or environmental hazards. Improved methods of protecting workers from chemical hazards have lowered the number of bladder tumors. Regular screening of those who have been exposed in the past is also helpful.
- Don't smoke.

WHAT TO EXPECT

DIAGNOSTIC MEASURES
- Your own observation of symptoms.
- Your health care provider will do a physical exam and ask questions about your symptoms.
- Medical tests include urine studies. A lighted optical instrument (cystoscope) may be used to see inside the bladder. It can also be used to remove a small piece of tissue, or even a small tumor, for viewing under a microscope (biopsy). The tumor may be cancerous or benign. X-ray, MRI, CT, or other tests may be done to see if a cancerous tumor has spread (called staging).

APPROPRIATE HEAL[...]
- Treatment may include s[...] chemotherapy (anticancer dru[...] therapy (body's immune system[...] cancer).
- Small tumors may be removed by f[...] This involves burning off the tumor by a [...] frequency electrical current (or with a laser) the cystoscope.
- Larger tumors are removed surgically. This may mean removal of part or all of the bladder (cystectomy) and other nearby body organs if needed. An alternate method of storing and removing urine may be needed.
- Radiation therapy may be combined with other types of treatment.

POSSIBLE COMPLICATIONS
- Spread of cancer to other places in the body, which can be fatal.
- Emotional stress about changes in body image.
- Side effects of treatments such as extreme fatigue.
- Treatment can lead to infertility for men and women.
- Anemia.
- Incontinence.

PROBABLE OUTCOME—When diagnosed early, treatment can be successful. However, tumors may return. Regular medical checkups are needed. If cancer has spread, the outcome will depend on many factors.

HOW TO TREAT

GENERAL MEASURES
- Counseling is helpful in learning to cope with having cancer.
- To learn more: American Cancer Society; (800) ACS-2345; website: www.cancer.org or National Cancer Institute; (800) 4-CANCER; website: www.cancer.gov.

MEDICATION—Anticancer drugs may be prescribed that are taken by mouth or given through a vein (IV). A catheter may be used to deliver drugs into the bladder itself (e.g., biologic therapy).

ACTIVITY—Resume your normal activities once your health care provider gives approval. This includes sexual relations.

DIET—No special diet.

CALL YOUR DOCTOR IF

- You or a family member has symptoms of a bladder tumor.
- Prescribed drugs produce unexpected side effects.

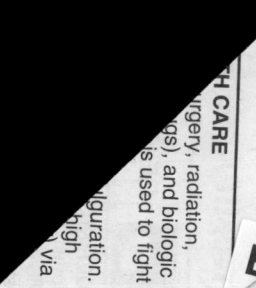

...IS

(...lastomycosis; Gilchrist's Disease)

...MATION

...rare
...s in the lungs.
...ugh the blood-
...specially the skin.
...se are found in parts of the south-central, south-eastern, and mid-western states and the Great Lakes area of the United States and Canada. It is also found in Central and South America and parts of Africa.

BODY PARTS INVOLVED—It can involve the lungs, mouth, skin (and tissue below the skin), and the prostate.

SEX OR AGE MOST AFFECTED—Both sexes, but most common in men from ages 20 to 40.

SIGNS & SYMPTOMS
- About 50% of those infected have no symptoms.
- Symptoms may begin slowly or may be sudden. They are often flu-like.
- Cough, either wet or dry.
- Chest pain.
- Chills, fever, and sweats.
- Shortness of breath.
- Fatigue, loss of appetite.
- May have bumps or sores on the skin.

CAUSES—Infection with *Blastomyces dermatitidis*. It is a fungus found in moist soil that has decomposing organic debris. The infection is spread by breathing in airborne spores of the fungus after disturbance of contaminated soil. Symptoms may appear between 3 and 15 weeks after exposure. Blastomycosis is not known to be transmitted from person to person. Animals such as dogs and cats can become infected also.

RISK INCREASES WITH
- Exposure to soils where the fungus is located (e.g., farmers, forestry workers, hunters, and campers).
- Weak immune system due to illness or drugs.

HOW TO PREVENT—Cannot be prevented at present.

WHAT TO EXPECT

DIAGNOSTIC MEASURES
- Your own observation of symptoms.
- Your health care provider will do a physical exam. Questions will be asked about your symptoms, medical history, and lifestyle.
- Medical tests may include blood tests and lab cultures (of the skin lesions, pus, saliva, or lung secretions). X-rays or a biopsy may be done. Biopsy is when a small amount of tissue is removed for viewing under a microscope.

APPROPRIATE HEALTH CARE
- Treatment is with drugs and other supportive care. Some patients with mild symptoms may require no treatment. The infection can clear on its own.
- Hospital care may be needed for severe symptoms.

POSSIBLE COMPLICATIONS
- Complications are more likely in those with weak immune systems due to illness or drugs.
- If not treated, it can spread to other body parts and lead to serious illness and even death. Most often, it involves the skin (and tissue below the skin). Small bumps develop and over time turn into open sores. Other complications can occur in the lungs, bones, scrotum, and prostate.
- Relapse can occur in up to 10% of patients.

PROBABLE OUTCOME—Cure rates are high, and the treatment (which may take months) is usually well tolerated.

HOW TO TREAT

GENERAL MEASURES—Keep follow-up appointments with your health care provider. It is important to monitor the treatment and watch for side effects or reactions from the drugs.

MEDICATION—An antifungal drug given orally is the treatment of choice for most forms of the disease. For more severe symptoms, the drugs may be given through a vein (IV).

ACTIVITY—Rest in bed if symptoms are more severe. Resume your activities slowly as strength returns.

DIET—No special diet.

CALL YOUR DOCTOR IF

- You or a family member has blastomycosis symptoms.
- Any of the following occur during treatment:
  - Weight loss.
  - Fever.
  - Diarrhea that is not controlled with self-care.
  - Severe headache and stiff neck.
  - Other new symptoms.

BLEPHARITIS

GENERAL INFORMATION

DEFINITION—Blepharitis is an inflammation (redness and soreness) of the eyelid edges.

BODY PARTS INVOLVED—Eyelids and eyelashes. It can also include the glands that lubricate the lid, and the white area of the eye.

SEX OR AGE MOST AFFECTED—Adults of both sexes.

SIGNS & SYMPTOMS
* Redness and greasy flakes on the eyelid edges.
* Small sores on the eyelid. Crusts may form on the edges of the eyelid.
* Discharge from the lids during sleep. Lids may be stuck together in the morning.
* A feeling that something is in the eye. This can cause itching, burning, redness, and swelling of the lid. May also have tearing and be sensitive to bright light.
* Eye may be irritated.
* Eyelashes that fall out.

CAUSES
* Seborrheic blepharitis is caused by a skin condition called seborrhea. It is similar to dandruff.
* Bacterial infection of the eyelash follicles and the glands that lubricate the eye. The infection cannot be spread from one person to another.
* Plugged glands on the eyelid.

RISK INCREASES WITH
* Dermatitis (skin infection).
* Acne rosacea.
* Allergen (substance that causes an allergy) exposure.
* Exposure to chemical or environmental irritants, such as smoke or smog.
* Work that keeps the hands dirty for most of the day.
* Elderly.
* Diabetes.
* Dry eye syndrome.

HOW TO PREVENT
* Wash hands often. Dry them with clean towel.
* Keep face, eyelids, and scalp clean.
* Avoid places where dust or air pollutants are heavy.
* Get treatment for any skin disorders.
* Control dandruff with anti-dandruff shampoos.

WHAT TO EXPECT

DIAGNOSTIC MEASURES
* Your own observation of symptoms.
* Your health care provider can diagnose blepharitis by an exam of the affected eyelid area.
* Other medical tests are not usually needed.

APPROPRIATE HEALTH CARE—Treatment will be prescribed for any problem that is causing the disorder or for any complications.

POSSIBLE COMPLICATIONS
* Styes or chalazia (blocked oil gland on eyelid).
* Conjunctivitis (eye inflammation).
* Loss of eyelashes or they grow in misdirected.
* Ulceration of the cornea (covering of the eye).
* Scarred eyelids.

PROBABLE OUTCOME—Symptoms can be improved with treatment. The condition is usually chronic and the symptoms come and go. If treatment is stopped, it tends to recur. It is usually not a serious condition. Complications are rare.

HOW TO TREAT

GENERAL MEASURES
* Warm soaks and keeping eyelids clean are usually advised for self-care.
  - For soaks, dampen a clean washcloth with warm water and place it over closed eyes. Do this four times a day, for about five minutes each time. Later on, you may apply the compress once a day, for a few minutes.
  - Cleansing the eyelids is important. Clean them twice a day with: warm water only, baby shampoo diluted with warm water, or a special product made for cleaning the lids. Dip a clean washcloth, cotton swab, or gauze pad into the cleaning solution. Gently wipe it across your lashes and lid margin. Rinse with cool water and dry the area.
* Avoid use of eye makeup until symptoms improve. When used, be sure to remove it each night at bedtime.
* Ask your health care provider about using contact lenses while you have the symptoms. You may need to temporarily stop their use.

MEDICATION
* Eye drops or ointment may be prescribed for use after the eyelid area is cleaned.
* Use artificial tears solution for dry eyes.
* Drugs to be taken by mouth may be prescribed in more severe cases.

ACTIVITY—No limits.

DIET—No special diet.

CALL YOUR DOCTOR IF

* You or a family member has symptoms of blepharitis.
* You have pain in the eye(s).
* Your vision changes.
* Symptoms recur after treatment.

BOILS
(Furuncles; Carbuncles)

GENERAL INFORMATION

DEFINITION—Boils (furuncles) are a painful, bacterial infection of a hair follicle. They are common and somewhat contagious. Carbuncles are clusters of boils that occur when the infection spreads.

BODY PARTS INVOLVED—They can occur anywhere on the skin, but most often appear on the neck, face, buttocks, and breasts.

SEX OR AGE MOST AFFECTED—Both sexes; all ages.

SIGNS & SYMPTOMS
- A domed nodule that is painful, tender, red, and is filled with pus. Boils can appear suddenly and ripen in 24 hours.
- Fever (rarely).
- Swelling of the closest lymph glands.

CAUSES—Infection, usually from *Staphylococcus aureus* bacteria. The bacteria (germs) normally live on the skin surface or in the nose. The germs may enter a damaged (such as from a razor cut) hair follicle and get into the skin's deeper layers.

RISK INCREASES WITH
- Poor nutrition or poor hygiene.
- Diabetes.
- Other skin problems (such as acne or skin infection).
- Weak immune system due to illness or drugs.

HOW TO PREVENT
- Keep the skin clean.
- If someone in the household has a boil, don't share towels, washcloths, or clothing with that person.
- If you have a chronic disease (such as diabetes), be sure to follow your medical care regimen.

WHAT TO EXPECT

DIAGNOSTIC MEASURES
- Your own observation of symptoms.
- Your health care provider can diagnose boils by an exam of the affected skin area.
- A laboratory culture may be made of the drainage (pus) from the boil.

APPROPRIATE HEALTH CARE
- Self-care.
- Your health care provider's treatment may include incision and drainage of the boil.

POSSIBLE COMPLICATIONS
- Spread of the infection to other skin surfaces or to other body parts.
- Scarring.
- Boils may recur.
- Family members may need treatment.

PROBABLE OUTCOME—Without treatment, a boil will heal in 10 to 20 days. With treatment, the boil should heal in less time, symptoms will be less severe, and new boils should not appear. Pus that drains when a boil opens on its own may infect nearby skin, causing new boils.

HOW TO TREAT

GENERAL MEASURES
- Do not squeeze the boil or pop it with a needle. Doing so may make the infection worse.
- You may be advised to gently soak the area with a warm, moist cloth. Do this 3 or 4 times daily for 20 minutes. If the boil starts to drain, wash the area with soap and apply a loose bandage. Wash your hands carefully after touching the boil.
- Prevent the spread of boils by using clean towels only once or using paper towels and discarding them.

MEDICATION—Antibiotics to be taken by mouth may be prescribed if infection is severe.

ACTIVITY—Usually no limits. Athletes involved in contact sports should ask their health care provider and their coaches about sports participation.

DIET—No special diet.

CALL YOUR DOCTOR IF

- You or a family member has a boil.
- The following occur during treatment:
  - Symptoms don't improve in 3 to 4 days, despite treatment.
  - New boils appear.
  - Fever.
  - Other family members develop boils.

BONE FRACTURE

GENERAL INFORMATION

DEFINITION—Bone fracture is a break in a bone. Different types of fractures can occur depending on the severity. A complete fracture means the bone is broken all the way through. An incomplete fracture means the bone is cracked. An open (or compound) fracture means the fractured bone sticks out through the skin. A stress fracture is a small crack in a bone due to overuse.

BODY PARTS INVOLVED—Bones.

SEX OR AGE MOST AFFECTED—Both sexes; all ages.

SIGNS & SYMPTOMS
- Pain, swelling, or tenderness at fracture site.
- Paleness and deformity (sometimes).
- Bleeding or bruising at the site.
- Weakness.
- Cannot bear weight.
- Numbness, tingling, or paralysis below the fracture (rare; this is an emergency).

CAUSES—The bone can't withstand a physical force exerted on it.

RISK INCREASES WITH
- Activities that carry the risk of injury.
- Reckless behavior that increases risks of an accident.
- Age. Older adults have bones that are more fragile and also tend to have more falls.
- Osteoporosis and osteopenia.
- Tumors of the bone or bone marrow.
- Sports activities.
- Stress fracture risk factors include: females, menstrual problems, poor physical condition, running or jumping sports, loss of bone density, and overweight.

HOW TO PREVENT
- May not always be preventable.
- Avoid high risk behaviors (e.g., drinking and driving).
- Wear seatbelts when in a motor vehicle.
- Wear proper protective gear for sports.
- Maintain healthy bones with diet and exercise. Talk to your health care provider about taking calcium and vitamin D supplements.
- Maintain a safe home. Take measures to prevent falls.

WHAT TO EXPECT

DIAGNOSTIC MEASURES
- Your own observation of symptoms.
- Your health care provider will do a physical exam of the injured area.
- X-rays will be done to confirm the bone fracture. In some cases, other tests are needed.

APPROPRIATE HEALTH CARE
- Treatment will depend on the specific fracture.
- Bone ends that have been displaced are maneuvered back into place (reduction). See Fracture Repair in Surgery section.
- Most fractures require casts, splints, or a special brace for healing. Crutches or other aids may be used to walk.
- Hospital care may be needed for severe fractures.
- Surgery may be needed. The fracture may be repaired with rods, plates, or screws.

POSSIBLE COMPLICATIONS
- Failure to heal (non-union).
- Shock from blood loss.
- Travel of a fat embolus (clump of fat cells) from the injury site to the lungs or brain.
- Obstruction of nearby arteries.

PROBABLE OUTCOME—Usually curable with treatment. Healing time varies. Recovery is complete when there is no bone motion at the fracture site, and x-rays show complete healing.

HOW TO TREAT

GENERAL MEASURES—Give first aid treatment for bleeding, cover any open wounds, move patient as little as possible. Then transport to hospital or other emergency facility.

MEDICATION—Pain relievers and muscle relaxants may be prescribed.

ACTIVITY
- Immobility of a bone for a long period of time can cause loss of muscle mass, stiffness in nearby joints, and edema (excess fluid in the tissues). Begin to use the affected part as soon as is safely possible.
- Physical therapy may be prescribed to maintain flexibility of the joint and provide strength to the muscles.
- Resume normal activities as soon as symptoms improve and your health care provider advises you to.

DIET—No special diet.

CALL YOUR DOCTOR IF

- You or a family member has symptoms of a bone fracture.
- The following occur after treatment:
  - Swelling above or below the fracture site.
  - Severe, persistent pain.
  - Blue or gray skin below fracture site (e.g., in fingernails); numbness or loss of feeling below fracture site.

BOTULISM

GENERAL INFORMATION

DEFINITION
- Botulism is a rare bacterial illness. Types are:
  - Foodborne botulism is a serious form of food poisoning that is usually caused by eating food contaminated with a botulinum toxin. This toxin affects both the central nervous system and the muscular system. Symptoms usually appear suddenly 18 to 36 hours (but can range anywhere from 2 hours to 1 week) after eating contaminated food.
  - Infant botulism is a special type that occurs in children less than 12 months of age.
  - Wound botulism occurs when the toxin in a wound spreads to other body parts.
  - Adult intestinal colonization botulism occurs in older children and adults with abnormal bowel condition (e.g., colitis).
  - Injection-related type and an inhalation type.

BODY PARTS INVOLVED—Central nervous system; muscular system.

SEX OR AGE MOST AFFECTED—All ages, but most common in adults.

SIGNS & SYMPTOMS
- Blurred or double vision and drooping eyelids.
- Dry mouth.
- Slurred speech.
- Trouble swallowing.
- Vomiting and diarrhea.
- Weakness of the arms and legs. Paralysis.
- No fever; no change in mental abilities.
- In infants: severe constipation, feeble cry, and unable to suck.

CAUSES
- A bacteria germ, *Clostridium botulinum* (other types may, rarely, be the cause). The germ may be found in contaminated or incompletely cooked foods. It can also be found in improperly canned foods. The germ generates a strong poison that is absorbed from the digestive tract. The poison spreads to the central nervous system.
- Foods likely to cause botulism include home-canned vegetables and fruits. Also, fish, smoked meats, milk products, and undercooked sausage.
- Honey or corn syrup may cause infant botulism.
- The bacteria may also contaminate a wound and produce the toxin.

RISK INCREASES WITH
- Infants.
- Home-canned foods.
- IV drug abuse (e.g., cocaine) for wound botulism.

HOW TO PREVENT
- If a can of food is bulging, don't even open it. If the contents of a can have a strange color or odor, don't even taste the food. Throw it away in a safe manner.
- Don't eat any foods that may not have been properly cooked or canned.
- Don't give infants under age 1 honey or corn syrup, not even a small taste.
- Get proper instructions about canning food.

WHAT TO EXPECT

DIAGNOSTIC MEASURES
- Your own observation of symptoms (especially if several persons eat the same food and become sick).
- Diagnosis and treatment involves emergency hospital care. Blood and stool studies can confirm the diagnosis.

APPROPRIATE HEALTH CARE
- For foodborne infection, vomiting may be induced, enemas given, or a washing out (lavage) of the stomach may be done to help rid the body of the toxin.
- Wound care will be given for infected wounds.
- Breathing support with a machine (ventilator) may be needed, along with other supportive-care measures.
- Fluids may be given through a vein (IV) or through a tube placed in the nose (nasogastric).
- Health care providers will report the disease to state or federal health agencies. They will remove any contaminated food from stores.

POSSIBLE COMPLICATIONS
- Long-lasting weakness.
- Nervous system problems (may last for a year).
- Lung infections, such as pneumonia.
- Respiratory failure caused by weak breathing muscles. It can lead to death.

PROBABLE OUTCOME—With prompt treatment, the outlook is good.

HOW TO TREAT

GENERAL MEASURES—If you suspect botulism, refrigerate some of the contaminated food for testing, if possible.

MEDICATION—A special drug (antitoxin) may be given by injection. It can prevent the symptoms from getting worse. It may be life-saving, but it has serious side effects.

ACTIVITY—Bed rest during treatment. Resume normal activities as your strength permits.

DIET—After treatment, no special diet is needed.

CALL YOUR DOCTOR IF

- You or a family member has symptoms of botulism. Call for medical help immediately.
- Any new symptoms develop after treatment.

BRAIN OR EPIDURAL ABSCESS

GENERAL INFORMATION

DEFINITION—A brain or epidural abscess is a collection of pus caused by infection. The abscess can develop in the brain or in the epidural space. This is the space between the covering (membrane) of the brain or spinal cord and the bones.

BODY PARTS INVOLVED—Brain; meninges (membranes that cover the brain); skull.

SEX OR AGE MOST AFFECTED—They can affect all ages and are more common in men than in women.

SIGNS & SYMPTOMS
- The following symptoms usually appear gradually over several hours. They resemble symptoms of a brain tumor or stroke:
  - Headache, usually severe.
  - Fever.
  - Stiff neck.
  - Confusion or delirium.
  - Seizures (convulsions).
  - Nausea and vomiting.
  - Pain in the back. It may occur if the infection is in the covering of the spinal cord.
  - One side of the body may feel numb or weak. The body may be paralyzed on one side.
  - Unable to walk normally.
  - Trouble speaking.

CAUSES
- An infection that spreads from another part of the head such as sinusitis or a middle ear infection.
- An infection due to a head injury or surgery.
- An infection that spreads through the blood from other infected organs. This includes the lungs, skin, heart valves, or dental infections.
- Infections, such as fungal or protozoan, that occur in people with weak immune systems.

RISK INCREASES WITH
- Head injury.
- Chronic illness, such as diabetes, AIDS, or cancer.
- Recent infection (in the ears, nose, eyes, or face).
- Weak immune system due to illness or drugs.
- IV drug abuse.
- Congenital (born with) heart disease.
- Tongue piercing.

HOW TO PREVENT
- None specific. To reduce risk factors:
  - Seek medical care for infections.
  - Wear protective headgear when you are involved in any activity that could lead to a head injury.

WHAT TO EXPECT

DIAGNOSTIC MEASURES
- Your health care provider will do a physical exam and ask questions about your symptoms and activities.
- Medical tests may include blood tests, CT, and MRI (see Glossary for both).

APPROPRIATE HEALTH CARE
- Medical or surgical treatment will depend on the location of the infection. Usually, surgery is needed to drain the infected area. Drugs will be given for the infection.
- Breathing support with a machine (ventilator) may be needed, along with other supportive-care measures. Fluids may be given through a vein (IV).

POSSIBLE COMPLICATIONS
- Seizures, coma, and death (without treatment).
- Rupture of the abscess.
- Brain hemorrhage.
- Brain damage that can lead to permanent disability or learning difficulties.
- Meningitis (more widespread infection).

PROBABLE OUTCOME—Treatment is usually successful with early diagnosis and treatment. Most people recover completely. Some may have mild speech, movement, or memory problems that may improve with time.

HOW TO TREAT

GENERAL MEASURES—The family should maintain an optimistic outlook, stay in contact with the patient's doctor and help by making their visits with the patient brief and supportive.

MEDICATION
- Antibiotic drugs will be given for the infection. They may be continued for several weeks.
- Drugs to prevent seizures may be prescribed.
- Following surgery, you may be given drugs to reduce swelling.

ACTIVITY—While in the hospital, you will need bed rest. After a 2 to 3 week recovery, you should be as active as your strength and feeling of well-being allow.

DIET—While you are in the hospital, essential fluids may be given through a tube in a vein. Following treatment, eat a normal, well-balanced diet.

CALL YOUR DOCTOR IF

- You or a family member has any symptoms of a brain abscess.
- New, unexplained symptoms develop.

BRAIN TUMOR

GENERAL INFORMATION

DEFINITION—A brain tumor is an abnormal cell growth in the brain. The growth may be benign (noncancerous) or malignant (cancerous). The symptoms can be caused by pressure as the tumor gets larger, or can be caused by the location, size, and type of tumor.

BODY PARTS INVOLVED—Brain; central nervous system.

SEX OR AGE MOST AFFECTED—All ages, but most common in adults ages 20 and 60.

SIGNS & SYMPTOMS
- Headache that is worse when lying down.
- Seizures (convulsions).
- Memory loss, confusion, and loss of concentration.
- Personality and behavior changes.
- Vomiting or nausea.
- Problems with vision. This includes double vision.
- Weakness on one side of the body.
- Lack of balance and dizziness.
- Loss of sense of smell and hearing.

CAUSES—Exact cause is unknown. There are genetic factors and environmental factors involved. Some tumors begin in the brain and are called primary. Other brain tumors are called secondary. They have spread (metastasized) from other cancers in the body. These include cancers of the breast, lungs, colon, or skin (melanoma).

RISK INCREASES WITH
- Unknown for most brain tumors.
- Radiation to the head for other cancer treatment.
- Rarely, certain types of tumors run in families.

HOW TO PREVENT—No specific preventive measures are known.

WHAT TO EXPECT

DIAGNOSTIC MEASURES
- Your own observation of symptoms.
- Your health care provider will do a physical exam and ask questions about your symptoms and activities.
- A variety of medical tests will be done to diagnose the tumor and to see if it has spread to or from other places in the body (called staging).

APPROPRIATE HEALTH CARE
- The treatment plan will be determined by the tumor's size, location, type, stage, and your age and health status. Because there are over 120 different types of brain tumors, treatment needs to be specific for each person.

- Treatment can include surgery, radiation, chemotherapy (anticancer drugs), and targeted drug therapy (kill specific cancer cells).
- Surgery is often needed. It may involve removal of all or part of the tumor and nearby tissue.
- Radiation may be used for certain stages of the tumor. It is normally not used for children under age 3.
- Immunotherapy uses the body's immune system to help fight the cancer.
- Treatment may involve steps to relieve symptoms and make you comfortable, rather than treating the tumor.

POSSIBLE COMPLICATIONS
- Long-term physical and mental side effects. They may be due to the effect of the tumor or to treatment.
- Tumor may recur after treatment.
- Death.

PROBABLE OUTCOME—The outcome depends on several factors. These include type of tumor, its size, location, spread of tumor, other cancer in the body, age and health of the patient, and the patient's response to treatment.

HOW TO TREAT

GENERAL MEASURES
- The more you can learn and understand about a disease, the more you will be able to make informed decisions about where to go for your care, the treatments available, the risks involved, side effects of therapy and expected outcome.
- To learn more: American Brain Tumor Association, 2720 River Road, Des Plaines, IL 60018; (800) 886-2282; website: www.abta.org or National Brain Tumor Foundation, 22 Battery Street, Suite 612, San Francisco, CA 94111; (800) 934-2873; website: www.braintumor.org.

MEDICATION
- Your health care provider may prescribe:
  - Drugs to reduce swelling of the brain tissue.
  - Drugs to control seizures.
  - Pain relievers.
  - Drugs that kill cancer cells (chemotherapy).
  - Targeted drugs to kill specific cancer cells.

ACTIVITY—Stay as active as your strength allows.

DIET—Eat a normal, well-balanced diet. You may need to take vitamins and minerals if you cannot eat normally.

CALL YOUR DOCTOR IF

- You or a family member has symptoms of a brain tumor.
- New, unexplained symptoms occur during treatment.

BREAST ABSCESS

GENERAL INFORMATION

DEFINITION—A breast abscess is an infected area of breast tissue that becomes filled with pus when the body fights the infection.

BODY PARTS INVOLVED—It involves breast tissue, nipple(s), milk glands, and milk ducts.

SEX OR AGE MOST AFFECTED—They almost always occur in a breast-feeding woman.

SIGNS & SYMPTOMS
- Breast pain.
- An area of the breast is tender, red, or hard.
- Fever and chills.
- Feeling ill.
- Tenderness in the area under the arm.

CAUSES—Bacteria that enter the breast through the nipple. This can happen if a nipple gets dry and cracked from breast-feeding.

RISK INCREASES WITH
- Breast infection, such as mastitis.
- Pelvic infection after delivery of a baby.
- Previous breast abscess.
- Diabetes.
- Rheumatoid arthritis.
- Use of steroid drugs.
- Heavy cigarette smoking. This is also a risk factor for women who are not breast-feeding.
- Lumpectomy with radiation.
- Some breast implants.

HOW TO PREVENT
- Clean the nipples and breasts carefully, before and after nursing.
- Lubricate the nipples after nursing. Use vitamin A & D ointment or another topical drug if recommended.
- Avoid clothing that irritates the breasts.
- Don't allow a nursing infant to chew nipples.

WHAT TO EXPECT

DIAGNOSTIC MEASURES
- Your health care provider will do a physical exam of the affected area. This is often all that is needed for diagnosis.
- Medical tests such as a culture of the pus and ultrasound may be done.

APPROPRIATE HEALTH CARE—The abscess may need to be drained. Draining of the abscess may be done with a needle inserted into the abscess or with a small incision. This will reduce pain and help clear up the infection.

POSSIBLE COMPLICATIONS—An abnormal opening (fistula) may develop between the breast and the outside of the body.

PROBABLE OUTCOME
- Usually curable in 8 to 10 days with treatment. Draining the abscess is sometimes needed to speed healing.
- You may or may not be able to keep breast-feeding with the affected breast. Your health care provider will help determine if this is possible. If you can't breastfeed, use a breast pump to remove milk from the infected breast until you can start nursing again on that side.

HOW TO TREAT

GENERAL MEASURES—Use a warm, moist compress on the breast to relieve pain, hasten healing, and help the flow of milk.

MEDICATION—Drugs for pain or antibiotics for infection may be prescribed.

ACTIVITY—After treatment, resume normal activity as soon as symptoms improve.

DIET—No special diet.

CALL YOUR DOCTOR IF

- You or a family member has symptoms of a breast abscess.
- Any of the following occur during treatment:
  - Fever.
  - Pain becomes more severe.
  - Infection seems to be spreading, despite treatment.
  - Symptoms don't improve in 72 hours.

BREAST CANCER

GENERAL INFORMATION

DEFINITION—Breast cancer is a malignant growth of breast tissue. It is the most common form of cancer in women other than non-melanoma skin cancers.

BODY PARTS INVOLVED—Breasts.

SEX OR AGE MOST AFFECTED—Breast cancer is rare before age 30, and is more common after the age of 50. Men can develop breast cancer also.

SIGNS & SYMPTOMS
- No symptoms in early stages. It may be detected by a mammogram or by feeling a breast lump.
- Swelling or lump in the breast.
- Vague discomfort in the breast without true pain.
- Inversion of the nipple.
- Distorted breast contour.
- Dimpled or pitted skin in the breast.
- Enlarged nodes under the arm (late stages).
- Bloody discharge from the nipple (rare).

CAUSES—The exact cause is unknown. Genetic, hormonal, and environmental factors probably play a role.

RISK INCREASES WITH
- Women and increasing age.
- Older age for having first child; never giving birth.
- Personal or family history of breast cancer (especially in mother, sister, or daughter).
- Changes in genes (BRCA1, BRCA2, others).
- Certain breast changes.
- Dense breast tissue (as seen on a mammogram).
- Early menstruation and/or late menopause.
- White women more than other racial groups.
- Previous radiation therapy to the chest area.
- Menopausal hormone therapy.
- Overweight or obesity (more so after menopause).
- Being physically inactive.
- Excess alcohol use.
- Women who used DES (diethylstilbestrol) between 1938 and 1971 and their daughters.
- Not having breastfed a child.

HOW TO PREVENT
- There is no sure way to prevent breast cancer. You can reduce certain risk factors.
- Maintain healthy weight, eat a low-fat diet high in vegetables and fruit, exercise daily, and avoid/limit alcohol.
- Consult your health care provider: about new breast symptoms or breast changes, mammogram screening, medical breast exams, and self breast exams.
- Avoid/limit hormone therapy after menopause.
- Women at high risk may have gene testing, take preventive drugs, or consider preventive surgery.

WHAT TO EXPECT

DIAGNOSTIC MEASURES
- Your own observation of symptoms.
- Your health care provider will do a breast exam and ask questions about your symptoms.
- Different medical tests will be done. The tests first help diagnose the cancer and then determine if it has spread (staging).

APPROPRIATE HEALTH CARE
- Treatment depends on the cancer type, location, and size; if it has spread; and your health, age, and preferences.
- Treatment may include surgery, drug therapy, and/or radiation therapy. The treatment choices are complex and often confusing. Be sure all options are discussed and that you understand the risks and benefits of each.
- Surgery can remove the lump (lumpectomy) or part or all of the breast (different degrees of mastectomy). Lymph nodes and supporting muscles may be removed also. Breast reconstruction surgery is an option.
- Radiation therapy may be used after surgery.
- Counseling may help you cope with cancer.

POSSIBLE COMPLICATIONS
- Cancer spreads in body or cancer recurs.
- Treatment side effects during/after treatment.

PROBABLE OUTCOME—Outcome depends on many factors for each individual.

HOW TO TREAT

GENERAL MEASURES
- The decision for treatment is very complex and often confusing. Learn about your options and understand the risks and benefits of each.
- To learn more: American Cancer Society, (800) 227-2345; website: www.cancer.org or Breast Cancer Network of Strength, (800) 221-2141; website: www.networkofstrength.org.

MEDICATION—Chemotherapy (anticancer drugs), hormone blockers, targeted therapy (attacks certain cancer cells), preventive drugs, or others may be prescribed.

ACTIVITY
- Treatments may limit activities temporarily.
- After treatment, daily exercise will help regain health. Physical therapy may be recommended.

DIET—Try to eat a healthy diet (appetite loss is common).

CALL YOUR DOCTOR IF

- You or a family member has breast changes.
- You have concerns or questions during or after treatment.

BRONCHIECTASIS

GENERAL INFORMATION

DEFINITION—Bronchiectasis is a lung disease in which the bronchi (airways in the lungs) become damaged and abnormally widened. Recurrent or severe lung infections occur. It may begin in childhood, but no symptoms appear until later in life.

BODY PARTS INVOLVED—Lungs; bronchi.

SEX OR AGE MOST AFFECTED—All ages, but most common in adults and older women.

SIGNS & SYMPTOMS
- Some people may have few or no symptoms.
- Frequent coughing. There may be foul-smelling mucus. The mucus may be green or yellow, and sometimes flecked with blood.
- Chest pain; wheezing; shortness of breath.
- Feeling tired and weak.
- Weight loss.

CAUSES—Over years, the walls of the bronchi (airways) become inflamed and damaged. Extra mucus builds up in the widened airways, which leads to infection and further airway damage. The extent of damage will vary and can affect one airway or many. There are a number of known underlying causes that can lead to the airway damage. In some cases, no cause is found.

RISK INCREASES WITH
- Certain hereditary disorders (e.g., cystic fibrosis, primary ciliary dyskinesia, and others).
- Lung infections (e.g., tuberculosis, whooping cough, measles, bronchitis, pneumonia, others).
- Airway obstruction (e.g., inhaled foreign body, tumor, or airway narrowing).
- Autoimmune disorders (e.g., rheumatoid arthritis).
- Complication of inflammatory bowel disease.
- Broncho-pulmonary aspergillosis.
- Inhaling backed up stomach acid or toxic gas.
- Weak immune system due to illness or drugs.

HOW TO PREVENT
- None specific. Avoid risk factors if possible.
- Obtain medical care for lung infections.
- Get childhood immunizations.
- Get vaccines for flu and pneumonia.
- Don't smoke.

WHAT TO EXPECT

DIAGNOSTIC MEASURES
- Your own observation of symptoms.
- Your health care provider will do a physical exam and ask questions about your symptoms.
- Medical tests may include studies of blood or sputum (material coughed up from the lung). Other tests may include CT, x-ray, bronchoscopy (looking in the airways with a lighted tube), and pulmonary function tests.

APPROPRIATE HEALTH CARE
- Treatment includes chest physical therapy (CPT) to remove lung secretions and drugs for symptoms and to prevent infections and to treat any underlying disorder.
- You will be instructed on chest physical therapy (called postural drainage) techniques. These help loosen mucus so it can be coughed up. They are done 3 or 4 times a day. There are several devices that can assist you with CPT. You may be taught certain breathing techniques that can also help loosen mucus.
- Oxygen therapy may be needed for severe symptoms.
- Surgery to remove areas of damaged lung tissue may be recommended if other treatments are not effective.

POSSIBLE COMPLICATIONS
- Chronic obstructive pulmonary disease.
- Repeated pneumonia or other infections.
- Cor pulmonale (heart disorder due to lung disease).
- Hospital care and breathing support may be needed.

PROBABLE OUTCOME—There is no cure. With treatment, many patients can lead nearly normal lives without major problems. In some cases, it will depend on the underlying cause.

HOW TO TREAT

GENERAL MEASURES
- Don't smoke. Find a way to quit. Smoking is not a direct cause, but can damage lungs.
- To learn more: American Lung Association, 61 Broadway, 6th Floor, New York, NY 10006; (800) 586-4872; website: www.lungusa.org.

MEDICATION
- Your health care provider may prescribe:
  - Antibiotic drugs for infections.
  - Inhaled steroids to reduce inflammation.
  - Bronchodilators to assist breathing.
  - Drugs to loosen or thin the mucus.
  - Drugs to treat any underlying disorder.

ACTIVITY—Remain as active as possible. Daily exercise such as walking is recommended. It helps loosen mucus also.

DIET—Eat a healthy diet. Drink plenty of fluids.

CALL YOUR DOCTOR IF

- You or a family member has signs of bronchiectasis.
- Symptoms of lung infection develop or fever occurs.
- Sputum contains blood, changes color, or thickens.
- Chest pain increases or you become short of breath.

BRONCHIOLITIS

GENERAL INFORMATION

DEFINITION—Bronchiolitis is an inflammation and infection of the smallest airways (bronchioles) of the respiratory tract. These airways normally carry air from the large bronchial tubes to tiny air sacs in the lungs. It is a common disorder.

BODY PARTS INVOLVED—Bronchioles.

SEX OR AGE MOST AFFECTED—It mainly affects infants and young children. Boys are affected more often than girls.

SIGNS & SYMPTOMS
- Often there is a mild common cold and cough before symptoms of bronchiolitis appear.
- Sudden trouble with breathing and wheezing.
- Rapid, shallow breathing.
- Chest and stomach are pulled in and out in seesaw movements with breathing.
- Grunting sounds while breathing in infants.
- Fever may occur or dehydration may develop.
- Blue skin or nails in severe cases.

CAUSES—Usually a viral infection. Respiratory syncytial virus (RSV) is the most common. Other viral infections may sometimes be the cause. Germs are spread by sneezing, coughing, or by contact of hands to nose, mouth, or eyes. Symptoms start 2 to 5 days after the exposure.

RISK INCREASES WITH
- Young children (usually under age 2).
- Winter and early spring seasons.
- Daycare centers.
- Crowded living conditions.
- Exposure to cigarette smoke.
- Children who were born premature, had low birth weight, were born with health problems (neurologic, heart, or lung), or have developed a lung disorder.
- Bottle fed baby more than breastfed baby.

HOW TO PREVENT
- No specific preventive measures.
- Wash hands often to prevent spread of germs.
- Avoid exposure to infected persons.
- Don't allow smoking around a baby or child.
- Children at risk for complications of RSV infections may be given therapy to prevent the infection.

WHAT TO EXPECT

DIAGNOSTIC MEASURES
- Your own observation of symptoms.
- Your health care provider will do a physical exam and ask questions about the symptoms and activities.
- Medical tests are usually not needed, but may be done to confirm the diagnosis.

APPROPRIATE HEALTH CARE
- There is no specific treatment for this disorder. Mild cases may be treated at home. Extra rest and drinking plenty of fluids is usually all that is needed.
- If the symptoms are more severe, hospital care may be required. Oxygen may be provided through a facemask. Some patients require breathing support with a ventilator (a device to help the lungs). Treatment to help remove lung secretions may be needed.

POSSIBLE COMPLICATIONS
- Respiratory failure.
- Chronic lung disease.
- Heart disorders.
- Bronchiolitis obliterans (collapse of part of the lung).
- Other infections.

PROBABLE OUTCOME—Mild cases may last for one or two days. Other cases may take 5 to 12 days for recovery. A few children who have other health problems may be more at risk for complications.

HOW TO TREAT

GENERAL MEASURES
- Use an ultrasonic, cool-mist humidifier if recommended by your health care provider. Clean the humidifier daily.
- A blocked-up nose may be suctioned with a rubber suction device or use saline nasal drops.

MEDICATION
- Hospital care may include drugs to relieve breathing problems, treat infections, and prevent complications.
- Acetaminophen may be used for fever.

ACTIVITY—Rest until symptoms have improved for 48 hours. Then gradually return to normal activities.

DIET—Offer a child clear fluids often. These include water, clear juice, clear broth, or others. Infants should continue to nurse or drink formula.

CALL YOUR DOCTOR IF

- You or a family member has bronchiolitis symptoms.
- The symptoms become worse. or temperature rises to 101°F (38.3°C) or higher.
- Breathing becomes more difficult.
- A cough begins that produces colored mucus.
- The skin, lips, or nails turn bluish in color.
- The child becomes drowsy and lacks energy.

BRONCHITIS, ACUTE

GENERAL INFORMATION

DEFINITION—Acute bronchitis is an inflammation of the mucous lining of the bronchi (main air passages) to the lungs. Symptoms of acute bronchitis may start suddenly and last just a few days. Chronic bronchitis is a different disorder that persists over a long period of time.

BODY PARTS INVOLVED—Trachea; bronchi; bronchioles.

SEX OR AGE MOST AFFECTED—It is a common disorder affecting all age groups.

SIGNS & SYMPTOMS
- A common cold or sore throat may occur prior to bronchitis.
- Cough that produces little or no mucus at first. Later, mucus may be produced.
- Low fever (usually less than 101°F/38.3°C).
- Burning feeling in chest. Feeling of pressure behind the breastbone.
- Wheezing. There may be trouble breathing.
- Feeling tired.

CAUSES
- Viral infection usually. Most cases begin with a cold virus in the nose and throat. The virus then spreads to the lungs. A bacterial infection may also cause bronchitis. Infection causes the mucous membranes to become inflamed and produce thick, sticky mucus. This narrows the airways and causes the symptoms.
- Irritative bronchitis is caused by allergies, chemicals, and other irritants in the environment.

RISK INCREASES WITH
- Chronic lung disease or chronic sinusitis.
- Smoking or secondhand smoke.
- Poor nutrition.
- Allergies.
- Areas with polluted air.
- Elderly and very young age groups.
- Gastroesophageal reflux disease (GERD).

HOW TO PREVENT
- Avoid close contact with people who have a cold or the flu. Wash hands often to avoid germs.
- Don't smoke.
- If you work around chemicals, dust, or other lung irritants, wear a special facemask.

WHAT TO EXPECT

DIAGNOSTIC MEASURES
- Your own observation of symptoms.
- Your health care provider will do a physical exam and use a stethoscope to listen to your lungs.
- Medical tests are usually not needed. A chest x-ray may be done if symptoms are more severe.

APPROPRIATE HEALTH CARE—Treatment is directed toward relieving the symptoms. Self-care is often all that is needed. Most cases will clear up on their own.

POSSIBLE COMPLICATIONS
- Pneumonia.
- Chronic bronchitis.
- Bronchiectasis (bronchial tubes become blocked).
- Pleurisy (swelling of the lining of the lungs).

PROBABLE OUTCOME—Usually curable in 1 week. Cases with complications are usually curable in 2 weeks, with drug therapy. In some people, the cough may continue for several weeks, even after the infection is gone.

HOW TO TREAT

GENERAL MEASURES
- If you are a smoker, don't smoke during your illness. Smoking makes it harder to recover. Nonsmokers should avoid secondhand smoke.
- Increase air moisture. Take warm showers. Use a room humidifier (clean it per instructions).
- To learn more: American Lung Association, 61 Broadway, 6th Floor, New York, NY 10006, (800) 586-4872; website: www.lungusa.org.

MEDICATION
- Use acetaminophen for fever and minor pain.
- Nonprescription cough suppressants (to ease coughing) or expectorants (to thin mucus) may be used to relieve symptoms. The mucus should be coughed up, so use cough suppressants with caution.
- Antibiotics may be prescribed for bacterial infection. They will not help a viral infection.
- Drugs may be prescribed for specific symptoms.

ACTIVITY—Get extra rest until symptoms improve. Then return to normal activities, as you feel better.

DIET—No special diet. Drink plenty of fluids each day. This helps makes mucus easier to cough up.

CALL YOUR DOCTOR IF

- You or a family member has symptoms of acute bronchitis.
- You develop a high fever and chills. You have chest pain. You cough up mucus that is thick, colored, or has blood in it. You feel short of breath, even when resting.

BRONCHITIS, CHRONIC

GENERAL INFORMATION

DEFINITION—Chronic bronchitis is an inflammation of the mucous lining of the bronchi (main air passages) to the lungs. It often occurs along with emphysema (damaged air sacs in the lungs).

BODY PARTS INVOLVED—Bronchial tubes (bronchi).

SEX OR AGE MOST AFFECTED—It usually affects adults over age 45 and women more than men.

SIGNS & SYMPTOMS—Symptoms don't start suddenly. They develop over time. They include: presence of a mucus-producing cough most days of the month, 3 months of the year, for 2 consecutive years.

CAUSES—Repeated irritation or infection in the bronchial tubes. The tubes begin to thicken and become more narrow. They begin to lose their elasticity. The main cause is smoking.

RISK INCREASES WITH
- Smoking.
- History of lung disorders.
- Family history of lung disease.
- Exposure to air pollutants or cigarette smoke.
- Work that involves exposure to high levels of dust and irritating fumes.

HOW TO PREVENT
- Don't smoke. This is the best prevention.
- Avoid fumes in the environment.
- Get prompt medical care for lung infections.

WHAT TO EXPECT

DIAGNOSTIC MEASURES
- Your own observation of symptoms.
- Your health care provider will do a physical exam and ask questions about your symptoms, smoking habits, and exposure to pollutants or irritants. Many lung and heart disorders cause symptoms identical to those of chronic bronchitis.
- Medical tests are used to confirm diagnosis.

APPROPRIATE HEALTH CARE
- Treatment can help relieve symptoms and help prevent complications. A treatment plan will be developed based on your individual needs.
- Your health care provider can teach you exercises to help improve your breathing.
- Supplemental oxygen may be required.
- Lung reduction surgery or lung transplantation may be recommended for advanced cases.

POSSIBLE COMPLICATIONS
- Pneumonia, emphysema, abnormal heart rhythms, or cor pulmonale (heart disorder).
- Respiratory failure (lungs fail to function properly).

PROBABLE OUTCOME—There is no cure for this disorder. Treatment can help relieve the symptoms and slow the progress of the disease. Smokers must stop smoking.

HOW TO TREAT

GENERAL MEASURES
- Stop smoking. Find a way to quit that works for you.
- Avoid areas with air pollution, dust, or fumes. Consider changing jobs if you need to.
- Install air-conditioning with a filter and humidity control in your home.
- Avoid shouting, laughing loudly, and crying if these make you cough.
- Get a pneumococcal vaccine and annual flu vaccine.
- To learn more: American Lung Association, 61 Broadway, 6th Floor, New York, NY 10006, (800) 586-4872; website: www.lungusa.org.

MEDICATION
- Don't take drugs to lessen your cough. They can make this condition worse.
- Antibiotics for infection may be prescribed.
- Oral or inhaled bronchodilator drugs may be prescribed to relax and open the airways in the lungs.
- Oral or inhaled steroids may be prescribed to reduce inflammation.
- Drugs to thin the mucous may be prescribed.

ACTIVITY
- Regular exercise is important. Long periods of being inactive can add to your disability.
- Avoid sudden temperature changes. Avoid cold, wet weather.
- Be careful when exercising or working. Work at a pace that does not make you cough.

DIET—No special diet. Drink plenty of fluids. This can help thin the mucus produced by your lungs.

CALL YOUR DOCTOR IF

- You or a family member has symptoms of chronic bronchitis.
- You have a fever or vomiting.
- Mucus gets thicker or has blood in it.
- Your chest pain gets worse.
- You feel short of breath even when you are resting or not coughing.

BRUCELLOSIS
(Undulant Fever; Bang's Disease)

GENERAL INFORMATION

DEFINITION—Brucellosis is an infection passed to humans from infected cows, pigs, sheep, or goats. The infection may be acute (short lasting) or chronic (persisting over months or years). It is a rare disease in the United States.

BODY PARTS INVOLVED—Blood-producing organs, including bone marrow, lymph glands, liver and spleen.

SEX OR AGE MOST AFFECTED—Both sexes and all ages, but most common in men between ages 20 and 60.

SIGNS & SYMPTOMS
- Sweating, chills, and fever (may come and go).
- Tiredness.
- Upset stomach.
- Tenderness along the spine.
- Headache.
- Muscle and joint aches.
- Constipation.
- Weight loss.
- Depression.
- In later stages of the infection, mental problems and seizures may occur.

CAUSES
- Infection from germs of the bacterial genus *Brucella*. The germs can be passed to humans by eating or drinking something that is contaminated. This most often involves milk and milk products such as cheese. Infection can also occur from breathing in germs in the air. Germs can enter the body through skin wounds. After a person is exposed, symptoms may develop in 1 to 8 weeks.
- Person-to-person spread is extremely rare. An infected mother may pass it through breast-feeding to an infant. Sexual transmission has been reported.
- Dogs can get infected with the germs, but it is unlikely to be passed to humans. However, persons with a weak immune system should not handle infected dogs.

RISK INCREASES WITH
- Persons who work with animals. This includes farmers, ranchers, meat processors, and veterinarians.
- Travel to some foreign countries.
- Biological warfare.

HOW TO PREVENT
- Don't drink milk from any source that has not been pasteurized.
- Protect yourself when working around animals. Use safety protection (gloves and mask) as needed.
- Farm animals should be immunized.

WHAT TO EXPECT

DIAGNOSTIC MEASURES
- Your own observation of symptoms.
- Your health care provider will do a physical exam and ask questions about your symptoms and activities. Be sure to discuss any contact with animals you have had in the last few months.
- Medical tests may include studies of blood, urine, and spinal fluid. X-ray, CT, heart tests, and others may be done depending on the symptoms.

APPROPRIATE HEALTH CARE
- Treatment usually consists of drugs for infection and getting extra rest.
- If symptoms are more severe, hospital care may be needed.

POSSIBLE COMPLICATIONS
- Endocarditis (heart inflammation).
- Complications can affect almost any body system.
- Brucellosis may recur.

PROBABLE OUTCOME—Can usually be cured in 3 to 4 weeks with treatment. Some muscle aches may continue for a period of time.

HOW TO TREAT

GENERAL MEASURES
- It usually is not necessary to keep the ill person away from others.
- Avoid contact with animals that may be the source of the infection.
- Family members who may have been exposed to the same infected food products should see their health care provider.

MEDICATION
- Antibiotic drugs will be prescribed for the infection. You usually need to take them for several weeks.
- Drugs to reduce swelling in severe cases and for relief of muscle pain may be prescribed.

ACTIVITY—Get extra rest until fever and other symptoms improve. Return to your normal activities slowly.

DIET—No special diet.

CALL YOUR DOCTOR IF

- You or a family member has symptoms of brucellosis.
- Fever or other symptoms return after treatment.
- New, unexplained symptoms develop. Drugs used in treatment may produce side effects.

BUERGER'S DISEASE
(Thromboangiitis Obliterans)

 GENERAL INFORMATION

DEFINITION—Buerger's disease is a blockage of small and medium arteries due to inflammation of blood vessels. The symptoms come on gradually over a period of time.

BODY PARTS INVOLVED—Arteries (and sometimes veins) in the extremities.

SEX OR AGE MOST AFFECTED—The disease is most common in men between ages 20 and 45 who are heavy cigarette smokers. However, it is now being diagnosed more in women.

SIGNS & SYMPTOMS
- Numbness and tingling in the legs, feet, arms, and fingers.
- Pain in the feet and legs while walking or during exercise. This pain occurs less often in the hands and fingers. Pain comes from not having enough blood flow to these areas of the body. Pain becomes persistent as disease progresses.
- Raynaud's phenomenon. A condition where the hands, fingers, feet, and toes turn white, blue, or red when exposed to cold.
- Painful sores (ulcers) and gangrene (dead tissue) on the toes and fingertips.

CAUSES—Unknown. The disease is probably triggered by smoking combined with an immune reaction in the body. Most patients are heavy smokers, but some are moderate smokers, and some use smokeless tobacco. Genetic factors are thought to be involved also. Israeli Jews of Ashkenazi have higher risk, as do people in the Middle East, Far East, and Asia.

RISK INCREASES WITH
- Smoking or using smokeless tobacco.
- Family history of Buerger's disease.

HOW TO PREVENT—There are no specific preventive measures, except never to smoke.

 WHAT TO EXPECT

DIAGNOSTIC MEASURES
- Your own observation of symptoms.
- Your health care provider will do a physical exam and ask questions about your symptoms and smoking history. This is often enough to make the diagnosis.
- Medical tests may be done to rule out other disorders and check for complications.

APPROPRIATE HEALTH CARE
- There is no effective drug or specific treatment for the disorder.
- Counseling may be recommended to help with lifestyle changes required to cope with the disease.
- If gangrene develops, amputation of the affected limb, toes, or fingers is likely.

POSSIBLE COMPLICATIONS
- Blood clots in the legs.
- Finger and toe ulcers, gangrene, and amputation.
- Life expectancy is shorter.

PROBABLE OUTCOME—This condition is currently considered incurable. Stopping smoking is the only effective treatment to stop the progress of the disease.

 HOW TO TREAT

GENERAL MEASURES
- Get treatment for any infection or injury that occurs.
- The disease will get worse if smoking continues, so stop smoking. Join a program to help you stop.
- Avoid exposure to the cold if possible. Cold causes blood vessels to constrict. This deprives your body of a normal blood supply. If you are going out in cold weather, wear warm footwear and gloves.
- Clip nails carefully to avoid injuring the skin.
- Wear shoes that fit well. Wear cotton or wool socks.
- Insert soft pads in your shoes to protect your feet.
- Don't go barefoot outdoors.

MEDICATION—Drugs that open the blood vessels may be prescribed. These drugs will not help if you continue smoking.

ACTIVITY—Stay as active as you can. Begin an exercise program to become as physically fit as possible.

DIET—No special diet.

 CALL YOUR DOCTOR IF

- You or a family member has symptoms of Buerger's disease.
- You have pain that cannot be controlled.
- Sores develop on your fingers or toes.
- New, unexplained symptoms develop. Drugs used in treatment may produce side effects.

BULIMIA

GENERAL INFORMATION

DEFINITION—Bulimia is an eating disorder. A person with bulimia eats larger amounts of food (called binging) than most people would eat in a short time. Then they purge (such as with self-induced vomiting or other methods) to rid themselves of the food and avoid weight gain. They may also use nonpurging methods such as fasting or exercising too much. There can be numerous symptoms including behavioral, physical, and emotional effects.

BODY PARTS INVOLVED—Brain and central nervous system; kidneys; liver; endocrine system; gastrointestinal tract.

SEX OR AGE MOST AFFECTED—Bulimia affects both sexes (women much more than men). It often starts in the teen years.

SIGNS & SYMPTOMS
- Episodes of binge eating. Eating in secret or in hiding.
- Denial of hunger.
- Self-induced vomiting that occurs after eating.
- Frequent trips to the bathroom after meals.
- Frequent use of laxatives, water or diet pills.
- Excess exercising.
- Consistently aspires to achieve or overachieve.
- Obsessed with body image, appearance, and weight.
- A "chipmunk" like appearance. It may include swelling of the cheeks, face, or salivary glands.
- Lack of menstrual periods.
- Depression, anxiety, or mood swings. Feeling out of control. Low self-esteem; poor self-identity.
- Heartburn, bloating, indigestion, constipation.
- Dental problems and sore throat.
- Weakness, tiredness, bloodshot eyes, dry skin.

CAUSES—There is no single known cause. Factors that play a role include emotional and psychological factors, genetics, and cultural pressures (e.g., feel pressured to be very thin).

RISK INCREASES WITH
- Young females, compulsive and perfectionistic type persons, dieters, and those overly concerned about weight.
- Stress, including lifestyle changes, such as moving, starting at a new school or job, or relationship breakup.
- Personality disorders.
- Sports, work, or artistic activities. These can include athletes, actors, television personalities, dancers, models, gymnasts, runners, boxers, and wrestlers.
- Homosexual males.

HOW TO PREVENT—No specific preventive measures. Early treatment may help keep it from progressing.

WHAT TO EXPECT

DIAGNOSTIC MEASURES
- Your own observation of symptoms. Many patients are secretive, and parents may be unaware of this condition.
- Your health care provider can often diagnose bulimia with a physical exam and by asking questions about your symptoms, eating habits, and weight concerns.
- There is no test to diagnose bulimia. Medical tests may be done to check for underlying disorders, physical problems, or complications.

APPROPRIATE HEALTH CARE
- Treatment goals include: education about the disorder, healthy eating patterns, maintaining normal weight, and preventing a relapse.
- Treatment may include counseling for the patient and the family, nutritional help, and drug therapy if needed. Care in a hospital or special facility may be required.
- A dental exam is usually recommended.
- Counseling can change how you think about food and how you handle feelings and emotions.

POSSIBLE COMPLICATIONS—Many mental and physical health problems can develop. They can be serious and life-threatening.

PROBABLE OUTCOME—Outcome varies. If patients desire to change, they can often be helped with therapy. For some patients, it may continue long-term. A few may have episodes of bulimia that occur only with life events and crisis.

HOW TO TREAT

GENERAL MEASURES
- Denial of the severity or even the existence of the problem is common in patients. Most resist treatment and behavior changes at first. Some want a quick, easy solution which is not possible.
- Support groups can often help patients.
- To learn more: National Eating Disorders Association, 603 Stewart St., Suite 803, Seattle WA 98101; (800) 931-2237; website: www.nationaleatingdisorders.org.

MEDICATION—Drugs for depression or anxiety and dietary supplements may be prescribed.

ACTIVITY—May be limited at first. Then choose activities for fun and fitness—not to lose weight.

DIET—A dietitian can help with meal planning.

CALL YOUR DOCTOR IF

- You have symptoms of bulimia or you suspect a family member has bulimia.
- Treatment does not improve bulimia behavior.

BUNION
(Hallux Valgus)

GENERAL INFORMATION

DEFINITION—A bunion is a bony swelling or bump that occurs along the side of the big toe joint.

BODY PARTS INVOLVED—Great (big) toe.

SEX OR AGE MOST AFFECTED—Bunions may start in the teenage years, but usually occur in the 20 to 30 age group. Three times as many women as men have bunions.

SIGNS & SYMPTOMS
- A big toe that points in, toward the other toes. This is called hallux valgus.
- Thickened skin over an enlarged, bony bump at the base of the big toe.
- Fluid may build up under the thickened skin.
- Foot pain and stiffness.
- The symptoms progress slowly over a period of years.

CAUSES—The big toe has been forced into an incorrect position. This causes the joint to stick out. The big toe may overlap one or more of the other toes.

RISK INCREASES WITH
- Family history of foot problems (inherited weakness in the toe joints).
- Flat feet.
- Arthritis.
- Shoes that have high heels and narrow toes that push the toes together.

HOW TO PREVENT
- Exercise daily to keep muscles of the feet and legs in good condition.
- Wear shoes that have wide toes and fit well. Don't wear high heels or shoes without room for toes in their normal position.

WHAT TO EXPECT

DIAGNOSTIC MEASURES
- Your own observation of symptoms.
- Your health care provider can diagnose a bunion by its appearance.
- An x-ray of the toe joint may be done.

APPROPRIATE HEALTH CARE
- Treatment usually involves self-care steps and surgery, if needed.
- Custom-made orthotics (shoe inserts) may be prescribed.
- Surgery (bunionectomy) may be recommended when bunion makes walking painful. The bunion is removed and the toe may be straightened. Specific instructions will be provided for self-care after surgery (see Bunion Removal in Surgery section).

POSSIBLE COMPLICATIONS
- Infection of the bunion, especially in persons with diabetes.
- Inflammation and arthritis in other joints caused by difficulty in walking. Arthritis can result from abnormal stress on the foot, hip, and spine.
- Bunion may grow back after surgery.

PROBABLE OUTCOME—A bunion is permanent unless surgery is performed to remove it. Self-care can help improve the symptoms.

HOW TO TREAT

GENERAL MEASURES
- Wear comfortable shoes that fit well.
- If there is swelling, redness, and pain, keep pressure off the affected toe.
- Before bedtime, separate the first toe from the others with a foam-rubber pad.
- Wear a thick, ring-shaped pad around and over the bunion. Use arch supports to relieve pressure on the bunion. These are available in drugstores or shoe-repair shops.

MEDICATION—Use nonprescription drugs such as aspirin or ibuprofen for pain, swelling, and soreness.

ACTIVITY—If you have surgery, resume your normal activities slowly after surgery. Recovery may take 2 months or more.

DIET—No special diet.

CALL YOUR DOCTOR IF

- You or a family member has a bunion that is interfering with normal activities.
- You develop signs of infection after treatment or surgery. Signs of infection include fever, tenderness, or pain.

BURNS

GENERAL INFORMATION

DEFINITION—A burn is an injury to the skin from contact with heat, radiation, electricity, sunlight, or chemicals. Sometimes internal organs may also be injured.

BODY PARTS INVOLVED—Skin; underlying tissue and respiratory system (sometimes).

SEX OR AGE MOST AFFECTED—Both sexes; all ages. The risk of damage is greatest with infants and young children.

SIGNS & SYMPTOMS
- Thin or superficial burns (1st-degree burns) are limited to the upper skin layer. They cause redness, tenderness, pain, and swelling.
- Partial thickness burns (2nd-degree burns) affect deeper skin layers. Symptoms are more severe and usually include blisters.
- Full thickness burns (3rd-degree burns) involve all skin layers. Skin is white and appears cooked. There may be no pain in the initial stages.

CAUSES
- Rise in skin temperature from heat sources such as fire, steam, or electricity. Open flame and hot liquid are the most common causes.
- Tissue injury caused by chemicals or radiation, including sunlight.
- Lightning strikes can cause internal burns with few external signs.

RISK INCREASES WITH
- Stress, carelessness, smoking in bed, or excess alcohol use. All of these make accidents more likely.
- Jobs involving exposure to heat or radiation (e.g., firefighting, police work, or factory work).
- Faulty electrical wiring.
- Hot water heaters set too high.

HOW TO PREVENT
- Fireproof your home. Install smoke alarms. Plan emergency exits and have regular fire drills.
- Wear protective gear around heat or radiation.
- Don't touch uncovered electric wires.
- Teach children safety rules for matches, fires, electrical outlets, cords, and stoves.
- Use extension cords only when necessary.
- If you have small children, put safety covers on outlets. Get rid of frayed cords.
- Buy flame-resistant sleepwear for children.
- Use sunscreen to prevent sunburn.
- Find safe shelter if in lightning storm.

WHAT TO EXPECT

DIAGNOSTIC MEASURES
- Your own observation of symptoms.
- A health care provider can diagnose burns by an exam of the skin.
- Medical tests will depend on type of injury.

APPROPRIATE HEALTH CARE
- Emergency care and a hospital stay are usually needed for severe burns. Problems such as lung damage from smoke may need treatment. There are special burn centers for the most serious cases.
- See your health care provider for burns that are less severe. The burn area will be examined and treatment given depending on the type of burn and size of the area affected.
- Self-care can be done for most minor burns.
- Special dressings and skin-care products may be prescribed.
- Surgery may be needed to graft skin, and rehabilitation may be needed after burns start healing (see Skin Graft in Surgery section).

POSSIBLE COMPLICATIONS
- Infection.
- Shock, due to loss of fluids from the body.
- Severe burns can cause serious health problems that can lead to death.

PROBABLE OUTCOME—With less severe burns, skin usually heals in 1 to 3 weeks. Most persons recover if the burns affect less than 50% of the body's surface.

HOW TO TREAT

GENERAL MEASURES
- For minor burns treated at home:
  - Place the burned area in cold water, hold it under running water, or use wet compresses on it for at least 5 minutes (longer for chemical burns). This will reduce pain and swelling. Don't use ice on a burn.
  - Use an aloe vera cream or antibiotic ointment (no butter). Wrap the area loosely with sterile gauze dressing to protect the area. Change the dressing each day.
  - Don't break blisters. This can cause infection.
  - Keep the burned area higher than the rest of the body, if possible.

MEDICATION
- You may use acetaminophen or ibuprofen for pain.
- Hospital care may include drugs to treat the burns, for pain, and to prevent infection. A tetanus booster is needed if it is not up to date.

ACTIVITY—Resume normal activity as soon as possible. This will help speed recovery.

DIET—No special diet unless advised.

CALL YOUR DOCTOR IF

- You or a family member has a burn that does not heal in 5 to 6 days.
- Child under age 2 has any burns.
- You develop chills, fever; increased pain, redness, swelling, or pus in the burn area.

BURSITIS

GENERAL INFORMATION

DEFINITION—Bursitis is the inflammation (swelling and pain) of a bursa. A bursa is a soft, fluid-filled sac that serves as a cushion between tendons and bones. There are over 150 bursa in the human body.

BODY PARTS INVOLVED—Bursae, especially near the shoulders, elbows, knees, pelvis, hips or Achilles tendons.

SEX OR AGE MOST AFFECTED—Both sexes; usually in adults.

SIGNS & SYMPTOMS
* Pain, swelling, tenderness, and limited movement in the affected joint. Pain may spread into nearby areas of the body.
* A feeling of warmth over the affected joint.

CAUSES—Inflammation can be caused by overuse, injury, disease, or infection. Sometimes no cause is found.

RISK INCREASES WITH
* Injury to a joint.
* Overuse of a joint.
* Exercising more than usual.
* Calcium deposits in shoulder tendons.
* Infection.
* Arthritis.
* Gout.
* People who suddenly increase their activity levels ("weekend warriors").
* Not stretching properly or over-stretching.

HOW TO PREVENT
* Avoid injuries when possible. Don't overuse muscles. Wear protective gear for contact sports.
* Warm-up before exercise. Cool-down after exercise.
* Stay physically fit.

WHAT TO EXPECT

DIAGNOSTIC MEASURES
* Your own observation of symptoms.
* See your health care provider if self-care does not help or symptoms are severe. Bursitis can be diagnosed by a physical exam.
* Medical tests are usually not done.

APPROPRIATE HEALTH CARE
* Your health care provider may sometimes drain fluid from the joint with a needle. Surgery is rarely needed.
* Physical therapy may be recommended to maintain flexibility, mobility, and strength of the joint.

POSSIBLE COMPLICATIONS
* Prolonged healing time if the activity that led to the problem is resumed too soon.
* Chronic bursitis may occur due to repeated injuries or recurrent attacks of bursitis.

PROBABLE OUTCOME—This is a common, but not serious problem. Symptoms usually improve in 7 to 14 days with treatment.

HOW TO TREAT

GENERAL MEASURES
* Self-care may be all that is needed.
  - Use RICE therapy (rest, ice, compression, and elevation). Rest the affected joint. Use an ice pack to massage the area several times a day. Use compression by wearing an elastic bandage. Elevate the affected joint by resting it on a pillow.
  - You may use heat, in addition to ice, if it feels better. Apply a hot, wet towel or use a heating pad. A deep-heating ointment may be helpful.

MEDICATION
* Use nonprescription acetaminophen or ibuprofen for mild pain.
* Your health care provider may prescribe:
  - Nonsteroidal anti-inflammatory drugs or creams.
  - Antibiotics (if the bursa is infected).
  - Prescription pain relievers for severe pain.
  - Injection with a local anesthetic mixed with a corticosteroid drug.

ACTIVITY
* Rest the affected joint as much as possible. It may help to wear a sling or a brace, or to use crutches until the pain becomes easier to bear. Begin normal, slow joint movement as soon as pain permits.
* Follow directions for any recommended home exercise routines.

DIET—No special diet.

CALL YOUR DOCTOR IF

* You or a family member has symptoms of bursitis that is severe or self-care methods do not help.
* New symptoms develop after treatment.

CALCIUM IMBALANCE
(Hypercalcemia; Hypocalcemia)

 GENERAL INFORMATION

DEFINITION—Calcium is a mineral that helps regulate the heartbeat, transmit nerve impulses, and contract muscles. It also helps form bone and teeth. Too much calcium (hypercalcemia) or too little calcium (hypocalcemia) can cause mild to serious medical problems. The problems can sometimes be life-threatening.

BODY PARTS INVOLVED—Most calcium is stored in the bones, but it is also found in the blood and cells. The parathyroid glands and parathyroid hormones regulate calcium absorption and utilization.

SEX OR AGE MOST AFFECTED—Both sexes; all ages.

SIGNS & SYMPTOMS
- Usually no symptoms unless calcium levels are very high or very low.
- Too little calcium:
  - Muscle spasms, twitching, or cramping.
  - Arms, hands, legs, and feet may tingle or feel numb.
  - Seizures (convulsion).
  - Heartbeat is irregular.
  - High blood pressure.
- Too much calcium:
  - Feeling tired and sluggish.
  - Loss of appetite.
  - Vomiting, diarrhea, dehydration, and thirst.
  - Heartbeat is irregular.
  - Low blood pressure.
  - Depression; mental changes (confused or delirious).
  - Seizures or coma (in severe cases).

CAUSES
- Too little calcium:
  - Parathyroid glands that are underactive (can be caused by disease or parathyroid damage).
  - Not getting enough calcium and vitamin D.
  - Problems with calcium absorption.
  - Severe burns or infections.
  - Problems with the pancreas.
  - Kidney failure.
  - Low levels of certain minerals in your blood.
- Too much calcium:
  - Parathyroid gland that is overactive.
  - Broken bones and long periods of bed rest.
  - Cancer of the bone marrow.
  - Tumors that destroy bone.
  - Certain drugs (e.g., thiazide diuretics).

RISK INCREASES WITH
- Too little calcium:
  - Use of certain drugs such as diuretics.
  - Injury, cancer, or surgery of the thyroid or parathyroid glands.
  - Excess alcohol use.
  - Poor nutrition.

- Too much calcium:
  - Diet that is too high in dairy products or excess use of antacids that contain calcium.
  - Kidney disease.
  - Being inactive or bed rest for long periods.

HOW TO PREVENT
- Eat a normal, well-balanced diet.
- Avoid alcohol or limit it to 1 to 2 drinks a day.
- Don't use nonprescription antacids on a regular basis.

 WHAT TO EXPECT

DIAGNOSTIC MEASURES
- Your own observation of symptoms.
- Your health care provider may do a physical exam.
- Medical tests can include blood studies of calcium levels, x-rays of bones, and heart study.

APPROPRIATE HEALTH CARE—Treatment involves correcting the problem or treating the disorder causing the imbalance. This may be all that is required. In other cases, treatment may be done to remove excess calcium or replace low calcium.

POSSIBLE COMPLICATIONS
- Heart attack.
- Bones may become weak and break easily.
- Kidney stones from high calcium.
- Ulcer from high calcium.

PROBABLE OUTCOME—Generally good, but the outcome will depend on the cause.

 HOW TO TREAT

GENERAL MEASURES—Follow the advice of your health care provider.

MEDICATION
- Drugs may be prescribed to raise or lower your calcium levels, depending on the need. Drugs may be given by mouth or through a needle placed in your vein (IV).
- For mild, low calcium level, calcium and vitamin D supplements may be recommended.
- Other drugs may be prescribed to treat a disorder causing the calcium imbalance.

ACTIVITY—Usually no limits unless symptoms are severe. Follow medical advice.

DIET—Be sure to eat a healthy, well-balanced diet. You will be advised if specific dietary changes are needed.

 CALL YOUR DOCTOR IF

- You or a family member has symptoms of calcium imbalance.
- Symptoms get worse or they don't improve.

CANDIDIASIS OF SKIN
(Moniliasis)

 GENERAL INFORMATION

DEFINITION—Candidiasis is a fungal (or yeast) infection in skin folds, or in areas of skin that touch other areas of skin.

BODY PARTS INVOLVED—It can affect the underarm area, spaces between fingers and toes, inner thighs, under the breasts, and over the base of the spine. It may affect the skin of the scrotum, vagina, and vaginal lips.

SEX OR AGE MOST AFFECTED—Both sexes; all ages.

SIGNS & SYMPTOMS
- Plaques (patches or flat areas) on skin.
- Bright-red patches with poorly defined borders. They are often 2.5 to 5 inches across, but may be larger.
- Patches may weep or ooze.
- Skin appears moist and crusted.
- Itching is usually severe.
- Smaller patches may surround larger patches. They sometimes form small white blisters with pus inside.

CAUSES—It is caused by *Candida*, a type of fungus. *Candida* fungi actually live on the skin and normally cause no harm. If skin is damaged or there is excess moisture and warmth, the fungus germs can grow and cause infection. The infection can be spread from one person to another by direct contact, and less often, by sexual contact. Germs are also spread by sharing damp towels or washcloths.

RISK INCREASES WITH
- Taking antibiotics.
- Use of any type of steroids.
- Diabetes.
- The elderly or infants (it causes diaper rash).
- Pregnant women or use of birth control pills.
- Using plastic pants for infants.
- Obesity.
- Existing skin infection or skin disorder.
- Weak immune system from illness or drugs.
- People who work in wet conditions.

HOW TO PREVENT
- Take antibiotics only when prescribed.
- Keep skin cool and dry.
- Avoid risk factors where possible.

 WHAT TO EXPECT

DIAGNOSTIC MEASURES
- Your own observation of symptoms.
- Your health care provider can diagnose the infection by an exam of the affected skin area.
- Medical tests may include a study of a skin scraping or pus.

APPROPRIATE HEALTH CARE
- Treatment involves drugs and self-care measures.
- Any skin condition that may have led to the candidiasis infection should be treated also.

POSSIBLE COMPLICATIONS
- Nail infection, causing them to thicken or crumble.
- Bacterial infection, in addition to the fungal infection.
- Infection spreading to the whole body (in those with weak immune systems).

PROBABLE OUTCOME
- Usually curable in 2 weeks with treatment. Without treatment, healing may be slow.
- It is common for these fungal infections to recur.

 HOW TO TREAT

GENERAL MEASURES
- Keep skin cool and dry. Expose affected skin areas to air as much as possible.
- Wear loose cotton clothing. Avoid synthetic or wool fabrics. Change socks often if feet are affected.
- To avoid spreading germs, don't go barefoot on wet floors where other people may walk. Don't share towels. Clean the bathtub or shower after you use it.
- Protect skin from injury, but don't bandage the affected skin.

MEDICATION—Antifungal drugs to be applied to the skin are usually prescribed. Gently massage a small amount into the affected area as directed. Use only enough to cover the affected area. Larger amounts don't help. In more severe cases, an antifungal drug taken by mouth may be prescribed.

ACTIVITY—No limits, except to avoid heat and sweating.

DIET—No special diet. Eating yogurt or taking probiotic supplements may or may not help prevent these infections (research is ongoing).

 CALL YOUR DOCTOR IF

- You or a family member has symptoms of candidiasis.
- During treatment, the infection continues to spread.
- Secondary bacterial infection develops (pain, tenderness, redness, warmth, and oozing).

CANKER SORES
(Aphthous Ulcers)

GENERAL INFORMATION

DEFINITION—Canker sores are painful ulcers (sores) that occur in the lining of the mouth. They cannot be spread from one person to another. They may be confused with herpes infections.

BODY PARTS INVOLVED—Mouth and adjacent areas.

SEX OR AGE MOST AFFECTED—Both sexes, but more common in women.

SIGNS & SYMPTOMS
* Ulcers are small, very painful, shallow, and covered by a gray membrane. Borders are surrounded by an intense red halo.
* Ulcers appear on lips, gums, inner cheeks, tongue, palate, and throat. Usually, 2 or 3 ulcers appear during an attack. As many as 10 to 15 ulcers is not uncommon.
* Ulcers may be so painful during first 2 or 3 days that they interfere with eating or speaking.
* Sometimes there is tingling or burning for 24 hours before the ulcer appears.
* In severe cases, fever, tiredness, or swollen lymph nodes may occur.

CAUSES—Exact cause is unclear.

RISK INCREASES WITH
* Emotional or physical stress, anxiety, or premenstrual tension.
* Injury to the mouth lining caused by rough dentures, hot food, toothbrushing, or dental work.
* Irritation from foods, such as chocolate, citrus, acidic foods (e.g., vinegar, pickles), salted nuts, or potato chips.
* Changes in the body's immune system.
* Family history of canker sores.

HOW TO PREVENT
* Brush teeth at least twice a day. Floss regularly to keep the mouth clean and healthy.
* Avoid risk factors where possible.
* Pay attention to your diet and when canker sores develop. Don't eat foods that seem to trigger the sores.

WHAT TO EXPECT

DIAGNOSTIC MEASURES
* Your own observation of symptoms.
* If you are concerned about the sores, see your health care provider. Canker sores can normally be diagnosed by an exam of the mouth.
* Medical tests may be done to rule out certain other disorders.

APPROPRIATE HEALTH CARE
* Medical care is usually not needed.
* If a canker sore is caused by a rough tooth, braces, or dentures, consult your dentist. The sore won't heal until the cause is treated.

POSSIBLE COMPLICATIONS—Rarely, dehydration may occur if eating and drinking are limited by the pain of the canker sores.

PROBABLE OUTCOME—Most will heal on their own in 2 weeks. It is common for them to recur. Recurrence can vary from a single canker sore 2 or 3 times a year, to frequent episodes of many sores.

HOW TO TREAT

GENERAL MEASURES—Rinse the mouth 3 or more times a day with a salt solution (1/2 teaspoon salt to 8 oz. water) if this isn't painful. You may try dabbing milk of magnesia on the canker sore several times a day. It can help relieve pain.

MEDICATION
* Nonprescription topical products are available that can help relieve canker sore discomfort.
* You may be prescribed an antibacterial mouth rinse, a corticosteroid ointment or rinse, a solution to control pain and irritation, or other drug therapy.

ACTIVITY—No limits.

DIET
* Avoid foods that irritate the sores. Drink lots of fluids. If possible, eat a well-balanced diet while healing.
* To avoid pain, sip liquids through straws. Foods that cause the least pain are milk, liquid gelatin, yogurt, ice cream, and custard.

CALL YOUR DOCTOR IF

* You or a family member has canker sores that don't improve in 2 weeks.
* Other symptoms occur at the same time as canker sores.

CARBON MONOXIDE POISONING

 GENERAL INFORMATION

DEFINITION—Carbon monoxide poisoning occurs after breathing in carbon monoxide (CO), a poison gas that has no color or smell. In the United States, it is the most common form of accidental poisoning. CO is produced when fuel such as gas, wood, oil, or coal is burned. Sources include motor vehicle or boat exhaust, space heaters, furnaces, charcoal grills, gas burning appliances or tools, propane-fueled equipment, and smoke from fires.

BODY PARTS INVOLVED—Total body.

SEX OR AGE MOST AFFECTED—Both sexes; all ages.

SIGNS & SYMPTOMS
- The first symptoms may be mild and flu-like.
- Headache; feeling dizzy and tired.
- Nausea and vomiting; stomach pain.
- Feeling like you might faint; trouble with walking.
- Difficulty breathing; chest pain; changes in heartbeat.
- Seizure.
- Vision changes.
- Confusion, depression, and other behavior changes.
- Coma (loss of consciousness).

CAUSES—Carbon monoxide is breathed into the lungs. It gets into the blood system and prevents the flow of oxygen that the body needs for survival.

RISK INCREASES WITH
- Furnaces or space-heating devices that do not work properly; a fireplace with a clogged chimney.
- Riding in the back of a pickup truck under a closed cover of some type.
- Poor venting (exhaust fumes escape into buildings or homes).
- Use of charcoal grill in enclosed place, such as a tent.
- Faulty motor vehicle exhaust system, or leaving a car running in a garage attached to a house.
- Winter months when heaters are in use and houses are more closed up.

HOW TO PREVENT
- Avoid the risk factors where you are able.
- Install a carbon monoxide alarm in your home. If it goes off, leave the house right away and call 911.
- Make sure the furnace, fireplaces, gas appliances, and heaters in your home work properly. Call your gas company if you think there may be a gas leak.
- Have a smoke alarm and fire extinguisher for each floor of your home. Develop an emergency exit plan.

 WHAT TO EXPECT

DIAGNOSTIC MEASURES
- If CO poisoning is suspected, move yourself or victim to fresh air. Seek emergency help.
- This type of poisoning cannot be treated at home. Medical care is needed.
- Your health care provider will do a physical exam and test your blood for carbon monoxide.
- Other medical tests may be done for more severe symptoms.

APPROPRIATE HEALTH CARE
- For mild cases, the symptoms usually disappear after you breathe in pure oxygen through a mask for a few hours.
- Some patients with more severe symptoms will require the use of breathing support in a hospital.
- Rarely, a patient is placed in a sealed chamber where high-pressure oxygen is used for treatment.

POSSIBLE COMPLICATIONS
- Poisoning can result in damage to the brain, heart, or lungs, and death. Children, the elderly, and those with lung disease are at high risk for adverse effects.
- Pregnant women may suffer miscarriage, early labor, fetal death, or a child with cerebral palsy.

PROBABLE OUTCOME
- In milder cases with quick treatment, recovery is complete and without complications.
- Some patients have delayed symptoms weeks later. They may feel extra tired, have memory problems, feel confused, or have mood and behavior changes.

 HOW TO TREAT

GENERAL MEASURES
- The source of the carbon monoxide needs to be found and repaired or replaced.
- To learn more: Consumer Product Safety Commission; (800) 638-2772; website: www.cpsc.gov or the Medline Plus website: www.nlm.nih.gov/medlineplus/carbonmonoxide poisoning.html.

MEDICATION—Usually not needed. Drugs may be used for seizures if they occur.

ACTIVITY—Depends on severity of symptoms.

DIET—No special diet.

☎ CALL YOUR DOCTOR IF

- You or a family member has carbon monoxide poisoning symptoms. Get emergency help!
- After recovery, any symptoms cause concern.

CARCINOID SYNDROME

GENERAL INFORMATION

DEFINITION—Carcinoid syndrome is a group of symptoms caused by a tumor (carcinoid). Carcinoids are called "cancers in slow motion" because of their slow growth. The tumors produce certain hormones (e.g., serotonin). When the tumor is within the intestine, the hormones are removed from the body by the liver. If the tumor has spread to the liver, it can no longer remove them. The hormones then travel through the body and cause the carcinoid syndrome symptoms. If the tumors occur outside the intestinal tract (e.g., lungs), carcinoid syndrome can develop without spread to the liver.

BODY PARTS INVOLVED—These tumors most often develop in the intestinal tract (e.g., small intestine, colon, or appendix) or lungs.

SEX OR AGE MOST AFFECTED—Adults (of both sexes) usually ages 50 to 70.

SIGNS & SYMPTOMS
• Because the tumors grow slowly, there may be no apparent symptoms.
• Symptoms may be triggered by physical or emotional stress, eating, and/or drinking hot liquids or alcohol.
• Flushing of head, neck, and chest. May last minutes or hours. Skin may be bluish afterwards.
• Diarrhea with abdominal cramps.
• Breathing problems (similar to asthma) and wheezing.
• Heart palpitations or irregular heartbeat.
• May have high or low blood pressure.
• Swelling of the face, hands, or feet.
• Weight loss.
• Intestinal obstruction may cause fever along with stomach pain and tenderness.

CAUSES—Unknown.

RISK INCREASES WITH
• Older adults.
• Family history of multiple endocrine neoplasia, type 1 (a hereditary disorder).

HOW TO PREVENT—No preventive measures.

WHAT TO EXPECT

DIAGNOSTIC MEASURES
• Your health care provider will do a physical exam and ask questions about your symptoms.
• Blood and urine studies are done to look for certain hormones and chemicals. Different imaging tests are done to locate the tumor and check for any disease spread.

APPROPRIATE HEALTH CARE
• Treatment varies and depends on the location and size of the tumor, person's health, age, and preferences.

• Surgery can bring [...] tumor is removed. If [...] removed, surgery can [...] portion as large as possi[...] symptoms.
• Hepatic artery embolizatio[...] cut off blood supply to the tum[...] frequency ablation uses heat to [...] cancer cells. Other procedures may be d[...]e depending on any complications.

POSSIBLE COMPLICATIONS
• Low blood pressure. It can increase risk of falls and injury.
• Carcinoid heart disease.
• Intestinal obstruction.
• Carcinoid crisis (a severe episode of the symptoms).
• Renal failure.

PROBABLE OUTCOME—In some patients, it can be cured with surgery. In others, the problem may progress, recur, or relapse.

HOW TO TREAT

GENERAL MEASURES
• Avoid emotional stress that can trigger symptoms.
• To learn more: American Cancer Society; (800) ACS-2345; website: www.cancer.org or National Cancer Institute; (800) 4-CANCER; website: www.cancer.gov.

MEDICATION
• Your health care provider may prescribe:
 - Antidiarrheal drugs.
 - Anticancer drugs (chemotherapy).
 - Drugs to prevent serotonin production.
 - Biologic therapy to stimulate the immune system.
 - Drugs to prevent flushed skin.
 - Multivitamins and niacin supplements.

ACTIVITY—Mild physical activity is usually not harmful. Avoid intense physical activity that can trigger symptoms.

DIET
• Increased protein intake in the diet is often advised.
• Avoid alcohol and foods that trigger symptoms.

CALL YOUR DOCTOR IF

• You or a family member has symptoms of carcinoid syndrome.
• Symptoms become worse or drugs used for treatment cause unexpected side effects.

BASAL CELL

DEFINITION—Basal cell carcinoma (BCC) is a cancer that develops in the skin's basal layer. The basal layer is at the bottom of the skin's outer layer (epidermis). BCC is the most common type of skin cancer.

BODY PARTS INVOLVED—It usually involves the skin exposed to sun (e.g., face, ears, backs of hands, shoulders, and arms).

SEX OR AGE MOST AFFECTED—Adults over age 40 are most often affected, and men more than women.

SIGNS & SYMPTOMS
- The skin cancer can vary in size and appearance. It usually grows slowly over months or even years.
- A sore that does not heal within 3 weeks or heals and recurs. It may bleed, ooze, or have a crust.
- An area or patch of skin that is reddish or irritated. It might have a crust.
- A shiny, pearly looking bump on the skin. The color is usually pink, red, or white. On some people, the color may be tan, black, or brown and look like a mole.
- A skin growth that is pink with a slightly raised, rolled border. The center is crusted and is lower than the border. Tiny blood vessels may be seen as it grows larger.
- An area that looks like a white or yellow scar; skin is shiny and looks tight (a more rare type).

CAUSES—Exact cause is unknown. Genetic and environmental factors play a role.

RISK INCREASES WITH
- Ultraviolet (UV) radiation from sun exposure. Tanning lamps or booths are also risks. UV rays damage the skin. The effect is cumulative over a lifetime.
- People with fair skin or sunburn easily.
- Living in area where there is lots of sunlight.
- Older adults and males more than females.
- Radiation therapy.
- Family history of skin cancers.
- Previous skin cancer.
- Other, more rare risk factors.

HOW TO PREVENT
- Limit exposure to sunlight. Protect skin with a hat, clothing, and sunscreen with SPF of 30 or more. Reapply sunscreen every 2 hours during sun exposure.
- Perform a skin self-exam once a month. Check for new growths or changes in other growths.

 WHAT TO EXPECT

DIAGNOSTIC MEASURES
- Your observation of symptoms.

- Your health care provider will examine the affected skin area. All or part of the affected skin tissue may be removed for a biopsy. The tissue is then viewed under a microscope to see if it is cancerous.

APPROPRIATE HEALTH CARE
- Treatment varies with appearance, location, and extent of the skin cancer. The method chosen is often decided by you and your health care provider together. Options can include:
  - Curettage and electrodesiccation—local anesthetic applied, then cutting out or shaving of the cancer, followed by high-frequency electrical current to destroy tissue with heat.
  - Surgical excision—local anesthetic is applied, skin is marked for surgery, and a scalpel is used for excision.
  - Moh's surgery—a special type of surgery used to treat high-risk cancers, especially on the head and face.
  - Cryosurgery—use of liquid nitrogen to freeze and kill the cells. A local anesthetic may be used.
  - Topical drug therapy—used in some cases.
  - Laser treatment—sometimes used.
  - Radiation treatment—used if cancer location requires it, such as near lips and eyelids.
  - Photodynamic therapy—uses drugs and special light.
- A skin graft or flap may be used to repair skin.

POSSIBLE COMPLICATIONS
- Rarely, skin cancer may recur or spread.
- Complications or scarring from the surgery.

PROBABLE OUTCOME—Curable in almost all cases with early diagnosis and treatment. People who have had skin cancer are at higher risk for new skin cancers elsewhere on the skin.

 HOW TO TREAT

GENERAL MEASURES
- Your health care provider will advise you of any follow-up care needed after treatment.
- To learn more: American Cancer Society; (800) ACS-2345; website: www.cancer.org or National Cancer Institute; (800) 4-CANCER; website: www.cancer.gov.

MEDICATION—Topical drugs (chemotherapy) may be prescribed.

ACTIVITY—No limits.

DIET—No special diet.

 CALL YOUR DOCTOR IF

- You or a family member has signs of skin cancer.
- After treatment, any new skin problems develop.

CARCINOMA, SQUAMOUS CELL

GENERAL INFORMATION

DEFINITION—Squamous cell carcinoma (SCC) is a cancer that develops in the skin's squamous cells. These cells make up the skin's outer layer (epithelium). SCC is the second most common type of skin cancer.

BODY PARTS INVOLVED—It usually involves the skin of the face, ears, backs of hands, shoulders, and arms.

SEX OR AGE MOST AFFECTED—Adults over age 40 are most often affected, and men more often than women.

SIGNS & SYMPTOMS
- A sore that does not heal within 3 weeks. It may bleed or ooze or have a crust.
- An area or patch of skin that is reddish or irritated. It might have a crust.
- A shiny, pearly looking skin bump. The color is usually pink, red, or white. On some people, the color may be tan, black, or brown and look like a mole.
- A skin growth that is pink with a slightly raised, rolled border. The center is crusted and is lower than the border. Tiny blood vessels may be seen as it grows larger.
- An area that looks like a white or yellow scar. The skin is shiny and looks tight. This type is more rare.

CAUSES—Exact cause is unknown. Genetic and environmental factors play a role.

RISK INCREASES WITH
- Ultraviolet (UV) radiation from sun exposure. Tanning lamps or booths are also risks. UV rays damage the skin. The effect is cumulative over a lifetime.
- People with fair skin or sunburn easily.
- Living in area where there is lots of sunlight.
- Older adults and males more than females.
- Radiation therapy.
- Family history of skin cancers.
- Previous skin cancer.
- Other, more rare risk factors.

HOW TO PREVENT
- Limit exposure to sunlight. Protect skin with a hat, clothing, and sunscreen with SPF of 30 or more. Reapply sunscreen every 2 hours during sun exposure.
- Perform a skin self-exam once a month. Check for new growths or changes in other growths.

WHAT TO EXPECT

DIAGNOSTIC MEASURES
- Your observation of symptoms.

- Your health care provider will examine the affected skin area. All or part of the affected skin tissue may be removed for a biopsy. The tissue is then viewed under a microscope to see if it is cancerous.

APPROPRIATE HEALTH CARE
- Treatment varies with appearance, location, and extent of the skin cancer. The method chosen is often decided by you and your health care provider together. Options can include:
  - Curettage and electrodesiccation—local anesthetic applied, then cutting out or shaving of the cancer, followed by high-frequency electrical current to destroy tissue with heat.
  - Surgical excision—local anesthetic is applied, skin is marked for surgery, and a scalpel is used for excision.
  - Moh's surgery—a special type of surgery used to treat high-risk cancers, especially on the head and face.
  - Cryosurgery—use of liquid nitrogen to freeze and kill the cells. A local anesthetic may be used.
  - Topical drug therapy—used in some cases.
  - Laser treatment—sometimes used.
  - Radiation treatment—used if cancer location requires it, such as near lips and eyelids.
  - Photodynamic therapy—uses drugs and special light.
- A skin graft or flap may be used to repair skin.

POSSIBLE COMPLICATIONS
- Rarely, skin cancer may recur or spread.
- Complications or scarring from the surgery.

PROBABLE OUTCOME—Curable in almost all cases with early diagnosis and treatment. People who have had skin cancer are at higher risk for new skin cancers elsewhere on the skin.

HOW TO TREAT

GENERAL MEASURES
- Your health care provider will advise you of any follow-up care needed after treatment.
- To learn more: American Cancer Society; (800) ACS-2345; website: www.cancer.org or National Cancer Institute; (800) 4-CANCER; website: www.cancer.gov.

MEDICATION—Topical drugs (chemotherapy) may be prescribed.

ACTIVITY—No limits.

DIET—No special diet.

CALL YOUR DOCTOR IF

- You or a family member has signs of skin cancer.
- After treatment, any new skin problems develop.

CARDIAC ARREST

GENERAL INFORMATION

DEFINITION—Cardiac arrest is the total loss of heart-pumping action. This stops blood flow to the rest of the body. Delay of treatment for only 3 to 5 minutes may cause death or permanent brain damage. Cardiac arrest is not the same as a heart attack which is due to a lack of blood flow usually from a blood clot. But in some cases, a heart attack can trigger cardiac arrest.

BODY PARTS INVOLVED—Heart.

SEX OR AGE MOST AFFECTED—Up to age 45, it is more common in men. After age 45, the incidence is equal in men and women.

SIGNS & SYMPTOMS
- Brief dizziness; then fainting and unconsciousness.
- No pulse. Usually breathing also stops.
- Skin color becomes bluish-white. The pupils of the eye may get bigger.
- Seizures.
- Loss of bowel and bladder control (sometimes). Simple fainting may seem like a cardiac arrest, but heartbeat and breathing continue.

CAUSES—Heart suddenly stops beating. This may be due to a heart that is beating too fast, too slow, or that has an irregular heartbeat. Other causes include electrical shock, drowning, choking, trauma, or respiratory arrest (lungs stop working).

RISK INCREASES WITH
- Heart attack or heart disease.
- Pulmonary embolism (a blood clot to the lung).
- Lack of blood circulation and profound shock caused by uncontrolled bleeding or overwhelming infection.
- Loss of oxygen from drowning, choking, or from anesthesia during surgery.
- Potassium or fluid imbalance in the blood.
- Diabetes.
- Use of certain heart medicines.
- Use of medicines that help with fluid retention. These can cause low potassium in the blood.
- Use of any drug that raises blood pressure in a heart patient. This can include cold capsules, decongestant tablets, and nasal sprays.
- Using drugs of abuse, such as cocaine and intravenous drugs.

HOW TO PREVENT
- Live a healthy lifestyle. Get regular exercise, eat a healthy diet, maintain ideal weight for height, and don't smoke.
- If you have heart disease or other risk factors, follow your treatment instructions carefully.
- Have family members and close friends learn CPR (cardiopulmonary resuscitation).

WHAT TO EXPECT

DIAGNOSTIC MEASURES—Your observation of symptoms. Once the patient is in the hospital, medical tests will confirm the diagnosis.

APPROPRIATE HEALTH CARE
- Rescuers should start CPR if the victim is unconscious, not moving, and not breathing. Even if the victim takes occasional gasps, rescuers should suspect cardiac arrest has occurred and should start CPR.
- Emergency medical care involves shocking the heart back into a normal heartbeat. This process is called defibrillation.

POSSIBLE COMPLICATIONS—Death or permanent brain damage if heart action cannot be resumed in 3 to 5 minutes. Most patients die before reaching an emergency care center.

PROBABLE OUTCOME—The person may survive if emergency medical treatment is given in the first few minutes. The outcome depends on what caused the cardiac arrest.

HOW TO TREAT

GENERAL MEASURES
- Ensure that you and your family members learn CPR. Call your local Red Cross or hospital for information. You may save a life.
- If you have heart disease or have risk factors, wear a medical alert identification (a bracelet or neck tag).
- Automated external defibrillators (AEDs) are being placed in public places (such as airports). They can be used by anyone to help a person who is having cardiac arrest.

MEDICATION—Drugs may be prescribed to treat the cause of cardiac arrest once the crisis is over.

ACTIVITY—After recovery, activities should be resumed gradually. Follow your health care provider's instructions.

DIET—Don't give fluids or foods to anyone with signs of cardiac arrest. He or she could choke.

CALL YOUR DOCTOR IF

- If the victim is not conscious and not breathing:
  - Call 911 (emergency) for an ambulance or medical help.
  - Yell for help. Don't leave the victim.
  - Perform CPR.
  - Don't stop CPR until help arrives.

CARDIOMYOPATHY

GENERAL INFORMATION

DEFINITION—Cardiomyopathy is the general term for conditions that cause the heart muscle to become enlarged, thick, or rigid, and rarely, scarred. The heart becomes weaker and is less able to pump blood through the body and maintain a normal rhythm. This can lead to heart failure or irregular heartbeat (arrhythmia). Some people who have cardiomyopathy have no signs or symptoms and need no treatment. For other people, it develops quickly with severe symptoms, and serious complications. The main types are dilated cardiomyopathy, hypertrophic cardiomyopathy, restrictive cardiomyopathy, and arrhythmogenic right ventricular dysplasia.

BODY PARTS INVOLVED—Heart muscle. May eventually affect lungs, liver, and blood vessels.

SEX OR AGE MOST AFFECTED—All ages, but more common in adults and males.

SIGNS & SYMPTOMS
- If the condition is severe enough to cause heart failure, these symptoms may occur:
  - Rapid and abnormal heartbeat.
  - Shortness of breath (may be worse when lying down or being physically active).
  - Swollen legs, feet, and ankles.
  - Feeling tired and weak.
  - Chest pain; cough.
  - Loss of appetite (yet, may have weight gain).
  - Dizziness or fainting.

CAUSES—Cardiomyopathy can be caused by a variety of health problems. Genetics play a role in some cases. Sometimes, no cause is found.

RISK INCREASES WITH
- Coronary artery disease.
- Alcoholism.
- Cancer treatment.
- Certain infections or other medical disorders.
- Chronic rapid heart rate.
- Family history of cardiomyopathy.
- Heart damage from a previous heart attack.
- Heart valve problems.
- Long-term high blood pressure.
- Metabolic disorder (e.g., thyroid disease or diabetes).
- Inflammation of the walls of the heart.
- Abuse of cocaine, heroin, organic solvents, etc.
- Nutritional deficiency.
- Pregnancy.

HOW TO PREVENT—No specific preventive measures. Avoid risk factors, where possible.

WHAT TO EXPECT

DIAGNOSTIC MEASURES
- Your own observation of symptoms.
- Your health care provider will do a physical exam and ask questions about your symptoms and activities and family health history.
- Medical tests may include chest x-ray, heart function studies, and blood tests. A tube-like instrument may be inserted into the heart and a biopsy (removal of a sample of heart tissue for testing) may be done.

APPROPRIATE HEALTH CARE
- The goals of treatment are to help the symptoms and to prevent complications. Treatment steps includes lifestyle changes, drug therapy, surgery, and/or other procedures.
- Lifestyle changes can include stopping the use of alcohol and cigarette smoking, diet changes, weight loss, and limiting physical activity.
- Surgery may include implanting a pacemaker to change the heart rate and pattern. Surgery to remove part of the thickened heart wall or replace heart valves may be needed.
- A heart transplant may be recommended if other treatments fail. A long wait for a transplant is normal. A mechanical device may be used to temporarily help the heart's pumping function.

POSSIBLE COMPLICATIONS—Heart failure, heart rhythm problems, blood clots, and cardiac arrest (all can be life-threatening).

PROBABLE OUTCOME—Varies widely depending on the cause and severity, and patient's age and general health. Treatment can improve symptoms and help in preventing complications. Some people live long, healthy lives with cardiomyopathy and some people don't even realize they have it.

HOW TO TREAT

GENERAL MEASURES
- Stop smoking. Avoid secondary smoke.
- Get regular medical and dental checkups.

MEDICATION—Drugs may be prescribed to improve heart function, to slow and regulate the heart rate, get rid of extra fluid, lower blood pressure, relax blood vessels, and suppress the immune system.

ACTIVITY—Follow medical advice about physical activity limits and when it is safe to resume sexual relations.

DIET
- Reduce your salt and fat intake. Avoid alcohol.
- Begin a weight-loss diet if you weigh more than is healthy for your body type.

CALL YOUR DOCTOR IF

- You or a family member has cardiomyopathy symptoms.
- Symptoms worsen despite treatment.
- You have chest pain. Get emergency help.

CARPAL TUNNEL SYNDROME

 GENERAL INFORMATION

DEFINITION—Carpal tunnel syndrome is a common nerve disorder that affects the hands and wrists. The carpal tunnel is a tunnel-like passageway located on the palm side of the wrist. It is made up of ligaments and bones. It surrounds the median nerve and tendons that go to the thumb and first two fingers.

BODY PARTS INVOLVED—It usually affects the thumb and first three fingers. In some cases, it may affect the 4th and 5th fingers only.

SEX OR AGE MOST AFFECTED—It usually affects adults and occurs in women much more often than men.

SIGNS & SYMPTOMS
• Symptoms usually start gradually and often affect the thumb and the index and middle fingers. The dominant hand is usually affected first.
• Tingling or numbness in part of the hand.
• Sharp pains that shoot from the wrist up the arm, especially at night.
• Burning sensations in the fingers.
• Morning stiffness or cramping of hands.
• Thumb weakness.
• Inability to make a fist.

CAUSES—It is often the result of a combination of factors that increase pressure on the median nerve and tendons in the carpal tunnel. The median nerve becomes irritated, which leads to the hand symptoms.

RISK INCREASES WITH
• Types of work that cause stress on the wrist (e.g., repetitive tasks, vibration, etc.) may increase risks. (Many people develop the condition regardless of the type of work they do.). Research is ongoing about the relationship of carpal tunnel syndrome and work.
• Women (possibly due to a smaller carpal tunnel).
• Certain medical or physical conditions may increase risk. These include arthritis, diabetes, hypothyroidism, alcoholism, obesity, menopause, pregnancy, or others.
• Wrist injury, fracture, dislocation, or other conditions that can cause wrist inflammation.

HOW TO PREVENT
• There are no specific preventive measures.
• Get treatment for any medical risk factors.
• Seek medical care at the onset of any hand symptoms.
• Reduce the risk of hand injury at work. Take frequent breaks. Learn ways to do the work with less stress on the hands and wrists. Use good posture. Relax the grip. Keep hands warm. Perform hand and wrist exercises.

 WHAT TO EXPECT

DIAGNOSTIC MEASURES
• Your own observation of symptoms. For a simple test, place the backs of your hands together with your fingers pointing straight down and your elbows pointing straight out to the side (wrists are at a 90° angle). If symptoms are brought on by you holding this position for one minute, you may have carpal tunnel syndrome.
• Your health care provider will examine your hand and wrist. Questions will be asked about your symptoms and daily activities.
• Medical tests may be done to see how well the median nerve is functioning or to check for an underlying disorder.

APPROPRIATE HEALTH CARE
• Treatment for any underlying condition will be prescribed. Conservative treatment for the carpal tunnel symptoms is usually tried first.
• Wearing a splint on the affected wrist for 4 to 6 weeks may be advised. The splint can keep the wrist in a neutral position at rest. Splints may be worn at night, during the day, or both day and night.
• Surgery to free the pinched nerve may be needed. The procedure may be done as an outpatient. Allow 2 weeks for healing. Physical therapy will then help rebuild wrist strength.

POSSIBLE COMPLICATIONS—If the condition is severe and untreated, permanent damage in the hand may occur.

PROBABLE OUTCOME—With treatment and time, most people will recover completely.

 HOW TO TREAT

GENERAL MEASURES
• Activities that are causing your symptoms need to be changed or stopped if at all possible.
• Use ice or warm and cold soaks if they help with symptoms.

MEDICATION
• You may take aspirin or ibuprofen to reduce pain and inflammation.
• Anti-inflammatory drugs or cortisone injections at the wrist to reduce inflammation may be prescribed.

ACTIVITY—Strengthening and stretching exercises for the wrist may be recommended.

DIET—Eat a normal, well-balanced diet.

 CALL YOUR DOCTOR IF

• You or a family member has symptoms of carpal tunnel syndrome.
• Symptoms aren't improving with treatment.

CATARACT

GENERAL INFORMATION

DEFINITION—A cataract is a clouding of the lens of the eye. The lens is a clear, flexible structure near the front of the eyeball. It helps to keep vision in focus and screens and refracts light. Cataracts may form in one or both eyes. If they form in both eyes, their growth rate may be very different. They can take several months or several years to develop. They do not spread from one eye to the other.

BODY PARTS INVOLVED—Lens of the eye(s).

SEX OR AGE MOST AFFECTED
- Adults over 60.
- Newborns (congenital form only).

SIGNS & SYMPTOMS
- Blurred vision. It may be worse in bright light. The blurring may first become apparent while driving at night, when lights seem to scatter or have halos.
- Difficulty reading.
- Faded colors.
- Poor night vision.
- Double or multiple vision.
- Opaque, milky-white pupil (advanced stages only).
- Frequent changes in prescription for eyeglasses

CAUSES
- The lens of the eye is made up of water and protein. The protein is arranged in a certain way that keeps the lens clear and lets light pass through it. A cataract forms when some of the protein clumps together and begins to cloud a small area of the lens. Over time, it grows larger and affects vision.
- Congenital (present at birth) cataracts can occur.

RISK INCREASES WITH
- Natural aging.
- Illnesses with high blood sugar, such as diabetes.
- Prolonged exposure to sunlight.
- Chronic eye disease.
- Exposure to some types of radiation.
- Family history of cataracts.
- Smoking.
- Use of steroid drugs.
- Surgery for other eye problems.
- Injury to the eye (cataract can occur years later).

HOW TO PREVENT—No specific preventive measures. Getting medical care for eye disorders, wearing sunglasses (that filter UV light) outside during the day, and not smoking may help reduce the risk or delay cataract development. Research is ongoing for methods to prevent cataracts.

WHAT TO EXPECT

DIAGNOSTIC MEASURES
- Your own observation of symptoms.
- Cataracts are usually diagnosed with an exam done by an eye doctor (ophthalmologist).

APPROPRIATE HEALTH CARE
- Treatment depends on amount of vision problems. Surgery to remove the cataracts is the only cure.
- Surgery to remove cataracts is recommended if vision loss interferes with daily activities, such as reading, watching television, or driving.
- Surgery may be done on an inpatient or outpatient basis. Usually one eye is operated on at a time (if cataracts are in both eyes). The eye lens is usually removed and replaced with an artificial lens. Different types of surgery are available. See Cataract Extraction in Surgery section.

POSSIBLE COMPLICATIONS
- Loss of vision.
- Postsurgery complications. These include inflammation, infections, bleeding, loss of vision, and light flashes. These can usually be treated successfully.

PROBABLE OUTCOME—Some cataracts never impair vision enough to require surgery. During the time cataracts are forming, frequent eyeglass changes may help vision. Cataracts that cause vision problems can be cured with surgery.

HOW TO TREAT

GENERAL MEASURES—If vision is not too badly affected, wear eyeglasses that provide maximum benefit. Wear sunglasses during the day for outside activities. Use a magnifying glass to read if needed. Improve the lighting in your home.

MEDICATION—Eye drops or drugs taken by mouth may be prescribed after your surgery.

ACTIVITY—No limits. Don't drive at night if your vision is poor.

DIET—Eat a healthy diet with plenty of fruits and green, leafy vegetables. It helps overall health and may help reduce risk of cataracts.

CALL YOUR DOCTOR IF

(Or call your eye care provider).
- You or a family member has symptoms of cataracts.
- Any eye symptoms develop after cataract surgery.

CAT-SCRATCH DISEASE

GENERAL INFORMATION

DEFINITION—Cat-scratch disease is a mild, infection caused by a scratch or bite or a lick from a cat (often a kitten). After a cat bite or scratch in a human, the infection spreads to lymph glands near the scratch by way of lymphatic vessels. It is not contagious from person to person. More than one family member can be infected at one time.

BODY PARTS INVOLVED—Skin and the lymph nodes.

SEX OR AGE MOST AFFECTED—Both sexes; all ages.

SIGNS & SYMPTOMS
- A lump, with or without pus or fluid, which starts on the scratched skin 3 to 10 days after the cat scratch.
- Swollen lymph nodes near the affected area.
- Fever of 99°F to 101°F (37.2°C to 38.3°C).
- Fatigue.
- Headache.
- Loss of appetite.
- AIDS patients or patients on immune-suppression drugs may have more severe symptoms.

CAUSES—A type of bacteria or germ (*Bartonella henselae*) carried in a cat's saliva. The cat can spread the bacteria to its paws by licking. The germs can then be transmitted to a human by way of a cat scratch or bite.

RISK INCREASES WITH—Owning or handling cats.

HOW TO PREVENT
- Teach children to avoid rough play with a cat or kitten.
- Cats may get the bacteria from fleas, so get rid of any fleas on pet cats.
- Don't pick up strange cats.

WHAT TO EXPECT

DIAGNOSTIC MEASURES
- Your own observation of symptoms.
- Your health care provider can usually diagnose the disorder by an exam of the affected skin, feeling the swollen lymph nodes, and knowing about the exposure to a cat.
- Medical tests may include skin or blood tests to rule out other disorders that can cause swollen lymph nodes.

APPROPRIATE HEALTH CARE
- Medical care is usually not needed. An antibiotic drug may be prescribed.
- Needle aspiration to drain the lymph gland is rarely needed.

POSSIBLE COMPLICATIONS—Unlikely to occur in otherwise healthy persons. People with weak immune systems may develop central nervous system problems.

PROBABLE OUTCOME—The condition normally heals on its own. The skin symptoms usually clear up in 1 to 3 weeks. Swollen lymph nodes may take 2 to 4 months (and sometimes longer) to heal.

HOW TO TREAT

GENERAL MEASURES
- Apply heat to affected areas; use warm soaks or use heating pad.
- It is not necessary to isolate the ill person because the disease is not transmitted from person to person.
- You may want to consult your veterinarian about the cat or kitten that caused the infection. Cats usually do not need treatment as the bacteria normally does not cause any health problems for them.

MEDICATION
- Antibiotics may be prescribed.
- To ease discomfort or soreness, use nonprescription acetaminophen or ibuprofen.

ACTIVITY—Get extra rest if you feel tired. Avoid activities that might cause injuries to swollen lymph nodes.

DIET—No special diet.

CALL YOUR DOCTOR IF

- You or a family member has symptoms of cat-scratch disease that cause concern.
- A swollen lymph gland becomes painful and red.

CELIAC DISEASE
(Gluten Enteropathy; Nontropical Sprue)

GENERAL INFORMATION

DEFINITION—Celiac disease is a digestive disorder that damages the intestines and prevents the body from getting nutrients from food. It occurs when foods that contain gluten, a protein found in grains (wheat, rye, and barley), cause an immune reaction in the body.

BODY PARTS INVOLVED—Digestive system.

SEX OR AGE MOST AFFECTED—Symptoms may begin at any age in a child or an adult. Symptoms often start during infancy or early childhood after the child begins eating food with gluten. In adults, symptoms may develop gradually over months or even years.

SIGNS & SYMPTOMS
- Symptoms vary from person to person and from one episode to another.
- Weight loss or slowed weight gain in an infant following the introduction of cereal to the diet.
- Poor appetite. Weight loss in older children or adults.
- Loose, pale, bulky, bad-smelling stools; frequent gas.
- Swollen abdomen; stomach pain. Muscle cramps.
- Mouth ulcers.
- Anemia or vitamin deficiency, with fatigue, pale skin, skin rash, or bone pain.
- Mildly bowed legs in children.
- Vague tiredness and weakness. Swollen legs.
- Irritability, depression, or anxiety.
- Adults tend to have fewer of the digestive symptoms and more of other, general types of symptoms.

CAUSES—The exact cause is unknown. It is an autoimmune disorder because the body's own immune system causes the damage to the lining of the small intestine. A person inherits the tendency to get celiac disease.

RISK INCREASES WITH
- Family history of celiac disease. A person's risk is about 10% if a first-degree relative has celiac disease.
- The disease may be triggered, or becomes active, after surgery, with pregnancy or childbirth, a viral infection, or severe emotional stress.

HOW TO PREVENT
- Cannot be prevented at present.
- Continuing to breast-feed at the time cereal is first given to an infant may help reduce the risk.

WHAT TO EXPECT

DIAGNOSTIC MEASURES
- Your own observation of symptoms.

- Your health care provider may do a physical exam and ask questions about your symptoms and diet.
- Medical tests may include blood, urine, and stool studies. A biopsy may be done (small sample of tissue is taken from the small intestine for viewing under a microscope). Sometimes, diagnosis is based on a person going on a gluten-free diet to see if the symptoms stop.

APPROPRIATE HEALTH CARE—The only treatment is a gluten-free diet.

POSSIBLE COMPLICATIONS
- If untreated, malnutrition and anemia can occur.
- Celiac disease patients are more likely to have other autoimmune disorders, diabetes, dermatitis herpetiformis, certain cancers, and other medical problems.

PROBABLE OUTCOME—With a strict, gluten-free diet, most persons with celiac disease can expect a normal life. Improvement of symptoms begins in 2 to 3 weeks.

HOW TO TREAT

GENERAL MEASURES
- Pay careful attention to the dietary instructions provided by your doctor or dietitian.
- To learn more: Celiac Sprue Association, PO Box 31700, Omaha, NE 68131; (877) 272-4272; website: www.csaceliacs.org or Celiac Disease Foundation, 13251 Ventura Blvd., Studio City, CA 91604; (818) 990-2354 (not toll free); website: www.celiac.org.

MEDICATION
- Iron and folic acid for anemia may be prescribed.
- Calcium and multiple-vitamin supplements for deficiencies may be recommended.
- Cortisone drugs to reduce the body's inflammatory response may be prescribed.

ACTIVITY—No limits.

DIET—Gluten-free diet. Gluten is found in wheat, rye, barley, and possibly oats. It is difficult to exclude gluten from the diet completely. Be patient while becoming familiar with the diet. A dietitian can help you with a diet plan.

CALL YOUR DOCTOR IF

- You or your child has symptoms of celiac disease.
- Symptoms don't improve after 3 weeks of gluten-free diet or they recur or a child fails to regain lost weight.

CELLULITIS

GENERAL INFORMATION

DEFINITION—Cellulitis is an inflammation of the skin and the tissues just below the skin (subcutaneous).

BODY PARTS INVOLVED—It is most likely to occur on the face, arms, lower legs, and anal area.

SEX OR AGE MOST AFFECTED—It can affect all age groups, including children.

SIGNS & SYMPTOMS
- Tenderness, warmth, swelling, and redness in an area of the skin. A thin red line may extend from the area toward the heart. Fluid or pus may leak out.
- Fever, chills, sweating, and a general ill feeling.
- Lymph glands near the area may be swollen.

CAUSES—Infection with bacteria, or rarely, a fungal infection. It can begin with a minor injury to the skin that is invaded by the bacteria. The infection leads to inflammation, which is the body's response to infection. Cellulitis cannot be passed from one person to another.

RISK INCREASES WITH
- Chronic illness, such as diabetes.
- Weak immune system due to illness or drugs.
- Any injury that breaks the skin.
- Use of drugs by injection.
- Burns.
- Surgical wound infection.
- Skin disorders (eczema or psoriasis) or infections that cause skin symptoms, such as chickenpox.
- Poor blood circulation.

HOW TO PREVENT
- Keep the skin clean.
- Avoid skin damage. Use protective clothing or proper gear for work or sports where injuries may occur.
- Wear shoes that fit well. Avoid going barefoot in areas where there may be risk of injury.
- If the skin is injured, wash the area with soap and water. Check the injured skin for the next few days to make sure it is healing. If not, seek medical care.
- Avoid swimming if you have any sores on your skin.

WHAT TO EXPECT

DIAGNOSTIC MEASURES
- Your own observation of symptoms.
- Your health care provider can usually diagnose the disorder by a physical exam of the affected area.

- Medical tests may include blood tests and study of a sample of fluid removed from the affected skin.

APPROPRIATE HEALTH CARE
- Treatment is with drugs for the infection, rest, and hospital care, if needed.
- If too much fluid is lost from the skin, you may need hospital care. Replacement fluids will be given through a tube into a vein under the skin.

POSSIBLE COMPLICATIONS
- Blood poisoning, if bacteria enter the bloodstream.
- Brain infection, if the condition occurs on the central part of the face.
- Infection of the bone, muscle, and tissue beneath the affected areas.
- Vein or lymph gland inflammation.

PROBABLE OUTCOME—With treatment, symptoms will begin to improve in 2 to 3 days, and complete recovery occurs in 7 to 10 days. Complications are rare, but may develop in those with chronic disease or weak immune systems.

HOW TO TREAT

GENERAL MEASURES
- Soak the area in warm water to help it heal. This may also reduce pain and swelling.
- Elevate the affected area. Rest the arm or leg on a pillow. Don't move that area of your body unless you have to. This can help reduce swelling.

MEDICATION
- Antibiotics will be prescribed for infection. They may be taken by mouth or injection. Complete the entire dose prescribed, even if symptoms disappear quickly.
- Use acetaminophen or ibuprofen for minor pain and fever.

ACTIVITY—Get extra rest until symptoms improve. Then return to your normal level of activity.

DIET—No special diet.

CALL YOUR DOCTOR IF

- You or a family member has symptoms of cellulitis.
- The following occur during treatment:
  - High fever and chills.
  - Pain, redness, or swelling increases.
  - Red streaks continue to extend, despite treatment.
  - Vomiting.
- New, unexplained symptoms develop. Drugs used in treatment may produce side effects.

CEREBRAL PALSY

GENERAL INFORMATION

DEFINITION—Cerebral palsy (CP) refers to a group of life-long disorders that affect muscle movement and body coordination. Cerebral refers to the brain and palsy refers to a disorder of movement. Most children with cerebral palsy are born with it, but symptoms may not appear for months or years. The number and severity of symptoms vary widely among children with CP.

BODY PARTS INVOLVED—Central nervous system; muscular system.

SEX OR AGE MOST AFFECTED—It is often diagnosed in the first 1 to 2 years of life.

SIGNS & SYMPTOMS
- Drooling, difficulty with sucking or swallowing.
- Lack of normal muscle tone (floppy).
- Slow development (holding head up, turning over, crawling, sitting, reaching with hand, walking, talking).
- Unusual body postures, stiffness, muscle spasms; uncontrolled and abnormal body movements; poor coordination or balance.
- Impaired hearing, vision, or speech. Crossed eyes.
- Convulsions (seizures).
- Dental problems.
- Bowel and bladder control problems.
- Normal or above normal intelligence or may have degrees of mental retardation.

CAUSES—Damage to motor areas of the brain that disrupts its ability to adequately control movement and posture. The reason for the damage is often unknown. In most cases, the damage occurs before birth, but it can occur during or after childbirth. CP is not inherited.

RISK INCREASES WITH
- Prematurity and low birthweight.
- Breech birth, multiple births (e.g., twins), complicated labor and delivery, maternal bleeding late in pregnancy, or mother exposed to toxins during pregnancy.
- Birth injury, including severe oxygen shortage.
- Congenital malformation of nervous system.
- Severe jaundice in an infant.
- Rh incompatibility (a blood disorder).
- Stroke in a fetus or newborn, or seizures in newborn.
- Low Apgar score (a rating scale done on newborns).
- An infection in the mother during pregnancy, such as rubella (German measles), toxoplasmosis, and others.
- Mothers who have thyroid problems, seizure disorder, mental retardation, or drug and alcohol abuse.
- Brain disease (meningitis or encephalitis) in infant.
- Head injuries during infancy or childhood.

HOW TO PREVENT—Most cases can't be prevented. Reduce risk where possible. Get good medical care during pregnancy and don't smoke, use alcohol, or abuse drugs. Protect infants and children from accidents or injuries.

WHAT TO EXPECT

DIAGNOSTIC MEASURES
- Your child's health care provider will do a physical exam and ask about medical history.
- Medical tests include testing motor skills and reflexes. Tests are also done to rule out other disorders.

APPROPRIATE HEALTH CARE
- You and your child's health care team will decide on a program of care based on your child's special needs. The program will change over time as the child matures and the needs change.
- The program can include drug therapy, physical therapy, occupational and speech therapy, behavior therapy, and emotional help. Braces, casts, mechanical aids, hearing aids, and surgery help some specific problems.

POSSIBLE COMPLICATIONS—Joint deformities; problems with nutrition, speech, vision, or hearing; mental retardation; or seizures.

PROBABLE OUTCOME—It is not progressive and children will vary widely in the severity of the condition. A child with CP may have high intelligence despite major muscular disability. Those with less-severe impairment can lead relatively normal, productive lives. Children with severe impairments may require special care.

HOW TO TREAT

GENERAL MEASURES
- Parents often join a support group to seek help.
- To learn more: United Cerebral Palsy Foundation, 1660 L St. NW, Suite 700, Washington, DC 20036; (800) 872-5827; website: www.ucp.org.

MEDICATION—Drugs may be prescribed to reduce abnormal movements, ease spasticity, for seizures, constipation, or other problems.

ACTIVITY—Limits or abilities will depend on degree of impairment.

DIET—Eating and swallowing may be difficult. Special diets and feedings may be needed.

CALL YOUR DOCTOR IF

- You are concerned about your child's development or suspect cerebral palsy.
- After diagnosis, you have any concerns.

CERVICAL CANCER

 GENERAL INFORMATION

DEFINITION—Cervical cancer is cancer of the cervix. This cancer develops slowly over time. The cervical cells first go through precancerous changes (called dysplasia). In these early stages, there are usually no symptoms. Cervical cancer screening is important. Abnormal cells can be found before cancer develops.

BODY PARTS INVOLVED—The cervix is about an inch long and is the narrow end of the uterus where it meets the vagina.

SEX OR AGE MOST AFFECTED—Average age at diagnosis is 50 to 55, but it can affect women of all ages.

SIGNS & SYMPTOMS
- As the cancer progresses, the following may occur:
  - Heavy or longer menstrual periods. Bleeding occurs between periods, after intercourse, or after menopause.
  - Vaginal discharge that has an odor.
  - Pelvic discomfort or pain during intercourse.
- Later stages or advanced disease:
  - May have appetite and weight loss or fatigue.
  - Swelling in one leg. Pain in the back, pelvis, or legs.
  - Bloody urine; constipation; other symptoms.

CAUSES—Human papillomavirus (HPV) plays a role. There are many different types of HPV. It is a sexually transmitted disease and a woman can have it for many years and not know it. Most HPV infections heal on their own and most women with HPV do not develop cancer. Other factors are involved in addition to an HPV infection that trigger cancer cells to grow.

RISK INCREASES WITH
- Early age of first intercourse.
- Multiple sex partners or sex with men who have had multiple sexual partners.
- Multiple pregnancies.
- Human papillomavirus infection.
- Use of oral contraceptives (birth control pills).
- Family history of cervical cancer.
- Weak immune system due to illness or drugs.
- Having sexually transmitted diseases.
- Low income women. Poor nutrition. Smoking.
- Daughters of mothers who took DES (diethylstilbestrol) to prevent miscarriage between 1938 and 1971.

HOW TO PREVENT
- Avoid the risks listed above as much as possible.
- Limit the number of sexual partners.
- Use condoms when you have sexual intercourse.
- Get regular pelvic exams, Pap smears, and HPV tests.
- Quit smoking or never start smoking.
- Ask your health care provider about HPV vaccine. It protects against most, but not all, HPV types that cause cancer. It is most effective when given before first sexual contact.

 WHAT TO EXPECT

DIAGNOSTIC MEASURES
- Your health care provider will do a physical exam and a pelvic exam.
- Medical tests will be done to diagnose the cancer and to see if it has spread (called staging).

APPROPRIATE HEALTH CARE
- Treatment will depend on the stage.
- Surgery may be done to remove the cancerous area. During early cancer stages, this may involve only a small area of the cervix. This will still allow childbearing. The surgery is usually done as an outpatient.
- The cancer cells may be frozen (cryotherapy), cut out with an electrical loop, burned away by laser, or removed in a cone biopsy. Your health care provider will explain these options and any risk factors involved.
- Advanced stages may require removal of reproductive organs and other tissue (hysterectomy). Chemotherapy and radiation therapy are also options.

POSSIBLE COMPLICATIONS
- Complications often occur from treatments.
- Cancer may recur. Advanced cancer can spread to other parts of the body (can be fatal).

PROBABLE OUTCOME—Usually curable with early diagnosis and treatment.

 HOW TO TREAT

GENERAL MEASURES
- Educate yourself about where to go for your care, treatments available, the risks involved, side effects of therapy, and expected outcome.
- To learn more: American Cancer Society; (800) ACS-2345; website: www.cancer.org or National Cancer Institute; (800) 4-CANCER; website: www.cancer.gov.

MEDICATION—Anticancer drugs (chemotherapy) may be prescribed.

ACTIVITY—Stay as physically active as you can.

DIET—Eat a well-balanced diet.

 CALL YOUR DOCTOR IF

- You or a family member has symptoms of cervical cancer.
- New symptoms develop after treatment.
- Pelvic exam, Pap smear, HPV test are due.

CERVICAL DYSPLASIA

GENERAL INFORMATION

DEFINITION—Cervical dysplasia is the growth of abnormal cells on or in the cervix. It may be mild, moderate, or severe, depending on the spread and type of the abnormal cells. Dysplasia is not cancer, but can become cancerous.

BODY PARTS INVOLVED—Cervix (the lower third of the uterus, which opens into the vagina).

SEX OR AGE MOST AFFECTED—Dysplasia occurs in females age 15 and over, and most often in those age 25 to 35.

SIGNS & SYMPTOMS—Usually no signs or symptoms occur. The diagnosis results from a routine Pap smear test.

CAUSES—Human papillomavirus (HPV) plays a role. There are many different types of HPV. It is a sexually transmitted disease and a woman can have it for many years and not know it. Most HPV infections heal on their own and most women with HPV do not develop cancer. Other factors are involved in addition to an HPV infection that trigger cancer cells to grow.

RISK INCREASES WITH
- Early age of first intercourse.
- Multiple sex partners or sex with men who have had multiple sexual partners.
- Multiple pregnancies.
- Human papillomavirus infection.
- Use of oral contraceptives (birth control pills).
- Family history of cervical cancer.
- Weak immune system due to illness or drugs.
- Having sexually transmitted diseases.
- Smoking.
- Women in low income groups. Poor nutrition.
- Daughters of mothers who took DES (diethylstilbestrol) to prevent miscarriage between 1938 and 1971.

HOW TO PREVENT
- Avoid the risks where possible.
- Limit the number of sexual partners.
- Use condoms when you have sexual intercourse.
- Get regular pelvic exams, Pap smears, and HPV tests.
- Quit smoking or never start smoking.
- Ask your health care provider about HPV vaccine. It protects against most, but not all, HPV types that cause cancer. It is most effective when given before first sexual contact.

WHAT TO EXPECT

DIAGNOSTIC MEASURES
- Your health care provider will do a pelvic exam.
- Medical tests include a Pap smear. A swab of cervical cells may be taken for exam to check for HPV. A colposcopy (exam of the cervix with an instrument with a lighted tip) may be done. It can be combined with a biopsy. A biopsy involves removal of any tissue that appears abnormal for viewing with a microscope. Other tests may be done if further diagnosis is needed. The results of these tests help classify the dysplasia.

APPROPRIATE HEALTH CARE
- Treatment will vary depending on the degree and extent of the cervical dysplasia. No treatment may be recommended in some cases. Follow up visits will be needed to be sure the dysplasia clears up on its own.
- The abnormal cells may be frozen (cryotherapy), cut out with an electrical loop, burned away by laser, or removed in a cone biopsy. Your health care provider will explain these options and any risk factors involved.

POSSIBLE COMPLICATIONS
- Some moderate or severe dysplasia may progress to cervical cancer. It can take years for this to happen.
- Dysplasia may recur after treatment. Recurrent dysplasia may be treated with a hysterectomy.
- Rarely, treatment may cause bleeding or infection.

PROBABLE OUTCOME—Most dysplasia is the mild form. Many of these cases resolve without treatment. Moderate to severe dysplasia can usually be cured with treatment.

HOW TO TREAT

GENERAL MEASURES
- Follow up care will depend on the treatment method.
- Follow-up Pap smears every 3 to 6 months, for 1 to 2 years, are usually recommended. This will verify the success of treatment and detect any recurrence. Be sure to schedule annual Pap smears after that time.

MEDICATION
- You may use nonprescription drugs, such as acetaminophen, for minor pain.
- Prescription pain drugs may be prescribed depending on the treatment procedure.

ACTIVITY—After treatment, resume daily activities, including work, as soon as you are able. Delay sexual relations until a follow-up medical exam shows that healing is complete.

DIET—No special diet.

CALL YOUR DOCTOR IF

- Pelvic exam, Pap smear, HPV test are due.
- New symptoms develop after treatment.

CERVICAL POLYPS

GENERAL INFORMATION

DEFINITION—Cervical polyps are a common disorder that involves a small growth on the cervix. The cervix is about an inch long and is the narrow end of the uterus where it meets the vagina. Polyps vary in size and look like a bulb on a thin stem. There may be one (usually) or groups of polyps. A polyp can't be seen or felt by a woman.

BODY PARTS INVOLVED—Endometrium (thin membrane lining the uterus); cervix (lower third of the uterus).

SEX OR AGE MOST AFFECTED—Women of all ages. They occur most often in women over age 20 who have had at least one child.

SIGNS & SYMPTOMS
- Polyps may cause no symptoms. They are often found on a routine pelvic exam.
- Bleeding between monthly menstrual periods.
- Heavier bleeding during periods.
- Spotting of blood after sexual intercourse.
- Vaginal discharge.

CAUSES—Exact cause is unknown. Inflammation of the cervix may be involved. This can be from infection, erosion, or other problems. The majority of polyps are benign (not cancerous). In very rare cases, they represent early cancer of the cervix. They are not contagious.

RISK INCREASES WITH
- Women over age 20 who have had one child.
- Recurrent vaginitis or cervicitis (inflammation or infection of the cervix).

HOW TO PREVENT
- No specific preventive measures.
- Get regular pelvic exams. This is the best way to identify cervical polyps.

WHAT TO EXPECT

DIAGNOSTIC MEASURES
- Your health care provider will do a pelvic exam.
- Medical tests are usually not needed.

APPROPRIATE HEALTH CARE
- Treatment involves surgery to remove the polyps. This can usually be done in a simple office procedure. All tissue removed is examined in a laboratory for any sign of cancer.
- Polyps are usually removed by gently twisting the stem with forceps to break them off.
- A dilation and curettage (D & C) may be done. This involves a scraping procedure.
- You may feel brief, mild pain during the procedure. Mild to moderate cramps may occur for several hours. Spotting of blood may last for a few days.
- If the polyp is large or has a thick stalk, it may require surgery that is more extensive. This may be done in a hospital.

POSSIBLE COMPLICATIONS
- Infection can develop following surgery.
- In very rare cases, cancer may first appear as a polyp.
- After treatment, polyps may grow again on another area of the cervix.

PROBABLE OUTCOME—Polyps are easily treated and seldom grow back.

HOW TO TREAT

GENERAL MEASURES
- Don't douche unless it is medically recommended.
- Use small sanitary pads to protect your clothing from creams or suppositories.

MEDICATION
- Use acetaminophen or ibuprofen for minor pain.
- Antibiotics may be prescribed if signs of an infection are present. Antibiotics can interfere with the effectiveness of some birth control pills. If you are currently taking birth control pills, discuss this with your health care provider.

ACTIVITY—No limits. Delay sexual relations until a follow-up pelvic exam confirms that healing is complete.

DIET—No special diet.

CALL YOUR DOCTOR IF

- You or a family member has symptoms of cervical polyps.
- The following occur after treatment:
  - Discomfort persists longer than 1 week.
  - Unexplained vaginal bleeding or swelling develops.

CERVICAL SPONDYLOSIS

GENERAL INFORMATION

DEFINITION—Cervical spondylosis is a disorder caused by the slow degeneration of bones and discs in the neck (cervical spine). There may be no symptoms or they may be very mild. It is a common disorder in people as they get older.

BODY PARTS INVOLVED
- 7 bones of the neck.
- Discs between the bones.
- Blood vessels to the head.
- Bladder and lower legs (advanced stages).

SEX OR AGE MOST AFFECTED—Usually adults ages 40 to 60 and affects men and women equally. Men tend to develop the disorder at an earlier age.

SIGNS & SYMPTOMS
- Stiff and painful neck. The pain may come and go and worsen with movement (e.g., lifting the head or chin), and over time. Pain may range from mild discomfort to severe.
- Pain may spread to the shoulder, arm, or chest.
- Headaches and trouble with sleeping.
- Arms, hands, legs, or feet have tingling, burning, or prickling sensations. Numbness and weakness may occur.
- Difficulty with walking or lack of coordination.
- Anxiety or depression due to decreased mobility.

CAUSES—Chronic wearing away (degenerating) of the vertebrae (bones of the spine) and the discs between these vertebrae. Bony growths called osteophytes (or spurs) can develop on the vertebrae. These changes can cause certain nerves to become compressed (pinched) and inflamed (called radiculopathy). The spinal cord may also be compressed (called myelopathy) and cause more severe symptoms.

RISK INCREASES WITH
- Aging. By age 60, 70% of women and 85% of men show signs of the disorder on x-ray.
- Previous neck injury may play a role. It can occur years before.

HOW TO PREVENT
- There are no specific preventive measures for cervical spondylosis. It comes with aging.
- You can prevent some neck injuries, which might help prevent the risk. Use seat belts in vehicles and keep headrests at proper height.
- For good health, keep as fit as possible.

WHAT TO EXPECT

DIAGNOSTIC MEASURES
- Your health care provider will do a physical exam and ask questions about your symptoms.

- X-rays, CT or MRI scans, or nerve function tests may be done to confirm the diagnosis and rule out other disorders.

APPROPRIATE HEALTH CARE
- Treatment usually involves conservative measures. These may include self-care, drugs, ultrasound therapy, physical therapy, or other types of therapy if needed.
- A soft cervical collar or neck brace may be prescribed for day wear to limit neck motion and ease nerve irritation. A soft cervical pillow may be recommended as a sleeping aid.
- Neck traction at home or in a hospital may be recommended.
- Surgery (sometimes) may be needed for more severe symptoms. Your health care provider will discuss the options and risks and benefits.

POSSIBLE COMPLICATIONS
- Chronic neck pain.
- Spinal cord dysfunction.
- Loss of control of the bladder or bowels.
- Symptoms may make it difficult to perform work activities, home care tasks, or recreational activities.

PROBABLE OUTCOME—Treatment does not cure the disorder, but does help improve the symptoms and prevent further problems.

HOW TO TREAT

GENERAL MEASURES
- Follow any instructions from your health care provider or try the treatment steps listed here.
- You can apply moist heat to relieve symptoms. Take warm showers or apply warm soaks to neck. Gentle massage may help.
- Improve your posture. Pull in the chin and abdomen when sitting or standing. Use a firm chair and sit with buttocks against the back.

MEDICATION
- For minor pain, you may use aspirin or ibuprofen.
- Stronger pain drugs, muscle relaxants, antidepressants, or cortisone injections may be prescribed.

ACTIVITY
- Walk, swim, do yoga or other low impact exercise on a regular basis.
- Physical therapy may help with flexibility, strength, and mobility.

DIET—No special diet.

CALL YOUR DOCTOR IF

- You or a family member has symptoms of cervical spondylosis.
- Symptoms persist or worsen despite treatment.

CERVICITIS

GENERAL INFORMATION

DEFINITION—Cervicitis is an inflammation of the cervix. The cervix is about an inch long and is the narrow end of the uterus where it meets the vagina. Cervicitis is common and occurs more often in women under age 25.

BODY PARTS INVOLVED—Cervix and mucous membranes covering the cervix.

SEX OR AGE MOST AFFECTED—Cervicitis is common and occurs in females of all ages, but more often in women under age 25.

SIGNS & SYMPTOMS
- Often there are no symptoms.
- Vaginal discharge. It may be thick and creamy, foamy and greenish-white, white and curd-like, or thin and grey.
- There may be bleeding after sexual intercourse.
- Pelvic pain may occur with severe infection.

CAUSES
- Infection. Cervicitis is most often caused by an infection (a sexually transmitted disease [STD]). Bacteria infections, *Neisseria gonorrhoeae* or *Chlamydia trachomatis,* are the most common. Herpes simplex or human papillomavirus (HPV) can also be the cause.
- Allergic reaction (such as to latex).
- Injury or irritation.

RISK INCREASES WITH
- Multiple sexual partners.
- Practicing unsafe sex.
- Women who begin having sex at an early age.
- History of sexually transmitted diseases.
- Having sexual partners who engage in high-risk sexual behavior or have an STD.

HOW TO PREVENT
- Practice safe sex. Begin sexual activity at a later age. Have sex with just one person.
- Avoid sexually transmitted diseases. Do not engage in sexual intercourse with an infected partner. Have your sexual partner use a condom during sexual activity.
- Avoid irritants to the cervix (e.g., douches or sprays).
- Have routine pelvic exams and Pap smears to detect cervicitis at an early stage.

WHAT TO EXPECT

DIAGNOSTIC MEASURES
- Your own observation of symptoms.
- Your health care provider will do a pelvic exam.
- Medical tests usually include a culture of the vaginal discharge and a Pap smear.

APPROPRIATE HEALTH CARE
- Treatment is with drugs to cure any infection. If a sexually transmitted disease caused the cervicitis, your sexual partner must also be treated.
- If the cause is other than infection, appropriate treatment will be provided.
- Repeated or prolonged cervicitis may require other treatment (e.g., surgery to treat infected cervix tissue).

POSSIBLE COMPLICATIONS
- Pelvic inflammatory disease (PID). The infection spreads to other parts of the reproductive system. PID sometimes does not cause symptoms. It can lead to infertility.
- Untreated or prolonged cervicitis may make it difficult or impossible for a woman to become pregnant.
- Pregnant women who develop cervicitis are at risk for miscarriage or preterm delivery. The newborn is at risk for serious infections.
- HPV infection is a risk factor for cervical cancer.

PROBABLE OUTCOME—Cervicitis typically heals with treatment.

HOW TO TREAT

GENERAL MEASURES
- Use sanitary pads instead of tampons during treatment.
- Don't douche unless it is recommended by your health care provider.

MEDICATION
- Oral, or sometimes injected, antibiotics will be prescribed for bacterial infection. Antibiotics may interfere with the effectiveness of some birth control pills.
- Antiviral drugs may be prescribed for viral infection.
- Topical drug therapy may be used in some cases.

ACTIVITY
- Avoid sexual relations for 7 days (or as advised) after treatment has started.
- If your partner needs treatment, do not have sexual relations until the treatment is completed.

DIET—No special diet.

CALL YOUR DOCTOR IF

- You or a family member has symptoms of cervicitis.
- During treatment, discomfort lasts longer than one week or symptoms worsen.
- Vaginal bleeding or swelling develops during or after treatment.

CHALAZION

GENERAL INFORMATION

DEFINITION—A chalazion (the plural is chalazia) is a lump (also called a cyst) on the eyelid. It may be so small that it is barely visible or as large as a pea. It results from inflammation of a gland that lubricates the edges of the eyelid. A chalazion is not a stye.

BODY PARTS INVOLVED—Eyelid.

SEX OR AGE MOST AFFECTED—Chalazia are more common in adults than children.

SIGNS & SYMPTOMS—A painless (most often), slow-growing, firm lump in the eyelid. Skin over the lump can be moved loosely. The upper eyelid is the one usually affected.

CAUSES—Blockage of a type of oil-producing gland (meibomian gland) in the eyelid. There are about 100 of these glands located near the eyelashes. A chalazion is usually not due to infection, but may become infected.

RISK INCREASES WITH
- Acne rosacea or seborrheic dermatitis.
- Chronic blepharitis (an eyelid and lash condition).

HOW TO PREVENT
- There are no specific preventive measures.
- Eyelid hygiene may help prevent problems such as blepharitis (a risk factor). Follow any instructions provided by your health care provider. These steps are one possibility:
  - Wash your eyelid area every day. Dilute baby shampoo with water. Use diluted solution with a washcloth or cotton swab. Gently scrub eyelid area with a back and forth motion with eyes closed. Rinse with warm water.
  - There are also commercial products available to clean eyelids.

WHAT TO EXPECT

DIAGNOSTIC MEASURES
- Your own observation of symptoms.
- See your health care provider if you are concerned about the problem. An exam will be made of the affected eyelid area.
- Medical tests are not required.

APPROPRIATE HEALTH CARE
- Self-care is often all that is needed.
- Medical treatment may involve drugs injected into the chalazion, drugs to be applied to the eyelid, or surgery to remove it.
- Surgery to remove the chalazion may be recommended. This is usually done in your health care provider's office. The area will be numbed before the lump is removed.

POSSIBLE COMPLICATIONS
- A chalazion may recur or become chronic.
- Complications are rare. They may include eye irritation, infection, or visual changes if a large chalazion presses on the cornea. Very rarely, a recurring chalazion may be a symptom of a type of cancer.

PROBABLE OUTCOME—A chalazion often heals by itself in a month or so. If not, it can be treated.

HOW TO TREAT

GENERAL MEASURES—Use warm-water soaks to reduce inflammation and hasten healing. Apply soaks for 10 to 15 minutes, 4 times a day. Gently massage the area several times a day. Do not squeeze or try to pop the chalazion.

MEDICATION
- Injection of a steroid drug into the chalazion may be recommended to reduce inflammation.
- Antibiotic ointment or drops may be prescribed for infection or following surgical treatment.
- Oral antibiotics may be prescribed for persons with a chronic or recurring chalazion.

ACTIVITY—No limits.

DIET—No special diet.

CALL YOUR DOCTOR IF

- You or a family member has symptoms of a chalazion that is not better after self-care.
- Chalazion recurs or other eye symptoms develop after treatment.

CHICKENPOX
(Varicella)

GENERAL INFORMATION

DEFINITION—Chickenpox is a very contagious disease caused by the herpes zoster virus. The symptoms are usually mild in children and may be more severe in adults.

BODY PARTS INVOLVED—Skin and mucous membranes.

SEX OR AGE MOST AFFECTED—Both sexes; all ages, but most common in children.

SIGNS & SYMPTOMS
- Fever, stomach pain, headache, or a general ill feeling that lasts 1 to 2 days (or longer).
- Itchy skin eruptions that appear almost any-where on the body, including the scalp, penis, and inside the mouth, nose, throat, or vagina. They may be scattered over large areas, and they occur least on the arms and legs. Blisters collapse within 24 hours and form scabs. New crops of blisters erupt every 3 to 4 days.
- Adults have other symptoms that resemble influenza.

CAUSES—Infection with the herpes zoster virus. It is spread from person to person by airborne droplets or contact with a skin eruption on an infected person. Symptoms may appear 7 to 21 days after exposure. A person is contagious 2 days before the rash appears until all the blisters have crusted over (usually takes 5 to 6 days).

RISK INCREASES WITH
- Weak immune system due to illness or drugs.
- Persons who have not been vaccinated or who have not had the infection.

HOW TO PREVENT
- Children and adults who have not had chickenpox should get a chickenpox (varicella) vaccine. Check with your health care provider.
- A newborn has some temporary immunity for chickenpox if the mother has had chickenpox. Breast-feeding an infant will provide some immunity.
- For persons not immune to chickenpox, varicella vaccine given within 3 days of exposure may prevent or limit an infection. An immune globulin may be used to prevent chickenpox in persons at risk for complications. Antivirals may also be used.

WHAT TO EXPECT

DIAGNOSTIC MEASURES
- Your own observation of symptoms.
- Your health care provider can diagnose chickenpox by the appearance of the skin rash.

- Medical tests are usually not needed, but a blood test or test of pox blisters may be done.

APPROPRIATE HEALTH CARE—Home care is usually all that is needed. Drug therapy may be prescribed for some patients.

POSSIBLE COMPLICATIONS
- Bacterial infection of chickenpox blisters. Scarring, if blisters become infected (rare).
- Pneumonia.
- Central nervous system complications (rare).
- Shingles many years later in adulthood (possibly).

PROBABLE OUTCOME
- Children usually recover in 7 to 10 days. Adults may take longer. Adults and persons with weak immune systems are more at risk for complications.
- After recovery, a person has lifelong immunity against a recurrence of chickenpox.
- After chickenpox runs its course, the virus sometimes remains dormant in the body (probably in the roots of nerves near the spinal cord). The same virus may cause shingles many years later.

HOW TO TREAT

GENERAL MEASURES
- Use cool-water soaks such as oatmeal baths or cool-water compresses to reduce itching.
- Keep the patient as quiet and cool as possible. Heat and sweat trigger itching.
- Keep the nails short to discourage scratching, which can lead to secondary infection.

MEDICATION
- To help decrease itching, use topical lotions such as calamine lotion or oral antihistamines.
- Use acetaminophen to reduce fever. Never give aspirin to children during a viral illness.
- An antiviral drug may be prescribed.

ACTIVITY
- Bed rest is not needed. Allow quiet activity in a cool environment (indoors or outdoors).
- Keep an ill child away from others, and from school, until all blisters have crusted and no new ones occur.

DIET—Blisters in the mouth may make eating and drinking painful. Fluid intake is needed to prevent dehydration. Try Popsicles, cool drinks, and bland foods.

CALL YOUR DOCTOR IF

- You or your child has chickenpox symptoms.
- Symptoms don't improve within a few days or they worsen or new symptoms develop.

CHILD ABUSE

GENERAL INFORMATION

DEFINITION—The major types of child abuse (or maltreatment) are:
• *Physical abuse* is physical injury (from minor injury to broken bones, or death). A child may be hit, bitten, shaken, punched, kicked, beaten, burned, or harmed in other ways.
• *Sexual abuse* includes touching a child's genitals, intercourse, forcing a child to watch sexual acts, having a child touch or look at an adult's genitals, watch or be in pornographic films, and any other sexual act.
• *Emotional abuse* harms a child's emotional growth or can destroy a child's confidence. Constant yelling and screaming, name-calling, threats, and not giving love and affection are forms of this abuse.
• *Child neglect* is when the child's basic needs are not met. This can include lack of proper food, clothes, school, hygiene, medical care, or leaving a child alone.

BODY PARTS INVOLVED—All.

SEX OR AGE MOST AFFECTED—All children.

SIGNS & SYMPTOMS
• All types of abuse will cause both physical and behavioral signs. Parents or other adults who know the child are unlikely to suspect child abuse. A child's injuries or behavior changes can result from other problems also.
• Physical signs. Any type of injury (mild or serious), pain when they urinate, genital bleeding, weight loss or no weight gain (in infants), stomach pain, headaches, or infections. Pregnancy in young adolescents.
• Behavioral signs. Avoiding family and friends, a change in eating habits, sleeping problems, emotional upsets, and poor school performance. Outgrown habits such as bed-wetting or thumb-sucking may recur. There may be inappropriate sexual behavior.
• Older children may abuse drugs or alcohol, talk about suicide, or behave in a reckless and destructive manner.

CAUSES—Abusers are more likely to be someone the child knows, rather than a stranger. Abusers may be parents, relatives, neighbor, babysitters, or other caregivers.

RISK INCREASES WITH
• Children:
  - A child of any age, sex, race, religion, rich or poor can be a victim of abuse.
  - Infants: under age one are high risk for injury.
  - Females: more likely to suffer sexual abuse.
• Adult abusers:
  - Parents who lack parenting skills or have financial, relationship, mental, emotional, or stress problems.
  - Adults who were victims of child abuse.

HOW TO PREVENT
• For children, education about abuse.
• If you suspect child abuse, report it right away.

WHAT TO EXPECT

DIAGNOSTIC MEASURES
• Children are often afraid to tell anyone about abuse. They feel they are at fault and no one will believe them.
• If your child tells you about abuse, stay calm and let the child know that he or she is believed. Take steps to protect the child. Take action to report the abuse. You may want to call the local Child Protective Service. If you are unsure what to do, ask someone you trust.
• Call your child's health care provider if you think your child has been abused. Treatment will be given for any injuries. The child may need hospital care. Health care providers must report any suspected or known cases of child abuse to the proper authorities.
• Mental health counseling for the child and the family can help everyone learn ways to cope.

APPROPRIATE HEALTH CARE
• Medical care as needed for any physical injury.
• Other therapy and counseling will be needed depending on each individual situation.

POSSIBLE COMPLICATIONS
• Physical injuries that could be fatal.
• Emotional and mental problems for the child.
• Risk of many types of problems later in life.

PROBABLE OUTCOME—The best hope for the child is early discovery of the problem, and prompt action and treatment.

HOW TO TREAT

GENERAL MEASURES
• To learn more. Childhelp USA, 15757 N. 78 Ave., Scottsdale, AZ 85260; (480) 922-8212 (not toll free); website: www.childhelp.org.
• To report abuse, call Local Child Protective Services or the national hotline (800) 422-4453.
• If you have abused a child or think you might, seek help. Call your health care provider or a local help line.

MEDICATION—Drugs may be needed to treat or prevent a sexually transmitted disease (STD), or to prevent a pregnancy.

ACTIVITY—No limits usually.

DIET—No special diet.

CALL YOUR DOCTOR IF

An abused child needs medical or emotional help. You suspect someone is abusing a child.

CHLAMYDIA

GENERAL INFORMATION

DEFINITION—Chlamydia is a bacterial infection that mainly affects the genitals of men and women. It is the most common reported bacterial sexually transmitted disease (STD) in the United States.

BODY PARTS INVOLVED—The urethra (the tube that allows urine from the bladder to pass outside the body), vagina, cervix, uterus, fallopian tubes, ovaries, penis, and anus.

SEX OR AGE MOST AFFECTED—It can develop in anyone who is sexually active. It affects females more often than males.

SIGNS & SYMPTOMS
- There are often no symptoms during the early stages.
- Vaginal discharge in women.
- Bleeding may occur between menstrual periods.
- Pain when urinating.
- Penis discharge in males.
- Men may have scrotal discomfort or burning or itching around opening of the penis.
- Genital, lower abdominal, or back discomfort or pain.
- Painful sexual intercourse in females.
- Infection in the rectum may cause rectal pain, discharge, or bleeding.

CAUSES
- *Chlamydia trachomatis* bacteria. Symptoms may appear 1 to 3 weeks after exposure. It is spread by:
    - Vaginal sexual intercourse.
    - Anal sexual intercourse.
    - Oral-genital contact.
    - Vaginal infection during delivery of a newborn, which may infect the newborn's eyes or lungs.

RISK INCREASES WITH
- Sexually active men and women.
- Unprotected sex, especially in young females.
- Having other sexually transmitted diseases.
- New or multiple sex partners.

HOW TO PREVENT
- Abstain from sex or have one sexual partner or limit the number of sexual partners. Use condoms for sexual activity to help reduce risk of infections.
- Talk to your health care provider about screening tests for chlamydia and other sexually transmitted diseases.
- Women should avoid douching.

WHAT TO EXPECT

DIAGNOSTIC MEASURES
- Your own observation of symptoms.
- Your health care provider may do a physical exam of the genital area.
- Medical tests can include urine tests or studies of the discharge from the cervix or penis. A Pap test or pregnancy test may be done in women. Testing for other sexually transmitted diseases is usually recommended.

APPROPRIATE HEALTH CARE
- Treatment is with antibiotic drugs. All sexual partners must be treated.
- A follow-up medical exam may be needed after completing the prescribed treatment.

POSSIBLE COMPLICATIONS
- Because the infection often has no symptoms, complications in a woman can occur even before she knows there is a problem.
- If untreated, the infection can cause:
    - Pelvic inflammatory disease (PID) in women (uterus and fallopian tubes become infected). It may result in infertility, chronic pelvic pain, and ectopic pregnancy.
    - Higher risk for HIV infection or cervical cancer in women.
    - Epididymitis in men.
    - Rarely, Reiter's syndrome (a type of arthritis).

PROBABLE OUTCOME—Complete cure with adequate antibiotic treatment.

HOW TO TREAT

GENERAL MEASURES
- Keep the genital area clean. Take showers rather than baths. Use plain unscented soap.
- To learn more: Centers for Disease Control and Prevention; website: www.cdc.gov/std or American Social Health Association, PO Box 13827, Research Triangle Park, NC 27709; (919) 361-8488 (not toll-free); website: www.ashastd.org.

MEDICATION—The infection is treated with an oral antibiotic. It may be with a single dose or taken more often for 7 days.

ACTIVITY—Avoid sexual relations until you and your sexual partner have been treated. This is usually 7 days after a single dose treatment or after completing a 7 day treatment (or as advised). A woman is at risk for re-infection if her sexual partner is untreated.

DIET—No special diet.

CALL YOUR DOCTOR IF

- You or a family member has symptoms of chlamydia.
- Symptoms worsen or last longer than a week.
- Unusual vaginal bleeding or swelling occurs or new unexplained symptoms develop.

CHOLECYSTITIS OR CHOLANGITIS

GENERAL INFORMATION

DEFINITION—Cholecystitis is inflammation of the gallbladder. It can be acute or chronic. Cholangitis is inflammation and infection of the bile ducts (tubes that carry bile from the liver to the gallbladder and small intestine).

BODY PARTS INVOLVED—Gallbladder (located under the liver, in the upper right abdomen); bile ducts in the liver, leading to the gallbladder.

SEX OR AGE MOST AFFECTED—The conditions usually occur in older adults (women more than men). They may rarely occur in children or teens.

SIGNS & SYMPTOMS
- Cramping pain in the upper right of the abdomen. Pain may also occur in the chest (imitating a heart attack), in the upper back, or the right shoulder. These symptoms frequently follow a meal rich in fats.
- Tenderness in the upper abdomen.
- Nausea, vomiting, or belching.
- Slight fever. High fever and chills if there is infection.
- Jaundice (yellow skin and eyes) may occur.
- Stools may change color.
- Cholangitis may cause mental status changes.

CAUSES
- Cholecystitis usually results when a gallstone blocks the outlet of the gallbladder and bile builds up. Chronic cholecystitis results from recurrent inflammation.
- Acalculous cholecystitis is inflammation not caused by gallstones. It may be due to severe illness, surgery, burns, or injury.
- In cholangitis, the main bile duct becomes blocked by one or more gallstones or a tumor. Bile builds up behind the blockage and leads to a bacterial infection.

RISK INCREASES WITH
- Older adults.
- Gallstones.
- Pregnancy.
- Hispanic populations and American Indians.
- Being overweight or rapid weight loss.
- Certain drugs (e.g., hormone therapy in women).
- Major surgery, severe trauma/burns, or critical illness.

HOW TO PREVENT—None specific.

WHAT TO EXPECT

DIAGNOSTIC MEASURES
- Your own observation of symptoms.
- Your health care provider will do a physical exam and ask questions about your symptoms and medical history.
- Medical tests usually include blood studies along with ultrasound and imaging techniques.

APPROPRIATE HEALTH CARE
- Specific treatment will depend on severity of symptoms, infection, and your general health. Hospital care is normally needed. Emergency surgery may be required for severe cases. Fluids may be given through a vein (IV).
- Treatment may include drugs for pain or other symptoms, antibiotics for infection, and diet changes (once patient can eat).
- Surgical removal of the gallbladder (cholecystectomy) is usually recommended for cholecystitis. It may be done using a laparoscope (an instrument placed into 4 small slits in the abdomen) or with open surgery (through an incision).

POSSIBLE COMPLICATIONS
- Peritonitis (inflammation of abdomen lining).
- Blood infection (sepsis).
- Liver, kidney, or pancreas problems.
- Gallstones may cause intestinal blockage.
- Treatments may cause complications.

PROBABLE OUTCOME
- With cholecystitis, some mild attacks clear up on their own. Recurrences are common. Attacks will stop after surgery to remove the gallbladder.
- Outcome is generally good in cholangitis. It depends on early diagnosis and treatment and patient's health.

HOW TO TREAT

GENERAL MEASURES—To learn more: National Digestive Diseases Information Clearinghouse, 2 Information Way, Bethesda, MD 20892; (800) 891-5389; website: www.niddk.nih.gov.

MEDICATION
- Drugs for pain or vomiting may be prescribed.
- Antibiotics are usually prescribed for infection.

ACTIVITY
- Rest as needed until symptoms disappear or recovery from surgery is complete.
- Other limits on activity depend on treatment.

DIET
- Food intake will be limited during hospital care.
- A low-fat diet may be recommended.

☎ CALL YOUR DOCTOR IF
- You or a family member has symptoms of cholecystitis or cholangitis. If symptoms are severe, call immediately!
- Symptoms recur after diagnosis or treatment.

CHOLESTEROL, HIGH
(Hypercholesterolemia)

GENERAL INFORMATION

DEFINITION—High cholesterol means there is too much cholesterol circulating in the blood. The medical term is hypercholesterolemia. Cholesterol is a lipid (similar to fat) carried in the blood. It has several important functions in the body, but too much of it can cause problems. The liver makes all the cholesterol the body needs. More cholesterol comes from foods, such as meat, dairy products, and eggs.

BODY PARTS INVOLVED—Blood vessels.

SEX OR AGE MOST AFFECTED—Adults of both sexes, but more common in men.

SIGNS & SYMPTOMS—High cholesterol in itself does not produce symptoms.

CAUSES—Total cholesterol is made up of LDL (low-density lipoprotein) cholesterol and HDL (high-density lipoprotein) cholesterol. A high level of LDL causes a fatty buildup in the walls of the arteries (blood vessels) and reduces the flow of blood and oxygen in the body. This can lead to heart disease, stroke, circulation problems, and kidney disease. LDL is called the "bad" cholesterol. HDL, the "good" cholesterol, seems to have a protective effect against heart disease. Triglycerides are another form of fat in the blood. High levels of triglycerides may increase the risk of disease.

RISK INCREASES WITH
- Excess saturated fat and cholesterol in diet.
- Being overweight.
- Not being physically active.
- Heredity. High cholesterol can run in families.
- Age. As people get older, cholesterol levels rise. For women, LDL levels tend to rise after menopause.

HOW TO PREVENT
- Eat a low-fat, healthy diet.
- Exercise on a routine basis.
- Maintain the proper body weight.
- Get cholesterol and triglyceride blood tests as advised. Early treatment is more effective.

WHAT TO EXPECT

DIAGNOSTIC MEASURES
- Your health care provider will have your blood tested for cholesterol levels. The blood test will check for levels of total cholesterol, LDL, HDL, and triglycerides.
- The test results must be looked at on an individual basis, and will take into account your other risk factors for heart disease. Cholesterol levels are measured in milligrams per deciliter (mg/dL).

- Desired level for total cholesterol is less than 200; 200 to 239 is borderline high risk; over 240 is high risk.
- LDL below 130 is the recommended level; below 100 is ideal; over 160 is high risk.
- HDL of 60 and above is good; under 40 for men and under 50 for women is high risk.
- Triglyceride of 150 is borderline high; 200 is high.

APPROPRIATE HEALTH CARE—You and your health care provider can decide on an action plan to reduce your risks of heart disease and stroke. This may include changes in diet, more exercise, weight loss, quitting smoking, and drug therapy.

POSSIBLE COMPLICATIONS
- Heart disease and stroke. Other factors that can increase their risk include smoking; stress; high blood pressure; obesity; lack of exercise, medical problems (e.g., diabetes, use of some drugs, men over 45, women over 55, and family history of early heart disease).
- Atherosclerosis (hardening of the arteries).
- May be some decrease of kidney function.
- Poor circulation.

PROBABLE OUTCOME—High cholesterol can be lowered to desired levels with changes in lifestyle, or drugs, if needed.

HOW TO TREAT

GENERAL MEASURES
- Diet and lifestyle changes do not mean you have to give up all the good things you enjoy.
- To learn more: American Heart Association, 7272 Greenville Ave., Dallas, TX 75231; (800) 242-8721; website: www.americanheart.org.

MEDICATION—Cholesterol-lowering drugs may be prescribed if diet and exercise changes are not effective, or if you are at high risk for heart disease.

ACTIVITY—Increase physical activity. Try to get at least 30 minutes of aerobic exercise (such as brisk walking) every day.

DIET
- Limit foods that contain saturated fats and high amounts of cholesterol.
- Eat a diet that is high in fiber with lots of fruits and vegetables.
- Begin a weight-loss diet if you are overweight.

CALL YOUR DOCTOR IF

You or a family member wants testing for cholesterol levels or wants help with diet and exercise planning.

CHRONIC FATIGUE SYNDROME

GENERAL INFORMATION

DEFINITION—Chronic fatigue syndrome (CFS) is a disorder that involves profound fatigue. The fatigue is not improved by bed rest. It may be worsened by physical or mental activity. Persons with CFS most often function at a much lower level of activity than they were capable of before the onset of illness.

BODY PARTS INVOLVED—Endocrine system, muscles, gastrointestinal system, central nervous system.

SEX OR AGE MOST AFFECTED—It is seen most often in young adults between 20 and 40. Women are diagnosed more often than men.

SIGNS & SYMPTOMS
• For diagnosis of CFS: a person has severe chronic fatigue of six months or longer and other known medical conditions have been ruled out; and at the same time, has 4 or more of the following: 1) Memory or concentration problems. 2) Sore throat. 3) Tender lymph nodes. 4) Muscle pain. 5) Multi-joint pain (no swelling or redness). 6) Headaches (new type, pattern, or severity). 7) Sleep disturbances. 8) Extreme tiredness that lasts more than 24 hours after physical or mental activities.
• Other symptoms may include: abdominal pain, alcohol intolerance, bloating, chest pain, chronic cough, diarrhea, dizziness, dry eyes or mouth, earaches, irregular heartbeat, jaw pain, morning stiffness, nausea, night sweats, psychological problems (depression, irritability, anxiety, panic attacks), shortness of breath, skin sensations, tingling sensations, and weight loss.

CAUSES—The cause is unknown. Infections and the immune, endocrine, and nervous systems may play roles.

RISK INCREASES WITH—Unknown.

HOW TO PREVENT—Unknown.

WHAT TO EXPECT

DIAGNOSTIC MEASURES
• Your health care provider will do a physical exam and ask questions about your symptoms. There is no one test to identify CFS.
• Medical tests are often done to rule out medical disorders that could be causing the symptoms. The guidelines used to help diagnose CFS are listed under Signs & Symptoms.

APPROPRIATE HEALTH CARE
• Steps in therapy may include a combination of lifestyle changes, starting a gradual exercise program, counseling, behavior therapy, and drug therapy.

• Lifestyle changes may include finding ways to cut back on work or other activities. This may help reduce physical and emotional stress. Stop smoking (find a way to quit that works for you).
• Counseling and/or behavior therapy may be helpful for coping with the emotional aspects of the disorder and learning how to reduce stress.
• Alternative therapies such as massage, yoga, muscle-relaxing techniques, or acupuncture may be helpful.

POSSIBLE COMPLICATIONS—The symptoms can lead to a variety of complications (e.g., depression, missing work, or loss of job).

POSSIBLE OUTCOME—CFS affects each person differently. Some people remain homebound. Other persons improve and are able to resume work and other activities, even though they continue to have symptoms. In general, improvement is slow and may take years.

HOW TO TREAT

GENERAL MEASURES
• Joining a CFS support group is helpful for some patients.
• Learn more: Chronic Fatigue & Immune Dysfunction Syndrome Association, PO Box 220398, Charlotte, NC 28222; (704) 365-2343 (not toll-free); website: www.cfids.org.

MEDICATION
• There is no specific drug to treat CFS. Drugs may be prescribed for depression, pain, low blood pressure, allergy-like symptoms, insomnia, or other specific symptoms.
• Other drugs are being studied and may prove to be helpful in treatment. Talk to your health care provider before taking herbal remedies or dietary supplements.

ACTIVITY
• Strenuous exercise should be avoided. Some exercise, however, is important. Begin a gradual program that may be just 3 to 5 minutes a day to start with. Increase the activity by about 20% every 2 to 3 weeks. Setbacks will sometimes occur, so don't be discouraged.
• Get enough sleep at night. Limit daytime napping.

DIET—Eat a healthy diet and drink plenty of fluids. Limit caffeine and avoid alcohol.

CALL YOUR DOCTOR IF

• You or a family member has symptoms of chronic fatigue syndrome.
• Symptoms worsen after treatment is started.

CHRONIC OBSTRUCTIVE PULMONARY DISEASE (COPD)

 GENERAL INFORMATION

DEFINITION—Chronic obstructive pulmonary disease (COPD) is a condition in which airflow in and out of the lungs is restricted. This causes breathing difficulty and other symptoms. The most common forms of COPD are chronic bronchitis and emphysema and patients usually have both disorders. Some also have asthma.

BODY PARTS INVOLVED—Lungs.

SEX OR AGE MOST AFFECTED—Women are more often affected by chronic bronchitis, while men are more often affected by emphysema.

SIGNS & SYMPTOMS
- Chronic bronchitis:
  - Frequent cough or coughing spasm. Mucus is usually present. It is thick and difficult to cough up. The mucus color and thickness may change according to whether infection is present.
  - Shortness of breath.
- Emphysema:
  - Often, no symptoms in the early stages.
  - Shortness of breath that worsens over time.
  - Lung infections.
  - Weight loss.
  - Some wheezing or coughing.
  - Little mucus is produced.

CAUSES—Years of exposure to irritants that cause inflammation and damage to the lungs and airways. Smoking is the usual cause.

RISK INCREASES WITH
- Cigarette smoking (less so—pipes or cigars).
- Secondhand smoke.
- Chronic exposure to dust, ozone, chemicals, smoke, traffic exhaust fumes, sulfur, and others.
- An inherited form of emphysema.
- Older adults and it may run in some families.

HOW TO PREVENT—Stop smoking (or never start). Avoid breathing secondhand smoke. Take preventive steps to protect lungs if work involves exposure to toxic fumes.

 WHAT TO EXPECT

DIAGNOSTIC MEASURES
- Your own observation of symptoms.
- Your health care provider will do a physical exam and ask questions about your symptoms and activities and exposure to lung irritants.
- Medical tests may include blood and sputum studies, x-rays, CT, and lung function testing.

APPROPRIATE HEALTH CARE
- Goals of treatment are to relieve symptoms, slow progression of the disorder, and prevent complications.

- Treatment may include drug therapy, lifestyle changes, supplemental oxygen, special exercises, and sometimes, surgery. You and your health care provider will discuss a treatment plan depending on your individual needs. Educate yourself about this disorder.
- Usually, you can be treated at home. Hospital care may be needed for infections or if symptoms get worse.
- Lung procedures, surgery, or a lung transplant may be an option for a few patients.

POSSIBLE COMPLICATIONS—Frequent infections, anxiety and depression, other lung diseases, heart problems, disability, and death.

PROBABLE OUTCOME—Stopping smoking improves outcome (more so in mild COPD). Other factors that affect outcome are severity of disease, other health problems, and frequency of flare-ups (exacerbations). They can become life-threatening. Treatment can help ease symptoms and reduce complication risks. Other treatments are undergoing research.

 HOW TO TREAT

GENERAL MEASURES
- If you smoke, stop now. This is the most important thing you can do. Avoid secondhand smoke and other lung irritants (air pollution, fumes, dust).
- Get vaccine for pneumonia and yearly flu shot.
- Follow your prescribed COPD treatment plan.
- Avoid excessive heat, cold, and very high altitudes. Talk to your health care provider about airplane travel.

MEDICATION
- Drugs may be prescribed to help symptoms. They can open narrowed airways, reduce inflammation, treat or prevent infections, and reduce the amount of mucus in your lungs.
- Drugs may be prescribed for depression or anxiety.
- Antibiotics will be prescribed for bacterial infections.

ACTIVITY
- Not being active for long periods of time can make your disability worse. Maintain a regular exercise program. Walking is a good activity.
- Your health care provider may prescribe physical therapy or special breathing exercises.

DIET—Eat healthy. Drink plenty of fluids daily (unless advised to limit fluid intake).

 CALL YOUR DOCTOR IF

- You or a family member has COPD symptoms.
- Symptoms worsen or an infection develops.

CHRONIC PAIN SYNDROME

GENERAL INFORMATION

DEFINITION—Chronic pain syndrome is pain that has lasted for months (usually 3 to 6). It is pain that is ongoing after a person has healed from an injury or illness. In some cases, the pain has no known cause. Pain symptoms vary and involve both the body and the mind. They affect your physical and emotional well-being. Chronic pain syndrome is common.

BODY PARTS INVOLVED—Any body part.

SEX OR AGE MOST AFFECTED—All ages (often older adults) and women more than men.

SIGNS & SYMPTOMS
- Pain affects one or more body parts (e.g., back, legs, neck, shoulders, hips, arms, head, stomach, or chest). It may spread or radiate (move) from one part to another.
- Pain may be mild, moderate, or severe and may vary at times. It may be constant pain or it may come and go.
- Pain is described as aching, shooting, burning, sharp, stabbing, cramping, throbbing, or other terms.
- Fatigue, trouble sleeping, or loss of appetite.
- Fear of more pain leads to avoiding activities.
- Problems in doing daily activities (e.g., work, school, or household tasks). Unable to enjoy life.
- Mood changes, low self-esteem, depression, anger, irritability, stressed, anxious, or thoughts of suicide.

CAUSES
- The exact cause is unclear. It is known that the pain is real. Factors may include:
  - Pain signals in the nerves and brain continue after normal healing from an injury or illness.
  - Pain control brain chemicals fail to function.
  - Nerves become damaged.
  - Emotional, mental, social, or behavioral aspects (called psychosocial).

RISK INCREASES WITH—None specific. Risk may be higher for women, people with anxiety (especially anxiety about health) or depression, or people who have certain psychological conditions.

HOW TO PREVENT—No preventives known.

WHAT TO EXPECT

DIAGNOSTIC MEASURES
- Your health care provider will ask questions about your pain and emotional symptoms, medical history, and your quality of life. You may be asked to fill out a form about the pain. A physical exam will be done.
- Medical tests may be done to find a cause. There is no test for chronic pain syndrome. It is diagnosed only after other causes are ruled out.

APPROPRIATE HEALTH CARE
- Treatment usually involves physical and behavioral therapies combined with drug therapy. The treatment plan will be a team effort—patient, family, health care provider, and other medical professionals.
- The goal is to manage the pain and have a reasonable quality of life. Several types of therapies help the body and the mind learn to cope with the pain symptoms.
- Therapies for the body can help improve physical mobility, enable you to perform daily living tasks, and help with issues involving work and social life.
- Therapies for the mind can help change the way you think about pain, teach you ways to relax, and help you learn how to control your body's responses.
- Counseling can help with specific problems (e.g., depression, stress, sleep, relationships, and others).
- Other treatments (e.g., massage, yoga, acupuncture, chiropractic, electrical stimulation) may be options.

POSSIBLE COMPLICATIONS
- Pain continues despite treatment.
- Side affects of drugs used for treatment.
- Family or marriage problems, job loss, or disability.
- Feelings of hopelessness and despair.
- Poor motivation to follow a treatment plan.
- Going from doctor to doctor in search of a cure.
- Dependence on or addiction to drugs for pain.

POSSIBLE OUTCOME—It depends on each person's response to treatment. There is no cure, but pain and emotional symptoms can be controlled so you can lead a more normal life.

HOW TO TREAT

GENERAL MEASURES—To learn more: American Chronic Pain Association; (800) 533-3231; website: www.theacpa.org.

MEDICATION—Drugs will be prescribed as appropriate for pain relief, depression, or other specific symptoms. The risks and benefits of any prescribed drug should be explained to you.

ACTIVITY—Exercise daily—a few minutes a day to start and increase slowly to 30 minutes. Walking is an excellent exercise.

DIET—Eat a healthy diet.

CALL YOUR DOCTOR IF

- You or a family member has symptoms of chronic pain syndrome.
- Symptoms don't improve or worsen during treatment.

CHRONIC PELVIC PAIN

GENERAL INFORMATION

DEFINITION—Chronic pelvic pain is any pain in the pelvic area that has lasted for at least 6 months. Pelvic pain is a common problem in women and the pain symptoms will vary for each woman.

BODY PARTS INVOLVED—Pelvic area, genitals, back and abdomen area.

SEX OR AGE MOST AFFECTED—Females, usually ages 18-50.

SIGNS & SYMPTOMS
- The main symptom is pain in the pelvic and lower stomach and back area. Other terms women use to describe the problem include discomfort, pressure, aches, tenderness, or a heavy feeling.
- The pain may be mild to severe. It may come and go, or it may be there all the time.
- The pain may occur before or during menstrual periods. Some women may have the pain when they have sex or when they exercise.
- Urination and bowel symptoms may occur, such as diarrhea or constipation.

CAUSES—There are many possible causes for this type of pain and sometimes the exact cause is not found. It may involve health problems that are both physical (such as with menstrual periods) and mental (such as stress).

RISK INCREASES WITH
- Prior health problem such as a pelvic infection or pelvic surgery.
- History of abuse as a child or adult.
- Having family members with chronic pelvic pain.

HOW TO PREVENT—No specific way to prevent.

WHAT TO EXPECT

DIAGNOSTIC MEASURES
- Diagnosis begins with a physical exam plus a pelvic exam by your health care provider. You will be asked questions about the pain symptoms you are having.
- Different tests may be ordered to help find the cause of your pain. These include blood and urine studies, a pregnancy test, and a Pap smear (to check the cells in your cervix). X-rays may be needed.
- Minor surgery using a laparoscope may be necessary. This is an instrument with a thin, lighted tube. It is inserted into the body through a small incision. It can help diagnose and sometimes treat the pain at the same time.

APPROPRIATE HEALTH CARE
- Treatment will depend on any medical problems that are diagnosed.
- Your health care provider will talk to you about the treatment options for chronic pain and what may work best for you. Options may include drugs (oral and injections), physical therapy, and possibly surgery. It may be helpful to consult a behavior counselor and learn how to relax and control stress in your life.
- If the cause for the pain is unclear, you may be asked to keep a pain diary for 2 or more months. This can help you and your health care provider see how the pain symptoms relate to what is going on in your life day to day.

POSSIBLE COMPLICATIONS
- Depression, sleep problems, poor appetite, and weight loss occur along with the pain.
- Pain limits your normal activities and lifestyle.

POSSIBLE OUTCOME—Pain symptoms can usually be helped with one or more types of treatment.

HOW TO TREAT

GENERAL MEASURES
- For self-care, apply a heating pad to the painful area. Soak in a bathtub.
- To learn more: National Women's Health Information Center; (800) 994-9662; website: www.womenshealth.gov or International Pelvic Pain Society, Two Woodfield Lake, 1100 E. Woodfield Rd., Ste 520, Schaumburg, IL 60173; (847) 517-8712 (not toll-free); website: www.pelvicpain.org.

MEDICATION
- You may use nonprescription pain relievers such as ibuprofen or naproxen.
- Drugs may be prescribed to treat any medical problems diagnosed or help control severe pain symptoms.
- Drugs may be used to stop your menstrual periods for two months to see if this helps stop the pain.

ACTIVITY
- Try to maintain a regular exercise program. It can help with the pain. It will also help you build strength and be more flexible.
- Physical therapy may be recommended.

DIET—No special diet is usually needed.

CALL YOUR DOCTOR IF

- You or a family member has symptoms of chronic pelvic pain.
- Your pelvic pain continues despite treatment.

CIRRHOSIS OF THE LIVER

 GENERAL INFORMATION

DEFINITION—Cirrhosis involves damage to the liver that develops gradually over months to years. This can lead to serious health problems because the body depends on the liver for many vital functions.

BODY PARTS INVOLVED—Liver and its major blood vessels.

SEX OR AGE MOST AFFECTED—It usually occurs in people ages 40 to 60. It is more common in men than women.

SIGNS & SYMPTOMS
- Early stages (some may not have symptoms):
  - Feeling tired and weak. Nausea may occur.
  - Loss of appetite and weight loss.
  - Pinhead-sized red spots on the skin.
- Later stages:
  - Yellow skin and eyes (jaundice).
  - Palms of hands may be reddish and blotchy.
  - Urine may be dark yellow or brown.
  - Loss of body hair and itchy skin.
  - Fluid build-up in the stomach (called ascites) and legs.
  - Stool may be black, bloody, or clay-colored.
  - Bleeding and bruising.
  - Mental/personality changes.
  - Men—testicles may shrink; breasts may swell.
  - Women—menstrual periods may stop or be irregular.

CAUSES—Liver damage is due to scar tissue that replaces healthy tissue. This blocks the flow of blood through the liver and decreases liver function. A number of disorders can lead to the liver damage.

RISK INCREASES WITH
- Alcoholism. People are all affected differently by alcohol. An amount that causes cirrhosis in one person may not be a problem for another. Nutrition may be a factor.
- Chronic hepatitis B, C, or D.
- Chronic autoimmune hepatitis.
- Blood vessel disease or chronic heart failure.
- Certain inherited disorders.
- Nonalcoholic steatohepatitis (NASH)—fat in the liver.
- Blocked bile ducts.
- Certain drugs, toxins, and infections.

HOW TO PREVENT
- Limit alcohol use, or avoid it entirely.
- Avoid other risk factors, where possible.

 WHAT TO EXPECT

DIAGNOSTIC MEASURES
- Your health care provider will do a physical exam and ask questions about your symptoms, activities, and use of alcohol.
- Medical tests may include blood and urine tests, liver function studies, CT, and ultrasound.
- A biopsy of your liver may be done. This involves removing a sample of liver tissue for viewing under a microscope.

APPROPRIATE HEALTH CARE
- Treatment may include drugs, diet and lifestyle changes, prevention or treatment of complications, and liver transplant. Your health care provider will devise a treatment plan based on your individual needs.
- Bleeding (hemorrhage) or excess fluid (ascites) may be treated with drugs or medical procedures.
- Liver transplant may be an option for severe disease.
- Counseling or a support group may help.

POSSIBLE COMPLICATIONS
- Continued alcohol use will lead to more liver damage.
- Cirrhosis can cause serious, sometimes fatal problems in any organ system in the body.

PROBABLE OUTCOME—It will vary due to the many causes and possible complications. Stopping alcohol use and treating the disorder that led to cirrhosis may slow or stop the progress of the disease.

 HOW TO TREAT

GENERAL MEASURES
- If the condition is caused by alcoholism, stop drinking. Ask for help from family, friends, or support group. Contact Alcoholics Anonymous.
- To learn more: American Liver Foundation, 39 Broadway, Suite 2700, New York, NY 10006; (800) 465-4837; website: www.liverfoundation.org.

MEDICATION
- Your health care provider may prescribe:
  - Drugs for the underlying disorder, to decrease excess fluid in the body, and to prevent bleeding.
  - Supplements, such as vitamins.
  - Drugs to help remove toxins from the body.
  - Drugs for complications, such as infection.
- Don't take other drugs without medical advice.

ACTIVITY—Stay as active as possible. Rest when you feel tired.

DIET—Eat a well-balanced diet. You will be advised about any limits for fat, salt, or protein.

 CALL YOUR DOCTOR IF

- You or a family member has symptoms of cirrhosis.
- Unusual bleeding, bloody vomit, fluid build-up, sudden weight gain, yellow skin or eyes, mental changes, fever, pain, or breathing problem occur.

CLAUDICATION

GENERAL INFORMATION

DEFINITION—Claudication is a feeling of muscle fatigue or cramp-like pain in one or both legs. The discomfort occurs with minimal exercise, such as a short walk, and is normally relieved by resting.

BODY PARTS INVOLVED—The calf is more frequently affected, but it can occur in the thighs, buttocks, hips or feet.

SEX OR AGE MOST AFFECTED—It is more common in men than women, particularly men over age 55.

SIGNS & SYMPTOMS
- Pain, tension, weakness, or cramping in the limb.
- Pain occurs while walking and stops when resting.
- Unable to walk distances.
- Loss of the hair on the toes or lower legs.
- Lameness or limping.
- Numbness in feet or legs.

CAUSES
- Blockage or narrowing of the arteries of the legs due to atherosclerosis.
- Rarer cause is spinal stenosis (pressure on nerve roots that pass into either leg).

RISK INCREASES WITH
- Being a male, women after menopause, age over 60.
- Smoking.
- Diabetes.
- Being sedentary (getting little or no exercise).
- High blood pressure.
- Overweight.
- Heart disease.
- High blood cholesterol.
- Family history of atherosclerosis or claudication.

HOW TO PREVENT
- Stop smoking (or never start).
- Weight loss, if overweight.
- Routine exercise program.
- Reduce the amount of saturated fats in diet.
- Seek medical care for treatable risk factors.

WHAT TO EXPECT

DIAGNOSTIC MEASURES
- Your health care provider will do a physical exam and ask questions about your symptoms and activities.
- A variety of medical tests, including an ultrasound (sometimes done with exercise) or MRI, may be ordered. These will help confirm the diagnosis and rule out other disorders that have similar symptoms.

APPROPRIATE HEALTH CARE
- You will be given exercises to do at home, and/or supervised exercises that are done on a treadmill.
- High blood pressure and high cholesterol may be treated with drugs.
- Various surgical procedures, depending on the site of the disease and the health of the patient, are available for more severe cases.

POSSIBLE COMPLICATIONS
- Complications are usually due to the effects of atherosclerosis, such as cardiovascular problems (e.g., heart attack or stroke).
- Symptoms may cause a reduced quality of life.
- Rarely, severe problems may lead to possible loss of the limb, leg ulcers, gangrene, and disabilty.

PROBABLE OUTCOME—With treatment, there is a gradual improvement in ability to walk distances without pain. Improvement may take 6 to 12 months. It is important to follow an exercise program.

HOW TO TREAT

GENERAL MEASURES
- Stop smoking. Find a way to quit that works for you.
- If diabetic, carefully follow your foot care plan.

MEDICATION
- Low doses of aspirin may be prescribed.
- Drugs to lower blood pressure and reduce cholesterol levels, and special drugs to increase blood flow may be prescribed.
- Avoid drugs that constrict blood vessels (e.g., pseudoephedrine).

ACTIVITY
- Begin an exercise program. Walking or riding an exercise bike is recommended. Stop and rest if the pain becomes more severe. Try for 30 to 60 minutes of exercise 3 to 5 days a week.
- Strength training for the arms and legs also helps to improve symptoms.

DIET—Eat a healthy diet (include fruits, vegetables, and fiber). Consider a weight-loss diet, if overweight is a problem.

CALL YOUR DOCTOR IF

- You or a family member has claudication symptoms.
- You experience chest pain, shortness of breath, or rapid heartbeat during exercise.
- Drugs used for treatment cause unexpected side effects.

COCCIDIOIDOMYCOSIS
(Valley Fever; San Joaquin Valley Fever)

GENERAL INFORMATION

DEFINITION—Coccidioidomycosis is a lung infection caused by a fungus (plural is fungi) that lives in soil. The infection is usually so mild that it produces no symptoms.

BODY PARTS INVOLVED—Lungs (most commonly), but the kidneys, lymph system, brain, and spleen can be affected.

SEX OR AGE MOST AFFECTED—Both sexes, all ages.

SIGNS & SYMPTOMS
• People may think they have a mild case of flu. In a few cases the symptoms may include:
  - Cough.
  - Fatigue.
  - Sore throat; chills; fever; chest pain.
  - Headache; muscle and joint aches.
  - Skin rash.
  - General ill feeling.
  - Sweating at night.
  - Weight loss.
  - Stiff neck (sometimes).

CAUSES—Infection by the fungus, *Coccidioides immitis*, which thrives in soil, especially soil that lines rodent burrows. A person becomes infected when they breathe the dust from such soil and the fungi lodge in the lungs. Symptoms may occur 1 to 4 weeks after exposure. It cannot be spread from person to person.

RISK INCREASES WITH
• Geographic location. The fungus is most common in the southwestern United States: California (e.g., San Joaquin Valley), Arizona, New Mexico, Nevada, Utah, and southwest Texas. It is also found in areas of Mexico, Central America, and South America.
• Work or environmental exposure to dust, such as farmers, construction workers, landscaping work, an archeology site, dirt biking, and others.
• Risk increases on windy days when the soil is dry and when the soil is disturbed, as with excavation. Outbreaks occur following dust storms or earthquakes. Cases increase during and after rainy seasons.

HOW TO PREVENT—Cannot be prevented at present.

WHAT TO EXPECT

DIAGNOSTIC MEASURES
• Your health care provider may do a physical exam and ask about your symptoms and activities.
• Medical tests may include blood studies, sputum cultures, chest x-ray, and others.

APPROPRIATE HEALTH CARE
• Treatment usually involves care at home and sometimes, drug therapy.
• Hospital care is required only for severe cases. Very rarely is surgery needed.

POSSIBLE COMPLICATIONS
• Spread of infection to other parts of the body, which can cause serious complications and could be fatal.
• Pneumonia.
• The disorder may become chronic.
• Risk factors for complications: weak immune system, pregnancy, African Americans or Filipinos, chronic medical disorders, and corticosteroid therapy.

PROBABLE OUTCOME—Most infected persons recover on their own in 3 to 6 weeks. Patients may continue to feel ill for 3 to 6 weeks after signs of infection disappear. After recovery, most people will have a life-long immunity to the infection.

HOW TO TREAT

GENERAL MEASURES
• Your health care provider will usually schedule follow-up visits to verify that your recovery is progressing as expected.
• To learn more: Valley Fever Center for Excellence; 1656 E Mabel St., PO Box 245215, Tucson, AZ 85724; (520) 629-4777 (not toll free); website: www.vfce.arizona.edu.

MEDICATION
• You may use nonprescription nonsteroidal anti-inflammatory drugs for pain, and antitussives for cough if needed.
• Antifungal drugs will usually be prescribed for severe infections. They may also be prescribed in some mild infections as determined by your health care provider.

ACTIVITY—Stay as active as your strength allows.

DIET—No special diet.

CALL YOUR DOCTOR IF

• You or a family member has symptoms of coccidioidomycosis.
• Continued weight-loss, fever, diarrhea that cannot be controlled, stiff neck with headache develop.

COLD, COMMON

 GENERAL INFORMATION

DEFINITION—A common cold is a contagious viral infection of the upper-respiratory tract.

BODY PARTS INVOLVED—Nose, throat, sinuses; ears, eustachian tubes, trachea, larynx, and bronchial tubes.

SEX OR AGE MOST AFFECTED—Colds affect all ages (often infants and children) and may occur 2 to 10 times in a year in an individual.

SIGNS & SYMPTOMS
- Stuffy or runny nose. Nasal discharge may be watery at first, becoming thick and yellow.
- Throat feels scratchy or sore.
- Coughing and sneezing.
- Loss of voice.
- Mild headache. Watering eyes.
- Fatigue.
- Low-grade fever.
- Cold symptoms start slowly. Flu symptoms are more sudden and include higher fever, major aches, chills, sweats, weakness, possible severe sore throat, cough, and chest discomfort.

CAUSES—Any of at least 100 viruses. Virus germs spread through the air or from person-to-person contact or by touching an object that has cold germs on it and then touching your eyes, nose, or mouth.

RISK INCREASES WITH
- Winter (most colds occur in cold weather).
- Children attending school or daycare.
- Household member who has a cold.
- Crowded or unclean living conditions.
- Stress, fatigue, and allergies.

HOW TO PREVENT
- To prevent spreading a cold to others, avoid contact if possible during the contagious phase (first 2 to 4 days).
- Wash hands often, especially after blowing your nose or before handling food.
- Avoid crowded places when possible, especially during the winter.
- Eat a well-balanced, healthy diet. Include plenty of citrus fruits and other sources of vitamin C.

 WHAT TO EXPECT

DIAGNOSTIC MEASURES
- Your own observation of symptoms.
- Diagnosis by a health care provider.

APPROPRIATE HEALTH CARE
- Self-care at home.
- Medical treatment (for complications only).

POSSIBLE COMPLICATIONS—Bacterial infections of the ears, throat, sinuses, or lungs.

PROBABLE OUTCOME—Most people with a cold will recovery in 7 to 14 days.

 HOW TO TREAT

GENERAL MEASURES
- There is no cure for a cold. Self-care and time are usually all that is needed for a cold. There are many remedies for cold symptoms. They include nonprescription cold preparations, getting extra rest, drinking plenty of fluids, and others that may be suggested by friends and family members. One or more of these may help you feel better until the body's defenses fight off the germs.
- Don't smoke. It can further irritate the nasal passages.
- For a baby too young to blow his or her nose, use an infant nasal aspirator. Don't insert cotton swabs into a child's nostrils.

MEDICATION—No drugs, including antibiotics, can cure the common cold. To help relieve symptoms, adults may use nonprescription drugs, such as acetaminophen, decongestants, nose drops or sprays, cough remedies, and throat lozenges. It is best to get a product that works for one symptom, such as a runny nose, rather than a multi-symptom product. If you take other drugs, talk to your health care provider or pharmacist about possible drug interactions. For colds in children, don't use any nonprescription product unless advised by a health care provider or the label states that it can be used for your child's age.

ACTIVITY—Bed rest is not needed, but try to get extra rest for the first few days of a cold.

DIET
- Regular diet. Drink extra fluids, including water, fruit juice, tea, and carbonated drinks.
- Hot fluids (e.g., chicken soup) may help keep nasal passages moist, soothe sore throat, and thin out mucus.

 CALL YOUR DOCTOR IF

- You have increased throat pain, or white or yellow spots on the tonsils or other parts of the throat.
- You have long coughing episodes. Your cough produces thick, yellow-green or gray sputum. You have a cough that lasts longer than 10 days.
- A fever lasts several days, or is over 101°F (38.3°C).
- You have chills, chest pain, or shortness of breath.
- You develop a painful earache or severe headache.
- You develop a skin rash or bruised skin.
- You feel pain in the teeth or over the sinuses.
- You have enlarged, tender glands in the neck.
- Infant with a cold unable to bottlefeed or breastfeed.

COLIC IN INFANTS

GENERAL INFORMATION

DEFINITION
- Colic in infants involves repeated episodes of excessive crying that cannot be explained. The baby is healthy and does not have a specific disorder, such as an ear infection. Colic is different in each baby.
- It may be defined as crying for 3 hours a day at least 3 days a week for 3 consecutive weeks.
- Infant colic can also be defined as whatever amount of crying seems excessive to the parent(s). This is affected by how successful they feel at soothing their baby. Babies who are difficult to soothe are more apt to be termed "colicky" even if their actual crying time is no different from another baby who cries a lot but can be easily consoled.

BODY PARTS INVOLVED—Possibly the lower intestinal tract.

SEX OR AGE MOST AFFECTED—Colic affects infants up to 5 months old and is more common in a first child and boys.

SIGNS & SYMPTOMS
- Crying ranges from being fussy to a high-pitched, loud cry. Crying periods usually occur in late afternoon or evening.
- Colic usually begins at 2 to 4 weeks and can last through several months.
- The infant's stomach may rumble, face may be flushed (red), and the child may draw up the legs as if in pain. There may be passing of gas.

CAUSES—Unknown. Some possible, but not proven, causes include an immature nervous or digestive system, food allergy or food intolerance, or the baby is extra sensitive to things going on in the home.

RISK INCREASES WITH—None known.

HOW TO PREVENT—None specific.

WHAT TO EXPECT

DIAGNOSTIC MEASURES
- Your own observation of symptoms.
- The baby's health care provider will examine the infant and ask questions about the crying, feeding, and other behaviors. Once any medical problems are ruled out, the diagnosis of colic can be made.

APPROPRIATE HEALTH CARE
- Home care.
- Medical treatment (rarely).

POSSIBLE COMPLICATIONS—There are usually none for the baby. In parents, it can cause distress, depression, sleep loss, marital problems, and a feeling that their parenting ability is lacking.

PROBABLE OUTCOME
- Parents can be assured that it is not something they are doing or not doing that is causing the colic.
- Colic will resolve on its own with time. It is a temporary condition. It peaks at about 4 to 6 weeks of age and then begins to improve slowly. It is almost always gone by 3 to 5 months of age. Colicky babies tend to eat well and gain weight and develop normally.
- Various soothing methods may or may not be of help.

HOW TO TREAT

GENERAL MEASURES
- No single treatment for colic has been shown to work for sure. Parents may try several methods. Your baby's health care provider may suggest certain techniques.
- Some babies may be soothed by being held close to a parent's chest and carried. A pacifier may help. Some babies like motion (rocking chair, cradle, stroller, swing, or a car trip). Others respond to a warm bath, or gentle massage, or being swaddled (wrapped snugly). Music or background noise (e.g., a vacuum or electric fan) may be of benefit.
- Do not overstimulate the baby. Babies under 3 months may cry less if a parent stops jiggling, patting, or generally making them too excited.
- Parents may find it helpful to seek out the support of other parents who have been through this before.
- Ask someone to take care of the baby in order to give you a break as often as possible. Parents need to get rest and try to avoid becoming too stressed.

MEDICATION—Drugs are usually not helpful for colic. Don't use any herbs or other supplements without medical approval.

ACTIVITY—No limits.

DIET
- Try burping the baby more often. Hold the baby in an upright position for 20 minutes after feeding.
- Breast-feeding mothers may try avoiding dairy, nuts, or foods that cause gas (e.g., beans, cabbage, etc.).
- A change in baby formula may be recommended.

CALL YOUR DOCTOR IF

- Your baby has colic and you are concerned about it.
- You fear that you are about to lose emotional control.

COLITIS, ULCERATIVE

GENERAL INFORMATION

DEFINITION—Ulcerative colitis (UC) is a chronic inflammatory disease of the colon (large intestine). The inflammation causes small sores or ulcers. UC is an inflammatory bowel disease (IBD) as is Crohn's disease. The two disorders have similar symptoms.

BODY PARTS INVOLVED—It usually affects the rectum (the lower end of the colon), but may affect the entire colon. Rarely, a portion of the small intestine is involved.

SEX OR AGE MOST AFFECTED—Both sexes and all ages (more common in young women).

SIGNS & SYMPTOMS
- Symptoms may be mild, moderate, or severe. They can come and go.
- Diarrhea. Blood and mucus may be present.
- Abdominal cramping, tenderness, or sounds (e.g., gurgling).
- Urgency to have a bowel movement.
- Later symptoms may include: appetite and weight loss, fever, and anemia (e.g., paleness and fatigue).

CAUSES—Unknown. Genetic, infectious, immunologic, and environmental (e.g., smoking) factors may be involved.

RISK INCREASES WITH—Family history of ulcerative colitis.

HOW TO PREVENT—No specific measures.

WHAT TO EXPECT

DIAGNOSTIC MEASURES
- Your health care provider will do a physical exam and ask questions about your symptoms.
- Medical tests may include stool and blood studies and x-ray of the colon (barium enema). A sigmoidoscopy or colonoscopy may be done. In these procedures, a thin tube with a lighted tip is used to view inside the colon and rectum and a small piece of tissue can be removed for biopsy.

APPROPRIATE HEALTH CARE
- Treatment will depend on the severity and extent of the inflammation. Treatment steps may include drug therapy, surgery, and, sometimes, diet changes.
- Hospital care may be needed if bleeding or dehydration develops. Fluids may be given through a vein (IV).
- Surgery to remove part of or the entire colon may be needed. This is done for severe symptoms (such as bleeding), rupture of the colon, cancer risk, failure of other treatments, or side effects of steroid drugs. The options for surgery and stool elimination will be explained to you.

- It is recommended that patients who have had UC for 6 to 7 years should start having a colonoscopy every 1 to 2 years for cancer screening purposes.
- Counseling may help with emotional aspects of the disease or the surgery. Try to decrease the stress in your life. It can worsen symptoms.

POSSIBLE COMPLICATIONS
- Toxic megacolon (a rare, severe inflammation which can be life-threatening).
- Profuse bleeding, dehydration, bowel perforation, or liver disease.
- Inflammation of joints, eyes, and skin.
- Colon cancer risk is greater.
- Delayed growth or sexual development in a child (due to nutritional problems or drug effect).

PROBABLE OUTCOME—The course of the disease varies. Symptoms tend to come and go throughout life. Treatment can help.

HOW TO TREAT

GENERAL MEASURES
- To reduce cramps, apply a hot-water bottle, warm moist towels or heating pad to the abdomen or try taking a warm bath.
- To learn more: Crohn's and Colitis Foundation of America, 386 Park Ave. South, 17th Floor, New York, NY 10016; (800) 932-2423; website: www.ccfa.org.

MEDICATION
- Drugs called 5-aminosalicylates (5-ASA) are often prescribed to help control inflammation.
- Cortisone drugs may be prescribed for more severe symptoms. They may be taken by mouth, injected, given through an enema, or as a suppository.
- Drugs called immunomodulators may be prescribed.
- Antibiotics for infection, antidiarrheals for diarrhea, or vitamin and mineral supplements (e.g., iron) may be prescribed.

ACTIVITY—Bed rest may be needed during acute attacks. Resume normal activity as soon as symptoms improve.

DIET—Eat a healthy diet. Some foods aggravate symptoms in different people. Keep a food diary to learn which foods cause you symptoms so you can avoid them.

CALL YOUR DOCTOR IF

- You or a family member has symptoms of ulcerative colitis.
- After diagnosis and treatment, fever and chills develop, the frequency of bowel movements or bleeding increases, jaundice (yellow eyes and skin with dark urine) develops, vomiting begins, or pain increases.

COLON CANCER
(Colorectal Cancer)

 GENERAL INFORMATION

DEFINITION—Colon cancer is cancer that grows in the colon or the rectum. They are part of the body's digestive system. It is also called colorectal cancer.

BODY PARTS INVOLVED—The colon (large intestine) is about 5 feet long and the rectum is the last 6 inches of the colon.

SEX OR AGE MOST AFFECTED—Both sexes; all ages; usually affects adults over age 50.

SIGNS & SYMPTOMS
- No symptoms in the early stages (frequently).
- Bloody or black, tarry stools or rectal bleeding.
- Cramping stomach pain; feeling of fullness.
- Change in bowel habits, such as diarrhea, constipation, or narrow stools.
- Unexplained weight loss.
- Anemia (pale skin and fatigue).
- Loss of bowel control (sometimes).
- Pain in the rectum (sometimes).

CAUSES—Exact cause is unknown. Genetic and environmental factors may contribute. There are known risk factors.

RISK INCREASES WITH
- Family history of colon cancer or colon polyps.
- Inherited genetic abnormality.
- Inflammatory bowel disease (ulcerative colitis).
- Intestinal polyps (benign growths).
- Having other cancer or prior colon cancer.
- Blacks and Ashkenazi Jews have higher risks.
- Diabetes.
- Diet high in fat and meat (both red and white).
- Age over 50, obesity, sedentary (not active physically) lifestyle, smoking, and/or alcohol use.

HOW TO PREVENT
- To reduce risk: exercise daily; eat a low-fat, high-fiber diet (lots of fruits and vegetables); control weight; don't smoke; and limit alcohol.
- Colon cancer screening tests.
- Genetic tests for family members at risk.
- Precancerous conditions should be treated.
- Vitamins, calcium, nonsteroidal anti-inflammatory drugs, folic acid, or female hormones may be recommended for some patients as preventive therapies.

 WHAT TO EXPECT

DIAGNOSTIC MEASURES
- Your health care provider will do a physical exam and ask questions about your symptoms.
- A number of medical tests will be done. The tests help diagnose the cancer and then determine if it has spread (staging).

APPROPRIATE HEALTH CARE
- Treatment depends on location and size of tumor, any spread of the cancer, your health, age, and your preferences.
- Treatment may include surgery, chemotherapy and/or radiotherapy, and targeted/biologic therapy.
- Chemotherapy uses anticancer drugs while radiotherapy uses radiation to kill cancer cells. Targeted/biologic therapy uses drugs to attack specific cancer cells.
- The goal of surgery is to remove as much of the cancer as possible. Part, or all, of the colon, rectum, and nearby organs may be removed. A colostomy to collect stool or an urostomy to collect urine may be needed to help the body get rid of these wastes.
- Treatment may involve steps to relieve symptoms and make you comfortable, rather than treating the cancer.
- Counseling may help you cope with having cancer.

POSSIBLE COMPLICATIONS
- Complications may occur due to treatments.
- Cancer recurs or spreads in the body (can be life-threatening).

PROBABLE OUTCOME
- Outlook varies. The earlier the cancer is diagnosed and treated, the greater the chances for recovery.
- After treatment, regular follow-up medical exams are important to check for recurrence or new cancers.

 HOW TO TREAT

GENERAL MEASURES—To learn more: American Cancer Society; (800) ACS-2345; website: www.cancer.org or National Cancer Institute; (800) 4-CANCER; website: www.cancer.gov.

MEDICATION—Your health care provider may prescribe anticancer drugs (chemotherapy), targeted/biologic therapies, and pain relievers.

ACTIVITY—You will be advised when to resume normal activities, including driving and sexual relations. After treatment, a follow-up exercise program may be recommended.

DIET—Eat small, healthy meals until digestive system returns to normal. Drink plenty of fluids each day. A dietitian can help with meal plans.

 CALL YOUR DOCTOR IF

- You or a family member has symptoms of cancer of the colon or rectum.
- New symptoms occur after treatment.

COLON POLYPS
(Colorectal Polyps)

GENERAL INFORMATION

DEFINITION
- Colon polyps are slow growing, fleshy growths on the lining of the colon (large intestine). Many adults, especially over age 40, have them. Most polyps (90%) are considered benign (harmless or noncancerous). A less common type of polyp may lead to cancer. The only way to find out if you have polyps and what type they are is with medical testing.
- Features of polyps:
  - A person may have just one polyp or several.
  - Most are small. They may range in size from smaller than a pea to golf ball size.
  - A polyp is called pedunculated if it grows on a stalk (like a mushroom). A flat-shaped polyp is called sessile.
  - Hyperplastic is the name for benign type of polyp.
  - Adenomas (or adenomatous) polyp is the type that may lead to cancers. Larger polyps increase the risk.

BODY PARTS INVOLVED—Colon.

SEX OR AGE MOST AFFECTED—Both sexes; and often affects adults over age 50.

SIGNS & SYMPTOMS—Most polyps cause no symptoms. If symptoms occur, they may include rectal bleeding, constipation or diarrhea, or decreased or bloody stools.

CAUSES—It is unknown why colon polyps develop. Dietary, genetic, and environmental factors may play a role.

RISK INCREASES WITH
- Age (starting at around 40).
- Your own history or a family history of colon polyps or colon cancer.
- Polyposis syndromes. These are rare, usually inherited disorders. Many polyps occur (hundreds to thousands). These patients will require special medical care.

HOW TO PREVENT
- No known specific preventive measures.
- Self-care methods may help with prevention.
  - Eat a low fat, high fiber diet.
  - Maintain a healthy body weight.
  - Avoid smoking and excess alcohol use.
  - Ask your health care provider about taking calcium, folate, aspirin, or other supplements to aid prevention.

WHAT TO EXPECT

DIAGNOSTIC MEASURES
- Get tested for colon polyps if you: are age 50 or older, have symptoms, or have a family history of polyps or cancer. Tests types:

- Fecal occult blood test (FOBT): a lab test to find blood in the stool. If blood is found, more tests are needed to find the cause (e.g., polyps).
- Barium enema: a liquid called barium is placed in the rectum. X-rays are taken of the large intestine. This test can detect polyps, but it cannot remove them.
- Colonoscopy: a lighted tube that has a camera on the end is used to see inside the entire length of colon. If a polyp is found, it is often removed (a polypectomy). Small polyps may be left as they carry very little risk of cancer. A biopsy (viewing the polyp tissue with a microscope) determines if it is benign (most likely), precancer, or cancer. Rarely, open surgery may be needed to remove large or multiple polyps.
- Flexible sigmoidoscopy: similar to a colonoscopy. It views just the rectum and lower end of the colon. If a polyp is found, it can be removed and biopsied. A follow-up colonoscopy is usually needed to look for and remove any polyps in the rest of the colon.
- Virtual colonoscopy: a screening test that uses a CT scan (or MRI) to view the colon. If polyps are found, a colonoscopy is needed.

APPROPRIATE HEALTH CARE—Further treatment and plans for future screening tests depend on the results of the completed tests. Your health care provider will discuss the options with you.

POSSIBLE COMPLICATIONS
- Polyps may cause bleeding, obstruction, or diarrhea.
- Colon cancer may develop.
- Rarely, a procedure to remove polyps can cause bleeding or perforation (hole in colon).

PROBABLE OUTCOME—Almost all colon polyps are benign and should cause no problems (even when not removed). Polyps can be removed safely. New polyps develop in about 30% of people who had them removed.

HOW TO TREAT

GENERAL MEASURES—None specific.

MEDICATION—Drugs to help you relax are used for some tests.

ACTIVITY—No limits unless advised.

DIET—May be restricted prior to a test.

CALL YOUR DOCTOR IF

You or a family member wants tested for colon polyps or symptoms occur after a test.

CONJUNCTIVITIS
(Pink Eye)

GENERAL INFORMATION

DEFINITION—Conjunctivitis is an inflammation (redness and soreness) of the conjunctiva.

BODY PARTS INVOLVED—The conjunctiva is a clear membrane that covers the white part of the eye and the inside of the eyelids.

SEX OR AGE MOST AFFECTED—Both sexes and all ages, but more common in children.

SIGNS & SYMPTOMS
- Symptoms vary depending on the cause.
- One or both eyes may be affected.
- Eye discomfort or pain.
- Gritty feeling in the eye (like there is a piece of sand in the eye).
- Redness of the eye (term "pink eye").
- Clear, green, or yellow eye discharge.
- After sleeping, crusts on lashes that cause eyelids to stick together.
- Swollen eyelids.
- Sensitivity to bright light.
- Intense itching (allergic type only).

CAUSES
- Bacterial or viral infection. Conjunctivitis may occur with colds or childhood diseases such as measles. An infection can be spread from one eye to the other. It can also be spread from one person to another.
- Chemical irritation or dust, smoke, chlorine, other types of air pollution, or home chemicals.
- Allergies caused by cosmetics, pollen, animal dander, or other allergens. (Both eyes are usually affected.)
- A blocked tear duct.
- Certain autoimmune disorders (e.g., Sjögren's).

RISK INCREASES WITH
- Children and the elderly.
- Contact lens wearers.
- Contact with an infected person.
- Newborns of mothers who are carriers of gonorrhea or chlamydia.

HOW TO PREVENT
- Wash hands often to avoid spreading germs.
- Avoid exposure to eye irritants.
- Newborns in hospital deliveries are routinely given antibiotic eye drops.
- Don't share eye makeup (discard after 4 to 6 months).

WHAT TO EXPECT

DIAGNOSTIC MEASURES
- Your own observation of symptoms.
- See your health care provider if you have any concerns about the symptoms. Your health care provider can diagnose conjunctivitis with an exam of the affected eye.
- A laboratory culture of fluid or discharge from the eye may be done to verify the cause.

APPROPRIATE HEALTH CARE—Treatment of conjunctivitis varies with the cause. Self-care may be all that is needed. Topical drugs for the eye or taken by mouth may be prescribed in some cases.

POSSIBLE COMPLICATIONS—Complications are rare, but may include other eye infections or problems of the cornea.

PROBABLE OUTCOME
- Most forms will heal on their own in 1 to 2 weeks with no serious harm.
- Allergic conjunctivitis can be cured if the allergen is removed. However, it is likely to recur.

HOW TO TREAT

GENERAL MEASURES
- Wash hands often with antiseptic soap, and use paper towels to dry. Don't touch the eyes. Gently wipe the discharge from the eye with disposable tissues. Use separate washcloths and towels for each family member.
- For infectious conjunctivitis, use warm-water compresses on the eye to reduce discomfort. Cool compresses feel better with allergic conjunctivitis. Apply for 5 to 10 minutes several times a day.
- For contact lens-related conjunctivitis, stop contact lens wear until a cause is found (e.g., allergy to solution or injury from the lens).
- Do not use eye makeup while symptoms are present.

MEDICATION
- You may use nonprescription artificial tears in the eyes to help relieve symptoms.
- Antibiotic eye drops or ointments may be prescribed for bacterial infection. Antibiotics taken by mouth may be prescribed for more severe cases.
- For other causes of conjunctivitis, topical or oral drugs may be prescribed.
- Use nonprescription anti-allergy eye drops for allergic conjunctivitis (unless otherwise advised).

ACTIVITY—Return to work or school once symptoms improve.

DIET—No special diet.

CALL YOUR DOCTOR IF

- You or a family member has signs of conjunctivitis that does not improve in 48 hours.
- Changes in vision or other symptoms occur.

CONSTIPATION

GENERAL INFORMATION

DEFINITION—Constipation may be defined as having fewer bowel movements than usual and difficulty in passing stools. In most people, constipation is harmless. In some, it can be a sign that something else is wrong with the body. People may think they are constipated when their bowel movements are actually regular. There is no right number of daily or weekly bowel movements. Everyone has different bowel patterns.

BODY PARTS INVOLVED—Colon.

SEX OR AGE MOST AFFECTED—Both sexes; all ages.

SIGNS & SYMPTOMS
- Hard, dry, or lumpy stools.
- Having to strain to have a bowel movement.
- Pain or bleeding with bowel movements.
- Feeling bloated or sluggish.
- Feeling like you still need to go after having a bowel movement.
- May have fewer than 3 bowel movements a week.

CAUSES—The slow movement of feces (stool) through the intestines—most often, the colon (large intestine). This results in a dry, hard stool.

RISK INCREASES WITH
- Constipation can be a symptom or a complication of many different medical disorders.
- Not getting enough fluids.
- Not enough fiber in the diet.
- Being inactive.
- Taking certain drugs (e.g., narcotic drugs for pain).
- Problems with the rectum.
- Laxative abuse.
- Travel-related constipation.
- Advancing age.
- Emotional factors (e.g., depression or anxiety).
- Pregnancy.

HOW TO PREVENT
- Eat a well-balanced diet. Include lots of fiber.
- Exercise regularly.
- Drink plenty of fluids every day.

WHAT TO EXPECT

DIAGNOSTIC MEASURES
- Your own observation of symptoms.
- If you have any concerns about constipation, see your health care provider. He/she may do a physical exam. Questions will be asked about your symptoms, diet, and activities.
- Medical tests may be done (for severe symptoms, if bowel habits change, or to find a cause).

APPROPRIATE HEALTH CARE
- Self-care may be all that is needed.
- Treatment will be prescribed for any specific cause. If a drug is the cause, the drug or dosage may be changed.

POSSIBLE COMPLICATIONS
- Hemorrhoids.
- Fecal impaction (hardened stool that won't pass).
- Anal fissure (tears in skin around anus).
- Chronic constipation.
- Becoming dependent on laxatives. A person should slowly stop using them. Normal bowel function will begin again in time.

PROBABLE OUTCOME—Constipation may go away on its own. It is usually curable with simple changes in diet or lifestyle.

HOW TO TREAT

GENERAL MEASURES
- In most cases, constipation can be helped with changes in diet and lifestyle (such as more exercise). Laxatives are usually not needed for mild constipation.
- Make a regular time each day for bowel movements. The best time is often within 1 hour after breakfast. Don't try to hurry. Sit at least 10 minutes, even if bowel movement doesn't occur.
- To learn more: National Digestive Disease Info.; (800) 891-5389; website: www.digestive.niddk.nih.gov.

MEDICATION
- Ask your health care provider about using laxatives for a short period of time. Avoid regular use as they can lead to laxative-dependence. Types of laxatives:
  - Stool softener (softens stools by mixing in fluids).
  - Bulk-former (adds bulk and water to stools).
  - Lubricant (coats stools so they pass easier).
  - Saline (draws fluid into bowels to soften stools).
  - Stimulant (helps the bowel to contract). Avoid these (unless prescribed) as they are more harsh.
- Fiber supplements may be recommended.

ACTIVITY—Get regular exercise and stay physically fit. This helps stimulate the bowel and helps maintain healthy bowels.

DIET—Drink plenty of fluid each day. Eat a high-fiber diet (beans, bran cereals, raw fruits, and vegetables). Avoid refined cereals and breads, pastries, and sugar.

CALL YOUR DOCTOR IF

Constipation is not helped with self-care or the following occur: sharp pain, bloody stools, fever, diarrhea, weakness, vomiting, or swelling.

COR PULMONALE
(Pulmonary Hypertension)

 GENERAL INFORMATION

DEFINITION—Cor pulmonale is a type of heart disease. It develops when the right side of the heart fails to function properly. This means the pumping power of the heart is weaker than normal. The condition is due to high blood pressure in the lungs. Cor pulmonale is usually chronic (ongoing), but may be acute (short term).

BODY PARTS INVOLVED—Lungs; heart; blood vessels.

SEX OR AGE MOST AFFECTED—Both sexes and all ages, but more common in adults over 50, and occurs in men more than women.

SIGNS & SYMPTOMS
- Early symptoms may be vague and mild.
- Shortness of breath with physical activity.
- Feeling weak and tired.
- Chest pain.
- Fainting or near fainting.
- Rapid heartbeat.
- Cough or wheezing.
- Swelling of the ankles, feet.
- Swelling of the stomach (ascites).
- Bluish color of the skin.
- Neck veins swollen (distended).

CAUSES—Lung disease or dysfunction leads to pulmonary hypertension (high blood pressure in the lungs). This slows or blocks blood flow in the lungs. This in turn causes an extra load on the right side of the heart as it tries to pump enough blood through the lungs. The heart muscle becomes overdeveloped (enlarged) and the load on the heart becomes too great, leading to heart failure.

RISK INCREASES WITH
- Chronic lung disease (e.g., chronic bronchitis, emphysema, silicosis, cystic fibrosis, and others).
- Blood clots in the lungs (pulmonary embolism).
- Extensive loss of lung tissue due to surgery or injury.
- Severe curvature of the spine.
- Severe obesity and sleep apnea.

HOW TO PREVENT
- Avoid risk factors for lung disease, such as smoking.
- Obtain medical care for any heart or lung disorder.

 WHAT TO EXPECT

DIAGNOSTIC MEASURES
- Your own observation of symptoms.
- Your health care provider will do a physical exam and ask questions about your symptoms and activities.
- Medical tests may include blood studies, lung scan, x-ray, lung function tests, and echocardiogram (heart study).

APPROPRIATE HEALTH CARE
- Treatment is directed at the illness that is causing cor pulmonale. Treatment steps usually include drug therapy, supplemental oxygen, and surgery (if needed). Hospital care may be required, especially if a blood clot is diagnosed.
- Supplemental oxygen is usually needed on a continuous basis. An oxygen therapist can arrange for the type of oxygen that allows you to be up and about.
- Surgery may be needed to correct heart defects.
- Lung transplant or heart-lung transplant may be recommended in some cases.

POSSIBLE COMPLICATIONS—Serious, sometimes fatal, heart failure.

PROBABLE OUTCOME—The outcome will depend on the underlying lung disorder. Symptoms can often be relieved or controlled with treatment.

 HOW TO TREAT

GENERAL MEASURES
- Avoid contact with people with infections.
- Avoid air irritants (e.g., smoke).
- To learn more: American Heart Association, local branch, or call (800) 242-8721; website: www.americanheart.org.

MEDICATION—Drugs may be prescribed to improve heart function, to slow and regulate the heart rate, get rid of extra fluid, lower blood pressure, thin the blood, relax blood vessels, and to treat any underlying disorder.

ACTIVITY—Be as active as your condition allows, but don't overexert. Rest between activities.

DIET—You may be advised to follow a low-salt and low fat diet and limit your fluid intake.

 CALL YOUR DOCTOR IF

- You or a family member has symptoms of cor pulmonale.
- The following occur during treatment:
  - Temperature of 101°F (38.3°C) or higher.
  - Weight gain of 3 to 4 pounds in 1 or 2 days.
  - Increased shortness of breath.
  - Increased swelling of the ankles or stomach.
  - Cough with mucus that is discolored or bloody.

CORN OR CALLUS

GENERAL INFORMATION

DEFINITION
- A corn is a thickening (bump) of the outer skin layer, usually over bony areas such as toe joints.
- A callus is a painless thickening of skin caused by repeated pressure or irritation.

BODY PARTS INVOLVED
- Corn: toe joints and skin between toes.
- Callus: any part of the body, especially hands, feet or knees, that endures repeated pressure or irritation.

SEX OR AGE MOST AFFECTED—Both sexes and all ages except infants.

SIGNS & SYMPTOMS
- Corn: a small, tender, and painful raised bump on the side or over the joint of a toe. Corns are usually 3 mm to 10 mm in diameter and have a hard center.
- Callus: a rough, thickened area of skin that appears after repeated pressure or irritation.

CAUSES—Corns and calluses form to protect a skin area from injury caused by repeated rubbing or squeezing. Pressure causes cells in the irritated area to grow at a faster rate, leading to overgrowth.

RISK INCREASES WITH
- Shoes that fit poorly. Socks that bunch up.
- Persons with jobs that involve pressure on the hands or knees, such as carpenters, writers, guitar players, or tile layers.
- Foot deformity.

HOW TO PREVENT
- Don't wear shoes or socks that fit poorly.
- Avoid activities that create constant pressure on specific skin areas.
- When possible, wear protective gear, such as gloves or knee-pads.
- Keep skin moisturized.

WHAT TO EXPECT

DIAGNOSTIC MEASURES
- Your own observation of symptoms.
- See your health care provider or a foot care provider if self-care is not effective. Diagnosis is done by an exam of the affected area.
- Medical tests are usually not needed, but an x-ray may be done.

APPROPRIATE HEALTH CARE—Medical care may involve shaving or cutting off the hardened area of skin, removing the corn or callus with a medicine used on the skin, and (rarely) surgery. Surgery does not remove the cause, and scarring from surgery is painful and may complicate healing.

POSSIBLE COMPLICATIONS
- Back, hip, knee, or ankle pain caused by a change in the way you walk due to foot pain.
- Infection and bleeding may occur from treatments such as cutting or shaving a corn or callus.
- Having diabetes increases the risks of bleeding or infection from a corn or callus.

PROBABLE OUTCOME—Usually curable if the problem that caused it can be removed. Allow 3 weeks for recovery. Corns and calluses are likely to recur, even with treatment, if the cause is not removed.

HOW TO TREAT

GENERAL MEASURES
- Remove the source of pressure, if possible. Get rid of shoes that do not fit well.
- Use corn and callus pads to reduce pressure on the irritated areas.
- Peel or rub the thickened area with a pumice stone to remove it. Don't cut it with a razor. Soak the area in warm water to soften it before peeling.

MEDICATION
- Peel the upper layers of the corn once or twice a day, and then apply a nonprescription 5% or 10% salicylic ointment. Cover with adhesive tape.
- Corn or callus may be injected with cortisone medicine to reduce swelling or pain.
- An antibiotic may be prescribed for skin infection.

ACTIVITY—Resume your normal activities as soon as symptoms improve.

DIET—No special diet.

CALL YOUR DOCTOR IF

- You or a family member has corns or calluses that do not heal, despite self-treatment.
- You develop signs of infection around a corn or callus. Signs of infection include redness, swelling, pain, heat, or tenderness.

CORNEAL ABRASION & ULCER

GENERAL INFORMATION

DEFINITION—An abrasion is a scratched, scraped, or torn area of the cornea. An ulcer is an open sore of the cornea.

BODY PARTS INVOLVED—Cornea (covering); conjunctiva (white of the eye); iris (colored part of the eye); and aqueous humor (fluid in the eyeball).

SEX OR AGE MOST AFFECTED—Both sexes; all ages.

SIGNS & SYMPTOMS
- Eye pain that may be severe.
- Eyes are sensitive to bright light.
- Feeling as if a foreign body is in the eye.
- Watering of the eye.
- Blurred vision.
- Redness in the white of the eye.
- Discharge from the eye.
- Clouding of the cornea.

CAUSES
- Corneal abrasion usually occurs from some type of injury to the eye. It may be a direct injury by a pencil, staple, pin, fingernail, or other object. It may be due to particles flying in the air, such as sand, dust, or from woodworking.
- Corneal ulcer usually occurs when the cornea has been injured and germs enter the injured area and cause an infection. The germs may be viral, bacterial, fungal, or a parasitic infection.

RISK INCREASES WITH
- Contact lens wear.
- Recent eye infection or injury, or other infection.
- Very dry eyes (lack of tearing).
- Small children playing with pointed objects.
- Athletes playing sports without using eye protection.
- Work or hobbies that use pointed tools or produce dust, and construction or farm workers.
- Weak immune system, such as with HIV.
- Severe allergies.
- Eyelids that do not close completely.

HOW TO PREVENT
- Avoid eye injury. Wear safety goggles or protective eye gear when using power tools or when participating in certain sports activities.
- Don't touch your eyes if you have cold sores.
- Handle contact lenses properly.
- Wash hands often to prevent spread of germs.

WHAT TO EXPECT

DIAGNOSTIC MEASURES
- Your own observation of symptoms.
- Usually, an eye doctor (ophthalmologist) will examine the eye using a slit lamp (an eye microscope). A yellow dye may be used in the eye to make it easier to see the affected area. Medical tests may include a vision test and a culture study of corneal scraping.

APPROPRIATE HEALTH CARE
- Treatment will depend on the underlying cause. This may involve removing any foreign object in the eye and drug treatment for the eye. Rarely, hospital care may be needed for severe corneal ulcers.
- If corneal ulcers cause scarring that affects vision, a corneal transplant may be needed.

POSSIBLE COMPLICATIONS—Scarring of the cornea, which can cause permanent partial or complete blindness.

PROBABLE OUTCOME—Abrasions are usually mild and heal on their own in a few days. Corneal ulcers are a more serious eye problem, but should heal in 2 to 3 weeks with treatment.

HOW TO TREAT

GENERAL MEASURES
- An eye patch may or may not be prescribed.
- Apply cool water compresses to the eye as often as they feel good.
- Wear sunglasses. They may help relieve pain.

MEDICATION
- Eye drops or ointments for an eye infection, pain, or inflammation may be prescribed.
- For minor pain, you may use an oral nonprescription drug such as acetaminophen or ibuprofen. Stronger pain drugs may be prescribed if needed.
- For an abrasion, nonprescription artificial tears or eye lubricants may help ease eye discomfort.
- A tetanus shot may be needed if it is not up to date.

ACTIVITY—Resting your eyes will help with healing. Avoid reading. Don't drive until you have medical approval.

DIET—No special diet.

CALL YOUR DOCTOR IF

- You or a family member has symptoms of a corneal abrasion or corneal ulcer. Seek medical care right away.
- After diagnosis, eye pain becomes more severe, vision changes (blurring or loss of vision), or eye becomes red.

CORONARY ARTERY DISEASE
(Coronary Atherosclerosis; Ischemic Heart Disease)

 ## GENERAL INFORMATION

DEFINITION—Coronary artery disease is due to hardening and narrowing of the coronary arteries that provide the blood supply to the heart. There are three main coronary arteries. When any or all become narrowed, they can no longer provide adequate oxygen for heart cells.

BODY PARTS INVOLVED—Blood vessels to the heart.

SEX OR AGE MOST AFFECTED—It often affects adults of both sexes over age 40. It is less common in women before menopause.

SIGNS & SYMPTOMS
- Usually no symptoms occur in early stages.
- Angina pectoris (burning, squeezing, heaviness, or tightness in the chest that may extend to the left arm, neck, jaw, or shoulder blade).
- Irregular heart rate.
- Shortness of breath with exercise or lying down. May sleep propped up on pillows.
- Swelling of feet or ankles.

CAUSES—Atherosclerosis. This is a build-up of plaque on the artery walls. Plaque is made up of fat (e.g., cholesterol), calcium, and other substances found in the blood.

RISK INCREASES WITH
- Increasing age.
- Smoking.
- Hypertension (high blood pressure).
- Diabetes.
- Family history of coronary artery disease, diabetes, high blood pressure, or atherosclerosis.
- Poor nutrition (e.g., too much fat in the diet).
- Previous heart attack or stroke.
- Lack of exercise. Overweight.
- Hostile or impatient personality type.
- Elevated cholesterol or LDL (low density lipoprotein) and/or low level of HDL (high-density lipoprotein).

HOW TO PREVENT
- Don't smoke. Exercise regularly. Eat a low-fat, low-salt, high-fiber diet.
- One aspirin a day (if medically advised).
- Reduce stress level when possible.
- If you have diabetes, hypertension, or high cholesterol, adhere to the treatment plan, including diet limits.
- Maintain ideal body weight.

 ## WHAT TO EXPECT

DIAGNOSTIC MEASURES
- Your health care provider will do a physical exam.

- Medical tests may include electrocardiogram (measures electrical activity of the heart), echocardiogram (measures sound waves), exercise-tolerance test, coronary calcium scoring, radionuclide stress test, blood studies, x-rays of the chest, and coronary angiogram (cardiac catheterization).

APPROPRIATE HEALTH CARE
- Treatment may include drug therapy, lifestyle changes, and surgery.
- Lifestyle changes include diet changes, losing weight, exercising, stopping smoking, and stress control.
- Counseling for stress problems may be helpful.
- Surgical treatment may be needed in some patients. Balloon angioplasty can open narrowed vessels. Vein graft bypass can help restore blood to the heart. A stent may be placed in the artery to keep it open.
- End-stage coronary artery disease can still be cured with a heart transplant (in rare cases).

POSSIBLE COMPLICATIONS
- Heart attack or stroke, congestive heart failure, kidney disease, or heartbeat irregularity problems.
- Sudden death.

PROBABLE OUTCOME—Following a treatment plan can help control symptoms and prevent complications.

 ## HOW TO TREAT

GENERAL MEASURES
- Stop smoking. Find an effective way to quit.
- To learn more: American Heart Association, local branch, or call (800) 242-8721; website: www.americanheart.org.

MEDICATION
- Nitroglycerin, anticoagulants, drugs for angina pectoris and blood-vessel spasms, and drugs to increase the blood supply to the heart may be prescribed.
- Cholesterol-lowering drugs are usually prescribed.
- Vitamin supplements may be recommended.

ACTIVITY—Follow medical advice. Usually, the goal is 30 to 60 minutes of physical activity daily.

DIET—Eat a low-fat, high-fiber diet that includes fruits and vegetables. Begin a weight loss diet, if overweight.

 ## CALL YOUR DOCTOR IF

- You or a family member has symptoms of coronary artery disease.
- After diagnosis, new or unexplained symptoms occur.

COSTOCHONDRITIS
(Tietze's Syndrome)

 GENERAL INFORMATION

DEFINITION—Costochondritis is an inflammation of the cartilage of one or more ribs, most commonly the second or third rib. The pain that results is often increased by movements that change the position of the ribs, such as lying down, bending over, coughing, or sneezing. Pain may mimic that of heart disease or digestive disorders. The term Tietze syndrome is often used for costochondritis.

BODY PARTS INVOLVED—Cartilage of one or more ribs.

SEX OR AGE MOST AFFECTED—It is more common in young adults and in females, but can occur in any age group.

SIGNS & SYMPTOMS
* Pain in the chest wall, usually sharp in nature.
* Pain worsens with movement.
* Pain may occur in more than one location and may radiate into the arm.
* Tightness in the chest.
* Affected area is sensitive to the touch.

CAUSES—Inflammation (soreness and swelling) of the cartilage where the ribs attach to the sternum. The cause of the inflammation is often unknown.

RISK INCREASES WITH
* Trauma, such as a severe blow to the chest.
* Unusual physical activity.
* Upper respiratory infection.

HOW TO PREVENT—Avoid activities that may strain or cause trauma to the rib cage.

 WHAT TO EXPECT

DIAGNOSTIC MEASURES
* Your own observation of symptoms.
* Your health care provider will do a physical exam and ask questions about your symptoms.
* There is no specific test that can diagnose costochondritis. An x-ray or other tests may be done to rule out other disorders.

APPROPRIATE HEALTH CARE—Self-care is usually all that is needed. Medical care may include drug therapy.

POSSIBLE COMPLICATIONS—None likely unless an underlying condition is the cause.

PROBABLE OUTCOME—The disorder usually heals on its own in 3 to 8 weeks. In some cases, mild discomfort may last longer.

 HOW TO TREAT

GENERAL MEASURES
* Use a heating pad or ice massage on the affected area. Use the one that feels better.
* Avoid sudden movements that will intensify the pain.
* Gently stretching the chest muscles several times a day may be helpful.

MEDICATION
* Mild pain drugs, such as ibuprofen or naproxen, may help relieve discomfort.
* Stronger pain drugs or steroid injections may be prescribed, but these are rarely needed.

ACTIVITY—Activities may need to be limited until symptoms improve. Get extra rest when you are able to.

DIET—No special diet.

 CALL YOUR DOCTOR IF

* You or a family member has symptoms of costochondritis.
* Pain continues or gets worse after treatment.

CROHN'S DISEASE
(Regional Enteritis)

GENERAL INFORMATION

DEFINITION—Crohn's disease is an inflammation (painful swelling) of the digestive tract. It can affect any part of the tract from the mouth to the anus, but most often affects the ileum. The ileum is the lower part of the small intestine. Crohn's is a type of inflammatory bowel disease (IBD). Symptoms can come and go. Periods between flare-ups vary from every few months to every few years. Sometimes, symptoms appear only once or twice, and then the disease disappears.

BODY PARTS INVOLVED—Ileum, colon and other parts of the gastrointestinal tract; regional lymph nodes; the mesentery (outside covering of the intestines).

SEX OR AGE MOST AFFECTED—It often starts between ages 15 to 35, and affects men and women equally.

SIGNS & SYMPTOMS
- Cramps and pain in the abdomen (stomach area). The pain is often in the lower-right part of the abdomen.
- Diarrhea.
- Loss of appetite and weight loss.
- Stools may be bloody or contain mucus.
- General ill feeling with fatigue.
- Fever may occur.
- Children with this condition may not grow at a normal rate, and have delayed puberty.

CAUSES—Unknown. The inflammation may result from the body's immune system overreacting to an infection. Genetic and environmental factors (such as diet) may play a role. Research is ongoing.

RISK INCREASES WITH
- Family history of Crohn's or other bowel disease.
- Smoking.
- History of allergies.
- People of Jewish and European ancestry.

HOW TO PREVENT—Cannot be prevented at present.

WHAT TO EXPECT

DIAGNOSTIC MEASURES
- Your own observation of symptoms.
- Your health care provider will do a physical exam and ask questions about your symptoms and activities.
- Medical tests may include blood and stool studies, special x-rays, CT, MRI, or ultrasound. A colonoscopy or capsule endoscopy may be done.

APPROPRIATE HEALTH CARE
- Treatment steps can include drugs, diet changes, and surgery. Hospital care may be needed for severe symptoms.
- Surgery may be required. It may improve the symptoms and delay progress of the disease.

POSSIBLE COMPLICATIONS
- Intestines may become blocked (obstruction).
- An abnormal opening (fistula) may develop between the bowel and nearby areas.
- Abscess (pus-filled sore).
- The bowel may burst or begin to leak.
- Higher risk of colon cancer.
- The body may not be able to absorb nutrients.
- Bleeding (can lead to low iron levels in blood).

PROBABLE OUTCOME—There is no cure for the disease, but patients can have a reasonable quality of life. Treatment can help relieve symptoms. Over time, the treatment usually becomes less effective, and many patients develop complications that require surgery.

HOW TO TREAT

GENERAL MEASURES
- For home care, use heat to relieve pain. Apply a heating pad or take warm-water baths. Check stool daily for signs of bleeding.
- To learn more: Crohn's and Colitis Foundation of America, 386 Park Ave. South, 17th floor, New York, NY 10016; (800) 932-2423; website: www.ccfa.org.

MEDICATION
- Your health care provider may prescribe:
  - Anti-inflammatories, steroids, or anti-TNF (tumor necrosis factor) drugs.
  - Drugs to relieve pain.
  - Antidiarrheals to control diarrhea.
  - Vitamin supplements.
  - Drugs that suppress the immune system.
  - Antibiotics for infection.

ACTIVITY—Remain as active as you can.

DIET
- Avoid foods that aggravate the condition. This may include alcohol, milk products, fatty foods, fiber, popcorn, nuts, and spices. Keep a food diary to find what foods you can and cannot eat.
- Eat small, frequent meals. Take small bites and chew food completely. Drink fluids with meals. Drink liquid nutrient formulas if it is difficult to eat regular food.

CALL YOUR DOCTOR IF

- You or a family member has symptoms of Crohn's disease.
- Symptoms get worse or new ones develop.

CROUP
(Laryngotracheobronchitis)

GENERAL INFORMATION

DEFINITION—Croup is a common infection that causes redness and swelling of the larynx (vocal cords). It may extend into the trachea (windpipe) and bronchi (airways in the lungs).

BODY PARTS INVOLVED—Larynx; throat; trachea (windpipe) and bronchi (airways in the lungs).

SEX OR AGE MOST AFFECTED—Children under age 5 are most often affected.

SIGNS & SYMPTOMS
- The infection can start gradually with a cold, cough, and low fever. Frequently, symptoms come on suddenly in the middle of the night.
- Barking cough. It may be worse when child cries.
- Trouble breathing, especially at night.
- Noisy breathing or wheezing (called stridor).
- Hoarseness.
- Throat discomfort with difficulty in swallowing.
- More severe symptoms include fast breathing, ribs that seem to pull in when breathing, paleness, and bluish skin around the mouth.

CAUSES—A contagious, viral infection is the usual cause. Croup often occurs in outbreaks in the winter and early spring months. Symptoms may begin 3 to 5 days after exposure, but time will vary depending on the type of virus.

RISK INCREASES WITH
- Repeated colds and lung infections or lung disease.
- Previous croup or family history of croup.
- Younger than age 3.

HOW TO PREVENT—No specific preventive measures. Wash your hands often to prevent the spread of any germs.

WHAT TO EXPECT

DIAGNOSTIC MEASURES
- Your own observation of symptoms.
- If symptoms are more severe or you are concerned about the symptoms, see your child's health care provider. A physical exam is usually all that is needed for diagnosis.
- Rarely, an x-ray may be done to rule out other disorders that cause breathing difficulty.

APPROPRIATE HEALTH CARE
- A child who has severe breathing problems may need hospital care. Oxygen may be given to help breathing.
- Most children can be treated at home using supportive care. There are no specific drugs to treat croup.

POSSIBLE COMPLICATIONS
- Recurrence of croup.
- Ear infection.
- Pneumonia.
- Lymph node inflammation.
- Rarely, a blocked airway.

PROBABLE OUTCOME—Croup can be frightening, because attacks usually happen at night and the child has trouble breathing. In almost all cases, croup is not serious and clears up in about a week or less. Complications are rare, but they may occur in children born prematurely or children with lung disease such as asthma.

HOW TO TREAT

GENERAL MEASURES
- Turn on the hot water in the bathroom shower and let the room fill with steam. Hold the child in your arms in the bathroom filled with steam for 10 to 15 minutes. Repeat this procedure if another attack occurs.
- Wrapping the child in a blanket and walking around outdoors may help. It is better if outdoor air is cool.
- Keep the child comfortable in a semi-seated position. Use TV, radio, or a story to distract the child so he or she can relax. Crying can aggravate symptoms.
- Use of a cool-mist humidifier if advised by your child's health care provider. Clean the humidifier as per instructions.

MEDICATION
- Since the cause is usually viral, antibiotics do not help. Cough medicines are also not helpful.
- Acetaminophen may be given to lower fever.
- Oral, injected, or nebulized drugs may be given to a child in the hospital. In severe cases, supplemental oxygen is given.

ACTIVITY—Rest until symptoms improve.

DIET—Usually, a child with croup is not as hungry as normal. It is important to drink plenty of fluids. Offer frequent small amounts of clear fluids or Popsicles.

CALL YOUR DOCTOR IF

- Your child is having trouble breathing and cannot swallow saliva or water. This is an emergency! Call 911 or take the child to the nearest emergency room.
- Nails or lips become bluish.
- Mild croup symptoms don't improve with home care.

CRYPTOCOCCOSIS
(Torulosis)

GENERAL INFORMATION

DEFINITION—Cryptococcosis is a fungal disease that usually affects the lungs, but may spread to other body parts. It is much more serious when there are underlying illnesses or risk factors. This condition has become more common due to HIV and AIDS.

BODY PARTS INVOLVED—Lungs, central nervous system, kidneys, bone, skin.

SEX OR AGE MOST AFFECTED—Both sexes and all ages. It is most common in men between ages 40 and 60.

SIGNS & SYMPTOMS
- Some people may have no symptoms or symptoms are mild and go unnoticed.
- Fever.
- Cough, sometimes with mucus.
- Headache, sometimes severe.
- Shortness of breath.
- Weight loss.
- Tiredness.
- Personality or mental changes if the infection affects the nervous system. This can include confusion or depression or being agitated.
- If the skin is infected, sores or ulcers may occur.
- The infection may cause symptoms in bones, the prostate, and the eyes.

CAUSES—Infection with *Cryptococcus neoformans*. A person gets the infection by breathing in air that contains the germs. The germs are found throughout the world, often in pigeon droppings. The infection is not passed from one person to another. Animals may also get the infection, but do not spread it to humans.

RISK INCREASES WITH
- Persons who have AIDS.
- Organ transplant.
- Drugs that suppress the immune system.
- Cancer (Hodgkin's disease, leukemia, myeloma, lung cancer, and others).
- Chronic lung disease, diabetes, cirrhosis, rheumatoid arthritis, lupus, and splenectomy (spleen removal).

HOW TO PREVENT—Avoid being in areas that have pigeon droppings.

WHAT TO EXPECT

DIAGNOSTIC MEASURES
- Your own observation of symptoms.
- Your health care provider will usually do a physical exam and ask questions about your symptoms and activities.
- Medical tests may include blood, urine, and spinal fluid studies. A chest x-ray and brain CT or MRI may be done.

APPROPRIATE HEALTH CARE
- Some patients require no treatment. Those with underlying disorders are usually treated with drug therapy.
- Hospital care may be needed for severe symptoms.

POSSIBLE COMPLICATIONS
- Infection or inflammation of the brain (encephalitis) or the membranes that surround the brain (meningitis).
- Permanent brain damage, vision loss, and death.

PROBABLE OUTCOME—In those with normal immune systems, the infection usually heals on its own or with treatment. In those with weak immune systems, treatment may control the disease, but not cure it. Lifelong drug therapy may be needed to prevent a relapse.

HOW TO TREAT

GENERAL MEASURES
- It is usually not necessary to isolate ill persons.
- Weigh daily and keep a weight chart. An unexplained weight loss might indicate that infection has spread.

MEDICATION—Antifungal drugs are often prescribed. One drug is usually given by injection at first, followed by another drug that is taken by mouth. People with HIV or AIDS will usually need to take an antifungal drug for life.

ACTIVITY—Get extra rest until the symptoms improve.

DIET—No special diet.

CALL YOUR DOCTOR IF

- You or a family member has symptoms of cryptococcosis, especially if you have a severe headache.
- Symptoms recur after treatment.
- New, unexplained symptoms develop.

CUSHING'S SYNDROME

GENERAL INFORMATION

DEFINITION—Cushing's syndrome is due to excess levels of cortisol, a hormone. Cortisol helps the body respond to stress and change.

BODY PARTS INVOLVED—Adrenal gland (located over the kidney) and pituitary gland (at the base of the brain) are involved in the production of cortisol.

SEX OR AGE MOST AFFECTED—Both sexes and all ages. It is most common in adults ages 20 to 50 and in women more than men.

SIGNS & SYMPTOMS
- Round (moon-like) face and puffy eyes.
- Thin, fragile skin; easy bruising.
- Weakness.
- Weight gain. Fat deposits, such as around the torso and the back of the neck.
- Growth of facial hair in women.
- Stretch marks (red/blue streaks on the skin).
- Mental, mood, and emotional changes.
- Menstrual changes (heavy, irregular, or absent).
- More infections. High blood pressure.
- Sexual and fertility problems.
- Children may have growth retardation, acne, or very early or very late puberty.

CAUSES
- It may result from an overproduction of cortisol by the adrenal glands due to a variety of medical disorders.
- It may result from long-term use of cortisol-like drugs (steroid hormones) to treat medical disorders (such as asthma, arthritis, and inflammatory bowel disease).

RISK INCREASES WITH
- An abnormal growth in the pituitary gland. This causes production of excessive ACTH (adrenocorticotropic hormone). This in turn stimulates the adrenal glands to secrete hormones. This is called Cushing's disease.
- Benign or cancerous tumor in adrenal gland.
- Tumors in other places in the body produce hormones that in turn cause the adrenal glands to produce excess cortisol.
- Prolonged use of steroid hormone drugs.

HOW TO PREVENT—If steroid hormone drugs are prescribed, take the lowest dose possible for the shortest time.

WHAT TO EXPECT

DIAGNOSTIC MEASURES
- Your health care provider will do a physical exam and ask questions about your symptoms and drug use.
- Medical tests may include blood and urine studies of hormone levels, pituitary and adrenal glands function tests, and CT, MRI, or x-rays.

APPROPRIATE HEALTH CARE
- Treatment will depend on the cause of the disorder.
- If it is due to steroid hormone use, the dosage may be slowly reduced (depending on the disease being treated). If the steroid hormone needs to be continued, other drugs may be taken to control the side effects.
- Pituitary gland tumors may be treated with surgery or radiation. If the pituitary gland is removed, hormone replacement therapy will be needed for life.
- Adrenal gland adenoma tumors are removed with surgery. The other adrenal gland is left in place and will eventually take over hormone production.
- Adrenal gland cancerous tumors can be cured if diagnosed early. Often, they are not diagnosed until they have spread beyond the adrenal gland. When this happens, they are not curable. Drugs can treat symptoms.
- Tumors in other places in the body may be treated with surgery, radiation, or chemotherapy. This may help improve the Cushing's syndrome.

POSSIBLE COMPLICATIONS
- Osteoporosis (can lead to bone fractures).
- Side effects of steroid hormones.
- Diabetes, high blood pressure, infections, kidney stones, or spread of cancerous tumors.

PROBABLE OUTCOME—It will depend on the cause of Cushing's syndrome, the degree of excess cortisol, the length of the disease, and the person's basic health. If the cause is treatable, the symptoms may resolve in 2 to 18 months.

HOW TO TREAT

GENERAL MEASURES—Wear or carry medical ID that shows your medical problem and the drugs you take.

MEDICATION
- Drugs to suppress adrenal gland function, cortisone drugs (if adrenal gland removed), or drugs to replace pituitary hormones may be prescribed.
- Drugs to lower blood pressure, to prevent bone loss, and to reduce blood sugar may be prescribed.

ACTIVITY—No limits. Energy will improve once treatment begins.

DIET—No special diet, unless advised.

CALL YOUR DOCTOR IF

- You or a family member has symptoms of Cushing's syndrome.
- New or worsening symptoms develop.

CYSTIC FIBROSIS

GENERAL INFORMATION

DEFINITION—Cystic fibrosis (CF) is an inherited disease affecting the body's glands that produce secretions such as mucus, sweat, tears, saliva, and digestive juices. These secretions are normally thin and slippery and act as a lubricant. In CF, the secretions are thick and sticky. This means the lungs, pancreas, intestines, and other organs become clogged.

BODY PARTS INVOLVED—Pancreas; lungs; sweat glands of the skin; gastrointestinal tract.

SEX OR AGE MOST AFFECTED—Children of both sexes.

SIGNS & SYMPTOMS
- Symptoms will vary in different patients.
- In a newborn, there are thick, sticky stools (meconium). May lead to intestinal obstruction.
- Delayed growth.
- Poor weight gain despite good appetite.
- Bad-smelling, large, fatty stools.
- Sometimes, because the air is chronically trapped in the chest, the child gets a barrel-chested appearance.
- Chronic cough or wheezing.
- Sticky, hard-to-cough-up sputum.
- Salty sweat.
- Polyps in the nose.
- Frequent chest and sinus infections.
- Rounding (clubbing) of the fingertips or toes.
- Rectal prolapse and intussusception (bowel disorder).

CAUSES—A defective gene. A person can carry the gene for cystic fibrosis, but not develop the disease. If both parents are carriers of the defective gene, there is a 25% chance that a child will have the disease, a 50% chance the child will be a carrier, and a 25% chance the child will not have the disease or be a carrier. Carriers have no symptoms of CF.

RISK INCREASES WITH—Family history of cystic fibrosis.

HOW TO PREVENT—If you have a family history of cystic fibrosis, seek genetic counseling and testing before starting a family.

WHAT TO EXPECT

DIAGNOSTIC MEASURES
- Your child's health care provider will do a physical exam.
- Medical tests include sweat tests (done twice). CF is diagnosed if sweat contains high amounts of salt. Very young infants may not produce enough sweat, so genetic blood studies may be done for diagnosis. Tests may be done on lung, pancreas, and liver functions.
- Testing of brothers and sisters of a child with CF is usually recommended even if they have no symptoms.

APPROPRIATE HEALTH CARE
- A medical team (for lung therapy, diet needs, and medical help) will provide treatment.
- Goals of therapy are to prevent and treat infections, keep lungs free of sputum, improve airflow, and provide adequate calories and nutrition.
- Transplants for lung and other organs are possible.

POSSIBLE COMPLICATIONS
- Repeated respiratory infections.
- CF can lead to various medical conditions such as delayed puberty, infertility, diabetes, osteoporosis, digestive problems, and lung and heart disorders.

PROBABLE OUTCOME—CF is a lifelong condition. It is currently considered incurable. Careful long-term care and treatment can help those affected lead reasonably normal and productive lives. Many live into their thirties or forties. Gene therapy is being studied. Medical research is ongoing to find a cure.

HOW TO TREAT

GENERAL MEASURES
- Learn as much as possible about CF. Parents may want to join a support group.
- You will be instructed on how to perform daily postural drainage to drain mucus from the lungs. This is done with clapping on the front and back of the chest. Mechanical aids and special vests are available to help.
- Keep your child's vaccines up-to-date.
- Avoid any exposure to secondhand smoke.
- To learn more: Cystic Fibrosis Foundation, 6931 Arlington Road, Bethesda, MD 20814; (800) 344-4823; website: www.cff.org.

MEDICATION—Drug therapy may include digestive enzymes to help with digestion, mucus-thinning drugs, antibiotics for infections, and bronchodilators to help open airways.

ACTIVITY—Exercise is vital to reduce the impact and progression of CF. A regular exercise program will be prescribed.

DIET—Provide a diet high in calories, fat, and protein. Vitamin supplements and supplemental nutrition may be needed.

CALL YOUR DOCTOR IF

- You suspect your child has cystic fibrosis.
- After diagnosis, symptoms worsen or change.

DECOMPRESSION SICKNESS
(Bends)

 GENERAL INFORMATION

DEFINITION—Decompression sickness is a condition caused by the formation of nitrogen bubbles in the blood or body tissues as the result of a sudden lowering of atmospheric pressure. It can develop in deep-sea divers, astronauts, and pilots ascending too quickly. Symptoms may occur right away or up to 24 hours after the pressure change.

BODY PARTS INVOLVED—Blood in all body parts.

SEX OR AGE MOST AFFECTED—Both sexes; all ages. Usually occurs in young males.

SIGNS & SYMPTOMS
- Mild to severe joint and/or muscle pain (arms, legs, or torso).
- Numbness, tingling, or burning sensation.
- Muscular weakness.
- Difficulty urinating.
- Unusual fatigue.
- Skin itch, blotchy rash.
- Dizziness, vertigo, tremors.
- Ringing in the ears.
- Shortness of breath.
- Paralysis, muscle weakness, staggering.
- Confusion, amnesia, personality changes, or bizarre behavior.
- Coughing up bloody, frothy sputum.
- Paralysis, collapse, or unconsciousness.

CAUSES—Formation of nitrogen bubbles in the blood. Nitrogen is a normal blood component. If the pressure around the body drops rapidly, as in surfacing too quickly while scuba diving, or climbing too rapidly in a non-pressurized aircraft, the nitrogen collects in bubbles in the blood vessels. This blocks the normal blood flow and deprives the body of blood and oxygen.

RISK INCREASES WITH
- Commercial diving or recreational scuba diving. Repeated dives in one day increase risk.
- Some kinds of high-performance aircraft.
- Working in compression chambers.

HOW TO PREVENT
- Get certified instruction before scuba diving.
- Don't dive if you are not in good general health. You are at risk if you are obese or have a medical history of:
  - Lung conditions, such as asthma.
  - Pneumothorax.
  - Heart disease.
  - Chronic sinusitis.
  - Alcoholism.
- Allow for a slow, gradual change to normal air pressure when scuba diving. (The U.S. Navy has tested and set up guidelines.)
- Avoid air travel for 24 hours after diving.

 WHAT T

DIAGNOSTIC MEA
- Your own or a div symptoms.
- Physical exam and medical tests by a health care provider.

APPROPRIATE HEALTH CARE
- Self-care is impossible for this condition. If you observe someone with symptoms of decompression sickness, get emergency medical care immediately.
- Treatment involves time in a decompression chamber to force nitrogen bubbles to dissolve into the blood.
- Treatment is best when it is done early. However, some patients may benefit even at 6 to 9 days after the incident. Medical care is critical even if symptoms resolve because 25% of patients will relapse.
- For assistance in locating the nearest treatment chamber in your area, call the emergency Divers Alert Network (DAN) at any hour, (919) 684-4326 (accepts collect calls). For non-emergency information, call (919) 684-2948; website: www.diversalertnetwork.org.

POSSIBLE COMPLICATIONS
- Arterial gas embolism (gas bubbles block airflow to vital organs such as the brain).
- Rarely, there may be permanent damage to the lungs, bones, brain, or heart, possible paralysis, or death.

PROBABLE OUTCOME—Usually good for patients who receive early treatment. In others, it depends on duration and severity of symptoms prior to treatment.

 HOW TO TREAT

GENERAL MEASURES—Follow medical advice.

MEDICATION—Drugs are usually not needed for this disorder. Don't take pain relievers. These may further decrease normal breathing function.

ACTIVITY—Resume your normal activities as soon as symptoms improve after treatment.

DIET—No special diet.

 CALL YOUR DOCTOR IF

You develop any symptoms of decompression sickness within 24 hours after scuba diving or rapid ascent without pressurization.

...ENERAL INFORMATION

...TION—Dehydration is excessive loss of ...from the body. The majority of the human ...dy is made up of water. A person routinely ...ses water with breathing, sweating, urinating, and bowel movements. The water is normally replaced by the intake of fluids. Dehydration is most dangerous in newborns, infants, and persons over 60. The dehydration may be mild, moderate, or severe depending on the percentage of body weight lost.

BODY PARTS INVOLVED—Blood; gastrointestinal tract; kidneys.

SEX OR AGE MOST AFFECTED—Both sexes; all ages.

SIGNS & SYMPTOMS
- Dry mouth and swollen tongue. Severe thirst.
- Decreased or no urination; urine color may be deep yellow. In infants, there may be no wet diapers.
- Sunken eyes and wrinkled skin.
- Inability to sweat.
- Infants may have no tears when crying.
- Fatigue.
- Headache.
- Low blood pressure.
- Increase in heart rate and breathing.
- Dizziness, confusion, coma.

CAUSES—Dehydration develops when the body is not able to function properly due to excess fluid loss, not enough fluid intake, or a combination of the two.

RISK INCREASES WITH
- Severe vomiting or diarrhea from any cause.
- Heavy sweating.
- Too much urine output.
- Not taking in a sufficient amount of food or water.
- Newborns, infants, and adults over 60.
- Illness with high fever.
- Not eating or drinking due to illness or mouth sores.
- Use of drugs, such as diuretics ("water pills").
- Excess exposure to sun or heat.
- Diabetes or kidney disease.
- Injuries to the skin, such as burns, can cause fluid loss through the damaged skin.

HOW TO PREVENT
- If you are vomiting or have diarrhea, take small sips of a fluid replacement product. This is important during an illness with a fever. Children need to be observed for any symptoms of dehydration.
- If you use diuretics, weigh yourself daily.
- Carry water with you to outdoor activities. Drink plenty of water while exercising. Avoid exercising outdoors in very hot weather.
- Avoid drinking alcohol in hot weather.

WHAT TO EXPECT

DIAGNOSTIC MEASURES
- Your own observation of symptoms.
- Your health care provider will do a physical exam and ask questions about your symptoms.
- Blood tests may be done to check electrolyte levels (these include sodium, potassium, and bicarbonate). Electrolytes are vital for the body to function normally. Other tests may be needed to find the specific cause of the dehydration.

APPROPRIATE HEALTH CARE
- Treatment will be aimed at restoring body fluids and treating any illness that is diagnosed.
- If the dehydration is severe, a hospital stay may be needed for fluid replacement.

POSSIBLE COMPLICATIONS
- Depends on any medical problems. Usually with mild to moderate symptoms, no complications are expected.
- Severe dehydration or electrolyte imbalance may lead to seizures, kidney failure, heart problems, shock, brain damage, or death.

PROBABLE OUTCOME—Curable with control of the underlying cause and replacement of necessary fluids.

HOW TO TREAT

GENERAL MEASURES
- For infants and children, replace lost fluids and electrolytes with products such as Pedialyte or Gastrolyte (follow directions on product label). Infants require more frequent feedings (breast or bottle).
- For adults, drink fluids and take in salt in soups and salted crackers. Eat frequent, small meals.

MEDICATION—Usually not needed.

ACTIVITY—Limit activity as needed until you recover. Get plenty of rest.

DIET—An age-appropriate, unrestricted diet is suggested. Eat complex carbohydrates, fresh fruits, lean meats, yogurt, and vegetables. Avoid carbonated drinks or commercial juices with a high concentration of simple carbohydrates.

CALL YOUR DOCTOR IF

You or a family member has symptoms of dehydration.

DELAYED ONSET MUSCLE SORENESS
(Postexercise Muscle Soreness)

 GENERAL INFORMATION

DEFINITION—Delayed onset muscle soreness (DOMS) occurs hours after an exercise is over. DOMS is not an injury as such, but can be painful. Nearly every healthy adult has had DOMS no matter what the person's fitness level is. The symptoms of DOMS are a normal response, and are part of the process that leads to improved strength once the muscles recover. You can expect a certain amount of DOMS when getting in shape.

BODY PARTS INVOLVED—Muscles.

SEX OR AGE MOST AFFECTED—Both sexes; all ages.

SIGNS & SYMPTOMS
• Symptoms start about 8 to 24 hours after the activity and end within 3 to 7 days. They may be worse the second day than they are the first day.
• Muscle pain, aches, soreness, stiffness, and swelling.
• The muscles may be less flexible.
• Muscle areas feel tender when touched.

CAUSES—Exact cause is not clear and there may be several factors involved including the buildup of lactic acid or the swelling of muscle cells in response to work. DOMS results from doing any new or changed exercise or activity.

RISK INCREASES WITH
• Too much exercise, or a change in activity from non-impact, such as biking, to high-impact (e.g., running).
• New or heavy strength exercises. Even if you exercise on a regular basis, any new type of activity may cause delayed soreness.

HOW TO PREVENT
• There are no sure ways to prevent DOMS. Some ways to help reduce the amount of soreness are listed here.
• Most reports show that stretching prevents DOMS. If you do stretch before or after exercising, do so slowly, and only to the point at which you feel slight discomfort. Hold the stretch for anywhere between 10 and 30 seconds.
• Warm-up before you start an activity. Do a few minutes of slow walking or biking.
• Give your muscles time to adjust to an activity. Make changes slowly (over several weeks if needed) to a new exercise program or new or different sports activity.
• Cool down after a workout.
• If you start a new weightlifting program, begin with weights you can lift easily, and then add weight slowly.
• Drink plenty of fluids to help clear lactic acid from the tissues.

 WHAT TO EXPECT

DIAGNOSTIC MEASURES—Your own observation of symptoms.

APPROPRIATE HEALTH CARE—Self-care is often all that is needed. If pain is severe, see your health care provider.

POSSIBLE COMPLICATIONS—None expected. There is no long-term damage or change in function of the muscles involved.

PROBABLE OUTCOME—The soreness is usually gone within 3 to 7 days. Your muscles will not get sore again if you keep doing the exercise or activity on a regular basis.

 HOW TO TREAT

GENERAL MEASURES
• Use ice massage. Fill a Styrofoam cup with water and freeze it. Tear a small amount of foam from the top so ice sticks out. Rub the ice gently over the painful area in a circle about the size of a softball. Do this for 15 minutes at a time, 3 or 4 times a day, and before workouts.
• After 72 hours, if muscle is still sore, apply heat, such as hot soaks, instead of ice if it feels better.
• Use your hands to massage the muscle gently and often. Massage will provide comfort and reduce swelling, but it won't speed the recovery.

MEDICATION
• For minor pain and inflammation, you may try aspirin (not for children) or ibuprofen, but they do not always work for DOMS.
• Nonprescription topical products may be used to soothe sore muscles.
• Drugs will not help to prevent DOMS.

ACTIVITY
• Keep on with some exercising. Perform low-impact aerobic exercise to increase blood flow to the muscles.
• If muscle soreness or pain increases after you begin exercising, stop and use ice on the muscles.

DIET—No special diet.

 CALL YOUR DOCTOR IF

You or a family member has delayed onset muscle soreness that is severe or has lasted more than a week.

DEMENTIA

GENERAL INFORMATION

DEFINITION—Dementia is a gradual loss of brain function. It leads to problems with memory, thinking, judgment, behavior, and motor skills. It interferes with a person's ability to function and take care of everyday tasks. Dementia can be caused by many different medical conditions. It is not a normal part of aging. Types of dementia include Alzheimer's disease, vascular dementia, Lewy body disease, and others (more rare).

BODY PARTS INVOLVED—Brain.

SEX OR AGE MOST AFFECTED—Usually affects adults over age 65.

SIGNS & SYMPTOMS
- Memory problems. Forgetfulness, such as about recent events or ordinary information such as birth date and address; not able to recognize family and friends.
- Confusion and poor judgment.
- Loss of interest in normal activities.
- Trouble speaking well.
- Disorientation, especially at night.
- Poor personal hygiene and appearance.
- Sleep problems.
- Personality changes.
- Anxiety, depression, being suspicious, agitation, wandering, verbal abuse, or being assaultive.
- Incontinence, hallucinations, delusions (later stage).

CAUSES—Nerve cells in the brain become damaged and die. Once the cells die, they cannot be replaced. The brain shrinks and brain function deteriorates. Most dementias are progressive (get worse with time) and cannot be cured. There are a few causes of dementia that may be potentially reversible.

RISK INCREASES WITH
- Inadequate blood supply to the brain. It may be due to blood clots, strokes, tumor, high blood pressure, or atherosclerosis (hardening of the arteries).
- Severe, or repeated, head injury (such as in boxing).
- Infections, such as AIDS or syphilis.
- Down syndrome, Parkinson's disease, Huntington's chorea, and some hereditary disorders.
- Metabolic disorders, such as thyroid disease.
- Certain nutritional deficiencies.
- Toxic causes (alcoholism, drugs, heavy metals).

HOW TO PREVENT—Most dementias are not preventable. Reducing risk factors may help. Maintain a healthy lifestyle, protect yourself from head injuries, and control chronic illnesses.

WHAT TO EXPECT

DIAGNOSTIC MEASURES
- Family members may notice early behavior changes and seek medical care. The health care provider will do a physical exam and ask questions about the symptoms.
- There is no specific test to diagnose dementia. Medical tests may include cognitive tests (answering questions), blood, urine, and spinal fluid studies, heart studies, CT, MRI, PET scans, or others. Testing helps rule out other disorders that may cause similar symptoms.

APPROPRIATE HEALTH CARE
- Treatment will depend on the severity of the symptoms and the underlying cause.
- Drugs to treat the behavior symptoms can help make a patient more comfortable and make their care easier.

POSSIBLE COMPLICATIONS—Each type of dementia has its own complications. Most have a downward course that leads to death.

PROBABLE OUTCOME—Most patients will worsen gradually over months to years.

HOW TO TREAT

GENERAL MEASURES
- A diagnosis of dementia is overwhelming, both for the patient and the family. Educate yourselves as much as possible about what to expect and how to plan for it. In early diagnosis, the patient can take part in making decisions.
- Caring for a family member with dementia is a difficult task. Caregivers need to take care of themselves. Joining a support group for caregivers may be helpful.
- To learn more: Alzheimer's Association, 225 N. Michigan Ave., Fl 17, Chicago. Il 60601; (800) 272-3900; website: www.alz.org.

MEDICATION
- Drugs may be prescribed to:
  - Help control behavior symptoms (anxiety insomnia, agitation, wandering, or depression).
  - Slow the progress of dementia.
  - Treat the underlying cause of dementia.

ACTIVITY—The patient's daily activities may require supervision at all times.

DIET—Feeding help will eventually be needed.

CALL YOUR DOCTOR IF

- You observe symptoms of dementia in a family member.
- Unexpected symptoms occur after diagnosis.

DEPRESSION

GENERAL INFORMATION

DEFINITION—Depression is a common mood disorder. The symptoms that occur (emotional and physical) interfere with everyday life for an extended period of time. Symptoms may be mild, moderate, or severe.

BODY PARTS INVOLVED—Nervous system.

SEX OR AGE MOST AFFECTED—Both sexes, but is more common in women; all ages.

SIGNS & SYMPTOMS
- Loss of interest in life, feeling bored and listless.
- Fatigue and lack of energy.
- Insomnia, excess sleep, or sleeping problems.
- Lack of pleasure, or withdrawal, from usual activities.
- Change in appetite that leads to weight gain or loss.
- Loss of sex drive.
- Difficulty making decisions; concentration difficulty.
- Unexplained crying bouts.
- Inappropriate guilt feelings, self-hate, lack of self-esteem, and feeling unworthy.
- Irritability, anger, and agitation.
- Headache or other aches and pains.
- Thoughts of suicide or death.

CAUSES—It is not fully known what causes depression. It appears to be a combination of factors. Chemical imbalances in the brain may cause or contribute to depression. Other factors may include biologic, genetic, psychological, environmental, and developmental events.

RISK INCREASES WITH
- Women are more at risk than men.
- Personal history or family history of depression.
- Advanced age.
- Compulsive, rigid, perfectionistic, or highly dependent personality.
- Other emotional or personality disorder.
- Substance abuse, such as alcoholism or drugs.
- Failure in job, marriage, or a personal relationship.
- Death or loss of a loved one.
- Recent, stressful life experience.
- Living alone, social isolation.
- Surgery, major illness, or disability.
- Passing from one life stage to another (e.g., retiring).
- Use of some drugs, not taking prescribed drugs, or side effect of drugs.
- Some chronic diseases.

HOW TO PREVENT—Depression is often not preventable. Reduce your risks where possible. If you have recurring depression, drugs may be prescribed for prevention.

WHAT TO EXPECT

DIAGNOSTIC MEASURES
- Your health care provider will do a physical exam and ask questions about your symptoms and activities.
- Screening tests for depression are helpful in diagnosis. Medical tests may be done to rule out other disorders.

APPROPRIATE HEALTH CARE
- Therapy consists of treating acute symptoms, avoiding a relapse, and preventing recurrence.
- Psychotherapy or counseling along with drug treatment appears to obtain the best results.
- Types of psychotherapy include cognitive therapy, behavioral therapy, and interpersonal therapy. Therapy may involve 12 to 20 sessions over 12 to 16 weeks.
- Hospital care or inpatient at a special treatment center may be required for severe depression.
- Electroconvulsive therapy or less common therapies may be used in some patients.

POSSIBLE COMPLICATIONS
- Alcohol or substance abuse.
- Problems with physical health.
- Loss of job, failure in school, and family or marital problems.
- Failure to improve with treatment.
- Suicide.

PROBABLE OUTCOME—Treatment helps most patients. Depression may sometimes recur or it may be a one-time episode.

HOW TO TREAT

GENERAL MEASURES
- Follow your treatment plan.
- Avoid alcohol and drugs of abuse.
- Seek support groups. Contact social agencies for help. Contact the National Mental Health Association; (800) 969-6642; website: www.nmha.org.

MEDICATION
- Antidepressant drugs will usually be prescribed. Multiple drugs are necessary in some cases. It will take 2 to 4 weeks or longer for improvement.
- Drugs for other symptoms may be prescribed.

ACTIVITY—Regular exercise helps depression.

DIET—Eat a normal, well-balanced diet.

CALL YOUR DOCTOR IF

You or a family member has symptoms of depression or symptoms don't improve with treatment or time.

DERMATITIS, ATOPIC
(Eczema)

GENERAL INFORMATION

DEFINITION—Atopic dermatitis is a common, chronic skin disorder. Dermatitis means skin inflammation (redness and soreness). Atopic refers to an allergic condition.

BODY PARTS INVOLVED—Skin.

SEX OR AGE MOST AFFECTED—It often affects infants and children, but can occur in all age groups. It affects males and females equally.

SIGNS & SYMPTOMS
* Itchy, dry skin. Scaling, redness, swelling, weeping, cracking, and crusting of the skin may occur. It often affects the skin creases of elbows, knees, neck, face, hands, feet, groin, genitals, and around the anus. It may also affect the skin around the eyes.
* Itching may be worse during the night.
* An itch-scratch cycle develops. The itch causes a person to scratch, which in turn worsens the itch.
* An infant may be irritable and restless.

CAUSES—Unknown. It may be a combination of environmental factors and genetic (hereditary) factors. It cannot be passed from one person to another.

RISK INCREASES WITH
* History of hay fever or asthma or food allergy.
* Family history of atopic dermatitis or other allergic disorders.
* Weak immune system due to illness or drugs.
* People living in dry climates.

HOW TO PREVENT
* No preventive measures for the original outbreak.
* Identify and then avoid the factors that may trigger an outbreak in an individual. These can include:
  - Emotional factors (stress and anger).
  - Irritants (wool, perfumes, fabric softeners, smoke, some soaps, etc.).
  - Allergens (substances that inflame the skin) such as pollen, or cat and dog dander.
  - Temperature or climate.
  - Skin infections.

WHAT TO EXPECT

DIAGNOSTIC MEASURES
* Your own observation of symptoms.
* Your health care provider will perform a skin exam and ask questions about your symptoms and medical history.
* There is no test to diagnose atopic dermatitis. Skin tests may be done to rule out other skin problems.

APPROPRIATE HEALTH CARE—Treatment for symptoms and preventing flare-ups can include drugs (topical and oral), phototherapy (use of ultraviolet light), skin care, and lifestyle changes.

POSSIBLE COMPLICATIONS
* Skin infections.
* Skin may become thick and leathery or scarred from scratching.
* Anxiety or depression due to a chronic disorder.
* Eye problems (blepharitis, cataracts, conjunctivitis).
* Herpes simplex infections are more severe in people with atopic dermatitis.
* Skin changes due to prolonged steroid use.

PROBABLE OUTCOME—The disorder can come and go throughout life. Symptoms may decrease with age. Treatment and self-care will help relieve symptoms in most people.

HOW TO TREAT

GENERAL MEASURES
* Moisturize the skin often and always after bathing. Ointments (e.g., petroleum jelly), oils, or creams are best.
* Bathe in cool to warm water (not hot) with products other than soap. Use cool-water soaks for crusting, oozing skin. These decrease itching and remove crusts.
* Wear loose fitting, cotton clothing. Avoid fabric softeners and anti-static laundry products.
* Use a humidifier to add moisture to room.
* Try to avoid emotional problems in your life, if possible (itching often increases with stress).
* To learn more: National Eczema Association, 4460 Redwood Hwy, Suite 16-D, San Rapheal, CA 94903; (800) 818-7546; website: www.nationaleczema.org.

MEDICATION
* To relieve minor itching, use a nonprescription topical steroid product or other anti-itch product.
* You may be prescribed stronger topical drugs, oral steroids (for short periods only), anti-histamines, antibiotics for infection, drugs to suppress the immune system, or other drugs.

ACTIVITY—Try to avoid sweating. Avoid prolonged exposure to hot climate.

DIET—If food allergy is suspected, ask your health care provider if a diet change will help.

CALL YOUR DOCTOR IF

* You or a family member has symptoms of atopic dermatitis.
* New or worsening symptoms occur.

DERMATITIS, CONTACT

GENERAL INFORMATION

DEFINITION—Contact dermatitis is a common skin inflammation caused by contact with an irritating or allergy-causing substance. Contact dermatitis cannot be spread from one person to another. The two types are referred to as irritant contact dermatitis and allergic contact dermatitis.

BODY PARTS INVOLVED—Skin, especially of the hands, feet and groin.

SEX OR AGE MOST AFFECTED—All ages and both sexes, but more common in women.

SIGNS & SYMPTOMS
- Itching, rash, redness, or swelling of the skin.
- Bright red weeping areas or blisters that break open, ooze, crust, or scale in some cases.
- Skin may have a feeling of warmth, a burning sensation, pain, or tenderness.
- Allergic reaction symptoms may appear hours or days after exposure.
- Some reactions worsen with sun exposure.

CAUSES
- The irritant type is more common and is due to injury or damage to the skin by multiple or prolonged exposures, or sometimes, a single exposure, to a skin irritant (e.g., strong soap).
- The allergic type is less common and is due to an acquired sensitivity of the skin to an allergen. When exposed to the allergen, the body's immune system reacts and causes symptoms.
- There are many substances that can trigger either type of contact dermatitis. It may take time and effort to find the exact cause for each person and sometimes the cause is not found. Also, the cause could be a mix of irritants and allergens, especially dermatitis on the hands.

RISK INCREASES WITH
- Irritants such as soaps, bleaches, detergents, solvents, pesticides, and frequent handwashing. Almost any substance can be an irritant.
- Allergic reactions may come from nickel (often found in jewelry); glues; house-hold cleansers; leather; paints; latex or rubber; chemicals (in hair dyes, cosmetics, deodorants, and perfumes); plants such as poison ivy, oak, or sumac; topical drugs such as antibiotics; and other substances.
- Personal history of allergies or eczema.
- Job or an activity that exposes the skin to irritants or allergens.
- Infants and the elderly.

HOW TO PREVENT
- Avoid contact with known irritants or allergens, especially if they have triggered a past reaction.
- If unable to avoid contact with an irritant or allergen substance (due to work or an activity):
  - Wear proper protective clothing, gloves, or other equipment as needed. Use topical skin barriers. Wash skin surfaces right after contact.
  - Follow preventive measures at workplace.

WHAT TO EXPECT

DIAGNOSTIC MEASURES
- Your own observation of symptoms.
- See your health care provider if self-help steps are not working. A skin exam is usually all that is needed for diagnosis. Questions will be asked about any contact with possible irritating and allergic substances to help find the cause.
- Skin allergy testing may be done.

APPROPRIATE HEALTH CARE—Self-care usually. Medical care for severe symptoms.

POSSIBLE COMPLICATIONS
- Chronic or recurrent contact dermatitis.
- Bacterial infection or other skin problems.
- A change of job may be necessary if work exposure is the cause.

PROBABLE OUTCOME—The skin will usually heal on its own in 2 to 4 weeks. Self-care steps or medical treatment may help ease symptoms. Once the irritant or allergen is known, take care to avoid it in the future to prevent recurrence.

HOW TO TREAT

GENERAL MEASURES
- Try to avoid scratching. Wrap or cover the affected area if needed.
- Apply cool moist compresses for 30 minutes 3 or more times a day to help relieve itching.
- Soak in a cool bath. Add a cup of baking soda or use oatmeal product (e.g. Aveeno) in water.
- Use of emollients, lubricants, or moisturizers may help symptoms and prevent skin dryness.

MEDICATION
- Use a nonprescription product such as calamine lotion to help relieve itching.
- Use a nonprescription corticosteroid cream, gel, spray, or ointment (e.g., 1% hydrocortisone) for the inflammation and itching.
- Nonprescription oral antihistamines may help relieve itching. Don't use topical antihistamines.
- Your health care provider may prescribe:
  - Stronger corticosteroid topical drugs or other types of topical drugs.
  - Oral or injected steroids for severe cases.
  - Antibiotics (topical or oral) for bacterial infection.

ACTIVITY—No limits. Take preventive measures as needed to avoid any triggers or risk factors.

DIET—No special diet.

CALL YOUR DOCTOR IF

- You or a family member has contact dermatitis and self-care is not working.
- Symptoms worsen or skin infection develops.

DERMATITIS HERPETIFORMIS

 GENERAL INFORMATION

DEFINITION—Dermatitis herpetiformis is a rare, chronic skin condition.

BODY PARTS INVOLVED—Skin of the elbows, knees, shoulders, arms, legs and over the bottom of the spine (sacrum).

SEX OR AGE MOST AFFECTED—It can occur at any age (more often ages 20 to 40) and affects men slightly more than women.

SIGNS & SYMPTOMS
• Small clusters of 5 to 20 blisters. Clusters appear at the same time on both sides of the body in the same places.
• Severe itching and burning of the affected areas.
• Dryness of the mouth in some patients.

CAUSES—It is an autoimmune disorder associated with gluten sensitivity. Gluten is a protein (found in wheat and other foods) that cannot be digested by some persons because of the sensitivity. Most gluten-sensitivity persons have gastrointestinal symptoms (called celiac disease or gluten-sensitive enteropathy). Many patients with dermatitis herpetiformis do not have the gastrointestinal symptoms of celiac disease.

RISK INCREASES WITH—Family history of dermatitis herpetiformis.

HOW TO PREVENT—Cannot be prevented at present.

 WHAT TO EXPECT

DIAGNOSTIC MEASURES
• Your own observation of symptoms.
• Your health care provider will do a physical exam of the affected skin area.
• A biopsy of the skin (removal of a small amount of skin tissue for viewing under a microscope) will verify the diagnosis.

APPROPRIATE HEALTH CARE—Treatment includes drugs and a gluten-free diet or both. It can take 6 or more months for symptoms to improve using a gluten-free diet. Drugs can improve the symptoms more quickly.

POSSIBLE COMPLICATIONS
• Gastrointestinal symptoms of gluten sensitivity.
• People with dermatitis herpetiformis are more at risk for other autoimmune disorders (e.g., thyroid disease and diabetes) or lymphoma (cancer of the lymph tissue).

PROBABLE OUTCOME—This is a chronic disease. Treatment can help control symptoms (including itching) but it will not cure the disease.

 HOW TO TREAT

GENERAL MEASURES—Soak in a bathtub of cool water or use cool-water compresses to reduce itching.

MEDICATION
• Dapsone or sulfapyridine (drugs to be taken by mouth) are often prescribed to relieve the symptoms.
• Your health care provider may suggest topical skin products that help relieve symptoms.

ACTIVITY—No limits unless advised otherwise.

DIET
• Avoid gluten in your diet. A dietitian can help with meal planning.
• Other diet changes may be recommended by your health care provider.

 CALL YOUR DOCTOR IF

• You or a family member has symptoms of dermatitis herpetiformis.
• New, unexplained symptoms develop.

DERMATITIS, SEBORRHEIC

GENERAL INFORMATION

DEFINITION—Seborrheic dermatitis is a common, chronic, inflammatory skin condition. Dandruff and cradle cap are both forms of seborrheic dermatitis.

BODY PARTS INVOLVED—Skin of the scalp, eyebrows, forehead, face, folds around the nose, behind ears, external ear canal or skin of the trunk, especially over the breastbone (sternum) or in skin folds.

SEX OR AGE MOST AFFECTED—It occurs more often in babies under age 3 months and adults ages 30 to 60.

SIGNS & SYMPTOMS
- Flaking, white scales over reddish patches on the skin. Scales stick to hair shafts. They may itch, but they are usually painless unless complicated by infection.
- Infants can have it on the scalp (cradle cap), or in the diaper or armpit areas.

CAUSES—The cause is unclear. It may involve genetic factors, an over production of a fungus (*Malassezia*) normally present on the skin, and an excess of natural skin oil (sebum). It cannot be spread from person to person.

RISK INCREASES WITH
- Oily skin or hair.
- Family history of seborrheic dermatitis.
- Neurological disorders (e.g., Parkinson's disease or stroke).
- Immune disorders (e.g., HIV infection).

HOW TO PREVENT—First episode cannot be prevented. After diagnosis, treatment can help prevent a recurrence.

WHAT TO EXPECT

DIAGNOSTIC MEASURES
- Your own observation of symptoms.
- See your health care provider if self-help steps are not working. A skin exam is usually all that is needed for diagnosis.

APPROPRIATE HEALTH CARE—Self-care is usually all that is needed. Medical care may include drug therapy.

POSSIBLE COMPLICATIONS
- Embarrassment and social discomfort.
- Skin infection in affected areas.

PROBABLE OUTCOME—This is a chronic condition that can be successfully treated with self-care or medical care (if needed). Symptoms often come and go. It does not cause hair loss.

HOW TO TREAT

GENERAL MEASURES
- Shampoo once a day. Loosen scales with your fingernails while shampooing.
- For infants, use mild baby shampoo to wash the hair and rinse completely. Brush the hair gently with a soft brush after shampooing and other times during the day.
- Avoid scratching affected area.
- Don't use harsh soaps on the skin.
- A recurrence may be triggered by stress, stressful events, fatigue, poor skin care, infrequent shampoos, hot or cold weather, or use of skin lotions that contain alcohol.

MEDICATION
- For dandruff, use nonprescription antidandruff shampoos. They may contain different types of ingredients, and all are effective. Follow instruction on the label.
- For seborrheic skin infections in teens and adults, a nonprescription cream or lotion may be used. These may contain a corticosteroid (e.g., hydrocortisone) or antifungal (e.g., ketoconazole).
- For more severe problems, shampoos that contain coal tar, scalp creams that contain cortisone, or an oral drug may be prescribed. Follow instructions that are provided with each product on how to apply to hair or skin.

ACTIVITY—No limits.

DIET—No special diet.

CALL YOUR DOCTOR IF

- You or a family member has symptoms of seborrheic dermatitis that don't respond to self-care.
- Patches of seborrheic dermatitis ooze, form crusts, or drain pus.

DIABETES FEET & SKIN PROBLEMS

 GENERAL INFORMATION

DEFINITION—Infections of the skin, often of the feet, are more common in people with diabetes than in nondiabetics. The skin and feet of a diabetic person are more prone to injury. Diabetes also impairs the healing process.

BODY PARTS INVOLVED—Feet and skin.

SEX OR AGE MOST AFFECTED—Both sexes; all ages.

SIGNS & SYMPTOMS
- Often there is no pain associated with infection or injury to the foot or skin.
- New sores on feet or ulcers (open sores) that take a long time to heal.
- Numbness, burning, or tingling in the feet.
- Blood or pus stains on shoes or socks.

CAUSES
- High blood sugar from diabetes causes damage to nerves in the legs and feet. With damaged nerves, a person may not feel pain, heat, or cold in the legs and feet. This lack of feeling is called peripheral neuropathy. Nerve damage can lead to a sore or an infection that can become severe before being noticed.
- Another problem happens when not enough blood flows to the legs and feet. Poor blood flow makes it hard for a sore or infection to heal. This problem is called peripheral vascular disease (PVD). Smoking when you have diabetes makes blood flow problems much worse.
- If blood sugar is high, the body loses fluid. With less fluid in the body, the skin becomes dry. Dry skin can be itchy, causing scratching and soreness. Dry skin can crack and allow germs to enter and cause infection. Dry skin can occur on legs, feet, elbows, and other places.

RISK INCREASES WITH
- Peripheral neuropathy.
- History of foot problems or foot deformity.
- Peripheral vascular disease.
- Poor glucose control.
- Diabetes complications (e.g., heart disease).
- Smoking.

HOW TO PREVENT
- Wash your feet in warm (not hot) water every day. Do not soak your feet. Carefully dry the feet and between the toes.
- Look at your feet every day to check for cuts, sores, blisters, redness, calluses, or other problems. Checking every day is even more important if you have nerve damage or poor blood flow. If you cannot bend over or pull your feet up to check them, use a mirror. If you cannot see well, ask someone else to check your feet.
- Rub lotion on your feet after you wash and dry them. Do not put lotion between your toes.
- File corns and calluses gently with an emery board or pumice stone (after a bath or shower).

- Cut your toenails once a week or as needed. Cut toenails when they are soft from washing. Cut them to the shape of the toe and not too short. File the edges with an emery board.
- Always wear slippers or shoes to protect feet from injuries. Always wear socks or stockings to avoid blisters. Do not wear socks or knee-high stockings that are too tight below your knee.
- Wear shoes that fit well. Shop for shoes at the end of the day when feet are bigger. Break in shoes slowly.
- Have a medical foot exam every year.
- For skin care, wash with a mild soap, make sure to rinse and dry completely. Check your skin after you shower or bathe. Make sure there are no dry, red, or sore spots that can lead to an infection. Use a lotion or cream after you wash. Wear all-cotton underwear. Cotton allows air to move around your body better.

 WHAT TO EXPECT

DIAGNOSTIC MEASURES
- Your own observation of symptoms.
- See your health care provider if new skin problems don't clear up in a day or two.

APPROPRIATE HEALTH CARE
- Self-care for preventive measures.
- Medical care may be needed if complications occur. This may include drug therapy, special wound care and dressings, surgery, use of aids for walking (such as crutches), and others.

POSSIBLE COMPLICATIONS—Without treatment, serious foot problems may develop (infections, ulcers, gangrene, and amputation).

PROBABLE OUTCOME—Using preventive measures and seeking early treatment of infections will help to avoid serious problems.

 HOW TO TREAT

GENERAL MEASURES—To learn more: American Diabetes Association, 1701 North Beauregard St., Alexandria, VA 22311; (800) 342-2383; website: www.diabetes.org.

MEDICATION—Drugs for infections may be prescribed.

ACTIVITY—Regular activities (unless foot problems interfere).

DIET—Follow prescribed diabetes diet.

 CALL YOUR DOCTOR IF

You or a family member has diabetes and has any concerns about a new foot or skin problem.

DIABETES HYPOGLYCEMIA

 GENERAL INFORMATION

DEFINITION—Hypoglycemia means low blood sugar. When blood sugar drops too far below normal, a group of symptoms usually develop. Symptoms can vary in different people. Get to know your symptoms. Daytime symptoms may differ from those occurring at night. Symptoms may change as years go by. Some people may have no symptoms of hypoglycemia (called hypoglycemia unawareness).

BODY PARTS INVOLVED—Endocrine and metabolic body systems.

SEX OR AGE MOST AFFECTED—Both sexes; all ages.

SIGNS & SYMPTOMS
- Mild:
  - Hunger; weakness.
  - Nervousness; sweating.
  - Emotional ups and downs.
  - Difficulty in concentrating.
  - Headache.
- Moderate:
  - Increased weakness; excessive sweating.
  - Skin that is cold and clammy to touch.
  - Numbness of the mouth or maybe, fingers.
  - Pounding of heart.
  - Loss of memory; confusion.
  - Double vision.
  - Staring expression.
  - Difficulty walking.
  - Unaware of surroundings.
- Severe:
  - Twitching of muscles.
  - Unconsciousness.
  - Convulsions.
  - Unaware of passing urine.

CAUSES—Hypoglycemia occurs when there is too much insulin in the body and not enough intake of food. It is more frequent in insulin-dependent type diabetes, but can occur in those who take oral drugs for diabetes.

RISK INCREASES WITH
- Eating meals at times other than regular hours.
- Skipping meals or eating only parts of meals.
- Dosing with too much insulin or other diabetic drugs.
- More exercise or activity than usual.
- Alcohol use.
- Other, rarer risk factors.

HOW TO PREVENT
- Follow your treatment plan of diet, drugs, and exercise, and do routine blood sugar tests.
- Take prompt action if early symptoms of hypoglycemia occur. Family, friends, and coworkers should know the symptoms and what to do in an emergency.
- Always carry some type of sugar with you.

 WHAT TO EXPECT

DIAGNOSTIC MEASURES
- Your own or other's observation of symptoms.
- Medical diagnosis if needed.

APPROPRIATE HEALTH CARE
- Self-care is usually all that is needed.
- Medical care for complications or if there is any doubt about the cause.

POSSIBLE COMPLICATIONS—Diabetic shock, seizures, unconsciousness (can be life threatening).

PROBABLE OUTCOME—Full recovery is the usual outcome. It depends on quick diagnosis and treatment.

 HOW TO TREAT

GENERAL MEASURES
- If hypoglycemia symptoms begin, eat or drink something that has sugar in it. This includes hard candy, fruit juice, or glucose tablets that you can buy at a drug store. If there are 30 minutes or more to the next meal, some protein and starch foods should also be eaten. They can help prevent another reaction.
- If the patient passes out, glucagon needs to be injected. Diabetic patients and their families should have glucagon at hand and know how to inject it.
- Check blood sugar about 15 to 20 minutes after treatment for hypoglycemia. Repeat treatment if needed.
- If no glucagon is at hand, get the patient to the nearest emergency center or telephone for emergency help.
- To learn more: American Diabetes Association, 1701 North Beauregard St., Alexandria, VA 22311; (800) 342-2383; website: www.diabetes.org.

MEDICATION—Try to find the cause of the hypoglycemia. Insulin dose or oral antidiabetic drug dose may need to be adjusted.

ACTIVITY—Rest until symptoms resolve.

DIET—Maintain your regular diet, unless eating habits are the cause of the hypoglycemia. Changes may need to be made in your diet.

 CALL YOUR DOCTOR IF

- You or a family member has diabetes hypoglycemia symptoms that cause concern. Call 911 for emergency help if needed.
- Hypoglycemia episodes recur frequently.
- Adjustments need to be made in insulin dosages.

DIABETES INSIPIDUS

 ## GENERAL INFORMATION

DEFINITION—Diabetes insipidus is a rare disorder of the hormone system, centered in the pituitary gland. It disrupts normal fluid regulation in the body. This condition has nothing to do with blood sugar levels or other types of diabetes.

BODY PARTS INVOLVED—Pituitary gland; endocrine system.

SEX OR AGE MOST AFFECTED—It can affect all ages and occurs equally in men and women.

SIGNS & SYMPTOMS
- Excessive thirst that is difficult to satisfy.
- Passing large amounts of diluted, colorless urine (up to 15 quarts a day).
- Involuntary urination.
- Dry hands.
- Constipation.

CAUSES—In one type (neurogenic or central), the pituitary gland in the brain does not make enough of an antidiuretic hormone (called ADH) needed for the body to function. In another type (nephrogenic), there is enough ADH hormone produced, but the kidneys don't work with the hormone as they should. Two other types involve an abnormal thirst (dipsogenic) and pregnancy (gestagenic). The cause for diabetes insipidus may be known or unknown.

RISK INCREASES WITH
- Tumor of the pituitary gland or other brain tumor.
- Head injury, with damage to the pituitary gland.
- Brain surgery.
- Brain infection, such as encephalitis or meningitis.
- Blockage of the arteries to the brain.
- Aneurysm or other blood vessel problems.
- Granulomas (chronic inflammation).
- Drugs, such as lithium.
- Kidney disorders.
- Family history of diabetes insipidus.

HOW TO PREVENT—No specific preventive measures.

 ## WHAT TO EXPECT

DIAGNOSTIC MEASURES
- Your own observation of symptoms.
- Your health care provider will do a physical exam and ask questions about your symptoms.
- Medical studies may include water-deprivation tests to determine levels of ADH. Blood and urine studies are usually done. If diabetes insipidus is diagnosed, a CT or MRI of the brain may be done to check for any problems.

APPROPRIATE HEALTH CARE—Treatment involves controlling fluid balance and preventing dehydration and identifying the cause of the diabetes insipidus.

POSSIBLE COMPLICATIONS
- Electrolyte imbalance, especially low levels of sodium or potassium. Either of these can cause heartbeat irregularity, fatigue, and congestive heart failure.
- Young children may have growth failure.

PROBABLE OUTCOME—The prognosis is generally good depending on the underlying disorder.

 ## HOW TO TREAT

GENERAL MEASURES
- Check weight daily and maintain a record.
- Wear or carry medical ID that show your medical problem and the drugs you take.
- To learn more: Diabetes Insipidus Foundation, 5203 New Prospect Dr., Ellicott City, MD 21043; (706) 323-7576 (not toll free); website: www.diabetesinsipidus.org.

MEDICATION
- Desmopressin (DDAVP) may be prescribed. It is a synthetic ADH and may be used in nose spray, by mouth, or in an injection form.
- Drugs may be prescribed to help the body balance salt (sodium) and water.

ACTIVITY—No limits.

DIET
- Monitor fluid intake as advised by your health care provider.
- A low sodium diet may be prescribed.

 ## CALL YOUR DOCTOR IF

- You or a family member has symptoms of diabetes insipidus.
- Symptoms don't improve with treatment.
- New, unexplained symptoms develop.

DIABETES TYPE 1

GENERAL INFORMATION

DEFINITION—Diabetes is a chronic condition in which problems with insulin lead to high blood glucose levels. Glucose, a sugar, is needed by the body to produce energy, but high blood glucose (hyperglycemia) can cause serious problems. Glucose levels are normally controlled by insulin, a hormone produced by the pancreas. In type 1 diabetes (insulin dependent or juvenile), the pancreas loses its ability to produce insulin. In type 2 diabetes (non-insulin dependent or adult onset), either too little insulin is produced or it cannot be used effectively, or both. Type 2 is the most common (about 90% to 95% of diabetes cases).

BODY PARTS INVOLVED
- Islet cells of the pancreas that produce insulin.
- All body cells that need insulin to convert food into chemicals the body can use.

SEX OR AGE MOST AFFECTED—It can develop at any age, but often occurs in children, teenagers, or young adults of both sexes.

SIGNS & SYMPTOMS
- Fatigue, excess thirst, and frequent urination.
- Increased appetite and weight loss.
- General ill feeling.
- Blurred vision.
- Increased risk of infections, such as urinary-tract infections and yeast infections of the skin, mouth, or vagina.

CAUSES—The exact cause is unclear. Type 1 diabetes is considered to be an autoimmune disorder in which the body's immune system mistakenly attacks healthy tissue and cells such as the insulin-producing cells of the pancreas. As a result, these cells are damaged and cannot produce the insulin needed to control glucose in the blood. Genetic factors and environmental factors (e.g., viral infections) appear to play a role also.

RISK INCREASES WITH—Family history of type 1 diabetes.

HOW TO PREVENT—Cannot be prevented at present.

WHAT TO EXPECT

DIAGNOSTIC MEASURES
- Your own observation of symptoms.
- Your health care provider will do a physical exam and ask questions about your symptoms.
- Medical tests can include fasting and random blood glucose tests, oral glucose tolerance test, hemoglobin A1C (HbA1c) test, blood tests for autoantibodies, urine studies, and others.

APPROPRIATE HEALTH CARE—Type 1 diabetes is treated with insulin, exercise, diet, and steps to prevent complications. Your medical team will help develop a treatment plan.

POSSIBLE COMPLICATIONS
- Cardiovascular (heart and blood vessel) disease, such as stroke, atherosclerosis, and coronary-artery disease.
- Damage to the kidneys, eyes, and nerves.
- Foot and skin problems.
- Sexual impotence in men.
- Hypoglycemia (low blood glucose).
- Hyperglycemia (high blood glucose).
- Ketoacidosis (a severe complication).

PROBABLE OUTCOME—There is no cure, but patients who follow a treatment plan can manage their diabetes and reduce risk of complications.

HOW TO TREAT

GENERAL MEASURES
- Educate yourself about diabetes. Learn the techniques of self-monitoring of blood glucose and monitor regularly. Learn the symptoms of high and low glucose levels and what to do.
- Get routine foot care and eye check-ups.
- Exercise daily; don't smoke; eat healthy; get to ideal weight; control blood pressure, cholesterol, and stress.
- Wear or carry medical ID to indicate you have diabetes and that you take insulin.
- Get medical care for any infection.
- To learn more: American Diabetes Association, 1701 North Beauregard St., Alexandria, VA 22311; (800) 342-2383; website: www.diabetes.org.

MEDICATION
- One or more types of insulin will be prescribed depending on each patient's needs. Insulin types are based on how fast they work, when they peak, and duration of action. Insulin can be delivered by injection with a needle or pen or by use of a pump. Other insulin delivery methods are being studied.
- Oral antidiabetic drugs may be prescribed in addition to insulin.
- Drugs to treat high cholesterol, high blood pressure, or other disorders may be prescribed.

ACTIVITY—Exercise helps control diabetes. Follow medical advice about daily exercising.

DIET—A healthy diet is part of treatment. Don't skip meals. A dietitian can help with meal plans.

CALL YOUR DOCTOR IF

- You or a family member has symptoms of diabetes.
- Problems with symptoms or treatment occur.

DIABETES TYPE 2

 GENERAL INFORMATION

DEFINITION—Diabetes is a chronic condition in which problems with insulin lead to high blood glucose levels. Glucose, a sugar, is needed by the body to produce energy, but high blood glucose (hyperglycemia) can cause serious problems. Glucose levels are normally controlled by insulin, a hormone produced by the pancreas. In type 2 diabetes (non-insulin dependent or adult onset), either too little insulin is produced or it cannot be used effectively, or both. Type 2 is the most common (about 90% to 95% of diabetes cases). In type 1 diabetes (insulin dependent or juvenile), the pancreas loses its ability to produce insulin.

BODY PARTS INVOLVED
- Islet cells of the pancreas that produce insulin.
- All body cells that need insulin to convert food into chemicals the body can use.

SEX OR AGE MOST AFFECTED—Both sexes; usually adults, but can occur in children.

SIGNS & SYMPTOMS
- There may be no symptoms. It is often diagnosed with routine blood screening tests.
- Fatigue and excess thirst.
- General ill feeling, increased appetite, weight loss, and frequent urination.
- Slow healing of cuts and bruises.
- Blurred vision.
- Impotence (erectile dysfunction).
- Increased risk of infections.

CAUSES—The exact cause is unclear. In type 2 diabetes, the pancreas either produces enough insulin, but the body is unable to use it effectively (insulin resistance) or it produces too little insulin (insulin deficiency). Genetic factors and environmental factors play a role.

RISK INCREASES WITH
- Family history of diabetes.
- Gestational diabetes (diabetes in pregnancy).
- Overweight (more so if fat is in the abdomen).
- High blood pressure; high cholesterol or high triglycerides.
- Prediabetes (above normal blood glucose).
- Sedentary lifestyle (lack of physical activity).
- Metabolic syndrome (a group of risk factors).
- African Americans, Native Americans, Hispanic Americans, Pacific Islanders, and Asian Americans.

HOW TO PREVENT
- To help prevent or delay onset of type 2 diabetes:
  - Control weight and lose weight if overweight.
  - Exercise regularly.
  - Eat a healthy diet.
  - Get treatment to control high blood pressure and high cholesterol levels.

 WHAT TO EXPECT

DIAGNOSTIC MEASURES
- Your health care provider will do a physical exam and ask questions about your symptoms.
- Medical tests can include fasting and random blood glucose tests, oral glucose tolerance test, hemoglobin A1C (HbA1c) test, blood tests for autoantibodies, urine studies, and others.

APPROPRIATE HEALTH CARE—Type 2 diabetes may be treated with lifestyle changes (e.g., exercise and diet) and drug therapy. Your medical team will help develop a treatment plan.

POSSIBLE COMPLICATIONS
- Cardiovascular (heart or blood vessel) disease.
- Damage to the kidneys, eyes, or nerves.
- Foot or skin problems.
- Hypoglycemia (low blood glucose).
- Hyperglycemia (high blood glucose).
- Ketoacidosis (a severe complication).

PROBABLE OUTCOME—There is no cure, but patients who follow a treatment plan can manage their diabetes and reduce risk of complications.

 HOW TO TREAT

GENERAL MEASURES
- Educate yourself about diabetes. Learn the techniques of self-monitoring of blood glucose and monitor regularly. Learn the symptoms of high and low glucose levels and what to do.
- Get routine foot care and eye check-ups.
- Exercise daily; don't smoke; eat healthy; get to ideal weight; control stress, blood pressure, and cholesterol. Get medical care for infections.
- Wear or carry medical ID to indicate you have diabetes and the drugs you take.
- To learn more: American Diabetes Association, 1701 North Beauregard St., Alexandria, VA 22311; (800) 342-2383; website: www.diabetes.org.

MEDICATION
- One or more types of oral antidiabetic drugs may be prescribed to help control glucose levels. Your health care provider will discuss the options with you. Insulin may also be prescribed.
- Drugs to treat high cholesterol, high blood pressure, or other disorders may be prescribed.

ACTIVITY—Exercise helps control diabetes.

DIET—A healthy diet is part of treatment. Don't skip meals. A dietitian can help you plan meals.

 CALL YOUR DOCTOR IF

- You or a family member has symptoms of diabetes.
- Problems with symptoms or treatment occur.

DIAPER RASH

GENERAL INFORMATION

DEFINITION—Diaper rash is a general term that describes skin irritation or inflammation (dermatitis) in the area of the body covered by a diaper. It is very common.

BODY PARTS INVOLVED—Skin of the genitals, rectum, buttocks, and abdomen.

SEX OR AGE MOST AFFECTED—Infants and young children who wear diapers.

SIGNS & SYMPTOMS
- Moist, painful, red, spotty, and sometimes itchy skin in the diaper area. The skin may be cracked and split.
- In male infants a red, raw, and sometimes bloody area may appear around the opening at the tip of the penis.

CAUSES
- It is most often due to a simple skin irritation caused by dampness, urine, or feces.
- Less often, it may be due to other skin disorders that can cause rashes. These are usually not serious unless other symptoms also occur.

RISK INCREASES WITH
- Not changing diapers often enough.
- Skin gets rubbed from rough or tight diaper.
- Cloth diapers may not be washed properly.
- Diarrhea.
- Hot, humid weather.
- Recent treatment with an antibiotic.

HOW TO PREVENT
- Change diapers often.
- Use diaper products that are breathable. These allow more air to circulate. Breathable disposable diapers, cloth diapers, and diaper covers are available.
- Avoid using plastic pants.
- Leave diaper off for 10 to 30 minutes between diaper changes for air exposure.

WHAT TO EXPECT

DIAGNOSTIC MEASURES
- Your own observation of symptoms.
- See your child's health care provider if you are concerned about the rash.

APPROPRIATE HEALTH CARE
- Home care is all that is usually needed.
- Medical care if home treatment fails to cure the rash.

POSSIBLE COMPLICATIONS—Skin infection in the rash area.

PROBABLE OUTCOME—Curable with treatment. The rash is rarely serious. Recurrence is common.

HOW TO TREAT

GENERAL MEASURES
- Keep the baby's skin clean and dry. Clean the skin under the diaper with warm water and mild soap that is not perfumed. Baby wipes may also be used, but they might irritate skin in some babies.
- Don't use talcum powder or cornstarch. Avoid use of plastic diaper covers.
- Apply small amounts of petroleum jelly, lanolin ointment, or zinc oxide ointment to the skin at the first sign of diaper rash, and thereafter 2 or 3 times a day.
- Leave the diaper off and expose the affected skin area to air as much as possible.
- Change diapers often, even at night, if the rash is more severe.

MEDICATION—Your child's health care provider may recommend medicated ointments or creams to be applied to the skin to help clear up the rash.

ACTIVITY—No limits.

DIET—No special diet. Avoid baby foods that cause diarrhea.

CALL YOUR DOCTOR IF

- Home treatment doesn't cure the diaper rash in 1 week.
- The following occur during treatment:
  - Fever.
  - Sores develop in the rash area.

DIARRHEA, ACUTE

GENERAL INFORMATION

DEFINITION—Acute diarrhea is an abnormal increase in the liquidity and frequency of stools. This is a symptom, not a disease.

BODY PARTS INVOLVED—Colon; small intestine.

SEX OR AGE MOST AFFECTED—Both sexes; simple diarrhea is common among all age groups.

SIGNS & SYMPTOMS
- Cramping abdominal pain and bloating.
- Loose, watery, or unformed bowel movements.
- Lack of bowel control (sometimes).
- Fever and nausea (sometimes).

CAUSES—Either the intestines produce too much fluid or not enough fluid is absorbed from the intestines. There are many risk factors including infections (viruses, bacteria, or parasites).

RISK INCREASES WITH
- Viral gastroenteritis (stomach "flu").
- Food intolerance or lactose intolerance.
- Emotional upsets or stress.
- Food poisoning.
- Eating large amount of certain foods, such as prunes or beans.
- Children in daycare.
- Food allergy.
- Disease or tumor of the pancreas.
- Diverticulitis, appendicitis, or fecal impaction.
- Excess alcohol use.
- Use of drugs, such as laxatives, antacids, antibiotics, quinine, or anticancer drugs.
- Radiation treatments for cancer.
- Recent illness.
- Inflammatory bowel disease.
- Crowded or unsanitary living conditions.
- Weak immune system due to illness or drugs.
- Travel to foreign country.
- Drinking contaminated water.

HOW TO PREVENT
- No specific preventive measures. Wash hands often to prevent spread of germs, especially after using the bathroom.
- Avoid undercooked or raw seafood, buffet or picnic foods left out for several hours, and food served by street vendors.

WHAT TO EXPECT

DIAGNOSTIC MEASURES
- Your own observation of symptoms.
- Your health care provider may do a physical exam.
- Medical tests may include studies of blood and stool.

APPROPRIATE HEALTH CARE
- In most cases, this disorder will be self-treated at home. There is no specific drug therapy.
- Medical care may be of help (if symptoms persist longer than 2 to 3 days).
- Hospital care may be needed, if dehydration is severe.

POSSIBLE COMPLICATIONS—Dehydration if diarrhea is prolonged, especially in infants.

PROBABLE OUTCOME—It typically goes away by itself and has no lasting effects. Most cases of diarrhea last 24 to 48 hours and a search for the cause may be unnecessary.

HOW TO TREAT

GENERAL MEASURES
- Treatment usually involves drinking plenty of fluids and extra rest as needed.
- It is not necessary to keep persons with diarrhea away from others in the family or household. Try to avoid close contact if possible. Wash hands often.

MEDICATION
- Drugs are usually not needed for treatment. If symptoms are severe or prolonged, adults may use drugs for nausea or diarrhea such as loperamide or Pepto-Bismol.
- Some infections may require specific drug treatment.
- If a drug you take is the cause of the problem, you may be advised to change drugs or stop taking the drug.

ACTIVITY—Get extra rest if needed. Be sure to have quick access to a toilet.

DIET
- For infants and children, replace lost fluids and electrolytes with products such as Pedialyte, Ceralyte, or Infalyte (follow product's directions). Infants require more frequent feedings (breast or bottle).
- Adults should drink fluids and take in salt in soups and salted crackers. Eat frequent, small meals.
- An age-appropriate, unrestricted diet is suggested. Eat complex carbohydrates, fresh fruits, lean meats, yogurt, and vegetables. Carbonated drinks or commercial juices with a high concentration of simple carbohydrates should be avoided.

CALL YOUR DOCTOR IF

- Diarrhea lasts more than 48 hours.
- Mucus, blood, or worms appear in the stool. Fever or severe pain occurs in stomach or rectum. Dehydration develops.(excess thirst, dry mouth, wrinkled skin, and little or no urination).

DIARRHEA, CHRONIC, NONSPECIFIC OF CHILDHOOD

 GENERAL INFORMATION

DEFINITION—Chronic nonspecific diarrhea is a common problem in young children. The condition is sometimes called toddler's diarrhea. It is not contagious. Diarrhea is defined as an increase in frequency, volume, and liquidity of stools as compared to a normal pattern. Diarrhea is called chronic when it lasts more than three weeks. Nonspecific means no specific cause has been found such as infection, food intolerance, or allergy. Most cases of diarrhea in children are acute and last less than 10 days.

BODY PARTS INVOLVED—Gastrointestinal system.

SEX OR AGE MOST AFFECTED—Usually affects otherwise healthy children ages 1 to 3.

SIGNS & SYMPTOMS
- Loose stools, sometimes watery.
- Stools are sometimes normal.
- Stools are more frequent than usual.
- Stools may have strong odor.
- Stool may contain undigested bits of food.
- May have mild pain in the stomach area.
- Occasional soreness of the anal area caused by having many bowel movements.

CAUSES—This type of diarrhea appears to result from a combination of an immature digestive tract (e.g., food may move too fast through the digestive system) and dietary factors (e.g., excessive intake of fluid or juices such as apple juice).

RISK INCREASES WITH—No specific risk factors.

HOW TO PREVENT—Cannot be prevented at present. Providing a healthy diet for your child and limiting fruit juices may decrease risk.

 WHAT TO EXPECT

DIAGNOSTIC MEASURES
- Your own observation of symptoms.
- Your child's health care provider will do a physical exam and ask questions about the symptoms. Information about your child's activities, and eating and drinking habits will help with the diagnosis.
- Medical tests may be done to rule out any specific cause.

APPROPRIATE HEALTH CARE—Treatment may include diet changes for your child.

POSSIBLE COMPLICATIONS—Usually no complications. Emotional problems such as anxiety may occur with parents and children.

PROBABLE OUTCOME—Despite the chronic diarrhea, affected children grow and develop normally. Diet changes can help resolve the diarrhea symptoms in some children. In others, bowel movements often become normal at about age 4.

 HOW TO TREAT

GENERAL MEASURES—Don't blame or criticize your child for this problem. Handle toilet training as you would with any child. Treat your child as normal and try to ignore the problem. Avoid tension. If the child becomes anxious about diarrhea, the problem may become worse or emotional problems may arise.

MEDICATION—Drugs are usually not needed for this disorder. Your child's health care provider may sometimes prescribe antidiarrheal drugs for a short period of time. Don't give your child herbal products or other dietary supplements without medical approval.

ACTIVITY—Your child should be physically active as appropriate for the age group.

DIET—Your child's health care provider will discuss possible diet changes with you. The goal is to achieve a healthy diet with regard to fat, fiber, fluids, and fruit juices. The diet changes may include increases in fat (e.g., whole milk), more whole grain foods and fruits, maintaining a normal fluid intake, and limiting fruit juices (especially clear juices).

 CALL YOUR DOCTOR IF

- Your child has diarrhea that lasts over 3 weeks.
- There is blood in the stool.
- Fever occurs.
- Your child becomes listless, refuses to eat, or cries loudly and nonstop, even when picked up.
- Your child begins to lose weight or is not growing as expected.

DIPHTHERIA

GENERAL INFORMATION

DEFINITION—Diphtheria is an acute, highly contagious respiratory infection. Incubation period is from 2 to 5 days. Diphtheria is rare in the United States because of immunizing children against it. It is more common in developing countries where immunization rates are low.

BODY PARTS INVOLVED—Throat; skin; heart; central nervous system.

SEX OR AGE MOST AFFECTED—Older children (5 years and up), adolescents and adults.

SIGNS & SYMPTOMS
- Early stages:
  - Sore throat.
  - Low fever.
  - Swollen neck glands.
- Late stages:
  - Airway obstruction and breathing difficulty.
  - Shock (low blood pressure, rapid heartbeat, paleness, cold skin, sweating, and anxious appearance).

CAUSES—A bacterial germ, *Corynebacterium diphtheriae*, infects the throat and sometimes the skin. The germ produces poisons that spread to the heart, central nervous system, and other organs.

RISK INCREASES WITH
- Adults over 60 and children under 5.
- Poor nutrition.
- Outbreak in the community.
- Crowded or unclean living conditions.
- Lack of up-to-date immunizations.
- Alcoholism or drug abuse.
- Weak immune system due to illness or drugs.

HOW TO PREVENT
- Immunization with diphtheria vaccine.
- Improved nutrition and standard of living.
- Notify the local health department of any case of diphtheria. Anyone having contact with the patient must be examined and treated.

WHAT TO EXPECT

DIAGNOSTIC MEASURES
- Your own observation of symptoms.
- Your health care provider will do a physical exam.
- Medical tests usually include a throat culture and blood studies.

APPROPRIATE HEALTH CARE—Hospital care and isolation of the patient are needed until fully recovered. Protect susceptible individuals (the non-immunized, very young, or elderly) from exposure. Patients may require mechanical assistance in breathing.

POSSIBLE COMPLICATIONS
- Heart inflammation and heart failure.
- Suffocation.
- Nerve inflammation.
- Misdiagnosis as a less-serious infection, resulting in dangerous delay of treatment.

PROBABLE OUTCOME—Usually curable in 1 week if treatment is begun promptly, followed by slow recovery for several weeks. A delay in treatment may result in death or long-term heart disease.

HOW TO TREAT

GENERAL MEASURES—Dispose of all secretions (nose and mouth) and excretions (urine and feces) in an acceptable manner. Call the local health department for instructions.

MEDICATION
- Diphtheria antitoxin to neutralize the diphtheria toxin will be given during hospital care.
- Antibiotics to fight remaining diphtheria germs will be prescribed.

ACTIVITY—Prolonged bed rest (2 to 3 months or until fully recovered), especially if the heart is involved.

DIET—Liquid to soft diet as tolerated.

CALL YOUR DOCTOR IF

- You or a family member has symptoms of diphtheria or you observe them in someone else.
- Anyone in your family is exposed to diphtheria.
- Your immunizations are not current.
- The following occur during treatment:
  - Temperature rises to 102°F (38.9°C).
  - Increasing difficulty breathing.
  - Increasing shortness of breath.
  - Confusion.

DISC, HERNIATED
(Ruptured or Slipped Disc)

GENERAL INFORMATION

DEFINITION—A herniated disc is a common back condition that occurs when a portion of a spinal disc pushes out of its normal space. Discs are pads with a soft gel-like center surrounded by a tough outer layer. They act as a cushion between each of the hard bones (vertebrae) of the spine (backbone) and normally help the back to flex and bend. Discs degenerate with age (e.g., get less flexible, begin to shrink, may bulge, and more prone to injury).

BODY PARTS INVOLVED—Spinal column, vertebrae, discs, nerves.

SEX OR AGE MOST AFFECTED—Usually affects adults of both sexes ages 30 to 50.

SIGNS & SYMPTOMS
- Some herniated discs cause no symptoms and may show up in tests for other problems.
- The symptoms may begin suddenly or slowly.
- Symptoms generally include pain in the lower back (most often), neck, or upper back (rare).
- Shooting pain travels down the leg (sciatica).
- Arm and shoulder pain if neck disc involved.
- Pain is worsened by sitting, after standing, at night, coughing, sneezing, or stool straining.
- Other symptoms may include numbness, tingling, burning, and muscle weakness.
- Bowel and bladder symptoms may rarely occur.

CAUSES—A herniated disk occurs when a tear or crack in a spinal disc's tough outer layer allows the gel-like inner part to leak (or squeeze out) into the spinal canal. This can put pressure on (or "pinch") spinal nerves and cause pain, inflammation, and possibly, a chemical irritation.

RISK INCREASES WITH
- Heavy lifting.
- Poor physical condition.
- Twisting violently or jumping hard.
- Overweight or obesity.
- Adults ages 30 to 65.

HOW TO PREVENT
- No specific measures. To reduce risk:
  - Use proper posture when lifting.
  - Exercise regularly to maintain muscle strength and flexibility. Maintain ideal weight.

WHAT TO EXPECT

DIAGNOSTIC MEASURES
- Your own observation of symptoms.
- Your health care provider will do a physical exam and ask questions about your symptoms and recent activities.
- Medical tests may include x-rays, other imaging studies, and nerve studies.

APPROPRIATE HEALTH CARE
- Treatment steps including drugs and/or other therapies can help relieve the symptoms.
- Treatment may include exercise, physical therapy, massage, acupuncture, manipulation, yoga, and other types of therapies. Your health care provider will discuss options with you.
- Surgery may be needed for severe symptoms or nerve damage. There are different options. (See Disc Removal in Surgery Section.)

POSSIBLE COMPLICATIONS
- Loss of bladder and bowel function.
- Chronic pain; muscle loss and weakness.

PROBABLE OUTCOME—The condition typically heals on its own. Pain decreases as the inflammation and nerve pressure subside. (Per medical studies, symptoms can improve no matter if the disc protrusion gets smaller, goes away, or remains.) For many patients, recovery begins within a week and may take about 1 to 2 months. Surgery can help severe cases.

HOW TO TREAT

GENERAL MEASURES—Use ice packs to the painful area during the first 72 hours. After that, try using heat. Take warm showers or baths. Use warm compresses or a heating pad. Be patient about your recovery.

MEDICATION
- For minor pain, use nonprescription drugs such as aspirin, acetaminophen, or ibuprofen.
- Other drugs may be prescribed:
  - Oral or injected pain reliever.
  - Muscle relaxant.
  - Drugs to reduce swelling.
  - Laxative to prevent constipation.

ACTIVITY
- Activities may need to be limited, but stay as active as you can (including your work). Avoid any activities that worsen pain. If needed, rest in bed for 1 to 2 days. Longer bed rest is not helpful in recovery.
- Follow any exercise or stretching program prescribed by your health care provider or physical therapist.
- Your health care provider will advise you about resuming sports or other physical activity.

DIET—No special diet. Drink plenty of fluids.

CALL YOUR DOCTOR IF

- You or a family member has symptoms of a herniated disc.
- During recovery you have increased pain or weakness, bladder or bowel problems, fever, or stomach pain.

DISLOCATION OR SUBLUXATION

GENERAL INFORMATION

DEFINITION—A dislocation is a joint injury in which the ends of the bones are forced from their normal position. They are no longer connected. If the bones still have some contact, it is called a subluxation. An injury may also affect the joint capsule, ligaments, and nerves.

BODY PARTS INVOLVED—Bones in joints, especially the jaw, shoulder, knee and spine. Some infants are born with a hip dislocation.

SEX OR AGE MOST AFFECTED—Both sexes; all ages.

SIGNS & SYMPTOMS
- Sudden joint pain, swelling, or an out-of-place joint after an injury. The shoulder is most often affected, but it may happen to any joint (e.g., elbow, finger, knee, ankle, toe, hip, or jaw).
- Limited or no movement around a joint.

CAUSES—Injury (e.g., fall or hit) that puts too much pressure on a joint. Less often, a dislocation may occur as a result of disease that affects the structure of the joint. A joint is where two or more bones come together in the body. Ligaments connect bones to bones.

RISK INCREASES WITH
- Contact sports.
- Sports or activities that require quick motion, twisting, or pivoting.
- Hypermobile (loose) joints that move beyond their normal range with little effort.
- Prior dislocation or subluxation of the joint.

HOW TO PREVENT
- For sports or recreational activities (such as skating), wear proper equipment to protect the joints.
- Use safety measures in the home to prevent falls or other accidents.
- Weight training will help strengthen muscles and joints.

WHAT TO EXPECT

DIAGNOSTIC MEASURES
- Your own observation of symptoms.
- Your health care provider will do an exam of the injured joint and ask questions about the activity that caused the injury.
- Medical tests usually include x-rays of the joint and nearby bones to check for fractures.

APPROPRIATE HEALTH CARE
- Treatment to realign the bones after a dislocation or subluxation is called reduction. It may include maneuvers to put the bones back into the normal position. In some cases, surgery may be needed.

- After reduction treatment, the joint may be put into a sling, splint, or cast. This allows it to heal.
- Frequent dislocations in the same joint may need surgery to correct or replace the joint.

POSSIBLE COMPLICATIONS
- Damage to nearby nerves or major blood vessels.
- Soreness and swelling may persist for many months.
- Repeated injuries in the joint may lead to arthritis.

PROBABLE OUTCOME—It often depends on the joint involved, but in general patients can with time expect a return to full function. The joint may require immobilization for 2 to 8 weeks. Full recovery after surgery may take up to 6 months.

HOW TO TREAT

GENERAL MEASURES
- Right after an injury:
  - An untrained person should not try to move the joint back into position. It could cause further injury.
  - Apply ice packs to the involved joint. Elevate it (prop it up) if possible to ease pain and prevent swelling.
  - If needed, use a splint or sling to prevent movement while taking the injured person to a medical facility.
- Crutches may be needed while the injury heals. Elevate the injured area on a pillow when you are resting.

MEDICATION
- Anesthesia or muscle-relaxing drugs may be used to make the joint realignment possible.
- Use acetaminophen or ibuprofen for mild pain.
- Stronger pain relievers may be prescribed.

ACTIVITY
- Physical therapy may be prescribed to restore normal strength and range of motion to the joint.
- Your health care provider will advise you about returning to sports and other physical activities.

DIET—No special diet.

CALL YOUR DOCTOR IF

- You or a family member has symptoms of a dislocation or subluxation.
- Difficulty moving a joint develops after injury.
- Any joint area becomes numb, pale or cold, after injury. This is an emergency!
- Dislocations occur repeatedly that you can "pop" back into normal position.

DISSEMINATED INTRAVASCULAR COAGULATION

GENERAL INFORMATION

DEFINITION—Disseminated intravascular coagulation (DIC) is a serious, life-threatening disorder that prevents a person's blood from clotting normally. DIC can cause excessive clotting or bleeding throughout the body. It is a complication of one or multiple medical conditions. DIC may be acute or chronic.

BODY PARTS INVOLVED—Blood vessels and blood in all parts of the body.

SEX OR AGE MOST AFFECTED—All ages and occurs equally in men and women.

SIGNS & SYMPTOMS
- Bleeding from any or several body parts, such as the nose or gums. Bleeding may be heavy. Common signs of bleeding include:
  - Vomiting up blood or material that looks like coffee grounds.
  - Red or black stools.
  - Vaginal bleeding.
  - Red or cloudy urine.
  - Bruising, pinpoint red spots on the skin, or bleeding under the skin (purpura).
- If organ damage occurs:
  - Shortness of breath from lung damage.
  - Low urine output from kidney damage.
  - Stroke from damage to the brain.
  - In severe cases, shock, with low blood pressure and widespread organ failure, may occur.
- In chronic DIC, the body is able to make up for the abnormal clotting. This form of DIC may produce no symptoms or only mild blood clotting or small amount of bleeding from the skin or mouth.

CAUSES—Normally, blood clots are formed in the body as a reaction to an injury. With DIC, there is an overproduction of clots in many blood vessels at the same time. This uses up all the body's clotting factors. As a result, excessive and uncontrolled bleeding can occur. The clots can also block blood flow to body organs causing them to malfunction or fail. DIC can be triggered by a variety of medical conditions.

RISK INCREASES WITH
- Widespread or major infection.
- Cancer.
- Certain types of surgery.
- Diseases such as arthritis, ulcerative colitis, Crohn's disease, sarcoidosis, Raynaud disease, and others.
- Burns or injuries.
- Pregnancy complications such as placental abruption, eclampsia, or retained dead fetus.
- Poisonous snakebite.
- Transfusion or blood disorders.
- Heart attack.
- Prosthetic devices, shunts, or heart assist devices.

HOW TO PREVENT—Obtain prompt medical care for any underlying cause.

HOW TO TREAT

GENERAL MEASURES
- Your own observation of symptoms.
- Patients with this condition are often very ill. Hospital care is needed for diagnosis and treatment. There is no single test that is used to diagnose DIC. Several different tests may be needed for an accurate diagnosis.

APPROPRIATE HEALTH CARE
- Treatment will be provided for the DIC symptoms such as bleeding, and for any underlying disorder.
- Blood transfusions or replacement of blood products may be needed.
- Oxygen may be provided through a face-mask. Some patients require breathing support with a ventilator (a device to help the lungs).
- Surgery for the underlying disorder (sometimes)

POSSIBLE COMPLICATIONS
- Kidney failure.
- Shock.
- Gangrene and amputation.
- Blood clots or hemorrhage (excess bleeding).
- Hemothorax (blood in the lungs).
- Death.

PROBABLE OUTCOME—Outcome depends on the underlying cause, severity of the DIC, age, and health status.

HOW TO TREAT

GENERAL MEASURES—None specific.

MEDICATION
- Drugs to prevent blood clots and to help control hemorrhage are usually prescribed.
- Drugs as needed to treat the underlying disorder or medical problem.

ACTIVITY—Bed rest.

DIET—Whatever type of diet is tolerated depending on patient's condition.

CALL YOUR DOCTOR IF

- You or a family member has symptoms of DIC. This is an emergency.
- Symptoms recur after treatment.

DIVERTICULAR DISEASE
(Diverticulosis; Diverticulitis)

GENERAL INFORMATION

DEFINITION
- Diverticular disease includes two main conditions:
  - Diverticulosis is the presence of small pouches (diverticula) in the wall of the colon. The diverticula may be present without any symptoms.
  - Diverticulitis occurs if diverticula become infected or inflamed. It can be a serious and dangerous disorder.

BODY PARTS INVOLVED—Left side of the large intestine.

SEX OR AGE MOST AFFECTED—Both sexes; adults (diverticula are present in 30% to 40% of those over age 50).

SIGNS & SYMPTOMS
- Diverticulosis symptoms:
  - No symptoms (usually). May be diagnosed with a colonoscopy (colon exam using a thin, lighted tube).
  - Mild cramping that comes and goes. Bloating or tenderness in the abdomen. Passing gas or bowel movements may relieve these symptoms.
  - Constipation or diarrhea.
- Diverticulitis symptoms:
  - Pain in the abdomen that becomes constant. Pain may be disabling from the start or may not become disabling for several days.
  - Areas of abdomen become tender to touch.
  - Fever, chills, nausea, and vomiting.
  - Blood in the stool.

CAUSES—Exact cause is unknown. A low-fiber diet and constipation may be factors that lead to diverticula. Stool or bacteria in the diverticula may lead to infection and inflammation.

RISK INCREASES WITH
- Low-fiber diet or diet high in fat.
- Constipation.
- Age over 50.
- Smoking. It is a risk factor for complications.

HOW TO PREVENT—To reduce risks, eat a high-fiber diet, avoid constipation, exercise daily, and don't smoke.

WHAT TO EXPECT

DIAGNOSTIC MEASURES
- Your own observation of symptoms.
- Your health care provider may do a physical exam and a digital rectal exam (a gloved, lubricated finger is inserted into the rectum). Questions will be asked about your symptoms, diet, and bowel habits.
- Tests include blood and stool studies, x-ray, CT, or colonoscopy.

APPROPRIATE HEALTH CARE
- If there are no symptoms, treatment may not be needed. For mild symptoms, treatment may include a change in diet and the use of stool softeners. For more severe symptoms, bed rest, drugs, hospital care, and surgery may be needed.
- Surgery may be done for complications. These include abscess, fistula, intestinal obstruction, perforation, or peritonitis. A part of the affected colon may be removed (resection) and the remaining sections rejoined. A colostomy involves creating a temporary hole (stoma) in the abdomen to remove stool.

POSSIBLE COMPLICATIONS
- Intestinal bleeding or infections.
- Perforation, tear, or blockage of the intestines.
- Abscess (pus-filled, infected area).
- Peritonitis (inflammation of abdominal lining).
- Recurrent attacks of diverticulitis.
- Fistula (abnormal tract through bowel wall).

PROBABLE OUTCOME—Most cases of diverticulitis are mild, respond well to treatment, and have no recurrence. If complications occur, they can usually be treated successfully.

HOW TO TREAT

GENERAL MEASURES
- For self-care:
  - Try to have a bowel movement at the same time each day. Allow about 10 minutes, and don't strain.
  - Check your stool for bleeding. Ask your health care provider if a sample is to be taken to the medical office.
  - To relieve mild pain, use a heating pad.
- To learn more: National Digestive Diseases Information Clearinghouse, 2 Information Way, Bethesda, MD 20892; (800) 891-5389; website: www.digestive.niddk.nih.gov.

MEDICATION
- Antibiotics will be prescribed for infections.
- Stool softeners may be recommended.
- Don't take laxatives, unless prescribed.

ACTIVITY—If you have fever or severe pain, stay in bed. Resume normal activity as soon as symptoms improve.

DIET—Eat a diet that is high in fiber. Drink plenty of fluids.

CALL YOUR DOCTOR IF

- You or a family member has symptoms of diverticular disease.
- Symptoms don't improve or they become worse.

DOMESTIC VIOLENCE
(Battering; Spousal Abuse)

 GENERAL INFORMATION

DEFINITION—Domestic violence is abuse, usually by a spouse or partner, in an intimate relationship. It may include physical, sexual, emotional, or financial abuse. The victim is usually a woman (95% of abuse cases). Because of shame and guilt, the victim may not report the abuse to police, medical care givers, or talk about it with family or friends. Cycles of abuse are: *honeymoon* (apology, affection), *tension building* (poor communication, fear), and *acting out* (abusive incidents). Abuse is common. It may occur in any race, age group, economic or educational level, or nationality.

BODY PARTS INVOLVED—May affect all.

SEX OR AGE MOST AFFECTED—Both sexes, all ages, but most victims are females.

SIGNS & SYMPTOMS
- In female victims:
  - Physical or sexual abuse injuries. These include broken bones, bruises, burns, choking, bites, rape, and others. Most injuries are to the head, neck, chest, abdomen, and breasts. Arm injuries may result from self defense.
  - Other symptoms may include chronic pelvic pain, sexual dysfunction, anxiety, depression, sleep disorders, post-traumatic stress disorder (PTSD), eating disorders, psychological problems, and thoughts of suicide.
- In male abusers:
  - Angry, suspicious, tense and/or moody behaviors. Can be very charming at times. They go from periods of abuse to periods of affection.
  - May display extreme jealousy and possessiveness. May not allow partner's friends/family to visit or call.
  - Makes threats of violence or legal threats (such as custody of the children). May play with guns or knives.
  - Limits access to money or other basic needs.

CAUSES—The cause is unknown. Multiple factors are involved.

RISK INCREASES WITH
- A history of abuse in a family. Many male abusers and, often, female victims, witnessed abuse or were victims.
- Male abusers tend to use alcohol or drugs, are often unemployed, and may be less educated. However, many educated, professional men are abusers.
- Males who are dependent on women, have money worries, feelings of inadequacy, and have traditional (or archaic) attitudes (such as about sex).
- Females lacking self-esteem and females who feel dependent and useless.
- Pregnant females.

HOW TO PREVENT—Victims should seek help at the first sign of abuse. Don't assume the abuser will change or stop the abuse.

 WHAT TO EXPECT

DIAGNOSTIC MEASURES—Exam by a health care provider and medical tests as needed.

APPROPRIATE HEALTH CARE
- Treatment steps for a victim:
  - Get medical care for any injuries.
  - Counseling is important. It helps a woman learn to cope and regain self-confidence, and ability to function.
- Treatment for the abuser:
  - Treatment is often resisted by an abuser. Educational and treatment groups have had some success.
  - Abusers must be confronted with the results of the behavior; that they can go to jail if they don't change.

POSSIBLE COMPLICATIONS—Years of emotional and physical abuse. Alcohol and drug abuse by a female victim. Murder or suicide.

PROBABLE OUTCOME
- For victims, help is available, if they seek it.
- Abusers are unlikely to change their behavior.

 HOW TO TREAT

GENERAL MEASURES
- If you are abused:
  - Protect yourself, especially the head and abdomen. Get away from the abuser and get help. Document the abuse with pictures, telling someone, or calling 911.
  - Have a personal safety plan set up. Have a place to stay, a way to get there, transportation, and survival funds. Have clothing and personal essentials packed.
  - Agencies and shelters exist that help abused women and children Call a local crisis line.
- To learn more: National Domestic Violence Hotline; (800) 799-7233; website: www.ndvh.org. Note: Be aware that an abuser may monitor mail, telephone, and internet communication. Take precautions as needed.

MEDICATION—Drugs may be prescribed for anxiety or depression.

ACTIVITY—No limits.

DIET—No special diet.

 CALL YOUR DOCTOR IF

You or a family member is a victim of domestic violence. Get emergency help if needed!

DOWN SYNDROME
(Trisomy 21)

 GENERAL INFORMATION

DEFINITION—Down syndrome is a genetic disorder that usually results in abnormal physical appearance, mental retardation, and other health problems. One in every 800 babies is born with Down syndrome. It can occur in people of all races and economic levels.

BODY PARTS INVOLVED—Central nervous system; heart; skeletal system.

SEX OR AGE MOST AFFECTED—Newborns.

SIGNS & SYMPTOMS
- Appearance (some may have only a few of the recognizable traits, while others may have many):
  - Lack of normal muscle tone. Child seems "floppy."
  - Head that is not shaped normally, including a small or odd-shaped skull.
  - Facial features may include small, flattened nose, small mouth, small chin, and large tongue.
  - Slanting, almond-shaped eyes. The inner corner of the eyes may have a rounded fold of skin (epicanthal fold). Iris may be abnormal.
  - Ears that are not of normal shape.
  - Broad hands with a large, single palm crease. The little finger curves inward in some.
  - Slow growth and development. The child typically never reaches full height.
- Other possible conditions:
  - Heart and gastrointestinal defects.
  - Mild to moderate mental retardation.

CAUSES—Genetic. An extra chromosome creates abnormalities. It is not yet known why this occurs. Research is ongoing.

RISK INCREASES WITH
- Many risk factors have been studied. The only proven one is the increasing age of the woman.
- If a woman has one Down syndrome baby, she has a 1% risk increase for a second.

HOW TO PREVENT
- It cannot be prevented. If you or your partner has a family history of Down syndrome, get genetic counseling before a pregnancy.
- If you are pregnant and over age 40, or you or your partner have a family history of Down syndrome, talk to your health care provider about any recommended medical tests.

 WHAT TO EXPECT

DIAGNOSTIC MEASURES—A Down syndrome baby may be diagnosed during pregnancy by medical testing or at birth by the baby's appearance. A chromosome test may be done on the newborn. It is an extremely difficult time for new parents. Counseling may be helpful. Some parents blame themselves and need help to cope with feelings of guilt.

APPROPRIATE HEALTH CARE
- Home care.
- Health care is important. Children with Down syndrome are more likely to get infections and other illnesses. Surgery may be needed to correct heart or intestinal disorders.

POSSIBLE COMPLICATIONS
- Risk of infections, leukemia, thyroid disease, heart defects, hearing and vision problems, obesity, or apnea.
- Dementia later in life.
- Early death due to health complications.

PROBABLE OUTCOME—There is no cure. With help, people with Down syndrome can reach their full potential and lead happy, loving, and useful lives. Life expectancy is about 50 to 60 years and continues to improve.

 HOW TO TREAT

GENERAL MEASURES
- Raising the child to his or her full potential should be the goal for parents of a child with Down syndrome.
- Learn all you can about programs in your city to help children with Down syndrome. Join a support group.
- Learning programs for these children begin in infancy and continue all through their lives. Some children can be taught in regular classrooms (with extra help), while others may need special education. They can take part in, and enjoy, sports, music, art, and other activities.
- As adults, they can hold jobs, live in group-homes, have social lives, and some may marry.
- To learn more: National Down Syndrome Society, 666 Broadway, New York, NY 10012; (800) 221-4602; website: www.ndss.org.

MEDICATION—Drugs are usually not needed unless an illness occurs.

ACTIVITY—Encourage the child to be as active as possible in a protected environment.

DIET—No special diet. Feeding an infant with Down syndrome may be a problem. Some have difficulty sucking or are not eager to eat.

 CALL YOUR DOCTOR IF

- You have a child with Down syndrome and have any questions or concerns.
- A child with Down syndrome develops an infection or other medical problem.

DROWNING, NEAR

GENERAL INFORMATION

DEFINITION—Near drowning results from being submerged in water or other fluid and almost dying.

BODY PARTS INVOLVED—Lungs; blood; heart.

SEX OR AGE MOST AFFECTED—Both sexes; all ages. Children under age 4, young adults (ages 15 to 24), and males are often the victims.

SIGNS & SYMPTOMS
- Difficulty breathing or shortness of breath.
- Fast or slow heartbeat.
- May be unconscious.
- Anxious appearance.
- Skin may be bluish-white, cold, and pale.
- Coughing or vomiting.
- May have breathed foreign material into lungs.

CAUSES—In most cases, a person under water attempts to breath and aspirates (breathes in) water into the lungs. In some cases, a spasm of the larynx (voice box) cuts off oxygen to the lungs. Both cases lead to a lack of oxygen in the body and can result in unconsciousness, cardiac arrest, and other major problems.

RISK INCREASES WITH
- Not able to swim or overestimating swimming ability.
- Alcohol or drug use; seizure, stroke, or heart problem during water activity.
- Accidents from diving, surfing, water skiing, boating, or scuba diving.
- Unsupervised children in or near water. This includes swimming pools, bathtubs, or pails of water (such as used for mopping).
- Falling through thin ice.
- Attempted suicide.

HOW TO PREVENT
- Learn cardiopulmonary resuscitation (CPR).
- Have all family members learn to swim.
- Adult supervision of children near water.
- Install a fence around a home swimming pool. Always be sure that pool gates are locked.
- Never swim alone.
- Don't drink alcohol or abuse drugs and swim.
- Wear life jackets in boats.
- Scuba divers need to be fully trained, use caution when diving, and avoid risky dives.

WHAT TO EXPECT

DIAGNOSTIC MEASURES—Emergency care usually includes supplemental oxygen, body temperature control, maintenance of the body's electrolytes and blood sugar levels, and prevention of complications. Treatment for any injuries will be provided.

APPROPRIATE HEALTH CARE
- Immediate cardiopulmonary resuscitation (CPR).
- Hospitalization for observation for delayed, serious reactions.

POSSIBLE COMPLICATIONS
- Pulmonary edema (fluid in the lungs).
- Lung infection.
- Permanent brain damage.
- Heart problems, including cardiac arrest and death.

PROBABLE OUTCOME
- With mild symptoms, patients are usually sent home after 6 to 8 hours in the emergency room/hospital. Complications are unlikely.
- More severe symptoms require extended time for treatment and could result in complications.

HOW TO TREAT

GENERAL MEASURES
- If the victim is unconscious and not breathing, yell for help. Have someone call 911 (emergency) for an ambulance or medical help. Don't leave the victim.
- Try to warm the person with whatever means are at hand (blankets, towels, jackets).
- Begin mouth-to-mouth breathing and CPR if needed.
- Don't stop rescue effort until medical help arrives.
- The near-drowning victim should be taken to the nearest hospital for intensive care even if the victim has become conscious.
Complications may occur several hours after the near drowning.

MEDICATION
- Drugs used for treatment may include:
  - Cortisone drugs, to prevent or treat inflammation of the lungs.
  - Antibiotics, to prevent lung infection.
  - Bronchodilators, to enable oxygen to enter the lungs.
  - Anticonvulsants, to prevent seizures.

ACTIVITY—Complete bed rest for at least the first 24 hours.

DIET—Nutrition may be provided through a vein (IV) while in the hospital. After recovery, no special diet is needed.

CALL YOUR DOCTOR IF

- Someone appears to have drowned. Call for emergency help immediately!
- Cough, shortness of breath, or fever develop after treatment.

DRUG ALLERGY
(Drug Hypersensitivity)

 GENERAL INFORMATION

DEFINITION—Drug allergy is an allergic reaction caused by drugs. The reaction may happen immediately after taking the drug or days to weeks later.

BODY PARTS INVOLVED—Skin; blood vessels; lungs.

SEX OR AGE MOST AFFECTED—Both sexes; all ages. Females are affected more often than males.

SIGNS & SYMPTOMS
- Symptoms vary and may be mild to severe.
- Rash (most common), hives (urticaria), and itching skin or eyes.
- Wheezing.
- Swelling (lips, tongue, and/or face).
- Anaphylaxis (a life-threatening reaction). It can cause difficult breathing with a wheeze, hives, swelling, fainting, lightheadedness, dizziness, confusion, rapid pulse, fast heart rate, diarrhea, nausea or vomiting, and stomach pain or cramping.

CAUSES—It is a reaction of the immune system in certain people. It leads to a misdirected response against a substance that does not cause a response in most people. The body becomes sensitized by the first exposure to the drug. The second or subsequent exposure causes an immune response (production of antibodies and release of histamine). Injected drugs are more of a risk than those taken by mouth or applied to the skin.

RISK INCREASES WITH
- Use of almost any drug. These are more likely:
  - Penicillin and cephalosporin antibiotics.
  - Sulfa drugs.
  - Vaccines.
  - Anesthetics applied to the skin.
  - Allergy extracts.
  - Iodine-containing compounds in some x-rays.
- Injected drugs, especially in high doses.
- Personal or family history of other allergies, such as hay fever, asthma, or eczema.
- Serious illness.
- Weak immune system due to illness or drugs.

HOW TO PREVENT
- Drug allergies cannot be prevented. Tell any health care provider you consult about the drug reactions you have had.
- Avoid drugs that have caused a past reaction.

 WHAT TO EXPECT

DIAGNOSTIC MEASURES
- Your own observation of symptoms.

- Your health care provider may do a physical exam. Questions will be asked about your symptoms and the drugs you take (including nonprescription, herbals, or other supplements). Usually, a diagnosis can be made based on the type of reaction, timing of the reaction, and that a drug you used is known to cause reactions.
- Skin tests or blood tests may be done.

APPROPRIATE HEALTH CARE
- The first step of treatment is to stop using the drug that caused a reaction. Usually, another drug can be safely substituted. Symptoms of the drug reaction may be treated with other drugs.
- If there is no substitute drug that can be used, other treatment steps may be taken. There are methods (called desensitizing) that gradually introduce a drug into the body in small doses.

POSSIBLE COMPLICATIONS
- Anaphylaxis (can be life-threatening).
- Serum sickness (a delayed type of reaction that occurs 1 to 3 weeks or more after exposure). It can occur with the first time use of a drug. Symptoms include fever, rash, joint pain, and nerve damage.
- Rarely, may affect internal organs.

PROBABLE OUTCOME—In many cases, stopping the drug is all that is needed. In other cases, symptoms can be relieved with treatment. Most symptoms should resolve in about 2 weeks.

 HOW TO TREAT

GENERAL MEASURES
- Wear or carry medical ID that shows you have the drug allergy.
- Keep an anaphylaxis kit at home, on your person, nearby at work, and in your car for emergency use if anyone in the family has had a severe drug reaction.

MEDICATION
- Cortisone drugs to decrease inflammation, antihistamines for the itching, and broncho-dilators for wheezing may be prescribed.
- Epinephrine may be injected to treat anaphylaxis.

ACTIVITY—No limits once symptoms improve.

DIET—No special diet.

 CALL YOUR DOCTOR IF

- You have symptoms of drug allergy or observe them in someone else.
- You or a family member has anaphylaxis symptoms. This is an emergency! Call 911. Get help immediately!

DRY EYE SYNDROME

GENERAL INFORMATION

DEFINITION
• Dry eye syndrome (DES) develops when the surface of the eye is not kept moist. It is caused by problems with tear production. Both eyes are usually involved (one eye may be worse). Some people have no symptoms. DES is a common condition and affects all ages.

BODY PARTS INVOLVED—Eyes.

SEX OR AGE MOST AFFECTED—Both sexes; (more often in women); older adults.

SIGNS & SYMPTOMS
• Eye itching, burning, stinging, or redness.
• Eye irritation, discomfort, pain, or excess tearing.
• Feels like something is in the eye.
• Blurred, changing, or decreased vision (symptoms may improve with blinking).
• Difficulty wearing contact lenses.
• May have mucus in or around the eyes.
• Sensitivity to light.

CAUSES
• A decrease in quantity or quality of tear production, or the tears evaporate too quickly. This can be caused by many conditions. Problems can develop in any of the three layers of the tear film—water, mucus, or oil—or in the tiny glands that produce tears.
• Two types of tears are produced in the eyes:
 - Lubricating tears keep the eye moist, clean, and fight infection. These tears are constantly produced and have three layers in their tear film—water, mucus, and oil. With each blink, the eyelids spread the tears over the eye. Excess tears flow into two tiny drainage ducts in the corner of the eye by the nose.
 - Reflex tears are produced in response to emotion, injury, irritation, or can be a response to dry eyes. They make tears more watery.

RISK INCREASES WITH
• Aging (decreased production or poor quality of tears).
• Women after menopause.
• Certain autoimmune diseases (e.g., Sjögren syndrome, rheumatoid arthritis, or lupus).
• Some drugs (e.g., antihistamines, antidepressants, beta-blockers, and oral contraceptives).
• Conditions such as stroke, Bell's palsy, or eyelid problems. They can make it difficult to close the eyes.
• Lack of vitamin A.
• Contact lens use.
• Eye surgery.
• Other, less common risk factors.

HOW TO PREVENT—No specific preventive measures. Avoid risk factors where possible.

WHAT TO EXPECT

DIAGNOSTIC MEASURES
• Your own observation of symptoms.
• Your health care provider or eye care provider will do an eye exam.
• You may be asked to fill out a form about the dry eye symptoms. Tests may be done to check on tear production.

APPROPRIATE HEALTH CARE
• Treatments may include artificial tear use, other eye or oral drugs, surgery, special eyewear, and self-care.
• Any underlying causes of dry eyes will be treated. If a drug is the cause, a different one may be prescribed.
• Moisture chamber spectacles or customized contact lenses may be recommended to help retain moisture.
• Surgery options may be recommended. In one, tiny plugs are placed in tear drainage ducts to help tears stay on the eye's surface. Eyelid disorders may need surgery.

POSSIBLE COMPLICATIONS—Rarely, scarring, decreased vision, or symptoms worsen.

PROBABLE OUTCOME—It is usually a chronic condition. Treatment can relieve symptoms.

HOW TO TREAT

GENERAL MEASURES
• Symptoms may increase with certain activities. Take breaks from computer work, reading, or TV to rest the eyes. Use a humidifier to moisten the air. Avoid smoke. Don't rub eyes. Remember to blink.
• Blepharitis (eyelid inflammation) may occur with dry eyes. Treat it with eyelid cleaning and warm soaks.

MEDICATION
• Use nonprescription artificial tears (drops, gel, or ointment) with or without preservatives. Try several to find what works best. Preservative-free type is recommended for sensitive eyes or if used more than every 2 hours.
• Other eye products or oral drugs may be prescribed for more severe dry eye symptoms.
• Omega-3 fatty acid supplements may be recommended.

ACTIVITY—Usually, no limits.

DIET—No special diet.

☎ CALL YOUR DOCTOR IF

• You or a family member has dry eye symptoms.
• Symptoms don't improve with treatment.

DUMPING SYNDROME

 GENERAL INFORMATION

DEFINITION—Dumping syndrome is a group of symptoms that are usually a complication of stomach surgery. Most patients experience the problem to a minor degree for 1 to 6 months after surgery. The symptoms are of 2 types—early dumping syndrome and late dumping syndrome. Symptoms of the first begin a few minutes to 45 minutes after every meal. Symptoms of the second begin 2 to 3 hours after eating. Most persons experience late dumping syndrome (you cannot have both types). People with a rare disorder called Zollinger-Ellison syndrome may also have dumping syndrome.

BODY PARTS INVOLVED—Gastrointestinal system; cardiovascular system.

SEX OR AGE MOST AFFECTED—Both sexes of adults following surgery on the stomach.

SIGNS & SYMPTOMS
- Early dumping syndrome:
  - Weakness and fainting.
  - Sweating.
  - Irregular or rapid heartbeat.
  - Decreased blood pressure.
  - Skin gets flushed (reddens).
  - Dizziness.
  - May become hard to breathe.
  - Vomiting.
  - Explosive diarrhea and stomach cramps.
- Late dumping syndrome:
  - Sweating, anxiety, and tremors.
  - Exhaustion and faintness.
  - Decreased blood pressure.
  - Headache.

CAUSES
- Early dumping syndrome: rapid entry of food and fluids directly into the small intestine, producing decreased blood pressure and increased blood flow to the intestines.
- Late dumping syndrome: low blood sugar caused by too much insulin being made by the body in response to sudden dumping of food and fluids into the intestine.

RISK INCREASES WITH—The larger the amount of stomach removed, the more severe the dumping syndrome.

HOW TO PREVENT—Cannot be prevented. Recurrence and severity can be reduced with changes in the diet.

 WHAT TO EXPECT

DIAGNOSTIC MEASURES
- Your own observation of symptoms.
- Your health care provider will do a physical exam and ask questions about your symptoms and surgery history.
- Medical tests may include glucose tolerance test, x-rays, and gastric emptying study.

APPROPRIATE HEALTH CARE
- Treatment includes diet changes and sometimes drugs.
- In ongoing severe cases of dumping syndrome, surgery may be considered.

POSSIBLE COMPLICATIONS
- Poor nutrition and weight loss.
- Anxiety.
- Electrolyte problems such as low potassium.
- Low blood sugar (hypoglycemia).

PROBABLE OUTCOME—The problem clears up on its own for most patients. Early dumping syndrome usually lasts 3 to 4 months. Late dumping syndrome usually lasts 1 year, but it may persist for many years.

 HOW TO TREAT

GENERAL MEASURES
- Lie down as soon as you finish any meal. This helps reduce the symptoms.
- To learn more: National Digestive Diseases Information Clearinghouse, 2 Information Way, Bethesda, MD 20892; (800) 891-5389; website: www.niddk.nih.gov.

MEDICATION
- Your health care provider may prescribe drugs to help with digestion or lower blood sugar.
- Vitamin and mineral supplements may be prescribed.

ACTIVITY
- Between symptoms, there are no limits.
- With symptoms, rest until they pass.

DIET—Diet control is the most important treatment. Eat a diet low in sugar and other simple carbohydrates. Increase fat and protein food items. Avoid milk and milk products. Avoid foods that are very hot or very cold. Eat 6 small, evenly spaced meals a day. Take meals dry without water or beverages and drink fluids only between meals.

 CALL YOUR DOCTOR IF

- You or a family member has symptoms of dumping syndrome not helped by diet changes.
- You vomit blood, have black, tarry stools, or other new symptoms occur.

DYSENTERY, BACILLARY
(Shigellosis)

GENERAL INFORMATION

DEFINITION—Bacillary dysentery is a bacterial infection of the intestinal tract. It often happens in epidemics (affects a large number of people at the same time).

BODY PARTS INVOLVED—Lower small intestine (ileum); large intestine (colon).

SEX OR AGE MOST AFFECTED—Both sexes; all ages. It occurs most often in young children.

SIGNS & SYMPTOMS
- Stomach cramps.
- Fever.
- Diarrhea (up to 20 or 30 watery bowel movements in one day). There may be small amounts of blood, mucus, or pus in the stool.
- Nausea or vomiting.
- Muscle aches or pain.

CAUSES—Bacteria called *Shigella bacillus* that attack the lining of the colon. It spreads from person to person, usually from germs on the hands. The infection is also spread from germs on objects such as toys, in food, in drinking water (in areas with poor sanitation), or in wading pools. Symptoms usually start 1 to 2 days after being exposed to germs.

RISK INCREASES WITH
- Travel to foreign countries.
- Crowded or unclean living conditions.
- Persons with poor health.

HOW TO PREVENT
- Wash hands after bowel movements and before handling food. Children need to be reminded often.
- Avoid contact with an infected person.
- Put soiled clothes and bedclothes in covered buckets of soap and water until they can be washed.
- Use safety precautions if traveling to high risk areas.

WHAT TO EXPECT

DIAGNOSTIC MEASURES
- Your own observation of symptoms.
- Your health care provider will do a physical exam and ask questions about the symptoms.
- Tests and culture of a stool sample may be done to confirm the diagnosis.

APPROPRIATE HEALTH CARE
- Home care.
- Treatment usually includes fluids (to replace those lost from diarrhea), a bland diet, and drug therapy.
- A hospital stay may be needed if patient is severely ill. This may happen with small children with dehydration or severe rectal bleeding.

POSSIBLE COMPLICATIONS—Severe cases may occur in the very young or the elderly. Symptoms include convulsions, severe dehydration, and disorders that cause kidney failure and a type of arthritis.

PROBABLE OUTCOME—The infection resolves on its own or with treatment in about 5 to 7 days. Rarely, it may last a month. Most *Shigella* infections are mild.

HOW TO TREAT

GENERAL MEASURES
- Watch for signs of dehydration. These include severe thirst, dry mouth and tongue, tiredness, sunken eyes, dry skin, being irritable, and less urination.
- Keep the patient away from others if possible.
- Use warm compresses on the stomach to help relieve pain.

MEDICATION
- Antibiotics may be prescribed in severe cases or for certain patients. They can help speed recovery and reduce risk of spreading germs. Be sure to take them for as long as prescribed.
- Don't use antidiarrhea drugs, unless they are prescribed. These may extend the illness.

ACTIVITY—The ill person should be at home and away from others when possible. A return to daycare, school, or work is permitted after taking antibiotics for 5 days.

DIET—Be sure to drink plenty of liquids. A soft or liquid diet may be recommended. Use special drinks (or popsicles) that replace body fluids quickly.

CALL YOUR DOCTOR IF

- You or a family member has symptoms of bacillary dysentery.
- The following occur during treatment:
  - Rectal bleeding or bloody stools.
  - Signs of dehydration appear.
  - Symptoms get worse despite treatment.

DYSMENORRHEA
(Menstrual Cramps)

 GENERAL INFORMATION

DEFINITION—Dysmenorrhea is pain that occurs with menstruation. In primary dysmenorrhea, there is no underlying pelvic condition. It is very common and typically occurs in women under age 20. Secondary dysmenorrhea is associated with pelvic conditions and occurs more often in women over age 20.

BODY PARTS INVOLVED—Female reproductive system, especially the uterus.

SEX OR AGE MOST AFFECTED—Women of childbearing age.

SIGNS & SYMPTOMS
- Severity of symptoms varies from woman to woman, and from one time to the next in the same woman.
- Cramping and, sometimes, sharp pains in the lower abdomen, lower back, and thighs. Pain usually begins with a menstrual period and lasts for hours to days. For some women, the pain may begin a week or more before her period and last for a few days after it stops.
- Other symptoms that may occur:
  - Nausea, vomiting, diarrhea, headache, and sweating.
  - Lack of energy.
  - Fainting.
  - Feeling irritable, anxious, or depressed.

CAUSES
- In primary dysmenorrhea, excess prostaglandin (a hormone-like substance) appears to be the cause. It stimulates uterine contractions.
- In secondary dysmenorrhea, the cause may be an underlying pelvic disorder or abnormality.

RISK INCREASES WITH
- Primary dysmenorrhea:
  - Family history of dysmenorrhea.
  - Age under 20; early menstruation; never being pregnant.
  - Obesity, smoking, and possibly alcohol use.
  - Behavior or psychological factors may also be involved. Some factors may lead to more severe dysmenorrhea symptoms.
- Secondary dysmenorrhea:
  - Endometriosis, pelvic inflammatory disease, ovarian cysts or tumors, fibroids, uterine polyps, adenomyosis, or other pelvic disorders.
  - Congenital (being born with) uterine or vaginal abnormalities.
  - Intrauterine device (IUD).

HOW TO PREVENT—Taking naproxen or ibuprofen just before period helps prevent primary type. Treating underlying cause may help prevent secondary type.

 WHAT TO EXPECT

DIAGNOSTIC MEASURES
- Your health care provider will do a physical exam and a pelvic exam. Questions will be asked about your menstrual history.
- Medical tests may include blood and urine studies, and an ultrasound.

APPROPRIATE HEALTH CARE
- Treatment often includes drugs to help pain.
- Transcutaneous electrical nerve stimulator (TENS) treatment, massage therapy, yoga, acupuncture, meditation, or other therapies may help in some cases.
- Counseling may be helpful if emotional problems such as stress are a concern.
- For secondary dysmenorrhea, treatment will depend on the cause. Drugs or surgery (such as removing fibroids) may be recommended.

POSSIBLE COMPLICATIONS
- Severe pain that interferes with daily life.
- Infertility from underlying cause.

PROBABLE OUTCOME
- For primary dysmenorrhea, symptoms can be helped with treatment. Symptoms improve or disappear with age and with childbirth.
- For secondary dysmenorrhea, the outcome depends on the cause and its treatment.

 HOW TO TREAT

GENERAL MEASURES—Heat helps relieve pain. Use a heating pad on the abdomen or back. Take a warm bath (for 10 to 15 minutes) as often as needed.

MEDICATION
- Use nonsteroidal anti-inflammatory drugs (NSAIDs) such as ibuprofen or naproxen starting 1 to 2 days before period begins.
- Antiprostaglandins (for painful menstrual periods) and oral contraceptives, which prohibit ovulation, may be prescribed.
- In severe cases, hormones (e.g., a gonadotropin-releasing hormone [Gn-RH]) can stop ovary function to relieve pain.
- Diet supplements may be recommended.

ACTIVITY—Exercise may help reduce the discomfort of menstrual cramps.

DIET—No special diet.

 CALL YOUR DOCTOR IF

- You or a family member has symptoms of dysmenorrhea that cannot be relieved.
- Pain worsens or you have excess bleeding.

DYSPAREUNIA

GENERAL INFORMATION

DEFINITION—Dyspareunia is pain that occurs with sexual intercourse. Dyspareunia and vaginismus (spasm of the pubic muscles of the lower vagina) may occur together in a woman.

BODY PARTS INVOLVED—Genital area, vaginal muscles, uterus (sometimes), brain.

SEX OR AGE MOST AFFECTED—Sexually active females of all ages. Dyspareunia also occurs in men, but less often.

SIGNS & SYMPTOMS
- Pain in the genital area during sexual activity. It can occur before, during, or after sexual intercourse.
- Women may have pain on entry or during intercourse (with deep thrusts of partner's penis).
- Men may have pain in the penis or testes.
- Pain may be mild or severe, and vary with different intercourse positions.

CAUSES
- The pain is a symptom that can be due to one or more factors such as:
  - Physical and medical problems.
  - Emotional, interpersonal, and environmental problems (called psychosocial problems).
  - It may be a combination of factors and sometimes no cause is found.

RISK INCREASES WITH
- Physical:
  - Infection, inflammation, or injury of the genitals or the urinary tract.
  - A lack of vaginal lubrication. This can be due to illness, drugs, or lack of estrogen (such as at menopause).
  - Vaginal scarring from surgery or radiation therapy.
  - Episiotomy scar (from repair after childbirth).
  - Intact hymen (covering of vaginal opening).
  - Allergy to diaphragms, condoms, or contraceptive foams and jellies.
  - Endometriosis or pelvic inflammatory disease.
  - Muscle spasms of the vagina (vaginismus).
  - Vulvodynia (chronic vulva pain).
  - Tilted or enlarged uterus.
- Emotional:
  - Lack of sexual arousal or sexual foreplay; unhappy with sexual partner; fatigue, or anxiety.
  - Lack of sexual experience or information.
  - Past sexual abuse (e.g., rape) or emotional trauma.
  - Fear of pregnancy.

HOW TO PREVENT
- Get medical care for genital infections.
- Avoid perfumed soaps, bubble baths, or toilet paper that is scented or colored. Don't douche.
- Get counseling for depression, stress, or anxiety.

WHAT TO EXPECT

DIAGNOSTIC MEASURES
- Your health care provider may do a physical exam and a genital exam. You will be asked about your symptoms and sexual history.
- Medical studies, such as a Pap smear and culture of vaginal discharge may be done to diagnose medical problems that can be treated.

APPROPRIATE HEALTH CARE
- Treatment will be directed to any physical or emotional cause that is diagnosed.
- In cases of scarring, problems with the hymen, or others, a minor surgical procedure may relieve symptoms.
- Instructions may be given for exercises or techniques to dilate (widen) the vagina. They involve use of fingers or dilators to condition the body and mind to the sensation of something being inserted into the vagina.
- Treatments for emotional causes will vary. They can involve education, counseling, sensate focus exercises, and teaching of appropriate foreplay techniques.

POSSIBLE COMPLICATIONS—Treatment may be long-term and may not always help. An intimate relationship with partner may suffer.

PROBABLE OUTCOME—Physical causes are often curable with treatment. Psychosocial causes may be helped with treatment.

HOW TO TREAT

GENERAL MEASURES
- Sitz baths help ease discomfort. Sit in a tub of warm water for 10 to 15 minutes, 3 times a day.
- Use a nonprescription lubricant, such as K-Y Lubricating Jelly, during sexual intercourse.
- Try different sexual intercourse positions. They may reduce penile penetration and lessen pain.
- Discuss the lack of sexual arousal with your partner, including ways to improve foreplay.
- To learn more: American College of Obstetricians and Gynecologists; website: www.acog.org.

MEDICATION—Drugs may be prescribed for infection or inflammation. Steroid creams or estrogen creams may be prescribed.

ACTIVITY—Regular exercise is helpful for general well-being.

DIET—No special diet.

CALL YOUR DOCTOR IF

- You or a family member has symptoms of dyspareunia.
- Symptoms do not improve with treatment.

DYSPHAGIA

GENERAL INFORMATION

DEFINITION—Dysphagia is difficulty or pain in swallowing. It may involve solid foods, liquids, or both. It is a common symptom with a wide variety of causes that can be benign or malignant. The risk of a serious disorder is rare.

BODY PARTS INVOLVED—Pharynx; esophagus.

SEX OR AGE MOST AFFECTED—Both sexes; all ages. It occurs more often in older adults.

SIGNS & SYMPTOMS
- Pain that occurs with swallowing.
- Sore throat.
- Feeling that food "gets stuck" as you swallow.
- Coughing or choking with eating or drinking (food may come back out through the nose).
- Drooling, belching, and bad breath.
- Pressure sensation in mid-chest.

CAUSES—The swallowing difficulty may involve the mouth, the throat, and the esophagus. There are numerous risk factors that may be the cause.

RISK INCREASES WITH
- Gastroesophageal reflux disease (GERD) or acid reflux.
- Tumors (benign or cancer).
- Stricture (narrowing of the passage).
- Inflammation (esophagitis) or infections.
- Recent head, neck, or throat surgery.
- Laryngitis, pharyngitis, or tonsillitis.
- Foreign object lodges at back of the throat.
- Scratch in throat lining due to a foreign object.
- Insufficient production of saliva.
- Esophageal spasm (loss of normal muscle movement).
- In children, it may be caused by delayed maturation, malformation, cerebral palsy, or muscular dystrophy.
- Hernia of part of the esophagus through a weak area in the surrounding muscle.
- Nervous system disorder (stroke, Alzheimer's disease, myasthenia gravis, Parkinson's disease, and others).
- Pressure on the esophagus (a goiter or aortic aneurysm).
- Emotional disorders (anxiety, fear, and others).
- Anemia.
- Smoking.
- Certain drugs (potassium chloride, some antibiotics, vitamin C, NSAIDs, some antipsychotics, and others).

HOW TO PREVENT—No specific preventive measures. Avoid risk factors where possible.

WHAT TO EXPECT

DIAGNOSTIC MEASURES
- Your health care provider will do an exam of the mouth, throat, head, and neck. You may be asked to chew and swallow so the action can be observed.
- Medical tests may be done to find the cause of the dysphagia. These may include blood tests, swallowing studies (endoscopy, esophageal manometry, barium x-ray exam), ultrasound, or CT scan.

APPROPRIATE HEALTH CARE
- Treatment will be provided for the cause of the dysphagia. Specific treatment for the swallowing difficulty may include diet changes and swallowing therapy.
- Hospital care may be needed in severe cases.
- Devices to dilate (widen) the esophagus or surgery may be needed for some disorders.

POSSIBLE COMPLICATIONS
- Dehydration or malnutrition due to not eating or drinking enough to meet the body's needs.
- Aspiration: food or liquid passes through the vocal folds ("going down the wrong way"). The food, liquid, (or vomit) may enter the lungs.

PROBABLE OUTCOME—Most causes are minor and easily treated. Other outcomes will vary depending on the cause.

HOW TO TREAT

GENERAL MEASURES
- Brush teeth twice daily for good oral hygiene.
- For dry mouth, chew gum or suck on lozenge.

MEDICATION—Drugs will be prescribed as needed for an underlying cause.

ACTIVITY
- Swallowing therapy may be prescribed. It can include exercises to strengthen the swallowing muscles or exercises that are done while swallowing.
- Posture changes may help swallowing: tilting or turning the head to one side, tucking the chin in, using a head-back position, or lying on one's side or back. You will be given instructions about using these positions.

DIET—May start with pureed foods, progress to soft food and semi-solids, and to regular diet.

CALL YOUR DOCTOR IF

You or a family member develops swallowing difficulty.

DYSPLASTIC NEVI

GENERAL INFORMATION

DEFINITION—Dysplastic nevi are moles that are atypical. This means they do not have the appearance of common moles. Nevi is another word for moles. Dysplastic nevi can increase the risk for melanoma, a serious type of skin cancer. A large number of dysplastic nevi increases the melanoma risk. The melanoma risk is even higher for a person with dysplastic nevi along with a family history of melanoma. This is called either familial atypical mole/melanoma (FAMM) or dysplastic nevus syndrome.

BODY PARTS INVOLVED—Skin.

SEX OR AGE MOST AFFECTED—Both sexes; late teens and adults.

SIGNS & SYMPTOMS
- Dysplastic nevi begin to appear at puberty.
- Borders are irregular and ill defined.
- Have both flat and elevated areas.
- Are larger than common moles.
- Color may range from tan to dark brown or have other various shades of color within them.
- They can appear anywhere on the body, but most often are found on the back, chest, buttocks, breast, and scalp. They are found in sun-exposed as well as sun-protected areas.
- A person may have one (nevus), or a few, or more than 100 dysplastic nevi. (An average person with common moles has 15 to 20.)

CAUSES—Dysplastic nevi are acquired. A person is not born with them. The exact cause is unknown. Sunlight damage may play a part, but is not always a factor. Dysplastic nevi can appear on the buttocks and female breasts, which are generally covered. The tendency to develop dysplastic nevi does run in families.

RISK INCREASES WITH—Family history of dysplastic nevi or melanoma.

HOW TO PREVENT
- There are no specific preventive measures.
- Routine use of sunscreens may help reduce risks. Use one with an SPF of 15 to 30 or higher and that protects against both ultraviolet A and ultraviolet B radiation. Be sure to read label on how to apply. Avoid tanning beds.
- If you have a family history of dysplastic nevi or skin cancer, get regular medical skin exams to detect any new moles or changes in existing ones. Exams may be as often as every 3 months for high-risk persons.
- Perform routine skin self-exams to check for any changes in skin appearance. Have a family member help check the areas of your body that you cannot see.

WHAT TO EXPECT

DIAGNOSTIC MEASURES
- Your own observation of symptoms.
- Your health care provider will do a physical exam of the skin.
- A biopsy may be done of a nevus (single mole) if skin cancer is suspected. Biopsy involves removing all or a portion of a nevus for viewing under a microscope. If the biopsy shows cancer, the whole nevus is removed.

APPROPRIATE HEALTH CARE
- Other dysplastic nevi may be removed or watched over time to see if they change. Most dysplastic nevi will not develop into melanoma; removing all of them is unnecessary. If the nevi look like melanoma, have changed over time, or are new and look abnormal, then removal may be the recommended treatment.
- In some cases, nevi may be removed because of bleeding, irritation, or they are a cosmetic concern.
- Removal usually involves excision (cutting out) of the nevi. The procedure is done in a medical office while the patient is under a local anesthetic. Sometimes stitches are required. A small scar may remain. If there are numerous nevi to be removed, it may be done over several office visits. Plastic surgery may be needed if the skin area involved is extensive.
- Color photographs may be taken of your body, so that on future office visits any changes can be verified.

POSSIBLE COMPLICATIONS—Melanoma may rarely develop in some cases.

PROBABLE OUTCOME—There is little risk for most people of developing melanoma. For those few at risk, prompt diagnosis and treatment, if needed, can help reduce their risk.

HOW TO TREAT

GENERAL MEASURES—Follow medical instructions for post-treatment care.

MEDICATION—Drugs are not normally needed.

ACTIVITY—Be sure to use sunscreens and protective clothing for any exposure to the sun. Avoid sun exposure between 10 a.m. and 3 p.m., if possible.

DIET—No special diet.

CALL YOUR DOCTOR IF

- You or a family member has nevi (moles) that have changed in appearance or new ones developed and cause concern.
- New nevi appear after treatment.

DYSTHYMIA
(Depression, Low-Grade)

GENERAL INFORMATION

DEFINITION—Dysthymia is a chronic, mild form of depression. The start of dysthymia often goes unnoticed. Many people are not aware of the change in their lives. Symptoms may begin in childhood or in adolescence and go on for years.

BODY PARTS INVOLVED—Nervous system.

SEX OR AGE MOST AFFECTED—Both sexes; late teens, young to middle-age adults. It affects females more than males.

SIGNS & SYMPTOMS
- The depressed mood has occurred for most of each day, for most days, for two years or more (one year for children/teens). There has been no more than two months without some of the symptoms listed and at least two of the symptoms should be present.
- Poor appetite or overeating.
- Sleeping too much or too little.
- Lack of energy; feeling tired all the time.
- Feelings of hopelessness.
- Low self-esteem.
- Trouble with concentration and making decisions.

CAUSES—It appears to be due to an imbalance of certain brain chemicals along with other factors. These can include genetic, developmental, medical problems, coping strategies, and social factors (such as job loss or divorce).

RISK INCREASES WITH
- Family history of depressive illnesses.
- Chronic stress or chronic illness.
- Stressful life events.
- Persons who have other psychiatric disorders.

HOW TO PREVENT—No specific preventive measures. A healthy lifestyle with good nutrition and exercise and having close friends and family and a job you enjoy may help reduce risk.

WHAT TO EXPECT

DIAGNOSTIC MEASURES
- Your own observation of symptoms.
- Your health care provider may do a physical exam, and will ask questions about your symptoms and activities.
- There is no medical test to diagnose dysthymia. Medical tests may be done to rule out other disorders.

APPROPRIATE HEALTH CARE
- Treatment usually includes some form of psychotherapy (counseling) and/or drug therapy.
- Cognitive-behavioral therapy is often recommended. The cognitive part teaches people how to change thoughts, behaviors, or attitudes. The behavior part teaches people ways to reduce anxiety, such as with deep breathing and muscle relaxation.
- Interpersonal therapy can help a patient identify personal relationship problems and how to correct them.
- Psychodynamic therapy resolves emotional conflicts.
- Job counseling may be recommended for some patients to be sure their work suits their temperament.

POSSIBLE COMPLICATIONS
- Dysthymia recurs after treatment.
- Major depression develops.
- Alcohol or substance abuse.
- Problems with school or work (e.g., decreased productivity or job loss).
- Problems and conflicts with personal relationships.
- Risk of suicidal behavior.

PROBABLE OUTCOME—Most people are helped by treatment. It may take several months before symptoms improve. Sometimes it isn't until a patient has been treated and is feeling better that they realize how depressed they were.

HOW TO TREAT

GENERAL MEASURES
- Join a support group. They help many people.
- Try to reduce emotional stress in your life. Learn techniques to cope with stress.
- Avoid alcohol abuse or drug abuse. If you need help stopping, ask your health care provider, or contact a support organization.

MEDICATION—An antidepressant may be prescribed for some patients. The drug will usually be needed for several months or several years. If one antidepressant doesn't work, another type can often help.

ACTIVITY—No limits. A daily exercise program is recommended. It can help improve well-being.

DIET—Eat a normal well-balanced diet.

CALL YOUR DOCTOR IF

- You or a family member has symptoms of dysthymia.
- Symptoms worsen or don't improve over time.
- Suicidal behaviors occur, get emergency help.

EAR INFECTION, MIDDLE
(Otitis Media)

GENERAL INFORMATION

DEFINITION—Middle ear infection is an infection and inflammation (redness and soreness) in the middle ear. The medical term is acute otitis media (AOM). Otitis media with effusion (OME) is fluid in the middle ear, but without the symptoms of infection. It often follows AOM.

BODY PARTS INVOLVED—Middle-ear space where nerves and small bones connect to the eardrum on one side and the eustachian tube on the other side.

SEX OR AGE MOST AFFECTED—Both sexes and all ages, but most common in infants and children ages 3 months to 3 years.

SIGNS & SYMPTOMS
- Earache.
- Feeling of fullness in the ear.
- Hearing may be reduced.
- Child is fussy or irritable.
- Fever.
- Dizziness.
- Discharge or leakage from the ear.
- Diarrhea or vomiting (sometimes).
- Pulling at the ear (small children).

CAUSES—The ear infection is usually caused by bacteria, and less often by a virus. The infection creates a build up of fluid or pus in the middle ear. Middle ear infections often occur after a cold or other illness of the nose or throat.

RISK INCREASES WITH
- Recent illness, such as a cold or sore throat.
- Having asthma, allergies, or previous ear infections.
- Family history of ear infections.
- Being in daycare.
- Winter and spring seasons.
- Being bottle-fed while lying down, and (possibly) use of a pacifier.
- Smoking in the household.
- Use of antibiotic drugs in the past 1 to 3 months.
- Genetic factors. American Indians and Eskimos seem to get more ear infections than is usual.

HOW TO PREVENT
- Bottlefeed or breastfeed infants in a sitting position with head up, never lying down. Breast-feeding reduces chances of child having ear infections.
- No smoking in household.
- Wash hands often to prevent spread of germs that can cause colds, sore throats, or other infections.
- Possibly, a pneumococcal vaccine.

WHAT TO EXPECT

DIAGNOSTIC MEASURES
- Your own observation of symptoms.
- Your health care provider can diagnose a middle ear infection by an exam of the ear.
- Other medical tests are normally not needed.

APPROPRIATE HEALTH CARE
- Treatment may include drugs and other steps to relieve pain. Not all infections need antibiotic treatment.
- If ear infections recur often, surgery may be done to put in plastic tubes through the eardrum to drain pus or fluid from the middle ear. Surgery may also be done to remove the adenoids.
- If the eardrum is bulging, a small cut may be made in it to relieve pressure and pain.

POSSIBLE COMPLICATIONS
- Middle ear infections often recur.
- Chronic otitis media (infection lasts over 6 weeks).
- Rarely, more serious ear problems, hearing loss, brain infection, or other complications may occur.

PROBABLE OUTCOME—The outcome is good in almost all cases.

HOW TO TREAT

GENERAL MEASURES
- Apply heat to the area around the ear to relieve pain. Use a warm washcloth.
- Avoid swimming until the infection clears up.

MEDICATION
- An oral antibiotic may be prescribed for 7 to 10 days. Take the full dose even if symptoms get better. In severe cases, antibiotic injections may be given.
- Ear drops may be prescribed for pain.
- You may use acetaminophen to reduce pain and fever. Do not give aspirin to children.
- Don't use cold remedies, decongestants, or antihistamines. They won't help an ear infection.

ACTIVITY—Reduce activity until healed.

DIET—No special diet.

CALL YOUR DOCTOR IF

- You or your child has symptoms of a middle ear infection.
- The following occur during or after treatment: fever, severe headache, earache that persists longer than 2 days despite treatment, swelling around the ear, twitching of the face muscles, or dizziness.

EAR INFECTION, OUTER
(Otitis Externa; Swimmer's Ear)

 GENERAL INFORMATION

DEFINITION—Outer ear infection is an infection and inflammation of the outer ear and ear canal. The ear canal extends from the eardrum to the outside opening of the ear. The medical term is otitis externa and it is also called swimmer's ear. It is very common.

BODY PARTS INVOLVED—Skin of the ear canal.

SEX OR AGE MOST AFFECTED—Both sexes; all ages.

SIGNS & SYMPTOMS
- Ear pain that worsens when the earlobe is pulled.
- Itching in the ear.
- Slight fever (sometimes).
- Discharge of pus from the ear.
- Temporary loss of hearing on the affected side.
- A small, painful lump or boil in the ear canal.

CAUSES
- Bacterial (most common) or fungal infection of the delicate skin lining of the ear canal. The infection often develops when water is trapped in the ear (such as from swimming).
- Injury to the ear canal.

RISK INCREASES WITH
- Swimming in dirty or polluted water.
- Excess moisture in the ear from any cause.
- Irritation from cotton swabs or metal objects, such as bobby pins.
- Previous ear infections.
- Disorders like diabetes that affect the immune system.
- Use of hair spray or hair dye that may enter the ear canal.

HOW TO PREVENT
- Dry your ears completely after they have become wet.
- Wear ear-plugs when swimming.
- Don't clean your ears with any object.
- If you have had otitis externa, ask your health care provider about keeping the prescribed eardrops on hand. If the ear canals get wet for any reason, such as swimming or shampooing, put drops in both ears at bedtime.

 WHAT TO EXPECT

DIAGNOSTIC MEASURES
- Your own observation of symptoms.
- Your health care provider can diagnose an outer ear infection by an exam of the ear.
- Other medical tests are normally not needed.

APPROPRIATE HEALTH CARE
- Treatment may involve your health care provider cleaning and draining the ear, drug therapy, and other steps to relieve pain.
- Self-care after diagnosis.

POSSIBLE COMPLICATIONS
- Chronic otitis externa. The infection persists or recurs often.
- Spread of infection to bones or cartilage. This is a rare, yet serious complication.

PROBABLE OUTCOME—Usually curable with treatment in 7 to 10 days.

 HOW TO TREAT

GENERAL MEASURES
- Apply heat to the area around the ear to relieve pain. Use a warm washcloth.
- Avoid swimming until the infection clears up.
- Gentle cleaning of the ear canal; remember that a small amount of ear-wax helps protect against infection.
- Keep the infected ear dry. Wear ear-plugs or shower cap for showering.

MEDICATION
- You may use acetaminophen or ibuprofen for minor pain. Don't give aspirin to children.
- Your health care provider may prescribe:
  - Eardrops for bacterial infections and cortisone drugs to help other symptoms. An ear wick may be used that allows the drug to reach the end of the ear canal.
  - Oral antibiotics for severe infection.

ACTIVITY—Resume your normal activities as soon as symptoms improve. Avoid getting water in the ears if possible. If you do, dry ears carefully.

DIET—No special diet.

 CALL YOUR DOCTOR IF

- You or a family member has symptoms of outer ear infection.
- Pain persists, despite treatment.

EARDRUM, RUPTURED
(Tympanic Membrane Perforation)

 GENERAL INFORMATION

DEFINITION—A ruptured eardrum is a hole or tear in the eardrum. The eardrum is involved in hearing.

BODY PARTS INVOLVED—The eardrum which is a thin membrane (called the tympanic membrane) that separates the inner ear from the outer ear.

SEX OR AGE MOST AFFECTED—Both sexes; all ages.

SIGNS & SYMPTOMS
- Sudden pain in the ear.
- Some loss of hearing.
- Bleeding or discharge from the ear (sometimes).
- Ringing in the ear.
- Dizziness.

CAUSES
- An infection of the middle ear. Fluid or pus builds up behind the eardrum and causes it to burst.
- Injury or trauma to the eardrum.

RISK INCREASES WITH
- Using a sharp object to clean the ear or relieve an itch. This can be a cotton swab, hairpin, or paperclip.
- Changes in air pressure due to scuba diving or during an airplane flight.
- A loud noise such as a nearby explosion.
- Injury to the head, such as a skull fracture.
- A blow or hit directly to the ear.
- Middle-ear infection (otitis media).

HOW TO PREVENT
- Don't put any object into the ear canal.
- Get prompt medical treatment for ear infections.

 WHAT TO EXPECT

DIAGNOSTIC MEASURES
- Your own observation of symptoms.
- Your health care provider can diagnose the problem by an exam of the ear.
- Fluid from the ear may be sent to the lab for a medical test.
- A hearing test may be performed.

APPROPRIATE HEALTH CARE
- Treatment may involve drugs to prevent infection and for pain.
- A patch may be used to repair the hole. In this procedure, a chemical is applied to the area to help the healing and a paper patch placed on the eardrum. This may need to be redone a few times until healing is complete.
- Surgery called tympanoplasty may be done to repair the hole if it doesn't heal within 2 months. This can be done in a medical office. Your health care provider will give you instructions for home care after surgery.

POSSIBLE COMPLICATIONS
- Ear infection, with fever, vomiting, and diarrhea.
- Mastoiditis. This is an infection of the mastoid (bony area just behind the ear).
- Permanent hearing loss (rare).

PROBABLE OUTCOME
- The eardrum will usually repair itself in 2 months. If it becomes infected, the infection is curable with treatment. Any hearing loss is usually short term.
- Surgery helps if the eardrum does not heal on its own.

 HOW TO TREAT

GENERAL MEASURES
- Try to avoid blowing your nose. If you must, blow gently.
- Keep the ear as dry as possible. Don't swim. Take baths instead of showers. If you do shower, wear a plastic shower cap and be sure the ear is covered.

MEDICATION
- Antibiotics to prevent or treat infections may be prescribed.
- Pain relievers. For minor pain, you may use nonprescription drugs such as acetaminophen.

ACTIVITY—Resume your normal activities as soon as symptoms improve.

DIET—No special diet.

 CALL YOUR DOCTOR IF

- You or a family member has symptoms of a ruptured eardrum.
- The following occur during treatment:
  - Fever.
  - Pain that persists, despite treatment.
  - Dizziness lasting longer than 12 to 24 hours.

EARWAX BLOCKAGE
(Cerumen Impaction)

 GENERAL INFORMATION

DEFINITION—Earwax blockage is an overproduction of earwax (cerumen), causing blockage of the external ear canal. Wax is produced by glands in the ear to protect the canal leading from the eardrum to the outside. The amount of wax produced varies from person to person. Some produce so little wax that it never accumulates. Others produce enough to block the canal every few months.

BODY PARTS INVOLVED—External ear canal on one or both sides.

SEX OR AGE MOST AFFECTED—Both sexes; all ages.

SIGNS & SYMPTOMS
- Decreased hearing.
- Ear pain.
- Plugged feeling in the ear.
- Ringing in the ear.

CAUSES—Overproduction of wax by glands in the external ear canal.

RISK INCREASES WITH
- Exposure to dust or debris.
- Family history of overproduction of earwax.
- Water in the ear, which can cause the wax to swell.
- Use of cotton swabs in an attempt to clean the ear canal.

HOW TO PREVENT
- Avoid areas where the air is dusty or filled with debris. This stimulates overproduction of earwax. Consider wearing earplugs if you must be in this type of environment.
- Monthly use of 1 to 2 drops of glycerin, olive oil, almond oil, or baby oil in the ear may soften the wax and prevent recurrent blockage.

 WHAT TO EXPECT

DIAGNOSTIC MEASURES
- Your own observation of symptoms.
- If concerned, see your health care provider. An ear exam can confirm the diagnosis.

APPROPRIATE HEALTH CARE
- Self-care. Sometimes wax can be removed easily at home with ear drops and irrigation of the ear canal.
- Medical care if the wax is difficult to remove.

POSSIBLE COMPLICATIONS
- Ear infection.
- Eardrum damage.

PROBABLE OUTCOME—Earwax can be removed, but stubborn cases require patience.

 HOW TO TREAT

GENERAL MEASURES
- Earwax can be removed at home:
- Buy wax-softening ear-drops at a drug store.
- Lie down with the affected ear toward the ceiling.
- Pull the top of the ear gently up and back toward the back of the head.
- Instill the ear-drops as directed by the instructions on the package.
- Leave the drops in the ear for 20 minutes or as directed. Continue to lie down, if possible. Plug the ear with cotton.
- Sit up, leaning a little toward the affected side.
- Use a soft, rubber bulb syringe to irrigate the ear canal gently with plain warm water.
- Repeat irrigations until the ear feels clear. If the ear doesn't clear, call your health care provider, so that wax can be removed using other methods.
- Don't try to remove wax with a stick or cotton swab. You may damage the eardrum or cause infection in the ear canal. Caution—if you have a perforated eardrum, don't try to remove wax; call your health care provider.
- Do not use ear candling (use of a lighted candle in the ear) for wax removal. It is not an effective treatment for removing wax and may cause injury.

MEDICATION—For minor pain, you may use nonprescription drugs such as acetaminophen.

ACTIVITY—No limits.

DIET—No special diet.

 CALL YOUR DOCTOR IF

- You or a family member has symptoms of an earwax blockage that does not clear, despite treatment described above.
- A child younger than 4 has an earwax blockage.
- Fever and ear pain accompany an earwax blockage. Do not irrigate the ear in this case.

ECTOPIC PREGNANCY

GENERAL INFORMATION

DEFINITION—An ectopic pregnancy is one that develops outside the uterus. The most common site is in one of the narrow fallopian tubes that connect each ovary to the uterus. Other sites include the ovary or outside the reproductive organs in the abdominal cavity or the cervix. About 1% to 2% of pregnancies are ectopic.

BODY PARTS INVOLVED—Female reproductive system; abdominal cavity.

SEX OR AGE MOST AFFECTED—Females of childbearing age.

SIGNS & SYMPTOMS
- Early stages:
  - Missed or late menstrual period.
  - Vaginal spotting or bleeding.
  - Pain and cramps in the lower abdomen.
  - Pain in the shoulder (rare).
- Late stages:
  - Sudden, sharp, severe pain in the abdomen.
  - Dizziness, fainting, and shock (paleness, rapid heartbeat, drop in blood pressure, and cold sweats). These may occur before or along with the pain.

CAUSES—An egg from the ovary is fertilized and becomes implanted outside the uterus. This usually occurs in a fallopian tube that has been damaged (resulting in blockage or narrowing). As the fertilized egg enlarges, the fallopian tube may stretch and rupture. This leads to life-threatening internal bleeding.

RISK INCREASES WITH
- Prior abdominal or pelvic infection.
- Pelvic inflammatory disease (PID).
- Pregnancy after a tubal ligation.
- Assisted reproduction techniques, such as in vitro fertilization.
- Adhesions (scar tissue) from prior abdominal surgery.
- Previous ectopic pregnancy.
- Previous tubal or uterine surgery.
- History of endometritis (inflammation of the endometrium, which is the lining of the uterus).
- Endometriosis.
- Malformed (abnormal) uterus.
- Use of an intrauterine device (IUD).
- Smoking.
- History of exposure to diethylstilbestrol (DES).
- Many women diagnosed with an ectopic pregnancy do not have a risk factor.

HOW TO PREVENT—It cannot be prevented.

WHAT TO EXPECT

DIAGNOSTIC MEASURES
- Your own observation of symptoms.

- Medical tests may include blood studies, ultrasound, laparoscopy (a telescope-like tool is used to look inside the abdomen), and other tests as needed.
- Diagnosis and treatment may be done on an outpatient basis. Hospital care may be needed for surgery and supportive care. A blood transfusion may be required.

APPROPRIATE HEALTH CARE
- Before rupture of the tube, a diagnosed ectopic pregnancy may be treated by using the laparoscope instrument or with injected drug.
- Surgery may be needed to remove the developing embryo, placenta, and any damaged tissue. The fallopian tube is removed if it cannot be repaired. Future pregnancy is possible with one fallopian tube.
- Weekly blood tests may be recommended to be sure treatment is successful. If persistent ectopic pregnancy is diagnosed, a drug may be prescribed for treatment.

POSSIBLE COMPLICATIONS
- Internal bleeding that can be life-threatening.
- Reduced fertility.
- Repeat ectopic pregnancy.

PROBABLE OUTCOME—An ectopic pregnancy is always going to be lost. It may resolve on its own before a period is missed. Rupture of an ectopic pregnancy is an emergency. Full recovery is likely with early diagnosis and treatment.

HOW TO TREAT

GENERAL MEASURES
- At home, use heat to relieve pain. Apply a heating pad to the abdomen or back. Warm baths help. Sit in a tub of warm water for 10 to 15 minutes. Repeat as needed.
- Counseling may help with emotional aspects.
- To learn more: www.ectopicpregnancy.org.

MEDICATION
- In some ectopic pregnancies, methotrexate may be prescribed for treatment. Specific guidelines and close follow-up care are needed when this drug is used.
- Post-surgery pain reliever may be prescribed.

ACTIVITY—Your obstetric provider will advise you when to resume normal activities, as well as sexual relations.

DIET—No special diet.

CALL YOUR DOCTOR IF

You or a family member has symptoms of ectopic pregnancy, especially a rupture (this is an emergency).

ECTROPION & ENTROPION

GENERAL INFORMATION

DEFINITION—Ectropion is a disorder of the eyelid in which it turns outward (inside out). Entropion is a disorder of the eyelid (usually the lower) in which it curls inward toward the eye.

BODY PARTS INVOLVED—Eyelids.

SEX OR AGE MOST AFFECTED—Both sexes; all ages, but most often in adults over age 40.

SIGNS & SYMPTOMS
- Ectropion:
  - Turning out of the eyelid, usually the lower.
  - Pain, redness, and swelling in the affected eyelid.
  - Poor eye lubrication, caused when lubricating tears run down the cheek instead of into the eye.
- Entropion:
  - Swelling, redness, pain, and excessive tears of the eye. This is caused by the eyelid turning inward and the lashes rubbing against the cornea.

CAUSES
- Ectropion:
  - Weakening of the muscles and tissues that normally support the lid against the eye.
  - Paralysis of the nerve going to the eyelid muscles.
  - Shrinking of scar tissue from burns, wounds, or surgery near the eye.
- Entropion:
  - Relaxation of the eyelid's supporting tissue along with the inward pull of the eyelid muscles.
  - Chronic eye inflammation (including allergy), creating scar tissue in the eyelid.

RISK INCREASES WITH—Older adults.

HOW TO PREVENT—Cannot be prevented at present.

WHAT TO EXPECT

DIAGNOSTIC MEASURES
- Your own observation of the symptoms.
- Your eye care provider can diagnose either disorder by an exam of the affected eye.

APPROPRIATE HEALTH CARE—Treatment involves minor surgery. See Ectropion Repair and Entropion Repair in Surgery Section.

POSSIBLE COMPLICATIONS
- Ectropion—corneal damage caused by dryness.
- Entropion—blister of the cornea from eyelash and eyelid irritation.

PROBABLE OUTCOME—Usually curable with surgery.

HOW TO TREAT

GENERAL MEASURES
- Apply warm compresses to the eyelids several times a day for swelling and pain. To prepare compresses:
  - Pour warm water into a clean bowl. Soak a clean cloth in the water. Wring it out until it is almost dry.
  - Apply the warm, moist cloth to the closed eye for 10 to 15 minutes. Rewet the cloth frequently.
- Wear protective glasses or goggles if you are exposed to wind or pollutants.

MEDICATION
- Artificial tears may be recommended until surgery can be performed.
- Antibiotics may be prescribed if infection is present.

ACTIVITY—No limits.

DIET—No special diet.

CALL YOUR DOCTOR IF

- You or a family member has symptoms of ectropion or entropion.
- The following occur after surgery:
  - Eye pain, redness, or sensitivity to light.
  - Changes in vision.

ECZEMA, DYSHIDROTIC
(Dyshidrosis; Pompholyx)

 GENERAL INFORMATION

DEFINITION—Dyshidrotic eczema is a skin condition that causes small blisters on the hands or feet. It is a type of dermatitis (inflammation of the skin).

BODY PARTS INVOLVED—Skin.

SEX OR AGE MOST AFFECTED—It affects all ages and women more than men.

SIGNS & SYMPTOMS
- Burning and itching in the hands and feet before the skin breaks out. Small blisters appear. They may be on the tips and sides of fingers, toes, palms, and soles of the feet.
- Blisters are nontransparent and deep; they are either even with the skin, or slightly raised. They don't break easily. Eventually, small blisters come together and form large blisters.
- Hands and feet may be wet with perspiration.
- Blisters may worsen after contact with soap, water, or irritating substances.

CAUSES—Unknown. Excessive sweating is not a cause of this problem, but is often linked with it.

RISK INCREASES WITH
- Women are more often affected than men.
- Family history of dyshidrotic eczema.
- Allergic reactions may play a role.
- Periods of anxiety, stress, anger, and frustration seem to play a role in outbreaks.

HOW TO PREVENT—No specific preventive measures are known.

 WHAT TO EXPECT

DIAGNOSTIC MEASURES
- Your own observation of symptoms.
- Your health care provider can diagnose the condition by an exam of the affected skin area.
- Medical tests are usually not needed, but may be done to confirm the diagnosis.

APPROPRIATE HEALTH CARE
- Treatment involves drugs and self-care measures.

POSSIBLE COMPLICATIONS
- Continued peeling and cracking of the involved skin.
- Bacterial skin infection may occur.

PROBABLE OUTCOME—Outcome varies for different patients. Some recover completely with or without treatment. Others may continue to have symptoms even with treatment.

 HOW TO TREAT

GENERAL MEASURES
- Keep heat and moisture away from the affected areas whenever possible.
- Wear heavy-duty, cotton-lined vinyl gloves when in contact with water, soap, detergent, and other chemicals. Dry insides of gloves after use. Throw away gloves if they develop a hole.
- Wear gloves when you peel or squeeze acid fruits and vegetables.
- Wear leather or heavy-duty fabric gloves for housework or gardening.
- Wear cotton or absorbent socks.
- Remove shoes and socks to allow feet to air.
- Avoid contact with irritating chemicals, such as paint; paint thinner; and polish for cars, floors, shoes, furniture, and metal.
- Use cool, moist compresses to help soothe the affected skin.
- Use lukewarm water and very little mild soap to shower or bathe.
- If emotional stress is a problem, try to identify the cause and find ways to control it. Counseling or learning stress management techniques may help.

MEDICATION
- Steroid creams or ointments are usually prescribed.
- Other topical drugs may be prescribed.
- Antihistamines may be prescribed to ease itching symptoms.
- Additional oral or topical drugs, ultraviolet light therapy, or other therapies may be prescribed.

ACTIVITY—Avoid activities or environments that lead to stress or excessive sweating. Sweating does not cause the disorder, but may aggravate it.

DIET—Usually no limits. In a few cases, a special diet such as low in nickel (avoiding cocoa, chocolate, nuts, whole grains, and other foods) may be recommended.

 CALL YOUR DOCTOR IF

- You or a family member has symptoms of dyshidrotic eczema.
- Signs of infection (swelling, redness, tenderness, or warmth) appear around blisters.
- Symptoms don't improve after 1 week, even with treatment.
- Symptoms recur after treatment.

ELECTRIC SHOCK

GENERAL INFORMATION

DEFINITION—An electric shock is an injury caused by electricity passing through the body.

BODY PARTS INVOLVED—Total body.

SEX OR AGE MOST AFFECTED—Both sexes; all ages.

SIGNS & SYMPTOMS
- Depends on where the current enters the body and the kind of electrical current. The following are the most common.
- Burns at areas of contact. The burns are often deep.
- Heart damage, including cardiac arrest.
- Severe muscle spasms that may cause fractures.
- Breathing paralysis.

CAUSES—Contact with electricity from downed power lines, exposed appliance wires, faulty electrical equipment, lightning strikes, or other electrical sources.

RISK INCREASES WITH
- Standing on wet ground or under a tree during an electrical storm.
- Mishandling of electrical equipment.
- Work involving electrical machinery or lines.

HOW TO PREVENT
- Inspect your house, especially the kitchen, bathroom and workshop, for hazards. Use grounded plugs wherever possible.
- Don't use hair dryers, radios or other electrical products in the bathroom where they can fall into a tub or sink.
- Use safety plugs in empty electrical outlets to prevent children from inserting metal objects.
- Don't try to repair electrical equipment unless you know how.
- Wear protective gloves and clothing for work that involves exposure to electricity.
- Replace worn cords or wiring in your home.
- Use ground fault electrical interrupters when possible.
- Go indoors during electrical storms. Lightning may strike several miles away from actual rainfall.

WHAT TO EXPECT

DIAGNOSTIC MEASURES—Diagnosis is usually obvious from the circumstances. A physical exam and medical tests will be done as needed to check for complications.

APPROPRIATE HEALTH CARE
- Self-care after diagnosis (minor burns only).
- Emergency care with cardiopulmonary resuscitation (CPR) at the time of injury, if the victim is unconscious and not breathing.
- Hospital care (sometimes) for moderate to severe injuries. Care at a special burn center may be needed.
- Fluid replacement is often required to replace lost fluids and electrolytes.
- Severe burns may require surgery and skin grafts.
- Counseling may be recommended for patients with severe burns.

POSSIBLE COMPLICATIONS
- Pneumonia.
- Permanent brain damage.
- Severe burns of the skin and underlying muscle.
- Blood vessel damage that can lead to amputation or other problems.
- Death from heart damage.
- Other medical problems such as kidney failure, muscle damage, or cataracts.

PROBABLE OUTCOME—Depends on the extent of injury. Full recovery is likely if major brain or heart damage does not occur.

HOW TO TREAT

GENERAL MEASURES
- If the victim is touching live electrical wires, shut off the power or remove the wires with a nonmetal object (such as a wooden broomstick) before giving aid. Don't electrocute yourself trying to help someone else.
- If the victim is unconscious and not breathing:
  - Yell for help. Don't leave the victim.
  - Dial 911 (emergency) for an ambulance or medical help. Begin mouth-to-mouth breathing immediately.
  - If there is no heartbeat, give external cardiac massage.
  - Don't stop cardiopulmonary resuscitation (CPR) until help arrives.
- If multiple persons are struck, give CPR first to victims who are not moving (those moving are likely to recover).

MEDICATION—Antibiotics may be prescribed to prevent infections.

ACTIVITY
- No limits, if the shock is mild.
- If the shock is severe, the victim may resume activities gradually as injuries heal.

DIET—Usually, no special diet.

CALL YOUR DOCTOR IF

- You or someone around you receives an electric shock severe enough to cause injury.
- The following occurs during recovery:
  - Irregular heartbeat.
  - Fever or cough with sputum.

EMPHYSEMA

GENERAL INFORMATION

DEFINITION—Emphysema is a chronic, progressive lung disease that leads to reduced lung function. It develops slowly over years. In the early stages, there are often no symptoms. Emphysema and chronic bronchitis together are the two main disorders that comprise COPD (chronic obstructive pulmonary disease).

BODY PARTS INVOLVED—Lungs, and eventually almost all body systems.

SEX OR AGE MOST AFFECTED—Both sexes (men more than women) and older adults.

SIGNS & SYMPTOMS
- Shortness of breath, especially with physical activity. Over time, the shortness of breath becomes constant.
- Ongoing cough (may produce mucus).
- Wheezing; tightness in chest.
- Weight loss, frequent infections (e.g., colds), anxiety, depression, or barrel chest (due to enlarged lungs).

CAUSES—Alveoli (small air sacs) in the lungs become damaged and enlarged. This reduces the normal exchange of oxygen and carbon dioxide. The lungs lose their elastic quality which causes difficulty in exhaling. This leads to over-inflation of the lungs and shallow breathing.

RISK INCREASES WITH
- The main risk factor is cigarette smoking.
- Long-term exposure to lung irritants. These include air pollution (both inside and outside air) and workplace dust or chemicals.
- Inherited alpha 1-antitrypsin (AAT) deficiency.
- Secondhand smoke.
- HIV infection.

HOW TO PREVENT
- Don't smoke. If you do smoke, quit now.
- Avoid lung irritants and secondhand smoke.

WHAT TO EXPECT

DIAGNOSTIC MEASURES
- Your health care provider will do a physical exam. You will be asked questions about your symptoms, activities, and smoking history.
- Medical tests can confirm the diagnosis and the extent of the disease. These may include blood tests, x-rays, CT, and lung function tests.

APPROPRIATE HEALTH CARE
- Treatment goals are to relieve symptoms, slow the disease, and prevent complications.
- Get counseling for depression, anxiety, and other emotional problems.
- Surgery for lung reduction or lung transplant may be considered (rarely).

POSSIBLE COMPLICATIONS
- Infections, failure, or collapse of the lungs.
- Anxiety, panic disorder, and depression.
- Disability. Decreased ability to perform basic daily activities (e.g., caring for self, cooking, or walking).
- Heart disease and other major health problems.

PROBABLE OUTCOME—Cannot be cured. Symptoms can be controlled to slow progress and severity of the disease. The disease shortens life expectancy, but patients live many years with it.

HOW TO TREAT

GENERAL MEASURES
- Don't smoke. Smoking will cause the disease to become worse, despite treatment. Find a way to quit.
- If you work in an area with severe air pollution, do all you can to reduce exposure. Change jobs, if necessary.
- Install air-conditioning and humidity control in your home. Stay inside during air pollution alert.
- Attend a pulmonary rehab program (if available).
- Avoid sudden temperature or humidity changes, loud talking, laughing, crying, or exertion, if these trigger coughing episodes.
- Avoid higher altitudes where the air is thin.
- Raise the foot of the bed with 4 to 5-inch blocks.
- Home oxygen use may be needed.
- To learn more: American Lung Association, 61 Broadway, 6th Floor, New York, NY 10006; (800) 586-4872; website: www.lungusa.org.

MEDICATION
- You may be prescribed:
  - Drugs to relax spasms of bronchial tubes.
  - Steroids to reduce lung inflammation.
  - Antibiotics to fight or prevent infections.
  - Vaccines against flu and pneumonia.
  - Drugs for depression, anxiety, or panic disorder.
  - Intravenous alpha 1-antitrypsin (if deficient).

ACTIVITY—Physical exercises and breathing exercises are usually prescribed. Both are important in improving symptoms.

DIET—Eat a healthy diet. Drink plenty of fluids each day.

CALL YOUR DOCTOR IF

- You or a family member has symptoms of emphysema.
- You have signs of infection (fever, chills, or aches); increased trouble breathing or chest pain; or changes in sputum occur.

EMPYEMA

GENERAL INFORMATION

DEFINITION—Empyema is a collection of pus in a body cavity. It usually occurs in the space around the lungs (pleural cavity).

BODY PARTS INVOLVED—Lungs. It may rarely occur in the gall bladder or the pelvic cavity.

SEX OR AGE MOST AFFECTED—Older adults (men more than women) and young children are more often affected.

SIGNS & SYMPTOMS
- Chest pain. Pain varies from slight discomfort to stabbing pain. It is often worse with coughing or breathing. Pain may extend to the lower chest wall or stomach.
- Rapid, shallow breathing.
- Chills.
- Fever.
- Sweating, especially night sweats.
- Extreme fatigue.
- Dry cough.
- Bad breath.
- Weight loss.

CAUSES
- Usually a complication of pneumonia. Infection causes pus to build up in the pleural cavity. The pus, which can amount to a pint or more, puts pressure on the lungs and causes breathing problems.
- Gallbladder empyema usually results from infection and inflammation.

RISK INCREASES WITH
- Lung or chest infections.
- Chest injury.
- Thoracic surgery.
- Infection from elsewhere in the body that has spread to the lungs.

HOW TO PREVENT—No specific preventive measures.

WHAT TO EXPECT

DIAGNOSTIC MEASURES
- Your own observation of symptoms.
- Your health care provider will do a physical exam and ask questions about your symptoms.
- X-ray, CT, or ultrasound tests may be done of the chest. A sample of the pus may be taken for testing by using a needle inserted through the back into the affected area.

APPROPRIATE HEALTH CARE
- Treatment is done in a hospital and usually involves giving drugs to treat infection and a procedure to drain the pus (fluid).
- The fluid may be drained by using a chest tube or other type of surgery depending on the extent of the infection. The options will be explained to you by the surgeon.

POSSIBLE COMPLICATIONS—Lung failure or severe infection. Complications are more likely in the elderly and very ill.

PROBABLE OUTCOME—Outcome will depend on several factors: severity of the infection, patient's health, any underlying disease, and how effective the treatment is. In otherwise healthy persons, the outcome is generally good.

HOW TO TREAT

GENERAL MEASURES—None specific.

MEDICATION—Antibiotics for infection are given through a vein (IV).

ACTIVITY—Gradually return to normal activity after treatment. Allow 2 months for recovery.

DIET—A special diet may be required while in the hospital. After treatment, resume a normal diet.

CALL YOUR DOCTOR IF

- You or a family member has symptoms of empyema.
- Following treatment, any signs of infection occur, such as fever, chills, aches, or pain.

ENCEPHALITIS, VIRAL

GENERAL INFORMATION

DEFINITION—Viral encephalitis is inflammation of the brain. It can be primary (the virus attacks the brain and spinal cord directly). It can be secondary (virus infects other body tissue and then spreads to the brain).

BODY PARTS INVOLVED—Brain; sometimes meninges (membranes that cover the brain).

SEX OR AGE MOST AFFECTED—It can occur at any age in both sexes, but most often affects the very young or the elderly.

SIGNS & SYMPTOMS
- In some cases, there may be no symptoms or they are mild and flu-like.
- Fever.
- Headache (may be mild to severe).
- Nausea and vomiting.
- In infants, a bulging of the soft spot of the skull.
- Lethargy or lack of energy.
- Stiff neck.
- Drowsiness.
- Eyes are sensitive to light.
- Confusion; behavioral or personality changes.
- Seizures.
- Speech, hearing, or vision problems.
- Muscle weakness or partial paralysis.
- Loss of consciousness; coma in severe cases.

CAUSES—Encephalitis can be caused by one of many types of viruses. In the United States, the most common is the herpes simplex virus (it causes cold sores). It can also be caused by arboviruses (which are transmitted by mosquitoes or ticks), viruses that cause mumps or measles or chickenpox, or the rabies virus (very rare), and others.

RISK INCREASES WITH
- Newborns and infants and adults over 60.
- Weak immune system due to illness or drugs.
- Living in areas with a large mosquito population.

HOW TO PREVENT
- Get medical care for viral infections.
- Take precautions to prevent mosquito bites.
- Get vaccines for mumps, measles, rubella, chickenpox, and the flu.

WHAT TO EXPECT

DIAGNOSTIC MEASURES
- Your own observation of symptoms.
- Your health care provider will do a physical exam and ask questions about your symptoms and activities.
- Medical tests may include studies of blood and spinal fluid, CT, MRI, and electroencephalogram (which records brain waves). A brain biopsy (removal of a small amount of tissue for viewing under a microscope) may be done.

APPROPRIATE HEALTH CARE
- Hospital care is usually needed, especially for severe symptoms. Supportive care will be provided for breathing or heart problems. Fluid and electrolyte levels will be monitored. Steps will be taken to prevent complications.
- If brain function is affected, physical therapy, speech therapy, and behavioral therapy may be recommended.

POSSIBLE COMPLICATIONS
- A very small number of people suffer permanent brain damage that impairs mental or muscle functions.
- Coma and death (rare).

PROBABLE OUTCOME—Mild viral encephalitis may go unnoticed. In other cases, symptoms last 3 to 5 days. Complications from encephalitis are more likely in infants and the elderly. People in other age groups usually recover completely, but it may take up to several months.

HOW TO TREAT

GENERAL MEASURES—The illness can be frightening, both to the patient and to the family. Most hospitals have social workers who are there for your support.

MEDICATION
- Your health care provider may prescribe:
  - Pain relievers for headache or fever.
  - Antiviral drugs for certain viral infections.
  - Drugs to reduce inflammation.
  - Drugs to control seizures if needed.

ACTIVITY—Reduce activity until the pain and fever are gone. Gradually return to normal activity. Allow 2 or more months for complete recovery.

DIET—No special diet. May require fluids given through a vein (IV) while in the hospital.

CALL YOUR DOCTOR IF

- You or a family member has symptoms of encephalitis.
- New, unexplained symptoms develop or symptoms recur after treatment.

ENCOPRESIS

GENERAL INFORMATION

DEFINITION—Encopresis is when a child regularly passes bowel movements (stools) into his or her underpants (or some other inappropriate place). The child is of an age (typically age 4 and over) when children can control their bowel movements. In most children, encopresis is involuntary. The child does not do it on purpose.

BODY PARTS INVOLVED—Bowels.

SEX OR AGE MOST AFFECTED—Both sexes (boys more than girls) of children over age 4.

SIGNS & SYMPTOMS
• Bowel movements in underwear. Sometimes the bowel movements may be on the floor or other places. They usually occur during daytime and rarely at night.
• Not able to control bowel movements.
• Passing large, hard stools that cause pain.
• Secretive behavior about bowel movements.
• Stomach pain or cramps.
• Odor due to stool in child's pants.

CAUSES
• It is often a symptom of chronic constipation.
  - Constipation is often caused by the passage of large, hard, and painful stools. To avoid the pain, a child avoids going to the toilet, which worsens the problem.
  - The longer the stool remains in the colon, the more difficult it is for the child to push out. When the colon becomes too full, soft or liquid stool can leak out.
  - Over time, the child no longer senses the normal urge to have a bowel movement. He or she may pass a bowel movement into the underwear and not be aware of it. They also become unaware of the odor.
• Emotional and developmental issues may be involved.
• In rare cases, a child may have been born with a physical disorder that leads to the problem.

RISK INCREASES WITH
• Boys more often than girls.
• Chronic constipation; painful or difficult stooling.
• Toilet training that may be harsh, too early, or lacking.
• Avoidance of school bathrooms.

HOW TO PREVENT
• Try to prevent chronic constipation. Provide a diet high in fiber with plenty of fruits and vegetables. Use whole-grain products for cereals and breads. Be sure your child drinks enough fluids. Help the child to establish regular bowel habits.
• Get medical advice about toilet training your child and treatment for constipation.

WHAT TO EXPECT

DIAGNOSTIC MEASURES
• Your own observation of symptoms.
• Your child's health care provider will do a physical exam. Questions will be asked about the symptoms and other areas of the child's life.
• Medical tests may be done to check for illness or a physical problem.

APPROPRIATE HEALTH CARE
• Treatment may involve a combination of medical measures and behavioral therapy. Each child is different and will respond to different treatment steps.
• Emptying the bowel may be the first step (with enemas, suppositories, or oral laxatives).
• To help establish regular soft and pain-free bowel movements, daily laxatives are usually recommended. They help the child to pass soft stools without pain.
• Other treatments may include biofeedback and helping the child learn to control the urges and muscles involved in bowel movements.

POSSIBLE COMPLICATIONS—Child may suffer from embarrassment, shame, guilt, and low self-esteem. Parents may feel frustrated and angry.

PROBABLE OUTCOME—Usually curable once the constipation is controlled. Parents need to be patient. It may take several months for the problem to get better. Relapses may occur.

HOW TO TREAT

GENERAL MEASURES
• Set regular times for going to the bathroom. Each day, the child should sit on the toilet for 5 to 10 minutes after breakfast and dinner.
• Behavioral techniques may involve positive reinforcement by rewarding the child for developing regular toilet habits. Don't punish the child for accidents.
• During treatment, keep a record of the child's bowel movements, laxative use, and behavioral rewards. This helps find what steps are working.

MEDICATION—Your child's health care provider will discuss the options for enemas, suppositories, and the different types of laxatives used for treatment.

ACTIVITY—No limits.

DIET—See How to Prevent.

☎ CALL YOUR DOCTOR IF

• Your child has encopresis, and it persists longer than 2 months, despite your efforts.
• Symptoms don't improve despite treatment.

ENDOCARDITIS
(Bacterial Endocarditis; Infective Endocarditis)

GENERAL INFORMATION

DEFINITION—Endocarditis is an infection and inflammation involving the endocardium (the inner lining of the heart chambers). It typically involves the heart valves also. It can develop slowly or suddenly.

BODY PARTS INVOLVED—Heart muscle; heart valves; endocardium.

SEX OR AGE MOST AFFECTED—Both sexes; all ages.

SIGNS & SYMPTOMS
- Fatigue and weakness.
- Recurrent fever, chills, and heavy sweating, especially at night.
- Loss of appetite and weight loss.
- Vague muscle aches and joint pains.
- Headache.
- Blood in the urine.
- Cough; shortness of breath.
- Swelling of the feet, legs, and stomach.
- Fast or irregular heartbeat.
- Red spots on the skin (e.g., fingers and toes).

CAUSES—An infection (usually bacterial, sometimes fungal) that enters the bloodstream and infects the heart valves. The infection may start with a skin disorder or injury, a medical or dental procedure, or a skin prick (as with an IV drug user).

RISK INCREASES WITH
- History of endocarditis or rheumatic heart disease.
- Congenital (being born with) heart disease.
- IV (intravenous) drug abuse.
- Heart valve problems.
- Weak immune system due to illness or drugs
- Artificial heart valves or other artificial devices in the heart, such as a pacemaker wire.

HOW TO PREVENT
- If you have heart-valve damage or a heart murmur, ask about antibiotic use before medical procedures that may bring bacteria into the blood. These include dental work, childbirth, and some surgeries.
- Once you have had endocarditis, follow your health care provider's advice to prevent relapse.
- Don't abuse IV drugs.

WHAT TO EXPECT

DIAGNOSTIC MEASURES
- Your health care provider will do a physical exam and ask questions about your symptoms.
- Medical tests may include blood studies, echocardiogram and electrocardiogram (heart function tests), x-rays, and CT.

APPROPRIATE HEALTH CARE
- Treatment usually involves drugs for the infection, supportive care for symptoms, and steps to prevent complications.
- Hospital care is normally needed during acute phase. Once stable, some patients can continue with treatment at home.
- Surgery may be done to replace an infected heart valve in some patients.
- IV drug abusers may require special medical care and should receive drug abuse counseling.

POSSIBLE COMPLICATIONS
- Heart problems, including heart attack, congestive heart failure, arrhythmias, and others.
- Blood clots may break off and travel to other places in the body, such as the brain or kidneys.

PROBABLE OUTCOME—Usually curable with early diagnosis and treatment. Recovery can take weeks. If untreated, or if treatment is delayed, heart function declines resulting in serious complications.

HOW TO TREAT

GENERAL MEASURES
- If you have damaged heart valves, tell any doctor or dentist who treats you.
- Ongoing dental hygiene is important to prevent infection.
- Wear or carry medical ID that shows your medical problem. Carry a wallet card listing the antibiotic regimens needed for medical and dental procedures.

MEDICATION—Antibiotics (for a bacterial infection) will be prescribed. They are normally needed for 2 to 6 weeks. Antibiotic treatment is often given through a vein (IV), but in some cases may be taken orally.

ACTIVITY
- Rest in bed until fully recovered. While in bed, move your legs often to help prevent clots from forming in deep veins.
- Resume your normal activities, including sexual relations, when strength allows or upon medical advice.

DIET—No special diet.

CALL YOUR DOCTOR IF

- You or a family member has symptoms of endocarditis.
- The following occur during or after treatment:
  - Weight gain without diet changes.
  - Blood in the urine.
  - Chest pain or shortness of breath.
  - Sudden weakness or numbness in muscles.

ENDOMETRIAL HYPERPLASIA
(Adenomatous Hyperplasia of the Uterus)

GENERAL INFORMATION

DEFINITION
- Endometrial hyperplasia is an excess growth of tissue in the endometrium (inner lining of the uterus). It is not cancerous, but some hyperplasia is known to be precancerous (called atypia). Types of hyperplasia include:
  - Simple or complex (adenomatous) hyperplasia without atypia.
  - Simple or complex (adenomatous) hyperplasia with atypia.

BODY PARTS INVOLVED—Endometrium.

SEX OR AGE MOST AFFECTED—Women nearing, or have reached, menopause.

SIGNS & SYMPTOMS
- Abnormal vaginal bleeding.
- Bleeding between normal menstrual periods.
- Heavy menstrual flow.

CAUSES—Excess estrogen (a female hormone) as compared with the amount of progesterone (another female hormone). This excess is caused internally, or from the use of hormone-containing drugs. Tamoxifen, a drug for breast cancer, is a risk factor for hyperplasia.

RISK INCREASES WITH
- Estrogen replacement therapy without progestin use.
- Diabetes.
- Obesity (25 or more pounds overweight).
- Women in the years around menopause.
- Polycystic ovary syndrome.
- Women with irregular or no menstrual periods.

HOW TO PREVENT
- If taking estrogen, take progesterone also.
- Weight loss, if obesity is a problem.
- Birth control pills (oral contraceptives) contain estrogen and a form of progesterone. They may help protect against endometrial hyperplasia in women who do not have regular periods.

WHAT TO EXPECT

DIAGNOSTIC MEASURES
- Your own observation of symptoms.
- Your health care provider will do a physical exam and a pelvic exam.
- Medical tests may include blood tests of hormone levels and Pap smear. A vaginal ultrasound, an endometrial biopsy, a D & C (dilatation and curettage) procedure, or a hysteroscopy (use of a telescopic instrument inserted through the vagina to look inside the uterus) may be done. They are used to diagnose the type of hyperplasia and to rule out cancer.

APPROPRIATE HEALTH CARE
- Treatment will be based on findings from the medical tests, your age, and desires about future pregnancy.
- Drugs are normally the first step in treatment. They will cause the lining to shed and prevent it from building up again. This will show up as vaginal bleeding or a menstrual period.
- For some women, a hysterectomy (surgery to remove the uterus) is recommended. It may help when hormone therapy has failed and precancerous cells are discovered.

POSSIBLE COMPLICATIONS
- Without treatment, women who have hyperplasia with atypia have a higher risk for endometrial cancer.
- Excessive, uncontrolled bleeding.

PROBABLE OUTCOME
- In most cases, hormonal treatment with progesterone (progestin) will reverse the hyperplasia caused by the excess estrogen.
- In other cases, it is often curable with D & C (dilatation and curettage) or a hysterectomy. If a woman chooses not to have surgery, hormone therapy usually controls symptoms.

HOW TO TREAT

GENERAL MEASURES
- Long-term follow-up with your health care provider will be required to help avoid a recurrence. Periodic endometrial biopsies, and possibly other tests, will be used to watch for complications of this condition.
- Use heat to relieve pain. Place a heating pad on your abdomen or back. Take warm baths.

MEDICATION—Progesterone (progestin), a female hormone, may be prescribed. It may be given by mouth or a skin patch.

ACTIVITY—No limits unless you have surgery. Then resume your activities gradually. You may resume sexual relations once medical approval is given.

DIET—Usually, no special diet is required. If you are overweight, losing weight might help decrease estrogen in the body.

CALL YOUR DOCTOR IF

- You or a family member has symptoms of endometrial hyperplasia.
- Any unexpected symptoms occur with treatment.

ENDOMETRIOSIS

GENERAL INFORMATION

DEFINITION—The inner lining of the uterus (called the endometrium) is made up of endometrial tissue. This tissue normally builds up during the menstrual cycle. It is then shed each month during the normal menstrual period. Endometriosis occurs when this tissue grows outside the uterus in places such as the fallopian tubes or the ovaries. Rarely, the tissue may grow in other areas of the body. There may be no symptoms.

BODY PARTS INVOLVED—Uterus; ovaries; fallopian tubes; outer layer of the intestines.

SEX OR AGE MOST AFFECTED—Females between puberty and menopause. The average age is between 25 to 29.

SIGNS & SYMPTOMS
- Symptoms may be sudden or develop over years.
- Pelvic pain that may occur at anytime. It may increase during menstrual periods, especially the last days.
- Pain with sexual intercourse.
- Premenstrual spotting, blood in the urine, or blood in the stool (sometimes).
- Back pain.
- Infertility.

CAUSES
- Unknown. Different theories exist and include:
  - Menstrual tissue spreads through the fallopian tubes into the abdomen, where it implants and grows.
  - Genetic, or certain families have risk factors.
  - It is an autoimmune disorder.
  - Endometrial cells spread via blood or lymph vessels.
  - Cells in the abdomen change into endometrial cells.
  - Environmental factors may be involved.

RISK INCREASES WITH
- Never giving birth or delaying childbirth.
- Women with family history of endometriosis.
- Medical disorder involving cervix or vagina.

HOW TO PREVENT—Unable to prevent.

WHAT TO EXPECT

DIAGNOSTIC MEASURES
- Your own observation of symptoms.
- Your health care provider will do a physical exam and a pelvic exam.
- Medical tests may include laparoscopy. A thin, lighted tube (called a laparoscope) is inserted through a small incision (cut) in the abdomen to view internal organs and to sometimes remove tissue. Open surgery (laparotomy) may be needed for diagnosis.

APPROPRIATE HEALTH CARE
- Treatment may include drug therapy, surgery, or both. Alternative treatments (such as acupuncture) may help. Treatment will vary depending on the severity of the disease and the patient's age and desire for pregnancy. A patient may desire pregnancy now, at a later time, or not at all.
- Different procedures are used for treatment. The options will be explained to you. A hysterectomy may be suggested for women who do not desire pregnancy.

POSSIBLE COMPLICATIONS
- Infertility.
- Severe pain that causes depression, stress, and problems with daily living activities.
- Adhesions (scar tissue) of pelvic organs.
- Endometriosis can recur after treatment.
- Cysts and pelvic masses called endometriomas.
- An increased risk of cancer is a possibility.

PROBABLE OUTCOME—It is an ongoing, long-term disorder that may get worse until menopause (when it usually stops). Symptoms can be relieved with treatment. Women with severe disease may have less success with treatment. The ability to become pregnant depends on factors such as severity of the disorder and success of treatment.

HOW TO TREAT

GENERAL MEASURES
- Use a heating pad or take warm baths to relieve pain. Cold therapy may help (use ice packs on the abdomen). Put a pillow under your knees when you rest or sleep.
- To learn more: Endometriosis Association, 8585 N. 76th Place, Milwaukee, WI 53223; (800) 992-3636; website: www.endometriosisassn.org.

MEDICATION
- You may use nonprescription drugs, such as nonsteroidal anti-inflammatory drugs, for pain.
- Stronger pain relievers may be prescribed.
- Hormonal drugs to stop ovulation may be prescribed.

ACTIVITY
- Exercise, such as walking, helps relieve pain.
- You may be taught to do Kegel exercises to help strengthen the pelvic floor muscles.

DIET—Some women have pain relief with diet changes. Ask your health care provider.

CALL YOUR DOCTOR IF

- You or a family member has symptoms of endometriosis.
- Severe pain occurs, or other symptoms recur.

EPIDERMOID CYST
(Sebaceous Cyst)

 GENERAL INFORMATION

DEFINITION—An epidermoid cyst is a closed sac beneath the skin filled with a thick, yellow substance called keratin. The cysts are typically benign and may occur along with acne.

BODY PARTS INVOLVED—Skin of the trunk, face, neck, and scalp.

SEX OR AGE MOST AFFECTED—Both sexes; all ages (most common in teens and adults).

SIGNS & SYMPTOMS
- The cyst has sloped sides or is dome-shaped, is firm, and has a smooth surface. It normally does not hurt.
- The cyst is whitish or skin-colored.
- If the cyst becomes injured or infected, it may become bright red, painful, and swollen.

CAUSES—Cysts likely form from several different mechanisms involving the skin cells. Blocked hair follicles, injury, and genetics may play a role.

RISK INCREASES WITH—No specific risk factors.

HOW TO PREVENT—Cannot be prevented at present.

 WHAT TO EXPECT

DIAGNOSTIC MEASURES
- Your own observation of symptoms.
- Your health care provider will diagnose the cyst based on its appearance.

APPROPRIATE HEALTH CARE
- If needed, cysts can be removed through a simple incision in the skin lying over the cyst. The sac is removed and the incision closed with stitches. If the entire cyst wall is removed, it should not recur.
- For infected cysts, an incision may be needed to drain the pus.

POSSIBLE COMPLICATIONS
- Infection of a cyst can turn into an abscess (be filled with pus).
- Cysts can recur after treatment.

PROBABLE OUTCOME—Most cysts do not cause symptoms and do not require any medical treatment. Some may disappear on their own.

 HOW TO TREAT

GENERAL MEASURES—Sometimes cysts can be irritated by clothes rubbing against them or by shaving. Cysts that are causing problems, are infected, or are injured can be treated.

MEDICATION
- Drugs are usually not necessary for this disorder.
- If a cyst becomes infected, antibiotics may be prescribed.
- For some small infected cysts, treatment may include an injection of a steroid drug.

ACTIVITY—No limits.

DIET—No special diet.

 CALL YOUR DOCTOR IF

- You or a family member has new skin growths or there is a change in any existing skin growth.
- After treatment, the treated skin becomes hot, red, and painful.
- The treated area does not appear to be healing well within one week.

EPIDIDYMITIS

GENERAL INFORMATION

DEFINITION—Epididymitis is inflammation of the epididymis. The epididymis is a long, tightly coiled tube located at the top of each testicle. It stores and carries sperm to the penis. Epididymitis may affect one or both testicles. It may be acute or chronic (lasts for 6 weeks or more).

BODY PARTS INVOLVED—Epididymis.

SEX OR AGE MOST AFFECTED—All ages, but often affects men ages 19 to 35.

SIGNS & SYMPTOMS
- Pain, heat, redness, and swelling at the back or top of one testicle (sometimes both).
- Fever and chills.
- Urinary urge, frequency, burning, or pain.
- Discharge from the penis (sometimes).
- Painful ejaculation.

CAUSES
- The most common cause is a bacterial infection. Germs can spread from the urethra or bladder through the vas deferens to the epididymis. The bacterial infection is often due to a sexually transmitted disease (STD).
- Other causes may be a viral infection (more often in children), certain drugs (e.g., amiodarone, a heart drug), tuberculosis, injury, or other medical disorders. Sometimes, no cause is found.

RISK INCREASES WITH
- Recent urethral or urinary tract infection.
- Abnormalities or recent surgery involving the genitals or urinary tract.
- Unsafe sexual practices that lead to STDs.
- Catheter (use of a tube to carry urine from the body).
- Strenuous physical activity, bicycle or motorcycle riding, or prolonged periods of sitting (e.g., at work or travel).
- Prostate problems.

HOW TO PREVENT
- Practice safe sex or abstain from sexual activity.
- Avoid risk factors where possible.

WHAT TO EXPECT

DIAGNOSTIC MEASURES
- Your own observation of symptoms.
- Your health care provider will do an exam of the genitals.
- Medical tests include urine or discharge studies to check for bacteria or sexually transmitted diseases. Blood studies, ultrasound, and other tests may be done.

APPROPRIATE HEALTH CARE
- The goal of treatment is to cure the infection and reduce pain and swelling. Treatment can usually be done at home with rest, drugs, and self-care.
- Surgery may be recommended in cases of blockage or narrowing of the urethra, or for an abscess.

POSSIBLE COMPLICATIONS
- Abscess (pus-filled area).
- May rarely impair fertility.
- The disorder may become chronic.
- Atrophy (shrinking) of the testicle.

PROBABLE OUTCOME—Usually curable with treatment. Pain often goes away in 1 to 3 days. Complete healing may take several weeks.

HOW TO TREAT

GENERAL MEASURES
- While sitting, support the weight of the scrotum and tender testicles. Roll a soft bath towel and place it or a pillow between the legs under the inflamed area.
- Apply an ice bag (wrapped in a cloth) to the inflamed parts to help reduce swelling and relieve pain. Do this for 10 to 15 minutes at a time several times a day. Don't use heat.
- Wear an athletic supporter or two pairs of athletic briefs when you return to normal activity.

MEDICATION
- Antibiotics will be prescribed for infection. They may be given by injection or taken orally. Sexual partners often require treatment also.
- Use ibuprofen or naproxen for mild pain and inflammation. Stronger drugs may be prescribed for more severe pain.

ACTIVITY—Rest in bed until fever, pain, and swelling improve. Avoid sexual intercourse until your health care provider determines the treatment is complete.

DIET—No special diet.

CALL YOUR DOCTOR IF

- You or a family member has symptoms of epididymitis.
- Pain is not relieved by treatment.
- You develop severe scrotal pain, urinary pain or a discharge, fever, chills, or you become constipated.

EPIGLOTTITIS

GENERAL INFORMATION

DEFINITION—Epiglottitis is a rare, life-threatening inflammation of the epiglottis. The epiglottis is a small flap of tissue in the back of the throat that keeps food and drink from going into the windpipe (trachea). Immediate treatment is needed as swelling of the epiglottis may lead to complete blockage of the airway within 12 hours of onset.

BODY PARTS INVOLVED—Epiglottis and surrounding tissue.

SEX OR AGE MOST AFFECTED—It is more common in young children (ages 2 to 4) and boys more than girls. It can occur in adults as well.

SIGNS & SYMPTOMS
- Muffled voice or cry.
- Sore throat.
- Fever.
- Swallowing is difficult and painful.
- Hoarseness.
- Drooling caused by difficulty in swallowing saliva.
- Increased breathing difficulty.
- Noisy, high-pitched, squeaky inhalations.
- Odd head posture. The person tilts the neck back and leans forward with the tongue stuck out and the nostrils flared, trying to inhale more air.

CAUSES
- In children, the cause is usually a bacterial infection. Types include *Haemophilus influenzae* type B (Hib), *Streptococcus pneumonia*, and others. The number of cases of epiglottitis has decreased steadily in the United States since the *Haemophilus influenzae* type B (Hib) vaccine became a routine childhood immunization in the late 1980s.
- In adults, it can be caused by bacterial, viral, or combined viral-bacterial infections.
- Other causes include thermal (heat) injury (e.g., from drinking hot liquids).

RISK INCREASES WITH
- Lack of childhood Hib immunization.
- Weak immune system due to illness or drugs.

HOW TO PREVENT—Immunize children and others who have weak immune systems against *Haemophilus influenzae*.

WHAT TO EXPECT

DIAGNOSTIC MEASURES
- Your own observation of symptoms.
- Hospital care is needed. Your health care provider will perform exams under special controls to prevent complications.
- Treatment usually involves supportive care, drug therapy, and supplemental oxygen to help breathing.
- A tube may be inserted in the throat to assist breathing (intubation). Surgery may be done to make an opening in the windpipe (trachea). Usually the tube is withdrawn or the opening is closed in 1 to 3 days.

APPROPRIATE HEALTH CARE—Intensive care will be provided. A tube may be inserted in the throat to assist breathing (intubation). Surgery may be done to make an opening in the windpipe (trachea). Usually the tube is withdrawn or the opening is closed in 1 to 3 days.

POSSIBLE COMPLICATIONS
- Spread of infection to elsewhere in the body.
- Without treatment, complete airway obstruction and death can occur within hours.

PROBABLE OUTCOME—Full recovery with prompt diagnosis and treatment.

HOW TO TREAT

GENERAL MEASURES—Follow medical advice.

MEDICATION
- Antibiotics will be prescribed for infection. Continue for a minimum of 10 days or as advised.
- Steroid drugs may be given to reduce inflammation.

ACTIVITY—Bed rest is needed until all symptoms disappear. Activities may then be resumed gradually.

DIET—Fluids only (usually through a vein) until the patient can swallow. Once the patient is home, return to a normal diet.

CALL YOUR DOCTOR IF

- You or a family member has symptoms of epiglottitis, especially breathing difficulty. Call 911 or go to a hospital. This is an emergency.
  - Don't try to look at the person's throat yourself.
  - Keep the person upright and quiet.

EPILEPSY
(Seizure Disorder)

GENERAL INFORMATION

DEFINITION—Epilepsy is a brain disorder involving recurrent seizures of all types. Seizures are episodes of disturbed brain function that cause changes in attention and/or behavior. The two main categories of seizures are generalized seizures (the whole brain is involved) and partial seizures (a limited area of the brain is involved). Each category has different seizure types.

BODY PARTS INVOLVED—Nervous system.

SEX OR AGE MOST AFFECTED—Epilepsy affects both sexes and all ages. It often begins between ages 2 and 14.

SIGNS & SYMPTOMS
- Generalized seizures types:
  - Tonic-clonic (grand mal)—complete loss of consciousness, falling, jerking movements, urine loss.
  - Absence (petit mal)—brief loss of consciousness.
  - Myoclonic—brief jerking movements.
  - Atonic—abrupt loss of muscle tone (can lead to falls).
- Partial seizures types:
  - Simple partial—stays conscious; weakness, numbness, unusual smells or tastes, muscle twitching, turning head to side, visual changes, or vertigo may occur.
  - Complex partial—altered consciousness, automatic repetitive behavior, uncontrolled laughing, unusual thoughts, hallucinations, fears, or smells odd odors.

CAUSES—Abnormal changes in how the cells in the brain send signals to each other. The causes are often unknown.

RISK INCREASES WITH
- Family history of seizure disorders.
- Head injury (such as from accidents).
- Stroke and other vascular diseases.
- Brain infection (e.g., meningitis) or brain tumor.
- Prolonged seizures in childhood due to high fevers.

HOW TO PREVENT—No specific preventive measures.

WHAT TO EXPECT

DIAGNOSTIC MEASURES
- Your own observation of symptoms.
- Your health care provider will do a physical exam.
- Medical tests usually include blood studies; one or more types of brain scans; and electroencephalogram (EEG), a study of the brain's electrical activity.

APPROPRIATE HEALTH CARE
- Treatment for epilepsy usually involves drug therapy.
- Vagus nerve stimulation may be an option. A device implanted in the neck provides mild electrical stimulation to the vagus nerve to help control seizures.
- Surgery may be helpful in a few cases. An area of the brain causing seizures may be removed, or certain nerve pathways in the brain may be interrupted.

POSSIBLE COMPLICATIONS
- Seizures continue despite treatment.
- Risk of injury if seizure occurs while driving, using equipment, swimming, or other activity.
- For some patients, epilepsy carries a stigma. It can lead to emotional problems, difficulty in social and family relationships, and problems in finding employment.
- Status epilepticus (a prolonged seizure state).
- Sudden, unexpected death (rare).

PROBABLE OUTCOME—There is no cure. Treatment prevents most seizures and allows a near-normal life.

HOW TO TREAT

GENERAL MEASURES
- Seizures may result from too little sleep, stress, not taking your drugs, menstrual periods, or flashing lights.
- Wear or carry medical ID that shows you have epilepsy (in case you have a seizure).
- To learn more: Epilepsy Foundation of America, 8301 Professional Dr., Landover, MD 20785; (800) 332-1000; website: www.efa.org.

MEDICATION—Anticonvulsant drugs will usually be prescribed. Dosage changes are often needed. If a person is seizure-free for 2 or more years, drug withdrawal may be an option.

ACTIVITY—No limits usually. Most states allow persons with epilepsy to drive a vehicle after being seizure-free for 1 year.

DIET
- Usually no special diet. Avoid alcohol.
- Ketogenic diet may be an option for some.

CALL YOUR DOCTOR IF

- You or a family member has symptoms of epilepsy.
- Drugs used in treatment produce unusual side effects.
- The pattern of seizure activity changes.
- Call 911 (emergency) if the seizure is prolonged, or other symptoms occur that require emergency care.

ERECTILE DYSFUNCTION
(Impotence)

 GENERAL INFORMATION

DEFINITION—Erectile dysfunction (ED) is the consistent inability to get or keep an erection as needed for sexual intercourse. Sexual drive and the ability to have an orgasm may not be affected. ED affects millions of men and can occur at any age. It is not a normal part of aging (though arousal may take longer).

BODY PARTS INVOLVED—Male reproductive system; central nervous system.

SEX OR AGE MOST AFFECTED—Male adults and adolescents; more common over age 45.

SIGNS & SYMPTOMS—Repeated inability or inconsistent ability to achieve an erection or inability to sustain an erection.

CAUSES—An erection requires a sequence of events. It starts with sexual stimulation in the brain, which sends nerve signals to the arteries and muscles of the penis. The penis fills with blood and grows firm and erect. After the stimulation ends, or ejaculation occurs, the blood leaves the penis, and it softens again. In erectile dysfunction, the sequence of events is disrupted. It can be due to physical (most often) or psychological (mental or emotional) factors.

RISK INCREASES WITH
- Physical factors may include:
  - Diabetes, endocrine, liver, or kidney disorder.
  - Atherosclerosis (hardening of the arteries), heart or blood vessel disease, or high blood pressure.
  - Some drugs (e.g., for high blood pressure).
  - Disorders or injuries of the central nervous system.
  - Alcoholism, smoking, or drugs of abuse.
  - Reduced blood flow to penis from any cause.
  - Surgery (such as for heart or blood vessels).
  - Prostate cancer treatment.
  - Hormone imbalance or deficiency.
- Psychological factors may include:
  - Fear of sexual failure or performance anxiety, low self-esteem, or lack of interest in sex.
  - Relationship problems with sexual partner.
  - Depression, anxiety, stress, anger, and guilt.
  - Fear of disease (e.g., sexual) or heart attack.
  - Other people are around.

HOW TO PREVENT
- No specific measures. General steps are listed.
- Maintain good health and proper weight.
- Avoid the risk factors where possible.
- Control any medical disorder such as diabetes.
- Ask about side effects before taking new drug.
- Have open communication with your sexual partner.
- Try to avoid worrying about sexual performance.

 WHAT TO EXPECT

DIAGNOSTIC MEASURES
- Your health care provider will do a physical exam and ask questions about your sexual history.
- Medical tests may be done to diagnose any underlying disorder.

APPROPRIATE HEALTH CARE
- Treatment steps may involve lifestyle changes, therapy for any illness diagnosed, erectile dysfunction drugs or devices, counseling, and surgery.
- Lifestyle changes may include cutting back on alcohol, smoking, or drug abuse. Reducing stress, diet changes, and increased exercise may be recommended.
- Counseling can help. It may be for emotional problems (such as stress, anxiety, or guilt). Counseling may involve a sex therapist for you and your partner.
- Use of a vacuum inflation device is an option.
- Surgery for an inflatable or non-inflatable penile implant may help if other methods fail.
- Surgery to improve blood flow to the penis may be an option if there are blood vessel problems.

POSSIBLE COMPLICATIONS
- Reduced quality of life for man and partner.
- Depression, anxiety, and low self-esteem.

PROBABLE OUTCOME—It is treatable in all age groups. Near normal sexual activity can often be achieved with treatment.

 HOW TO TREAT

GENERAL MEASURES
- Stop smoking.
- Find ways to enjoy non-sexual and sexual activities without intercourse with your partner.

MEDICATION
- Drugs for erectile dysfunction (taken by mouth, self-injected, or by suppository) are often prescribed. Follow instructions provided.
- If a drug you take is the cause, a change in drugs or a dosage change may be made.
- Drugs may be prescribed for an underlying disorder.

ACTIVITY—No limits. Exercise daily for health.

DIET—Eat a healthy diet. Limit alcohol use.

 CALL YOUR DOCTOR IF

- You or a family member has erectile dysfunction.
- Treatment is not helping erectile dysfunction.

ERYTHEMA INFECTIOSUM
(Fifth Disease)

 GENERAL INFORMATION

DEFINITION—Erythema infectiosum is an infectious, mild, viral illness that occurs in outbreaks (often during the winter and spring months). The word erythema means skin redness, and infectiosum means infectious. The name fifth disease comes from its place on a list made up many years ago of the five most common childhood infections.

BODY PARTS INVOLVED—Skin and body as a whole.

SEX OR AGE MOST AFFECTED—It most often affects children ages 5 to 14, and is rare in infants and adults.

SIGNS & SYMPTOMS
- The illness begins with a headache, stuffy or runny nose, and sometimes, a low-grade fever and feeling of fatigue. These symptoms may get better.
- From 3 to 10 days later, a rash appears. It is called "slapped cheeks appearance" because it starts as a rash on the cheeks. The rash spreads to the trunk, buttocks, and limbs. It has a lace-like pattern, and it may be itchy.
- Rarely, other symptoms may occur such as sore throat, red eyes, diarrhea, and swollen glands.
- In adults, there may be mild joint pain or swelling.
- About 20% of infected people will have no symptoms.

CAUSES—A virus called parvovirus B-19. The germs come from fluids in the nose, mouth, and throat of someone who has the infection. When an infected person coughs or sneezes, the germs are spread into the air. The period of time from exposure to the germs until symptoms begin is 4 to 28 days with an average of 16 to 17 days. Once the rash appears, the germs are no longer being spread.

RISK INCREASES WITH—Children in school and daycare centers.

HOW TO PREVENT
- No specific preventive measures. Outbreaks can last for months, so there is no need to keep a child out of school or daycare.
- A pregnant woman should avoid daycare centers and schools if there is an outbreak.
- Wash hands often to prevent spread of any germs.

 WHAT TO EXPECT

DIAGNOSTIC MEASURES
- Your own observation of the symptoms.
- Call your health care provider if you have concerns about the symptoms, or if you or a child has a chronic illness. Pregnant women should call their obstetric provider if they have been exposed or if they have any symptoms of the illness.
- Your health care provider will examine the skin rash to diagnose the infection.
- In a few cases, a blood test is done to confirm the diagnosis.

APPROPRIATE HEALTH CARE—Home care is usually all that is needed for treatment.

POSSIBLE COMPLICATIONS
- None expected in most cases. In patients with disorders such as sickle-cell anemia or a weak immune (body's germ-fighting) system, the illness can cause a serious anemic reaction.
- In pregnant women there is a small risk of miscarriage if the infection occurs during the first 20 weeks of pregnancy. There is no evidence that it causes birth defects.

PROBABLE OUTCOME—Complete recovery. The rash usually clears in 10 days to 2 weeks. Once you have had the infection, you are immune (you cannot get it again).

 HOW TO TREAT

GENERAL MEASURES
- For home care, use Aveeno (an oatmeal bath product) for a cool, soaking bath. This can help with the itching.
- The rash may become redder, or it may come back again after it seemed to clear up, after spending time in the sun, taking a warm bath, getting excited, or exercising. This is no cause for concern.

MEDICATION
- There are no drugs for treating the illness. You may use acetaminophen for fever. Don't give a child younger than 18 aspirin for fever.
- If the rash itches, use plain calamine lotion.
- Your health care provider may prescribe other drugs.

ACTIVITY—No limits usually. If needed, get extra rest during the illness. Use sun protection when outdoors.

DIET—No special diet. Drink plenty of fluids.

 CALL YOUR DOCTOR IF

- If you or your child has symptoms of erythema infectiosum and you have concerns.
- Symptoms don't improve or worsen.
- You are pregnant and have been exposed to erythema infectiosum.

ERYTHEMA MULTIFORME

GENERAL INFORMATION

DEFINITION—Erythema multiforme is an inflammatory disorder of the skin and, sometimes, the mucous membranes (thin, moist linings of body cavities). It is called erythema multiforme minor (80% of the cases) when only the skin is involved. It is called erythema multiforme major when the mucous membranes are also involved. More severe forms of the disorder are Stevens-Johnson syndrome and toxic epidermal necrolysis.

BODY PARTS INVOLVED—Skin and mucous membranes (thin, moist linings of body cavities).

SEX OR AGE MOST AFFECTED—Erythema multiforme affects children and teens, as well as adults of both sexes.

SIGNS & SYMPTOMS
- Rash spots that are red and evenly shaped. They often appear in rings like bull's-eyes.
- Rash usually appears on palms, soles, and other areas of arms and legs. It may spread to the face and the rest of the body.
- Rash is sometimes painful, may have burning sensation, and is usually not itchy.
- Rash develops into blisters, hives, or becomes ulcerated (open sores).
- With erythema multiforme major, the mucous membranes of the mouth, eyes, and genitals may become inflamed. Fever, headache, sore throat, or diarrhea may also occur.

CAUSES—It is thought to be an immune response. The most common cause is a preceding herpes simplex virus (the same virus that causes cold sores). It is less often caused by drug reactions, cancer, radiation, other viruses, or bacteria. Sometimes, no cause is found.

RISK INCREASES WITH
- Previous history of erythema multiforme.
- Drugs such as sulfonamides, tetracyclines, barbiturates, metronidazole, nonsteroidal anti-inflammatories, oral contraceptives, pseudoephedrine, bupropion, and others. The reaction to the drug may not occur until days or weeks after first using it.
- Cancer.
- Radiation therapy.

HOW TO PREVENT—Therapy to prevent herpes simplex virus outbreaks may be recommended in some cases.

WHAT TO EXPECT

DIAGNOSTIC MEASURES
- Your health care provider may diagnose the disorder by the appearance of the skin rash.

- A biopsy may be done (involves removing a small piece of the affected skin for viewing under a microscope). Blood tests or other skin tests may be done.

APPROPRIATE HEALTH CARE
- Medical treatment may involve drug therapy.
- In some cases, no treatment is needed.
- Self-care after diagnosis may be all that is needed for mild cases.
- If a drug is the cause of the disorder, it will normally be discontinued.

POSSIBLE COMPLICATIONS
- May progress from the minor form to the major form of erythema multiforme.
- Recurrence of the disorder.

PROBABLE OUTCOME—The rash develops over 1 to 2 weeks. It usually clears up in 2 to 3 weeks, but some cases may take 5 to 6 weeks.

HOW TO TREAT

GENERAL MEASURES
- Wet dressings and soaks or lotions may help to soothe the skin. Bathing in lukewarm to cool water three times a day for 30 minutes is also helpful.
- If mouth sores are present, good oral hygiene is important to reduce risk of infection and to relieve discomfort.

MEDICATION
- Corticosteroids (topical or oral) may be prescribed to reduce inflammation and irritation.
- Antivirals may be prescribed to treat viral infection such as herpes simplex virus.
- Antibiotics will be prescribed for bacterial infection.
- If mouth sores are present, topical drugs or mouthwashes may be prescribed.
- If eyes are involved, eyewashes or other topical drugs may be prescribed.
- Pain remedies, sedatives, or antihistamines may be prescribed to help provide relief of symptoms.

ACTIVITY—As tolerated by the symptoms.

DIET
- Usually no special diet is needed.
- If mouth sores are present, a soft or liquid diet may be better tolerated.

CALL YOUR DOCTOR IF

- You or a family member has symptoms of erythema multiforme.
- Symptoms worsen during treatment.

ERYTHEMA NODOSUM

GENERAL INFORMATION

DEFINITION—Erythema nodosum is an inflammatory disorder of the skin and the tissue under the skin. It is not contagious.

BODY PARTS INVOLVED—Skin of the legs, especially areas over the large bone in the lower leg. The disease occasionally involves the arms or other areas.

SEX OR AGE MOST AFFECTED—Both sexes and all ages, but more likely in females (ages 20 to 45).

SIGNS & SYMPTOMS
- A flu-like infection may precede the skin symptoms by 1 to 2 weeks. There may be a period of feeling generally unwell and fever. Joint aches may occur, especially of the knee.
- Red lumps (also called lesions or nodules) appear on the shins or about the knees or ankles. They vary in size from a cherry to a grapefruit. There may be 2 to 50 or more.
- The lumps are raised slightly above the skin. They are hot and painful. The color is bright red to start, then purple, and then fades to a bruise-like color.
- Other, smaller, red lumps may appear on the outer arms, face, and neck.
- Lumps continue to appear for about 10 days or more.
- Conjunctivitis (eye inflammation) may occur.

CAUSES—It can be a hypersensitivity reaction to different causes (e.g., infection, use of certain drugs, or other factors). Often, no cause is found (idiopathic).

RISK INCREASES WITH
- Drugs, such as birth-control pills (especially those high in estrogen), sulfonamides, iodides, and bromides.
- A preceding infection, including *Streptococcus* (most common), coccidioidomycosis, histoplasmosis, sarcoidosis, blastomycosis, tuberculosis, and *Yersinia* infections.
- Autoimmune disease.
- Chronic bowel inflammation.
- Cancer.
- Pregnancy.

HOW TO PREVENT—No specific ways to prevent. Remove or treat the cause if it can be identified.

WHAT TO EXPECT

DIAGNOSTIC MEASURES
- Your health care provider will do an exam of the affected skin.
- Medical tests are not needed to diagnose erythema nodosum, but they may be done to diagnose an underlying disorder.

APPROPRIATE HEALTH CARE
- Erythema nodosum often heals on its own. Symptoms may be treated with drug therapy.
- Treatment may be provided for an underlying disorder. If a drug is the cause of the disorder, it will normally be discontinued.

POSSIBLE COMPLICATIONS
- None expected from erythema nodosum.
- Less than 20% of cases recur.
- Other complications can arise depending on the underlying cause.

PROBABLE OUTCOME—Lumps diminish in size and tenderness and heal in about 3 to 6 weeks. Complete healing may take several months. It does not leave scars. In some cases, joint aches may continue for months to years.

HOW TO TREAT

GENERAL MEASURES—For self-care:
- Elevate the legs whenever possible.
- Use elastic wrap or support stockings.
- Soak the affected areas in water. Warm-water soaks are usually more soothing for pain or inflammation. Cool-water soaks feel better for itching.

MEDICATION
- For minor discomfort, use nonprescription drugs such as aspirin (not for children) or other nonsteroidal anti-inflammatory drugs.
- Potassium iodide may be prescribed.
- Corticosteroids may be prescribed in very severe cases.
- Topical drugs for the skin usually do not help.

ACTIVITY—Rest in bed as much as possible with the legs elevated. This may help prevent new lumps from developing. When symptoms improve, resume normal activity.

DIET—No special diet.

CALL YOUR DOCTOR IF

- You or a family member has symptoms of erythema nodosum.
- Any new symptoms arise that you think may be due either to the disorder or the drugs prescribed.

ESOPHAGEAL STRICTURE

GENERAL INFORMATION

DEFINITION—Esophageal stricture is a narrowing of the tube (esophagus) that connects the throat to the stomach. The narrowing interferes with swallowing.

BODY PARTS INVOLVED—Esophagus.

SEX OR AGE MOST AFFECTED—Both sexes; all ages.

SIGNS & SYMPTOMS
- A gradual decrease in the ability to swallow. At first, it becomes difficult to swallow solid foods. Then it becomes difficult to swallow liquids.
- Uncomfortable feeling when swallowing.
- Food feels like it gets stuck in the throat.
- Stomach acid washing back into mouth.
- Vomiting (sometimes with mucus or blood).

CAUSES—Scarring of the lining of the esophagus. As the scar tissue builds up, it forms a ring that narrows the opening of the esophagus. The scarring most often results from excessive gastric acid in the stomach backing up (called reflux) into the esophagus. This causes repeated inflammation (esophagitis), which damages the lining of the esophagus. Other risk factors may also lead to scarring.

RISK INCREASES WITH
- Gastroesophageal reflux disease (GERD).
- Hiatal hernia (part of the stomach protrudes through the diaphragm).
- Prolonged use of feeding (nasogastric) tubes.
- Swallowing of corrosive (e.g., acid or lye) chemicals.
- Infections of the esophagus.
- Radiation injury to the esophagus.
- Injury from an endoscope (a tube-like device used to examine the internal organs).
- Cancer of the esophagus.
- Certain drugs that can irritate the esophagus.

HOW TO PREVENT
- Get medical care for any problems that involve difficulty swallowing or acid reflux.
- Keep dangerous products out of children's reach.
- Don't swallow any substance that may harm the esophagus.

WHAT TO EXPECT

DIAGNOSTIC MEASURES
- Your own observation of symptoms.
- Your health care provider may do an endoscopy. This is a medical test using an instrument with a lighted tip (endoscope) that is inserted into the esophagus. A small amount of tissue may be removed for testing (biopsy) to make sure the stricture is benign. A special type of x-ray of the esophagus may be done.

APPROPRIATE HEALTH CARE
- Treatment will be provided for any underlying disorder, such as gastroesophageal reflux disease.
- Treatment for the stricture usually involves a medical procedure to widen (dilate) the esophagus. Different types of procedures are available. They are normally done with the patient sedated. Your health care provider will explain the options to you.
- Surgery to remove the stricture may be recommended, if other treatments fail.

POSSIBLE COMPLICATIONS
- Not able to eat and drink enough foods and fluids.
- Perforation (hole) in the damaged esophagus.
- Inflammation that may lead to internal bleeding.
- Stricture recurs after treatment.
- Aspiration, which is the passage of food or liquid through the vocal folds ("going down the wrong way"). The food, fluid, or vomit may enter the lungs.

PROBABLE OUTCOME—Treatment can help relieve the stricture, but treatment may need to be repeated.

HOW TO TREAT

GENERAL MEASURES
- Stop smoking. Smoking may make symptoms worse.
- See your dental care provider to be sure dentures and oral prostheses fit well and are not loose.

MEDICATION—Drugs for reflux problems may be prescribed (e.g., proton pump inhibitors).

ACTIVITY—Usually no limits.

DIET
- Eat a soft or liquid diet after treatment, until normal swallowing is possible. Avoid spicy foods that irritate the esophagus.
- A diet that will help avoid acid reflux may be recommended.

CALL YOUR DOCTOR IF

- You or a family member has symptoms of esophageal stricture.
- The following occur during treatment:
  - Chest pain or fever.
  - Inability to speak.
  - Swallowing problems do not improve.

ESOPHAGUS CANCER

GENERAL INFORMATION

DEFINITION—Esophagus cancer is a malignant (cancerous) tumor of the esophagus. This is the tube connecting the mouth to the stomach.

BODY PARTS INVOLVED—Esophagus.

SEX OR AGE MOST AFFECTED—This type of cancer usually affects adults over age 60 and both sexes, but is more common in men.

SIGNS & SYMPTOMS
- Early cancer does not usually cause symptoms.
- Swallowing difficulty that gradually gets worse.
- Pain when swallowing.
- Rapid weight loss.
- Chronic cough. May cough up blood.
- Hoarseness.
- Feeling weak and tired.
- Nausea and vomiting.

CAUSES—Unknown. Risk factors for one type of cancer are due to smoking or alcohol use. Risk factors for a second type of cancer are due to esophageal conditions. Most esophagus cancers are primary (they begin there). Some are secondary (they spread from cancer elsewhere in the body).

RISK INCREASES WITH
- Ages over 60 and male.
- Smoking (including cigarettes, pipes, or cigars) or smokeless tobacco.
- Excess alcohol use.
- Barrett's esophagus (a precancerous condition).
- Previous esophagus, head, or neck cancer.
- Hiatal hernia.
- Esophageal stricture.
- Chronic gastric reflux (gastroesophageal reflux disease or GERD).
- Previous radiation therapy to the chest.
- Obesity (may be due to link with reflux disease).
- Celiac disease or human papilloma virus infection.
- Family history of cancer.

HOW TO PREVENT
- None specific. Avoid risk factors where possible.
- Don't smoke or use other tobacco products. Avoid alcohol or limit its use. Lose weight if overweight.
- Obtain medical care for any gastrointestinal disorders.

WHAT TO EXPECT

DIAGNOSTIC MEASURES
- Your own observation of symptoms.
- Your health care provider will do a physical exam and ask questions about any symptoms.
- A number of medical tests will be done. The tests first help diagnose the cancer and then determine if it has spread (staging).

APPROPRIATE HEALTH CARE
- Treatment varies and depends on the location and size of the tumor, any spread of the cancer, your health, age, and preferences.
- Treatment may include chemotherapy (anticancer drugs) and/or radiation therapy, immunotherapy, surgery, photodynamic therapy, and others.
- Chemotherapy uses drugs and radiation therapy uses radiation to attack the cancer cells. Immunotherapy uses the body's immune system to fight cancer. Photodynamic therapy combines drugs with laser use.
- Surgery may be performed to remove the tumor if the cancer has not spread in the body. Procedures can be done to allow passage of food and liquids.
- Treatment may involve steps to relieve symptoms and make you comfortable, rather than treating the cancer.
- Counseling may help you cope with diagnosis.

POSSIBLE COMPLICATIONS—If treatment is delayed, esophagus cancer can spread rapidly to the lungs, liver, brain, and bones.

PROBABLE OUTCOME—Recovery improves if diagnosed at an early stage. The diagnosis often comes too late for effective treatment, but symptoms can be relieved or controlled. Research into causes and treatment continues.

HOW TO TREAT

GENERAL MEASURES
- Stop smoking or using any tobacco product.
- To learn more: Esophageal Cancer Awareness Assn., PO Box 55071 #15530; Boston, MA 02205; (800) 801-0613; website: www.ecaware.org.

MEDICATION—Your health care provider may prescribe: anticancer drugs, pain relievers, antianxiety drugs, and drugs for esophageal spasms. Drugs for immunotherapy or photodynamic therapy may be used.

ACTIVITY—Remain as active as possible.

DIET—Eating may be difficult, but good nutrition is vital for healing. A dietitian can help.

CALL YOUR DOCTOR IF

- You or a family member has symptoms of esophagus cancer such as difficulty swallowing.
- Pain or symptoms get worse despite treatment.

ESSENTIAL TREMOR

GENERAL INFORMATION

DEFINITION—Essential tremor is a type of movement disorder. Movement disorders affect the ability to produce and control movement. Parkinson's disease is a different type of movement disorder.

BODY PARTS INVOLVED—Nervous system.

SEX OR AGE MOST AFFECTED—It is a common problem in people aged 60 and older. Men and women are affected equally.

SIGNS & SYMPTOMS
- The main symptom is a fairly slow, regular tremor, which is a trembling or an up-and-down movement. The tremor may be noticed when doing simple tasks such as holding a glass of water. The tremor may occur in the hands, arms, head, and voice. Rarely, it affects the trunk and legs.
- Walking in an unsteady manner.
- The symptoms start on a gradual basis, usually in mid-to-late life. In a few cases, symptoms begin in childhood, go away for many years, and then start up again.
- Being tired, feeling anxious, or being in hot climates can make the symptoms worse.
- Symptoms usually disappear when you sleep or rest.

CAUSES—The exact cause is unknown. In about half of the cases, a genetic factor appears to be involved. Familial tremor is the term used when it affects more than one person in a family. In other cases, the cause is unknown. Environmental (e.g., toxins) and aging factors may play a role.

RISK INCREASES WITH
- Family history of essential tremor.
- Age. Most often, the disorder occurs in older people.

HOW TO PREVENT—At present, there is no known way to prevent.

WHAT TO EXPECT

DIAGNOSTIC MEASURES
- Your own observation of symptoms.
- Your health care provider will do a physical exam, and ask questions about your symptoms and your activities. You may be asked to write, drink from a glass, or hold a piece of paper so that the tremor can be observed.
- There are a variety of medical problems that can involve similar symptoms. Medical tests on blood and urine are usually done to rule out other disorders.

APPROPRIATE HEALTH CARE
- Treatment may not be needed if the symptoms are mild and are not causing other problems.
- Treatment steps may include exercises using weights for your hands and arms. These will be taught to you by a physical therapist. You can then continue doing them at home.
- Counseling may help if you are having emotional problems in coping with the changes in your life brought on by the symptoms.
- Surgery is rare, but may help if symptoms are more severe.

POSSIBLE COMPLICATIONS
- The tremor makes it difficult to do everyday tasks at work or in the home, perform hobbies, or do other activities you enjoy.
- Feeling embarrassed about the tremor may lead to an avoidance of social activities.

PROBABLE OUTCOME
- In many people, the disorder may not get worse and the tremor may be mild throughout life.
- Others may have symptoms that get worse as they get older. There are treatments that can help relieve the symptoms.

HOW TO TREAT

GENERAL MEASURES
- Joining a support group may help some people. Ask your health care provider about groups in your area.
- To learn more: We Move, 5731 Mosholu Ave., Bronx, NY 10471; website: www.wemove.org.

MEDICATION—There are several different classes of drugs that are used to treat tremors. Your health care provider will discuss the options with you and decide if they are appropriate.

ACTIVITY—Try to maintain an active lifestyle. Exercise each day to the extent possible.

DIET
- Avoid caffeine in coffee, tea, and soft drinks. It may make the symptoms worse.
- Avoid alcohol, or use it on a limited basis. It may help the tremors short term, but it is not wise to use it as a form of treatment.

CALL YOUR DOCTOR IF

- You or a family member has symptoms of essential tremor.
- Symptoms get worse despite treatment.

EYE CONTUSION OR LACERATION

GENERAL INFORMATION

DEFINITION—Two types of eye injuries are blunt injury (contusion) or cut (laceration).

BODY PARTS INVOLVED—Eyeball; eyelid; bones around the eyeball (eye socket); muscles attached to the eyeball.

SEX OR AGE MOST AFFECTED—Both sexes; all ages.

SIGNS & SYMPTOMS
- Swelling, redness, tenderness, pain, bleeding, or bruising ("black eye") in or around the eye. A black eye may take 1 to 2 days to develop.
- Change in ability to see clearly.

CAUSES—A blunt or sharp blow or cut to the eye or the area around the eye.

RISK INCREASES WITH
- Doing work that may risk injury to the eyes. This includes bartending (opening bottles), carpentry, or construction work.
- Paintball, BB guns, rifles, or slingshot usage.
- Sports such as baseball, softball, basketball, soccer, football, or hockey.
- Using a rotary lawn mower.
- Fist fights. Eye injuries may occur in fights. Fights are more likely with alcohol use.

HOW TO PREVENT—When possible, wear appropriate eye protection for any activity that may lead to eye injury. This can include eye coverings or face shields.

WHAT TO EXPECT

- For most eye injuries, or if you are unsure if it is serious, see your health care provider. Seek emergency care if the injury is severe.
- If you have any blurred vision, you must see a health care provider.
- Your health care provider can diagnose the problem with an exam of the injured eye area.

APPROPRIATE HEALTH CARE—Treatment may involve stitches to repair cuts, or other surgical procedures.

POSSIBLE COMPLICATIONS
- Permanent vision loss.
- Infection.
- Cataract.

PROBABLE OUTCOME—Some injuries are mild and heal on their own. Others are usually curable with treatment. Allow 2 weeks for complete healing.

HOW TO TREAT

GENERAL MEASURES
- For a minor contusion (black eye) during the first 24 hours, use ice packs to reduce swelling. The next day, make a warm compress by folding a clean cloth in several layers. Dip in warm water, wring out slightly, and put on the eye. Dip the compress often to keep it moist. Apply compress for an hour, rest an hour, and repeat.
- For a minor cut or scrape around the eye, apply pressure to stop any bleeding. Use a clean cloth to clean the wound. Cover with a bandage if a cut or scrape is large.
- At home, sleep with the head raised with two pillows until symptoms get better.
- Protect eyes from bright light or sunlight by wearing dark glasses until healing is complete.

MEDICATION
- Antibiotics (oral or eyedrops) to prevent infection may be prescribed.
- Eyedrops to reduce inflammation may be prescribed.
- Use acetaminophen for pain relief.

ACTIVITY—For minor injury, resume normal activities after healing. For other injuries, your health care provider will give you specific advice about work or sports activities.

DIET—No special diet.

CALL YOUR DOCTOR IF

- You have a cut or other eye injury. This may be an emergency.
- The following occur after eye injury: fever, vision changes, or eye pain that persists after treatment.

EYE, FOREIGN BODY IN

GENERAL INFORMATION

DEFINITION—A foreign body in the eye can include a small speck of metal, wood, stone, sand, paint, an eyelash, or other material.

BODY PARTS INVOLVED—Eye, usually the conjunctiva (outer eye covering).

SEX OR AGE MOST AFFECTED—Both sexes; all ages.

SIGNS & SYMPTOMS
- Eye pain, irritation, watering, and redness.
- Eye is sensitive to light.
- Foreign body (object) that can be seen when the eye is examined. Sometimes the object is very small, trapped under the eyelid, and cannot be seen except with a medical exam.
- Scratchy feeling when blinking.
- Blurred vision or loss of vision in affected eye.

CAUSES—Accident.

RISK INCREASES WITH
- Windy weather.
- Jobs or activity, such as carpentry or grinding, in which fine pieces of wood or other materials fly loose in the air.

HOW TO PREVENT—Wear protective eye coverings if your job or hobby involves the risk of eye injury.

WHAT TO EXPECT

DIAGNOSTIC MEASURES
- Your own observation of symptoms.
- Most eye injuries should be seen by your health care provider. Ask someone else to drive you to the medical office or emergency center. Don't try to drive yourself. Keep the eye closed, if possible, until the exam.
- Your health care provider will do an exam of the injured eye. It may include staining the eye with a harmless substance to outline the object, examining the eye through a magnifying lens, and/or use of a special ultraviolet light. This helps rule out any abrasion or scrape on the surface of the eye.

APPROPRIATE HEALTH CARE
- The procedure to remove the object will depend on its size and location within the eye.
- An eye patch may be applied to help keep the eye closed.
- Follow-up exam will be done in 1 to 2 days.

POSSIBLE COMPLICATIONS
- Infection, especially if the object is not removed completely.
- Permanent vision damage.

PROBABLE OUTCOME—Most objects can be removed simply with self-care, in a health care provider's office, or in an emergency room.

HOW TO TREAT

GENERAL MEASURES
- For small foreign bodies, be sure not to rub the eye. Try to flush the eye with water (or saline solution) using one of these options:
  - Gently pour warm (not hot) water from a small pitcher over the eye. Keep eye open.
  - Stand at a sink with warm water running and cup your hands and put your face in the running water.
  - Use an eye dropper with warm water.
  - If outside, use a garden hose, but don't use high pressure. A water fountain may also be used to flush out the eye.
  - Check the eye often to see if the object is gone.
  - If flushing is not working, you may consider trying to remove the object with the tip of a tissue or cotton-tipped swab. Lift upper or lower eyelid (someone else may need to help you). Be extremely careful to not touch the eye itself with the swab. You could injure the cornea.
- If you removed the object, but it was large, or the patient is a child, a health care provider should be seen for follow-up check.
- Use moist compresses to relieve discomfort after removal of particle. Prepare by folding a clean cloth in several layers. Dip in warm water, wring out slightly, and apply to the eye. Dip the compress often to keep it moist. Do this for 1 hour, rest 1 hour, and then repeat.

MEDICATION
- Antibiotic eyedrops may be prescribed to prevent infection.
- Pain relievers may be prescribed.

ACTIVITY—Resume your normal activities gradually after removal of the foreign body and the patch, if one is applied.

DIET—No special diet.

CALL YOUR DOCTOR IF

- You or a family member has a foreign body in the eye that you are concerned about. If it is an emergency, call 911 to get emergency help right away.
- The following occur after removal:
  - Pain increases or does not disappear in 2 days.
  - Fever develops.
  - Vision changes.

FAILURE TO THRIVE

GENERAL INFORMATION

DEFINITION—Failure to thrive is actually a group of symptoms, rather than a specific disorder. The term is used to described infants or children who do not grow or gain weight at the expected rate.

BODY PARTS INVOLVED—Whole body.

SEX OR AGE MOST AFFECTED—Children under 5, usually infants, ages 3-6 months.

SIGNS & SYMPTOMS
- Height and weight do not progress normally, as measured on standard growth charts.
- Physical skills may be slow to develop. This includes rolling over, sitting, crawling, standing, or walking.
- Mental and social skills may be delayed. This includes talking, interactions, or self-feeding.
- Child lacks energy, has small muscles, rash or other skin changes, swollen arms or legs, and changes in hair.
- Other symptoms (they may be due to a medical condition).

CAUSES—It may be due to medical conditions (sometimes called organic failure). It may involve psychosocial and environmental causes, such as family concerns or problems in the home (sometimes called nonorganic failure). It may also be a combination of the two.

RISK INCREASES WITH
- Pregnancy problems (such as alcohol use or intrauterine growth restriction) or premature infants or children with chromosomal abnormalities.
- Children who have trouble eating, are unable to suck, have vomiting or reflux problems, or have infections.
- Children who are unable to absorb nutrients or need extra nutrients, due to certain medical disorders.
- Children with chronic illness (cystic fibrosis, asthma).
- Child neglect, abuse, or lack of attention by parents.
- Not providing enough food for a child. Child who refuses to eat, or problems with weaning.
- Parents who lack parenting skills.
- Dysfunctional family, difficult parent-child interactions, or lack of support (family or friends).
- Depression, alcohol or drug abuse in a parent.
- Poverty of parents (unable to provide needed foods).

HOW TO PREVENT
- Arrange for parenting classes if you are new parents. Get instructions on proper nutrition for a new baby.
- Get regular "well-baby" checkups for child.

WHAT TO EXPECT

DIAGNOSTIC MEASURES
- Your child's health care provider will do a physical exam. The child's height and weight will be compared to standard growth charts to determine if there is delayed growth.
- Medical tests may include blood and urine studies. To help pinpoint a cause for growth delay, questions may be asked about the pregnancy and birth, the child's behavior and eating habits, other family members, stress problems, and other concerns.

APPROPRIATE HEALTH CARE
- Treatment will depend on the cause. Organic causes may be treated medically. Nonorganic causes may be treated with counseling, education, and other help for the parents. The main goal of any treatment is to be sure your child has the proper nutrition.
- Hospital care may be needed in some cases.
- If child neglect or abuse is suspected, child protective services or other authorities may become involved.

POSSIBLE COMPLICATIONS—Ongoing mental, emotional, and physical delays.

PROBABLE OUTCOME—If the problem is short-term and the cause can be corrected, normal growth and development may resume. Recovery may take several months. In other cases, the outcome will depend on the underlying condition.

HOW TO TREAT

GENERAL MEASURES
- Home visits from a nurse may be scheduled.
- Community programs that help mothers and children are available. Other help can be provided to get financial aid (such as food stamps), medical benefits, parenting classes, or counseling for emotional problems.

MEDICATION—Drugs may be prescribed for an underlying disorder.

ACTIVITY—No limits.

DIET
- Changes in your child's diet will be prescribed. Specific instructions will be provided. Be sure to follow the instructions carefully.
- Tube feedings may be needed for severe cases. These can often be done at home.

☎ CALL YOUR DOCTOR IF

- You are concerned that your child is not developing properly or growing as expected.
- You have any concerns about your child.

FAINTING
(Syncope)

GENERAL INFORMATION

DEFINITION—Fainting is a sudden, temporary loss of consciousness due to a decrease in the supply of blood and oxygen to the brain. Fainting may be a symptom of a health problem or a one-time event. Syncope is the medical term for fainting.

BODY PARTS INVOLVED—Circulatory system (heart and blood vessels); brain.

SEX OR AGE MOST AFFECTED—Both sexes; all ages.

SIGNS & SYMPTOMS
- Before fainting, a person may have:
  - Paleness and sweating.
  - Sudden lightheadedness.
  - General weakness.
  - Blurred vision (sometimes).
  - Nausea (sometimes).
  - Rapid heartbeat and rapid breathing.
- Unconsciousness with fall to ground. A return to consciousness occurs quickly.

CAUSES
- The heart cannot pump enough blood for the body to function properly. This occurs with heart disease and blood vessel disorders.
- The blood volume (amount of blood) is low. This can be due to bleeding or dehydration.
- Stimulation of the vagus nerve (in the neck, chest, and intestine) may slow the heart. This can happen with pain, fear, distress, vomiting, having a large bowel movement, and even urinating.
- Blood flow returning to the heart is reduced. It occurs with straining when coughing, passing a stool, or in older men when trying to urinate (called micturition).
- Standing up or sitting down too quickly causes a sudden change in blood pressure. This is called orthostatic hypotension. Standing for long periods on a hot day can cause a similar problem due to lack of leg muscle use.
- Very rapid breathing or hyperventilating due to anxiety. Too much carbon dioxide is exhaled which then causes blood vessels in the brain to narrow.
- Other causes may be due to stroke, seizures, anemia, low blood sugar, lung problems, and others.
- In some cases, the cause of fainting is unknown.

RISK INCREASES WITH
- Heart disease or certain other chronic disorders.
- Certain drugs, such as those that slow the heartbeat or lower blood pressure.
- Being elderly.

HOW TO PREVENT
- Fainting cannot always be prevented. If you feel faint, lie down with feet up or sit in a chair and bend over.
- Avoid the problems that can cause fainting if possible. Try not to get overly anxious. Get treatment for any medical disorder and avoid constipation. Men can urinate while sitting down if standing causes fainting. Avoid sudden changes in physical activity, such as when getting up from a chair or bed (move slowly).

WHAT TO EXPECT

DIAGNOSTIC MEASURES
- See your health care provider after any fainting event. A physical exam may be done and questions asked about your symptoms and activities.
- Medical tests may be done to check for heart problems or other underlying cause of fainting.

APPROPRIATE HEALTH CARE—Sometimes, no treatment is needed. In other cases, treatment may be prescribed for a diagnosed problem. Rarely, hospital care is needed.

POSSIBLE COMPLICATIONS
- Injury while fainting, such as from a fall.
- Complications of a disorder that led to the fainting.
- Recurrent fainting can have a major impact on a person's lifestyle. It may prevent driving a motor vehicle.

PROBABLE OUTCOME—A person will recover from simple fainting in 1 or 2 minutes. There are normally no long-term effects.

HOW TO TREAT

GENERAL MEASURES—If you are subject to frequent fainting spells, avoid activities in which fainting may endanger your life or others. This includes climbing ladders, driving motor vehicles, or operating dangerous machinery. Make your home safe in case of falls.

MEDICATION—Drugs are usually not needed for fainting.

ACTIVITY—You can usually resume normal activities right away unless advised differently by your health care provider.

DIET—No special diet.

CALL YOUR DOCTOR IF

You or a family member has a fainting event even if it seems mild. It may be a symptom of a medical disorder.

FATTY LIVER
(Steatosis)

GENERAL INFORMATION

DEFINITION
• Fatty liver means there is excess fat in your liver. It is a common condition. There are two types of fatty liver. One type is NAFLD (nonalcoholic fatty liver disease) in non-alcohol users. The other type is ALD (alcoholic liver disease) in alcohol users.
• Fatty liver may cause no damage (be harmless). The medical name is steatosis. Some people with fatty liver also develop inflammation of the liver. This is either called NASH (nonalcoholic steatohepatitis) or alcoholic steatohepatitis depending on alcohol use. The inflammation can lead to other liver problems (e.g., fibrosis and cirrhosis).

BODY PARTS INVOLVED—Liver.

SEX OR AGE MOST AFFECTED—Both sexes; all ages.

SIGNS & SYMPTOMS
• Most often, there are no symptoms. Fatty liver may be found during routine medical tests.
• If symptoms occur, they may be vague (e.g., tiredness or mild pain in abdomen).

CAUSES—It is unclear just how the liver becomes fatty. A fatty liver does not process, break down, and store fats as it normally should. Insulin resistance and genetics may play a role. Why liver inflammation develops in some people with fatty liver is also unclear.

RISK INCREASES WITH
• Alcoholism.
• Obesity and overweight.
• Diabetes.
• High level of blood fats (cholesterol and triglycerides).
• Metabolic syndrome (a cluster of risk factors).
• Bypass surgery for obesity.
• Other rare risk factors for fatty liver include: certain prescribed drugs, toxins (such as organic solvents), nutrition problems (e.g., rapid weight loss), pregnancy complication, and some other diseases or disorders.

HOW TO PREVENT
• Reduce your risks where possible. There are no specific preventive measures.
• Get medical care for treatable risk factors.
• Maintain a healthy weight. Exercise daily.
• Avoid excess alcohol.

WHAT TO EXPECT

DIAGNOSTIC MEASURES
• Your health care provider may suspect fatty liver if routine lab tests show abnormal liver function or a slightly enlarged liver is felt in a physical exam. Questions will be asked about your medical history, diet, and alcohol use.
• Medical tests help rule out other liver disorders. Tests may include blood studies, ultrasound, CT scan, or MRI. A biopsy may be needed to confirm liver inflammation.

APPROPRIATE HEALTH CARE
• For nonalcoholic liver inflammation (or NASH), a cure has not been found. Certain treatments may help. These include weight loss and an increase in exercise. Patients need to control their diabetes and lower the blood fats in the body with diet and/or drugs. Weight loss surgery may be an option in a few cases.
• For alcohol-related fatty liver and alcoholic hepatitis, you will be advised to stop alcohol use. This will help prevent further liver damage. Other treatments are like those for NASH (e.g., diet, exercise, etc.).
• If fatty liver is due to drug, toxin, or other rare cause, treatment will be aimed at that problem.

POSSIBLE COMPLICATIONS
• Fibrosis and cirrhosis (liver scarring and hardening).
• Liver failure, cancer, or need of liver transplant.

PROBABLE OUTCOME
• In NAFLD, simple fatty liver is usually harmless. It is still important to maintain a healthy lifestyle. Lose weight if needed and increase your exercise levels.
• In ALD, stopping alcohol may reverse simple fatty liver.
• Patients with liver inflammation can take steps to help prevent or reverse some liver damage.

HOW TO TREAT

GENERAL MEASURES—All patients with liver disorders should have regular medical check ups to monitor the liver function.

MEDICATION
• Drugs may be prescribed for an underlying cause.
• Research is ongoing to study the benefits of new or existing drugs and diet supplements.

ACTIVITY—Get regular exercise (daily is best). Plan a program that fits your lifestyle.

DIET
• Eat a healthy diet.
• If overweight, a gradual weight loss is a must.

CALL YOUR DOCTOR IF

After diagnosis of fatty liver, you or a family member has questions, concerns, or needs help with treatment.

FEBRILE SEIZURE

 GENERAL INFORMATION

DEFINITION—A febrile seizure is a convulsion that occurs with a fever in infants or small children. The fever may be from many causes, such as a cold or ear infection. Febrile seizures are common in young children. For many children, a febrile seizure occurs just one time. About one-third of the children will have recurrent febrile seizures. Only a few children have more than three febrile seizures.

BODY PARTS INVOLVED—Nervous system, circulatory system (heart and blood vessels), and musculoskeletal system.

SEX OR AGE MOST AFFECTED—Both sexes; infants and young children.

SIGNS & SYMPTOMS
- Repeated rhythmic jerking or stiffening of your child's arms and legs. The child may first cry out.
- Eyes roll back in the child's head.
- Lack of consciousness.
- Twitches in only a part of the body, such as an arm or a leg, or only on the right or the left side.
- Usually occurs on the first day of a fever. Parents may not even know the child is ill.
- Rectal temperatures higher than 102°F (38.9°C).
- Simple febrile seizure—stops by itself within a few seconds to 10 minutes. Complex febrile seizure—lasts longer than 15 minutes, occurs in one part of the body, or recurs during the same illness.
- Child may be confused or drowsy after seizure.

CAUSES—Exact cause is unknown. The high fever, and possibly one that rises quickly, may trigger a brain disturbance.

RISK INCREASES WITH
- Children ages 6 months to 5 years.
- Slightly more common in boys than girls.
- Very high fever or a rapidly rising temperature.
- A history of febrile seizures in other family members.
- Rarely, fever and seizure occurs after a vaccination.
- Risk factors for recurrent seizures include:
  - Young age (less than 15 months) for the first seizure.
  - Family members with a history of febrile seizures.
  - Fever was below 102°F (38.9°C) at time of first seizure.

HOW TO PREVENT
- None for a first febrile seizure. There is no way to know for sure if a child is at risk.
- Fever-reducing drugs may help reduce future risk.
- Certain children with recurrent febrile seizures are sometimes given preventive drugs.

 WHAT TO EXPECT

DIAGNOSTIC MEASURES
- Medical care may include emergency room treatment or seeing your child's health care provider. Either way, your child will be examined and questions asked about the seizure symptoms.
- Medical tests may be done to be sure there is not a more serious illness causing the fever.

APPROPRIATE HEALTH CARE
- Sometimes, no treatment is needed.
- Reassurance to parents about the benign nature (not serious) of the seizure should help ease concerns.

POSSIBLE COMPLICATIONS
- Injury may result from bumping or falling into objects.
- There is a very small risk that certain children who have febrile seizures will develop epilepsy.

PROBABLE OUTCOME
- Outcome is usually excellent, with no lasting effects.
- The child will not be aware of having had the seizure.
- Most children who have febrile seizures will outgrow them by four to five years of age.
- Febrile seizures do not cause brain damage.

![plus] **HOW TO TREAT**

GENERAL MEASURES
- If a febrile seizure recurs:
  - Stay calm!
  - Do not put anything in your child's mouth.
  - Place your child on his/her side to help drain saliva from the mouth. Don't try to hold your child still.
  - Loosen clothing.
  - Move objects away from child to avoid injury.
  - Support child's head with a pillow or other soft object.
  - Try to watch a clock to time the seizure.

MEDICATION
- Drugs may be prescribed for any infection.
- Rarely, preventive drugs may be prescribed.
- Ask your child's health care provider about giving acetaminophen or ibuprofen for fevers. Don't give aspirin to children under age 18.

ACTIVITY—Child can rest or sleep after seizure.

DIET—No special diet.

 CALL YOUR DOCTOR IF

- Your child has another febrile seizure.
- A febrile seizure lasts more than 15 minutes.
- Child's symptoms cause you any concern.

FECAL IMPACTION

GENERAL INFORMATION

DEFINITION—A fecal impaction is a large, firm amount of stool that cannot be passed voluntarily. In most cases, the impacted stool is in the rectum, which is the lowest end of the bowels. Sometimes, the impaction may extend further up in the bowels.

BODY PARTS INVOLVED—Lower colon; rectum.

SEX OR AGE MOST AFFECTED—Both sexes; all ages.

SIGNS & SYMPTOMS
- Lack of normal bowel movements.
- Sense of fullness in the rectum, but unable to pass stool.
- Pain or cramps in the stomach or abdomen area (often after meals).
- Thin, watery discharge from the rectum.
- Headache, nausea, vomiting, loss of appetite.
- General sick feeling.

CAUSES—Irregular bowel function causes dry, hardened feces to remain in the colon or rectum.

RISK INCREASES WITH
- Long term constipation.
- Rectal disorders that make normal bowel movements uncomfortable, such as painful hemorrhoids or fissures.
- Rectal or colon cancer.
- Swallowing substance for x-rays of the intestinal tract.
- Nerve problems in the colon or rectum, as with a spinal-cord injury, stroke, Parkinson's disease, or multiple sclerosis.
- Being elderly or bedridden (such as after surgery).
- Disorders such as hypothyroidism, hypercalcemia, or chronic kidney disease.
- Use of some drugs, such as narcotic pain remedies.
- Being immobile or inactive.
- Living in a nursing home or adult care home.

HOW TO PREVENT
- Increase the fiber in the diet. Drink adequate amounts of fluid each day. Begin a program of regular exercise.
- Set aside a regular time each day for bowel movement (within an hour after breakfast is best). Don't try to hurry. Sit at least 10 minutes.
- If mild constipation develops, use a stool softener or a suppository.

WHAT TO EXPECT

DIAGNOSTIC MEASURES
- Your own observation of symptoms.
- Your health care provider will do an exam of the abdomen area and a digital rectal exam. The rectal exam is done with a gloved finger inserted into the rectum.
- Medical tests such as x-ray and others may be done to confirm the diagnosis and check for complications.

APPROPRIATE HEALTH CARE—The impacted mass may be removed partially by your health care provider. This is done as with the rectal exam. A gloved finger (sometimes two) is inserted into the rectum and the mass is broken up. The rest of the stool may be removed with the use of a suppository. In some cases, water irrigation with a special instrument inserted into the rectum is used.

POSSIBLE COMPLICATIONS
- Injury to the rectum.
- If the impaction is not removed, the problem can worsen and surgery may be required.

PROBABLE OUTCOME—Usually curable with treatment. Impaction may recur, unless the underlying cause is removed.

HOW TO TREAT

GENERAL MEASURES—See Constipation (in Illness section) for suggestions to improve bowel habits.

MEDICATION—After treatment, stool softeners may be prescribed.

ACTIVITY—No limits. Be as active as your health permits. Good physical fitness improves bowel function.

DIET
- Eat a normal, well-balanced diet that is high in fiber.
- Drink plenty of fluids each day.

CALL YOUR DOCTOR IF

- You or a family member has symptoms of a fecal impaction.
- Your normal bowel pattern changes.

FEMALE ATHLETE TRIAD

 GENERAL INFORMATION

DEFINITION
• Female athlete triad is a result of three related conditions. It can occur in females of any age, or athletic skill level. An athlete may have one, two, or all three of these conditions that make up the triad:
   - Energy deficit/disordered eating (imbalance between energy consumed [nutrition] and the energy expended during exercise).
   - Menstrual disorders (e.g., amenorrhea—no menstrual period for 3 months or more).
   - Low bone mineral density (e.g., weakened bones and osteoporosis).

BODY PARTS INVOLVED—Reproductive system, musculoskeletal system, and gastrointestinal system.

SEX OR AGE MOST AFFECTED—Females, usually early teens to late 20s.

SIGNS & SYMPTOMS
• Weight loss.
• Fatigue (sometimes).
• Not having monthly periods or irregular periods.
• Young females may not start their first period.
• Stress fractures (bones break for no apparent reason).
• Injuries to muscles.
• Eating only small amounts of food. May overeat (binge) and then throw up or use laxatives (purge).

CAUSES—Not eating enough food for the energy being spent. Muscles and bones soon start wearing down. Estrogen hormone levels decrease, causing problems with menstrual periods and loss of bone density.

RISK INCREASES WITH
• Compulsive exercising. Workouts become the most important part of life.
• Overly concerned with reaching goals or extremely competitive.
• Pushed by coach(es) or parents to lose weight for improved performance.
• Stress (emotional as well as physical).
• Activities where low body weights and thin body shape seem to be important. These include track and field, swimming, rowing, cycling, basketball, body-building, ballet, figure skating, and gymnastics.

HOW TO PREVENT
• Eat a healthy, well-balanced diet. Don't skip meals.
• Maintain a healthy body weight for your height.
• Keep track of your menstrual periods.
• Do not over exercise or over train.

 WHAT TO EXPECT

DIAGNOSTIC MEASURES
• Your health care provider will do a physical exam and may do a pelvic exam. You will be asked about your diet, weight changes, your exercise routine, and menstrual-cycle history.
• Blood and urine tests and a bone density test may be done.

APPROPRIATE HEALTH CARE
• Any injuries (e.g., stress fractures) will be treated first.
• You, your health care provider, your parents (important with adolescents), dietitians, mental health provider, along with physical trainers and coaches may all be involved in treatment plans. Your health care provider will monitor your progress on a regular basis.
• Treatment steps will depend on each person's needs. They will focus on lifestyle changes. These can include healthy eating, counseling, and modifying physical activities. Small changes may be all that is needed.
• Seeing a mental health provider for any stress or emotional problems may help.

POSSIBLE COMPLICATIONS
• A decrease in athletic performance.
• Permanent bone loss and bone fracture risk.
• Severe medical problems (can be life-threatening).

PROBABLE OUTCOME—Outcome will vary for each individual. With prompt diagnosis and early treatment, menstrual periods can return to normal, and further bone loss can be halted.

 HOW TO TREAT

GENERAL MEASURES—The treatment steps are not easy and will take time.

MEDICATION
• Hormones may be prescribed to stop bone loss and to help regulate menstrual periods.
• Calcium and vitamin D are often prescribed.

ACTIVITY—Try for a balance in activity levels that will still allow you to train, compete, and achieve your goals while not harming health.

DIET—It is vital to get adequate calories, protein, and calcium and eat foods you enjoy. Proper nutrition can enhance athletic performance. Consult a dietitian for help.

☎ CALL YOUR DOCTOR IF

• You or a family member has symptoms that make up the female athlete triad.
• Symptoms don't improve after a few months of treatment.

FERTILITY PROBLEMS IN MEN

GENERAL INFORMATION

DEFINITION—Infertility is the inability to achieve pregnancy after 1 year of sexual activity without contraception. Infertility affects 10% to 15% of reproductive-age couples. Causes of infertility are about equal in men and women (35% in each). In 20% of couples, both have problems, and in 10%, the cause is unknown.

BODY PARTS INVOLVED—Genitals; endocrine system; brain.

SEX OR AGE MOST AFFECTED—Males after puberty.

SIGNS & SYMPTOMS—Failure to impregnate a fertile woman.

CAUSES—In males, it is due to low sperm counts, poor sperm quality, or both. There are known risk factors (e.g., chronic illness), but in many cases, no cause is found.

RISK INCREASES WITH
- Certain physical problems of the penis or testicles (e.g., blockage in certain tubes or undescended testes).
- Antisperm antibodies (immune system targets sperm in error).
- Retrograde ejaculation (sperm go backward instead of forward).
- Urinary-tract infection or injury to the genitals.
- Hormone, metabolic, or endocrine disorders.
- Some surgeries (e.g., bladder or prostate).
- Mumps.
- Some genetic disorders (e.g., Klinefelter's syndrome).
- Excess alcohol use or substance abuse.
- Use of some drugs, such as antihypertensives, cytotoxic drugs, male hormones, and MAO inhibitors.
- Sexually transmitted disease, such as syphilis and nonspecific urethritis that causes scarring.
- Varicose veins in the testicles (varicocele).
- Overheating of the testicles.
- Intercourse problems (e.g., poor timing with menses, premature withdrawal, too infrequent).
- Exposure to insecticides or industrial chemicals.
- Aging, poor nutrition, or poor general health.
- Smoking.
- Cancer and its treatments.
- Obesity.
- Excess stress (both mental and physical).

HOW TO PREVENT—Preventive measures depend on the cause.

WHAT TO EXPECT

DIAGNOSTIC MEASURES
- Your own observation of symptoms.
- Diagnosis begins with a detailed medical history and general physical exam.
- Medical tests may include blood and urine studies and semen analysis (to check on quality, quantity, form, and motility). More testing may be done depending on these results.

APPROPRIATE HEALTH CARE
- A fertility treatment plan will be developed that is based on each couple's needs. It may include lifestyle changes, medical therapy (e.g., drugs or surgery), or assisted reproductive techniques (ART). ART can help many couples who are unable to conceive. The different ART options will be explained to you.
- A medical fertility specialist may be recommended for help and guidance.
- Counseling may be helpful for stress, sexual therapy techniques, marriage problems, or alcoholism.

POSSIBLE COMPLICATIONS—Emotional stress caused by feelings of guilt, inadequacy, and loss of self-esteem.

PROBABLE OUTCOME—Some fertility problems are minor and reversible. Often, no clear cause for infertility is found. Each patient should approach treatment with optimism.

HOW TO TREAT

GENERAL MEASURES
- To increase chances of conception, have intercourse every other day starting a few days before ovulation. (Sperm live for up to 72 hours.) Don't use lubricants.
- Try some lifestyle changes:
  - Stop smoking. It can reduce sperm counts and impair sperm motility.
  - Avoid alcohol or any substances of abuse.
  - Avoid hot baths or showers or hot tubs.
- To learn more: Resolve, 1760 Old Meadows Rd., Ste 500, McLean, VA 22102; (703) 556-7172 (not toll-free); website: www.resolve.org or American Fertility Assn., 305 Madison Ave., Suite 449, New York, NY 10165; (888) 917-3777; website: www.theafa.org.

MEDICATION
- Drugs may be prescribed to treat a cause of infertility.
- Dietary supplements may be recommended.

ACTIVITY—Usually no limits.

DIET—Eat a well-balanced diet. Begin a weight loss diet if overweight is a problem.

CALL YOUR DOCTOR IF

You or a family member has concerns about infertility.

FERTILITY PROBLEMS IN WOMEN

GENERAL INFORMATION

DEFINITION—Infertility is the inability to achieve pregnancy after 1 year (or 6 months for women over age 35) of sexual activity without use of birth control. Infertility affects 10% to 15% of reproductive-age couples. Causes of infertility are about equal in women and men (35% in each). In 20% of couples, both have problems, and in 10%, the cause is unknown.

BODY PARTS INVOLVED—Genitals; endocrine system; brain.

SEX OR AGE MOST AFFECTED—Females between puberty and menopause.

SIGNS & SYMPTOMS—Inability to conceive.

CAUSES—Infertility can be caused by a wide variety of factors, and sometimes the cause is unknown. In women, the causes are often due to ovulation problems or blocked or damaged tubes.

RISK INCREASES WITH
- Endometriosis (disorder of the uterine lining).
- Pelvic inflammatory disease.
- Ovulatory problem (unable to release eggs).
- Physical problems of the reproductive system.
- Repeated weight-gain/weight-loss cycles.
- Obesity.
- Hormone problems (such as thyroid).
- Vaginitis (inflammation of the vagina).
- Disorder of the cervix, such as infection, laceration or tearing from previous childbirth, or narrowing of the cervical opening for any reason.
- Amenorrhea (no menstrual periods).
- Chemical changes in the cervical mucus.
- Ovarian cysts.
- Smoking.
- Tumors.
- A genetic disorder (e.g., Turner syndrome).
- Emotional stress.
- Use of some drugs.
- Intrauterine device (IUD) may be a cause.
- Diabetes.
- Compulsive or excessive exercising.
- Marriage problems and infrequent sexual intercourse.
- Age. Female fertility decreases with age.
- Drugs of abuse, such as heroin or cocaine.
- Alcohol use.

HOW TO PREVENT
- Preventive measures depend on cause.
- Suggestions that may help you conceive:
  - Keep a basal body-temperature chart to become familiar with your ovulation pattern.
  - Have intercourse every other day starting a few days before ovulation. (Sperm live for up to 72 hours.) Don't use lubricants.
  - Your partner should withdraw his penis quickly from your vagina after ejaculation.
  - After partner's ejaculation, place pillows under your buttocks to allow sperm easier access.
  - Live a healthy lifestyle. Reduce stress. Eat a well-balanced diet. Exercise in moderation.
  - Avoid alcohol, drugs of abuse, and smoking.
  - Get counseling for emotional or marital problems.

WHAT TO EXPECT

DIAGNOSTIC MEASURES
- The first diagnostic tests may include a health history, blood tests, and a pelvic exam.
- Further testing may then be done. Multiple tests are available to study specific aspects of reproduction. You may be referred to a fertility specialist. Causes of infertility can be complex.

APPROPRIATE HEALTH CARE—A fertility treatment plan will be developed that is based on each couple's needs. It may include lifestyle changes, medical therapy (e.g., drugs or surgery), or assisted reproductive techniques (ART). ART can help many couples who are unable to conceive. The different ART options will be explained to you.

POSSIBLE COMPLICATIONS
- Emotional stress, including feelings of guilt, inadequacy, and loss of self-esteem.
- Treatment costs are high and often not covered by insurance.
- Long-term effect of fertility drugs is unknown.

PROBABLE OUTCOME—Some fertility problems are minor and reversible. Other problems may be helped with treatment.

HOW TO TREAT

GENERAL MEASURES—To learn more: Resolve, 1760 Old Meadows Rd., Ste 500, McLean, VA 22102; (703) 556-7172 (not toll-free); website: www.resolve.org or American Fertility Assn., 305 Madison Ave., Suite 449, New York, NY 10165; (888) 917-3777; website: www.theafa.org.

MEDICATION
- Drugs may be prescribed to treat a cause of infertility.
- Ovarian stimulating drugs may be prescribed.
- Begin taking folic acid. This will reduce the risk of birth defects once you become pregnant.

ACTIVITY—Regular exercise is important. Over-exercising may contribute to infertility.

DIET—Eat a well-balanced diet. If overweight, try to lose weight. Avoid caffeine and alcohol.

CALL YOUR DOCTOR IF

You or a family member is unable to become pregnant.

FETAL ALCOHOL SYNDROME

GENERAL INFORMATION

DEFINITION—Fetal alcohol syndrome (FAS) is a combination of irreversible birth abnormalities resulting from alcohol abuse by the mother during pregnancy. Fetal alcohol syndrome has been reported in babies of women who drank 2 mixed drinks or 2-3 bottles of beer or glasses of wine a day. Lesser degrees of alcohol abuse can result in less severe birth defects. There appears to be no safe level of alcohol during pregnancy.

SEX OR AGE MOST AFFECTED—Newborns.

SIGNS & SYMPTOMS
* Newborn behaviors:
  - Poor sucking ability; poor sleeping habits.
  - Irritability; effects of alcohol withdrawal.
* Possible physical abnormalities:
  - Small head; small eyes; unusually short stature.
  - Epicanthic folds (vertical folds of skin that go from upper eyelid to the side of nose).
  - Small jaw; protruding forehead.
  - Cleft palate.
  - Small brain; heart defects.
  - Hip dislocation; other joint deformities.
* Later:
  - Mental retardation; growth retardation.
  - Poor coordination; learning disabilities.
  - Speech and language difficulties; minimal brain dysfunction; hyperactivity; other behavioral problems.
* Adolescence to adulthood:
  - Maladaptive behaviors (social withdrawal, failure to consider consequence of actions, inappropriate emotional responses, excessive unhappiness, conduct problems).

CAUSES—Chronic (and probably binge-type) alcohol consumption during pregnancy. Alcohol intake can affect the unborn child during the first trimester by interfering with organ development, in the second trimester with mental retardation and the third trimester, retardation of fetal growth.

RISK INCREASES WITH
* The greater the alcohol consumption, the greater the risk for severe birth defects.
* Pregnant women not receiving prenatal health care.

HOW TO PREVENT
* Pregnant women (or those likely to become pregnant) should not drink any alcoholic drinks or abuse drugs. There is insufficient evidence that indicates an occasional glass of wine or beer is dangerous, but complete abstinence is recommended.
* If you are concerned about your alcohol consumption, seek help from your doctor, Alcoholics Anonymous or other support groups.
* Get early and continuing prenatal care.

WHAT TO EXPECT

DIAGNOSTIC MEASURES
* There is no diagnostic test that can determine an infant born with fetal alcohol syndrome. Some defects will be apparent at the time of birth; other defects will show up later.
* The diagnosis is difficult to confirm once the child is older. The mother may not remember if she drank during pregnancy or how much she drank. The child's academic performance may be blamed on behavior problems.

APPROPRIATE HEALTH CARE
* For the pregnant woman, get prenatal care.
* For the child, early diagnosis and recognition of a child at risk. A referral to medical professionals who can start immediately on special programs designed to enhance motor skills, improve communication skills and develop social interactions.

POSSIBLE COMPLICATIONS—The defects are generally irreversible. The complications may be mild or severe and include one or several of the problems listed in Signs and Symptoms.

PROBABLE OUTCOME—Since the effects of fetal alcohol syndrome can vary a great deal, the outcome is unpredictable.

HOW TO TREAT

GENERAL MEASURES
* If you are pregnant and continuing to drink alcohol, call your doctor to discuss the problem.
* If you know a family member or friend who is pregnant and continues to drink alcohol, talk to her about your concern and the risk she is taking with her unborn child.
* If you are the parent of a child with fetal alcohol syndrome, get the appropriate help needed for the child's development. Get help for yourself if the alcohol problem is continuing or if you need other psychological support.

MEDICATION—Drugs are usually not needed for this disorder.

ACTIVITY—Will depend on child's symptoms.

DIET—Usually no special diet is needed.

CALL YOUR DOCTOR IF

* You are pregnant or think you might be pregnant and have not had a check-up.
* You are concerned about your newborn's behavior, physical development or appearance.

FEVER OF UNKNOWN ORIGIN

 ## GENERAL INFORMATION

DEFINITION—Fever of unknown origin (FUO) is a diagnosis given in cases where a person has had a fever (off and on) for at least 3 weeks, and no cause has been found after a basic medical evaluation. It is a frustrating and challenging diagnosis for patients and their health care providers.

BODY PARTS INVOLVED—Any body organs or system may be the source of a fever-producing condition.

SEX OR AGE MOST AFFECTED—Both sexes; all ages.

SIGNS & SYMPTOMS
- Temperature above 101°F (38.3°C) on several occasions over a 3-week period.
- Muscle aches, chills, and headaches may occur in some cases.

CAUSES
- There are many possible causes (more than 200 disorders) for fever of unknown origin. Eventually, a specific cause is often determined, but in some cases, no cause is found.
- Likely causes of FUO in infants and children:
  - Infections.
  - Collagen or autoimmune diseases.
  - Tumors and cancer, especially leukemia.
- Likely causes of FUO in adults:
  - Infections.
  - Collagen or autoimmune diseases.
  - Tumors and cancer, especially kidney cancer, leukemia, and lymphoma.
  - Self-induced (in some emotionally unstable persons).
  - Adverse reaction of some drugs.

RISK INCREASES WITH
- Weak immune system due to illness or drugs.
- Chemical or environmental exposure to polluted water or air.
- Travel in areas with unsanitary conditions.
- Exposure to others with infectious diseases.
- Elderly persons.
- Drug abuse.

HOW TO PREVENT—There are no specific preventive measures.

 ## WHAT TO EXPECT

DIAGNOSTIC MEASURES
- Your own observation of symptoms.
- Your health care provider will do a physical exam and ask about your symptoms and activities.
- Because a fever may be the first evidence of a serious condition (in its early stages), careful medical testing may be done. This may include blood studies and a urine culture, x-rays of the chest, CT scan, an ultrasound, echocardiogram (heart function test), thyroid studies, liver function tests, an HIV antibody test, and others.

APPROPRIATE HEALTH CARE
- Treatment will depend on the underlying cause that is found.
- Hospital care may be recommended for elderly patients, patients with weak immune systems, and those with a serious chronic illness.

POSSIBLE COMPLICATIONS—Depends on the underlying condition causing the fever.

PROBABLE OUTCOME
- The outcome often depends on successful diagnosis and treatment of the underlying disorder.
- Some patients recover without having a diagnosis. It may take several months for the fever to resolve.

 ## HOW TO TREAT

GENERAL MEASURES—When at home, keep a daily temperature chart. Rectal temperatures are most accurate.

MEDICATION
- Acetaminophen or ibuprofen may be prescribed, to lower the fever.
- Until the cause is found, other prescription drugs may be withheld to avoid masking symptoms of the underlying disorder.
- In certain patients, antibiotics, steroids, or other drugs may be prescribed prior to a specific diagnosis.

ACTIVITY—Get extra rest while you have a fever.

DIET—No special diet. Drink extra fluids while you have a fever.

 ## CALL YOUR DOCTOR IF

- You or a family member has an unexplained fever that lasts longer than 24 hours.
- New symptoms develop. They may provide a clue about the underlying cause of the fever.

FIBROCYSTIC BREAST CHANGES

 GENERAL INFORMATION

DEFINITION—Fibrocystic changes are the most common cause of breast lumps in women. Over 50% of women have these changes at some point in their lives. The changes are not cancerous and are not a threat to health.

BODY PARTS INVOLVED—Breasts.

SEX OR AGE MOST AFFECTED—They can affect females from puberty to around age 50.

SIGNS & SYMPTOMS
- The changes may affect one or both breasts. Single lumps may occur, but multiple lumps are common.
- Lumps may offer resistance when pressed with fingertips and they may feel tender. They often enlarge before menstrual periods and shrink afterward.
- Breasts may be swollen and engorged.
- Mild to severe breast pain. It may be constant, on or off, irregular, or occur just before menstrual periods.
- Some women develop cysts, which are fluid-filled sacs that feel smooth and firm.
- Lumps come in different sizes. When the lumps are relatively large and near the surface, they can be moved freely within the breast.

CAUSES—The cause is unclear. Ovarian hormones appear to play a role. Fibrocystic changes may be caused by abnormal hormone levels or by an increased response of breast tissue to normal hormone levels.

RISK INCREASES WITH—Women who have not had children, have irregular menstrual cycles, or have a family history of fibrocystic breast changes or breast cancer. Studies on other risk factors are ongoing.

HOW TO PREVENT—Specific preventive measures are unknown. It may help to eat a low-fat diet and avoid smoking.

 WHAT TO EXPECT

DIAGNOSTIC MEASURES
- Your own observation of symptoms.
- Your health care provider will do a breast exam and examine the underarm area.
- Medical tests may include mammogram, ultrasound, and surgical diagnostic procedures, such as cyst aspiration.

APPROPRIATE HEALTH CARE
- The breast changes may get better without treatment. If symptoms continue, diet changes may help and drug therapy may be an option. Keep a pain diary for 2 to 3 months to determine the pattern of the pain.

- Some cysts can be aspirated (removing the fluid). This is done in a health care provider's office. Removing the fluid should cause the lump to disappear. If the lump does not disappear, further diagnostic testing is done.

POSSIBLE COMPLICATIONS—Only about 5% of fibrocystic breast changes have atypical cells that are a risk factor for developing cancer.

PROBABLE OUTCOME—Women with fibrocystic breast changes continue to have breast lumps that appear and dissolve. Some remain permanently. Treatment may help relieve symptoms. The condition often disappears after menopause (unless estrogen-replacement therapy is used).

 HOW TO TREAT

GENERAL MEASURES
- Apply heat in some form or cold compresses to the breasts to help any discomfort.
- Wear a well-fitting, supportive bra.
- Stop smoking. Find a way to quit.
- Examine your breasts carefully each month. Report new lumps or any changes in lumps that have been diagnosed previously.
- Get routine mammogram studies as advised.
- Visit your health care provider at least every year for a breast exam. If you have a family history of cancer, more frequent follow-up visits may be recommended.

MEDICATION
- Birth control pills may be prescribed to help control hormone levels. For more severe symptoms, danazol or bromocriptine may be prescribed.
- Use nonprescription pain remedies for pain.
- Some women take vitamin A, vitamin B-6, vitamin E, or evening primrose oil to relieve symptoms. Ask your health care provider about these supplements.

ACTIVITY—No limits. A regular exercise program is usually recommended. Avoid activities that cause breast discomfort.

DIET
- Avoiding beverages that contain caffeine (coffee, tea, and some soft drinks) may help relieve symptoms.
- Eat a low-fat diet. Reducing salt and sugar may help.

 CALL YOUR DOCTOR IF

- You or a family member has undiagnosed lumps in the breast.
- Lumps change, or new lumps appear.

FIBROMYALGIA
(Fibrositis)

GENERAL INFORMATION

DEFINITION—Fibromyalgia is a painful condition that involves muscles, tendons, and ligaments. It may affect the muscle areas of the low back, neck, shoulder, chest, arms, hips, and thighs. It is a chronic problem that can come and go for years.

BODY PARTS INVOLVED—Muscular areas of the low back, neck, shoulder, chest, arms, hips and thighs.

SEX OR AGE MOST AFFECTED—It occurs in both men and women in all age groups, including children. It most often affects women ages 20 to 50.

SIGNS & SYMPTOMS
- Pain and aches in the muscles, often described as "hurting all over all the time."
- Fatigue and sleep problems.
- Certain areas of the body are tender to the touch (tender points). Common tender points are in the knees, thighs, elbows, chest, hip joints, and around the neck.
- Feeling stiffness in mornings; swollen joints; hands and feet may be numb and tingly.
- Headache, anxiety, and depression.
- Other symptoms may also occur, such as digestion, bowel, and urinary problems; vision changes; emotional or mental changes; allergies; dry eyes and mouth; and painful menstrual periods.
- Symptoms may be brought on by a change in the weather, being in cold or damp places, stress, hormone changes, or in response to activity.

CAUSES—The cause is unknown. Genetics and other factors (e.g., severe physical or emotional trauma or an illness) may play a role.

RISK INCREASES WITH
- Females ages 20 to 50.
- Having a relative with the condition. It appears to run in families.

HOW TO PREVENT—There are no steps that will prevent fibromyalgia.

WHAT TO EXPECT

DIAGNOSTIC MEASURES
- Your own observation of symptoms.
- There is no special test to diagnose fibromyalgia. Your health care provider will do a physical exam, check the tender points in your body, and ask about all the symptoms you have. Similar symptoms occur in other health problems and these need to be ruled out.
- Medical tests (e.g., blood studies and x-rays may be done).

APPROPRIATE HEALTH CARE
- There is no cure for fibromyalgia. Taking steps to reduce the symptoms is the main goal.
- Treatment steps vary. They may include prescribed drugs and injections, exercise, physical therapy, acupuncture, chiropractic care, or massage therapy.
- Counseling can help reduce stress and anxiety and promote well-being.

POSSIBLE COMPLICATIONS
- Limits to activities of daily living.
- Disability in a few cases.

PROBABLE OUTCOME—The symptoms vary and may improve on their own or can be helped with treatment. The condition does not lead to more serious illness, nor is it life-threatening.

HOW TO TREAT

GENERAL MEASURES
- Make changes in your life as needed to help you cope day-to-day. Maintain your social life and contact with friends.
- Join a local support group so you can talk with others about self-help ideas that work.
- Get as much sleep as you need.
- Don't smoke. Find a way to quit.
- To learn more: National Fibromyalgia Assn., 2121 S. Towne Centre Pl., Suite 300, Orange, CA 92806; (714) 921-0150 (not toll-free); website: www.fmaware.org.

MEDICATION
- For minor pain, use nonprescription drugs such as acetaminophen or ibuprofen.
- Oral drugs may be prescribed for symptoms of pain, depression, anxiety, and sleep problems. They will take a few weeks to work.
- Injections into tender points may be prescribed.

ACTIVITY
- To help maintain muscle tone and reduce pain and stiffness, begin a daily, low-impact exercise program (e.g., water aerobics). Start slowly; increase gradually.
- Physical therapy may be recommended.
- Keep activity levels about the same each day.

DIET
- Limit or avoid caffeine and alcohol.
- Eat a healthy diet. Your health care provider or a dietitian can help you plan a diet.

CALL YOUR DOCTOR IF

- You or a family member has some of the symptoms of fibromyalgia.
- Symptoms continue or worsen despite treatment or new symptoms develop.

FLUID & ELECTROLYTE DISORDERS

GENERAL INFORMATION

DEFINITION—A fluid and electrolyte disorder is an imbalance of the fluids and electrolytes in the body. Electrolytes are minerals found in the body that maintain many important body functions. The major electrolytes are sodium, calcium, potassium, magnesium, bicarbonate, phosphate, and chloride.

BODY PARTS INVOLVED—All.

SEX OR AGE MOST AFFECTED—Both sexes; all ages.

SIGNS & SYMPTOMS
- Dry mouth and wrinkled skin.
- Increased, decreased, or no urination.
- Fatigue.
- Muscle weakness, cramping, or twitching.
- Puffy legs, hands, face, or stomach.
- Lung congestion. Problems with breathing.
- Changes in mental status, depression, irritability.
- Fast or slow heartbeat.
- Constipation, nausea, and vomiting.
- Seizures or coma.

CAUSES—A variety of diseases and medical problems can lead to an imbalance. When the body loses fluids (such as with diarrhea) or retains fluids (such as with heart failure), the electrolyte balance is affected. Electrolytes may be too low (hypo-) or too high (hyper-).

RISK INCREASES WITH
- Diarrhea and/or vomiting.
- Heavy sweating.
- Serious burns, wounds, or other injuries.
- Heart or kidney disorders.
- Excess fluid intake.
- Use of diuretics (water pills).
- Laxative abuse.
- Certain types of prescription drugs.
- Diabetes.
- Endocrine diseases.
- Bone disorders.
- Milk-alkali syndrome (excess calcium intake).
- Fever.
- Unusual or extreme diets, or eating disorders.
- Alcoholism.
- Infants, young children, and people over 60. These people lose fluids very quickly when sick.

HOW TO PREVENT
- Avoid risk factors, where possible.
- Get medical care for chronic medical disorder.

WHAT TO EXPECT

DIAGNOSTIC MEASURES
- Your health care provider may do a physical exam and ask questions about your symptoms and activities.

- Medical tests include blood studies of electrolyte levels.

APPROPRIATE HEALTH CARE
- Treatment will depend on the underlying cause. This may include changes in diet or fluid intake, changes in drugs that may have caused the problem, prescribing new drugs, or other therapies as needed.
- Treatment steps include correcting the fluid and electrolyte imbalance. Electrolytes that are too low will be replaced. Electrolytes that are too high will be reduced. Hospital care may be needed for some patients to provide IV (intravenous) treatment. Patients with milder symptoms may be cared for at home.
- Dialysis (use of a machine to filter wastes) may be needed for some patients with kidney disorders.

POSSIBLE COMPLICATIONS—Severe imbalances can cause serious and life-threatening disorders.

PROBABLE OUTCOME—Treatment is usually effective. A long-term outlook depends on the underlying cause.

HOW TO TREAT

GENERAL MEASURES—None specific.

MEDICATION
- Electrolyte replacements may be prescribed. They may be given through a vein (IV) or taken orally.
- Drugs to reduce high electrolyte levels may be prescribed.
- Drugs to treat an underlying disorder may be prescribed.

ACTIVITY—Limit activities and avoid exercise until treatment is complete. Resume normal activities gradually.

DIET
- For a severe imbalance, solid food may be withheld until fluids and electrolytes return to normal.
- Diet changes may be recommended by your health care provider to help prevent problems in the future.

CALL YOUR DOCTOR IF

- You or a family member has symptoms of a fluid and electrolyte imbalance or dehydration.
- Your weight increases or decreases several pounds in one day.

FOLIC ACID DEFICIENCY

GENERAL INFORMATION

DEFINITION—Folic acid deficiency occurs when the body does not have enough folic acid (folate). Folic acid is one of the B vitamins. It has important functions in the body, including making red blood cells. The folic acid in the body is normally acquired from foods in the diet. A folic acid deficiency can develop due to a number of health problems.

BODY PARTS INVOLVED—All.

SEX OR AGE MOST AFFECTED—Both sexes; all ages. Elderly persons and pregnant women are more often affected.

SIGNS & SYMPTOMS
- It may take months before any symptoms are obvious. The deficiency leads to anemia and its symptoms.
- Fatigue and weakness.
- Loss of appetite and weight loss.
- Red, sore tongue.
- Mouth sores.
- Headache.
- Paleness of skin.
- May have forgetfulness, irritability, or trouble with concentration.
- Nausea, vomiting, and diarrhea.
- Infants and children can have slow growth rate.

CAUSES
- The deficiency can be caused by:
  - Not enough folic acid foods in the diet.
  - The folic acid is not absorbed by the body.
  - The body cannot use the folic acid that is absorbed.
  - There is an increased need for folic acid.
  - The body excretes or destroys more folic acid than is normal.

RISK INCREASES WITH
- Adults over 60.
- Poor nutrition or malabsorption.
- Excess alcohol use.
- Pregnancy. A pregnant women needs eight times more folic acid than usual with pregnancy.
- Chronic illness or recent surgery.
- Deficiency of vitamin B-12 or vitamin C.
- Smoking.
- Use of certain drugs.

HOW TO PREVENT
- No specific preventive measures.
- Limit or avoid alcohol use.
- Eat a healthy diet.
- Don't smoke.
- Have regular medical checkups during pregnancy and take prenatal vitamins as prescribed.

WHAT TO EXPECT

DIAGNOSTIC MEASURES
- Your health care provider may do a physical exam and ask questions about your symptoms and diet.
- Medical tests usually include blood studies of folic acid levels and vitamin B-12 levels.

APPROPRIATE HEALTH CARE—Treatment consists of folic acid supplement and treating or eliminating any underlying cause.

POSSIBLE COMPLICATIONS
- Megaloblastic (pernicious) anemia.
- Pregnant women have increased risk of premature birth, low birth weight baby, and baby with neural tube defects (defects of the spinal cord and nervous system).
- Increased homocysteine levels (a possible risk for heart problems or cognitive decline).
- May increase risk of cancer.

PROBABLE OUTCOME—Usually curable in 2 weeks to 2 months with an adequate folic acid intake. It will also depend on the underlying cause.

HOW TO TREAT

GENERAL MEASURES—If you smoke, find a way to quit.

MEDICATION—Folic acid will be prescribed. It may be taken for a few months. In some people, it may be taken for life.

ACTIVITY—Fatigue can occur. Schedule regular rest periods until you are able to resume normal activity.

DIET
- Eat foods daily that are high in folic acid. Green, leafy vegetables, citrus fruits, beans, and whole grains are good sources.
- Avoid or limit alcohol use.

CALL YOUR DOCTOR IF

- You or a family member has symptoms of folic acid deficiency.
- Symptoms don't improve in a few weeks, despite treatment.

FOLLICULITIS

GENERAL INFORMATION

DEFINITION—Folliculitis is an inflammation of the hair follicles. Follicles are where the roots of body hair grow. Folliculitis can involve the hair on the skin anywhere on the body.

BODY PARTS INVOLVED—It usually affects the face (such as the beard area in men), scalp, legs, armpits, and groin area.

SEX OR AGE MOST AFFECTED—Both sexes; all ages.

SIGNS & SYMPTOMS
* Small groups of bumps (called papules or pustules) develop, usually with a hair in the middle of each bump. The bumps are small, and yellow-white in color, with a red area around them.
* Itchiness, tenderness, pain, redness, or swelling of the skin may occur.

CAUSES—Most often it is an infection of the hair follicles with *Staphylococcus* or *Pseudomonas* bacteria. It may also be caused by a fungal infection or irritation. Folliculitis may be superficial (on the surface of the skin) or deep in the hair follicle.

RISK INCREASES WITH
* Diabetes.
* Weak immune system due to illness or drugs.
* Excess sweating (hyperhidrosis).
* Eczema or dermatitis.
* Skin injuries, abrasions, surgical wounds, or draining abscess.
* Shaving, waxing, or plucking hairs.
* Poor hygiene.
* Obesity.
* Poorly cleaned swimming pools or hot tubs.
* Use of certain skin care products or overuse of topical steroids.
* Long-term antibiotic use.

HOW TO PREVENT
* Wash hands often to prevent spread of any germs.
* Frequent bathing. Keep fingernails short and clean.
* Wash towels and linens often to prevent spread of germs.
* Avoid risk factors where possible.

WHAT TO EXPECT

DIAGNOSTIC MEASURES
* See your health care provider if you have concerns about the disorder. A health care provider can diagnose folliculitis by an exam of the affected area.
* A culture of fluid from the pustule or other tests may be done.

APPROPRIATE HEALTH CARE—Treatment involves supportive care of the skin. Drug therapy may be used.

POSSIBLE COMPLICATIONS
* May progress to other types of skin problems.
* Scarring may occur.
* Folliculitis may recur or become chronic.

PROBABLE OUTCOME—Most cases clear up within 2 weeks. Some may take longer.

HOW TO TREAT

GENERAL MEASURES
* Don't scratch the affected area. The germs can be transferred from under the fingernails to other parts of the body.
* Use warm-water soaks to relieve itching and help healing.
* Clean area with antibacterial soap. Shampoo daily if the scalp is involved.
* Avoid using oils or greasy-type ointments on the skin.
* If you shave, change razor blades daily or use an electric razor.
* If folliculitis recurs or becomes chronic, shaving may need to be discontinued for a period of time.

MEDICATION
* If there are only a few bumps, you may use nonprescription, topical antibiotics (such as mupirocin) or anti-itch creams. Apply as directed.
* Oral or topical antibiotics or antifungals may be prescribed.
* A topical antibiotic drug applied into the front of the nose may be prescribed. The nostrils are a source of bacteria that can be spread to other parts of the body.
* Other drugs may be prescribed if a cause other than bacterial or fungal is diagnosed.

ACTIVITY—No limits.

DIET—No special diet. A weight-loss diet may be recommended for overweight patients.

CALL YOUR DOCTOR IF

* You or a family member has symptoms of folliculitis.
* You develop a boil or signs of spreading infection or folliculitis recurs after treatment.

FOOD ALLERGY

GENERAL INFORMATION

DEFINITION—Food allergy is a reaction of the body's immune system to some foods. Many people think they have a food allergy when it is food intolerance. Intolerance is caused by digestion problems, such as lactose or milk intolerance. A food allergy can cause severe symptoms. Food intolerance symptoms are rarely serious. It is important to know which one you have. Your health care provider can help you with the diagnosis.

BODY PARTS INVOLVED—Skin, lungs, gastrointestinal, central nervous system.

SEX OR AGE MOST AFFECTED—Males more often than females; all ages; food allergies are more common in children.

SIGNS & SYMPTOMS
- Symptoms begin in minutes to 2 hours after eating.
- Skin hives, rash (called eczema), itching, redness, and swelling of hands, feet, face, and lips.
- Diarrhea, stomach pains, nausea, or vomiting.
- Cough, wheezing, or sneezing; runny nose.
- Infants may have blood in the stool or colic.

CAUSES
- The immune system reacts to certain proteins found in foods. It treats them as harmful to the body and tries to fight them off by releasing chemicals and histamines. This is what starts the allergic symptoms. Why it occurs in some people is unknown.
- Just about any food can cause an allergic reaction. Most common are milk, eggs, wheat, soy, peanut, tree nuts (walnuts and pecans), fish, and shellfish. Chocolate is not a common cause.

RISK INCREASES WITH
- People who have other allergy problems.
- Having family members with a food allergy.
- Young children (food allergy is more common).

HOW TO PREVENT—Food allergy cannot be prevented. A reaction can be prevented once the food causing it is known.

WHAT TO EXPECT

DIAGNOSTIC MEASURES
- Your own observation of symptoms.
- For diagnosis, your health care provider will ask questions about your symptoms and your diet, and may include a physical exam. Testing might involve skin and blood allergy tests, a food challenge test, or an elimination diet that you do at home.

APPROPRIATE HEALTH CARE—Once you know for sure that you have a food allergy, the treatment is to avoid the food or foods involved.

POSSIBLE COMPLICATIONS—None expected as long as the foods are avoided. Rarely, anaphylaxis (a severe, life-threatening reaction) occurs. Symptoms come on very quickly. They can include those listed above plus trouble breathing, fast heart rate, and loss of consciousness. Seek emergency help.

PROBABLE OUTCOME
- Infants will often outgrow food allergy by 2 to 4 years.
- Adults with food allergy (particularly to milk, fish, shellfish, or nuts) are more likely to have their allergy for many years.
- Research is ongoing so new methods for treatment and prevention may become available.

HOW TO TREAT

GENERAL MEASURES
- Often, the food allergy is in a young child. Parents will need to discuss the allergy with any people who will be caring for, teaching, or working with the child. They need to know what foods are involved and how to handle a severe reaction if one occurs. Once a child is older, parents can begin to teach the child how to take control of the allergy.
- Wear or carry medical ID about food allergy.
- To learn more: Food Allergy & Anaphylaxis Network, 11781 Lee Jackson Hwy, Suite 160, Fairfax, VA 22033; (800) 929-4040; website: www.foodallergy.org.

MEDICATION
- Drugs will not cure a food allergy. Drugs may be prescribed to relieve some of the symptoms such as an antihistamine for itching or rash.
- If your food allergy is severe, you should carry a kit with a self-injecting device that contains the drug epinephrine. It can be used if the food is eaten by mistake and a reaction occurs. Know how to use the device. In addition, your family or others need to know how to give the injection if you are unable to do so.

ACTIVITY—No limits.

DIET
- Read labels carefully on food products.
- Use a food allergy cookbook to plan meals.
- Ask waiters in restaurants for details about foods and other items on the menu.

CALL YOUR DOCTOR IF

You or a family member has symptoms of food allergy.

FOOD POISONING

GENERAL INFORMATION

DEFINITION—Food poisoning is a term used to describe illnesses suspected of being caused by contaminated food (or beverages). Outbreaks can affect several members of a household, customers who dined at the same restaurant, nursing home patients, cruise ship passengers, university students, children in daycare, or shoppers who bought contaminated food in a store.

BODY PARTS INVOLVED—Gastrointestinal.

SEX OR AGE MOST AFFECTED—Both sexes; all ages.

SIGNS & SYMPTOMS
- Symptoms can begin within hours to days after eating the food. It depends on the cause of the contamination and how much food was ingested (eaten).
- Nausea and vomiting.
- Abdominal cramps or pain.
- Diarrhea.
- Bloody stools.
- Fever, chills, headache, and weakness may occur.
- In severe cases, shock and collapse can occur.

CAUSES
- Bacteria such as *Campylobacter*, *Escherichia coli*, *Salmonella*, and others. Botulism is a rare, life-threatening food poisoning.
- Virus infection such as Norwalk virus (a common contaminant of shellfish), adenovirus, and rotavirus.
- Chemical causes such as contamination with insecticide or food served in a lead-glazed dish.
- Eating plants or animals that contain a naturally occurring poison, such as mushrooms or toadstools. Shellfish may contain a toxin that is not destroyed by cooking.

RISK INCREASED WITH
- Eating improperly prepared or stored foods.
- Lack of good hygiene when preparing food.
- Drinking water or eating raw foods when traveling in a foreign country.

HOW TO PREVENT
- Avoid raw seafood, meat, or dairy products.
- Avoid unpasteurized food products.
- Properly cook and store foods.
- Keep cooking areas and utensils clean.
- Throw food items away that are old, have an "off" smell, or those in bulging tin cans.
- Always wash hands before preparing food.

WHAT TO EXPECT

DIAGNOSTIC MEASURES
- Your health care provider may do a physical exam. Questions will be asked about your symptoms and recent foods you have eaten, and if other people have eaten the same foods.
- Tests may be done on vomit, blood, urine, or stool samples. If some of the food that made you sick is available, you may be asked to bring it in for testing.

APPROPRIATE HEALTH CARE
- The main treatment is to replace fluid and electrolytes (salts and minerals) lost through vomiting or diarrhea.
- Hospital care may be needed if symptoms are severe. Fluids may be given through a vein (IV).
- If several persons are affected, contact the local health department. They can investigate and take steps to control any outbreaks and prevent more cases.

POSSIBLE COMPLICATIONS—Dehydration is the most common complication. More serious complications are rare but they can be life-threatening, especially in very young or elderly patients or persons with weak immune systems.

PROBABLE OUTCOME—Most cases are mild and clear up within a few days.

HOW TO TREAT

GENERAL MEASURES—In mild cases, self-care may be all that is needed. See a health care provider if symptoms are other than mild.

MEDICATION
- Drugs are not needed to treat food poisoning. They may be prescribed for certain symptoms.
- Antibiotics may be prescribed.
- Don't take drugs for diarrhea unless they are prescribed. They may prolong the symptoms.

ACTIVITY—Get extra rest until symptoms improve.

DIET
- Suck ice chips or drink small amounts of clear fluids often. Replace lost fluids and electrolytes with products such as Pedialyte or Ricelyte for infants and children, and diluted rehydration fluids (Gatorade) for adults.
- Once the symptoms improve, try a diet of complex carbohydrates (rice, wheat, potatoes, bread, cereal, and lean meat such as chicken). Milk and dairy products usually do not need to be limited.
- Avoid high-sugar foods or fatty foods for a few days.

CALL YOUR DOCTOR IF

You or a family member has signs or symptoms of food poisoning that cause concern or are not improving.

FROSTBITE

GENERAL INFORMATION

DEFINITION—Frostbite is the destruction of body tissue from exposure to temperatures or wind chill below freezing. Other nonfreezing cold injuries include: frostnip, chilblains, and immersion foot (a cold and wet exposure).

BODY PARTS INVOLVED—Arms and legs (especially fingers and toes); face (especially nose and ears).

SEX OR AGE MOST AFFECTED—Both sexes; all ages (more common in males ages 30 to 49).

SIGNS & SYMPTOMS
- In milder cases, there may be burning, numbness, tingling, itching, or coldness in the affected area. Skin may be white and frozen in appearance, and may have some resistance when pressed.
- In more severe cases of frostbite, there may be no sensations in the affected area. Swelling and blood-filled blisters may appear. Skin may be white or yellow, look waxy, and turn purple as it is rewarmed. The area is hard when it is pressed. The affected area can look blackened and dead.
- Hypothermia (low body temperature) can cause uncontrolled shivering, weakness, and confusion.

CAUSES—Frostbite occurs when ice crystals form in skin and blood vessels, which leads to destruction of the cells. Further damage can occur upon rewarming when blood flow resumes into the damaged blood vessels.

RISK INCREASES WITH
- Car accidents or car breakdowns in bad weather (especially in remote areas).
- Drinking too much alcohol or abusing drugs.
- Elderly persons.
- Diabetes, blood-vessel diseases, or smoking.
- Persons with mental disorders.
- Homeless persons.
- High-altitude travel or activities.
- Poor conditioning, inadequate clothing, clothing that is wet and tight, dehydration, malnutrition, and fatigue.

HOW TO PREVENT
- Dress for the cold weather. Dress in layers. Carry extra gear (e.g., jacket, gloves, socks, hat, and blankets).
- Avoid smoking and alcohol.
- Travel with someone, in case help is needed.

WHAT TO EXPECT

DIAGNOSTIC MEASURES—An exam by a health care provider is done to check for life-threatening problems and to diagnose frostbite or other types of cold injury, such as frostnip.

APPROPRIATE HEALTH CARE
- Rewarming for frostbite is usually done in a warm bath until the thaw is complete. It can be a painful process. Fluids are often given through a vein (IV). Supplemental oxygen may be needed.
- Hospital care may be required to treat skin damage, assess the extent of injury, and to prevent infection. Whirlpool bath therapy may be done to remove dead tissue. The affected area may be elevated and splinted.
- It may take months to see if the affected tissue will be healthy or permanently damaged. Surgery may be done to remove damaged tissue, including amputation.

POSSIBLE COMPLICATIONS
- Minor complications, such as pain, changes in sensitivity of the affected area, and skin color changes.
- Major complications, such as amputation.

PROBABLE OUTCOME—For milder cold injuries, complete recovery is expected. More severe frostbite may have complications. Full recovery can take months.

HOW TO TREAT

GENERAL MEASURES
- Emergency care for frostbite:
  - Call for help. Arrange for transport to a hospital.
  - Move patient to a warm area. Keep the affected area elevated. Keep the person warm to prevent hypothermia. Remove tight clothing or jewelry (they may block blood flow).
  - Don't rewarm the affected area if there is a chance it may freeze again. Don't rewarm it using an open fire or dry heat. Put the affected area in warm (not hot) water.
  - Give warm fluids to drink (no alcohol or caffeine).
  - Never massage (rub) the affected areas.
  - Cover the area with soft, cloth bandages.
  - Place cloth or cotton between toes/fingers to prevent rubbing.

MEDICATION—You may be prescribed drugs for pain relief, antibiotics to prevent infection, and/or a tetanus booster.

ACTIVITY—Will depend on extent of damage. Physical therapy may be needed.

DIET—Warm fluids to start with, as tolerated thereafter.

CALL YOUR DOCTOR IF

You or a family member has symptoms of frostbite or cold injury, or you observe them in someone else.

GALLSTONES
(Cholelithiasis)

GENERAL INFORMATION

DEFINITION—Gallstones are hard objects (stones) that form in the gallbladder and its ducts.

BODY PARTS INVOLVED—Gallbladder (body organ that stores bile); bile ducts.

SEX OR AGE MOST AFFECTED—They can affect young people and adults of both sexes, and are more common in women.

SIGNS & SYMPTOMS
- No symptoms in about 40% of cases.
- Sharp pain in the upper-right stomach area, between the shoulder blades, or in the right shoulder.
- Nausea, vomiting, bloating or belching.
- Fever (sometimes).
- Fatty foods cause indigestion.
- Jaundice, which causes yellow skin and eyes.

CAUSES—Bile is a liquid made by the liver and stored in the gallbladder. Its use in the body is to help with digestion. Gallstones form when substances in the bile liquid harden. This may be due to too much cholesterol or bilirubin, or not enough bile salts, or the gallbladder not emptying as it should. Stones may be small like a grain of sand or as large as a golf ball. There may be one or hundreds of tiny stones.

RISK INCREASES WITH
- Ages over 60 and women more than men.
- Family history of gallstones.
- Some ethnic groups (e.g., Hispanics and Native Americans).
- Overweight.
- Diabetes.
- Excess estrogen in the body (e.g., from birth control pills, pregnancy, or estrogen therapy).
- Rapid weight loss or fasting.
- Diet high in fat and cholesterol and low in fiber.
- Drugs that lower cholesterol can actually increase the cholesterol in the bile, which can lead to gallstones.
- Stomach reduction surgery.

HOW TO PREVENT—No known way to prevent.

WHAT TO EXPECT

DIAGNOSTIC MEASURES
- Your own observation of symptoms.
- Your health care provider will do a physical exam and ask questions about your symptoms.
- Medical tests may include blood tests and an ultrasound, which can detect the stones by sound waves. Other tests may be done to confirm diagnosis or check for complications.

APPROPRIATE HEALTH CARE
- There are several ways to treat gallstones that are causing symptoms. They include surgery, shockwave treatment, and sometimes drugs or diet changes.
- Cholecystectomy is surgery to remove the gallbladder. For most people, this will relieve the symptoms. Surgery options include:
  - Laparoscopic procedure. This procedure uses tiny incisions through the skin and a special instrument to remove the gallbladder.
  - Open surgery. A more serious procedure that requires a longer incision to remove the gallbladder.
- Less often, treatment involves shockwave (lithotripsy) to break up (shatter) the stones or chemicals passed into the gallbladder via a catheter to dissolve the stones.

POSSIBLE COMPLICATIONS
- A stone becomes lodged in a duct. Ducts are tubes that carry bile to and from the gallbladder. A lodged stone can cause serious problems with the gallbladder, pancreas, or liver.
- Gallstones may recur if treatment does not include removing the gallbladder.

PROBABLE OUTCOME—Gallstones that cause no symptoms can safely be left alone. They are unlikely to cause problems. For those who do have symptoms, treatment is available.

HOW TO TREAT

GENERAL MEASURES
- Diet changes may help symptoms for a while, but not permanently.
- To learn more: National Digestive Diseases Information Clearinghouse, 2 Information Way, Bethesda, MD 20892; (800) 891-5389; website: www.digestive.niddk.nih.gov.

MEDICATION—Less common treatment is the use of drugs taken by mouth to dissolve stones. It is used for certain types of stones and can require up to 2 years to be effective.

ACTIVITY—You will be advised of limits depending on the type of treatment. Get extra rest while you recover.

DIET—A low-fat or weight loss diet may be recommended.

CALL YOUR DOCTOR IF

- You or a family member has symptoms of gallstones.
- Fever or pain occurs that lasts for more than 3 hours.

GANGRENE

GENERAL INFORMATION

DEFINITION—Gangrene is dead tissue. It forms when a wound becomes infected or tissue is destroyed by an accident.

BODY PARTS INVOLVED—Any body part, but the most common sites are toes, feet, legs, fingers, hands and arms. It can also affect internal organs. The most dangerous areas are abdominal organs.

SEX OR AGE MOST AFFECTED—Both sexes; all ages.

SIGNS & SYMPTOMS
- Skin may be pale at first, then turn red or bronze, and finally, a purple or blue-black color.
- Crackling of the skin. This feels like pressing on air bubbles under the skin.
- Swelling of the skin tissue.
- Pain or loss of sensation in affected area.
- Bad-smelling discharge from the dead tissues.
- Fever, sweating, and fast heartbeat.

CAUSES—Gangrene occurs when blood flow to a section of the body is blocked or reduced. There are two types. Dry gangrene is when there is no infection and is often caused by a blood clot or frostbite. Wet gangrene occurs when a wound becomes infected with bacteria. Gas gangrene is a type of wet gangrene.

RISK INCREASES WITH
- Infection with bacteria.
- Body injury caused by accidents, surgery, or deep puncture wounds.
- Crush injury that cuts off blood supply.
- Blood clot in an artery.
- Hardening of the arteries.
- Prolonged frostbite.
- Diabetes.
- Smoking.
- Excess alcohol use.
- Poor blood circulation.
- Elderly.

HOW TO PREVENT
- Avoid any risk factors where possible.
- If you have diabetes, stick closely to your program to control diabetes. Check your feet often for signs of unhealthy tissue.
- Seek medical advice for signs of infection (warmth, swelling, redness, pain, or tenderness) in a skin injury.

WHAT TO EXPECT

DIAGNOSTIC MEASURES
- Hospital care is needed for treatment. Your health care provider will do an exam of the affected area.

- Medical tests will be done to determine the extent of the problem. These may include blood studies and a culture of the fluid from the wound. Imaging tests such as x-ray, CT, or MRI may help with diagnosis.

APPROPRIATE HEALTH CARE
- Treatment will be given for any medical problem that is causing the gangrene, and to help restore blood flow to the affected area.
- You may need oxygen supplied through a mask or into the nose to help you breathe.
- You may be placed in a sealed chamber (hyperbaric) where high-pressure oxygen is used for treatment.
- Amputation of an infected body part may be needed to keep the infection from spreading. This often involves part of an arm or leg. Instructions will be provided for ongoing home care and physical therapy following surgery.

POSSIBLE COMPLICATIONS
- Liver damage, kidney failure, shock, and coma.
- Limb removal (amputation).
- Gangrene can be fatal, even with treatment.

PROBABLE OUTCOME—Outcome will vary depending on severity of gangrene. Early diagnosis and aggressive treatment can improve prognosis.

HOW TO TREAT

GENERAL MEASURES—The family should maintain an optimistic outlook, stay in close contact with the patient's doctor and help by making their visits with the patient as supportive as possible.

MEDICATION—In the hospital, you will be given antibiotics, pain relievers, and, usually, blood thinners to prevent blood clotting. Additional drugs may be needed to treat other disorders diagnosed.

ACTIVITY
- Rest in bed until healing begins. Your health care provider will advise you of any limits to your activities.
- Physical therapy may be needed after an amputation.

DIET—Usually no special diet unless advised.

CALL YOUR DOCTOR IF

- You or a family member has symptoms of gangrene.
- Pain continues, despite drugs and treatment.
- Fever or infection develops during recovery.

GAS & GAS PAIN

GENERAL INFORMATION

DEFINITION—Expelling gas (flatulence) from the rectum is a byproduct of the digestive process. It is normal and most people pass gas 10 to 20 times a day. People may think they have too much gas when they actually have normal amounts. Belching is another way of passing gas, but is not discussed in this topic.

BODY PARTS INVOLVED—Digestive system.

SEX OR AGE MOST AFFECTED—All ages and both sexes.

SIGNS & SYMPTOMS
- Voluntary or involuntary passing of gas. It can be odorless or bad smelling; and quiet or loud.
- Cramps, discomfort, or pain in the abdomen. (These symptoms may disappear once gas is passed.)
- May have bloating (swelling and tightness in abdomen).

CAUSES—Swallowed air and normal breakdown of certain undigested foods by harmless bacteria normally present in the large intestine (colon). Gas is mostly made up of odorless vapors—carbon dioxide, oxygen, nitrogen, hydrogen, and sometimes methane. The unpleasant odor of gas that passes through the rectum comes from bacteria in the large intestine that release small amounts of gases containing sulfur.

RISK INCREASES WITH
- Many different foods or drinks (e.g., carbonated beverages) can cause gassiness. The amount of gas they produce varies from person to person.
- Swallowing too much air.
- Certain medical conditions (e.g., diverticulitis, ulcerative colitis, or Crohn's disease).
- Excess use of laxatives.
- Constipation.
- Food intolerances (e.g., lactose or gluten intolerance).
- Artificial additives or artificial sweeteners (e.g., sorbitol and mannitol).

HOW TO PREVENT—Passing gas is a normal body function and can't be entirely prevented. Avoiding risk factors and making some diet and lifestyle changes can help reduce the amount of gas you produce.

WHAT TO EXPECT

DIAGNOSTIC MEASURES
- Your own observation of symptoms.
- See your health care provider if you have concerns. A physical exam may be done. Asking questions about your symptoms, diet, and life-style usually determines cause of gas problems.
- You may be asked to keep a diary for a period of time about the foods and drinks consumed and your gas symptoms.
- Medical tests may be done to rule out conditions that are more serious.

APPROPRIATE HEALTH CARE
- If gas pains are caused by a health problem, treating that condition may provide relief.
- Most often, gas symptoms are self-treated with diet and lifestyle changes.

POSSIBLE COMPLICATIONS—None expected. An underlying condition may cause complications.

PROBABLE OUTCOME—In most cases, the amount of gas passed is normal. If a person is concerned or feels embarrassed, simple treatment steps can often help reduce the amount of gas passed each day.

HOW TO TREAT

GENERAL MEASURES
- Avoid swallowing too much air (e.g., from being nervous, eating too fast, chewing gum, sucking on candy, drinking through a straw, poorly fitting dentures, or smoking).
- Try to control stress in your life. It may cause some people to produce more gas.

MEDICATION
- Nonprescription digestive aids, digestive enzymes, activated charcoal, or probiotics may help some people.
- Your health care provider may prescribed drugs for certain medical conditions.
- Avoid excess use of laxatives.

ACTIVITY
- Get regular exercise. It improves digestion.
- To help pass painful gas, lie on back or side and bring knees to chest.

DIET
- Identify foods or drinks that trigger your gas symptoms and avoid or limit their intake.
  - There are many possibilities. Each person responds differently and will need to find specific foods or drinks causing their symptoms.
  - Some vegetables and fruits, fiber, and sugar are the more likely foods to cause gas.
  - Do maintain a healthy diet as you make any changes and adjustments.
- Eat several small meals each day.

CALL YOUR DOCTOR IF

- You or a family member has symptoms of gas that cause concern.
- Gas or gas pains are severe and interfere with daily life or new symptoms occur along with gas.

GASTRITIS

GENERAL INFORMATION

DEFINITION—Gastritis is an inflammation of the stomach lining. Inflammation causes pain, swelling, redness, and heat. Gastritis may start as a sudden (acute) attack, or develop slowly (chronic) over a period of time.

BODY PARTS INVOLVED—Stomach.

SEX OR AGE MOST AFFECTED—Both sexes; all ages.

SIGNS & SYMPTOMS
- Stomach pain and cramps.
- Black stool or bloody vomit due to stomach bleeding.
- Appetite loss.
- Fever.
- Weakness.
- Swollen stomach.
- Sharp, dull, or annoying pain in the chest.
- Acid taste in the mouth.
- Mild nausea and diarrhea (rare).
- Belching or gas.
- Hiccups.

CAUSES—The inflammation is a reaction to injury, infection, or irritation of the stomach lining. It can be brought on by a number of different factors. Sometimes the cause is unknown.

RISK INCREASES WITH
- Excess alcohol use.
- Use of nonsteroidal anti-inflammatory drugs such as aspirin, ibuprofen, or naproxen.
- Bacteria infection (e.g., *Helicobacter pylori*).
- Illness that has weakened the body.
- Surgery and being in the hospital for other problems.
- Serious injury or severe burns.
- Smoking.
- Pernicious anemia, immune problems, and chronic bile reflux.
- Emotional or physical stress.

HOW TO PREVENT
- Eat and drink moderately.
- Don't skip meals or eat irregularly.
- Avoid foods you find hard to digest.
- Don't smoke.
- Avoid drugs that irritate your stomach, if possible.

WHAT TO EXPECT

DIAGNOSTIC MEASURES
- Your own observation of symptoms.
- Your health care provider will do a physical exam and ask questions about your symptoms.
- Diagnosis is made by examining the stomach through a tube passed down the throat to the stomach. A small amount of tissue may be taken for a test.
- Blood and stool tests may be done.

APPROPRIATE HEALTH CARE
- Goals of treatment are to relieve the symptoms and get rid of the gastric irritant or other cause.
- A hospital stay may be necessary if excess bleeding occurs.

POSSIBLE COMPLICATIONS
- Bleeding is an uncommon but dangerous complication, especially in the elderly.
- Increased risk of stomach cancer in some cases.

PROBABLE OUTCOME—Usually cured in several days with treatment, and if the cause is taken away.

HOW TO TREAT

GENERAL MEASURES
- Consider lifestyle changes if they are contributing to symptoms.
- Smoking and alcohol drinking should be stopped. Your health care provider can help you find the plan that will work for you.

MEDICATION
- Drugs are usually prescribed to reduce stomach acid. Acid irritates the stomach lining.
- Take acetaminophen for minor pain. Don't use aspirin.
- Other drugs, such as antibiotics for infection, may be prescribed.
- A drug you take may be causing the problem. Your health care provider may stop the drug, change the dose, or prescribe a new drug.

ACTIVITY—Resume normal activities as soon as symptoms improve.

DIET—Don't eat solid food on the first day of the attack. Drink liquids often, preferably milk or water. Resume a normal diet slowly. Avoid hot and spicy foods, alcohol, coffee, and acidic foods until symptoms are gone.

CALL YOUR DOCTOR IF

- You or a family member has symptoms of gastritis.
- You vomit blood.
- Bowel movements become black or tarry.
- Pain becomes severe.
- Signs of dehydration, such as a dry mouth, wrinkled skin, excess thirst, or decreased urination, develop.

GASTROENTERITIS
(Stomach Flu)

 GENERAL INFORMATION

DEFINITION—Gastroenteritis is an irritation and inflammation of the stomach and intestines. It is a general term and is often used when there is a nonspecific, uncertain, or unknown cause.

BODY PARTS INVOLVED—Stomach; small intestine; colon.

SEX OR AGE MOST AFFECTED—Can affect all ages and both sexes, but is most severe in young children (1 to 5 years). Adults usually have mild cases, sometimes with no symptoms.

SIGNS & SYMPTOMS
- Diarrhea is the main symptom, and sometimes, the only one. Diarrhea may range from 2 or 3 loose stools to many watery stools.
- Nausea and vomiting.
- Stomach cramps, pain, or tenderness.
- Fever or chills.
- Appetite loss; weakness; dehydration.

CAUSES
- Viral infections are the most common cause. They are spread by contact with an infected person or by touching an object that has germs on it. Contaminated food or water is another source for infection.
- Other causes are bacterial or parasitic infections, food-borne toxins, shellfish and marine animal poisoning, food intolerance, drug-caused diarrhea, and colitis.

RISK INCREASES WITH
- Children in daycare centers.
- Crowded living or working conditions.
- Older adults in nursing homes.
- Schools, dormitories, camps, or cruise ships.
- Weak immune system due to illness or drugs.
- Use of drugs, such as antibiotics, laxatives, or antacids.
- Contaminated food or water.
- Travel to foreign countries.

HOW TO PREVENT
- No specific preventive measures.
- Wash hands often to prevent spread of germs.
- Don't share eating utensils or towels.
- Use safety steps in storing and cooking foods.
- If traveling in foreign countries, take care to eat food and drink water that is known to be safe.
- Vaccines against some viruses are being studied.

 WHAT TO EXPECT

DIAGNOSTIC MEASURES
- Call your health care provider if symptoms are severe or if they cause you any concern.

- Your health care provider may do a physical exam. Medical tests may include studies of blood and stool.

APPROPRIATE HEALTH CARE
- Care at home is usually all that is needed.
- Hospital care may be needed for severe dehydration.

POSSIBLE COMPLICATIONS—Serious dehydration that requires special treatment. Other complications are rare.

PROBABLE OUTCOME—The prognosis is excellent. Diarrhea and other symptoms usually clear up in 2 to 5 days. Adults may feel somewhat weak and fatigued for about a week.

 HOW TO TREAT

GENERAL MEASURES
- Treatment usually involves rest and fluids. There is no specific drug for viral infections.
- It is not necessary to keep persons with gastroenteritis away from others in the family or household. Try to avoid close contact if possible.

MEDICATION
- Drugs are usually not needed for treatment. Antibiotics do not work for viral infections.
- If symptoms are severe or prolonged, your health care provider may recommend nonprescription drugs for vomiting or diarrhea.
- Some infections may require specific drug treatment.
- If a drug you take is the cause of the problem, you may be advised to change drugs or stop taking the drug.

ACTIVITY—Get extra rest until diarrhea, nausea, vomiting, and fever are improved. Be sure to have access to a toilet or bedpan.

DIET
- Suck ice chips or drink small amounts of clear fluids often. Replace lost fluids and electrolytes with products such as Pedialyte for infants and children, and diluted rehydration fluids (e.g., Gatorade) for adults.
- Once the symptoms improve, try a diet of complex carbohydrates (rice, wheat, potatoes, bread, cereal, and lean meat such as chicken). Milk and dairy products usually do not need to be limited.
- Avoid high-sugar foods or fatty foods for a few days.

 CALL YOUR DOCTOR IF

- Symptoms of gastroenteritis last longer than 2 days.
- Symptoms continue or worsen after treatment.
- Blood or mucus appears in the stool.

GASTROESOPHAGEAL REFLUX DISEASE (GERD)

 GENERAL INFORMATION

DEFINITION—Gastroesophageal reflux disease (GERD) is a condition that occurs when acids from the stomach move backward (reflux) into the esophagus (the food pipe that carries food from the mouth to the stomach).

BODY PARTS INVOLVED—Gastrointestinal.

SEX OR AGE MOST AFFECTED—All ages, but most common in adults.

SIGNS & SYMPTOMS
- Persistent heartburn (stomach acid touches the lining of the esophagus and causes a burning sensation in the chest). You can have GERD without having heartburn.
- Regurgitation (taste of acid in the back of the mouth).
- Hoarseness in the morning.
- Difficulty swallowing. Burning in the mouth.
- Feels like you have food stuck in your throat, like you are choking, or your throat is tight.
- Dry cough and bad breath.
- Excessive clearing of the throat.
- Infants and children may have repeated vomiting, coughing, and other respiratory (lung) problems. Most babies grow out of GERD by their first birthday.

CAUSES—The problem occurs when the lower esophageal sphincter (LES) does not close properly. This allows stomach contents to leak back, or reflux, into the esophagus. The LES is a ring of muscle at the bottom of the esophagus. It acts like a valve between the esophagus and stomach.

RISK INCREASES WITH
- Hiatal hernia may contribute. It occurs when part of the stomach moves above the diaphragm.
- Alcohol use or smoking.
- Overweight.
- Pregnancy.
- Use of certain drugs.
- Certain foods can trigger symptoms (caffeine, chocolate, fatty and fried foods, garlic, onions, mint, spicy foods, spaghetti, chili, pizza, citrus).

HOW TO PREVENT—Follow steps listed in General Measures.

 WHAT TO EXPECT

DIAGNOSTIC MEASURES
- Your health care provider will do a physical exam and ask questions about your symptoms, diet, and activities.
- Medical tests may be done at this time or after simple treatment measures are tried.

APPROPRIATE HEALTH CARE
- Treatment depends on how severe your GERD is. It may involve lifestyle changes, drugs, further medical testing, or surgery.
- If lifestyle changes and drugs don't help, one or more medical tests may be done to check for other problems:
  - Barium swallow (a type of x-ray).
  - Endoscopy. A thin, flexible plastic tube with a tiny camera is used to see inside esophagus.
  - A device may be inserted into the esophagus that measures acid reflux. The device remains for 24 or 48 hours while you go about your regular activities.
- Surgery is an option when drugs and lifestyle changes do not work. Surgery may also be an alternative to a lifetime of drugs and discomfort.

POSSIBLE COMPLICATIONS
- Inflammation of the esophagus (esophagitis).
- Ulcers.
- Scars (from tissue damage) narrow the esophagus.
- Barrett's esophagus (disorder that can lead to cancer).
- Erosion or weakening of the teeth.
- Asthma, chronic cough, and pulmonary fibrosis may be worsened or even caused by GERD.

PROBABLE OUTCOME—Symptoms can be improved with treatment. GERD may come and go for weeks or months, or it may persist.

 HOW TO TREAT

GENERAL MEASURES
- If you smoke, stop. Find a way to quit.
- Make changes in your diet.
- Avoid tight clothes (e.g., waist, chest, and stomach).
- Avoid lying down or stooping or bending over for 3 hours after a meal.
- Raise the head of your bed 6 to 8 inches.

MEDICATION—Nonprescription antacids, or drugs that stop acid production and/or help the muscles that empty your stomach, may be prescribed. Your health care provider will help you decide which ones will work best for you.

ACTIVITY—No limits.

DIET—Do not drink alcohol. Lose weight, if needed. Eat small meals. Avoid the foods that trigger symptoms.

 CALL YOUR DOCTOR IF

- You or a family member has GERD symptoms.
- Symptoms continue despite treatment.

GENITOURINARY INJURY
(Bladder Injury; Kidney Injury; Urethra Injury; Ureter Injury; Penis or Testis Injury)

GENERAL INFORMATION

DEFINITION—A genitourinary injury may result from a variety of causes.

BODY PARTS INVOLVED—Kidney (organ that filters the blood and excretes waste products); bladder (the organ that stores urine); ureter (two tubes that carry urine from the kidneys to the bladder); urethra (the tube through which urine travels from the bladder to the outside); penis; scrotum.

SEX OR AGE MOST AFFECTED—Both sexes; all ages.

SIGNS & SYMPTOMS
- Severe abdominal pain.
- Shock (sweating; faintness; nausea; panting; rapid pulse; pale, cold, moist skin).
- Painful urination or inability to urinate.
- Pain or tenderness in the back, just below the ribs on the injured side.
- Fever (sometimes).
- Blood in the urine.
- If you have severe pain with large amounts of blood in your urine, one or both kidneys may be seriously injured.

CAUSES—Forceful or penetrating blow or wound to lower abdomen (gunshot or stab wounds, pelvic surgery, pelvic fracture, straddle injuries, kicks, penis amputation).

RISK INCREASES WITH
- Excess alcohol consumption.
- Hazardous occupations.
- Motor vehicle accidents.
- Sexually abused children.
- Medical treatments including surgery, shock waves, laser therapy, instrument use, radiation.
- Physical combat or physical violence.
- Penile rings.
- Excessive trauma during intercourse or other sexual activity.

HOW TO PREVENT
- Protect yourself from injury whenever possible.
- Buckle your automobile seat belt to minimize internal injury in case of accident.
- Don't drink and drive.
- Avoid alcohol or limit amount you consume.

WHAT TO EXPECT

DIAGNOSTIC MEASURES
- Your own observation of symptoms.
- Your health care provider will do a physical exam.
- Medical tests may include urine studies, x-rays of the urinary tract, ultrasound, intravenous urography, and cystography (the last two special x-rays used to see inside the kidneys and bladder).

APPROPRIATE HEALTH CARE
- Emergency care and/or hospital care.
- Surgery may be needed to repair any wounds, control bleeding and repair damage to the organs involved. A temporary catheter may be needed for urinary drainage while the body heals.
- Injury to external male genitalia may require skin grafts.
- An amputated penis may be re-implanted using microsurgical techniques.

POSSIBLE COMPLICATIONS
- Internal bleeding.
- Urine leakage into the abdomen, causing abdominal inflammation or infection.
- Recurrent infections from scars in the urethra that narrow the urinary passage.
- Scarring and narrowing of the injured ureter.
- Atrophy of testes following a rupture injury.

PROBABLE OUTCOME—A genitourinary tract injury usually requires emergency treatment. Most cases heal with bed rest, time, supportive treatment, or surgery.

HOW TO TREAT

GENERAL MEASURES—Follow medical advice.

MEDICATION
- Your health care provider may prescribe:
  - Antibiotics to prevent infection.
  - Pain medicine as required.
  - Anticholinergics for spasms.

ACTIVITY—Stay as active as your strength allows. Allow 1 month for recovery. Don't return to work or resume sexual relations until healing is complete.

DIET—No special diet.

CALL YOUR DOCTOR IF

- You or a family member has any symptoms of genitourinary injury.
- During or after treatment, you develop any new or recurring symptoms.

GESTATIONAL DIABETES
(Gestational Carbohydrate Intolerance)

 GENERAL INFORMATION

DEFINITION—Gestational diabetes (GD) is a type of diabetes that occurs only in pregnant women (about 2% to 5% of all pregnancies).

BODY PARTS INVOLVED—Pancreas.

SEX OR AGE MOST AFFECTED—Females of childbearing age.

SIGNS & SYMPTOMS
• Usually no symptoms are apparent. A prenatal exam may find that the fetus is larger than normal for the stage of pregnancy.
• Diagnosis is based on glucose testing done during the 24th to 28th week of pregnancy for nondiabetic mothers. Earlier testing is often done for patients diagnosed with GD in a previous pregnancy, a birth weight over 9 pounds in a previous infant, or for other risk factors.

CAUSES—Your body isn't able to use the sugar (glucose) in your blood as well as it should, so the level of sugar in your blood becomes higher than normal (hyperglycemia). Why gestational diabetes develops is unknown.

RISK INCREASES WITH
• Previous pregnancy with GD.
• Obesity (especially if excess fat is around the waist).
• Mother over age 30.
• Polycystic ovarian syndrome (PCOS).
• Family history of diabetes.
• Excess weight gain in pregnancy.
• Previous birth of a baby weighing over 9 pounds.
• Four or more previous pregnancies.
• History of an unexplained fetal death or stillbirth.
• Some population groups, such as Native Americans, Mexican-Americans, Asians, and East Indians.

HOW TO PREVENT—There are no specific preventive measures. Weight loss in overweight women prior to pregnancy may help. Careful attention to diet and exercise in pregnant women with risk factors may help.

 WHAT TO EXPECT

DIAGNOSTIC MEASURES—Your obstetric provider will do a glucose test.

APPROPRIATE HEALTH CARE
• Treatment will include diet changes, an exercise program, and drug therapy, if needed.

• You will learn how to monitor your glucose levels. At first, glucose checks may need to be done up to 4 to 6 times daily. Once glucose levels are in the desired range and diet changes are made, glucose checks may be reduced with your obstetric provider's approval.

POSSIBLE COMPLICATIONS
• Excess amniotic fluid (polyhydramnios).
• Premature labor.
• May need to have labor induced.
• Preeclampsia.

PROBABLE OUTCOME
• Successful treatment and a healthy baby often depend on the mother's motivation and ability to change her lifestyle. For some, dietary control is sufficient. Others may require drug therapy.
• In most cases, labor occurs naturally, and the birth is usually vaginal. Cesarean section may be required if the fetus is considered too large for vaginal birth.
• Gestational diabetes usually clears up with delivery.

 HOW TO TREAT

GENERAL MEASURES—To learn more: Contact the local or national office of the American Diabetes Association, Attention: National Call Center, 1701 Beauregard St., Alexandria, VA 22311; (800) 342-2383; website: www.diabetes.org.

MEDICATION
• Drugs are usually not needed if glucose control is achieved with diet and exercise.
• Insulin injections or oral antidiabetic drugs may be prescribed for some patients.

ACTIVITY—A program of moderate, non–weight-bearing exercise is usually recommended. Exercising for even small time periods can have major benefits. Follow any prescribed exercise program carefully.

DIET
• Diet changes are an important part of the treatment. Specific diet instructions will be provided. Following this diet will decrease the risks to the mother and her unborn child.
• The diet changes will involve increased fiber intake, fat limits, avoiding sweets, and monitoring caloric intake to prevent excess weight gain.

 CALL YOUR DOCTOR IF

• You are 24 to 28 weeks pregnant and have not been tested for gestational diabetes.
• After diagnosis, you develop any new signs or symptoms that cause you concern.

GIARDIASIS

 GENERAL INFORMATION

DEFINITION—Giardiasis is an intestinal infection caused by a parasite. It is a frequent cause of diarrhea. It may occur in clusters or outbreaks, affecting many persons at a time.

BODY PARTS INVOLVED—Gastrointestinal tract, especially the small bowel.

SEX OR AGE MOST AFFECTED—All ages and both sexes, but most common in children.

SIGNS & SYMPTOMS
- Often, there are no symptoms.
- Symptoms can be mild and recurrent, persisting for months, or longer.
- Sudden diarrhea and stomach cramping. Some persons have only mild diarrhea and upset stomach.
- Stools may have a foul smell and be greasy.
- Nausea and vomiting.
- Slight fever (rare).

CAUSES—A parasite, *Giardia lamblia*. The germs may be spread in food or water contaminated by feces from infected animals or humans. Germs can be spread from one person to another due to poor hygiene. Symptoms begin in 1 to 3 weeks after being infected.

RISK INCREASES WITH
- Drinking from a water supply that is contaminated.
- Drinking unsafe water while camping or hiking.
- Swimmers who swallow contaminated water.
- Weak immune system due to illness or drugs.
- Children or workers at preschool or daycare center.
- Foreign travel.
- Oral or anal sex.

HOW TO PREVENT
- Don't drink unsafe water. Boil or treat it first.
- Avoid uncooked foods that may have been rinsed in contaminated water.
- Wash hands often to prevent spread of germs.
- Keep children with diarrhea away from others.
- To avoid spreading the germs, don't swim if you have diarrhea.
- If traveling in foreign countries, take care to eat food and drink water that is known to be safe.
- Practice safe sex.

 WHAT TO EXPECT

DIAGNOSTIC MEASURES
- Your health care provider may do a physical exam. Questions will be asked about your symptoms and activities. Health providers are often aware if there is an outbreak of giardiasis in the community.
- Medical tests may include stool studies to detect the parasites.

APPROPRIATE HEALTH CARE
- Giardiasis responds well to drugs. Treatment is usually done at home. Drug therapy may be recommended for family members who are infected, but have no symptoms. Pregnant women may require special treatment.
- Hospital care to replace lost fluids may be required for patients with severe diarrhea and dehydration.

POSSIBLE COMPLICATIONS
- Dehydration.
- Chronic giardiasis.
- Malabsorption (unable to absorb nutrients from food) and weight loss.

PROBABLE OUTCOME—Complete recovery is expected within 1 to 2 weeks with treatment. Symptoms may go away for periods of time even without treatment, but a person can carry the germs for weeks or months.

 HOW TO TREAT

GENERAL MEASURES
- Prevention is the best treatment. Be cautious when away from normal drinking-water supplies.
- Practice careful personal hygiene if you, or others around you, have diarrhea.

MEDICATION—Antiparasitic drugs such as metronidazole (Flagyl) and others may be prescribed. Alcohol interacts with metronidazole to cause stomach cramps and nausea, so don't drink alcohol during this treatment.

ACTIVITY—No limits.

DIET
- Maintain an adequate fluid intake (at least 8 glasses of water or liquid a day).
- Some persons develop lactose intolerance. A lactose-free diet may be recommended.

 CALL YOUR DOCTOR IF

- You or a family member has symptoms of giardiasis.
- New, unexplained symptoms develop. Drugs used in treatment may produce side effects.

GILBERT'S SYNDROME
(Hyperbilirubinemia)

 GENERAL INFORMATION

DEFINITION—Gilbert's syndrome is a disorder that causes increased blood levels of bilirubin. Bilirubin is a yellow chemical that results from red-blood-cell breakdown. Gilbert syndrome is usually a chance finding of routine testing.

BODY PARTS INVOLVED—Blood.

SEX OR AGE MOST AFFECTED—It affects both sexes, but is most common in men. It is present from birth, but symptoms may not appear until ages 20 to 40.

SIGNS & SYMPTOMS
- Usually there are no symptoms.
- Mild jaundice (yellow skin and eyes) may occur in some patients. It may come and go.
- Some patients have symptoms that are nonspecific. These include stomach cramps, tiredness, and general ill feeling. They may be related to anxiety in some cases.

CAUSES—It is an inherited condition that leads to reduced production of an enzyme involved in processing bilirubin. This leaves above-normal levels of bilirubin in the blood. If blood levels are high enough, jaundice may appear.

RISK INCREASES WITH—Family history of Gilbert's syndrome.

HOW TO PREVENT—No specific preventive measures.

 WHAT TO EXPECT

DIAGNOSTIC MEASURES
- Your own observation of symptoms (sometimes). The minor jaundice may be unnoticeable.
- Your health care provider will usually do a physical exam.
- Blood tests of bilirubin and tests of liver function will be done to help confirm the diagnosis.

APPROPRIATE HEALTH CARE—No treatment is necessary. Your health care provider will explain that the syndrome is benign and will not cause health problems or affect lifestyle.

POSSIBLE COMPLICATIONS—No known complications.

PROBABLE OUTCOME—The condition is harmless.

 HOW TO TREAT

GENERAL MEASURES—Be alert to the symptoms of jaundice. It may be brought on by dehydration, fasting, illness, menstrual periods, missing sleep, and emotional stress. The jaundice usually clears up on its own and no treatment is needed. It is recommended that you try to avoid the situations, where possible, that lead to jaundice.

MEDICATION—Drugs are not necessary for this disorder.

ACTIVITY—No limits.

DIET—No special diet.

 CALL YOUR DOCTOR IF

You or a family member has symptoms of Gilbert's syndrome. This usually involves skin that looks a bit yellow.

GINGIVITIS

GENERAL INFORMATION

DEFINITION—Gingivitis is an inflammation (redness, soreness, swelling) of the gums (gingiva). This is a mild form of gum disease, but it can lead to more serious problems.

BODY PARTS INVOLVED—Gum tissue around teeth.

SEX OR AGE MOST AFFECTED—All ages, but most common in adults.

SIGNS & SYMPTOMS
- Gums that have become swollen, tender, red, and soft around the teeth. Gums may bleed easily.
- Bad breath.
- Gums may be tender.
- Fever (rarely).

CAUSES—Plaque. It is a sticky substance made up of food particles, germs, and mucus that builds up on the teeth.

RISK INCREASES WITH
- Poor dental hygiene, other tooth problems, and mouth infections.
- Poor nutrition. This can include eating too much sugar or vitamin deficiencies.
- Adverse reactions to drugs, such as phenytoin and barbiturates.
- People with diabetes, gastroesophageal reflux disease (GERD), or osteoporosis.
- Disorders that affect the immune system such as arthritis, lupus, and AIDS.
- Smoking.
- Pregnancy.
- Female hormones can affect the gums.
- Family history of dental disease.

HOW TO PREVENT
- Maintain good oral hygiene.
  - Brush teeth twice a day or after each meal. Use a soft bristle toothbrush or a power toothbrush. A fluoride toothpaste is often recommended.
  - Floss teeth at least once a day with waxed or unwaxed dental floss or use an interdental cleaner. An oral irrigator may be used in addition to flossing.
  - A tongue scraper can be used to clean the tongue.
  - Use an antiseptic mouthwash if desired.
  - Get dental check up and cleaning every six months; more often if you are prone to plaque or gingivitis.
- Eat a well-balanced diet. Take vitamin supplements if you are unable to eat well-balanced meals.
- Quit smoking. Find a way to stop.

WHAT TO EXPECT

DIAGNOSTIC MEASURES
- Your own observation of symptoms.
- Your dental health care provider can diagnose gingivitis with an exam of your teeth and gums. A special tool is used to check the depth of pockets in the gums.
- X-rays of the teeth help reveal any bone loss.

APPROPRIATE HEALTH CARE
- Treatment usually includes cleaning the teeth by a dental hygienist or other dental health care provider. There are different techniques depending on the degree of plaque build-up.
- Other dental work may be needed. Teeth may need straightening, cavities filled, or missing teeth replaced.
- Surgery may be needed to remove infected gum tissue, if other treatment fails.

POSSIBLE COMPLICATIONS—Without treatment, gingivitis can lead to more serious gum disease, infections, and tooth loss.

HOW TO TREAT

GENERAL MEASURES—To learn more: American Dental Association, 211 E. Chicago Avenue, Chicago, IL 60611, (312) 440-2500 (not toll free); website: www.ada.org.

MEDICATION
- Antibiotics may be prescribed to fight infection. They may be taken by mouth (orally) or applied to the gums with special devices.
- Fluoride mouthwash may be recommended.

ACTIVITY—No limits.

DIET—No special diet. Avoid candy, sweet drinks, or sweet snacks. Sugar stimulates the production of acid, which attacks normal teeth.

CALL YOUR DOCTOR IF

OR CALL YOUR DENTIST
- You or a family member has symptoms of gingivitis.
- The following occur after treatment:
  - Bleeding increases or there is more pain.
  - Fever of 101°F (38.3°C) or higher.
  - Neck or face is swollen, or it is hard to swallow.

GLAUCOMA, ANGLE-CLOSURE

GENERAL INFORMATION

DEFINITION—Glaucoma is a group of disorders that lead to damage to the optic nerve (the nerve connecting the eye to the brain). Angle-closure glaucoma is one of the two main types of glaucoma, and is more rare. (Open-angle glaucoma is the more common and frequently occurring type.) Angle-closure glaucoma symptoms can occur suddenly (acute), or develop over time (chronic).

BODY PARTS INVOLVED—Eye.

SEX OR AGE MOST AFFECTED—Adults of both sexes. It occurs more often in people over 55 and in women more than in men.

SIGNS & SYMPTOMS
- Acute angle-closure glaucoma (symptoms are sudden, and often occur in a darkened room, such as a movie theater, or during periods of stress):
  - Severe, throbbing eye pain; eye gets red.
  - Blurred vision.
  - May see halos around lights.
  - Nausea, vomiting, and headache.
- Chronic angle-closure glaucoma (not acute):
  - There may be no symptoms.
  - Slightly blurred vision, mild eye pain, or seeing halos around lights. These symptoms may come and go.

CAUSES—Normal eye pressure (intraocular pressure or IOP) is maintained by a balance of fluid (aqueous humor) that flows into the front of the eye and then drains out. The angle of the eye (where the iris and cornea meet) is where the drains (called trabecular meshwork) are located. With angle-closure glaucoma, the angle of the eye is not as wide (or open) as it should be. When the pupil dilates (gets larger), it pushes or pulls up the iris and narrows the angle even more so the drain is blocked or covered over. In acute cases, this happens suddenly. In chronic cases, it occurs over time. The blocked drain causes a buildup of fluid and pressure in the eye. The pressure can damage the optic nerve, sometimes within hours, and lead to vision loss.

RISK INCREASES WITH
- Adults over 55; females more than males.
- Family history of glaucoma.
- Having small eyes or farsighted eyes.
- Asian or Eskimo descent.
- One eye has had acute angle-closure glaucoma.
- Use of certain drugs or certain eye diseases.

HOW TO PREVENT
- Get regular eye exams (depends on general health, age, and risk factors for eye problems).
- Get medical care for any changes in your vision.

WHAT TO EXPECT

DIAGNOSTIC MEASURES
- Your own observation of symptoms.
- Your eye health care provider (ophthalmologist) will perform eye tests. These may include tonometry (measures pressure), gonioscopy (a test to check the angle of the eye), slit lamp exam (to look inside the eye), optic nerve imaging, or others as needed.

APPROPRIATE HEALTH CARE
- An acute angle-closure glaucoma attack is an emergency situation. Chronic angle-closure glaucoma may be diagnosed on a routine eye exam. Treatment of either is with drugs and/or surgery.
- Laser iridotomy surgery to reduce fluid pressure is often done. An iridectomy is surgery done with miniature instruments. A small opening is made in the iris so that the aqueous humor (fluid in the eye) can drain. It may be done in the other eye as a preventive measure.

POSSIBLE COMPLICATIONS
- With acute angle-closure, decreased or loss of vision in the affected eye. Acute attack may occur in other eye.
- With chronic angle-closure, decreased or loss of vision in the affected eye.

PROBABLE OUTCOME—Usually favorable in both acute and chronic types with IOP control.

HOW TO TREAT

GENERAL MEASURES—To learn more: Glaucoma Foundation, 80 Maiden Lane, Suite 700, New York, NY 10038; (212) 285-0080 (not toll-free); website: www.glaucomafoundation.org.

MEDICATION
- For emergency care, drugs are given to constrict the pupil and to reduce the fluid production of the eye. The drugs may be taken by mouth (oral), injected into a vein (IV), or topical drops into the eye.
- Eye drops may be prescribed to lower pressure inside the eye. Follow the instructions and schedule carefully.

ACTIVITY—No limits after treatment, unless advised otherwise.

DIET—No special diet.

CALL YOUR DOCTOR IF

- You or a family member has symptoms of acute angle-closure glaucoma. This is an emergency!
- Other vision or eye problems develop.

GLAUCOMA, OPEN-ANGLE

GENERAL INFORMATION

DEFINITION—Glaucoma is a group of disorders that lead to damage to the optic nerve (the nerve connecting the eye to the brain). Open-angle glaucoma is the most common type of glaucoma. It typically occurs in both eyes and is a chronic, progressive condition that can lead to loss of vision. It is often referred to as chronic open-angle glaucoma (COAG) or primary open-angle glaucoma (POAG). It is called secondary open-angle glaucoma when a known cause is found (such as an eye injury).

BODY PARTS INVOLVED—Eye.

SEX OR AGE MOST AFFECTED—Adults of both sexes and all ages, but occurs more often in people over 40.

SIGNS & SYMPTOMS
• Usually, there are no warning symptoms.
• Later stages of the disease include loss of peripheral vision in small areas, blurred vision, halos around lights, blind spots, and poor night vision.

CAUSES
• The exact cause of optic nerve damage in open-angle glaucoma is not certain. Increased internal eye pressure (intraocular pressure or IOP) is the main factor. IOP is maintained by a balance of fluid (aqueous humor) that flows into the front of the eye and then drains out. For unknown reasons, the drains become clogged or too much fluid is produced. The fluid builds up over time and eye pressure (IOP) increases. This causes damage to the optic nerve, which leads to vision loss.
• In some cases, the IOP remains normal, but optic nerve damage occurs due to decreased blood flow. This is called normal tension glaucoma.

RISK INCREASES WITH
• History of increased intraocular pressure.
• Adults over 45.
• Family history of glaucoma.
• Certain medical conditions (e.g., diabetes and high blood pressure).
• Myopia (nearsightedness).
• Previous eye injury or other eye disorders.
• Regular, long-term steroid use.
• African Americans over age 40.

HOW TO PREVENT
• Get regular eye exams. Your eye care provider will recommend a routine depending on your age, general health, and your risk factors for eye problems.
• Get medical care for any changes in your vision.

WHAT TO EXPECT

DIAGNOSTIC MEASURES
• An eye exam is usually done by an eye doctor (ophthalmologist). It includes a tonometry exam (measures pressure within the eyeball) and visual field test (to see how your vision is affected).
• An ophthalmoscope is used to see into the eye to view the optic nerve. A person has glaucoma if their eye exam shows changes to the optic nerve and blind spots.

APPROPRIATE HEALTH CARE
• There is no cure. The goal is to protect the optic nerve from future damage and possible loss of vision. Treatment may include drug therapy, laser surgery, eye operations, or a combination of methods.
• Laser surgery can help improve the draining of the excess fluid. Other eye surgery may be done to open up the draining area and relieve pressure.

POSSIBLE COMPLICATIONS—Optic nerve damage that cannot be reversed. A permanent vision loss can occur.

PROBABLE OUTCOME—The disorder can usually be controlled with treatment to prevent further vision loss.

HOW TO TREAT

GENERAL MEASURES—To learn more: Glaucoma Foundation, 80 Maiden Lane, Suite 700, New York, NY 10038; (212) 285-0080 (not toll-free); website: www.glaucomafoundation.org.

MEDICATION—One or more types of eye drops to lower pressure inside the eye will be prescribed. Follow the instructions and schedule carefully, even if symptoms improve. If eye drops do not control the pressure, oral drugs (taken by mouth) will usually be prescribed.

ACTIVITY—No limits.

DIET—No special diet.

CALL YOUR DOCTOR IF

• You or a family member has symptoms of glaucoma.
• Any sign of eye infection develops.
• Pain begins in the eye.
• Redness occurs in the eye.
• Vision changes suddenly.

GLOMERULONEPHRITIS

 GENERAL INFORMATION

DEFINITION—Glomerulonephritis is a group of disorders that cause inflammation of the glomeruli. These are the blood vessel structures in the kidneys that help filter out waste products and water and salt from the blood. Glomerulonephritis can be acute (occurs suddenly) or chronic (develops over time). The inflammation can lead to loss of kidney function.

BODY PARTS INVOLVED—Kidneys.

SEX OR AGE MOST AFFECTED—Both sexes; all ages.

SIGNS & SYMPTOMS
- There may be no symptoms. The disorder may be diagnosed during a routine urine study.
- Blood in urine (may be dark-colored like the color of tea or a cola drink).
- Reduced urine output.
- Swelling of face, hands, feet, or stomach. This is due to retained fluid (edema).
- Frothy or foamy urine.
- Chronic type: tiredness, dry skin, itching, headache, nausea or vomiting, poor appetite, high blood pressure, or muscle cramps.

CAUSES—There are many possible causes for the inflammation, and often the cause is unknown. It may be due to immune reaction to infections such as *Streptococcus* (e.g., strep throat). Other causes are genetic disorders, immune diseases (e.g., lupus), diabetes, high blood pressure, blood vessel inflammation (vasculitis), or infections (e.g., virus, bacteria, or protozoa).

RISK INCREASES WITH
- Family history of glomerulonephritis.
- Persons diagnosed with any of the possible causes.

HOW TO PREVENT—No specific preventive measures. Get treatment for any possible cause to help reduce risks.

 WHAT TO EXPECT

DIAGNOSTIC MEASURES
- Your own observation of symptoms.
- Your health care provider will do a physical exam and ask questions about your symptoms and recent illnesses.
- Medical tests may include blood and urine studies, x-rays, ultrasound, or CT. A kidney biopsy may be done. This involves removal of a small amount of kidney tissue for viewing under a microscope.

APPROPRIATE HEALTH CARE
- Treatment will depend on whether the disease is acute or chronic, any underlying cause, and severity of symptoms.
- Treatment steps may involve drugs, diet changes, and/or other therapies (e.g., dialysis or plasmapheresis).
- Temporary dialysis may be prescribed to remove excess fluid or to control high blood pressure.
- Plasmapheresis is a special blood filtering process.

POSSIBLE COMPLICATIONS
- Progressive kidney disease.
- Kidney failure. It may lead to dialysis (use of a machine to filter body waste) and a kidney transplant.
- Complications can occur depending on the cause.

PROBABLE OUTCOME
- Mild cases often recover on their own. Others are helped with treatment. Symptoms usually improve in 2 weeks to several months.
- In cases caused by certain medical problems, the outcome will vary depending on the underlying cause.

 HOW TO TREAT

GENERAL MEASURES
- None specific.
- To learn more: National Kidney Foundation, 30 E. 33rd St., Suite 1100, New York, NY 10016; (800) 622-9010; website: www.kidney.org.

MEDICATION
- Your health care provider may prescribe:
  - Antibiotics for bacterial infection.
  - Drugs for high blood pressure.
  - Diuretics, to help remove excess fluid.
  - Steroids, to reduce inflammation.
  - Drugs, to suppress the immune system.
  - Drugs to treat an underlying disorder.

ACTIVITY—Activity level is as tolerated. Your health care provider will advise you of any specific limits.

DIET—Diet changes may be advised to help reduce the work of the kidneys. These may include eating less salt, potassium, and protein.

 CALL YOUR DOCTOR IF

- You or a family member has symptoms of glomerulonephritis.
- Urine changes color or urine output is decreased.
- New symptoms occur during treatment.

GONORRHEA

GENERAL INFORMATION

DEFINITION—Gonorrhea is an infection caused by a sexually transmitted disease (STD). Gonorrhea can affect anyone (even a child) who has sexual contact with an infected person.

BODY PARTS INVOLVED—In males, it usually involves the urethra (urine canal). In females, it usually involves the cervix and, sometimes, the urethra. In both sexes, the rectum, throat and other body parts may be involved.

SEX OR AGE MOST AFFECTED—Both sexes and all ages. It most often occurs in younger persons (ages 15 to 29), and in men more than in women.

SIGNS & SYMPTOMS
- Symptoms usually begin 2 to 5 days, or up to 30 days after being exposed. Females have few or no symptoms. Males usually have symptoms.
- Burning sensation when urinating.
- White to yellow-green discharge from the urethra.
- Rectal discomfort and discharge (sometimes).
- Sore throat (mild).
- Females may have abdominal cramps.
- Conjunctivitis (eye inflammation). This occurs when the person touches infected genitals and then the eyes.
- If the infection spreads to other body parts: joint pain, low fever, rash, headache, neck pain, and stiffness.

CAUSES—Infection from *Neisseria gonorrhoeae*, a bacteria. It grows easily on delicate, moist tissue. The bacteria is transmitted sexually (vaginal, anal, or oral sex). It can be spread from mother to child during birth.

RISK INCREASES WITH
- Any sexually active persons.
- Having sex with an infected person.
- Multiple sexual partners, whether heterosexual or homosexual.
- Child sexual abuse.
- Passage of newborn through the infected birth canal of the mother.

HOW TO PREVENT
- Abstain from sexual activity.
- Avoid sexual partners whose health practices and status are uncertain.
- Use a latex condom during sexual intercourse.

WHAT TO EXPECT

DIAGNOSTIC MEASURES
- Your health care provider will do a physical exam and a pelvic exam.
- Medical tests may include blood and urine studies and studies of the discharge from the vagina, urethra, rectum, throat, or eyes.

- Tests for other sexually transmitted diseases are usually done. Additional tests may be done if complications are suspected.

APPROPRIATE HEALTH CARE
- Treatment is with antibiotic drugs. Follow-up tests may be done to confirm a cure.
- If the eyes are involved, an eye doctor (ophthalmologist) should be consulted.
- Hospital care may be needed for severe symptoms.

POSSIBLE COMPLICATIONS
- Persons who have no symptoms are at risk for complications and can unknowingly spread the infection.
- Spread from mother to child during birth. This can cause serious complications in a newborn.
- Blood poisoning (gonococcal septicemia).
- Infectious arthritis.
- Pelvic inflammatory disease in females (PID), which can lead to infertility.
- Heart inflammation or infection around the liver.
- in males, epididymitis (can lead to infertility), prostate problems, and urethral scarring.
- Risk of getting HIV is higher.

PROBABLE OUTCOME—Usually curable in 1 to 2 weeks with treatment.

HOW TO TREAT

GENERAL MEASURES
- Inform all sexual contacts so they can seek treatment.
- For self-care:
  - Use separate towels, washcloths, and disposable eating utensils during treatment.
  - Wash hands often, especially after using the bathroom.
  - Don't touch your eyes with your hands.
- To learn more: Centers for Disease Control & Prevention (CDC); website: www.cdc.gov/std.

MEDICATION
- Antibiotics will be prescribed. Take complete dosage.
- You may take nonprescription drugs, such as acetaminophen or aspirin (for adults), to reduce discomfort.

ACTIVITY—No limits on physical activity. Don't resume sexual activity until treatment is complete.

DIET—No special diet.

CALL YOUR DOCTOR IF

- You or a family member has symptoms of gonorrhea.
- Symptoms don't improve with treatment.

GOUT

GENERAL INFORMATION

DEFINITION—Gout is a disorder that affects the body's joints, especially the base of the big toe. It is a form of arthritis.

BODY PARTS INVOLVED—Any joint; often the base of the big toe; may also involve the elbow, knee, hand, foot, ankle, arm or shoulder.

SEX OR AGE MOST AFFECTED—Adults of both sexes but it is more common in men than women, until after menopause.

SIGNS & SYMPTOMS
- Sudden onset of severe pain (usually at night) in the inflamed joint (e.g., base of the big toe).
- Involved joints may be hot, swollen, and very tender. Skin over the joint is red and shiny.
- Fever, chills, or fatigue (sometimes).

CAUSES—It is usually due to high levels of uric acid in the blood. The body may produce too much or not eliminate enough in the urine. High uric acid leads to formation of crystals in the joints which cause inflammation.

RISK INCREASES WITH
- Family history of gout.
- Males over age 40.
- Overweight or obesity.
- Excess alcohol use.
- Kidney disease, thyroid disorders, high blood pressure, leukemia, or lymphoma.
- Use of certain drugs, such as diuretic drugs (water pills), high blood pressure drugs, aspirin, drugs that treat gout, and others.
- Starvation or dehydration.
- Eating large amounts of foods that contain purines. These include anchovies, sardines, sweetbreads, kidney, liver, tongue, and large amounts of red meat, shellfish, peas, lentils, and beans.
- Diet high in fructose-rich foods or drinks.

HOW TO PREVENT—Avoid risk factors, where possible.

WHAT TO EXPECT

DIAGNOSTIC MEASURES
- Your own observation of symptoms.
- Your health care provider will do an exam of the joints.
- Medical tests may include blood and urine levels of uric acid and studies of fluid removed from the joint. An x-ray may be done.

APPROPRIATE HEALTH CARE
- Goals of treatment are to control the symptoms, prevent a recurrence, and to lower uric acid levels. Treatment usually involves drug therapy, lifestyle changes, and rarely, surgery.
- Lifestyle changes may include diet changes and weight loss (if overweight).

- Surgery is rare, but may be recommended if the disorder was untreated or treated late.

POSSIBLE COMPLICATIONS
- Crippled, deformed joints.
- Kidney stones or kidney disease.
- Continued gout attacks (if untreated).
- Uric acid deposits called tophi develop in soft tissue, cartilage tissue, and tendons.

PROBABLE OUTCOME—The first attack may last a few days up to a week. Recurrent attacks are common unless the uric acid level in the blood is reduced. Treatment relieves symptoms and helps prevent long-term health problems.

HOW TO TREAT

GENERAL MEASURES—For home care—use warm or cold compresses on painful joints. Keep the weight of bedclothes off any painful joint. Make a frame to raise sheet off the feet.

MEDICATION
- Nonsteroidal anti-inflammatory drugs or colchicine to control inflammation and pain are usually prescribed.
- Steroids (e.g., prednisone) may be prescribed.
- Lifelong treatment with drugs to decrease uric acid production or to increase the kidneys' excretion of uric acid may be needed. Your health care provider will explain the risks and benefits.

ACTIVITY
- During an attack, rest and take care to avoid joint injury, and elevate the foot (if toe involved). Wear shoes that fit properly.
- When able, exercise daily.

DIET
- Drink plenty of water and other liquids daily. Fluids keeps the urine diluted (helps prevent kidney stones).
- Don't drink alcoholic beverages (especially beer). They can worsen or trigger an attack.
- If you are overweight, begin a medically approved weight-loss diet. Do not go on a crash diet, as rapid weight loss may bring on a gout attack.
- A diet low in seafood, red meat, organ meat, fructose, and purine may be recommended. A dietitian can help with meal planning.
- Increase low-fat dairy products. They may reduce the risk of gout symptoms.

CALL YOUR DOCTOR IF

- You or a family member has symptoms of gout.
- Pain gets worse, or fever and chills occur.
- New, unexplained symptoms develop.

GRANULOMA ANNULARE

GENERAL INFORMATION

DEFINITION—Granuloma annulare (GA) is a common and chronic skin disorder. The skin area affected may be small (localized) or widespread (generalized) over the body.

BODY PARTS INVOLVED—Skin on the bottoms of feet and backs of fingers, hands, arms, elbows, legs and knees.

SEX OR AGE MOST AFFECTED—It can affect all ages but is more common in children and young adults. Females are more often affected than males.

SIGNS & SYMPTOMS
- Small, raised bumps (lesions) on the skin.
- Bumps have a domed or slightly flat shape. Their color may vary on different people. Bumps may be skin-colored, reddish, bluish, or yellowish.
- They don't hurt, and usually don't itch.
- The bumps cluster in a ring. Bumps around the ring border are close, but don't grow completely together. This gives the border a beaded appearance. The ring's center is often darker than the edge.
- The appearance may change in size and shape over a few weeks to 6 months.

CAUSES—Unknown.

RISK INCREASES WITH—May be associated with diabetes.

HOW TO PREVENT—No specific preventive measures.

WHAT TO EXPECT

DIAGNOSTIC MEASURES
- Your own observation of symptoms.
- Your health care provider can diagnose the disorder by an exam of the affected skin area.
- In some cases, medical tests are done to confirm the diagnosis.

APPROPRIATE HEALTH CARE
- In many cases, the disorder is mild and treatment is not needed.
- Treatment options include drug therapy, PUVA, or cryotherapy. Currently, there is no effective treatment that works for everyone. Your health care provider will discuss the different options with you.
- Cryotherapy uses liquid nitrogen to freeze the bumps. It may be used for localized GA.

POSSIBLE COMPLICATIONS—No complications are expected.

PROBABLE OUTCOME—The disorder will heal on its own, but it usually takes months to years. The disorder may also recur with no apparent cause or timing.

HOW TO TREAT

GENERAL MEASURES—You may use cosmetics or fake-tan products to help hide the affected skin areas.

MEDICATION
- Steroid creams or ointments to be applied to the skin may be prescribed.
- Your health care provider may inject steroids directly into the bumps.
- One or more types of oral drugs may be prescribed for moderate to severe cases.
- A treatment called PUVA may be recommended. It combines a special light with a cream applied to the skin.

ACTIVITY—No limits.

DIET—No special diet.

CALL YOUR DOCTOR IF

- You or a family member has symptoms of granuloma annulare.
- The disorder recurs.

GRANULOMA INGUINALE
(Donovanosis)

GENERAL INFORMATION

DEFINITION—Granuloma inguinale is a sexually transmitted disease (STD) generally affecting people living in tropical climates. It is becoming more common in the U.S., especially in the south and southwest regions. Incubation period is 8 to 12 weeks.

BODY PARTS INVOLVED—Genitals.

SEX OR AGE MOST AFFECTED—Both sexes; all ages.

SIGNS & SYMPTOMS
- Formation of a nonpainful lesion (cyst, papule, or nodule) in the genital area that does not readily heal. This lesion ulcerates (becomes open and runny) and may spread so that it involves most of the vulva, and sometimes the buttocks and lower abdomen.
- Marked discomfort occurs if the ulceration spreads to the urethra or anal area. Walking, sitting and sexual intercourse become painful.
- Vaginal discharge that has unpleasant odor.

CAUSES—An organism, *Calymmatobacterium granulomatis* (Donovan body), that is spread via sexual intercourse with an infected person.

RISK INCREASES WITH
- Multiple sexual partners.
- Unprotected intercourse.
- Infection with other sexually transmitted diseases.

HOW TO PREVENT
- Monogamous sexual relationship.
- Having the male partner use a latex condom.
- Cleansing of the genital area before and after sex. Douching is usually not effective.
- If there has been good possibility of exposure, seek medical care immediately. Early treatment may head off the infection.

WHAT TO EXPECT

DIAGNOSTIC MEASURES
- Diagnosis is confirmed with laboratory studies of scrapings or biopsies of the lesions.
- Testing (screening) for other sexually transmitted diseases is often recommended.

APPROPRIATE HEALTH CARE
- Treatment is with drug therapy.
- A follow-up medical examination after treatment is important to verify that healing is complete.

POSSIBLE COMPLICATIONS
- Secondary bacterial infection.
- Relapse may occur.
- Scars may form where infection occurred.

PROBABLE OUTCOME—With treatment, healing should begin within a few days, but complete resolution will take up to 3 weeks.

HOW TO TREAT

GENERAL MEASURES
- Sitz baths frequently relieve soreness. Sit in a tub of hot water for 10 to 15 minutes. Repeat baths as often as 3 or 4 times a day.
- Sexual partners should be examined for infection.
- To learn more: Sexually Transmitted Diseases Hotline, (800) 227-8922.

MEDICATION—An antibiotic, such as trimethoprim-sulfamethoxazole, doxycycline, ciprofloxacin or erythromycin will be prescribed. If lesions do not respond within the first few days of therapy, another drug may be added to the treatment. Do not discontinue treatment until healing is complete or when advised to by your health care provider.

ACTIVITY—Avoid sexual intercourse during the active phase of the infection.

DIET—No special diet. If taking tetracycline, avoid dairy products within 3 hours of taking the medicine.

CALL YOUR DOCTOR IF

- You or a family member has symptoms of granuloma inguinale.
- Symptoms don't start improving within a few days after starting medication.
- Symptoms worsen despite treatment.
- New, unexplained symptoms develop. Drugs used in treatment may produce side effects.

GRANULOMA, PYOGENIC

GENERAL INFORMATION

DEFINITION—Pyogenic granuloma is a fairly common type of skin growth. It is not contagious or cancerous.

BODY PARTS INVOLVED—Skin anywhere on the body. It often affects the head, neck, upper trunk, and fingers. It can also affect the gums and other mucous membranes of the mouth.

SEX OR AGE MOST AFFECTED
- Children of both sexes (ages 5 to 15).
- Pregnant women.

SIGNS & SYMPTOMS
- Papule (small, raised bump on the skin). Usually, a single one is present, but in rare cases, there may be multiple papules.
- It first appears as pinhead-sized, but it grows rapidly over a period of a few weeks to about a half inch in size.
- The color is scarlet, brown, or blue-black.
- Will bleed easily when injured.
- They don't hurt or itch.
- May ulcerate (become an open sore) and form a crust.

CAUSES—Unknown. Possible factors include hormones, injury, infection, drug-caused, and others.

RISK INCREASES WITH
- Pregnancy.
- Recent injury (may develop at an injured site).
- Use of certain drugs (such as oral contraceptives, retinoids, or protease inhibitors).

HOW TO PREVENT
- Cannot be prevented at present.
- Because pyogenic granuloma resembles melanoma (skin cancer), medical diagnosis can be important.

WHAT TO EXPECT

DIAGNOSTIC MEASURES
- Your own observation of symptoms.
- Your health care provider will diagnose the disorder by an exam of the affected skin area.
- Medical tests may include a skin biopsy (removal of a small amount of tissue for viewing under a microscope).

APPROPRIATE HEALTH CARE
- Often, they are scraped off with an instrument called a curette and then cauterized (using heat to heal tissue). This helps to decrease the chance that they will regrow.
- Laser surgery can be used to destroy the growth.
- In some cases, they may be treated with chemicals (such as silver nitrate).
- The growth may be removed by surgical excision and closed with stitches.
- If a drug is the cause of the pyogenic granuloma, stopping the drug may lead to healing.

POSSIBLE COMPLICATIONS—Recurrence is common.

PROBABLE OUTCOME—Some heal on their own (such as in pregnancy). Others can be successfully treated.

HOW TO TREAT

GENERAL MEASURES—Follow medical advice for self-care after any treatment procedure.

MEDICATION—In some cases, topical drugs may be used for treatment.

ACTIVITY—No limits, except to avoid injury to the area while it is healing.

DIET—No special diet.

CALL YOUR DOCTOR IF

- You or a family member has symptoms of pyogenic granuloma.
- The wound bleeds after surgery, and applying pressure for 10 minutes cannot stop it.
- The wound shows signs of infection, such as redness, swelling, pain, or increased tenderness.

GRIEF
(Bereavement)

GENERAL INFORMATION

DEFINITION—Grief is the emotional reaction following the death of a loved person, a divorce, loss of a body part or its function, loss of self-esteem (such as losing a job), or other significant loss. Grief is a normal, appropriate reaction to loss. It comes in many forms. Grieving people gradually adjust to their loss and begin to make positive plans for the future. There are no guidelines for the normal time for grieving. Sometimes, grief is serious or long-lasting enough that medical help is needed.

BODY PARTS INVOLVED—Sometimes all.

SEX OR AGE MOST AFFECTED—Both sexes; all ages.

SIGNS & SYMPTOMS
● Feelings of sadness, numbness, pain, anger, despair, or guilt. These feelings can come and go for months, and may be overwhelming at times, especially on anniversaries of important or memorable dates.
● Sudden crying spells.
● Hallucinations (such as a sense of having seen or heard the dead person).
● Anxiety and depression.
● Being unwilling to accept the loss; for example, keeping the dead person's room or clothing as if he or she is expected to return.
● Unable to sleep.
● Nervousness and being overactive.
● Stomach problems.
● Tiredness, agitation, tearfulness.
● Increased use of alcohol and other drugs.

CAUSES—Grief naturally follows a loss.

RISK INCREASES WITH—Existing emotional problems can affect how a person responds to loss. This includes depression, social aloneness, strong feelings of guilt, self-blame, or anger due to one's relationship with the dead person.

HOW TO PREVENT—Grieving should not be prevented or denied. It is a normal and expected response to a loss.

WHAT TO EXPECT

DIAGNOSTIC MEASURES
● Your own observation of symptoms.
● See your health care provider if the feelings of grief are severe, or continue interfering with your daily life and/or work. A physical exam may be done and questions asked about your symptoms and feelings.

APPROPRIATE HEALTH CARE—Grief counseling may be recommended.

POSSIBLE COMPLICATIONS
● Difficulty maintaining relationships and jobs.
● Excess use of alcohol or other drugs.
● Chronic anxiety and depression.
● Symptoms that may need medical help include:
  - Severe depression, panic attacks, chronic anxiety.
  - Strong feelings of guilt, bitterness, or remorse.
  - Grief continues for 2 years or more. A person may build a life around the grief and never accept the loss.
  - Talk about or threats of suicide.

PROBABLE OUTCOME
● Don't expect your feelings of grief to follow any pattern or a particular timetable.
● With time, the grief lessens and adjustment begins. Your mind, body, and spirit will begin to heal. The feelings of grief may come and go, and will probably recur occasionally for years.
● The four stages of grief that people typically experience are: shock and disbelief, awareness, depression, and reconciliation and recovery.

HOW TO TREAT

GENERAL MEASURES
● Express your feelings following the loss. Don't keep them "bottled up" inside. Look to family and friends for help and support.
● Religious or spiritual help may be of benefit to some people. Talk to your pastor or other religious professional about your feelings.
● Join a grief support group. They are available in most areas. People often find comfort in sharing their feelings with others who have had similar experiences.
● Slowly begin to rebuild your life. Interest yourself in things you have enjoyed in the past or try some new activities.
● Avoid the overuse of alcohol or drugs to suppress the emotions that you are feeling.

MEDICATION—You may be prescribed drugs, such as sedatives or antidepressants, for a short time. In most cases, drugs are not needed.

ACTIVITY—Normally, no limits. Try to do some physical activity daily.

DIET—Eat a normal, well-balanced diet.

CALL YOUR DOCTOR IF

● You or a family member has symptoms of grief that are getting worse or not getting better with time.
● Any of the Possible Complications occur.

GUILLAIN-BARRÉ SYNDROME
(Infectious Polyneuropathy)

 GENERAL INFORMATION

DEFINITION—Guillain-Barré is a rare, inflammatory condition involving the peripheral nerves. These are nerves outside the brain and spinal column. It causes rapid weakness and loss of sensation.

BODY PARTS INVOLVED—Central nervous system.

SEX OR AGE MOST AFFECTED—Both sexes; all ages, but is more common in young adults and the elderly.

SIGNS & SYMPTOMS
- Muscle weakness or tingling starting in the lower limbs (feet and legs) and ascending (moving up) to the abdomen and chest, and to the arms and hands. The weakness spreads over days to weeks.
- Facial weakness and drooping, double vision, and difficulty in speaking and in swallowing.
- Pain, often in the back and legs; muscle cramps and tenderness; numbness, tingling, or burning sensations.
- Irregular heartbeat, high or low blood pressure.
- Shortness of breath.
- Complete paralysis (sometimes) for weeks or months.

CAUSES—The cause is unclear. It may be an autoimmune disorder. It sometimes follows a bacterial or viral infection.

RISK INCREASES WITH—Recent illness, such as a respiratory infection or gastroenteritis (stomach flu).

HOW TO PREVENT—No preventive measures.

 WHAT TO EXPECT

DIAGNOSTIC MEASURES
- Your own observation of symptoms.
- Your health care provider may be able to diagnose the disorder by the symptoms and with a physical exam.
- Medical tests may be done, such as lumbar puncture for spinal fluid analysis, electromyography (studying nerve and muscle disorders by recording electrical activity of muscles), and lung function tests.

APPROPRIATE HEALTH CARE
- Hospital care is needed in an intensive care unit so the condition can be closely monitored. There is no specific treatment for the disorder. Care involves supportive measures and methods to help speed recovery.
- A respirator (breathing machine) may be needed if muscles of respiration become greatly weakened. A tracheotomy (opening in the throat for breathing) may be required.

- Immunotherapy may be used to help shorten the duration and severity of the disease. It involves either plasmapheresis or IV immune globulin (injections).
- Plasmapheresis is a procedure where blood plasma is withdrawn from the patient, treated to remove antibodies, and then returned to the body by transfusion.
- Rehabilitation will begin as soon as it is feasible. It may involve physical therapy, occupational therapy (to promote self-care), speech therapy (to help with speaking and swallowing problems), and recreational therapy (helps the patient adjust to any disability).

POSSIBLE COMPLICATIONS
- A relapse may occur after initial improvement.
- Respiratory failure.
- Permanent muscle weakness or numbness.
- Permanent total or partial paralysis (rare).
- Pneumonia.
- Deep vein thrombosis.
- Contractures of joints.

PROBABLE OUTCOME
- Complete recovery without any lasting effects in many cases. Adults recover better than children. For some persons, symptoms clear in 15 to 20 days. Others require a year or more. Many mechanical devices can aid mobility until the person recovers.
- Some patients will have moderate lasting effects, and a few will have severe disabilities.

 HOW TO TREAT

GENERAL MEASURES
- Support group, if available, can help you cope.
- To learn more: GBS-CDIP Foundation, Holly Bldg, 104½ Forrest Ave., Narberth, PA 19096; (866) 224-3301; website: www.gbs-cidp.org.

MEDICATION
- IVIG (IV immune globulin) may be prescribed.
- Drugs as needed for symptoms, such as pain.

ACTIVITY
- Remain as active as muscle strength permits. Have a family member or physical therapist passively move and stretch muscles.
- Ongoing physical therapy will be needed to rebuild strength.

DIET—A feeding tube may be needed for patient with severe swallowing problem.

 CALL YOUR DOCTOR IF

- You or a family member has symptoms of Guillain-Barré syndrome.
- New symptoms occur after a patient returns home.

HAND, FOOT & MOUTH DISEASE

GENERAL INFORMATION

DEFINITION—Hand, foot and mouth disease is a common childhood infection with symptoms that begin in the mouth and throat.

BODY PARTS INVOLVED—Throat; tonsils; skin; gastrointestinal tract; central nervous system.

SEX OR AGE MOST AFFECTED—It most often affects children under the age of 10. Adults may get the infection, but it is less common.

SIGNS & SYMPTOMS
- Sore throat with blisters and sores in the mouth and throat lining.
- Sudden fever that is usually mild.
- Rash with blisters on the hands, feet, and groin.
- Refusal to eat.
- Stomach pain or headache (sometimes).

CAUSES—Viral infection commonly caused by coxsackieviruses. The germs are spread from person to person or by touching an object (such as a toy) that has the germs on it. It takes about 3 to 6 days after exposure for the symptoms to start. Outbreaks may occur in nursery schools or child-care centers.

RISK INCREASES WITH—Summer and fall seasons.

HOW TO PREVENT
- No specific preventive measures.
- Try to prevent exposure of infants and young children to anyone with an infection. Wash hands often to prevent spread of germs.
- Pregnant women should consult their obstetric provider if they are exposed to an infected person.

WHAT TO EXPECT

DIAGNOSTIC MEASURES
- Your own observation of symptoms.
- See your health care provider if you are concerned about the symptoms.
- Your health care provider can diagnose the infection by an exam of the affected mouth and skin area.
- Medical tests are normally not needed.

APPROPRIATE HEALTH CARE
- Home care is usually all that is required for this infection.
- There is no specific treatment for the infection, but treatment may help relieve pain and fever symptoms.

POSSIBLE COMPLICATIONS
- The infection may be more serious in some infants and dehydration can occur.
- Other complications are rare.

PROBABLE OUTCOME—The infection is usually mild and complete recovery occurs in about a week. It rarely recurs once someone has had the infection.

HOW TO TREAT

GENERAL MEASURES
- Rinse the mouth with salt water (1/2 teaspoon salt to 1 cup water) after eating, if the child is old enough to rinse without swallowing.
- Use separate dishes or disposable plates and cups to help avoid spreading the infection to other children in the family.

MEDICATION
- To reduce high fever or for pain, you may use nonprescription drugs such as acetaminophen. Don't use aspirin in young children. Antibiotics are not effective for this infection.
- For mouth pain, use oral numbing products such as sore throat sprays.

ACTIVITY—Have the child get extra rest at home until any fever is gone. Children may return to school or daycare while they still have the rash.

DIET—Encourage the child to increase their fluid and soft food intake. This may include milk, liquid gelatin, ice cream, custard, or special products that you can buy at grocery or drug stores.

CALL YOUR DOCTOR IF

- Your child has symptoms of hand, foot and mouth disease that cause you concern.
- Symptoms get worse or do not improve.

HANTAVIRUS
(Hantaviral Pulmonary Syndrome)

 GENERAL INFORMATION

DEFINITION—Hantavirus (named after a place in Korea) causes an illness called hantavirus pulmonary syndrome (HPS). Hantavirus has probably caused people to get sick for years in the United States, but it was not known about until recent years.

BODY PARTS INVOLVED—Respiratory system.

SEX OR AGE MOST AFFECTED—Both sexes; all ages.

SIGNS & SYMPTOMS
- Early symptoms are flu-like:
  - Chills.
  - Fever.
  - Muscle aches.
  - Headaches.
  - Nausea and vomiting.
  - Cough.
  - General ill feeling.
  - Feeling tired; lack of energy.
  - Somewhat short of breath.
- Later symptom (frequently occurs after 1 or 2 days of improvement):
  - Extreme difficulty in breathing.

CAUSES—Several types of mice can carry the hantavirus without getting ill. Where they nest, they leave the germs in their urine, feces (droppings), and saliva. If the nests are disturbed, the germs can get into the air as dust. When humans breathe in the air containing the germs, they can become infected. Infection may also come from a mouse bite, or from germs in food, water, or on something you touched. It may take a few days to 6 weeks for symptoms to appear once a person is exposed to the germs. The germs are not passed between humans.

RISK INCREASES WITH—No known specific risk factors.

HOW TO PREVENT
- Avoid exposure to rodent urine and feces.
- Use caution in cleaning areas where mice nests might be located.
- Keep a clean home. This includes clearing out potential nesting sites and maintaining a clean kitchen.

 WHAT TO EXPECT

DIAGNOSTIC MEASURES
- Your own observation of symptoms.
- The breathing problems progress very quickly and treatment must occur in the hospital. Usually this is in an intensive care unit. Your health care provider will do a physical exam and discuss the possible exposure to rodents.
- A number of medical tests will be done to confirm the diagnosis.

APPROPRIATE HEALTH CARE
- The main treatment is to help with any breathing problems.
- Supplemental oxygen is used to help the breathing. In severe cases, a machine may be needed to assist with the breathing.
- Blood oxygenation may be needed. The patient's blood is pumped through a machine to remove carbon dioxide and add oxygen.

POSSIBLE COMPLICATIONS—Hantavirus pulmonary syndrome is a serious infection, and is fatal in about 50% of cases.

PROBABLE OUTCOME—The outcome will vary for each patient. To date, there is no treatment to stop the infection once it sets in. But steps can be taken to help control the symptoms while your body fights off the infection.

 HOW TO TREAT

GENERAL MEASURES—The family should maintain a hopeful outlook, and be as supportive as possible.

MEDICATION
- Your health care provider will prescribe drugs as needed to help control any bleeding and improve lung function.
- An antiviral drug (ribavirin) may be used in some cases.

ACTIVITY—Bed rest for acute illness; resume normal activities gradually.

DIET—May require feeding through a vein (IV) while in the hospital. Then return to a regular diet with recovery.

 CALL YOUR DOCTOR IF

You or a family member has symptoms of hantavirus pulmonary syndrome, especially if you live in an area, or have traveled to an area, where the virus is present.

HAY FEVER
(Allergic Rhinitis)

 GENERAL INFORMATION

DEFINITION—Hay fever is an allergic response to an allergen in the air. The name is confusing since hay does not cause an allergic reaction and there is no fever. Attacks flare up in pollen season. Allergens in the air that cause an allergic sensitivity include: pollen (from weeds, flowers, grasses, and trees), mold, dust, mites, tobacco smoke, and other air pollutants.

BODY PARTS INVOLVED—Hay fever affects the eyes, nose, sinuses, throat, and bronchial tubes in the lungs.

SEX OR AGE MOST AFFECTED—Both sexes; all ages.

SIGNS & SYMPTOMS
- Itching, watery eyes.
- Frequent sneezing; stuffy nose with a clear discharge.
- Itching in the roof of the mouth.
- Ears may feel plugged up.

CAUSES—The body's immune system produces antibodies that release a chemical called histamine. Histamine in turn produces swelling and irritation in certain areas (nose, sinuses, eyes). The development of hay fever in a person appears to be a combination of both genetic and environmental factors.

RISK INCREASES WITH
- Having other allergic reactions, such as eczema or asthma.
- Family history of allergies.

HOW TO PREVENT—There is no way to prevent having allergies. You can take steps to help prevent having symptoms.

 WHAT TO EXPECT

DIAGNOSTIC MEASURES
- Your own observation of symptoms.
- Your health care provider will do a physical exam and ask questions about your symptoms.
- Medical tests such as blood and allergy skin tests may be recommended, but are usually not required for diagnosis.

APPROPRIATE HEALTH CARE—Medical care may include drugs and desensitizing treatment.

POSSIBLE COMPLICATIONS
- Difficulty in sleeping and chronic fatigue.
- Increased risk for other infections.

PROBABLE OUTCOME—Symptoms can be controlled with treatment, but the condition persists over a lifetime. It is usually more troublesome than disabling.

 HOW TO TREAT

GENERAL MEASURES
- Try to remove as many allergens from your home or the yard area as possible.
- Prepare your bedroom as follows:
  - Empty the room of furniture, rugs or carpet, and drapes or curtains. Clean the walls, floors, and woodwork with a damp mop. Wax the floor.
  - Cover box springs, mattress, and pillows with plastic covers. Use bedclothes that can be washed often.
  - Use throw rugs that can be washed easily.
  - Use wood or plastic chairs (not stuffed).
  - Use window shades or blinds, not drapes/curtains.
  - Use vacuum cleaner, damp rags, and a damp or oiled mop to clean bedroom once a week.
- Other preventive measures:
  - Keep windows and doors closed, if possible.
  - Don't handle objects that are very dusty, such as books or stored clothing.
  - Don't keep stuffed animals or toys in the house.
  - Remove all pets (except fish) from the house or keep them out of the bedroom.
  - Wear a filter face-mask during exposure to allergens, including during housecleaning.
  - Install an air-purification unit in your home's heating and air-conditioning system, preferably a high-efficiency particulate (HEPA) filter.
  - Drive an air-conditioned car.
  - Have someone else mow the lawn.

MEDICATION
- You may be prescribed:
  - Antihistamines; decongestants; eyedrops (cortisone, antihistamine, or anti-inflammatory); cortisone nasal spray; cortisone tablets (severe cases only); cromolyn nasal spray; or cromolyn nose drops. These drugs relieve symptoms, but they don't cure hay fever.
  - Desensitization injections for known allergens for severe or year-round cases. Once allergens are known (through skin or blood tests), small amounts are injected over a period of time. This helps block the immune system from releasing the histamine. This process may take months or years for effective results.

ACTIVITY—No limits. Avoid areas with known allergens.

DIET—No special diet.

 CALL YOUR DOCTOR IF

- You or a family member has symptoms of hay fever that are interfering with normal activities.
- Symptoms don't improve with treatment.

HEAD INJURY
(Traumatic Brain Injury; Concussion)

 GENERAL INFORMATION

DEFINITION—A head injury involves trauma to the scalp, skull, or brain. It can be minor (e.g., bump on the head) to severe (e.g., traumatic brain injury). A concussion is a less serious type of brain injury.

BODY PARTS INVOLVED—It involves the scalp, skull, or brain.

SEX OR AGE MOST AFFECTED—Males more than females and ages under 35.

SIGNS & SYMPTOMS
- Head injury symptoms may occur right away, or hours or days later. Older persons can develop symptoms up to 6 months after an injury. Signs and symptoms can include one or more of the following effects.
- Swelling and/or bleeding at the site of injury.
- Fracture of the skull.
- Loss of consciousness (short time or for long period).
- Abnormal breathing.
- Clear or bloody fluid from nose, mouth, or ear.
- Drowsiness, confusion, irritability, or loss of memory.
- Unable to feel or control muscle function.
- Black-and-blue color around the eyes.
- Vomiting and nausea; dizziness.
- Changes in vision or speech; pupils of different sizes.
- Pain, such as headache or stiff neck.
- Seizure.

CAUSES—Head injuries may be external (closed) or internal (penetrating). The brain can be damaged by a fractured skull or damaged due to brain swelling. Head injuries can cause physical problems, cognitive (thinking) dysfunction, emotional changes, and be life-threatening.

RISK INCREASES WITH
- Accidents (motor vehicle, work-related, sports, falls, physical assault, outdoor activities, and in the home).
- Child abuse or shaken baby syndrome.
- Alcohol or substance abuse.
- Contact sports (e.g., football, soccer, or boxing).
- Prior head injury or having a seizure disorder.
- Illnesses that affect balance or walking ability.
- Not using seat belts or not wearing helmets.

HOW TO PREVENT
- Don't drink or use mind-altering drugs and drive (or ride in a car with an impaired driver).
- Wear protective headgear when head injury is a risk.
- Use your auto seatbelt always. Place young children in approved safety car seats.
- If you are unsteady, use a walker or a cane.

 WHAT TO EXPECT

DIAGNOSTIC MEASURES
- Your own observation of symptoms.
- Medical care starts with checking the person's ABCs (airway, breathing, and circulation). Any visible head injuries will be treated.
- Medical test for alertness and an x-ray, CT, or MRI are often done to check for brain damage.

APPROPRIATE HEALTH CARE
- A person with a mild head injury can be sent home after initial medical care. Someone must stay with the person and watch for serious symptoms over the next 24 hours. Instructions may include waking the patient every 2 to 3 hours to check for alertness. Get medical help if you cannot awaken or arouse the person.
- In other head injuries, the treatment will depend on the severity. Hospital care may be needed for a period of time, and then rehabilitation care may be required.

POSSIBLE COMPLICATIONS—Permanent physical or mental disabilities, and social and economic problems (such as loss of job).

PROBABLE OUTCOME—The outcome will vary depending on a variety of factors (e.g., age, type of injury, severity of symptoms, and treatment). Many head injuries are mild and heal on their own with no lasting effects. Others can be treated successfully. Some may require long-term hospital care and rehabilitation.

 HOW TO TREAT

GENERAL MEASURES
- Self-care is sometimes done for mild injuries. Get medical help right away if any of the symptoms listed occur or other head injury symptoms cause concern. Give first aid if needed. Call 911 for emergency help.
- To learn more: Brain Injury Association, 1608 Spring Hill Rd., Suite 110, Vienna, VA 22182; (800) 444-6443; website: www.biausa.org.

MEDICATION—For self-care, you may use acetaminophen for pain or discomfort. Avoid aspirin. It can increase bleeding risk.

ACTIVITY—Follow your health care provider's instructions about resuming normal activity.

DIET—Food intake will depend on injury.

 CALL YOUR DOCTOR IF

- You or a family member has symptoms of a head injury. Get emergency help if needed!
- After head injury, symptoms cause concern.

HEADACHE, CLUSTER

 ## GENERAL INFORMATION

DEFINITION—A cluster headache typically causes severe pain on one side of the head, behind the head, or around one eye. The headaches occur in groups or clusters usually over weeks or months.

BODY PARTS INVOLVED—Central nervous system.

SEX OR AGE MOST AFFECTED—Adults over age 30, and men more than women.

SIGNS & SYMPTOMS
- Sudden onset of headache. It often occurs at night while sleeping.
- Headache reaches a peak within 15 minutes and lasts about 2 to 3 hours.
- Pain around the eye.
- Severe, piercing, or boring pain.
- Teary eyes.
- Swollen and droopy eyelid.
- Stuffy or runny nose.
- Sweating.
- Feeling agitated and restless during an attack.
- Episodic cluster headaches tend to recur at the same time each day for several days or weeks, separated by attack-free weeks or months.
- The more rare, chronic type occur almost daily with headache-free periods lasting about 2 weeks.

CAUSES—The cause is unknown. It may be a combination of factors, such as dilating blood vessels in the head, disturbance of the trigeminal nerve, or abnormal activity in part of the brain (hypothalamus).

RISK INCREASES WITH
- Male, age over 30.
- Previous head injury.
- Family history of cluster headache.
- Other possible factors include smoking, alcohol abuse, sleep disturbances or sleep apnea (periods of not breathing at night), stressful job, or history of migraines.

HOW TO PREVENT—Since the cause is unknown, no specific measures to prevent first episode.

 ## WHAT TO EXPECT

DIAGNOSTIC MEASURES
- Your own observation of symptoms.
- Your health care provider can usually diagnose the disorder based on the history of the headache patterns and symptoms.
- Medical tests are normally not required, but may be done to rule out other conditions.

APPROPRIATE HEALTH CARE
- Treatment goals are to treat the symptoms and prevent or abort future attacks. It may involve drug therapy, use of oxygen, and lifestyle changes.
- Surgical treatments may be considered when drug therapy is not helpful. Surgery has limited effectiveness.

POSSIBLE COMPLICATIONS—Cluster headaches do not cause complications or lead to other disorders. They are debilitating and can interfere with daily activities.

PROBABLE OUTCOME—There is no cure. The cluster headache attacks may come and go, or be ongoing. Many people are headache-free for a year or more, but then they may start up again. Various therapies are available that can help prevent and treat the headache attacks.

 ## HOW TO TREAT

GENERAL MEASURES
- During cluster periods, avoid bright light or glare, alcohol, excessive anger, stressful activity, or excitement. These can trigger attacks. Keeping a headache diary may be useful to help identify other triggers.
- Don't smoke. It may hinder drug therapy.
- Some patients also have sleep apnea. Treating the apnea (with a mechanical device) may help headaches also.
- To learn more: National Headache Foundation, 820 N. Orleans, Suite 217, Chicago, IL 60610; (888) 643-5552; website: www.headaches.org.

MEDICATION
- Your health care provider may prescribe one or more drugs to treat the headache and for prevention:
    - Drugs called triptans (by mouth or injection).
    - Dihydroergotamine (Migranal) by injection.
    - Ergotamine tartrate, in a tablet, suppository, aerosol, or injection form.
    - Verapamil or prednisone by mouth.
    - Oxygen therapy for home use.
    - Lidocaine nasal spray or nasal drops.
    - Other drugs to help treat/prevent cluster headaches.

ACTIVITY—Physical exercise may help bring relief in some patients.

DIET—Avoid alcohol and foods containing nitrates (such as smoked meat).

 ## CALL YOUR DOCTOR IF

- You or a family member has symptoms of cluster headache.
- Attacks continue after treatment is started.

HEADACHE, MIGRAINE

GENERAL INFORMATION

DEFINITION—Migraine is a severe type of headache that involves more than just the headache pain. There are five stages that may occur with a migraine. Prodrome (warning signs), aura (beginning symptoms), headache itself, resolution (pain stops), and postdrome (tiredness and other symptoms).

BODY PARTS INVOLVED—Central nervous system.

SEX OR AGE MOST AFFECTED—Both sexes, (more common in females); children and adults.

SIGNS & SYMPTOMS
- The nature of attacks varies between persons and from time to time in the same person.
- Prodrome (hours/days before attack). It can include changes in mood, behavior, energy, and appetite.
- Aura (minutes or an hour before attack). It affects vision, hearing, or smell.
  - The most common symptoms are the inability to see clearly and seeing bright spots and zig-zag patterns.
  - Visual disturbances may last several minutes or hours. They stop once headache begins.
- Headache. Dull, boring pain in the temple that spreads to the entire side of the head.
  - Pain gets more intense and throbs. Nausea, vomiting, and/or sensitivity to light and sound.
  - Headaches can last from 4 to 72 hours.
- Postdrome (may occur after an attack and last for hours or days). It includes exhaustion, weakness, lethargy, and elation (in some cases).

CAUSES—Exact cause is unknown. It may be due to a central nervous system disturbance that sets off a chain of events in the body. Genetic factors are involved also.

RISK INCREASES WITH
- Females and/or family history of migraines.
- Other disorders (such as asthma, allergies, *H. pylori* infection, epilepsy, and fibromyalgia).

HOW TO PREVENT—No preventive steps for first attack. After diagnosis, take steps to help prevent future attacks. Try to avoid the triggers of migraines (such as some foods and drugs, bright lights, weather changes, high altitudes, alcohol, skipping meals, and emotional stress). Keep a diary to learn your own specific triggers.

WHAT TO EXPECT

DIAGNOSTIC MEASURES
- Your own observation of symptoms.
- Your health care provider can usually diagnose the disorder based on the history of the headache pattern and symptoms.
- Medical tests are normally not required.

APPROPRIATE HEALTH CARE
- Treatment is usually with drug therapy and self-care.
- Hospital care may be needed for severe attack.
- Counseling, behavior therapy, or stress reduction techniques may be recommended.

POSSIBLE COMPLICATIONS
- Interferes with day-to-day life (work, family, or social).
- Status migraine (lasts over 72 hours) or stroke (rare).

PROBABLE OUTCOME—People with migraines tend to have them over many years. They can often be controlled with treatment. Migraines may end when a person gets older.

HOW TO TREAT

GENERAL MEASURES
- For self-care at first sign of a migraine attack:
  - Apply a cold cloth to your head and lie down in a quiet, dark room. Relax and sleep if you can.
  - Minimize noise, light, and odors (such as cooking odors and tobacco smoke). Don't read.
- To learn more: National Headache Foundation, 428 West St. James Pl., 2nd Flr., Chicago, IL 60614; (888) 643-5552; website: www.headaches.org

MEDICATION
- No single drug works best for everyone. A variety of drugs can be prescribed for symptoms and prevention.
- Triptans—subcutaneous (under the skin) self injection, oral tablet, or nasal spray.
- Ergot preparations in a tablet, suppository, aerosol, or injection form.
- Nonprescription drugs such as ibuprofen, or aspirin (for over age 18), or acetaminophen.
- Narcotics or butalbital alone or with other drugs.
- Antihistamines to expand blood vessels.
- Antiemetics to decrease nausea and vomiting.
- Vasoconstrictors to narrow blood vessels.
- Beta-adrenergic, calcium channel blockers, or anti-depressants to prevent attacks.
- Note: overuse of drugs can cause a "rebound" into another headache.

ACTIVITY—Exercise daily to maintain fitness.

DIET—Keep a diary to see if certain foods trigger migraines.

CALL YOUR DOCTOR IF

- You or a family member has migraine symptoms.
- Treatment is not helping the migraines.

HEADACHE, TENSION

GENERAL INFORMATION

DEFINITION—Tension headaches are the most common type of headache. These headaches may occur 15 or more days out of a month (chronic) or less often (episodic).

BODY PARTS INVOLVED—Sensory nerves in the skin, scalp, blood vessels and muscles of the head.

SEX OR AGE MOST AFFECTED—Both sexes; all ages.

SIGNS & SYMPTOMS
- Dull, steady pain on both sides of the head. The pain may be mild to severe. It usually comes on gradually.
- Tight feeling or tenderness in the muscles of the head, neck, or scalp. "Like a band around the head."
- Some people may clench their teeth.
- Tension headaches are different from migraines, which cause intense pain, usually on one side of the head. Migraines also cause nausea and light sensitivity.

CAUSES—The cause is not clearly understood. It may be a problem of the central nervous system and changes in brain chemicals. It may involve stress and tension that puts strain on the muscles of the neck, scalp, face, and jaw.

RISK INCREASES WITH
- People who might get tension headaches:
  - Women (more often affected than men).
  - Those with a family history of headaches.
  - Those who are overworked on a continuous basis.
  - Those with chronic poor posture or sleep disorders.
  - Those who suffer from depression, stress, anxiety, or have certain chronic medical problems.
  - Those who abuse alcohol or other substances.
- Things that might bring on (trigger) tension headaches include:
  - A stressful event.
  - Not eating on time; caffeine withdrawal.
  - Intense physical exercise.
  - Taking certain drugs.
  - Hormone changes in women.
  - Eyestrain, fatigue, or having a cold or the flu.
  - Certain foods or drinks (for some people).

HOW TO PREVENT—Avoid any of the risk factors when possible.

WHAT TO EXPECT

DIAGNOSTIC MEASURES
- Your own observation of symptoms.

- Self-care is often effective for handling the headache. If that doesn't work, or the pain gets worse, or headaches occur often, see your health care provider.
- Your health care provider will do a physical exam, and ask questions about your symptoms and your lifestyle.
- Medical tests and blood studies may be done to be sure no other medical problem is involved.

APPROPRIATE HEALTH CARE
- Chronic tension headaches may be treated with different methods for stress reduction and relaxation techniques, and prescribed drugs. Drugs that have been overused for headache pain may need to be withdrawn.
- There are more treatment options that you and your health care provider may discuss. These may include physical therapy, massage therapy, acupuncture, hypnosis, and others.

POSSIBLE COMPLICATIONS
- None expected for a simple headache.
- Chronic tension headaches may require trying several types of therapy. Headaches continue if risk factors are not changed or treated.
- Time lost from work. Reduced quality of life.
- Overuse, dependence, or addiction to therapy drugs.

PROBABLE OUTCOME—Most tension headaches can be relieved with treatment, and do not disrupt home or work activities.

HOW TO TREAT

GENERAL MEASURES
- Self-care can include mild pain relievers. If possible, stop what you are doing and try to relax. Take a hot bath or shower. Lie down. Place a warm or cold cloth, whichever feels better, over the aching area.
- To learn more: National Headache Foundation, 820 N. Orleans, Suite 217, Chicago, IL 60610, (888) 643-5552; website: www.headaches.org.

MEDICATION
- Use nonprescription pain relievers such as ibuprofen, naproxen, aspirin, or acetaminophen.
- Stronger drugs for pain and drugs to prevent chronic tension headaches may be prescribed.

ACTIVITY
- Exercise daily and get enough sleep.
- Get medical advice about exercises to stretch and strengthen neck and shoulder muscles.

DIET—Eat a normal, healthy diet.

CALL YOUR DOCTOR IF

- You or a family member has tension headaches and self-care steps are not working.
- Headaches recur or get worse.

HEARING IMPAIRMENT OR LOSS
(Deafness)

GENERAL INFORMATION

DEFINITION
• Hearing loss may be partial or total. It may develop gradually or suddenly. It may occur at any age. There are two types of hearing loss:
- Conductive loss. It is caused by anything that blocks the conduction of sound from the outer ear through to the inner ear.
- Sensorineural loss. It results from damage to the inner ear such as to the auditory nerve or hair cells of the cochlea. This type includes the gradual hearing loss that occurs with aging called presbycusis.
- Mixed loss involves both types of hearing loss.

BODY PARTS INVOLVED—Middle-ear bones that conduct sound; branches of the 8th cranial nerve that transmit sound to the brain.

SEX OR AGE MOST AFFECTED—Both sexes; all ages.

SIGNS & SYMPTOMS
• In an infant, there is a lack of response to sounds.
• Trouble understanding speech. Misunderstanding others and responding inappropriately.
• Difficulty in hearing a phone ring, or problem hearing over the phone.
• Difficulty hearing in a group of people or when there is background noise.
• Avoiding social activities (may feel embarrassed).
• Turning up the volume of television.
• Asking others to repeat themselves.
• Ringing in the ears, dizziness, or pain.

CAUSES—Hearing loss occurs when any part of the hearing system is unable to function. A wide variety of conditions can cause hearing loss. Sometimes, no cause is found.

RISK INCREASES WITH
• Conductive:
- Middle ear infection (otitis media).
- Collection of fluid in middle ear (glue ear).
- Blockage of the outer ear by wax.
- Damage to the eardrum from infection or injury.
- Otosclerosis (growth of spongy tissue in ear).
- Rarely, rheumatoid arthritis affects ear joints.
• Sensorineural:
- Aging (hearing starts decreasing in the 30s and 40s).
- Noise exposure (repeated and continuous).
- Viral infection such as mumps.
- Ménière's disease.
- Certain drugs (aspirin, quinine, some antibiotics).
- Acoustic neuroma (benign tumor).
- Brain infection, inflammation, or tumor.

- Multiple sclerosis or a stroke.
- Congenital (present at birth). A family history of hearing loss is also a risk factor.

HOW TO PREVENT—Avoid the risk factors where possible. Get medical care for any infections or any symptoms of hearing loss.

WHAT TO EXPECT

DIAGNOSTIC MEASURES
• Your health care provider will do an exam of the ears and ask questions about your symptoms.
• Hearing tests may include tests done with a tuning fork and an audiogram (to measure hearing levels). Other hearing studies and speech testing may be done.

APPROPRIATE HEALTH CARE
• Treatment will depend on the cause, the extent of hearing loss, and if it is conductive or sensorineural.
• It may involve simple procedures (like earwax removal). Other options include drug therapy, surgical treatments, and sound amplification (e.g., hearing aids).
• You may be referred to a health care provider who specializes in hearing problems.
• Cochlear implant may be an option to help severe deafness. It is a surgically placed electronic device.
• If the hearing loss is related to drugs, changes in dosage or stopping the drug may help.

POSSIBLE COMPLICATIONS
• Complete loss of hearing (deafness).
• Language delay or learning problems in a child.
• Emotional, social, and work-associated problems.

PROBABLE OUTCOME—The outcome depends on the cause. The hearing loss may be temporary, treatable, or manageable.

HOW TO TREAT

GENERAL MEASURES—To learn more: National Institute on Deafness; (800) 241-1044; website: www.nidcd.nih.gov/health/hearing.

MEDICATION—Drugs may be prescribed for any treatable disorder that is diagnosed.

ACTIVITY—No limits.

DIET—No special diet.

CALL YOUR DOCTOR IF

You or a family member has hearing problems.

HEART ATTACK
(Myocardial Infarction)

 GENERAL INFORMATION

DEFINITION—A heart attack occurs when there is a severe blockage in an artery that carries blood to the heart muscle. It is a life-threatening event.

BODY PARTS INVOLVED—Coronary arteries; heart muscle; platelets and clotting factors circulating in the blood.

SEX OR AGE MOST AFFECTED—Adults over age 40, and men more than women (after age 70, they are equally affected).

SIGNS & SYMPTOMS
- Chest pain or "heavy, squeezing, or crushing" feeling in the chest.
- Pain that radiates from the midchest over the breastbone to the jaw, neck, either arm, the area between the shoulder blades, or upper abdomen (sometimes).
- Feeling of impending doom.
- Shortness of breath.
- Nausea, vomiting, and sweating.
- Dizziness and/or weakness.
- Choking sensation.
- In some cases, no symptoms occur (called silent heart attack). It may be diagnosed during a routine exam.

CAUSES—An artery carrying blood to the heart becomes blocked due to plaque (fatty material) or a blood clot. Without blood, the affected heart muscle becomes damaged and heart function is decreased. A more rare cause is a artery spasm that stops blood flow.

RISK INCREASES WITH
- Men over age 45 and women over age 55.
- Coronary artery disease (plaque in arteries).
- Prior heart attack; family history of heart disease.
- Smoking, excess alcohol use, obesity/overweight, high blood pressure, diabetes, or stress.
- High LDL cholesterol levels or low HDL cholesterol levels or high triglycerides. (These are all blood fats.)
- Sedentary lifestyle (lack of physical activity).

HOW TO PREVENT—Exercise daily. Maintain a healthy weight. Eat a healthy diet. Don't smoke. Get medical care for diabetes, high blood pressure, and high cholesterol. A daily, low-dose aspirin may be prescribed by your health care provider.

 WHAT TO EXPECT

DIAGNOSTIC MEASURES—Diagnosis and treatment of a heart attack begins when emergency medical personnel arrive after you call 911. In the hospital emergency room, health care providers will work fast to find out if you are having or have had a heart attack and to give you treatment.

APPROPRIATE HEALTH CARE
- If you are having a heart attack, treatment is done to restore the blood flow to the heart, and to monitor your vital signs to detect and treat complications.
- Long-term treatment after a heart attack may include cardiac rehabilitation, checkups and tests, lifestyle changes (such as stopping smoking or weight loss), and drug therapy. To prevent another heart attack or complications, always follow all your prescribed therapies.

POSSIBLE COMPLICATIONS—Cardiac arrest (heart stops beating), shock, heart failure, heart rupture, irregular heart rhythms, pericarditis (heart lining inflammation), aneurysm, blood clots, another heart attack, or depression.

PROBABLE OUTCOME—The damage from a heart attack depends on how much of the heart is affected, how soon treatment begins, and other factors. Recovery will take 4 to 8 weeks. A full active life is possible after a heart attack.

 HOW TO TREAT

GENERAL MEASURES
- If you have symptoms of a heart attack, seek medical help right away. Don't drive yourself.
- If you suspect heart attack symptoms in someone, call 911 for help.
- To learn more: American Heart Association, 7272 Greenville Ave., Dallas, TX 75231; (800) 242-8721; website: www.americanheart.org.

MEDICATION
- Drugs to dissolve and/or prevent blood clots may be used for emergency care.
- After a heart attack, drugs may be prescribed to help the heart function, treat high blood pressure, prevent clots, or to lower cholesterol.

ACTIVITY
- Resume your normal activities gradually during recovery. An exercise program will usually be recommended.
- You will be advised about when to return to work, resume sexual relations, or drive a car.

DIET—Eat a low-fat, high-fiber diet. Lose weight if overweight.

 CALL YOUR DOCTOR

- You or a family member has symptoms of a heart attack. This is an emergency!
- New symptoms occur during recovery.

HEART BLOCK
(Atrioventricular Block)

 GENERAL INFORMATION

DEFINITION—Heart block is a persistent disruption (either mild or major) in transmission of electrical signals between the heart's upper and lower chambers. Contractions of the atria (upper heart chambers) lose synchronization with those of the ventricles (lower heart chambers). The heartbeat is no longer regulated normally to quicken under exertion or stress and slow down at other times.

BODY PARTS INVOLVED—Heart's electrical system that controls heartbeats.

SEX OR AGE MOST AFFECTED—All ages, but most common in men over 40 and women after menopause.

SIGNS & SYMPTOMS
- No symptoms may occur in mild forms.
- Slow, irregular heartbeat.
- Sudden loss of consciousness.
- Convulsions (sometimes).
- Attacks of dizziness, weakness or confusion.

CAUSES
- Coronary artery disease, a result of atherosclerosis (hardening of the arteries).
- Congenital heart abnormalities.
- Excessive digitalis and some other drugs.

RISK INCREASES WITH
- Adults over 60.
- Stress.
- Improper diet that is high in fat and salt.
- Obesity.
- Smoking.
- Diabetes.
- Heart disease, including atherosclerosis, congestive heart failure or heart-valve disease.
- High blood pressure.
- Previous electrolyte imbalance.
- Use of some drugs, such as digitalis, quinidine or beta-adrenergic blockers.

HOW TO PREVENT
- Obtain medical treatment for any underlying disease.
- Don't smoke.
- Exercise regularly.
- Eat a diet that is low in fat and low in salt and high in fiber.

 WHAT TO EXPECT

DIAGNOSTIC MEASURES
- Your own observation of symptoms.
- Your health care provider will do a physical exam.
- Medical tests may include electrocardiogram (ECG). The ECG provides information about the degree of heart block (1st, 2nd or 3rd) and will help decide what treatment, if any, is needed. Heart monitoring may be done while you go about your daily activities by wearing a special recording device (e.g., Holter monitor).

APPROPRIATE HEALTH CARE
- Some heart blocks require no treatment.
- Surgery is usually done to implant an artificial pacemaker. It provides a regular, mild electric stimulus that maintains a normal heartbeat.

POSSIBLE COMPLICATIONS—Uncontrolled slow, rapid or irregular heartbeat and cardiac arrest.

PROBABLE OUTCOME
- Heart blocks that do not bring on symptoms usually require no treatment.
- More serious heart blocks can be controlled with surgery to implant a pacemaker.

 HOW TO TREAT

GENERAL MEASURES
- Wear a medical alert bracelet or pendant showing the name of your condition.
- To learn more: American Heart Association, 7272 Greenville Ave., Dallas, TX 75231; (800) 242-8721; website: www.americanheart.org.

MEDICATION
- Atropine may be prescribed for a short term therapy.
- Don't take drugs to relieve allergy or nasal congestion without medical approval. They can worsen symptoms.

ACTIVITY—Don't think of yourself as an invalid. Mild exercise is helpful for most patients. Begin a regular exercise program (walking is ideal).

DIET
- Lose weight if you are overweight.
- Avoid excess use of alcoholic beverages. Alcohol depresses the heartbeat.

 CALL YOUR DOCTOR IF

- You or a family member has symptoms of heart block, especially an episode with loss of consciousness.
- After diagnosis, symptoms recur.

HEART FAILURE

GENERAL INFORMATION

DEFINITION—Heart failure (congestive heart failure [CHF]) develops when the heart has lost some of its ability to pump blood. Blood flow is backed up causing congestion in the body's tissues. This can lead to fluid build up and swelling (edema).

BODY PARTS INVOLVED—Heart; blood vessels; lungs; kidneys; liver; extremities.

SEX OR AGE MOST AFFECTED—Older adults and affects men more than women.

SIGNS & SYMPTOMS
- Feeling short of breath with activity or after lying down for a while.
- Feeling tired and weak.
- Coughing or wheezing.
- Sleep problems (e.g., sleep apnea).
- Swollen legs, ankles, and stomach.
- Appetite loss. A weight gain is due to retained water.
- Muscle wasting (loss of muscle mass).
- Swollen or protruding neck veins.
- Less urine, and a need to urinate at night.
- Less mentally alert, or unable to concentrate.

CAUSES—Over time, various disorders cause the muscles, valves, and blood vessels of the heart to become damaged and weak. The heart is not able to pump enough blood, oxygen, and nutrients to other organs in the body that they need in order for them to function properly.

RISK INCREASES WITH
- High blood pressure, coronary artery disease, heart attack, or heart valve disease.
- Aging, males, African Americans, family history of heart failure.
- Cardiomyopathy (enlarged heart).
- Congenital (being born with) heart disease.
- Abnormal rhythm or irregular heartbeat.
- Risk factors for heart disease that can lead to heart failure include: smoking, obesity, high levels of fats in the blood, use of certain drugs, diet high in fat or salt, diabetes, alcohol abuse, and lack of physical activity.

HOW TO PREVENT—If you have a condition that can lead to congestive heart failure, get medical care. Follow your treatment plan. Eat a diet high in fiber, and low in fat and salt. Don't abuse alcohol and don't smoke. Exercise regularly.

WHAT TO EXPECT

DIAGNOSTIC MEASURES
- Your own observation of symptoms.
- Your health care provider will do a physical exam and ask questions about your symptoms and activities.

- Medical tests may include blood studies and x-rays. Studies may be done of heart activity, function, and size. They help determine if there has been a heart attack and extent of any heart damage.

APPROPRIATE HEALTH CARE
- The goal of treatment is to improve the heart's pumping function. A treatment plan will be based on your individual needs. It may include drugs, lifestyle changes, treating underlying conditions. implantable devices, medical procedures, or surgery.
- Hospital care may be needed for severe cases.
- Supplemental oxygen may be used to help breathing.
- A heart transplant may be an option for patients not responding to other treatments.

POSSIBLE COMPLICATIONS—Heart attack, cardiac arrest, severe heart rhythm problems, pulmonary edema (fluid in the lungs), side effects of drugs, total heart failure, and death.

PROBABLE OUTCOME—Symptoms may be relieved with treatment. Long-term outcome depends on each individual patient and the severity of heart failure.

HOW TO TREAT

GENERAL MEASURES
- Don't smoke. Find an effective way to quit.
- Wear or carry medical ID listing this condition, drugs you take, and any implanted device.
- To learn more: American Heart Association local branch, or call (800) 242-8721; website: www.americanheart.org.

MEDICATION—Drugs may be prescribed to improve heart function, to slow and regulate the heart rate, remove extra fluid, lower blood pressure, relax blood vessels, suppress the immune system, and to treat any underlying disorder.

ACTIVITY
- Exercise daily. A plan will be prescribed for you.
- Resume driving and sexual relations as advised.

DIET
- Eat a diet that is low in salt and fat. Avoid alcohol.
- Go on a weight loss diet if your weight is a problem.

CALL YOUR DOCTOR IF

- You or a family member has symptoms of congestive heart failure.
- After diagnosis, any new symptoms occur that cause concern, or other symptoms worsen.

HEART MURMURS

GENERAL INFORMATION

DEFINITION—Heart murmurs are not a disease or illness. They involve the sounds, as heard through a stethoscope, of blood flowing through the heart. With murmurs, there is an extra sound (sometimes described as "swishing") in addition to the normal sounds (described as "lub-dup") of the heartbeat. Most heart murmurs are harmless or "innocent" and are detected at a routine physical or well-baby examination. Murmurs are heard in many healthy people.

BODY PARTS INVOLVED—Heart.

SEX OR AGE MOST AFFECTED—All ages, both sexes; more often heard in children and teenagers.

SIGNS & SYMPTOMS—People with heart murmurs have no symptoms, unless associated with other disorders.

CAUSES—The stethoscope picks up sounds made when the ventricles of the heart contract and the 4 heart valves snap shut. Most extra sounds caused by turbulent blood flow are known as murmurs. What causes innocent type heart murmurs is unknown.

RISK INCREASES WITH
• Congenital heart defects.
• Rheumatic fever.
• Myocarditis.
• Children with anemia.
• Pregnancy.

HOW TO PREVENT—There are no preventive measures.

WHAT TO EXPECT

DIAGNOSTIC MEASURES
• Heart murmurs are detected by a health care provider listening to the heart sounds through a stethoscope. By listening to these sounds, a trained person can judge by their quality, intensity, location and timing that the murmur is insignificant (most cases).
• In a few cases, the sounds that are heard may indicate a need for more testing in order to determine the cause. Chest x-ray, ECG and echocardiography may be done.

APPROPRIATE HEALTH CARE—No medical treatment is necessary for an innocent heart murmur.

POSSIBLE COMPLICATIONS
• None expected with innocent heart murmurs.
• If there is any underlying organic heart problem, it can usually be corrected surgically.

PROBABLE OUTCOME—Most innocent heart murmurs detected (particularly in children) disappear or become undetectable over time. People with these murmurs live a completely normal life.

HOW TO TREAT

GENERAL MEASURES—If your child has an innocent type heart murmur, treat him or her like any other healthy child. Parents sometimes become concerned about the idea of a heart murmur and become over-protective. This can cause problems for the child's emotional well-being.

MEDICATION—No drugs are needed.

ACTIVITY—Do not limit activity.

DIET—No special diet.

CALL YOUR DOCTOR IF

You need further assurance about heart murmurs.

HEART RHYTHM IRREGULARITY
(Arrhythmia)

 GENERAL INFORMATION

DEFINITION—A heart rhythm irregularity (arrhythmia) involves a change in the regular beat of the heart. They are common, and many are mild and require no treatment. Almost all adults have some amount of irregular heartbeats.

BODY PARTS INVOLVED—Heart; nerves that transmit impulses to coordinate heart muscle contractions.

SEX OR AGE MOST AFFECTED—Both sexes; all ages, but most likely over age 65.

SIGNS & SYMPTOMS
- A fluttering in the chest; the heart seems to skip a beat, or beat irregularly, or beat very fast or slowly.
- Shortness of breath and/or mild chest pains.
- Faintness, dizziness, or weakness.
- Feeling anxious.
- No symptoms (frequently).

CAUSES—The heart has an electrical system that controls its rate and contractions. The average heart beats at a rate of 60 to 100 times per minute. With arrhythmias, the electrical system does not function as it should. There are different types of arrhythmias depending on what part of the heart is involved. They can be due to a number of causes. In some cases, no cause is found.

RISK INCREASES WITH
- Older adults.
- Heart diseases. This includes rheumatic fever, congenital heart disease, cardiomyopathy, previous heart attack, or heart-muscle inflammation.
- Endocrine disorders, such as thyroid and adrenal gland diseases.
- Fluid and electrolyte imbalance, such as too little or too much potassium.
- Use of certain prescribed and nonprescription drugs.
- Overdose of certain drugs, including antidepressants, caffeine, marijuana, cocaine, and methamphetamine.
- Postoperative effects following chest or heart surgery.
- Chronic kidney disease.
- High blood pressure.
- Smoking or excess alcohol use.
- Stress.
- Sleep deprivation (lack of sleep) or sleep apnea.

HOW TO PREVENT—Avoid risk factors where possible and get treatment for those that are treatable.

 WHAT TO EXPECT

DIAGNOSTIC MEASURES
- Your health care provider will do a physical exam and listen to the heart with a stethoscope.
- Medical tests usually include an electro-cardiogram (ECG) or you may be asked to wear a Holter monitor (a portable ECG) for 1 to 5 days. These aid in diagnosing heart diseases by measuring the electrical activity of the heart. Other tests may be done to see if the cause is a heart disease.

APPROPRIATE HEALTH CARE
- Treatment, if needed, will depend on the cause.
- You may require cardioversion (brief electric shock to the heart) to restore normal rhythm.
- Surgery may be needed to correct some heart problems (coronary-artery bypass, to replace damaged heart valve, or insertion of a pacemaker or atrial defibrillator).
- Counseling may be helpful if stress is a major factor.

POSSIBLE COMPLICATIONS
- Complications may arise from the heart disease that is causing the arrhythmia.
- Some arrhythmias can lead to complications if they are untreated.

PROBABLE OUTCOME—Irregular heartbeats that occur only occasionally are typically harmless and require no treatment. Other arrhythmias can usually be controlled with treatment.

 HOW TO TREAT

GENERAL MEASURES
- Wear or carry medical ID that shows you have this condition.
- To learn more: American Heart Association, 7272 Greenville Ave., Dallas, TX 75231; (800) 242-8721; website: www.americanheart.org.

MEDICATION—Antiarrhythmic drugs may be prescribed. You may need to try several to find the most effective one. Certain arrhythmias may also require anticoagulant drug therapy.

ACTIVITY—Your health care provider will advise you if there are any limits.

DIET—Avoid caffeine and alcohol (if advised).

 CALL YOUR DOCTOR IF

- You or a family member has symptoms of heart-rhythm irregularity.
- New, unexplained symptoms develop.

HEARTBEAT, RAPID
(Tachycardia)

GENERAL INFORMATION

DEFINITION—A rapid heart rate (or heartbeat) is one that is faster than 100 beats a minute. A normal heart rate is between 60 and 100 beats per minute. Tachycardia is the medical term for rapid heart rate. Most people have occasional rapid heart rates due to emotional conditions (e.g., stress), exercise, fever, or anxiety. It is abnormal when it occurs while a person is at rest or there is no logical cause.

BODY PARTS INVOLVED—Heart muscle; electrical system of the heart.

SEX OR AGE MOST AFFECTED—Both sexes; all ages; more often in older adults and men.

SIGNS & SYMPTOMS
- Some people may have no symptoms.
- Heart palpitations.
- Lightheadedness or dizziness.
- Feeling faint or fainting.
- Anxiety.
- Chest pain, being short of breath, or sweating.

CAUSES—It is due to an interruption in the heart's electrical system, which normally keeps the heart rate regular. When the electrical system is interrupted, the heart rate can become too rapid and may not be able to supply all the blood and oxygen needed by the body. There are known risk factors for a rapid heart rate, but sometimes the cause is unknown. There are two main types—supraventricular tachycardia (upper heart) and ventricular tachycardia (lower heart). Sinus tachycardia is a fast heart rate in a normal functioning heart.

RISK INCREASES WITH
- Older adults; males more than females.
- Family history of heart disease.
- Congenital (being born with) heart disorders.
- Heart attack, coronary artery disease, high blood pressure, heart valve disease, heart failure, and others.
- Thyroid disease, certain lung disorders, electrolyte imbalances, adrenal tumor, and alcohol or drug abuse.
- Pain, exercising, being nervous, emotional changes (e.g., stress or anger), use of certain drugs (e.g., some allergy and asthma drugs), having a fever, smoking, or too much caffeine.

HOW TO PREVENT—May not always be preventable. Avoid the risk factors where possible. Get treatment for treatable disorders.

WHAT TO EXPECT

DIAGNOSTIC MEASURES
- Your own observation of symptoms.
- Your health care provider will do a physical exam and ask questions about your symptoms and activities.
- Tests may be done to measure the heart's electrical activity. Other tests may be done to check for medical problems that could cause the rapid heart rate.

APPROPRIATE HEALTH CARE
- In milder cases, no treatment may be required. Other treatment steps depend on the cause or severity.
- A few patients may require immediate treatment, including electrical shock (cardioversion) or IV drugs to stop the rapid heart rate.
- Radiofrequency ablation (uses radio waves to destroy abnormal heart tissue) or heart surgery may be options.
- In some cases, a small electrical device called implantable cardioverter-defibrillator (ICD) may be implanted under the skin. It can detect irregular heartbeats and shock the heart back into normal rhythm, when needed.

POSSIBLE COMPLICATIONS—Some tachycardias can lead to life-threatening heart problems.

PROBABLE OUTCOME—The outcome will depend on the type of tachycardia and the cause. In the majority of cases, the rapid heart rate can be controlled.

HOW TO TREAT

GENERAL MEASURES
- Ways to reduce stress in your life or reduce other risk factors may be recommended.
- You may be taught techniques to slow the heart rate. This may include the Valsalva maneuver: hold your nostrils closed and blow gently through the nose, making eardrums pop.
- To learn more: American Heart Association, 7272 Greenville Ave., Dallas, TX 75231; (800) 242-8721; website: www.americanheart.org.

MEDICATION
- For repeated attacks, one or more drugs to control heart rate may be prescribed.
- Drugs may be prescribed for an underlying condition.

ACTIVITY—Exercise daily (with medical approval).

DIET—Avoid caffeine and alcohol (if advised).

CALL YOUR DOCTOR IF

- You or a family member has a rapid, irregular heartbeat that lasts more than 4 or 5 minutes.
- Shortness of breath or chest pain develops.

HEARTBURN

GENERAL INFORMATION

DEFINITION—Heartburn (also known as acid indigestion) is a symptom, not a disease, and has nothing to do with the heart. The symptoms are sometimes mistaken for a heart attack. When heartburn occurs often or complications develop, the problem is known as GERD (gastroesophageal reflux disease).

BODY PARTS INVOLVED—Gastrointestinal system.

SEX OR AGE MOST AFFECTED—Both sexes; all ages. It is most common in adults over 60.

SIGNS & SYMPTOMS
- Belching or backward flow of stomach contents into the mouth and throat. This produces an acid taste.
- Heavy burning, discomfort, or pain in the chest.
- It may be difficult to swallow.
- Mild stomach pain or bloated feeling.

CAUSES—Heartburn is caused by a backflow of acid from the stomach into the esophagus. The esophagus is the tube that goes from the mouth to the stomach. The muscles that close off the upper stomach become lax (loose). This allows stomach juices to enter the esophagus and irritate its lining.

RISK INCREASES WITH
- Improper diet or overeating.
- Overweight.
- Smoking or excess alcohol use.
- Use of certain prescription drugs.
- Eating spicy or acidic (citrus, tomatoes) foods.
- Drinking carbonated beverages or caffeine-containing drinks.
- Exercise, lying down, bending over, or straining too soon after a meal.
- Pregnancy.
- Hiatal hernia, some autoimmune disorders, diabetes, disorders of the gastrointestinal tract, or respiratory disorders such as asthma.

HOW TO PREVENT
- Avoid smoking.
- Don't overeat or drink too much alcohol.
- Reduce amount of fats, fried foods, spices, coffee, tea, and tomato products in your diet.
- Don't bend over or lie down right after eating.
- Avoid tight clothes around the waist and stomach.
- Raise head of the bed with 4 to 6 inch blocks.
- Lose weight if you are overweight.

WHAT TO EXPECT

DIAGNOSTIC MEASURES
- Your own observation of symptoms.

- If the problem gets worse or self-care is not working, see your health care provider. A physical exam will be done and questions asked about your symptoms.
- Medical tests are usually not needed, but may be done to help diagnose any complications.

APPROPRIATE HEALTH CARE
- Treatment usually consists of self-care and drug therapy if needed.
- Rarely, surgery may be recommended when other treatment steps are not helping the symptoms.

POSSIBLE COMPLICATIONS—GERD (gastro-esophageal reflux disease). Rarely, bleeding or inflammation, or more rare esophageal cancer.

PROBABLE OUTCOME—Symptoms usually clear up on their own. In other cases, symptoms can be relieved with treatment.

HOW TO TREAT

GENERAL MEASURES
- Heartburn usually begins within about an hour after eating and may continue for several hours. Self-care involves preventive steps and heartburn drugs, if needed, to control symptoms.
- Stop smoking. Find a way that works for you.
- To learn more: National Heartburn Alliance, 303 East Wacker Drive, Suite 440, Chicago, IL 60601; (877) 471-2081; website: www.heartburnalliance.org.

MEDICATION
- For mild discomfort, you may use any of the heartburn preventive drugs available without a prescription. Different ones work for different people. If one type does not work for you, a different type may help.
- A stronger type of heartburn drug may be prescribed.
- If a drug you take is causing heartburn, a change in dosage or a new drug may be prescribed.

ACTIVITY—Symptoms may limit some activity, but daily exercise is important for good health.

DIET
- Avoid foods and beverages that cause excess stomach acid, such as spicy dishes, coffee, acidic fruit juice, or alcohol. Avoid chocolate, and eat less high-fat foods.
- Eat small, frequent meals.

CALL YOUR DOCTOR IF

- If you or a family member has heartburn that continues or worsens despite self-care.
- If symptoms are severe, get medical help right away. They could be warnings of a heart attack.

HEARTBURN DURING PREGNANCY

GENERAL INFORMATION

DEFINITION—Heartburn is the term used to describe a burning pain in the chest and upper abdomen. It is common for pregnant women to have the symptoms of heartburn. It usually comes and goes until delivery. Although it can cause you some discomfort, heartburn will not hurt your baby.

BODY PARTS INVOLVED—Gastrointestinal system.

SEX OR AGE MOST AFFECTED—Pregnant women.

SIGNS & SYMPTOMS
- Burning pain in the center of the chest and upper abdomen. It is often causes an unpleasant taste in the mouth.
- Belching (burping).

CAUSES
- Heartburn is not a heart disorder. It is caused by a backflow of acid from the stomach into the esophagus. The esophagus is the tube that goes from the mouth to the stomach. The muscles that close off the upper stomach become lax (loose), allowing stomach juices to enter the esophagus and irritate its lining.
- Changes caused by pregnancy include an increase in the amount of stomach acid. It also takes longer for the stomach to empty.
- During late pregnancy, the enlarged womb presses on the stomach and may increase the symptoms.

RISK INCREASES WITH
- Overeating or eating and then lying down.
- Smoking.
- Excess use of alcohol.

HOW TO PREVENT—Can't always be prevented. Avoid risk factors listed above.

WHAT TO EXPECT

DIAGNOSTIC MEASURES—Heartburn is usually self-diagnosed. Your obstetric provider can usually make the diagnosis from the symptoms you describe. Medical tests are seldom required.

APPROPRIATE HEALTH CARE—Treatment usually consists of self-care.

POSSIBLE COMPLICATIONS—Heartburn may affect your ability to eat a healthy diet. Low food and fluid intake might cause problems for the mother and the baby.

PROBABLE OUTCOME—The heartburn goes away after the baby is born unless the cause is not related to pregnancy. There are normally no complications.

HOW TO TREAT

GENERAL MEASURES
- General treatment suggestions:
  - Avoid bending over or lying down right after eating.
  - Don't wear tight clothing or belts.
  - Place books or blocks under the head of your bed to raise it about 4 to 6 inches.
  - Don't smoke.

MEDICATION
- While medicine is not usually needed for this disorder, in some cases it may be of benefit. Simple antacid mixtures or tablets, such as magnesium trisilicate, may be helpful. These drugs should be used only with your obstetric provider's approval. Other drugs may be prescribed if simple measures don't help the symptoms.
- Don't take any herbal remedies without asking your obstetric provider.
- If you can live with the symptoms, try to avoid use of drugs.

ACTIVITY—Stay active. Avoid exercises that require bending over.

DIET
- Eat small, frequent meals.
- Don't rush through your meals; eat slowly.
- Avoid drinking large quantities of fluids during meals.
- Don't eat before bedtime.
- Avoid highly seasoned food.
- Don't drink alcohol.
- Avoid very hot or very cold beverages.
- Avoid eating while lying down.
- Chewing gum may be helpful for some women.

CALL YOUR DOCTOR IF

- You or a family member has symptoms of heartburn during pregnancy. This should be diagnosed.
- The following occur after diagnosis:
  - Simple measures don't bring relief.
  - You begin vomiting late in pregnancy.
  - You vomit material that has blood in it or looks like coffee grounds.
  - You have black or tarry stools.

HEAT STROKE OR HEAT EXHAUSTION
(Sunstroke)

GENERAL INFORMATION

DEFINITION—Heat exhaustion and the more serious heat stroke are conditions that develop when the body is unable to cope with heat. They are caused by a breakdown in the body's natural cooling system.

BODY PARTS INVOLVED—Total body.

SEX OR AGE MOST AFFECTED—Both sexes; all ages, more common in older adults and young children.

SIGNS & SYMPTOMS
* Heat exhaustion:
  - Dizziness, nausea or vomiting, faintness, fatigue, thirstiness, or headache.
  - Skin that is pale and clammy.
  - Sweating.
  - Pulse may be rapid and weak.
  - Body temperature is normal or mildly raised.
  - Muscle cramps.
  - In some, the symptoms develop over days.
* Heat stroke:
  - Often follows heat exhaustion and its symptoms.
  - Skin that is hot, dry, and flushed.
  - High body temperature; usually no sweating.
  - May be hyperventilating (rapid breathing).
  - Rapid heartbeat.
  - Confusion.
  - Convulsions or loss of consciousness.

CAUSES
* Heat exhaustion is due to the body's loss of fluid and salts (electrolytes). It occurs with extreme heat and excessive sweating without sufficient fluid intake.
* Heat stroke occurs when the body's cooling system (controlled by the brain) stops working. It may be preceded by heat exhaustion. Body temperature is high (over 105°F [40.5°C]). Types of heat stroke are exertional (from strenuous exercise in a hot environment) and nonexertional or classic (which can affect the sick, elderly, or very young persons during a heat wave).

RISK INCREASES WITH
* Elderly or very young.
* Hot, humid weather; heavy clothing.
* Poor health, mental illness, obesity, or chronic illness (e.g., high blood pressure, diabetes, or heart disease).
* Exercise or work in a hot, humid location. This can be indoors or outdoors.
* Loss of body fluids—from sweating and failure to drink enough fluids.
* Certain drugs.
* Excess alcohol use or drug abuse.
* High fever.

HOW TO PREVENT
* Wear light, loose-fitting clothes in hot weather.
* Drink water often; even if not thirsty.
* Drink extra water if you sweat a lot. If urine output decreases, increase your water intake.
* If you become overheated indoors, open a window or use a fan or air conditioner. This helps sweat dry up, which cools the skin.
* Take precautions when going outside in hot weather.

WHAT TO EXPECT

DIAGNOSTIC MEASURES
* Your own observation of symptoms.
* Your health care provider will do a physical exam and ask questions about the symptoms and activities.

APPROPRIATE HEALTH CARE—Medical treatment depends on severity of the symptoms. Special cooling techniques may be required.

POSSIBLE COMPLICATIONS—Untreated heat exhaustion can lead to heat stroke. Heat stroke can cause damage to major organ systems (heart, lungs, kidneys, or brain) or may be fatal.

PROBABLE OUTCOME—Expect full recovery from heat exhaustion. Heat stroke recovery depends on a person's health and symptoms.

HOW TO TREAT

GENERAL MEASURES
* For someone with symptoms of heat stroke, move person to a cool location out of the heat. Call 911 for emergency help. Wrap person in damp sheet or spray with cool water. If able, have person drink cool water.
* For someone who has symptoms of mild heat exhaustion, lie the person down in a cool place and loosen clothing. Apply cool water to skin. Give them cool water (not iced) to sip or a sports drink containing electrolytes. If needed, seek medical advice for proper care.

MEDICATION—Drugs are usually not needed, but may be used for complications that develop.

ACTIVITY—Rest with legs elevated while symptoms are present. Normal activity may be resumed after symptoms improve.

DIET—No special diet.

CALL YOUR DOCTOR IF

You or a family member has symptoms of heat stroke or heat exhaustion, or observe them in someone else. Call immediately! These conditions may be serious or fatal.

HEEL PAIN
(Heel Contusion; Heel Spur; Heel Bursitis) *Joe*

GENERAL INFORMATION

DEFINITION
• Heel pain or heel discomfort can be caused by several conditions.
- Contusion or bruise of the heel bone. This causes inflammation of the tissue (periosteum) that covers the heel bone (calcaneus).
- Heel spur. A hard, bony sliver or needle that develops on the heel. It can cause inflammation or other problems in foot tendons and ligaments.
- Heel bursitis. This is inflammation of the connective tissue that surrounds a joint.

BODY PARTS INVOLVED—Heels.

SEX OR AGE MOST AFFECTED—Adults. The conditions are fairly common among runners and other athletes.

SIGNS & SYMPTOMS—Pain and tenderness in the heel and sole of the foot under the heel bone. Pain often occurs after resting or after rising in the morning. There may be no pain when sitting. One or both feet can be affected.

CAUSES—Heel pain is usually a result of putting too much stress on the heel bone and the soft connective tissues (called the fascia) that attach to it.

RISK INCREASES WITH
• Running, jogging, or fast walking.
• Previous, or recent, foot or leg injury.
• Poorly cushioned shoes; lack of arch support.
• Prolonged standing; sciatica (leg nerve pain).
• Overweight.
• Walking barefoot on hard surfaces.

HOW TO PREVENT
• Avoid activities that put constant strain on the foot. Switch to swimming or cycling.
• Wear a shoe with inserts.
• Wear athletic shoes with good shock support in the heels, good flexibility, and good support to control side-to-side motion.
• No more than 1.5-inch heels on everyday shoes.

WHAT TO EXPECT

DIAGNOSTIC MEASURES
• Your own observation of symptoms.
• Your health care provider will do a physical exam of the foot and ankle area. Questions will be asked about your symptoms and activities.
• Medical tests such as an x-ray are rarely needed.

APPROPRIATE HEALTH CARE
• Most people try self-care first.
• Medical care may include physical therapy, casts, taping, night splints, injections, ultrasound, orthotics, or surgery. Treatment steps will depend on the symptoms.

POSSIBLE COMPLICATIONS—Soreness and arthritic changes in the heel that place extra stress on joints, such as those in the knee, hip, and spine.

PROBABLE OUTCOME—Usually curable with treatment. Different types of treatment work for different people.

HOW TO TREAT

GENERAL MEASURES
• Use ice massage, or soak the heel in ice water. Do this for 15 minutes at a time, 3 or 4 times a day.
• Lightly massage the heel and calf before getting out of bed. Apply heat with a heating pad if it feels good.
• Taping helps some people. Apply athletic tape as directed on the product's instructions.
• Try heel cushions or lifts, arch supports, or medial wedge supports (available at sporting-goods stores and drug stores). Use products in both shoes so that other problems don't develop. Custom orthotics (inserts designed for an individual) may be helpful.
• Purchase shoes that fit well. Sandals help some people. Break in new shoes slowly by wearing them a few minutes per day to start.
• Stretching exercises will help.

MEDICATION
• To relieve minor pain, you may use ibuprofen or aspirin (adults only).
• Stronger anti-inflammatory drugs or injections of a steroid drug into the heel to reduce inflammation may be prescribed.

ACTIVITY—Stay off your feet as much as possible, especially at the beginning of treatment.

DIET—No special diet, unless you are overweight. If so, lose weight to reduce stress on the foot.

CALL YOUR DOCTOR IF

You or a family member has heel pain that isn't helped by self-care.

HEMOPHILIA

GENERAL INFORMATION

DEFINITION—Hemophilia is an inherited bleeding disorder. The two main types of hemophilia occur only in boys. The disorder is passed via a gene from mother to son. Most mothers who pass the gene on are carriers of hemophilia and have no symptoms of it.

BODY PARTS INVOLVED—All body parts.

SEX OR AGE MOST AFFECTED—It affects 1 in 10,000 males and appears early in childhood.

SIGNS & SYMPTOMS
- Symptoms often don't occur until the baby starts to crawl or walk. Sometimes, a circumcision procedure causes excess bleeding and this is the first symptom.
- Painful, swollen joints, or swelling in the leg or arm when bleeding occurs.
- Bruising (bruises may be large, deep, or slow to heal).
- Heavy bleeding from small cuts.
- Nosebleeds.
- Blood in the urine or stool.

CAUSES—Lack of a blood-clotting (coagulation) factor. Clotting is the process by which blood changes from a liquid to a solid substance in order to stop bleeding. There are 13 clotting factors in the body. Hemophilia occurs in three of them. Hemophilia A lacks enough clotting factor VIII. Hemophilia B lacks enough clotting factor IX. Hemophilia C (rare in the United States) lacks enough clotting factor XI.

RISK INCREASES WITH—Family history of the disorder.

HOW TO PREVENT
- Cannot be prevented at present. If your family has a history of this disorder, get genetic counseling before having children. If you are pregnant, talk to your obstetric provider about a test to see if the baby has inherited hemophilia.
- Testing for a female to check her hemophilia carrier status is done with a blood study. Blood studies of other family members are usually done.

WHAT TO EXPECT

DIAGNOSTIC MEASURES
- Your own observation of symptoms.
- Your child's health care provider will do a physical exam and ask questions about the symptoms and activities.
- Blood tests can diagnose blood-clotting problems.

APPROPRIATE HEALTH CARE
- Family education about the disorder is the first step. Parents need to learn how to recognize signs and symptoms of bleeding and how to provide therapy. They need to learn ways to

keep a child safe and appropriate physical activities. Vaccines need to be current.
- Bleeding episodes can usually be controlled with home care by self-administered replacement therapy.
- Hospital care to control bleeding may be needed when the bleeding is heavy or unusual.

POSSIBLE COMPLICATIONS
- Bleeding events needing emergency care.
- Joint damage and problems due to bleeding.
- Adverse reaction to clotting-factor treatment.
- Risk of getting other diseases through donated blood. Risk is less with genetically produced clotting products.

PROBABLE OUTCOME
- The disorder is not curable, but it is not fatal. With treatment, patients can have a near-normal life span.
- The disorder may be mild, moderate, or severe. It depends on amount of the clotting factor produced.

HOW TO TREAT

GENERAL MEASURES
- Parents need to make sure anyone (sitters, relatives, teachers) taking care of a child with hemophilia knows what to do in an emergency.
- Use good dental hygiene to avoid problems that can cause bleeding, such as pulling a tooth.
- Wear or carry medical ID that shows you they have hemophilia.
- To learn more: National Hemophilia Foundation, 116 West 32nd St., 11th Floor, New York, NY 10001; (800) 424-2634; website: www.hemophilia.org.

MEDICATION
- Bleeding can be controlled by injections of clotting factor. It can be taken as a preventive measure. Patients can be trained to give themselves the treatment.
- Desmopressin (DDAVP) may be injected into veins or given as a nasal drug. It can help to stimulate a release of the body's own clotting factor.
- Drugs to reduce joint pain may be prescribed.
- Avoid aspirin and other nonsteroidal anti-inflammatory drugs. They can increase bleeding.

ACTIVITY—Exercise daily. Avoid activities that can cause injury, such as contact sports. Swim, bicycle (wear a helmet), or walk instead.

DIET—No special diet.

CALL YOUR DOCTOR IF

- A child has symptoms of hemophilia.
- Bleeding or other symptoms cause any concern.

HEMORRHOIDS

GENERAL INFORMATION

DEFINITION—Hemorrhoids are swollen veins of the rectum or anus. Hemorrhoids may be located inside of the anal canal, or at the anal opening. They may be present for years, but go unnoticed until bleeding occurs.

BODY PARTS INVOLVED—Veins under the rectal or anal membrane.

SEX OR AGE MOST AFFECTED—Adults of both sexes.

SIGNS & SYMPTOMS
- Rectal bleeding. Bright-red blood may show as streaks on toilet paper or be a part of a bowel movement. Blood may be a slow trickle for a short while following bowel movements. It almost always colors the toilet water.
- Pain, itching, or discharge after bowel movements.
- A lump or swelling that can be felt in the anus.
- A feeling that the rectum has not emptied completely after a bowel movement.

CAUSES—Repeated pressure on the anal or rectal veins, which causes them to stretch.

RISK INCREASES WITH
- Chronic constipation or diarrhea.
- A diet that lacks fiber.
- Prolonged sitting or standing.
- Overweight people.
- Pregnancy.
- Loss of muscle tone in older adults.
- Rectal surgery or episiotomy.
- Liver disease.
- Anal sex.
- Colon cancer.

HOW TO PREVENT
- Don't try to hurry bowel movements, but do try to avoid straining and prolonged sitting on the toilet.
- Lose weight if you are overweight.
- Include plenty of fiber in your diet.
- Drink plenty of fluids each day.
- Exercise regularly.

WHAT TO EXPECT

DIAGNOSTIC MEASURES
- Your own observation of symptoms.
- Your health care provider can diagnose hemorrhoids by a physical exam of the rectal area.
- Medical tests may be done to check for complications.

APPROPRIATE HEALTH
- Treatment is aimed at easi usually involves diet and lifestyl
- Medical procedures or surgery recommended when simple treatmen measures are not helping the symptom health care provider will explain the option

POSSIBLE COMPLICATIONS
- Anemia, if there is a lot of blood loss.
- Severe pain caused by a blood clot in a hemorrhoid.
- Infection or inflammation of a hemorrhoid.

PROBABLE OUTCOME—Hemorrhoids often go away with diet and lifestyle changes, but symptoms may come and go. For more severe symptoms, medical procedures or surgery are available.

HOW TO TREAT

GENERAL MEASURES
- Never strain to push your stool out.
- When sitting on the toilet, place feet on a low footstool to aid bowel movement.
- Clean the anal area gently with soft, moist paper after each bowel movement.
- To relieve pain, sit in 8 to 10 inches of warm water for 10 to 20 minutes several times a day.

MEDICATION
- For minor pain, itching, or to reduce swelling, you may use topical drug products to relieve symptoms of hemorrhoids. If these symptoms occur during pregnancy, ask your obstetric provider which drugs are safe to use.
- Use a stool softener, if a laxative is needed.
- Other drugs may be prescribed for complications.

ACTIVITY—Get 30 minutes of exercise on a daily basis. Bowel function improves with good physical fitness.

DIET
- To prevent constipation, eat a well-balanced diet that contains many high-fiber foods.
- Drink 6 to 8 glasses of fluid daily.
- Go on a weight loss diet if you are overweight.

CALL YOUR DOCTOR IF

- You or a family member has symptoms of hemorrhoids.
- Hemorrhoids continue to cause severe pain.
- A hard lump develops where a hemorrhoid has been.
- Rectal bleeding is heavy.

...RMATION

...n inflammation
...pes. The most
...type C. Others

...er.

SEX OR AGE MOST AFFECTED—Both sexes; all ages.

SIGNS & SYMPTOMS
• There may be no symptoms, or symptoms may take weeks to months to appear. A person may first have flu-like symptoms, such as fever, fatigue, nausea, vomiting, diarrhea, and loss of appetite.
• Jaundice (yellow eyes and skin) caused by a buildup of bile pigment in the blood.
• Dark urine and light, "clay-colored," or whitish stools.
• Pain in the upper-right abdomen.

CAUSES
• Types A and E: the virus usually enters the body through water or food (especially raw shellfish) that has been contaminated by sewage (fecal-oral contact).
• Type B: usually sexually transmitted (contact with body fluids of an infected person), or by blood transfusions contaminated with the virus, or from injections with non-sterile needles or syringes. An infected mother can pass it to her newborn. Cause may be unknown.
• Type C: usually spread through intravenous (IV) drug use, blood transfusions, and other exposures to contaminated blood or its products. Cause may be unknown.
• Type D: occurs with infection of hepatitis type B.

RISK INCREASES WITH
• Alcoholism, blood transfusions (especially if before 1992), kidney disease, blood-clotting disorders, organ transplants, having prior sexually transmitted diseases.
• Daycare centers (children and workers; especially those who change diapers).
• Infants born to mothers with hepatitis B or C.
• Health care workers.
• Jobs or work involving contact with body fluids.
• Close contact with an infected person.
• Getting a tattoo or body piercing.
• People who engage in anal sex, and persons who have multiple sexual partners.
• IV drug abuse or intranasal cocaine use.
• Travel to countries where hepatitis is common.

HOW TO PREVENT
• Avoid the risk factors listed above if possible.
• If exposed to someone with hepatitis, seek medical advice about receiving gamma-globulin injections to prevent or decrease the risk of some types of hepatitis.
• Persons at risk for hepatitis should get hepatitis A and B vaccines (other vaccines are being studied) and immune globulin in addition to vaccine. Your health care provider can advise you if you are in a risk group.
• Routine hepatitis B vaccine for all newborns.

WHAT TO EXPECT

DIAGNOSTIC MEASURES
• Your health care provider will do a physical exam.
• Medical tests may include blood and urine studies and liver function tests. A liver biopsy may be done by using a needle to remove liver tissue for microscopic exam.

APPROPRIATE HEALTH CARE
• Acute (short term) hepatitis usually requires little or no treatment.
• Chronic hepatitis is treated with drugs.
• Hospital care may be needed for severe cases.

POSSIBLE COMPLICATIONS
• Liver disorders that could be life-threatening. This includes liver cancer.
• Chronic hepatitis. Some patients look and feel well and do not know they are infected. They can still pass the infection on to others. Some patients have symptoms that lead to liver damage (this can take 20 years).

PROBABLE OUTCOME—Most people recover fully in 1 to 4 months.

HOW TO TREAT

GENERAL MEASURES
• Most patients can be cared for at home. Keeping apart from others is not needed. If you have hepatitis or are caring for someone with it, wash your hands often.
• To learn more: Centers for Disease Control & Prevention (CDC) hotline: (888) 443-7232; website: www.cdc.gov/hepatitis/.

MEDICATION—Interferon, steroids, or antivirals may be prescribed.

ACTIVITY
• Extra rest may be helpful. People differ widely in returning to normal activity.
• Avoid contact sports until medically approved.
• Food handlers should seek medical advice about return to work.

DIET—Small, nutritious meals may help recovery. Drink plenty of water. Avoid alcohol.

CALL YOUR DOCTOR IF

• You or a family member has symptoms of hepatitis or has been exposed to hepatitis.
• After diagnosis, symptoms cause concern.

HEPATOCELLULAR CARCINOMA
(Liver Cancer, Primary; Hepatoma)

 GENERAL INFORMATION

DEFINITION—Hepatocellular carcinoma is a malignant tumor that begins in the liver. This is a primary liver cancer. Cancers that develop elsewhere in the body (such as the breast) and spread to the liver are secondary liver cancers.

BODY PARTS INVOLVED—Liver.

SEX OR AGE MOST AFFECTED—Adults of both sexes (more common in men after age 40).

SIGNS & SYMPTOMS
- There may be no symptoms.
- Hard lump in the right upper abdomen.
- Weight and appetite loss.
- Jaundice (yellow skin and eyes).
- Abdominal pain that feels like a pulled muscle.
- Low blood sugar (weakness, sweating, hunger, tremor, and headache).
- Fever.
- Fluid in the abdomen; enlarged spleen.
- Unusual bleeding.

CAUSES—This cancer is most often associated with liver disease, but they can develop in persons without known risk factors.

RISK INCREASES WITH
- Cirrhosis of the liver.
- Chronic hepatitis B virus infection.
- Chronic hepatitis C virus infection.
- Alcoholic liver disease; nonalcoholic steatohepatitis.
- Hemochromatosis (excess iron in the body).
- Long-term diet exposure to fungal aflatoxins (mostly found in foods in Asia and Africa).
- Obesity, diabetes.
- There are other known, but more rare risk factors.

HOW TO PREVENT
- No specific preventive measures. Steps can be taken to reduce a person's risk factors.
- Avoid alcohol or drink no more than 1 or 2 alcoholic drinks a day.
- Vaccine to prevent hepatitis B in high-risk persons.
- Screening tests for high-risk persons to diagnose and treat cancer at an early stage.

 WHAT TO EXPECT

DIAGNOSTIC MEASURES
- Your own observation of symptoms.
- Your health care provider will do a physical exam and ask questions about your symptoms.
- Medical tests may include blood studies and liver function tests. Other tests are usually done to confirm the diagnosis and to determine if cancer has spread (called staging).

APPROPRIATE HEALTH CARE
- Treatment will depend on the stage of the cancer, your health, and your preferences. Treatments may involve surgery (such as for small or slow-growing tumors), chemotherapy (anticancer drugs), and radiation (less often used). Alternative treatment methods include embolization, radiofrequency ablation, cryotherapy, injections of alcohol, and others. Your health care provider will discuss the options with you.
- Liver transplantation may be recommended for certain patients.
- Counseling may help in coping with this disorder.

POSSIBLE COMPLICATIONS
- Liver failure.
- Internal bleeding.
- Spread to other organs, especially the lungs, adrenal glands, and bones.

PROBABLE OUTCOME—The outcome depends on the stage (extent) of the cancer and also the patient's health and age. Smaller tumors along with early diagnosis and treatment can provide a better outcome. Outcome is poorer with later diagnosis and larger tumors.

 HOW TO TREAT

GENERAL MEASURES
- Educate yourself about this disorder. You will then be able to make informed decisions about where to go for your care, the treatments available, the risks involved, side effects of therapy, and expected outcome.
- To learn more: American Cancer Society; (800) ACS-2345; website: www.cancer.org or National Cancer Institute; (800) 4-CANCER; website: www.nci.nih.gov.

MEDICATION
- For minor discomfort, use nonprescription drugs such as acetaminophen. Stronger pain relievers will be prescribed as needed.
- Anticancer drugs may be prescribed.

ACTIVITY—Stay as active as your strength allows.

DIET—No special diet. Don't drink alcohol.

 CALL YOUR DOCTOR IF

- You or a family member has symptoms of hepatocellular carcinoma.
- Signs of bleeding develop, especially from the gastrointestinal tract. Signs include bloody vomit or vomit that contains black material resembling coffee grounds, blood in the stool, or black, tarry stools.

HERNIA

GENERAL INFORMATION

DEFINITION
- A hernia occurs when a part of a body organ or tissue protrudes (pokes out) through the muscle wall that normally holds it in place. The most common types involve the lower torso (abdominal wall area). They include:
  - Inguinal hernia and femoral hernia (both involve muscles in the groin).
  - Incisional hernia (involves muscles at the site of a prior surgery).
  - Umbilical hernia (in newborns, involves muscles around the navel).
  - Epigastric hernia (occurs in the upper abdomen, between the breastbone and the navel).
  - Periumbilical hernia (develops around the navel, more common in women).

BODY PARTS INVOLVED—Muscles.

SEX OR AGE MOST AFFECTED—Both sexes; all ages.

SIGNS & SYMPTOMS
- A swelling, lump, or bulge in the abdomen. It may be more apparent when standing or coughing. It may reduce in size when pushed back into the abdomen or when lying down.
- Heavy feeling, discomfort, or pain may occur in the abdomen, especially when bending over or lifting.
- May have constipation, nausea, or urinating difficulty.

CAUSES—Weakness in muscle wall or connective tissue (called fascia). The weakness may be present at birth or acquired later in life. Incisional hernias result from a prior surgery.

RISK INCREASES WITH
- Premature infants.
- Adults over 60.
- Chronic cough or chronic lung disease.
- Obesity or overweight.
- Pregnancy.
- Straining, as with chronic constipation.
- Family history of hernias.
- Heavy lifting.

HOW TO PREVENT
- Most hernias cannot be prevented.
- Maintaining proper weight and regular exercise to keep muscles toned may help prevent some types of hernias.
- Seek medical help if constipation or a chronic cough are problems.

WHAT TO EXPECT

DIAGNOSTIC MEASURES
- Your own observation of symptoms.
- Your health care provider will usually diagnose the hernia with a physical exam.
- An x-ray or ultrasound may be done if any complications are suspected.

APPROPRIATE HEALTH CARE
- Surgery is usually advised to repair the hernia (called a herniorrhaphy). Many hernia repairs can now be done by laparoscopy. In most cases, the surgery is elective (performed by choice), but there may be an emergency if the hernia is strangulated.
- Watchful waiting may be an option.
- If the hernia is causing only mild discomfort and can readily be pushed back, a supportive garment or truss may be used for treatment. This may be done if surgery is not possible or surgery needs to be delayed.

POSSIBLE COMPLICATIONS
- Strangulated hernia (loses its blood supply). It may cause serious complications.
- Hernia may recur after surgery.
- Surgery complications may develop.

PROBABLE OUTCOME—Most hernias are successfully treated with surgery. In some cases, hernias may be treated with methods other than surgery. Umbilical hernias usually heal on their own by age 4 and rarely require surgery.

HOW TO TREAT

GENERAL MEASURES
- For an explanation of surgery and post-operative care, see Hernia (in Surgery section).
- If surgery is not done, see your health care provider for periodic exams of the hernia.

MEDICATION—For minor discomfort, you may use nonprescription drugs such as ibuprofen or acetaminophen.

ACTIVITY
- Speed of recovery will depend on general heath and the type of hernia repaired. Work and regular activities can often be resumed in a week (or as advised). Complete recovery can take 4 to 6 weeks. Avoid heavy lifting for about 3 months.
- Your health care provider will advise you about returning to sports or exercise activities.

DIET
- Eat a diet high in fiber to avoid constipation.
- Maintain ideal weight.

CALL YOUR DOCTOR IF

- You or a family member has symptoms of a hernia.
- If you have vomiting, fever, severe pain, or are unable to have a bowel movement. Call immediately! This can be an emergency.

HERPANGINA

GENERAL INFORMATION

DEFINITION—Herpangina is a viral infection of the mouth and throat. It may be mistaken for canker sores, strep throat, or herpes.

BODY PARTS INVOLVED—Soft palate (back of the mouth and tonsil area).

SEX OR AGE MOST AFFECTED—It most often affects young children of both sexes ages 3 to 10 years.

SIGNS & SYMPTOMS
- Fever.
- Sudden sore throat, with redness, swelling, and painful swallowing.
- Tiny blisters in the affected areas. The blisters become small ulcers (open sores).
- General ill feeling.
- Vomiting and stomach pain (sometimes).
- Decreased appetite.
- If blisters appear on the palms or soles, it is a different disorder called hand, foot, and mouth disease.

CAUSES—Infection from a virus (usually coxsackie) that is spread from person to person. Symptoms appear from 2 to 14 days (average time is 3 to 5 days) after being exposed.

RISK INCREASES WITH
- Summer and early fall seasons.
- Children in daycare or school where the infection is occurring.

HOW TO PREVENT
- Cannot be prevented at present.
- Wash hands carefully to prevent its spread.
- Avoid close personal contact with infected persons, such as kissing or sharing food.

WHAT TO EXPECT

DIAGNOSTIC MEASURES
- Your own observation of symptoms.
- Your health care provider usually diagnoses the disorder by an exam of the blisters in the mouth and throat.

APPROPRIATE HEALTH CARE—Home care. Usually no treatment is necessary other than simple pain relievers.

POSSIBLE COMPLICATIONS—There are usually no complications.

PROBABLE OUTCOME—Rapid recovery in a few days to a week.

HOW TO TREAT

GENERAL MEASURES—Careful handwashing and sanitary disposal of excretions is important.

MEDICATION
- You may use nonprescription drugs, such as acetaminophen or ibuprofen, to relieve pain and fever. Don't give aspirin to children under age 18.
- Antibiotics do not help a viral infection such as this.

ACTIVITY
- Extra rest until the fever and sore throat disappear.
- A child may be kept at home from daycare or school for a few days if symptoms are present.

DIET—No special diet. Drink extra fluids, such as water, fruit ices, ice chips, or cool-gelatin solutions. Avoid acidic fruit juices, which irritate inflamed tissues.

CALL YOUR DOCTOR IF

You or a family member has symptoms of herpangina.

HERPES, GENITAL

GENERAL INFORMATION

DEFINITION—Genital herpes is an infection caused by one of two types of herpes simplex virus (HSV). Herpes type 2 virus (HSV-2) is the usual cause of genital herpes. Herpes type 1 virus (HSV-1) causes common cold sores around the mouth, but can also cause genital herpes.

BODY PARTS INVOLVED—Penis; vagina; cervix; thighs; buttocks (sometimes).

SEX OR AGE MOST AFFECTED—Both sexes and all ages of sexually active persons.

SIGNS & SYMPTOMS
• Person may not realize they are infected. No symptoms may occur or may not be noticed.
• Early symptoms may include itching or burning in the genital or anal area. This may be followed by pain. Women may have vaginal discharge.
• Within a few days, sores appear in the vaginal area, on the penis, around the anal opening, on the buttocks, thighs, or the mouth. Sores start as red bumps, then turn into a cluster of blisters that open and cause pain. They then crust over and heal. There is no scarring.
• First episode may include a general ill feeling, difficult and painful urination, swollen lymph glands, and fever.
• Symptoms can recur since the virus permanently remains in the body. Future outbreaks may be milder. They may occur several times a year in some, but others may have only one or two outbreaks in a lifetime.

CAUSES—Having sex (intercourse or oral sex) with someone who is having a herpes outbreak. An outbreak means that HSV is active and usually causes visible sores in the genital area. The sores shed the virus that can infect another person. In some cases, a person may have an outbreak with no visible sores. They can still shed the virus and infect the other person.

RISK INCREASES WITH—Anyone who is sexually active.

HOW TO PREVENT—Avoid sexual intercourse, oral or anal sex, or skin-to-skin contact if either partner has blisters or sores. Use a latex (rubber) condom during intercourse if either sex partner has inactive genital herpes.

WHAT TO EXPECT

DIAGNOSTIC MEASURES
• Your own observation of symptoms.
• Your health care provider can usually diagnose the disorder by an exam of the affected area.
• Medical tests may include blood studies or studies of fluid taken from the sores.

APPROPRIATE HEALTH CARE
• Treatment goals are to relieve the symptoms and prevent recurrences. Treatment steps may include drugs and self-care.
• Consider counseling for problems of emotional stress.
• If you are pregnant and have herpes, be sure to advise your obstetric provider so any safeguards can be taken.
• Women should have routine pelvic exam and Pap smear as medically advised.

POSSIBLE COMPLICATIONS—Complications are rare in otherwise healthy persons. A person with a weak immune system may have more severe and prolonged outbreaks.

PROBABLE OUTCOME—Genital herpes cannot be cured. During symptom-free periods, the virus returns to its dormant (inactive) state. Symptoms recur when the virus is reactivated. The symptoms vary from person to person and from time to time in the same person. Symptoms and recurrence can be relieved with treatment.

HOW TO TREAT

GENERAL MEASURES
• For self-care, keep the affected area clean and dry. Avoid touching the sores, but if you do, wash your hands right away. Warm or cool baths may ease some of the discomfort.
• Certain "triggers" can lead to outbreaks. They include skin friction, sex, stress, wind, fever, sunlight/sunburn, surgery, menstruation, infection, and some drugs. A person will begin to know the triggers and take care to avoid them when possible.
• To learn more: American Social Health Association, P.O. Box 13827, Research Triangle Park, NC 27709; (919) 361-8488 (not toll-free); website: www.ashastd.org.

MEDICATION—Antiviral drugs in oral form are often prescribed for treatment and prevention of outbreaks. A topical form is available, but it is not as effective.

ACTIVITY
• No limits on daily activities.
• Avoid sexual relations until symptoms disappear.

DIET—No special diet.

CALL YOUR DOCTOR IF

• You or a family member has symptoms of genital herpes.
• Symptoms don't improve in 1 week, despite treatment.

HERPES SIMPLEX VIRUS TYPE 1
(Cold Sore; Fever Blister)

 GENERAL INFORMATION

DEFINITION—Herpes simplex virus type 1 (HSV-1) is a common viral infection that affects the skin. The main symptom is a cold sore.

BODY PARTS INVOLVED—Lips, and less often, nostrils, cheeks, inside mouth.

SEX OR AGE MOST AFFECTED—Both sexes, all ages.

SIGNS & SYMPTOMS
• The first time a person (usually a child) is infected, symptoms may include mouth sores, sore throat, fever, aching, tiredness, problems with eating, and swollen glands.
• Cold sores usually involve the lips. In some cases, they occur on nostrils, cheeks, or inside the mouth. Prior to a cold sore, the skin area may feel itchy, tingly, or sensitive.
• A cluster of small, painful, fluid-filled blisters appear in the affected area. The blisters break and ooze. A yellow crust forms and sloughs off, leaving pink skin and no scarring.

CAUSES
• Herpes simplex virus type 1 infection. It begins on the skin and then the virus moves into certain nerve cells and stays in the body. It can be inactive for months or years, until an active infection occurs and symptoms appear. People often become infected with the virus in childhood (e.g., being kissed by an adult with the virus). The blisters and open sores can spread the virus, but the virus can also spread even if sores are not present.
• Another type, herpes simplex virus type 2., is the cause of genital herpes. However, either type can cause sores on mouth or genitals.

RISK INCREASES WITH
• Everyone is at risk for a first HSV-1 infection. It can come from contact with fluid from a cold sore, saliva, contact with an item that has the germs on it, or sharing food or drinks with an infected person.
• Risk factors that may trigger a later outbreak:
  - Physical or emotional stress.
  - Illness, including a cold, flu, or fever.
  - Menstrual periods.
  - Dental treatment that stretches the mouth.
  - Weak immune system due to illness or drugs.
  - Exposure to the sun.
  - Certain foods or drugs.
  - Eczema (a skin infection).
  - In daycare settings, sharing toys that children put in their mouths.

HOW TO PREVENT—No specific way to prevent a first HSV-1 infection. Do avoid close contact or sharing food or items with person with cold sores. If infected, wash hands often.

 WHAT TO EXPECT

DIAGNOSTIC MEASURES
• Your own observation of symptoms.
• See your health care provider if you have concerns about the symptoms. An exam of the infected area can confirm the diagnosis. Rarely, a medical test is done on fluid from the sore.

APPROPRIATE HEALTH CARE—Medical care may include prescription drugs.

POSSIBLE COMPLICATIONS—Rarely, infection spreads to other places in the body (e.g., eyes and brain). Prompt treatment is vital.

PROBABLE OUTCOME—Recovery takes a few days to a week. Recurrence will vary for different people. Cold sores may recur often or rarely. Complications are unlikely.

 HOW TO TREAT

GENERAL MEASURES
• Most people use self-care to treat cold sores:
  - Apply ice to the affected area, or use nonprescription products for cold sores, to ease discomfort.
  - Don't squeeze or pick at the blisters. Avoid touching them except to apply cream or ointment. Then wash hands carefully. Be careful about touching other places in the body, especially the eyes and genital area, where the infection could spread.
  - Don't share lip products, or cups and other utensils.

MEDICATION
• Use aspirin, acetaminophen, or ibuprofen to relieve minor pain. Don't give aspirin to children under 18.
• Nonprescription creams or ointments for cold sores may be used.
• Antiviral drugs may be prescribed. They can be taken by mouth or applied to the skin.

ACTIVITY—No limits on physical activity. Avoid close contact with others, especially newborns and persons who have weak immune systems.

DIET—No special diet.

 CALL YOUR DOCTOR IF

• The following occur with a cold sore:
  - The cold sore does not heal in a week.
  - Signs of infection, such as fever or pus, instead of clear fluid in the blister. Sores occur on the genitals, or the eyes become infected.
  - You have a weak immune system due to illness or drugs.

HERPES ZOSTER
(Shingles)

GENERAL INFORMATION

DEFINITION—Herpes zoster is a condition that causes pain, rash, and blisters on the skin. You get it only if you have had chickenpox in the past.

BODY PARTS INVOLVED—Sensory nerves of the skin on one side of the body.

SEX OR AGE MOST AFFECTED—Both sexes and all ages (most common in adults over 50).

SIGNS & SYMPTOMS
- Starts with pain, tingling, or burning on the skin.
- A rash appears a few days after the first symptoms begin. It appears as a band of reddened skin on one side of the chest, neck, or face. The rash turns into fluid-filled blisters. These may itch or be very painful. The blisters then begin to dry out and crust over within several days.
- Mild chills and fever.
- General ill feeling.
- Mild nausea, stomach ache cramps, or diarrhea.
- Chest pain, face pain, or burning pain in the skin of the stomach (depends on affected area).

CAUSES—Herpes zoster is caused by the varicella-zoster virus, the same virus that causes chickenpox. After a chickenpox infection, the virus remains inactive in nerve cells in the body. In some people, the virus becomes active again and causes zoster. Why this happens is unknown.

RISK INCREASES WITH
- Anyone who has had chickenpox.
- Adults over 50.
- Cancer.
- High stress situations.
- People who have a weak immune system due to drugs or illness.

HOW TO PREVENT—A vaccine is available to help prevent shingles. Ask your health care provider about its use.

WHAT TO EXPECT

DIAGNOSTIC MEASURES
- Your own observation of symptoms.
- Your health care provider can usually diagnose the disorder by a skin exam of the affected area and asking questions about your pain symptoms. If the rash has not appeared, it is more difficult to diagnose.
- Medical tests are usually not needed.

APPROPRIATE HEALTH CARE
- Goals of treatment are to relieve the itching and the pain as much as possible. This is usually done with topical and oral drugs.
- The nerve pain that remains after the skin clears up is the most difficult to treat.

POSSIBLE COMPLICATIONS
- Skin infection in the herpes zoster blisters.
- Post-herpetic neuralgia which involves chronic pain. It can last for months or years in the nerves where the blisters have been.
- Zoster spreads over the body or to internal organs.
- If the face is affected, eye problems can occur.
- When blisters are present, herpes zoster patients can spread the virus and cause chickenpox in people who have never had it. Avoid physical contact with pregnant women, infants, and those with weak immune systems.

PROBABLE OUTCOME—The rash usually clears in 14 to 21 days. The nerve pain may last for a month or longer. One attack usually provides immunity against herpes zoster, but a few persons have had more than one attack.

HOW TO TREAT

GENERAL MEASURES
- For self-care:
  - When bathing, wash blisters gently.
  - Don't bandage the blistered area.
  - Try applying cool, moist compresses to help decrease the pain.
  - Soak in a tub of water to which cornstarch or an oatmeal product (e.g., Aveeno) has been added.

MEDICATION
- Use calamine lotion or capsaicin ointment for the blisters. For minor pain and discomfort, you may use drugs such as ibuprofen or naproxen.
- Oral antihistamines may help itching.
- You may be prescribed one or more drugs to help treat the symptoms. Antiviral drugs can help if the disorder is diagnosed early. Injections of a nerve block may be recommended in severe and long-lasting cases.
- Other drugs for pain may be prescribed. Different types may need to be tried, as they are not always effective for every person.

ACTIVITY—No limit, except those caused by the symptoms.

DIET—Maintain a healthy diet.

CALL YOUR DOCTOR IF

- You or a family member has symptoms of herpes zoster.
- Pain gets worse, despite treatment.
- New symptoms develop. Drugs may have side effects.

HIATAL HERNIA

GENERAL INFORMATION

DEFINITION—A hiatal hernia develops when a part of the stomach protrudes (pokes) through the diaphragm upward into the chest. The diaphragm is a thin muscle between the chest and the stomach. The esophagus (the tube from the mouth) connects to the stomach through an opening in the diaphragm called the hiatus. A hiatus may become weak and allow part of the stomach to push up through the weak area and into the chest. This becomes a hiatal hernia. It is a common problem.

BODY PARTS INVOLVED—Esophagus; stomach; diaphragm.

SEX OR AGE MOST AFFECTED—Both sexes; all ages, but more often affects older adults and males.

SIGNS & SYMPTOMS—Hiatal hernias do not usually cause symptoms. A person with a hiatal hernia may be more likely to have reflux or it may make existing reflux worse. Reflux occurs when stomach acid backs up into the esophagus. This can lead to heartburn symptoms such as burning in the chest after a meal.

CAUSES—A person may be born with a hiatal hernia or develop one as they get older. Why they occur is unclear. Genetic factors may be involved.

RISK INCREASES WITH
- Aging.
- Males more than females.
- Prior surgery of esophagus or stomach area.
- Pressure in the abdomen, such as with heavy lifting, obesity, or pregnancy.

HOW TO PREVENT—No specific preventive measures.

WHAT TO EXPECT

DIAGNOSTIC MEASURES
- Your health care provider will usually do a physical exam and ask about your symptoms and eating habits.
- Medical tests may include x-rays of the esophagus and stomach. An endoscopy (the passing of a tube with a camera on the end into the esophagus) may be done.

APPROPRIATE HEALTH CARE
- No treatment may be needed if there are no symptoms.
- Lifestyle changes and drug therapy may be prescribed for reflux or heartburn treatment.
- Surgery to repair the hernia may be an option for certain patients with severe GERD or other health problems, such as chronic lung disease.

POSSIBLE COMPLICATIONS
- Esophageal complications.
- Gastroesophageal reflux disease (GERD).
- Bleeding, anemia, or reduced blood to stomach.

PROBABLE OUTCOME—Reflux and heartburn symptoms can usually be relieved with treatment. Surgery may help in certain patients.

HOW TO TREAT

GENERAL MEASURES
- For reflux or heartburn symptoms:
  - Raise the head of your bed 4 to 6 inches. This allows gravity to keep stomach acid away from the hernia.
  - Don't smoke. Find a way to stop that works.
  - Don't wear tight pantyhose, undergarments, belts, or pants.
  - Don't strain with bowel movements or urination.

MEDICATION
- Antacids in tablet or liquid form. These are most effective for some persons when they take them 1 hour before meals and at bedtime. Others find them more helpful 1 to 2 hours after meals and at bedtime. Try both ways to find the best schedule for you.
- Use stool softeners to prevent constipation.
- Nonprescription or prescription drugs called H2-receptor blockers or proton pump inhibitors are often prescribed for symptoms.
- Drugs that help the stomach empty more quickly may be prescribed.

ACTIVITY—No limits. Don't bend over or lie down immediately after a meal.

DIET
- Avoid large meals. Eat 6 small meals a day instead. Eat slowly. Don't eat anything 1 to 2 hours before bedtime.
- A diet with more fiber may help prevent constipation.
- Lose weight, if you are overweight.
- Avoid alcohol, caffeine-containing drinks (coffee, tea, cocoa, cola drinks), and any other food, juice, or spice that may cause symptoms.

CALL YOUR DOCTOR IF

- You or a family member has symptoms of heartburn which could indicate a hiatal hernia.
- Call immediately if pain occurs along with shortness of breath, sweating, or nausea.
- Symptoms don't improve in 1 month with treatment.

HICCUP
(Hiccough; Singultus)

GENERAL INFORMATION

DEFINITION—Hiccups are a symptom, not a disease. Hiccups involve the diaphragm (the large, thin muscle that separates the chest from the abdomen) and the phrenic nerve (the nerve that connects the diaphragm to the brain).

BODY PARTS INVOLVED
- Diaphragm (big muscle which separates the chest from the abdomen).
- Phrenic nerve (nerve that connects the diaphragm to the brain).

SEX OR AGE MOST AFFECTED—Both sexes; all ages. Almost everybody gets hiccups, even unborn babies.

SIGNS & SYMPTOMS—A sharp, quick sound produced from the mouth by a spasm of the diaphragm. The spasm closes muscles in the back of the throat.

CAUSES—Irritation of nerves that control breathing muscles, especially the diaphragm. The cause of short hiccup episodes is usually unknown. Prolonged or recurrent hiccup episodes may be caused by many different medical problems.

RISK INCREASES WITH
- Swallowing hot or irritating substances.
- Diseases of the pleura (thin membrane layers that cover the lung).
- Pneumonia.
- Uremia (a blood infection).
- Alcoholism.
- Disorders of the stomach, esophagus, bowel, or pancreas.
- Pregnancy.
- Bladder irritation.
- Hepatitis of the liver.
- Spread of cancer from another part of the body to the liver or part of the pleura.
- Recent surgery, especially abdominal surgery.
- Emotional causes.
- Use of drugs, such as those that irritate the stomach.
- Full stomach.
- Laughter or intense emotions.
- Changes in temperature.
- Alcohol use.
- Noxious fumes (bad smells in the air).

HOW TO PREVENT—Cannot be prevented at present.

WHAT TO EXPECT

DIAGNOSTIC MEASURES
- Your own observation of symptoms.

- See your health care provider if hiccups continue or recur often. A physical exam will be done and questions asked about your symptoms and activities.
- Medical tests are usually not needed, but may be done to check for a medical problem.

APPROPRIATE HEALTH CARE
- Self-care almost always.
- In rare cases, drugs or nerve surgery may be needed for severe, persistent hiccups.

POSSIBLE COMPLICATIONS—None, unless hiccups are prolonged, which may indicate a medical problem.

PROBABLE OUTCOME—Short hiccup episodes usually don't indicate disease. They will go away on their own or with treatment. Continued hiccups can be a problem and require medical care to find and treat the cause.

HOW TO TREAT

GENERAL MEASURES
- These instructions are for short hiccup episodes. Prolonged hiccups require medical care. Try one or more methods to see which works best for you.
  - Hold your breath and count to 10.
  - Breathe into a paper bag, and rebreathe air in the bag. Don't use a plastic bag because it may cling to nostrils.
  - Insert your thumb between your teeth and upper lip; press the upper lip with your index finger just below the right nostril.
  - Press a forefinger into each ear for about 20 seconds.
  - Drink a glass of water rapidly.
  - Swallow dry bread or crushed ice.
  - Pull gently on the tongue.
  - Close eyelids and apply gentle pressure to the eyeballs.
  - Swallow a teaspoon of dry sugar.

MEDICATION—Usually no drugs are needed for this disorder. In some severe or prolonged cases, drugs may be prescribed to help control the hiccups.

ACTIVITY—No limits.

DIET—Avoid overeating or drinking carbonated drinks.

CALL YOUR DOCTOR IF

- Hiccups persist longer than 8 hours.
- You suspect a prescription drug may be the cause of hiccups.

HIDRADENITIS SUPPURATIVA

GENERAL INFORMATION

DEFINITION—Hydradenitis suppurative is a chronic, recurrent, inflammatory skin disease. Hydradenitis means inflammation of the sweat glands. Suppurative means pus-forming. The skin symptoms vary widely in different persons.

BODY PARTS INVOLVED—The armpits are usually affected, but it can occur on the buttocks, groin, or under the breasts in females.

SEX OR AGE MOST AFFECTED—It develops after puberty, usually in people ages 20 to 40, and affects females more than males.

SIGNS & SYMPTOMS
- It can begin with a cluster of 2 or 3 blackheads.
- Red, tender bumps (called lesions) develop.
- The lesions fill with pus which leads to abscesses (or boils). Draining pus causes a foul odor.
- Abscesses can grow to be as large as an orange or can be as small as a green pea. They are usually hot, tender, and painful to the touch.
- The abscesses heal incompletely and cause cord-like scars on the skin.
- The infection can progress under the skin in tracts linking the abscesses. These can be very painful and restrict movement of affected area.

CAUSES—The exact cause is unclear. It looks similar to acne and may be caused by the formation of keratin plugs in the hair follicles. It occurs in areas that contain apocrine (sweat) glands, so it may be caused by a blockage of the apocrine gland. In either case, the plugged gland or follicle becomes larger, ruptures, and becomes infected. It is not contagious.

RISK INCREASES WITH
- Family history of the disease.
- Females more than males (hormones may play a role).
- Obesity, acne vulgaris, cigarette smoking, disorders such as inflammatory bowel disease may play a role.
- Flare-ups may be caused by stress, sweat, clothing friction, and heat and humidity. It is a hygiene issue.

HOW TO PREVENT—No specific preventive measures.

WHAT TO EXPECT

DIAGNOSTIC MEASURES
- Your own observation of symptoms.
- Your health care provider can usually diagnose the disorder by an exam of the affected area.
- Medical tests may be done to check for infection or other problems.

APPROPRIATE HEALTH CARE
- Treatment depends on the severity (called stages) of the disease. It usually involves self-care measures, drug therapy, surgery, or other procedures. No specific therapy works for all patients.
- Surgery to drain or remove affected area may be recommended. Other medical procedures may be options.

POSSIBLE COMPLICATIONS
- Distress and embarrassment about the symptoms.
- Lesions may not respond to treatment.
- Scarring (may limit mobility in affected area).
- Skin cancer or medical problems due to infection, inflammation, or lack of treatment.

PROBABLE OUTCOME—There is no cure, but treatment can relieve symptoms and prevent progression. Different treatments may need to be tried. Recurrence is common.

HOW TO TREAT

GENERAL MEASURES
- For self-care:
  - Avoid tight or skin-irritating clothing.
  - Wash with antibacterial soap. Don't shave the area.
  - Avoid stress if you can. It may worsen symptoms.
  - Stop smoking. Find a way to quit.
  - Use cool-water soaks for itching or warm-water soaks for pain and inflammation.
- To learn more: Hydradenitis Suppurative Foundation, 7895 Via Belfiore #4, San Diego, CA 92129; website: www.hs-foundation.org.

MEDICATION
- You may be prescribed:
  - Oral or topical antibiotics to fight infection.
  - Hormones or retinoids to help with healing.
  - Anti-inflammatory drugs for pain and

WHAT TO EXP

DIAGNOSTIC MEASURES
- Your own observation of symptoms.
- Your health care provider will do a phys
exam.
- Medical tests include x-rays of the hip.

HOW TO
- Mo contact
- Protect aga
- Drug therapies
- Daily exercise p
strength and improve
- Sufficient intake of ca

HIP FRACTURE
(Femoral Neck Fracture)

GENERAL INFORMATION

DEFINITION—A hip fracture is a complete break or partial break in the femur. The femur is the major bone in the hip joint.

BODY PARTS INVOLVED—Femur, including muscles and tendons that attach the head of the femur to the acetabulum (hip socket).

SEX OR AGE MOST AFFECTED
- Breaks from common injuries affect both sexes and all ages.
- Spontaneous (occurs without an injury) breaks, and breaks from minor injuries, affect mostly older people.
- Nine out of 10 hip fractures occur in persons over 65, and 3 out of 4 occur in women.

SIGNS & SYMPTOMS
- Severe pain when trying to walk.
- Pain may occur in the groin or thigh.
- Swelling, tenderness, and bruising in hip area.
- Deformed hip appearance.

CAUSES—Hip fractures are usually caused by injuries (trauma) such as falls, other types of accidents, and sports injuries. Weakened bones are more at risk of a fracture.

RISK INCREASES WITH
- Female, over age 65, and white.
- Osteoporosis, especially in women after menopause.
- Decreased bone mineral density; fragile bones.
- Falls. Risk of falls increases with muscle weakness, problems with walking or balance, use of certain drugs, disorders such as stroke and Parkinson's, poor eyesight, foot problems, arthritis, previous falls, and home risks.
- Self-reported poor health.
- Family history of hip fracture.
- Sedentary (lack of physical activity) lifestyle.
- Previous fractures of any kind.
- Previous hyperthyroidism.
- Motor vehicle accidents, physical activities, and sports for younger hip fracture patients.

PREVENT
- against falls, especially in the home.
- to improve bone density.
- program for bone and muscle balance.
- calcium and vitamin D.

EFFECT

ical

APPROPRIATE HEALTH CARE
- Hospital care with surgery is the main treatment. Nonsurgical therapy, such as traction, may be used if surgery is too risky for a patient.
- A femoral neck fracture is treated either by hip pinning (using screws) or hip hemiarthroplasty (hip replacement). The choice depends on patient's age and severity of fracture.
- An intertrochanteric hip fracture is repaired with a metal plate and screws or a rod inserted down the center of the bone.
- After surgery, time is spent in a rehab center to regain mobility and functions of daily living.
- Ongoing physical therapy may be needed to help rehabilitate the muscles, bones, and joints.

POSSIBLE COMPLICATIONS
- Surgical-wound infection, incomplete healing, and other surgery complications.
- Long-term bed rest can lead to blood clots, pulmonary embolism, pneumonia, and weak muscles.
- Loss of mobility (may require wheelchair use), loss of independence, reduced quality of life, and depression.

PROBABLE OUTCOME—Outcome depends on the age and health of the patient and the location of the fracture. In older persons, there is often a loss of ability to function as they did before the fracture. The function loss may be mild to severe.

HOW TO TREAT

GENERAL MEASURES—See Hip Nailing for Hip Fracture in Surgery section.

MEDICATION
- Pain relievers as needed may be prescribed.
- Antibiotics for infection or drugs to prevent blood clots may be prescribed after surgery.
- Stool softeners help prevent constipation.
- Drugs to increase bone mass and to prevent bone loss may be prescribed.

ACTIVITY
- After surgery, move the unaffected leg often to decrease risk of blood clots. Most patients are urged to get up and move about as soon as able.
- Physical therapy can take several months. A walker or crutches will be used at first.
- Resume your normal activities to the extent possible as healing progresses.

DIET—Usually no special diet.

CALL YOUR DOCTOR IF

- You or a family member has symptoms of a hip fracture. Call right away.
- Any new symptoms develop after surgery.

HIRSUTISM

GENERAL INFORMATION

DEFINITION—Hirsutism is increased growth of hair on the face and body in women. It usually occurs gradually over an extended period of time. It may begin with puberty. Hirsutism is a benign condition and is mostly a cosmetic problem. When it occurs along with signs of masculinity (maleness), a more serious disorder may be involved.

BODY PARTS INVOLVED—Endocrine system.

SEX OR AGE MOST AFFECTED—Post-pubescent females.

SIGNS & SYMPTOMS
• Excessive growth of thick, dark hair in body areas of women where hair growth is normally absent or minimal. It grows in a male pattern (beard, moustache, chest, around the nipples, genitals, and other places).
• Hair growth may occur along with irregular or absent menstrual periods, acne, deepening of the voice, and infertility problems.

CAUSES—It may be due to high levels of androgens (male hormones). All females make small amounts of androgens, but certain conditions can cause an excess. In other cases of hirsutism (idiopathic), the cause is unknown.

RISK INCREASES WITH
• Family history of hirsutism.
• Dark-haired persons, especially those of Hispanic, African American, Mediterranean, or Indian ancestry.
• Use of certain drugs such as testosterone, steroids, and others.
• Polycystic ovarian syndrome.
• Adrenal disorders.
• Adrenal or ovarian tumor.
• Anorexia, acromegaly, hypothyroidism, or porphyria.

HOW TO PREVENT—No specific preventive measures.

WHAT TO EXPECT

DIAGNOSTIC MEASURES
• Your health care provider will do a physical exam and ask questions about the hair growth.
• A variety of medical tests may be done to help diagnose any disorder that could be the cause of the hair growth.

APPROPRIATE HEALTH CARE
• The treatment depends on the cause of the hirsutism. A mild case of hirsutism with no menstrual problems may not require treatment. For others, treatment sometimes depends on the patient's desire for pregnancy.
• Treatment may involve drugs, surgery, and hair removal techniques.

• Tumors may be treated with surgery.
• Permanent hair removal may be done with electrolysis or thermolysis. These use an electric current to remove hair. Multiple treatments are needed. It is time-consuming, can be costly, and cause some discomfort.
• Permanent hair removal may be done with a laser. Larger areas can be treated with minimal discomfort. Multiple treatments are needed.
• Other forms of hair removal include pulsed light and photodynamic (use of a topical drug and special light).
• The various forms of hair removal can cause skin irritation, folliculitis (inflamed hair follicles), skin color changes, and, rarely, scarring.

POSSIBLE COMPLICATIONS
• Poor self-image. A woman may feel unattractive, stressed, anxious, and find social activities with other people difficult.
• Complications occur from underlying disorder.

PROBABLE OUTCOME—Diagnosis and treatment of the cause can often halt further hair growth. Excess hair may be removed by various methods.

HOW TO TREAT

GENERAL MEASURES—Cosmetic treatments of hirsutism include covering up with makeup, bleaching, and removal with physical methods. These include cutting, shaving, plucking, threading, or waxing. Chemical depilatories are designed to use on specific body locations. Home hair-removal devices are available. All methods are temporary (effects lasting from hours to days) and have certain drawbacks.

MEDICATION
• There are a variety of drugs used to treat the underlying cause of hirsutism. They may take 3 to 6 months for results. They can help decrease new hair growth. They will not change the amount of hair you already have.
• Eflornithine (Vaniqa), a topical drug, may be prescribed for reducing facial hair growth.
• If skin gets irritated, use nonprescription 1% hydrocortisone cream.
• If a drug causes hirsutism, it may be stopped.

ACTIVITY—Usually no limits.

DIET—No special diet. If you are overweight, losing weight may help.

CALL YOUR DOCTOR IF

• You or a family member has symptoms of hirsutism.
• New, unexplained symptoms develop.

HISTOPLASMOSIS

GENERAL INFORMATION

DEFINITION—Histoplasmosis is a fungal infection that occurs throughout the world. In the United States, it normally affects people who live in the eastern and midwestern states. Almost all cases are mild and go undiagnosed.

BODY PARTS INVOLVED—Lungs usually; central nervous system; gastrointestinal system.

SEX OR AGE MOST AFFECTED—Both sexes; all ages.

SIGNS & SYMPTOMS
- Usually no symptoms are present.
- Cold or flu-like symptoms (cough, fever, chills, chest or stomach pain, tiredness, and weight loss). In chronic cases (occurs in those with lung disease), there may be shortness of breath, sweating, and increased chest pain.
- In rare disseminated cases (infection spreads throughout the body), the symptoms will vary.

CAUSES—Infection by the fungus, *Histoplasma capsulatum*. People become infected by breathing dust that contains fungus spores. The fungus is found in soil contaminated by feces of birds and bats that carry the fungus. This soil is most often found in pigeon lofts, barns, chicken houses, and in damp areas under bridges, along streams, and in caves.

RISK INCREASES WITH
- Geographic location. The disease is normally found in the western Appalachian slopes and the Mississippi, Missouri, and Ohio River valleys. Millions of people living in these areas have been infected, but never have symptoms or they are so mild that they go unnoticed.
- Working in construction-related activities that disturb contaminated soil (e.g., bulldozing or demolition).
- Spelunking (cave exploring).

HOW TO PREVENT—No specific preventive measures. Wear protective masks for work in areas that might be contaminated.

WHAT TO EXPECT

DIAGNOSTIC MEASURES
- Your own observation of symptoms.
- Your health care provider will do a physical exam and ask about your symptoms and activities.
- Medical tests may include sputum culture, blood studies, skin tests, and chest x-ray.

APPROPRIATE HEALTH CARE—Treatment is with supportive care and drugs (if needed). Hospital care may be required for patients with severe symptoms.

POSSIBLE COMPLICATIONS
- People with weak immune systems or middle-aged smokers are more at risk for complications.
- Spread of infection to other organs. This is rare, but it can be fatal.
- Histoplasmosis often recurs in AIDS patients.
- Eye problems (they may take years to develop).

PROBABLE OUTCOME
- Mild cases usually resolve on their own. Most people only feel tired or "bad" for several weeks.
- Severe cases are treatable with antifungal drugs.

HOW TO TREAT

GENERAL MEASURES
- Isolation is not necessary. The disease is not transmitted from person to person.
- Don't smoke.
- Use warm compresses or a heating pad on the chest to relieve pain.

MEDICATION
- For mild cases, no medicine is usually necessary.
- For more-severe cases, antifungal drugs will be prescribed. Some may be given intravenously (IV).
- Anti-inflammatory drugs for inflammation may be prescribed.
- For certain patients, continued therapy with antifungal drugs will be necessary.

ACTIVITY—Activity levels will depend on the symptoms. The disorder is not contagious.

DIET—No special diet.

CALL YOUR DOCTOR IF

- You or a family member has histoplasmosis symptoms.
- The following occur during treatment:
  - Weight loss continues.
  - Fever rises to 101°F (38.3°C) orally.
  - Severe headache and stiff neck occur.

HIV & AIDS
(Human Immunodeficiency Virus; Acquired Immunodeficiency Syndrome)

GENERAL INFORMATION

DEFINITION—Human immunodeficiency virus (HIV) is a virus that gradually destroys the body's ability to fight infection and certain cancers. Acquired immunodeficiency syndrome (AIDS) is a secondary immunodeficiency syndrome resulting from HIV infection.

BODY PARTS INVOLVED—Lungs; central nervous system; gastrointestinal system.

SEX OR AGE MOST AFFECTED—Both sexes; all ages; more often occurs in younger males.

SIGNS & SYMPTOMS
- HIV infection may produce no symptoms.
- Early symptoms clear up on their own and may include: fatigue, sore throat, fever, nausea/vomiting, swollen glands, muscle ache, headache, and joint pain.
- HIV symptoms may recur after several years: swollen and sore lymph glands, fatigue, chills, fever, night sweats, persistent headache, weight loss, diarrhea, cough, white coating on tongue (thrush), or persistent vaginal yeast infections.
- In later stages, multiple symptoms can occur.

CAUSES—HIV is a virus that invades and destroys cells of the body's immune system. It is passed from person to person via body fluids (blood, semen, and vaginal fluid). A person with HIV infection is not a risk for spreading the infection to the general population.

RISK INCREASES WITH
- Sexual contact with HIV-infected person.
- Having high-risk partners (e.g., has sex with other men, has multiple sex partners, or injects drugs).
- Having unprotected sex with multiple partners.
- IV drug abusers using contaminated needles.
- Children born to an HIV-infected mother.
- Having a sexually transmitted disease (STD).

HOW TO PREVENT
- Abstain from sex or have sex with only one person who is known to be free of HIV.
- Avoid sexual contact with HIV-affected persons or known IV drug users.
- Use a new latex (or polyurethane) condom for each act of vaginal, anal, or oral intercourse if partner has unknown HIV status.
- Avoid IV drugs. Do not share needles.
- Avoid untested blood products in other countries.
- Health care workers need to use precautions in handling needles and blood products.
- If you are HIV-positive: do advise sexual partners and health care providers, do practice safe sex, don't donate blood/organs, don't share certain items (needles, syringes, razor, or toothbrush).

WHAT TO EXPECT

DIAGNOSTIC MEASURES
- Early diagnosis is helpful. If you are at risk, get a medical test even if you feel well. If you plan to be, or are pregnant, HIV testing can be helpful.
- Your health care provider will do a physical exam and ask questions about your sexual history and any IV drug use.
- Medical tests may include routine blood studies and an HIV antibody blood test. It takes 1 to 3 months (sometimes up to 6 months) after HIV exposure for antibodies to be detected in the blood. Tests for other sexually transmitted diseases and infections are usually done.

APPROPRIATE HEALTH CARE
- Treatment includes drug therapy and self-care. Hospital care may be needed in some cases.
- Counseling helps you cope with having HIV.

POSSIBLE COMPLICATIONS—Serious infections, cancer, or death.

PROBABLE OUTCOME—There is no cure and the outcome will vary for each person. With proper treatment, many patients are living longer and with basically good health.

HOW TO TREAT

GENERAL MEASURES
- Advise past/present sexual partners to get HIV tests.
- Get regular medical and dental check-ups. Tell any health care provider you consult that you have HIV.
- Avoid exposure to people with infections.
- Join a support group.
- To learn more: Centers for Disease Control; (800) 232-4636; website: www.cdc.gov/hiv.

MEDICATION—Drugs to treat HIV and AIDS, and drugs to treat infections or complications will be prescribed.

ACTIVITY—Fatigue or infections can limit some activities. Get the rest you need, but try to exercise to the extent possible.

DIET—Poor eating habits, changes in metabolism, and weight loss may develop. Consult a dietitian for advice on diet.

CALL YOUR DOCTOR IF

- You or a family member has HIV symptoms.
- Any infections occur after diagnosis. Symptoms include fever, cough, and diarrhea.
- Other new symptoms develop (e.g., side effects from drugs used in treatment).

HIVES
(Urticaria)

GENERAL INFORMATION

DEFINITION—Hives is an allergic reaction that involves the skin. Urticaria is the medical name for hives. Hives are very common.

BODY PARTS INVOLVED—Hives may occur anywhere on the body, but the arms, legs, and trunk are most often affected.

SEX OR AGE MOST AFFECTED—Both sexes; all ages.

SIGNS & SYMPTOMS
- Raised, irregular, red areas on the skin. They may be referred to as wheals or welts. They usually itch, but they may also burn or sting. The size may range from small spots to the size of a dinner plate. They can sometimes cause the whole lip or eyelid to swell.
- Wheals can join together quickly and form large, flat plaques. These are raised, skin-colored areas.
- Wheals and plaques change shape, go away, and come back in minutes or hours.

CAUSES—Release of histamines. These are chemicals in the cells of the human body that are released during an allergic reaction. They may be released due to a specific reaction or in some cases for unknown reasons.

RISK INCREASES WITH—People who have had hives, angioedema, other allergic reactions, certain disorders (e.g., lupus, thyroid disease, or lymphoma), or family history of hives.

HOW TO PREVENT
- There are no specific preventive measures to stop the first outbreak of hives. Once you have had hives and know the cause (trigger), you need to avoid it in the future.
- Possible triggers for hives include:
  - Eating eggs, fruits, nuts, and shellfish. Other foods may cause hives in infants but not in adults. Certain food additives may cause hives.
  - Drugs. Nearly all drugs can cause hives in some persons.
  - Insect stings.
  - Pollens.
  - Exposure to cold, heat, water, sunlight, or pressure on skin.
  - Exercise-induced.
  - Exposure to animals, especially cats.
  - Recent infection or blood transfusion.
- Your health care provider may advise you to keep an emergency kit handy if you have had severe reactions.

WHAT TO EXPECT

DIAGNOSTIC MEASURES
- Your own observation of symptoms.
- See your health care provider if the hives are more severe or cause concern. Your health care provider will do a physical exam of the affected skin. Questions will be asked to help identify the cause.
- Medical tests are usually not needed.

APPROPRIATE HEALTH CARE
- Most persons will treat hives at home. Try to identify the cause of the hives.
- Treatment usually involves antihistamines and avoiding the cause of the hives when known (such as a drug or food). If the reaction is severe, hospital care may be needed.

POSSIBLE COMPLICATIONS
- Other allergic reactions may occur with hives:
  - Angioedema (face, throat, and tongue swelling).
  - Anaphylaxis (severe reaction that causes shock and difficulty in breathing).

PROBABLE OUTCOME—Hives usually clear up within hours or days (even if the cause is unknown). They can be uncomfortable, but normally they cause no complications. A few cases become chronic and may last for weeks.

HOW TO TREAT

GENERAL MEASURES
- Don't wear tight clothing. Any skin irritation may trigger new outbreaks.
- Don't take hot baths or showers.
- Apply cold-water compresses or soaks.
- Try to relax and not become over-stressed.

MEDICATION
- Use nonprescription antihistamines for itching.
- Prescription antihistamines, steroids, or other drugs to relieve symptoms may be prescribed.
- Epinephrine by injection may be used for severe symptoms.

ACTIVITY—Decrease activities until several days after hives disappear. Avoid getting hot, sweaty, or overly excited.

DIET—If foods are suspected as a cause, keep a food diary to help identify the offending food.

CALL YOUR DOCTOR IF

- You or a family member has hives that aren't helped by self-care or last for more than 2 days.
- If reaction is severe, seek emergency help!

HODGKIN'S DISEASE

GENERAL INFORMATION

DEFINITION—Hodgkin's disease is a rare cancer that involves the lymphatic system (part of the body's immune system). It is a type of lymphoma (the other type, non-Hodgkin's lymphoma, is more common).

BODY PARTS INVOLVED—The lymphatic system is made up of the lymph nodes (glands), spleen, thymus gland, and bone marrow. Lymph nodes are found throughout the body and are connected by vessels (called lymphatics).

SEX OR AGE MOST AFFECTED—All ages and both sexes, but most common in young adults and older persons. It is rare in children under 10.

SIGNS & SYMPTOMS
- Swollen, non-tender, rubbery, distinct lymph nodes (glands) anywhere in the body, but most commonly in the neck, armpit, or groin.
- Intermittent fever and night sweats.
- Itching all over the body.
- Weight loss and loss of appetite.
- Jaundice (yellow skin and eyes).
- General ill feeling.
- Cough.

CAUSES—Unknown. Research is ongoing.

RISK INCREASES WITH
- Young adults and older adults.
- Males more than females.
- Past infection with Epstein-Barr virus (e.g., infectious mononucleosis).
- Having a first-degree relative with Hodgkin's disease.
- People with weak immune systems due to illness or drugs.

HOW TO PREVENT—No specific preventive measures.

WHAT TO EXPECT

DIAGNOSTIC MEASURES
- Your own observation of symptoms.
- Your health care provider will do a physical exam and ask questions about your symptoms and activities.
- Different medical tests are done to verify the diagnosis and to determine if the cancer has spread to other places in the body (called staging).

APPROPRIATE HEALTH CARE
- Treatment will depend on the stage of the disease, patient's age and health status, and whether patient is pregnant.
- Treatment usually combines chemotherapy (anticancer drugs) and radiation therapy. Less often, each one may be used alone. Treatment using a stem cell transplant may be an option in certain patients. Your health care provider will discuss your options with you.
- Males receiving therapy may want to consider sperm-banking in case of sterility. Females may want to store fertilized eggs.
- Counseling may help a person to cope with having cancer.

POSSIBLE COMPLICATIONS
- Spread of cancer to other places in the body.
- Infertility in males and females.
- Heart or lung disorders, anemia, hypothyroidism, and infections.
- Cancer may return after treatment.

PROBABLE OUTCOME—Often curable if diagnosed and treated early. The outcome will vary for patients with advanced stage disease. The treatment can also have long term effects.

HOW TO TREAT

GENERAL MEASURES
- Try to remain optimistic about your treatment and chances for cure. A good mental attitude is a powerful ally.
- Supports groups can be helpful for persons coping with cancer.
- To learn more: American Cancer Society; (800) ACS-2345; website: www.cancer.org or National Cancer Institute; (800) 4-CANCER; website: www.cancer.gov.

MEDICATION
- Anticancer drugs (chemotherapy) are usually prescribed. These may cause side effects or adverse reactions in some people.
- Steroid drugs may be prescribed for short periods.

ACTIVITY—Remain as active as your strength allows. Regular exercise can help both physical and emotional health.

DIET—No special diet.

CALL YOUR DOCTOR IF

- You or a family member has symptoms of Hodgkin's disease.
- Any new symptoms develop or other symptoms get worse during treatment.

HYPERALDOSTERONISM
(Aldosteronism)

 GENERAL INFORMATION

DEFINITION—Hyperaldosteronism is an endocrine disorder caused by too much aldosterone, a hormone made by the adrenal glands. These glands are attached to the upper part of the kidneys. Excess aldosterone causes the kidneys to take in too much sodium and water, and eliminate too much potassium (called hypokalemia).

BODY PARTS INVOLVED—Adrenal glands, kidneys, and fluids and electrolytes in the bloodstream and body cells.

SEX OR AGE MOST AFFECTED
- Both sexes, but more common in females.
- All ages, but most common in adults between ages 30 and 50.

SIGNS & SYMPTOMS
- Often, there are no symptoms. It may be diagnosed when checking for the cause of high blood pressure.
- Symptoms that occur may include fatigue, muscle cramps or weakness, heart palpitations, frequent urination, headache, and temporary paralysis (sometimes).
- High blood pressure (hypertension).

CAUSES
- Primary hyperaldosteronism:
  - Is often caused by an aldosterone-producing adenoma (APA). This is a noncancerous (benign) tumor of the adrenal gland.
  - It may also be caused by idiopathic hyperaldosteronism or IHA (also referred to BAH or bilateral adrenal hyperplasia).
  - There are other, more rare causes including an inherited condition and cancer.
- Secondary hyperaldosteronism is caused by conditions outside of the adrenal glands. These include high blood pressure, cirrhosis of the liver, heart failure, or nephrotic (kidney) syndrome.

RISK INCREASES WITH
- High blood pressure.
- Disorders listed above that can lead to secondary hyperaldosteronism.
- Family history of hyperaldosteronism.

HOW TO PREVENT—There are no known preventive measures.

 WHAT TO EXPECT

DIAGNOSTIC MEASURES
- Your own observation of symptoms.
- Your health care provider will do a physical exam and ask questions about your medical history.

- Medical tests usually include checking the levels of sodium and potassium in the blood. Other blood studies may be done to measure the levels of aldosterone and renin (an enzyme released by the kidneys). A CT or MRI of the adrenal glands may be done.

APPROPRIATE HEALTH CARE
- Treatment depends on the cause. It may include surgery, drug therapy, diet changes, and other lifestyle changes.
- An adrenal adenoma is usually removed with laparoscopic surgery (called adrenalectomy). This can cure or improve high blood pressure in most patients.
- Other causes of primary hyperaldosteronism and the underlying causes of secondary hyperaldosteronism are usually treated with drugs and diet changes.

POSSIBLE COMPLICATIONS
- Poorly controlled high blood pressure. It can lead to cardiovascular (heart and blood vessels) complications and kidney disease or failure.
- Long-term drug therapy in men may lead to impotence or enlarged breasts (gynecomastia).

PROBABLE OUTCOME
- With early diagnosis and treatment of primary hyperaldosteronism, the outcome is good.
- With secondary hyperaldosteronism, the outcome will vary depending on the cause.

 HOW TO TREAT

GENERAL MEASURES
- Don't smoke. Find a way to quit that works.
- Wear or carry medical ID that shows this medical condition and any drugs that you take.

MEDICATION
- Drugs for high blood pressure and to reduce the aldosterone effect may be prescribed.
- Drugs may be prescribed for underlying causes.

ACTIVITY
- If surgery is needed, your health care provider will advise you of any limitations.
- Get regular exercise to maintain good health.

DIET
- You may be prescribed a low salt diet.
- Maintain a healthy weight. If overweight is a problem, a weight-loss diet may be advised.
- Limit or avoid alcohol use.

 CALL YOUR DOCTOR IF

- You or a family member has symptoms of hyperaldosteronism.
- New, unexplained symptoms develop.

HYPEREMESIS GRAVIDARUM

GENERAL INFORMATION

DEFINITION—Hyperemesis gravidarum is severe, persistent nausea and vomiting in a pregnant woman. It is more serious than the typical nausea and vomiting (morning sickness) in pregnancy. Hyperemesis gravidarum usually occurs before the 20th week of pregnancy; often between the fourth and twelfth week.

BODY PARTS INVOLVED—Gastrointestinal tract; vomiting center in the brain.

SEX OR AGE MOST AFFECTED—Pregnant females.

SIGNS & SYMPTOMS
- Severe and frequent nausea and vomiting.
- Fatigue, weakness, and feeling faint or lightheaded.
- Sleep problems.
- Smell and taste changes. Excessive saliva.
- Dehydration (less urine; pale and dry skin).
- Failure to gain weight, or there is weight loss.
- Unable to eat and maintain proper nutrition.
- Some affected women may have a distinct odor to their breath (ketonic odor).
- Often unable to work, perform daily household tasks and routines, or care for young children.
- Fast heartbeat (sometimes).
- Mood changes, anxiety, depression, irritability, or loss of concentration.
- Symptoms may start, stop, and then recur.

CAUSES—The exact cause is unclear. Multiple factors are likely involved including changes in hormone levels.

RISK INCREASES WITH
- First pregnancy.
- Multiple-pregnancy (more than one fetus).
- Hyperemesis gravidarum in a previous pregnancy or a family history of the disorder.
- Overweight.
- Trophoblastic disease (pregnancy-related condition).
- Some chronic medical conditions.

HOW TO PREVENT
- There is no specific prevention. Women who take a multivitamin at the time of conception and in early pregnancy may have a reduced risk.
- Pregnant women who have had hyperemesis gravidarum in a prior pregnancy should discuss possible preventive measures with their obstetric provider.

WHAT TO EXPECT

DIAGNOSTIC MEASURES
- Your own observation of symptoms.
- Your obstetric provider will usually do a physical exam and ask questions about your symptoms.

- Medical tests may be done to check for other health problems.

APPROPRIATE HEALTH CARE
- Hospital care may be needed to replace lost fluids and electrolytes (substances needed for body function). Fluids are given through a vein (IV) to provide nutrition and relieve dehydration. Other forms of nutritional support may be required (e.g., tube feeding).
- If symptoms are not too severe, home care with diet instructions and rest may be recommended. In some cases, home IV fluids are a part of the treatment.
- You and your obstetric provider may discuss alternate treatments for nausea and vomiting. These can include acupressure wristbands or nerve stimulation device (used to help motion sickness), hypnosis, or others.

POSSIBLE COMPLICATIONS
- Severe dehydration and weight loss that can cause complications for mother and baby.
- May increase the risk of preterm birth and baby having a lower than normal birth weight.
- Problems with social or psychological (mental) issues may be associated with this disorder.

PROBABLE OUTCOME—Usually curable with time and treatment. Pregnancy can continue to the successful delivery of a healthy baby.

HOW TO TREAT

GENERAL MEASURES
- Weigh daily. Report unusual changes to your obstetric provider.
- To learn more: Hyperemesis Education and Research Foundation, 932 Edwards Ferry Rd., #23, Leesburg, VA 20176; website: www.helpher.org.

MEDICATION
- Intravenous (IV) fluid, vitamins, and electrolyte replacement may be required.
- Other drugs may be prescribed for nausea.
- Don't use nonprescription drugs or herbal products for vomiting without medical advice.

ACTIVITY—Increased rest helps most patients.

DIET
- Eat when hungry. Eat small, frequent, and bland meals. High-protein snacks may help. Avoid fatty or spicy foods.
- Drinking seltzer or sparkling water may help.
- Eat dry toast or crackers first thing in morning.
- Avoid foods and odors that trigger symptoms.

CALL YOUR DOCTOR IF

- You or a family member has symptoms of hyperemesis gravidarum.
- Symptoms continue despite treatment.

HYPERHIDROSIS

GENERAL INFORMATION

DEFINITION—Hyperhidrosis is a condition of excessive sweating. It usually begins in childhood or adolescence. The excessive sweating may occur for no apparent reason.

BODY PARTS INVOLVED—Skin, especially of the underarms, palms and soles.

SEX OR AGE MOST AFFECTED—Both sexes and all ages.

SIGNS & SYMPTOMS
- Heavy sweat from underarm area, soles, palms, and other body parts.
- Sweating occurs without warning or cause.
- The amount of sweating, body parts involved, and when it occurs differs in different people.
- An odor, which is caused by bacteria in sweat.

CAUSES
- Primary focal hyperhidrosis is the term used when there is no physical cause for the excessive sweating. Sweating is normally regulated by the body's sympathetic nervous system. In some people, this system becomes overactive. Why this occurs is unknown.
- Secondary generalized hyperhidrosis results from a specific factor such as diabetes.

RISK INCREASES WITH
- Unknown for primary focal type.
- Secondary type may be caused by:
  - Diabetes.
  - Hyperthyroidism.
  - Menopause.
  - Some cancers.
  - Some drugs, such as narcotics.
  - Obesity.
  - Certain psychiatric conditions.
  - Chronic alcoholism.

HOW TO PREVENT—No specific measures to prevent primary type hyperhidrosis. Steps may be taken to help control the sweating. Preventing secondary type depends on cause.

WHAT TO EXPECT

DIAGNOSTIC MEASURES
- Your own observation of symptoms.
- Your health care provider will do a physical exam and ask questions about your symptoms and activities.
- Medical tests may be done to identify any disorder that is causing the excessive sweating.

APPROPRIATE HEALTH CARE
- Treatment for an underlying condition will be provided.
- Counseling, if stress is a major factor.
- Drug therapy may be recommended.

- Electrical devices that temporarily reduce sweating of palms or feet may be recommended.
- Surgery to remove sweat glands or sever nerves to major sweat areas, may be an option in more serious cases.

POSSIBLE COMPLICATIONS
- Emotional distress caused by embarrassment.
- Rashes from deodorants or antiperspirants.

PROBABLE OUTCOME—Primary type can be helped with a variety of treatment options. No single treatment works for everyone. Secondary type can often be controlled with treatment of the underlying condition.

HOW TO TREAT

GENERAL MEASURES
- Bathe daily. Use an antibacterial soap. Dry carefully.
- Change clothes often.
- Wear loose-fitting clothes made of natural fibers, such as cotton.
- Use underarm sweat shields.
- Use antiperspirants (some contain a deodorant to reduce odor). Use an unscented product that contains aluminum chloride. Apply it at night for better results.
- Use drying powders.
- Wear cotton socks.
- Change shoes often. Use absorbent shoe inserts.
- Shave underarm hair.
- Learn and practice relaxation techniques.
- To learn more: International Hyperhidrosis Society, Suite 6121-A, Kellers Church Road, Pipersville, PA 18947; website: www.sweathelp.org/english.

MEDICATION
- Drugs to reduce activity of the central nervous system may be prescribed. Side effects can be a problem.
- Prescription antiperspirants may be prescribed.
- Botulinum toxin (Botox) injections may be prescribed. It helps reduce or stop sweating for 3 to 6 months.
- Other drugs may be prescribed to be taken by mouth or applied to the skin.

ACTIVITY—No limits.

DIET—Avoid hot drinks, alcohol, or spices that make you sweat.

CALL YOUR DOCTOR IF

- Excessive sweating is causing you problems at work or in social situations.
- Treatment for excessive sweating is not working.

HYPERLIPIDEMIA

GENERAL INFORMATION

DEFINITION
- Hyperlipidemia is the medical term used to describe having high amounts of lipids in the blood. Lipids, such as cholesterol and triglycerides, are fat or fat-like substances that maintain important body functions. They travel in the bloodstream attached to proteins. The lipid-protein combinations are called lipoproteins. Lipoproteins help the lipids get absorbed by the body's cells. Hyperlipidemia is called primary if it is inherited and secondary if it is caused by illness or other health problem. Subcategories of hyperlipidemia include:
    - Hypercholesterolemia (high levels of cholesterol).
    - Hypertriglyceridemia (high levels of triglycerides).

BODY PARTS INVOLVED—Blood and arteries.

SEX OR AGE MOST AFFECTED—Both sexes; all ages, but most common in adults. Different types appear at different ages.

SIGNS & SYMPTOMS
- There are usually no symptoms. It may be discovered on routine blood studies.
- There may be pinkish-yellow deposits of fat in the skin beneath eyes, elbows, and knees, and in tendons.

CAUSES
- There are five types of lipoproteins—defined by size and density. Two types carry cholesterol and the other three types carry triglycerides.
    - Cholesterol is carried through the blood by high-density lipoproteins (HDL) and low-density lipoproteins (LDL). High levels of LDL and/or low levels of HDL can increase the risk of heart disease and stroke.
    - Triglycerides are carried by three lipoproteins. These are very low-density lipoprotein (VLDL), intermediate density lipoproteins (IDL), and chylomicrons. High triglyceride levels may increase the risk of heart disease and stroke.
- Guidelines suggest that to reduce risks, HDL should be above 40, LDL should be below 130, and triglycerides should be below 150, for most people.

RISK INCREASES WITH
- Hereditary factors.
- Diet high in fat, cholesterol, and sugar.
- Illness or medical problems, such as diabetes, hypothyroidism, nephrotic syndrome, alcoholism, or obstructive liver disease.
- Sedentary lifestyle (lack of physical activity).
- Age. Males over 40 and females over 55.

HOW TO PREVENT
- Exercise daily. Maintain a healthy weight. Eat a healthy diet.
- Don't smoke. Avoid or limit a
- Get a medical test to check you of cholesterol and triglycerides.

WHAT TO EXPECT

DIAGNOSTIC MEASURES
- Your health care provider may do a physical exam and ask questions about any symptoms.
- For diagnosis, a blood study will be done to measure blood lipids.

APPROPRIATE HEALTH CARE
- Treatment will depend on the results of your blood studies, your health risks, and other medical problems.
- For some patients, an altered diet and lifestyle changes may be sufficient for treatment. Others may require drugs to reduce blood lipids.

POSSIBLE COMPLICATIONS—Coronary heart disease and stroke

PROBABLE OUTCOME—Usually treatable or controllable with diet and drugs.

HOW TO TREAT

GENERAL MEASURES
- Emotional stress can increase the risk of heart disease. Look for ways to reduce stress in your life. Learn relaxation methods.
- Quit smoking. Find a way to stop that works.

MEDICATION
- Several different drugs are now prescribed to control blood lipids. Your health care provider will discuss the options with you.
- Drugs to treat diseases, such as high blood pressure, diabetes, or thyroid conditions may be prescribed.

ACTIVITY—Regular exercise is helpful for reducing weight, staying fit, and controlling stress. It might help in increasing the body's ability to clear fat from the blood after meals.

DIET
- Eat a diet that is low in fat (avoid saturated fat). Eat a high fiber diet with plenty of fruits and vegetables. Reduce intake of simple carbohydrates (e.g., sugar and white flour). Consult a dietitian for advice if needed.
- Lose weight, if you are overweight. The more overweight you are, the more lipids your body produces.
- Reduce alcohol intake.

CALL YOUR DOCTOR IF

- You or a family member has symptoms or a family history of hyperlipidemia.
- New, unexplained symptoms develop.

...ORMATION

...roidism occurs ...s become overactive ...athyroid hormone (P...) ...are four pea-sized glands loc... ...e thyroid gland in the neck. PTH help... ...ain the body's levels of certain minerals. Excess PTH leads to high calcium levels (hypercalcemia) and low phosphorous levels in the blood.

BODY PARTS INVOLVED—Parathyroid glands; teeth; blood, which affects all body tissues—especially the heart, blood vessels, bones, kidneys, gastrointestinal tract, central nervous system, and skin.

SEX OR AGE MOST AFFECTED—Both sexes and all ages, but more common in older adults and in women more than men.

SIGNS & SYMPTOMS
* There may be no symptoms, or the symptoms may be mild to severe. It comes on over years and may be diagnosed on routine blood tests.
* Feeling tired, depressed, or forgetful.
* Muscle weakness and bone and joint pain.
* Loss of appetite, thirst, frequent urination, weight loss, or constipation.
* Nausea, vomiting.
* Severe side (flank) pain caused by kidney stones.
* Easy bone fractures due to osteoporosis.
* High blood pressure.
* Pain in the upper abdomen caused by a peptic ulcer or pancreatitis (inflammation of the pancreas).

CAUSES
* Primary hyperparathyroidism begins in the parathyroid itself. It is often caused by a benign tumor (adenoma) that grows in one or two of the parathyroid glands. Why the tumors occur is unknown. Enlargement of the glands (hyperplasia) is another cause, and why this occurs is also unknown. Rarely, cancer or a hereditary disorder is the cause.
* Secondary hyperparathyroidism is due to disorders (e.g., kidney failure) that affect parathyroid function.

RISK INCREASES WITH
* Older adults; females over age 50.
* Severe vitamin D or calcium deficiency, kidney disease, certain cancers, malnutrition, or malabsorption.
* Family history of hyperparathyroidism and certain inherited conditions.
* Radiation therapy that affected the neck.
* Use of the drug lithium.

HOW TO PREVENT—No specific preventive measures.

WHAT TO EXPECT

DIAGNOSTIC MEASURES
* Your own observation of any symptoms.
* Your health care provider will usually do a physical exam and ask questions about any symptoms.
* Urine and blood studies are done to check levels of calcium, phosphorus, and PTH. Bone scans may be done.

APPROPRIATE HEALTH CARE
* Severe symptoms may require hospital care.
* Primary hyperparathyroidism:
  - Surgery is usually the best form of treatment. The parathyroid gland or glands that are producing the excess hormones are removed. There are different types of operations that are done and they will be explained to you.
  - In mild cases, or if there are no symptoms, or surgery is not desired, watchful waiting may be an option. This means monitoring the patient for a time to see if the disorder worsens.
* Secondary hyperparathyroidism:
  - Treatment depends on the underlying cause and may include drug therapy and/or surgery.

POSSIBLE COMPLICATIONS
* Weak bones (osteopenia and osteoporosis), kidney problems, ulcers, pancreatitis, or heart problems.
* Rarely, surgery complications may occur.

PROBABLE OUTCOME
* Surgery usually resolves primary type.
* With secondary type, outcome depends on the cause. It can require parathyroid surgery if it no longer responds to treatment (tertiary hyperparathyroidism).

 ## HOW TO TREAT

GENERAL MEASURES—None specific.

MEDICATION
* Estrogen for postmenopausal females may be prescribed.
* Bone-building drugs or vitamin D may be prescribed.

ACTIVITY—Follow medical advice about resuming activities after surgery.

DIET
* Drink extra water helps prevent complications.
* Your health care provider will discuss the needed amount of daily calcium intake.

 ## CALL YOUR DOCTOR IF

* You or a family member has symptoms of hyperparathyroidism.
* New symptoms occur with treatments.

HYPERTENSION
(High Blood Pressure)

 GENERAL INFORMATION

DEFINITION—Hypertension (high blood pressure) is a common disorder and often affects adults over age 60. Blood pressure measures the force of blood as it flows through the arteries. Stroke and heart attack risks begin to increase as blood pressure rises. Adult blood pressure is normal at less than 120/80. The first number is systolic pressure, which measures pressure as the heart contracts (pumps). The second number is diastolic, which measures pressure when the heart is relaxed (between beats). Hypertension is when the blood pressure reading is higher than 140/90. Prehypertension is when the blood pressure is between 120/80 and 139/89.

BODY PARTS INVOLVED—Heart and blood vessels.

SEX OR AGE MOST AFFECTED—Both sexes; all ages, but most common in adults.

SIGNS & SYMPTOMS
• Usually no symptoms occur. It is often discovered when blood pressure is measured.
• Vague, mild symptoms such as headache, dizziness, blurred vision, or nausea may occur.

CAUSES—Mostly unknown (called primary or essential hypertension). In some cases, it results from certain medical problems (called secondary hypertension).

RISK INCREASES WITH
• Aging and hardening of the arteries.
• Prehypertension.
• Chronic kidney disease or thyroid dysfunction.
• Narrowing of the aorta (major artery of the heart).
• Adrenal gland disorders.
• Alcoholism.
• Hormone problems of adrenals or pituitary glands.
• Overweight; smoking; stress.
• Sedentary (lack of physical activity) lifestyle.
• Sensitivity to sodium (salt).
• Genetic factors (it is common in African Americans).
• Family history of hypertension.
• Use of certain drugs. These include birth-control pills, steroids, diet pills, and decongestants.

HOW TO PREVENT—No specific preventive measures. Avoid risk factors where possible. Maintain a healthy weight, be physically active, eat a healthy diet (limit salt), drink little or no alcohol, and don't smoke. If you have a family history of hypertension, have frequent blood-pressure checks.

 WHAT [...]

DIAGNOSTIC MEASURES
• Your health care provider will do [...] exam and measure your blood pressu[...] separate occasions). Questions will be as[...] about your lifestyle and family medical history.
• Medical tests may include blood and urine studies. Other tests may be done to find a cause for the high blood pressure.

APPROPRIATE HEALTH CARE
• Treatment steps will depend on each person's health status. You and your health care provider will decide on a treatment plan.
• Steps may involve diet changes, weight loss, stopping smoking, increasing exercise, limiting alcohol use, reducing stress, and taking drugs.

POSSIBLE COMPLICATIONS—Without treatment, high blood pressure can lead to heart attack, stroke, congestive heart failure, pulmonary edema, and kidney failure. High blood pressure is called the "silent killer."

PROBABLE OUTCOME—Outlook is good if blood pressure can be controlled.

 HOW TO TREAT

GENERAL MEASURES
• Ask your health care provider before trying alternate forms of treatment.
• Don't smoke. Find a way to quit.
• Find ways to manage your stress levels.
• Learn to check blood pressure at home.

MEDICATION
• One or more antihypertensive drugs to reduce blood pressure may be prescribed. Do not stop drugs unless advised by health care provider.
• Avoid nonprescription decongestant drugs. They may raise blood pressure.

ACTIVITY—Increase physical activity. Exercise moderately hard for 30 minutes, most, if not all, days of the week. It helps reduce stress, control body weight, and lowers blood pressure. Get medical advice about an exercise plan.

DIET—Eat a healthy diet, high in fiber, fruits, and vegetables. Limit fat and salt use. If overweight, limit calories. Avoid or limit alcohol.

 CALL YOUR DOCTOR IF

• You or a family member has blood pressure concerns.
• Blood pressure increases or drugs used for treatment cause unexpected side effects.
• Call 911 if symptoms of a heart attack or stroke occur.

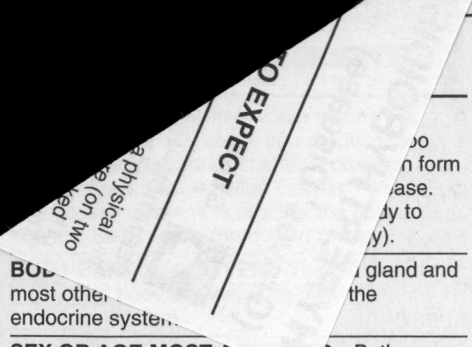

EXPECT

...a physical
(on two
...

...o
...n form
...ase.
...dy to
...y).

BO... gland and
most othe... the
endocrine syste...

SEX OR AGE MOST AF...**D**—Both sexes
(mostly women); adults ages 2... to 50.

SIGNS & SYMPTOMS
- Anxiety, nervousness, and restlessness.
- Feeling warm or hot all the time; sweating; itchy skin.
- Heart palpitations.
- Weight loss, even though appetite increases.
- Sleeplessness, fatigue, and weakness.
- Frequent bowel movements.
- Women may have less menstrual flow.
- Eyes appear to bulge out, there is swelling around the eyes, and may have vision changes.
- Goiter (visibly enlarged thyroid) may occur.
- Hair loss.
- Tremor of the hands.
- High blood pressure.

CAUSES
Graves' disease is an autoimmune disorder. In these disorders, the immune system by mistake attacks the body itself in different ways. In Graves' disease, abnormal antibodies from the immune system cause the thyroid to produce more hormone. Other causes of hyperthyroidism may be due to thyroid disorders.

RISK INCREASES WITH
- Thyroid nodules or tumors.
- Thyroiditis (inflammation of thyroid gland).
- Personal or family history of thyroid or autoimmune diseases.
- Radiation treatment.
- Females more than males.
- Excess iodine intake.
- Stress may be a contributing factor.

HOW TO PREVENT
No known way to prevent.

 ## WHAT TO EXPECT

DIAGNOSTIC MEASURES
- Your health care provider will do a physical exam.
- Medical tests include blood studies for thyroid levels. Radioactive iodine studies may be done.

APPROPRIATE HEALTH CARE
- Treatment usually involves drugs to reduce thyroid hormone levels. Permanent treatment involves use of radioactive iodine or surgery. With these two treatments, thyroid hormone production is decreased. Sometimes, hypothyroidism (too little thyroid hormone) occurs, which will need to be treated.
- Radioactive iodine treatment is usually done as an outpatient. The iodine (taken by mouth) causes the thyroid gland to shrink over a period of months.
- Surgery to remove part of the thyroid (called a thyroidectomy) may be advised in some cases.
- For eye symptoms, an exam and follow-up care by an eye specialist (ophthalmologist) is often prescribed.

POSSIBLE COMPLICATIONS
- Thyroid eye disease (e.g., visual loss or double vision).
- Heart problems.
- Bone mineral loss (osteoporosis).
- Dermopathy (a skin disorder).
- Hypothyroidism (low thyroid hormone levels).
- Thyroid crisis (rare and possibly fatal complication).

PROBABLE OUTCOME
Treatment is effective in controlling the disorder. It may take 6 months for thyroid levels to return to normal.

 ## HOW TO TREAT

GENERAL MEASURES
Follow medical advice.

MEDICATION
- Antithyroid drugs to depress thyroid activity are usually prescribed. Follow-up blood tests are done to adjust the dosage until thyroid hormone levels are normal.
- Beta blockers to treat the heart and nervous system symptoms may be prescribed.
- Thyroid replacement drugs may be prescribed if the thyroid gland becomes underactive due to treatment.
- Avoid drugs or supplements that contain iodide. It may interfere with drugs used in treatment.

ACTIVITY
Usually no limits in otherwise healthy persons. In older persons or those with heart problems, decrease activity until thyroid levels are normal.

DIET
No special diet.

 ## CALL YOUR DOCTOR IF

- You or a family member has symptoms of hyperthyroidism.
- Symptoms worsen or new symptoms occur.

HYPERTROPHIC CARDIOMYOPATHY

GENERAL INFORMATION

DEFINITION—Hypertrophic cardiomyopathy (HCM) is a chronic heart condition that produces an enlarged heart muscle. It can obstruct the blood flow from the heart (obstructive cardiomyopathy) and cause symptoms. If blood flow is normal (called nonobstructive cardiomyopathy), the condition can go undetected for years.

BODY PARTS INVOLVED—Heart.

SEX OR AGE MOST AFFECTED—Both sexes; all ages, but is more common in young adults.

SIGNS & SYMPTOMS
- Many patients have no symptoms. Symptoms that occur are often felt after exercising or exertion.
- Chest pain (called angina pectoris).
- Heart palpitations or fluttering.
- Faintness.
- Shortness of breath (may awaken person from sleep).
- Fatigue.
- Dizziness or lightheadedness.

CAUSES—Thickening of the heart muscle (myocardium). This is caused by a defect in the genes and often runs in families. The thickened walls obstruct the flow of blood, and the heart may be unable to pump enough blood for the needs of the body.

RISK INCREASES WITH—Family history of HCM. It is the most common inherited heart defect.

HOW TO PREVENT—It cannot be prevented. If you have a family history of HCM, ask your health care provider about genetic counseling before starting a family.

WHAT TO EXPECT

DIAGNOSTIC MEASURES
- Your health care provider will do a physical exam and listen to your heart with a stethoscope. Questions will be asked about your symptoms and family medical history.
- Medical tests include an echocardiogram and ECG (electrocardiogram) to check the structure and function of the heart. Other heart tests will be done as needed.

APPROPRIATE HEALTH CARE
- Treatment may include drugs, lifestyle changes, pacemaker or defibrillator insertion, or surgery. Treatment depends on the individual patient. Certain patients are more at risk of sudden death than others.
- Lifestyle changes may involve reducing activity levels and diet changes.

- An electronic cardiac pacemaker may be inserted. It helps relieve symptoms by changing the pattern of the heartbeat.
- An implantable-cardioverter defibrillator may be inserted. It can help prevent sudden death.
- A procedure that uses alcohol injected into an artery may be recommended. It can help to reduce obstruction and improve symptoms.
- Surgery may be recommended to reduce the obstruction, if other treatments do not control the problem.
- Heart transplantation may be an option.
- Counseling may be helpful in adjusting to emotional effects of chronic illness.

POSSIBLE COMPLICATIONS
- Abnormal heart rhythms.
- Heart failure or stroke.
- Mitral valve problems.
- Sudden death.

PROBABLE OUTCOME—Many patients continue without symptoms for years (some may be over age 70). In others, symptoms may progress with age. Symptoms can often be controlled with treatment and life-style changes. Lifelong medical follow-up is needed.

HOW TO TREAT

GENERAL MEASURES
- Wear or carry medical ID to indicate you have this disorder.
- Don't smoke. Find a way to quit.
- Screening tests for HCM should be performed for close relatives of a patient with HCM.
- Family members should learn CPR (cardio-pulmonary resuscitation) in case of emergency.

MEDICATION
- Drugs to prevent heartbeat irregularities will be prescribed for most patients.
- Anticoagulant drugs may be prescribed.

ACTIVITY
- Instructions will be provided about how much physical activity is ideal. Your ability to increase activity is dependent on your individual situation.
- Avoid high-intensity competitive sports.

DIET
- Usually no special diet. A low-salt diet or reduced fluid intake may be recommended.
- Avoid alcohol.
- If overweight, losing weight can help heart function and lessen risks of surgery.

CALL YOUR DOCTOR IF

- You or a family member has symptoms of hypertrophic cardiomyopathy.
- New, unexplained symptoms develop.
- Family members need screening tests.

HYPOCHONDRIASIS

GENERAL INFORMATION

DEFINITION—Hypochondriasis is a disorder that causes a person to feel that he or she has a serious or fatal disease, even though there is no medical evidence of this. A person with the disorder may be aware and admit that the fear of having a serious disease is unfounded, excessive, or unreasonable.

BODY PARTS INVOLVED—Brain.

SEX OR AGE MOST AFFECTED—It occurs equally in men and women. It may begin at any age, but is most common in early adulthood.

SIGNS & SYMPTOMS
- Preoccupied for over 6 months with the fear of having a serious disease. There may be constant thought about the possibility of heart disease or cancer.
- Anxiety and reports of symptoms involving any body part. Symptoms may be vague or specific.
- Symptoms may change, but the person's belief that a serious condition exists does not.
- Person may have periods of hypochondriasis for months and years, and then go months and years without hypochondriasis.

CAUSES—The cause is uncertain. There may be childhood developmental factors or predisposing factors and others. Social position or education level or marital status do not appear to be risk factors.

RISK INCREASES WITH
- Some people may be more at risk:
  - Those who have anxiety disorder, depression, panic disorder, or other mental health conditions.
  - Having family members with hypochondriasis.
  - Had a serious illness or a form of abuse in childhood.
  - A belief that good health means no symptoms occur.
- Symptoms may be triggered by certain events:
  - Family member or others develop a serious disorder.
  - Death of a relative or close friend.
  - Periods of increased emotional stress.

HOW TO PREVENT—No specific measures known.

WHAT TO EXPECT

DIAGNOSTIC MEASURES
- Your health care provider will do a physical exam and ask questions about your symptoms.
- Medical tests may be done as needed. A mental (emotional) health exam may be done.

APPROPRIATE HEALTH CARE
- Your health care provider will assure you that the diagnosis of the symptoms shows there is no threat to life or risk of disability. Regular follow-up medical appointments may be scheduled for further assurance.
- Behavior therapy can help a patient understand what generates the symptoms and how to overcome worrisome thoughts.
- Interpersonal therapy can help a patient identify personal relationship problems and how to correct them.
- Group therapy can help some patients.
- Patients should depend on one health care provider for their treatment. Avoid going to different health care providers and having repeat medical tests.

POSSIBLE COMPLICATIONS
- Can affect all aspects of a person's life (e.g., work, social, and personal relationships).
- A real illness may be overlooked.
- Becoming dependent on pain relievers or sedatives.
- Patients tend to "doctor shop." They feel rejected if they aren't believed about the symptoms.
- Taking unneeded medical tests that are dangerous or could result in complications.

PROBABLE OUTCOME—Outcome varies. Some are helped with treatment, in others, the symptoms persist, and a few recover completely.

HOW TO TREAT

GENERAL MEASURES—Having the diagnosis of hypochondriasis is hard for anyone to accept. Feelings of anger, sadness, or frustration are normal. Education about the disorder for you and your family may help you cope. Your health care provider is the first source. Then learn what you can from books, researching on the Internet, or support groups.

MEDICATION
- Antidepressants may be prescribed for anxiety or depressive symptoms.
- Other drugs may be prescribed for symptoms such as mood disorders or stress.

ACTIVITY—Exercise daily. This can improve physical fitness as well as having a positive affect on mental health. It helps improve mood, reduce tension, and improve sleep.

DIET—Eat three regular, healthy meals daily. Avoid alcohol or caffeine.

CALL YOUR DOCTOR IF

You or a family member has symptoms of this disorder and wants help with the problem.

HYPOGLYCEMIA, REACTIVE

GENERAL INFORMATION

DEFINITION—Reactive hypoglycemia is a low level of blood sugar (glucose) in the body. It is usually a reaction to eating. It is not the type of hypoglycemia that diabetic patients often have.

BODY PARTS INVOLVED—Pancreas.

SEX OR AGE MOST AFFECTED—Both sexes; all ages.

SIGNS & SYMPTOMS
- Frequency and severity of symptoms vary.
- Headache.
- Nervousness or anxiety.
- Sweating.
- Dizziness.
- Fast heartbeat.
- Weakness or faintness.
- Fatigue.
- Shaking muscles.
- Hunger.
- More severe symptoms are less likely. They may include being forgetful, poor concentration, confusion, poor coordination, or slurred speech.

CAUSES—There is some debate about the actual cause. The amount of sugar (glucose) in the blood normally increases for one to two hours after a meal, especially a high-carbohydrate meal (sugars and starches). In some people, the rapid rise in blood sugar will cause a release of too much insulin, causing a rapid drop in the blood sugar. It will then rise back again to normal levels. Most of these people do not have any symptoms from the drop in glucose levels. In a few, the symptoms of hypoglycemia occur for unknown reasons.

RISK INCREASES WITH
- Improper diet.
- Obesity.
- Smoking, alcohol, stress, or other emotional or mental problems may contribute.

HOW TO PREVENT
- Follow instructions under Diet.
- Get treatment for emotional problems such as stress.
- Don't smoke.
- Don't drink alcohol.
- Recognize early symptoms and drink or eat something that contains sugar.

WHAT TO EXPECT

DIAGNOSTIC MEASURES
- Your health care provider may do a physical exam.
- Medical tests may include blood-sugar and glucose-tolerance studies to rule out other medical problems.

APPROPRIATE HEALTH C
- Treatment usually involves d
- Counseling or other therapy m learn to cope with stress or emotio

POSSIBLE COMPLICATIONS—No expected.

PROBABLE OUTCOME—The immedia symptoms usually clear up on their own (o glucose) in a very short period of time. A change in diet may help prevent symptoms fr occurring in the future.

HOW TO TREAT

GENERAL MEASURES—Short-term treatment during an episode can raise blood sugar more quickly. This includes drinking juice or eating candy to raise the glucose level. Take a protein food, such as milk or cheese, at the same time. This helps the body slowly absorb the glucose and avoid a "seesaw" effect of glucose levels.

MEDICATION—Drugs are not usually needed for treatment.

ACTIVITY—Regular exercise may improve blood-sugar control. It can help to reduce stress and build self-esteem. It helps to control and maintain an ideal weight. It also helps improve heart and lung function, lower blood pressure, improve blood circulation, and lower cholesterol levels.

DIET
- Eat several smaller meals a day that are low in simple carbohydrates, moderate in fats, and high in protein.
- Don't skip meals.
- Between-meal snacks should include protein, such as chicken, eggs, cheese, nuts, or skim milk, rather than carbohydrates.
- Avoid sugar and foods containing sugar (especially on an empty stomach).
- Weight-loss diet will help if being overweight is a problem.
- Limit or avoid alcohol.
- Avoid caffeine (coffee, tea, or soft drinks).

CALL YOUR DOCTOR IF

- You or a family member has symptoms of reactive hypoglycemia.
- Symptoms continue even with treatment.

...ORMATION

...m occurs
...produce
...PTH helps
..., and vitamin
...parathyroidism (an
...ore common disorder.

...S INVOLVED—Parathyroid glands
...sized glands located on the back and
...side of the thyroid gland); teeth; blood, which
affects all body tissues, especially the heart,
blood vessels, bones, kidneys, gastrointestinal
tract, central nervous system and skin.

SEX OR AGE MOST AFFECTED—Both sexes;
all ages. It affects children more than adults.

SIGNS & SYMPTOMS
• Symptoms are due to low calcium levels. A
decrease in PTH leads to low levels of calcium
in the blood (hypocalcemia).
• Tingling or burning (paresthesias) in fingertips,
toes, and lips. Twitching of the facial muscles.
• Muscle cramps or pain (legs, feet, abdomen,
or face).
• Muscle spasms called tetany (often around
the mouth, but also in hands, arms, and throat).
In the throat, they may interfere with breathing.
• Fatigue or weakness.
• Painful menstruation.
• Dry hair and patchy hair loss.
• Dry, coarse skin; brittle nails.
• Anxiety, nervousness, depression, mood
swings, or memory problems.
• Headaches.

CAUSES
• Most often, the cause is an injury to the
parathyroid glands during neck surgery.
Symptoms may begin days or up to years after
the surgery.
• There are other more rare causes and in some
cases, the parathyroids are absent from birth.

RISK INCREASES WITH
• Surgery on the parathyroid glands, the thyroid
glands, or other neck tissues.
• Autoimmune disorders.
• Rarely, radiation of the thyroid gland.
• Family history of parathyroid diseases.
• Low magnesium level in the body.

HOW TO PREVENT—No specific preventive
measures.

WHAT TO EXPECT

DIAGNOSTIC MEASURES
• Your own observation of symptoms.
• Your health care provider will do a physical
exam and ask questions about your symptoms
and surgery history.

• Medical tests include blood and urine studies.
An ECG (electrocardiogram—method of
diagnosing heart diseases), CT, and x-rays of
bones may be done.

APPROPRIATE HEALTH CARE
• Treatment typically involves vitamin D and
calcium supplements. Diet changes may be
recommended.
• If symptoms are severe, hospital care may be
needed for calcium injections for quick relief.

POSSIBLE COMPLICATIONS
• Overtreatment with calcium or vitamin D.
• Cataracts, seizures, heart problems, or kidney
stones.
• In children may lead to stunted growth,
malformed teeth, and slow mental development.

PROBABLE OUTCOME—With early diagnosis
and treatment, the outlook is good. It is a
chronic disorder, so lifelong treatment is
needed. In some cases, outcome depends on
underlying cause.

HOW TO TREAT

GENERAL MEASURES
• Get periodic medical tests to check calcium
levels in your blood. It is important to remember
to have these tests done on time. Get regular
eye exams.
• Wear or carry medical ID that shows you have
hypoparathyroidism.

MEDICATION
• Vitamin D and calcium supplements are
normally prescribed. A lifelong course of these
drugs is necessary.
• Intravenous (IV) calcium may be given for
severe muscle spasms.
• Other drugs for treating muscle spasms may
be prescribed.

ACTIVITY—No limits.

DIET—A high-calcium, low-phosphorus diet
may be helpful. Your health care provider will
advise you of special diet needs.

CALL YOUR DOCTOR IF

• You or a family member has
hypoparathyroidism symptoms.
• Symptoms do not improve with treatment.
• Illnesses that cause diarrhea occur or you are
unable to take prescribed supplements by
mouth.
• Severe symptoms develop (numbness,
tingling, cramping-spasms, especially of the
toes and fingers or mouth), seek emergency
care.

HYPOTHERMIA

GENERAL INFORMATION

DEFINITION
• Hypothermia is an abnormally low body temperature (normal is around 98.6°F [37°C]). It can occur indoors due to lack of heat, outside in cold weather, or from being in water.
  - Primary hypothermia occurs in healthy persons and is caused by exposure to cold and/or damp conditions.
  - Secondary hypothermia is due to a medical illness that affects the body's heat-balancing mechanisms. It can develop in milder cold and damp conditions.

BODY PARTS INVOLVED—All major organ systems, including decreased blood flow through the kidneys and brain.

SEX OR AGE MOST AFFECTED—Both sexes; all ages, but most common in adults over 60.

SIGNS & SYMPTOMS
• Symptoms can take several hours or even several days to develop.
• Poor muscle coordination.
• Cold hands, feet, and face; cold and pale skin.
• Shivering.
• Weakness; drowsiness.
• Mental confusion; disoriented; irritable attitude.
• Slurred speech.
• Slowed, shallow breathing and/or slow heart rate.
• Rigid muscles.
• Loss of consciousness.

CAUSES—More heat is lost than the body can generate. This starts affecting many different functions of the body.

RISK INCREASES WITH
• Adults over 60 or infants.
• Mentally impaired.
• Poorly heated homes.
• Outdoor work or activities in cold weather.
• Certain medical conditions.
• Homeless persons.
• Excess alcohol use or drug abuse.
• Malnutrition.

HOW TO PREVENT
• In cold weather, wear windproof clothing in many loose layers, including a scarf, hat, and mittens. If your clothes get wet, change clothes or dry them quickly.
• Avoid alcohol use if you are going out into the cold.
• If camping, walking, or hiking in a cold climate, carry emergency gear for use if stranded or injured. Travel with a partner.
• Be sure the home is heated adequately.

• Persons who are unable to care for themselves fully, such as the elderly, the mentally impaired, or the alcoholic, should be visited, supervised, or monitored during cold weather.

WHAT TO EXPECT

DIAGNOSTIC MEASURES—Diagnosis is done in the emergency care center. Medical tests are often needed to check for any complications.

APPROPRIATE HEALTH CARE—In the hospital or emergency center, the process of rewarming will be started. The patient will be treated until the temperature returns to normal.

POSSIBLE COMPLICATIONS—Many complications can occur depending on the patient's health and the length of the exposure to cold.

PROBABLE OUTCOME—The outcome is usually good if the patient is otherwise healthy and treatment is started quickly. Some children have been revived despite being in ice water for an hour or more.

HOW TO TREAT

GENERAL MEASURES
• Urgent medical care is needed. Transport to the nearest emergency center right away.
• The following may be helpful in taking care of someone while waiting for emergency care:
  - Remove cold, wet clothing. Keep the person lying down and cover them with a warm blanket. Use your own body heat to aid warming if needed.
  - If the person is outdoors, move them inside. If unable to do so, put a blanket under and over them. Cover the head, but not the face.
  - Do not rub or massage their skin. Do not use heating pad or electric blanket. Do not put person in hot bath.
  - Warm fluids may be given if the patient is able to swallow. Don't give the person any alcohol to drink.

MEDICATION—Drugs will be provided as needed for any complications.

ACTIVITY—After treatment, normal a[...] should be resumed gradually.

DIET—No special diet is neede[...]

CALL YOU[...]

You or a family me[...]
hypothermia or [...]
someone. Thi[...]

HYPOTHYROIDISM

 GENERAL INFORMATION

DEFINITION—Hypothyroidism means the thyroid gland is underactive and produces too little thyroid hormone. The thyroid is a small butterfly-shaped gland in the neck. Just about all chemical reactions in the body are affected by the thyroid hormone.

BODY PARTS INVOLVED—Thyroid gland and the endocrine system.

SEX OR AGE MOST AFFECTED—Adults of both sexes , but more common in women.

SIGNS & SYMPTOMS
- You will have some, but not all, of these symptoms.
- Feeling cold (especially hands and feet).
- Decrease in sweating.
- Dry, itchy skin; paleness.
- Loss of appetite, but a weight gain occurs.
- Constipation.
- Loss of energy, feeling tired or sluggish.
- Coarse, dry, brittle hair, or hair loss.
- Muscle aches.
- Blurred vision; hearing loss.
- Sleepiness or insomnia.
- Emotional or mental changes and mood swings.
- Puffy skin around the eyes.
- Decreased sex drive.
- Changes in menstrual cycle.
- Deepened or hoarse voice.

CAUSES—A variety of medical disorders or health problems can damage, inflame, enlarge, shrink, or otherwise affect the thyroid gland and cause it to be underactive.

RISK INCREASES WITH
- Autoimmune disorder (e.g., Hashimoto's thyroiditis). The body's immune system functions abnormally and attacks the thyroid gland.
- Treatment for hyperthyroidism (e.g., surgery, iodine).
- Drugs (e.g., lithium) that cause thyroid dysfunction.

 WHAT TO EXPECT

DIAGNOSTIC MEASURES
- Your own observation of symptoms.
- Your health care provider will do a physical exam and ask questions about your symptoms.
- Blood tests will be done for thyroid hormone and TSH (thyroid-stimulating hormone) levels.

APPROPRIATE HEALTH CARE
- Treatment for hypothyroidism involves restoring thyroid blood levels to normal with synthetic thyroid hormone.
- Rarely, hospital care may be needed if emergencies occur, such as myxedema coma.
- Pregnancy will require careful monitoring and additional thyroid replacement as the pregnancy advances.

POSSIBLE COMPLICATIONS
- Risk of infections, heart disease, and pituitary tumors.
- Infertility and risk of miscarriage in pregnant women.
- Myxedema coma (rare life-threatening complication).

PROBABLE OUTCOME—Normal thyroid levels can be achieved with treatment. Most people will need to take thyroid hormones for life.

 HOW TO TREAT

GENERAL MEASURES
- Follow-up is usually needed for several months to be sure of the correct dose of thyroid replacement. Then the follow-ups may be less frequent but still done on a regular basis.
- To learn more: American Thyroid Association; (800) 849-7643; website: www.thyroid.org.

MEDICATION—Thyroid hormone replacement is often prescribed. Dosage will depend on age, weight, capacity of thyroid function, other drugs you take, and intestinal function.

ACTIVITY—No limits. Stay as active as possible.

DIET—No special diet for hypothyroidism. Avoid constipation by eating a high-fiber diet. A weight-loss diet is recommended if you are overweight.

 CALL YOUR DOCTOR IF

- You or a family member has symptoms of hypothyroidism.
- Symptoms don't improve after 3 weeks of treatment, or new, unexplained symptoms develop.
- Coma or seizures occur. Call for emergency help immediately!

IMMUNODEFICIENCY DISEASE

 GENERAL INFORMATION

DEFINITION
• Immunodeficiency disease involves defects in the body's immune system. This means a person is more likely to develop infections. A healthy immune system protects the body against germs (bacteria, viruses, and fungi), cancer (partial protection), and any foreign material that enters the body.
- Primary immunodeficiency is most often inherited. Nearly 100 forms have been recognized (from mild to severe). One form is common variable immunodeficiency (CVID). A rare form is severe combined immune deficiency (SCID).
- Secondary immunodeficiency is acquired. It occurs in persons who previously had a normal immune system. Note: AIDS (acquired immuno-deficiency syndrome) is not discussed here.

BODY PARTS INVOLVED—Immune system (blood, bone marrow, lymph tissue, liver, spleen and thymus gland).

SEX OR AGE MOST AFFECTED—Both sexes; all ages.

SIGNS & SYMPTOMS
• Repeated, severe, and hard to cure infections, illnesses, and other health problems.
- Ear infections (otitis media), and sinus or other respiratory infections, such as pneumonia. Yeast infections, such as candidiasis, and eczema (a skin disorder).
- Cancer, especially leukemia and lymphoma.
- Bleeding disorders.
- Other immune disorders (anemia, arthritis).
- Meningitis or encephalitis (brain infections).
- Heart, digestive, or nervous system disorders.

CAUSES
• Primary: Being born with a faulty immune system is the main cause. One or more or all of the essential parts of the immune system are missing due to a genetic defect.
• Secondary: Caused by diseases or other health problems that affect the immune system.

RISK INCREASES WITH
• Surgical removal of the spleen.
• Use of drugs that suppress immune system.
• Radiation treatment or severe burns.
• Some cancers, such as leukemia.
• Viral infections, such as measles or influenza.
• Malnutrition (severe nutrient deficiency).
• Blood transfusion or intravenous (IV) drug use.
• Family history of immunodeficiency disease.

HOW TO PREVENT
• No preventive measures for primary type. If you have a family history, get genetic counseling before starting a family.
• Prevention of secondary type may or may not be possible. It depends on the cause.

 WHAT TO EXPECT

DIAGNOSTIC MEASURES
• Your own observation of symptoms, especially repeated infections in children.
• Your health care provider will do a physical exam.
• Medical tests may include blood studies of antibodies, microscopic exams of blood and tissue cells, skin tests, chest x-rays of the thymus gland, and radioactive studies of immune function.

APPROPRIATE HEALTH CARE
• Specific treatment will depend on the type of immune deficiency. General treatment involves preventing and treating infections. Your health care provider will discuss your individual treatment steps.
• Surgery to transplant bone marrow or the thymus gland may be recommended.
• Hospital care for treatment of serious infection may be required.

POSSIBLE COMPLICATIONS
• Infections and other diseases that may not respond to treatment.
• Complications can occur due to specific deficiency.

PROBABLE OUTCOME—Primary type patients can have near normal life if diagnosed early and infections treated properly. For secondary type patients, it depends on under-lying cause, but treatment improves outlook.

 HOW TO TREAT

GENERAL MEASURES
• Avoid exposure to persons with infections. Don't get any type of vaccine without medical advice. Wear or carry medical ID that shows you have this condition and any drugs you take.
• To learn more: Immune Deficiency Foundation, 40 W. Chesapeake Ave., Suite 308, Towson, MD 21204; (800) 296-4433; website: www.primaryimmune.org.

MEDICATION—Antibiotics for infection, transfusion of blood components, and gamma globulin injections may be prescribed.

ACTIVITY—Activity will depend on the type of deficiency. A risk of bleeding may limit activities.

DIET—Eat a healthy diet.

 CALL YOUR DOCTOR IF

• You or a family member has symptoms of immunodeficiency disease.
• After diagnosis, signs of infection or illness or injury, or unexplained symptoms occur.

IMPETIGO
(Pyoderma)

GENERAL INFORMATION

DEFINITION—Impetigo is a very common and highly contagious bacterial skin infection. The two forms of impetigo are called bullous (less common) and nonbullous.

BODY PARTS INVOLVED—It usually involves the skin of the face (often around the mouth and nose), arms, and legs.

SEX OR AGE MOST AFFECTED—Both sexes; all ages, but most common in infants and children.

SIGNS & SYMPTOMS
- Small red sores that change to blisters. Some blisters contain pus, and yellow-brown crusts form when they break. The blisters don't hurt, but they may itch.
- Slight fever (sometimes).

CAUSES—*Staphylococcus aureus* or *streptococcus pyogenes* (or both) bacteria growing in the upper skin layers. It is usually spread from person to person, or from germs on something an infected person has touched. The time from exposure to the germs and the start of symptoms is 1 to 3 days. Person is contagious when the rash is crusting or oozing pus.

RISK INCREASES WITH
- Contact with an infected person.
- Skin that is sensitive to sun and irritants, such as soap and makeup.
- Other skin problems, such as bites, burns, infections, sores, or injuries.
- Poor general health.
- Warm, moist weather.
- Children in daycare.
- Poor hygiene.

HOW TO PREVENT
- Can't always be prevented.
- Avoid contact with an infected person.
- Maintain good general health and good hygiene.

WHAT TO EXPECT

DIAGNOSTIC MEASURES
- Your own observation of symptoms.
- Your health care provider can diagnose impetigo by an exam of the infected skin.
- Medical skin tests are usually not needed.

APPROPRIATE HEALTH CARE—Treatment is with drugs used for bacterial infection.

POSSIBLE COMPLICATIONS
- Can rarely lead to other skin conditions and scarring.
- Kidney disorder (rare).

PROBABLE OUTCOME—It can clear up on its own, but your health care provider may recommend treatment to help prevent any complications. It may recur in young children.

HOW TO TREAT

GENERAL MEASURES
- Self-care steps include:
  - Wash sores with gauze using soap and water and pat dry. If crusts are difficult to remove, soak them in warm, soapy water and scrub gently.
  - Cover impetigo sores with gauze and tape to keep hands away from them.
  - Keep fingernails short. Don't scratch the blisters. Scratching can spread infection to other parts of the body.
  - If there is an outbreak in the family, urge all members to wash hands often with antibacterial soap. Antibacterial wipes may be used.
  - Do not share towels, washcloths, sheets, pillows, clothes, or toys with an infected person. Wash items in hot water before using them again.
  - Men should shave around sores on the face, not over them. Use an aerosol shaving cream and change razor blades each day. Don't use a shaving brush; it may have germs on it. Don't share razors with other people.

MEDICATION
- An antibiotic ointment or cream is usually prescribed.
- Oral antibiotics may be prescribed.

ACTIVITY—No limits. Children can return to school or daycare as soon as they are not contagious.

DIET—No special diet.

CALL YOUR DOCTOR IF

- You or your child has symptoms of impetigo.
- Fever occurs.
- Sores continue or don't begin to heal in 3 days, despite treatment.

INCONTINENCE, FECAL

GENERAL INFORMATION

DEFINITION—Fecal incontinence is the loss of bowel control. It can be due to several problems. Bowel control requires normal function of the rectum, anus, and nervous system. Bowel control also requires that a person be mentally alert and physically able to get to a bathroom. It greatly affects a person's quality of life. They won't leave home in fear of an accident. They avoid talking about the problem with their health care provider. Urinary incontinence (lack of bladder control) often occurs along with fecal incontinence.

BODY PARTS INVOLVED—Rectum, anus, and nervous system.

SEX OR AGE MOST AFFECTED—It can affect anyone over age four. It occurs more often in older adults and women.

SIGNS & SYMPTOMS
• Unable to control the passage of gas or stool.
• It can range from an occasional stool leakage to a complete loss of bowel control.
• Cramping, bloating, constipation, or diarrhea.

CAUSES
• The muscles of the anus (called sphincters) can become weak or damaged.
• Nerves in the anus or rectum are damaged.
• The rectum loses its ability to hold stool.
• Weakness of the pelvic floor muscles that hold the rectum in place.

RISK INCREASES WITH
• Older adults; females more than males.
• Obesity and/or lack of physical activity.
• Childbirth; episiotomy
• Muscle or nerve injury; pelvic surgery or radiation.
• Diabetes, fecal impaction, irritable bowel syndrome, inflammatory bowel disease, constipation, or diarrhea.
• Physical disability (e.g., bedridden) or cognitive disorder (e.g., stroke, dementia, or Alzheimer's disease).
• Chronic laxative use. Use of certain weight loss drugs.

HOW TO PREVENT
• Cannot always be prevented. Get medical care for treatable risk factors. Maintain healthy weight. Exercise regularly.
• Avoid episiotomy during childbirth if possible. After giving birth, pelvic floor muscle training and biofeedback may help prevent future problems.
• Avoid routine use of laxatives.

WHAT TO EXPECT

DIAGNOSTIC MEASURES
• Your own observation of symptoms.

• Your health care provider may do a physical exam of the anal area. A pin or probe can be used to check for nerve damage. A digital rectal exam (inserting a finger into the rectum) checks for muscle strength. Questions will be asked about your symptoms, diet, and activities.
• Medical tests may include ultrasound, nerve and muscle studies, sigmoidoscopy, or others.

APPROPRIATE HEALTH CARE
• Treatment depends on the cause, how severe the symptoms are, and the patient's physical and mental health. Steps may include treating an underlying cause, diet changes, drugs, bowel training, biofeedback, surgery, or other specific therapy.
• Bowel training can involve strengthening muscles or training the bowels to empty at a specific time of day.
• Biofeedback is a type of behavior change therapy. It helps you learn to control bodily functions.
• Surgery to repair sphincter muscles may be an option.
• Other types of treatment may be discussed. They can include injections in the anus, anal plugs, nerve stimulation, an artificial bowel sphincter, surgical procedures, or other therapy.

POSSIBLE COMPLICATIONS
• Embarrassment and shame. Avoiding social activities.
• Surgical treatment may lead to complications.
• Irritated skin around the anus.

PROBABLE OUTCOME—Simple treatment measures help many patients improve bowel function and restore their quality of life. Surgery helps symptoms in others, but may fail with time.

HOW TO TREAT

GENERAL MEASURES—Wear disposable underwear or pads if needed.

MEDICATION
• Drugs may be prescribed for diarrhea or constipation.
• Fiber supplements may be recommended.
• Protective creams can prevent skin irritation.

ACTIVITY—No limits. Pelvic floor muscle exercises (called Kegel) may be prescribed.

DIET
• Eat several, small meals each day. Eat more high fiber foods. Eat and drink at different times.
• Keep a food diary to see if foods are a cause.

CALL YOUR DOCTOR IF

• You or a family member has symptoms of fecal incontinence.
• Symptoms don't improve with treatment.

INCONTINENCE, STRESS

GENERAL INFORMATION

DEFINITION—Stress incontinence is the involuntary leaking of urine that occurs with sudden increased pressure on the bladder. It is a very common problem.

BODY PARTS INVOLVED—Kidneys and urinary system.

SEX OR AGE MOST AFFECTED—It can affect both sexes (males rarely) and all ages. It is most common in older women.

SIGNS & SYMPTOMS—Leaking of urine. This may happen with lifting, sneezing, singing, coughing, laughing, exercising, sports activity, crying, or straining to have a bowel movement. It may also occur with small movements such as rolling over in bed or standing up from a sitting position.

CAUSES—It is usually due to pelvic floor muscle or sphincter muscle problems. Pelvic floor muscles support the bladder. Sphincter muscles keep the opening of the bladder closed until it is time to urinate, and then they relax. When these muscles become weak or don't function properly, urine can leak out from the bladder.

RISK INCREASES WITH
- Older adults; females; pregnancy and childbirth.
- Obesity.
- Surgery or radiation of the genitals or urinary tract.
- Chronic cough (may be due to smoking) or asthma.
- Prostate problems in men.

HOW TO PREVENT
- There are no specific preventive measures. To reduce your risks: maintain a healthy weight, exercise daily, don't smoke, and limit alcohol and caffeine intake. Get medical check up to detect early problems.
- Strengthen pelvic floor muscles with Kegel exercises.
  - First step is to identify pelvic floor muscles. When urinating, stop the flow by squeezing the pelvic floor muscles. Another way is to insert a finger into vagina (women) or rectum (men), then tighten the muscles around the finger. Repeat each method until you are sure you can feel which muscles are involved.
  - The exercises can be done any time and any place, lying down or sitting up. Start by emptying the bladder.
  - Tighten the pelvic floor muscles and hold for a count of 10.
  - Relax the muscles completely for a count of 10.
  - Perform 10 exercises, 3 times a day (morning, afternoon, and night). Don't do more than this.
  - It may take 6 weeks to 3 months for improvement.

WHAT TO EXPECT

DIAGNOSTIC MEASURES
- Your health care provider will do a physical exam and ask questions about your symptoms.
- Medical tests of blood and urine may be done to check for other conditions. Additional tests may be done to help diagnose specific urinary-tract problems. You may be asked to keep a diary about your urination patterns.

APPROPRIATE HEALTH CARE
- Treatment may involve weight loss, stopping smoking, suppressing cough, Kegel exercises, drugs, pessary, other therapy, or surgery.
- Other therapies include biofeedback, electrical stimulation, bladder training, magnetic innervation, or special weights to strengthen pelvic muscles. These options will be explained.
- A pessary (support device) to fit inside the vagina to support the uterus is helpful for some women. Other types of devices include urethral plugging or stenting.
- If other methods fail, surgery to tighten relaxed or damaged muscles that support the bladder helps some. Even with surgery, some leakage may continue.

POSSIBLE COMPLICATIONS—Medical problems are rare. It can affect quality of life.

PROBABLE OUTCOME—Kegel exercises can be effective for mild stress incontinence. With more severe incontinence, other treatment steps can help improve symptoms.

HOW TO TREAT

GENERAL MEASURES
- Learn and practice Kegel exercises. Try to use the squeezing technique just before any sneeze or a cough.
- Try to schedule toilet trips.
- Wear special underwear or incontinence pad.
- To learn more: National Association for Continence; (800) 252-3337; website: www.nafc.org.

MEDICATION
- Drugs to help sphincter muscles may be prescribed.
- Estrogen therapy may be prescribed.

ACTIVITY—No limits. Exercise daily for health.

DIET—Start a weight loss diet if overweight. No need to limit fluid intake unless advised.

CALL YOUR DOCTOR IF

- You or a family member has symptoms of stress incontinence.
- Symptoms don't improve with treatment.

INCONTINENCE, URGE

GENERAL INFORMATION

DEFINITION—Urge incontinence involves a need or urge to urinate followed by an involuntary loss of urine. The condition may be referred to as overactive bladder.

BODY PARTS INVOLVED—Kidneys and urinary system.

SEX OR AGE MOST AFFECTED—Both sexes, more common in older women.

SIGNS & SYMPTOMS
• Loss of urine right after feeling an urge to urinate. It may be a few drops to complete bladder emptying. It may occur with sudden change in position or activity, hearing or touching running water, drinking a small amount of liquid, and during sleep.
• Key-in-lock syndrome may occur. This happens when you rush home, put a key in the door lock, and experience a sudden bladder contraction and urine leakage.

CAUSES—The usual cause is a spasm or contraction of the bladder muscle. It squeezes at the wrong time, earlier than it should, and causes the leakage. The spasm may result from bladder nerve damage, other nerve problem, or problem of the bladder muscles. The bladder may be described as spastic, overactive, or unstable.

RISK INCREASES WITH
• Repeated vaginal childbirth.
• Adults over 60. Women more than men.
• Hormonal change in women after menopause.
• Obesity.
• Surgery or radiation of genitals or urinary tract.
• Urinary-tract infection, stone, cancer, or obstruction; prostate problems in men.
• Some neurological (nervous system) disorders.

HOW TO PREVENT
• There are no specific preventive measures. To reduce your risks: maintain a healthy weight, exercise daily, don't smoke, and limit alcohol.
• Do Kegel exercises to strengthen pelvic floor muscles:
  - First step is to identify pelvic floor muscles. When urinating, stop the flow by squeezing the pelvic floor muscles. Another way is to insert a finger into vagina (women) or rectum (men), then tighten the muscles around the finger. Repeat each method until you are sure you can feel which muscles are involved.
  - The exercises can be done any time and any place, lying down or sitting up. Start by emptying the bladder.
  - Tighten the pelvic floor muscles and hold for a count of 10.
  - Relax the muscles completely for a count of 10.
  - Perform 10 exercises, 3 times a day (morning, afternoon, and night). Don't do more than this.
  - It may take 6 weeks to 3 months for results.

WHAT TO EXPECT

DIAGNOSTIC MEASURES
• Your health care provider will do a physical exam and ask questions about your symptoms.
• Medical tests of blood and urine may be done to check for other conditions. Additional tests may be done to help diagnose specific urinary-tract problems. You may be asked to keep a diary about your urination patterns.

APPROPRIATE HEALTH CARE
• Treatment may involve drugs for bladder spasms or infection, weight loss, smoking cessation, Kegel exercises, pessary, other types of therapy, or surgery.
• Therapies include bladder training, electrical stimulation, biofeedback, magnetic innervation, or special weights to strengthen pelvic muscles.
• Learn and practice Kegel exercises. Try to use the squeezing technique just before any activity that brings on the urinary urge (running water or drinking water).
• A pessary (support device) to fit inside the vagina to support the uterus or other devices including urethral plugging or stenting may help.
• If other methods fail, surgery helps some. Even with surgery, some leakage may continue.

POSSIBLE COMPLICATIONS—Medical problems are rare. It can affect quality of life.

PROBABLE OUTCOME—Treatment can help reduce symptoms.

HOW TO TREAT

GENERAL MEASURES
• Have quick access to a toilet. Urinate on schedule. Learn and practice Kegel exercises.
• Wear special underwear or incontinence pad.
• To learn more: National Association for Continence; (800) 252-3337; website: www.nafc.org.

MEDICATION
• Drugs to control bladder spasms may be prescribed.
• Estrogen therapy may be prescribed for women.
• Drugs for infection if needed.

ACTIVITY—No limits. Exercise daily for health.

DIET
• Start a weight-loss diet if overweight.
• No need to limit fluid intake unless advised.

☎ CALL YOUR DOCTOR IF

• You or a family member has symptoms of urge incontinence.
• Symptoms don't improve with treatment.

INDIGESTION
(Dyspepsia)

GENERAL INFORMATION

DEFINITION—Indigestion is the term used to describe pain or discomfort in the upper abdomen or chest usually following meals. The medical term is dyspepsia. Almost everyone will experience indigestion at one time or another. Some people have it every day, others may have it occasionally.

BODY PARTS INVOLVED—Stomach; esophagus; small intestine.

SEX OR AGE MOST AFFECTED—Both sexes; all ages.

SIGNS & SYMPTOMS
- Bloated or full feeling after eating.
- Upper abdomen pain, discomfort, or burning.
- Stomach feels full soon after starting a meal.
- Mild nausea or upset stomach.
- Gas or belching.
- Acid taste in the mouth; may have bad breath.

CAUSES—It may be due to a specific medical disorder. In many cases, the exact cause is unclear. This is often referred to as functional dyspepsia. It may involve problems of the muscles and nerves of the digestive system, infection, or psychological and social factors.

RISK INCREASES WITH
- Peptic ulcer disease.
- Gastrointestinal reflux disease (GERD).
- Esophagitis (inflammation of esophagus).
- *Helicobacter pylori* (a bacteria infection).
- Other, less common medical causes.
- Some drugs tend to cause indigestion:
  - Nonsteroidal anti-inflammatories (such as aspirin or ibuprofen).
  - Antibiotics, iron supplements, steroids, bisphosphonates (for bone loss), and others.
- Triggers that cause symptoms in some people:
  - Eating too much and eating too quickly.
  - Eating food with a high fat content, spicy foods, or gas-forming foods (e.g., beans).
  - Smoking.
  - Alcohol, carbonated drinks, or caffeine.
  - Stress or anxiety or other emotional problem.
  - Swallowing too much air when chewing.

HOW TO PREVENT—Avoid risk factors where possible.

WHAT TO EXPECT

DIAGNOSTIC MEASURES
- If symptoms persist or cause concern, see your health care provider. A physical exam may be done and questions asked about symptoms.
- Medical tests may include breath, blood and stool studies; x-rays; and others as needed.

APPROPRIATE HEALTH CARE
- Many people will self-treat this disorder.
- Medical care may include drug therapy or other treatment for an underlying condition.

POSSIBLE COMPLICATIONS—Usually does not cause complications. It can be a symptom of another disorder that could be more serious.

PROBABLE OUTCOME—Symptoms can often be helped with treatment, but they may recur. Treatment of an underlying disorder can improve or even cure indigestion.

HOW TO TREAT

GENERAL MEASURES
- Don't smoke. Find a way to quit.
- Relax after meals, but don't lie down.
- Find ways to control stress or anxiety in your life. Try relaxation techniques or other types of therapy. Ask your health care provider for advice.
- Avoid things that make you swallow air, such as chewing gum or drinking carbonated drinks.

MEDICATION
- You may use nonprescription antacids to neutralize the stomach acid. Use H2 antagonists (such as cimetidine or ranitidine) or proton pump inhibitors (such as omeprazole) to reduce stomach acid.
- Other types of drugs may be prescribed if needed for symptoms or underlying condition.
- Avoid nonsteroidal anti-inflammatory drugs or other drugs that may cause symptoms. Ask your health care provider about options.

ACTIVITY—Do get enough rest. Daily exercise (such as 30 minute walk) helps promote good health. Don't exercise right after a meal or just before bedtime.

DIET
- Eat small meals. Don't eat near bedtime.
- Avoid foods that cause discomfort.
- Eat slowly. Chew food carefully and entirely.
- Try avoiding alcohol, caffeine, or carbonated drinks for a while to see if symptoms improve.
- Losing weight if overweight may help improve symptoms.

CALL YOUR DOCTOR IF

- You or a family member has symptoms of indigestion that persist, are severe, or cause concern.
- Other symptoms occur along with indigestion, such as chest pain, shortness of breath, rapid weight loss, bloody vomit or stools, or trouble with swallowing.

INFLUENZA (Flu)

GENERAL INFORMATION

DEFINITION—Influenza (flu) is a contagious infection caused by a virus that affects the nose, throat, and lungs. The two main flu virus types are called A and B. Each type has different strains that tend to change each year. Flu outbreaks occur in the late fall and winter with varying degrees of severity. An outbreak may be epidemic (occurs in a set geographic area) or pandemic (occurs worldwide).

BODY PARTS INVOLVED—Upper-respiratory system.

SEX OR AGE MOST AFFECTED—Both sexes; all ages.

SIGNS & SYMPTOMS
- Moderate-to-high fever and chills.
- Headache; joint or muscle aches.
- Sore throat; dry cough; runny or stuffy nose.
- Skin may feel warm or hot.
- Fatigue and weakness; vomiting or diarrhea.

CAUSES—The flu virus germs are spread when an infected person coughs, sneezes, or speaks. The germs get into the air, and nearby persons breathe them in. It is also spread by touching a surface that has the virus germs on it and then touching your nose, mouth, or eyes. Symptoms start 1 to 5 days after exposure. Adults are contagious 1 day before symptoms and up to 7 days after getting sick. Children may be contagious for more than 7 days.

RISK INCREASES WITH
- Schools and day care centers.
- Infants, children, elderly, and pregnant women.
- Nursing homes or long-term care centers.
- Chronic heart or lung disease, or diabetes.
- Weak immune system due to illness or drugs.
- Health care workers.

HOW TO PREVENT
- Have a yearly influenza vaccine injection or a nasal spray flu vaccine. A different vaccine is made every year because strains of the virus change from year to year. Sometimes, an unpredicted new strain appears and you may still get the flu, but it is usually a milder case.
- Some antiviral drugs may help prevent flu.
- Wash hands often to prevent the spread of germs or use alcohol-based hand cleaner. Avoid crowds. Get medical advice about the use of a facemask/respirator.
- Follow guidelines set by public health officials.

WHAT TO EXPECT

DIAGNOSTIC MEASURES
- Call your health care provider about your symptoms and if you need to be seen at an office visit.

- Your health care provider may do a physical exam. A diagnosis of flu can usually be made based on the symptoms.
- Medical tests may be done to verify the flu type or check for complications.

APPROPRIATE HEALTH CARE
- Many people who get the flu can use self-care methods at home.
- Treatment steps include getting extra rest, drinking plenty of fluids, flu remedies, or prescribed drugs.

POSSIBLE COMPLICATIONS—Pneumonia, kidney failure, swelling of the brain, and death. In children, sinus problems or ear infections.

PROBABLE OUTCOME—Most people who get the flu get better in a week. A cough or tired feeling may last a little longer. Elderly persons, young children, pregnant women, and people with chronic illness are more at risk for complications.

HOW TO TREAT

GENERAL MEASURES
- For nasal congestion, use salt-water drops in the nose. Mix one-quarter teaspoon of salt in four ounces of water.
- To help a sore throat, gargle often with warm or cold double-strength tea or salt water (mix one-half teaspoon of salt in one cup of water).
- Use a cool-mist humidifier (if advised).
- Don't smoke. Avoid second-hand smoke.
- Avoid spreading germs. Cover your mouth and nose when you cough. Use a tissue and then throw it into the trash. Avoid close contact with others if possible. All household members should wash their hands often with soap and water or use alcohol-based hand cleaner.

MEDICATION
- Use nonprescription drugs, such as acetaminophen, ibuprofen, cough syrups, decongestants, or nasal sprays for specific symptoms. Do not give aspirin to children under age 18. Consult your health care provider about giving drugs to a child age 6 or younger.
- Antiviral drugs may be prescribed.

ACTIVITY—Get extra rest. Wait 7 days after symptoms begin (or 24 hours after symptoms clear up) before going back to work or school.

DIET—You may just want liquids at first. Then progress to small meals of bland starchy foods.

CALL YOUR DOCTOR IF

- You or a family member has symptoms of influenza that seem severe or cause concern.
- Symptoms don't improve, get worse, or new symptoms develop.

INFLUENZA, H1N1

 ## GENERAL INFORMATION

DEFINITION—H1N1 influenza (sometimes referred to as swine flu) is a respiratory infection caused by a virus. it first appeared in 2009.

BODY PARTS INVOLVED—Upper-respiratory system.

SEX OR AGE MOST AFFECTED—Any age, but occurs more often in people under age 25. People over age 64 are less often affected.

SIGNS & SYMPTOMS
- Fever, cough, and sore throat.
- Runny or stuffy nose.
- Body aches and headache.
- Chills and fatigue.
- Diarrhea and vomiting (sometimes).

CAUSES—An influenza A virus (H1N1). Virus germs are easily spread when an infected person coughs or sneezes and a nearby person breathes in the germs. Infection can also be spread by touching something (such as a surface or object) with germs on it and then touching your mouth, nose, or eyes. Infected people shed virus germs and may infect others from 1 to 2 days before symptoms appear and up to 7 to 10 days after becoming ill.

RISK INCREASES WITH
- Exposure to an infected person.
- Ages 5 to 25.

HOW TO PREVENT
- Get flu vaccine that protects against H1N1.
- Wash hands often with soap and water. Alcohol-based hand cleaners are also effective. Avoid touching your eyes, nose, or mouth. Germs spread this way.
- Try to avoid close contact with sick people.
- If you are sick with flu-like illness, keep away from others as much as possible. Cover your nose and mouth with a tissue when you cough or sneeze, throw tissue in the trash, and then wash your hands. If no tissue is available, cough into your elbow. Stay home until well.
- Virus germs may survive for 2 to 8 hours on objects and surfaces. Clean with chlorine, hydrogen peroxide, or detergents.
- A facemask may help an infected person or their caregiver from spreading germs to others.

 ## WHAT TO EXPECT

DIAGNOSTIC MEASURES
- If the symptoms are more severe or you or your child is at risk for complications, consult your health care provider.
- Your health care provider may do a physical exam and ask questions about symptoms and exposure to infected persons. Nasal and throat swabs may be taken for a lab test.

APPROPRIATE HEALTH CARE
- Many people who get the flu can use self-care methods at home.
- Medical treatment may include drug therapy and supportive care. Hospital care may be needed for certain persons with more severe symptoms.

POSSIBLE COMPLICATIONS
- Severe complications will vary. They may affect the lungs, heart, brain, muscles, and other body systems.
- Underlying chronic medical conditions may worsen.
- People at risk for serious flu complications (age 65 and older, children under age 5, pregnant women, and people with certain chronic medical conditions).

PROBABLE OUTCOME—Most people who become ill with this virus recover completely in about 7 to 10 days without medical treatment.

 ## HOW TO TREAT

GENERAL MEASURES—Most people with mild symptoms will treat the illness at home. Treatment involves getting extra rest and maintaining fluid intake. Drugs are seldom needed. Follow suggestions in How to Prevent to limit spreading germs. As a precaution, you may want to contact your (or your child's) health care provider to be sure no additional treatment is needed.

MEDICATION
- Antiviral drugs (pills, liquid, inhaled powder, or injected) may be prescribed or given in a hospital. They can be used for treatment and prevention. Antiviral drugs work best for treatment if taken within 2 days of getting sick.
- Drugs for fever, coughing, or specific symptoms may be recommended by your health care provider.

ACTIVITY
- Get extra rest while symptoms are present. Resume normal activities gradually after recovery.
- It is recommended that flu-infected persons stay home until 24 hours after the fever and cough are gone.

DIET—Drink plenty of fluids while ill. Eating pork will not give anyone this infection.

 ## CALL YOUR DOCTOR IF

- You or a family member has symptoms of influenza that seem severe or cause concern.
- Symptoms don't improve, get worse, or new symptoms develop.

INSECT BITES & STINGS

GENERAL INFORMATION

DEFINITION—Insect bites and stings are usually harmless and cause mild symptoms. Less often, they cause serious reactions or infections. Bites or stings can come from insects (having 6 legs), such as mosquitoes, fleas, chiggers, bedbugs, ants, bees, wasps, hornets, or from arachnids (having 8 legs), such as spiders and scorpions.

BODY PARTS INVOLVED—Skin on any part of the body.

SEX OR AGE MOST AFFECTED—Both sexes; all ages.

SIGNS & SYMPTOMS
- Redness, swelling, spots, or lumps on the skin. These symptoms may occur within minutes or be delayed.
- Pain, such as from bee stings.
- Itching, such as from mosquitoes or fleas.
- May feel a burning, tingling, or numbness.
- Rare, severe allergic reaction includes facial swelling, red blotches, wheezing, or shortness of breath.

CAUSES—The symptoms are caused by the body's immune system response to the bite or sting. The response may be immediate or delayed (usually occurs within 48 hours). Stings are most often the cause of allergic reactions. Bites rarely cause an allergic reaction, but can lead to other disorders, such as malaria or Lyme disease. Certain bites or stings (e.g., brown recluse spider bites) carry a toxin that can cause serious complications.

RISK INCREASES WITH
- Areas with heavy insect infestations.
- Warm weather in spring and summer.
- Lack of protective measures.
- Wearing perfumes or colognes.

HOW TO PREVENT
- Apply insect repellent with diethyltoluamide (DEET) to the skin.
- Wear protective clothing. Apply permethrin to clothing to repel insects and ticks.
- Keep yards free of standing water. Use tight-fitting door and window screens.

WHAT TO EXPECT

DIAGNOSTIC MEASURES
- Your own observation of symptoms.
- See your health care provider if any symptoms cause you concern.

APPROPRIATE HEALTH CARE—For severe reactions to a bite or sting, get emergency help right away. They can be life-threatening.

POSSIBLE COMPLICATIONS
- A bacterial infection at the site of the bite.
- Anaphylaxis (life-threatening allergic reaction) for certain super-sensitive persons.
- Scarring on the skin.
- Disorders carried by certain insects. These include Lyme disease, Rocky Mountain spotted fever, West Nile virus, malaria, and others.

PROBABLE OUTCOME—Most of the symptoms are mild and go away in 2 to 3 days. Scratching may occur for several weeks. Treatment helps, but it doesn't cure quickly.

HOW TO TREAT

GENERAL MEASURES
- Self-care is often all that is needed for most bites and stings. For severe reaction, get medical help right away.
- Remove stinger. Scrape it out. Don't use tweezers.
- For bee, wasp, yellow-jacket, or hornet stings, rub a paste of meat tenderizer and water on site.
- For ant bites rub the bite with ammonia; repeat as often as necessary.
- For spider or scorpion bites, capture the insect, if possible, and seek medical help.
- For a tick, use a tweezer to remove it. Put it in a jar with alcohol to kill it. Save it in case more medical problems develop.
- Clean the wound. Apply an ice pack.
- Elevate and rest the affected body part.
- Warm-water soaks help soothe minor pain. Cool-water soaks feel better for itching.
- If you have had a severe allergic reaction following an insect sting, carry a special kit to treat it in the future.

MEDICATION
- Use nonprescription products:
  - Topical and oral antihistamines, calamine lotion, or topical anesthetics for itching or pain
  - Topical steroid drugs to reduce redness, soreness, and itching.
- For serious symptoms, you may be prescribed:
  - Stronger topical steroids or oral steroids.
  - Drug injection to treat/prevent anaphylaxis.
- A tetanus shot, if needed, for some patients.

ACTIVITY—No limits.

DIET—No special diet.

CALL YOUR DOCTOR IF

- You or a family member has an insect bite or sting and has a severe reaction. This is an emergency!
- Symptoms don't improve after 2 to 3 days of treatment or new symptoms develop.

INSOMNIA

GENERAL INFORMATION

DEFINITION—Insomnia involves problems falling asleep, staying asleep, waking early, or a combination of these. Insomnia is often described by how long it has gone on. Transient is a few days, short-term is less than 3 weeks, and chronic is more than 3 weeks.

BODY PARTS INVOLVED—Whole body.

SEX OR AGE MOST AFFECTED—Both sexes; all ages; more often in older adults and women.

SIGNS & SYMPTOMS
- Difficulty falling asleep.
- Brief period of sleep followed by wakefulness.
- Normal sleep until very early in the morning, then wakefulness (often with frightening thoughts).
- Daytime fatigue, tiredness, and sleepiness.
- Lack of sleep causes problems with social, work, family, and other areas of one's life.

CAUSES—Physical, mental, biological, and environmental factors are involved. Insomnia can be primary (not due to other health problem) or secondary (is due to other health problem). Short term and transient insomnia often result from reaction to life changes or stresses.

RISK INCREASES WITH
- Older adults and women more than men.
- Chronic medical disorder (e.g., those causing pain, shortness of breath, nerve problem, reflux).
- Mood or mental health disorder (e.g., anxiety, depression, bipolar disorder, or schizophrenia).
- Odd work hours, such as swing shifts.
- Sleep disorders (e.g., restless leg syndrome).
- Sleep-related breathing problem (e.g., apnea).
- Family history of insomnia.
- Daytime napping.
- Noise (including a snoring partner).
- Frequent need to urinate at night.
- Night sweats or disorders that cause itching.
- Sexual problems.
- Drinking caffeine drinks (coffee, tea, or cola).
- Life events (e.g., recent illness or death in close contact, new job or school, deadlines, new environment or location, or jet lag after travel).
- Use of some drugs.
- Smoking, alcoholism, or drug abuse, including overuse of sleep-inducing drugs.

HOW TO PREVENT—Not always preventable. Avoid risk factors where possible. Try ideas listed under General Measures.

WHAT TO EXPECT

DIAGNOSTIC MEASURES
- See your health care provider if self-care isn't helping. A physical exam may be done and questions asked about your symptoms, sleep habits, and activities.

- Medical tests may be done to check for health problems. A sleep study may be prescribed.

APPROPRIATE HEALTH CARE
- Cognitive behavioral therapy may help insomnia. Counseling for depression or other mental health problem may be recommended.
- Treatment as needed for any medical problem.

POSSIBLE COMPLICATIONS—Insomnia can cause impaired thinking, and health and emotional problems that affect all aspects of life.

PROBABLE OUTCOME—Insomnia can usually be relieved by treating the cause, using self-care steps, or with other medical treatment.

HOW TO TREAT

GENERAL MEASURES
- You may try these self-care steps:
  - Try to reduce tension, stress, or anxiety in your life.
  - Don't turn your bedroom into an office or den.
  - Bedroom should be dark and quiet.
  - Create a comfortable sleep setting.
  - Relax in a warm bath before bedtime.
  - After 15 to 20 minutes of trying to sleep, get up and do some relaxing activity. Don't watch television.
  - Turn off your mind. Worries about life's stresses can turn into worries about sleeping. Focus on peaceful and relaxing thoughts. Play soft music or relaxation tapes.
  - Set a strict sleep schedule and keep to it.
  - Use ear plugs, eye shades, or an electric blanket.
  - Avoid clock-watching while trying to sleep.

MEDICATION
- Drugs called hypnotics may be prescribed. Some may be used short-term due to a concern for dependence. Others may be used longer term. They can help you fall asleep and/or stay asleep.
- Drugs for depression or anxiety or other underlying medical disorder may be prescribed.

ACTIVITY
- Exercise daily to create healthy fatigue, but not within 2 hours of going to bed.
- Have sexual relations, if they are satisfying and fulfilling, before going to sleep.

DIET—Avoid alcohol or a heavy meal within 3 hours of bedtime. Avoid caffeine or chocolate within 8 hours of bedtime. Try a light snack with milk at bedtime.

CALL YOUR DOCTOR IF

- You or a family member has had insomnia for over 4 weeks or it is interfering with your ability to function.
- Treatment is not relieving insomnia.

INTERSTITIAL CYSTITIS

GENERAL INFORMATION

DEFINITION—Interstitial cystitis (IC) is a chronic bladder disorder. It is also referred to as painful bladder syndrome (PBS). Symptoms are similar to cystitis (an infection of the urinary tract), but no apparent infection is found with IC.

BODY PARTS INVOLVED—Bladder.

SEX OR AGE MOST AFFECTED—The average age of onset is 40, but it affects all ages, women more commonly than men.

SIGNS & SYMPTOMS
- Symptoms vary greatly for each person.
- Pelvic pain and a feeling of pressure.
- Urgent need to urinate day and night (up to 60 times a day). This also causes sleep problems.
- Bladder does not feel like it empties completely when you urinate.
- Pain during sexual intercourse.
- Burning when urinating.
- Vaginal and rectal pain.

CAUSES—The exact cause is unknown. A breakdown or dysfunction of the bladder's lining (bladder wall) appears to be involved. There actually may be several causes, or there may be different disorders, rather than just one.

RISK INCREASES WITH
- Females ages 20 to 60.
- A family history of IC.

HOW TO PREVENT—No preventive measures.

WHAT TO EXPECT

DIAGNOSTIC MEASURES
- There are a number of medical problems that cause similar symptoms. They include kidney stones, urinary or vaginal infection, cancer, and others. Your health care provider will perform tests to rule out these other causes of the symptoms.
- A physical exam will be performed and urine tests are needed to check for infection. A cystoscopy may be done. In this test, a thin, tube-like device with a camera is used to see inside the bladder. The test can be uncomfortable because the bladder is stretched. A drug (anesthetic) will be used to stop pain. A stretched bladder holds more urine so this test helps symptoms also. A tissue sample may be removed for a biopsy.

APPROPRIATE HEALTH CARE
- There are a variety of treatment options. It is important to find out what works for you.
- Bladder instillation (a bladder wash or bath) is done at the medical office. It involves stretching the bladder by filling it with a solution for about 15 minutes.

- Bladder training involves teaching yourself to urinate at certain times.
- Counseling or behavior training. Learn how to relax and cope with stress, anxiety, or depression.
- A TENS (transcutaneous electrical nerve stimulation) device uses mild electric pulses to help block pain.
- Surgery is rarely needed. It may be done as a last resort when other methods have failed.

POSSIBLE COMPLICATIONS
- The symptoms may come and go over days, weeks, or months, sometimes years, even with treatment.
- Chronic symptoms can lead to problems with your work, friends, family, and sexual activity.

PROBABLE OUTCOME—Treatments can help control or relieve the symptoms, but they do not cure the disorder. It may take time to find the treatments that work best for you.

HOW TO TREAT

GENERAL MEASURES
- Don't smoke. Smoking makes symptoms worse.
- Learn about the disorder. Consider a support group.
- To learn more: The Interstitial Cystitis Association (ICA), PO Box 17522, Baltimore, MD 21209; (800) 435-7422; website: www.ichelp.org.

MEDICATION
- You may use nonprescription pain relievers.
- You may be prescribed drugs to treat the symptoms of IC. Several may be tried to find what works best for each individual.
- Other drugs may be prescribed for sleep problems, depression, anxiety, and severe pain.

ACTIVITY
- No limits unless limited by the symptoms.
- Regular exercise may help patient feel better.

DIET—Diet changes help some patients. Avoid drinks with caffeine, alcohol, or artificial sweeteners; spicy foods, chocolate, soda/carbonated beverages, citrus fruits, and tomatoes.

CALL YOUR DOCTOR IF

- You or a family member has symptoms of interstitial cystitis.
- Treatment is not helping the pain or other symptoms.
- New symptoms occur. Drugs may cause side effects.

INTESTINAL OBSTRUCTION

GENERAL INFORMATION

DEFINITION—An intestinal obstruction is a partial or complete blockage of the intestines. The material in the bowel cannot move pass the blockage. This causes the symptoms and also upsets the body's electrolyte balance.

BODY PARTS INVOLVED—Small and large (colon) intestines.

SEX OR AGE MOST AFFECTED—Both sexes; all ages.

SIGNS & SYMPTOMS
- Cramping abdominal pain.
- Nausea and vomiting. In the advanced stages, vomit resembles feces.
- Weakness, dizziness, or fainting.
- Little or no urine due to fluid loss.
- Failure to pass stools or gas.
- Audible noises from the abdomen in early stages; later, no sounds are audible.
- Abdominal bloating, swelling, and gas.
- Fever (sometimes).
- Diarrhea (partial obstruction only).
- Passing jelly-like mucus or bloody mucus.

CAUSES—A mechanical obstruction occurs when the bowel is physically blocked. Nonmechanical obstruction (called ileus) occurs when peristalsis (wavelike motion of the intestine) stops.

RISK INCREASES WITH
- Mechanical:
  - Adhesions (constricting bands of fibrous tissue that result from previous surgery).
  - Intestinal hernias.
  - Intestinal inflammation or tumors (either benign or cancerous).
  - Tumors in adjacent organs that cause pressure on the intestines.
  - Inflammatory bowel disease.
  - Foreign objects inside the intestines (gallstones, swallowed objects or parasites such as worms).
  - Bowel telescopes into itself (intussusception).
  - In newborns or infants, it may be caused by a birth defect.
  - Twisted bowel (volvulus).
  - Fecal impaction.
- Nonmechanical:
  - Certain drugs, such as narcotics.
  - Decreased blood supply to intestines due to injury or other problem.
  - Complication of abdominal surgery.
  - Infection of the lining of the abdominal cavity.
  - Kidney or thoracic (chest cavity) disease.
  - Metabolic problems, such as low potassium.

HOW TO PREVENT
- There are no specific preventive measures. Suggestions listed may help in prevention.
- Eat a diet high in fiber and drink plenty of fluids each day to avoid constipation or fecal impaction.
- Obtain medical treatment for hernias.
- See your health care provider if your bowel habits change significantly for longer than 7 days. It may be an early sign of bowel cancer.

WHAT TO EXPECT

DIAGNOSTIC MEASURES
- Your own observation of symptoms.
- Your health care provider will do a physical exam and ask about your symptoms.
- Medical tests include blood and urine studies. Other tests may include a barium enema or air enema (either one may also resolve the problem by straightening the intestine). X-ray, CT, and ultrasound may be done.

APPROPRIATE HEALTH CARE
- Emergency care is usually needed. A nasogastric tube is used to suction out the contents of the stomach and/or intestines above the blockage. Fluid and electrolyte replacement will be provided by IV (intravenous).
- Surgery to remove the obstruction is necessary in some cases.

POSSIBLE COMPLICATIONS
- Obstruction may recur after treatment.
- Dehydration, shock, and sepsis.
- Bowel complications such as gangrene, perforation, abscess, or peritonitis.

PROBABLE OUTCOME—With proper diagnosis and treatment, the outcome is good.

HOW TO TREAT

GENERAL MEASURES—Intestinal obstruction usually develops rapidly into an emergency. Home remedies are of no value and some, such as enemas or laxatives, may be harmful.

MEDICATION—Antibiotics are often prescribed to prevent infection.

ACTIVITY—You will be advised about limits depending on the treatment.

DIET—Don't eat or drink anything until the obstruction is corrected. You will probably receive intravenous nourishment until then.

CALL YOUR DOCTOR IF

- You or a family member has symptoms of intestinal obstruction. This is an emergency!
- Your bowel habits change.

INTUSSUSCEPTION

GENERAL INFORMATION

DEFINITION—Intussusception is an intestinal obstruction in which the bowel telescopes (folds into itself), forming a tube within a tube.

BODY PARTS INVOLVED—Intestine, usually the large intestine.

SEX OR AGE MOST AFFECTED—Both sexes; all ages, but most common in infants and children between 2 months and 6 years. It is more common in boys. It is rare in adults.

SIGNS & SYMPTOMS
• Cramping pain in the abdomen. Infants cry out, bring the legs up to the abdomen. They become pale and sweaty during an attack. Attacks of pain may occur 10 to 20 minutes apart.
• Vomiting.
• May have stool that is mixed with blood and mucus.
• Weakness and lack of energy.
• Swollen abdomen.
• Mass in the abdomen that can be felt.
• Later symptoms: increased weakness, fever, shock (rapid heartbeat, weak pulse, rapid breathing).

CAUSES
• Unknown for infants. The disorder may be caused by a virus infection, but this is unproven.
• In older children (usually over age 3) or in adults, it may be due to an intestinal problem.

RISK INCREASES WITH
• Infants and boys more than girls.
• Certain intestinal disorders.
• Season of the year (for unknown reasons). It is most common in late spring, early summer, and midwinter.

HOW TO PREVENT—No specific preventive measures.

WHAT TO EXPECT

DIAGNOSTIC MEASURES
• Yours or your child's health care provider will do a physical exam with careful attention to the abdomen. Medical tests may include blood, urine, and stool studies; x-rays; or ultrasound.
• A barium or air enema may be done for diagnosis and treatment. In this procedure, a liquid containing barium is given with a tube into the rectum and special x-rays are taken. Barium helps show the intussusception on the x-ray. In many cases, the pressure of the barium unfolds the bowel and cures the problem. An air enema can work in the same way.

APPROPRIATE HEALTH CARE—Surgery to correct the problem may be needed. This is done if the child is too ill for the enema procedure or it was done and did not provide a cure. Surgery involves pushing out the telescoped portion of the intestine. In a few cases, a part of the bowel must be cut out.

POSSIBLE COMPLICATIONS
• Dehydration and shock.
• Intestinal perforation.
• Tissue damage that cannot be reversed.
• An infection may occur after surgery.
• The disorder may recur after barium treatment.
• Without treatment, complications are life-threatening (rare).

PROBABLE OUTCOME—Outcome for most patients is very good. With early diagnosis and treatment, complications are unlikely to develop In adults, the outcome may depend on the underlying condition.

HOW TO TREAT

GENERAL MEASURES—Follow medical advice.

MEDICATION
• Drugs are usually not needed for this disorder unless infection develops. Then antibiotics may be prescribed.
• Don't use home remedies or nonprescription drugs, such as laxatives, for this condition. They may be dangerous.

ACTIVITY—The patient should rest in bed until the obstruction is cleared. Activities may then be resumed gradually.

DIET—Don't feed a patient who has signs of intestinal obstruction. Intravenous (through a vein) fluids are given in the hospital until the person can eat again.

CALL YOUR DOCTOR IF

• You or a family member has signs or symptoms of intussusception. This condition changes quickly from a curable one to a life-threatening one.
• Any new symptoms develop after treatment.

IRITIS
(Uveitis, Anterior)

GENERAL INFORMATION

DEFINITION—Iritis is an inflammation of the iris. The iris is the colored ring that surrounds the eye's pupil. The disorder is also called anterior uveitis. It may sometimes be confused with pink eye (conjunctivitis).

BODY PARTS INVOLVED—Eye.

SEX OR AGE MOST AFFECTED—Both sexes; all ages.

SIGNS & SYMPTOMS
- Symptoms may develop suddenly and affect one or both eyes.
- Eye pain.
- Photophobia (sensitivity to light).
- Eye redness.
- Smaller pupil in the affected eye (sometimes).
- Tears.
- Blurred vision; may see dark, floating spots in the field of vision.

CAUSES
- In many cases, no cause is found.
- It may be caused by:
  - Trauma (injury) to the eye.
  - An infection (such as tuberculosis, herpes, and others).
  - Sometimes, it is one of the symptoms of a systemic disease (one that affects numerous parts of the body).
  - A genetic alteration makes some people more at risk for certain autoimmune disorders that have iritis as a symptom.

RISK INCREASES WITH
- Sarcoidosis.
- Behçet syndrome.
- Inflammatory bowel disease.
- Juvenile idiopathic arthritis.
- Rheumatoid arthritis.
- Ankylosing spondylitis.
- Reactive arthritis (Reiter's syndrome).
- Multiple sclerosis.
- Herpes virus infections.
- Syphilis.
- HIV.
- Histoplasmosis.
- Toxoplasmosis.
- Tuberculosis.
- Lyme disease.
- Cytomegalovirus.
- Injuries.

HOW TO PREVENT
- No specific preventive measures known.
- For people at risk for recurrence of iritis, steroid eyedrops may be prescribed to be used if symptoms occur.

WHAT TO EXPECT

DIAGNOSTIC MEASURES
- Iritis can be diagnosed by your eye care provider using special equipment to look into the eye.
- Other medical tests may be needed to help diagnose any health problem that is associated with iritis.

APPROPRIATE HEALTH CARE
- Treatment goals are to reduce pain and redness, prevent complications, and treat other health problems that are diagnosed.
- Treatment usually involves drug therapy.

POSSIBLE COMPLICATIONS
- Glaucoma, cataracts, other eye problems, or possible vision loss.
- Recurring or chronic iritis.

PROBABLE OUTCOME—With prompt diagnosis and treatment, the outcome is generally good. Iritis due to trauma usually heals in 1 to 2 weeks. In other cases, healing may take 6 to 8 weeks.

HOW TO TREAT

GENERAL MEASURES
- For comfort, wear dark glasses (even indoors) until treatment is complete.
- Follow-up eye exams are needed to be sure that healing is complete.

MEDICATION
- Dilating eyedrops (cycloplegics) that dilate the pupil and prevent scarring are usually prescribed. You may need to use eyedrops for a long time.
- Oral cortisone drugs or cortisone eyedrops to reduce inflammation may be prescribed.
- Antibiotic eye drops may be prescribed for bacterial infection.
- Drugs for other medical problems diagnosed may be prescribed.

ACTIVITY—No limits (unless advised).

DIET—Eat a normal well-balanced diet.

CALL YOUR DOCTOR IF

- You or a family member has symptoms of iritis. Call immediately.
- Vision changes in any way.
- New, unexplained symptoms develop. Drugs used in treatment may produce side effects.

IRRITABLE BOWEL SYNDROME
(Spastic Colon; Mucous Colitis)

GENERAL INFORMATION

DEFINITION—Irritable bowel syndrome (IBS) is a disorder of the large intestine (bowel). It can cause a variety of symptoms and episodes may last for days, weeks, or months. It is not contagious, inherited, or cancerous.

BODY PARTS INVOLVED—Intestines.

SEX OR AGE MOST AFFECTED—Often begins in adolescents or young adults; twice as likely to affect women as men.

SIGNS & SYMPTOMS
- Cramp-like pain in the middle or to one side of the lower abdomen. A bowel movement relieves the pain.
- Diarrhea or constipation; frequently alternating.
- Swollen or bloated (distended) abdomen; gas.
- Mucus in the stools.
- Straining to have bowel movement.
- Urgency to have bowel movement.
- Feeling that the bowels still have to be emptied after having a bowel movement.

CAUSES—Exact cause is unknown. The nerves and muscles in the bowel seem to be extra-sensitive in people with IBS. Nerves can cause pain and discomfort if they become irritated. Muscles that contract to pass food through the intestines may contract too much and cause cramping and diarrhea. The bowel can overreact to food, stress, exercise, and hormones. Stress may trigger symptoms if you have IBS, but it doesn't cause IBS.

RISK INCREASES WITH
- Under age 50.
- Women more than with men.
- Other family members with similar bowel problems.
- People who have panic disorder, or similar disorders.
- People who have had a history of sexual, physical, or emotional abuse.

HOW TO PREVENT—No specific measures to prevent IBS. After it is diagnosed, you can find ways to help prevent symptoms.

WHAT TO EXPECT

DIAGNOSTIC MEASURES
- Your health care provider may do a physical exam and ask questions about your symptoms and activities.
- Medical tests may include blood and stool studies, as well as other tests to exclude more serious disorders. A mental health exam may be done also.

APPROPRIATE HEALTH CARE
- Treatment may involve a combination of lifestyle changes and drugs, if needed.
- Counseling for emotional or personal problems or stress may be recommended.

POSSIBLE COMPLICATIONS
- IBS can affect all aspects of life. It can interfere with work schedules, limit physical activities, disrupt personal relationships, and cause a restricted social life. It may lead to depression and/or anxiety.
- IBS does not lead to serious disease or cancer.

PROBABLE OUTCOME—The condition is usually recurrent throughout life. Symptoms may be mild to severe and may come and go. Most people can be helped with treatment. No specific treatment works best for everybody. You may need to try several to see what works.

HOW TO TREAT

GENERAL MEASURES
- Reduce stress in your life. Try various techniques that can help you relax. Meditation, self-hypnosis, or biofeedback may help. Keep a stress and symptom diary so you know who or what may trigger an episode.
- Quit smoking. Nicotine may add to problem.
- Join a support group. They can be reassuring.
- To learn more: National Digestive Diseases Information Clearinghouse; (800) 891-5389; website: www.digestive.niddk.nlh.gov.

MEDICATION
- Antispasmodics to relieve severe cramps and drugs to treat the constipation form of IBS may be prescribed.
- Drugs for depression or anxiety may be prescribed.
- Antidiarrheals or laxatives need to be used with caution. Get medical advice before using.

ACTIVITY—Daily exercise helps bowel function, keeps you fit, and reduces stress.

DIET
- Increase fiber in the diet to promote good bowel function. Add fiber to your diet slowly. Too much fiber can cause gas.
- Avoid foods or drinks that can worsen symptoms. These include fatty foods, milk products, chocolate, alcohol, caffeine, and carbonated drinks. Keep a food diary to help find the foods that cause you problems.
- Avoid large meals, but eat regularly.

CALL YOUR DOCTOR IF

- You or a family member has IBS symptoms.
- Symptoms don't improve with treatment.

JET LAG

GENERAL INFORMATION

DEFINITION—Jet lag results from east-west travel between different time zones. (North-south travel does not cause jet lag.) The degree of severity depends on the number of time zones crossed and the direction traveled. Most people find traveling eastward and adapting to a shorter work day is more difficult than traveling westward and adapting to a longer work day.

SEX OR AGE MOST AFFECTED—Both sexes; all ages.

SIGNS & SYMPTOMS
- Extreme fatigue.
- Sleep disturbances.
- Loss of concentration.
- Malaise.
- Disorientation.
- Sluggishness.
- Stomach upset.
- Loss of appetite.
- Swollen feet.

CAUSES—Disturbance in the body's physiological processes that control not only sleep and wakefulness, but also alertness, hunger, digestion, urine production, temperature and hormone secretion.

RISK INCREASES WITH—Frequent travel in short periods of time.

HOW TO PREVENT
- Avoid alcohol.
- There are many jet lag prevention methods that have been proposed, written about, and discussed among travelers. There is no one method that works for everyone. You may want to try one or more prevention methods to see what might work for you. Check in bookstores, libraries, and the Internet for information.

WHAT TO EXPECT

DIAGNOSTIC MEASURES—Your own observation of symptoms.

APPROPRIATE HEALTH CARE—No medical care is necessary for typical cases of jet lag.

POSSIBLE COMPLICATIONS—Usually, no complications develop.

PROBABLE OUTCOME—Symptoms usually resolve themselves after a short period of time in the same geographic location.

HOW TO TREAT

GENERAL MEASURES
- Plan destination activities to accommodate for time differences.
- Spend some time every day in natural sunlight.
- Adjust your bed and mealtimes to the new timetable as soon as possible.
- Set your watch to local time as soon as possible after takeoff.

MEDICATION
- Drugs for insomnia may be prescribed for a short period of time. You might try them before you leave to see how they effect you and if they cause any unwanted side effects.
- The hormone melatonin has been used for this condition, but long-term data are lacking.

ACTIVITY
- Continue with any regular exercise program once you arrive at your destination. Do not exercise close to bedtime.
- Don't operate motor vehicles or swim alone if you feel tired.

DIET
- Eat a normal well-balanced diet, even if you have no appetite.
- Drink plenty of liquids, but avoid alcoholic drinks.

CALL YOUR DOCTOR IF

You or a family member has symptoms of jet lag and they don't improve after one week.

KAPOSI SARCOMA

 GENERAL INFORMATION

DEFINITION—Kaposi sarcoma (KS) is a form of skin cancer that is found most often in patients with advanced HIV (human immunodeficiency virus) infection. A second form of Kaposi sarcoma is associated with some immunosuppressive drugs. A third form, referred to as classic KS, is found in elderly men of Mediterranean and Eastern European ancestry. A fourth form affects adults and children in Africa.

BODY PARTS INVOLVED—Skin.

SEX OR AGE MOST AFFECTED—Usually adult males.

SIGNS & SYMPTOMS
* Skin lesions (sores) usually on the face, arms, and trunk. They may also be found in the mouth, lymph nodes, and other areas.
* The color may be brown, reddish-purple, or purple-black. Usually don't itch or cause pain.
* Lesions in the mouth may interfere with eating or swallowing.
* Lesions on the feet may interfere with walking.
* Swelling of the face, scrotum, and lower extremities if the lymph nodes are affected.
* May cause internal bleeding if the stomach is affected
* May have breathing problem if lungs affected.

CAUSES—A herpesvirus (HHV-8, Kaposi sarcoma herpesvirus [KSHV]) is believed to be the cause. It is spread mainly in saliva, blood, or semen. It can be passed during sexual contact, kissing, blood transfusions, organ transplantation, or from mother to her unborn child.

RISK INCREASES WITH
* Weak immune system due to HIV-AIDS infection.
* Elderly men of Mediterranean and Eastern European descent. People of central African ethnicity.
* Weak immune system due to drug therapy (e.g., for organ transplantation).

HOW TO PREVENT—People at risk for Kaposi sarcoma should talk to their health care provider about screenings exam and preventive therapy.

 WHAT TO EXPECT

DIAGNOSTIC MEASURES
* Your own observation of symptoms.
* Your health care provider will do an exam of the affected skin areas. Tissue from a sore will be used for a biopsy. Medical tests may be done to confirm the diagnosis and to see if the disorder has spread to other places in the body (staging).

APPROPRIATE HEALTH CARE
* For AIDS-related KS:
 - If there are only a few skin lesions, they may be followed up for a period of time rather than being treated.
 - Treatment usually includes antiretroviral drugs.
 - Skin lesions can be treated in other ways. They can be frozen (cryotherapy), treated with radiation, cut out surgically, or drugs that are injected into the skin or used on the skin.
 - Cosmetic cover-up products can be used on the skin to camouflage the lesions.
 - If lesions have spread to the inside (internal organs) of the body, drugs are used for treatment.
* Classic KS does not usually need treatment, but radiotherapy may be used in some cases.
* Transplant KS can be treated by stopping, changing, or reducing drugs.
* African KS may be treated with chemotherapy.

POSSIBLE COMPLICATIONS—Other cancers, lymphedema, infections, internal bleeding, or recurrence of KS after therapy. It can be fatal.

PROBABLE OUTCOME
* There is no cure. It is a lifelong condition.
* For AIDS-related KS, the outcome depends on the extent and location of the lesions and the immune system status. In some cases, treatment may stabilize or reverse the condition.
* For KS due to an immune-suppressing drug, it often improves if drug or dosage is changed.
* For classic type KS, outcome varies. It grows slowly. Elderly patients may die of other causes.
* African KS can spread rapidly. Premature death may result, even with treatment.

 HOW TO TREAT

GENERAL MEASURES—To learn more: American Cancer Society, (800) 227-2345; website: www.cancer.org; or National Cancer Institute, (800) 422-6247; website: www.nci.nih.gov.

MEDICATION
* Highly active antiretroviral therapy (HAART) is usually prescribed if they not taken already.
* Anticancer or other drugs may be prescribed.

ACTIVITY—As tolerated.

DIET—You may need a special diet if the mouth is affected.

 CALL YOUR DOCTOR IF

* You or a household member has symptoms of Kaposi sarcoma.
* New skin lesions or other symptoms develop.

KELOIDS

GENERAL INFORMATION

DEFINITION—Keloids are an overgrowth of fibrous tissue (scar) on the skin.

BODY PARTS INVOLVED—Anywhere on the skin, but most commonly appear on the earlobes, chest, upper back, and shoulders.

SEX OR AGE MOST AFFECTED—Both sexes; all ages. Keloids are more frequent in black people than in white people and occur more often in young women.

SIGNS & SYMPTOMS
- Keloids begin as a small bump. The lump grows and turns into firm, raised, hard scars that are slightly pink.
- Scars may continue to grow over time.
- Keloids may have itchiness, burning sensation, pain, or tingling.
- They may become a cosmetic problem.
- May become irritated from rubbing on clothing.

CAUSES—Keloids probably occur due to a defective healing process. An excess of collagen forms at the site of a healing scar. Keloids usually arise in an area of injury (such as after a burn or from severe acne), but sometimes arise from a very minor scratch. Why they occur in certain people is unknown.

RISK INCREASES WITH
- Certain persons:
  - Family history of keloids.
  - Personal history of keloids.
  - Darkly pigmented skin (Blacks, Hispanics, Asians).
  - During pregnancy or puberty.
- Other risk factors:
  - Surgical wound or burn injury (especially if healing is delayed more than 3 weeks).
  - Acne.
  - Body piercing.
  - Vaccination or biopsy.
  - Insect bite.
  - Folliculitis barbae (inflammation of a hair follicle).

HOW TO PREVENT—People who tend to form keloids should avoid skin injury, body piercing, and surgery if possible. When surgery is needed, consult your health care provider about keloid preventive measures.

WHAT TO EXPECT

DIAGNOSTIC MEASURES
- Your own observation of symptoms.
- Your health care provider can diagnose keloids by their appearance on the skin.
- Medical tests are usually not needed, but may be done to rule out any other skin problem.

APPROPRIATE HEALTH CARE
- No single treatment is best for all keloids. There are a variety of treatment options and the options can be combined. Your health care provider will discuss them with you.
- Treatment may include injections into the scars.
- Occlusive dressings include silicone gel sheets and dressings, nonsilicone sheets, and a clear surgical tape.
- Compression therapy includes different products that are used to apply pressure to the keloids.
- Laser therapy or radiotherapy (radiation) are options.
- Cryotherapy involves freezing the affected area with liquid nitrogen.
- Surgery (excision) may be done if other treatments are not successful. Surgery is usually combined with pressure therapy, injections, or radiotherapy.
- Other therapies are being researched.

POSSIBLE COMPLICATIONS
- They may recur, despite treatment.
- Emotional distress.

PROBABLE OUTCOME—Keloids are difficult to treat. The response to different treatments varies among patients. Treatment may soften, flatten, lighten color, decrease size, or improve texture of the keloids. Keloids are generally considered harmless and noncancerous.

HOW TO TREAT

GENERAL MEASURES—There is no self-treatment for keloids. Follow medical advice for follow-up measures after treatment.

MEDICATION
- Injection of corticosteroid drugs directly into the keloid. May be repeated every 3 to 4 weeks until desired degree of flattening and softening has been achieved.
- Other types of injections or topical drugs may be prescribed.

ACTIVITY—No limits.

DIET—No special diet.

CALL YOUR DOCTOR IF

- You or a family member has signs of keloids.
- Keloids recur after treatment.

KERATITIS

GENERAL INFORMATION

DEFINITION—Keratitis is an inflammation (redness and swelling) of the cornea.

BODY PARTS INVOLVED—The cornea is the clear membrane on the front of the eye that covers the iris and the pupil.

SEX OR AGE MOST AFFECTED—Both sexes; all ages.

SIGNS & SYMPTOMS
- Symptoms may be mild to severe. One eye is usually affected, but it may occur in both eyes.
- Eye pain.
- Redness and itching of the eye.
- Feeling that there is something in the eye.
- Photophobia (sensitivity to light).
- Tearing or discharge of the eye.
- Blurry vision.

CAUSES—There are many causes and types of keratitis. In many cases, an injury to the cornea has allowed an infection to occur. Infections include bacteria, fungi, parasites, or viruses. Prompt treatment is important.

RISK INCREASES WITH
- Contact lens use. Wearing soft lenses overnight can increase the risk.
- Eye trauma (injury). It may be due to foreign body, chemical, radiation, heat, or other problem.
- Eye surgery.
- Use of topical steroids in the eyes.
- Weak immune system due to illness or drugs.
- Dry eyes, eyelid disorders, ingrown eyelashes, or conjunctivitis (pink eye).
- Vitamin A deficiency (rare in normal diet).

HOW TO PREVENT
- Follow instructions provided with contact lenses for cleaning and length of wearing time.
- Wear protective glasses or goggles if work or sports activity involves eye hazards.
- Get treatment for eye injury or other eye disorders.
- For dry eyes, use eyedrops recommended by your health care provider.
- Avoid rubbing the eyes if you have cold sores.

WHAT TO EXPECT

DIAGNOSTIC MEASURES
- Your own observation of symptoms.
- Your health care provider or eye specialist (ophthalmologist) will ask questions about your symptoms.
- Diagnosis often begins with a special eye exam (slit lamp) and a test of vision acuity. Blood tests may be done to check for an infection in the body. A corneal scraping sample can be used for lab tests to determine the type of infection.

APPROPRIATE HEALTH C
- Eye medications are used to and to help prevent complications
- An eye shield (patch) may be pres some cases to protect eye from light a ease discomfort.
- Don't wear contact lenses or eye makeup while the eye is inflamed.
- Rarely, surgery may be needed to replace the cornea.

POSSIBLE COMPLICATIONS
- Glaucoma and/or cataract.
- Permanent scarring of the cornea.
- Some degree of vision loss.
- Herpetic keratitis (caused by the herpes virus) can recur.

PROBABLE OUTCOME—Depends on the type and cause. With early treatment, most types of keratitis are curable. It may take several months.

HOW TO TREAT

GENERAL MEASURES—Cool compresses applied to the closed eye may help symptoms.

MEDICATION
- Antibiotic, antifungal, antiviral, or antiparasitic eyedrops or ointments are prescribed depending on the infection.
- Other types of eyedrops may be prescribed.
- Use nonprescription oral pain relievers for pain. If pain is severe, stronger drugs may be prescribed.
- Don't treat any eye inflammation without medical advice. Don't use nonprescription eyedrops containing topical corticosteroids. These may worsen the condition or cause eyeball perforation.

ACTIVITY—Limit activities as needed by your symptoms. Extra rest may be helpful at start of treatment.

DIET—No special diet.

CALL YOUR DOCTOR IF

- You or a family member has symptoms of keratitis. Get treatment right away.
- Your vision changes in any way.

...RMATION

...oses are
...e skin. They are
...ncer.

...ey often affect
...breasts in females,
back, face, and/or arms.

SEX OR AGE MOST AFFECTED—Adults of both sexes. By age 50, almost everyone has a few seborrheic keratoses.

SIGNS & SYMPTOMS
- Growths are raised, thick bumps. They are flat-topped with well-defined borders.
- Newer growths are relatively flat and light brown. Older ones are dark brown or black.
- Growths are wider than tall. They appear "stuck on."
- They may itch or bleed if they get irritated. They do not cause any pain.
- There may be only I or 2 growths, or there may be as many as 100.

CAUSES—Unknown. They cannot be spread from one person to another.

RISK INCREASES WITH
- Aging.
- Family history of the disorder.

HOW TO PREVENT—No specific preventive measures.

 WHAT TO EXPECT

DIAGNOSTIC MEASURES
- Your own observation of symptoms.
- See your health care provider as advised for routine skin exams or if you have concerns about a skin growth. Seborrheic keratoses can be diagnosed with a skin exam.
- In some cases, a growth may be removed for viewing under a microscope to confirm the diagnosis.

APPROPRIATE HEALTH CARE
- Usually, no treatment is needed.
- The growths can be removed if they are unsightly, are irritated by clothing, or cause problems with shaving. Removal methods include cryosurgery (freezing), chemocautery, light electrosurgery, shave biopsy, or topical drugs. Laser therapy may be an option. Your health care provider will discuss treatments.
- Seborrheic keratoses on the eyelid borders may require special treatment.

POSSIBLE COMPLICATIONS
- None expected from the growths.
- Complications may sometimes occur from treatment procedure such as scars, keloids, or hyper- or hypopigmentation (changes in skin color in treated area).

PROBABLE OUTCOME—The number of growths usually increases with age. Each growth is permanent unless removed. Seborrheic keratosis are harmless and require no treatment. People may want them removed (especially if they are unsightly or irritated by clothing).

 HOW TO TREAT

GENERAL MEASURES—After removal, a blister (sometimes with blood) will develop at the treatment site. The top of the blister will come off spontaneously in about 2 weeks. You should have little or no scarring. Wash and use makeup or cosmetics as usual. If clothing irritates the blister, cover it with a small adhesive bandage.

MEDICATION
- Use nonprescription topical corticosteroids to help relieve itching.
- Topical skin creams may be prescribed.

ACTIVITY—No limits.

DIET—No special diet.

 CALL YOUR DOCTOR IF

- You or a family member has symptoms of seborrheic keratoses and are concerned.
- You want unsightly seborrheic keratoses removed.
- Treated areas become infected (sore, red, feels warm).
- You have a sudden increase in number or size of seborrheic keratoses.

KERATOSIS, ACTINIC

GENERAL INFORMATION

DEFINITION—Actinic keratosis (AK; also called solar keratosis) is an area of sun-damaged skin. It is the most common sun-related skin growth. It is considered a precancerous condition.

BODY PARTS INVOLVED—Skin of exposed areas, especially the scalp, face, ears, lips, arms and hands.

SEX OR AGE MOST AFFECTED—Adults of both sexes; more common in adults over age 50 and occurs in men more than women.

SIGNS & SYMPTOMS
- Rough, dry, scaly lesions (patches) on exposed areas of the skin (such as the scalp, face, ears, lips, arms, and hands).
- They have an irregular shape and can be flat or slightly raised. Can range in size from a pinhead to larger than a quarter. May grow into a horn-like appearance.
- There may be single or multiple lesions.
- Color can be pink to red, brown, or skin colored.
- They are usually painless, but may sometimes itch or have a tender sensation.

CAUSES
- Prolonged exposure to the sun's radiation is the most common cause. It may develop years after the person's most intense sun exposure.
- Exposure to tanning devices, or very rarely to x-rays or certain industrial chemicals may be a cause.

RISK INCREASES WITH
- Outdoor athletic activities and sports.
- Outdoor occupations, such as farming.
- Ages over 50 and men more than women.
- Light (fair) complexion and blue, gray, or green eyes.
- Weak immune system due to illness or drugs.
- Living at higher elevations.

HOW TO PREVENT
- Protect yourself against direct sun exposure. When outdoors, wear a hat and protective clothing. Use sunscreen lotions and creams with SPF ratings of 15 or more. Avoid sun between 10 AM and 4 PM if possible.
- Do skin self-exams on a regular basis (each month).

WHAT TO EXPECT

DIAGNOSTIC MEASURES
- Your own observation of symptoms.
- Your health care provider can diagnose the condition by an exam of the skin.
- A skin biopsy may be done. This involves removing a sample of skin tissue for viewing under a microscope.

APPROPRIATE HEALTH C
- Several treatment options
health care provider will disc
work best for you, depending o
the condition, your health, and you
- Cryosurgery (the most common treatment) is the application of liquid nitrogen to the skin.
- Curettage is the scraping away of the lesions with a sharp instrument.
- Excisional (cutting) surgery removes the lesions.
- Laser surgery may be used to destroy the cells.
- Dermabrasion is a treatment where the top layers of the skin are ground away.
- Photodynamic therapy. Medicine is applied to the affected skin, and then it is exposed to a special light.
- Chemical peels may be used for facial lesions.

POSSIBLE COMPLICATIONS
- Skin damage.
- Some risk of skin cancer if untreated. This is usually squamous cell carcinoma, which is curable when treated early.

PROBABLE OUTCOME—There are several types of effective treatment, and outcome is usually excellent. New outbreaks do sometimes occur following treatment.

HOW TO TREAT

GENERAL MEASURES
- Minimize direct sun exposure.
- See your doctor for routine checkups to ensure early detection and treatment of skin cancers.

MEDICATION—There are different topical drugs used for treating AK lesions. Treatment time will vary and can take 2 to 12 weeks. Each drug has risks and benefits that your health care provider will discuss with you.

ACTIVITY—No limits.

DIET—No special diet.

CALL YOUR DOCTOR IF

- You or a family member has signs of actinic keratosis. Even though this causes no symptoms, it can be a risk for cancer.
- Any new or unexpected symptoms develop during treatment with drugs or after a treatment procedure.

GENERAL INFORMATION

DEFINITION—Keratosis pilaris is a common, benign (noncancerous) disorder that involves rough bumps on the skin.

BODY PARTS INVOLVED—It usually involves the skin on the backs of upper arms, fronts of thighs, or buttocks. Less often, it may affect the face and be mistaken for acne.

SEX OR AGE MOST AFFECTED—Both sexes; may start in childhood, around age 2 or 3; affects many teenagers, and some adults.

SIGNS & SYMPTOMS
* Skin bumps that are small and firm. They may be skin-colored, white, or sometimes red. They have a dry "sandpaper" or "goosebumps" texture.
* They are located at the openings of hair follicles.
* The condition is usually worse in winter months when a person's skin is dryer.
* Bumps usually don't itch or cause pain.

CAUSES—The openings of the hair follicles become filled with hard plugs (made up of keratin). Why it occurs is unknown. It does run in families. It often occurs along with other skin disorders such as ichthyosis (an inherited dry skin condition). The condition cannot be spread from one person to another.

RISK INCREASES WITH
* Family history of keratosis pilaris.
* Ichthyosis (dry and scaly skin disorder).
* Atopic dermatitis.

HOW TO PREVENT—Cannot be prevented at present.

WHAT TO EXPECT

DIAGNOSTIC MEASURES
* Your own observation of symptoms.
* If you are concerned about the skin rash, see your health care provider. The condition can be diagnosed by an exam of the affected area.

APPROPRIATE HEALTH CARE
* Treatment usually involves self-care.
* Topical drugs may be prescribed.
* Medical-office treatment procedures such as peels or dermabrasion or laser treatments have mixed results. Ask your health care provider about these options.

POSSIBLE COMPLICATIONS—Complications are unlikely. A skin infection may occur if the affected area is scratched or overly treated with abrasive methods.

PROBABLE OUTCOME—Keratosis pilaris is a chronic, harmless skin problem with no permanent cure. The bumps may come and go over a period of time. Many cases clear up on their own as a person gets older. Cosmetic appearance and rough skin texture are often bothersome to patients.

HOW TO TREAT

GENERAL MEASURES
* Maintain a daily skin care program. Avoiding dry skin is the main goal.
  - Use a mild non-soap cleanser when bathing. Regular soap may cause dryness. Pat skin dry.
  - Apply lubricating ointments or creams to the affected areas 2 or 3 times a day. The most useful time is immediately after bathing to help skin retain moisture.
  - Nonprescription medicated creams containing urea, salicylic acid, or alpha-hydroxy acid may be used twice a day. These can be irritating to the skin, so use with caution.
  - Exfoliation may help. After a soaking bath or shower, go over the affected skin area with a course washcloth, loofah sponge, pumice stone, or brush to gently loosen the plugs.

MEDICATION—Your health care provider may prescribe a topical retinoid or steroid drug or other drugs to be applied to the skin. Treatment may take months and bumps are likely to return once treatment is stopped.

ACTIVITY—No limits.

DIET—No special diet.

CALL YOUR DOCTOR IF

* You or a family member has signs of keratosis pilaris and are concerned about them.
* Appearance of the affected area changes. There may be a skin infection.

KIDNEY CANCER
(Renal Cell Carcinoma; Hypernephroma)

GENERAL INFORMATION

DEFINITION—Kidney cancer is a growth of malignant cells in the kidney. The most common type is renal cell carcinoma. Other types are less common. The kidneys normally help remove waste products from the blood.

BODY PARTS INVOLVED—Kidney.

SEX OR AGE MOST AFFECTED—Both sexes; (men more than women); ages 50 to 80.

SIGNS & SYMPTOMS
- No symptoms may occur in early stages.
- Appetite and weight loss.
- Low-grade fever may come and go.
- Night sweats.
- Abdominal, side, or back pain.
- Red or smoky urine caused by bleeding from the tumor.
- Lump in the abdomen.
- General ill feeling.

CAUSES—Unknown. Certain risk factors are known.

RISK INCREASES WITH
- Smoking.
- Males; older adults.
- Obesity (especially in women).
- Estrogen therapy without progestin.
- High blood pressure and its treatment.
- Occupational exposure to certain toxins.
- Cystic kidney disease.
- Dialysis therapy.
- Kidney transplant.
- Certain inherited disorders.
- Family history of kidney cancer.

HOW TO PREVENT
- Cannot be prevented at present.
- Reduce risk factors where possible, especially, avoid smoking. Maintain ideal weight. Avoid exposure to toxins.

WHAT TO EXPECT

DIAGNOSTIC MEASURES
- Your own observation of any symptoms.
- Your health care provider will do a physical exam and ask questions about your symptoms.
- Medical tests may include blood studies and liver-function tests. Other tests are usually done to confirm the diagnosis and to determine if cancer has spread (called staging).

APPROPRIATE HEALTH CARE
- Treatment will depend on the stage of the disease, your health, and your preferences.
- Treatment may include surgery, biologic therapy, targeted therapy, chemotherapy, and radiation.
- Surgery may involve removal of all or part of the kidney. If surgery isn't possible, other procedures may be done to destroy cancer cells.
- Biologic therapy uses the body's immune system to fight cancer. Targeted therapy attacks specific cancer cells. Chemotherapy uses drugs and radiation therapy uses radiation to attack the cancer cells.

POSSIBLE COMPLICATIONS
- Spread to other organs, especially the liver, lungs, brain, and bones. This may occur before diagnosis.
- Kidney failure.
- Cancer recurs after treatment.
- Side effects of therapy.

PROBABLE OUTCOME—Outcome will depend on different factors. May be curable with treatment, if the tumor is detected before it spreads to other body parts. Other outcomes depend on the spread of the cancer and success of treatment.

HOW TO TREAT

GENERAL MEASURES
- Joining a support group helps many patients.
- To learn more: American Cancer Society, (800) ACS-2345; website: www.cancer.org; or National Cancer Institute, (800) 4-CANCER; website: www.nci.nih.gov.

MEDICATION—Your health care provider may prescribe anticancer drugs (chemotherapy), drugs to stimulate the immune system (biologics), targeted therapy, pain relievers, and others if needed.

ACTIVITY
- Follow medical advice about returning to normal activities after treatment.
- Stay as active as your strength allows.

DIET—Eat a low-fat, high-fiber diet.

CALL YOUR DOCTOR IF

- You or a family member has symptoms of kidney cancer.
- New symptoms occur during or after treatment.

KIDNEY DISEASE, POLYCYSTIC

GENERAL INFORMATION

DEFINITION
- Polycystic kidney disease (PKD) is an inherited disorder in which cysts develop in the kidneys. Cysts are benign, round sacs that contain water-like fluid. The cysts replace normal kidney tissue and reduce kidney function. There are two forms of PKD.
  - Autosomal dominant PKD (ADPKD) is the more common form. It is one of the most common inherited disorders in humans. Symptoms often don't occur until ages 30 to 40, but may begin in childhood.
  - Autosomal recessive PKD is more rare and begins early in life. It is not covered in this topic.

BODY PARTS INVOLVED—Kidneys.

SEX OR AGE MOST AFFECTED—Both sexes; all ages.

SIGNS & SYMPTOMS—A person with ADPKD often has no symptoms. Routine physical exams and blood and urine tests may not diagnose the disease in the early stages. Symptoms that occur may include pain in the side, back, or abdomen; increase in size of abdomen; less urine; blood in the urine; and high blood pressure.

CAUSES—It is an inherited disorder. Autosomal dominant means if one parent has the disease, there is a 50% chance the disease gene will pass to a child. Two genes are known—called PKD1 (more severe disease) and PKD2. In a few cases, the disease results from a spontaneous gene mutation (non-inherited PKD).

RISK INCREASES WITH—Family history of PKD.

HOW TO PREVENT—Cannot be prevented. If polycystic kidney disease runs in your family, get medical advice about tests to discover if you have kidney cysts. If you have a family history of polycystic kidney, seek genetic counseling before starting a family. Women with PKD can have a successful pregnancy, but some may develop preeclampsia.

WHAT TO EXPECT

DIAGNOSTIC MEASURES
- Your health care provider will do a physical exam and ask questions about your family medical history.
- Medical tests may include blood studies, CT, MRI, and ultrasound. Genetic tests may be done.

APPROPRIATE HEALTH CARE
- There is no specific treatment for the disorder. Treatment goal is to prolong life, maintain kidney function, and manage complications.
- Treatments include drug therapy, lifestyle changes, surgery, and medical check-ups.
- Surgery may be needed if kidney cysts rupture, large cysts cause pain, or if cysts in the liver cause problems.
- Once kidney failure develops, dialysis or surgery to perform a kidney transplant may be recommended.

POSSIBLE COMPLICATIONS
- High blood pressure.
- Aneurysms (ballooning of weak places in arteries).
- Infection or rupture of cysts.
- Cysts in the liver and other organs.
- Heart valve problems.
- Chronic pain.
- Colon problems such as diverticulosis.
- Kidney failure and end-stage renal disease (ESRD).
- Need for dialysis or kidney transplantation.

PROBABLE OUTCOME—There is no cure for polycystic kidney disease. Medical care may slow the progressive kidney damage and improve quality of life.

HOW TO TREAT

GENERAL MEASURES
- Check your blood pressure each day and keep a record.
- Prompt treatment of any infection is important.
- To learn more: PKD Foundation, 9221 Ward Parkway, Suite 400, Kansas City, MO 64114; (800) 753-2873; website www.pkdcure.org.

MEDICATION
- Antibiotics for infection, drugs to control high blood pressure, and drugs for pain are often prescribed.
- Most drugs are removed from the body by the kidneys. If you have chronic kidney failure and take prescription drugs, the dose may need adjusting.
- Avoid nonprescription drugs unless medically approved.

ACTIVITY
- Get rest as needed. Otherwise, stay as active as your strength allows. Try to exercise on a regular basis.
- Avoid contact sports (to prevent kidney injury).

DIET—You will be advised about the need for any special diet and amount of fluids to drink.

CALL YOUR DOCTOR IF

- You or a family member has symptoms of polycystic kidney.
- You have symptoms of kidney failure, signs of infection, severe headache, urination decreases, or blood appears in urine.

KIDNEY INFECTION, ACUTE
(Pyelonephritis, Acute)

GENERAL INFORMATION

DEFINITION—Acute kidney infection is an infectious, inflammatory disorder of the kidneys. The symptoms may begin suddenly and can range from mild to severe. It is called uncomplicated or complicated depending on a person's health status.

BODY PARTS INVOLVED—Kidneys; urinary tract.

SEX OR AGE MOST AFFECTED—Both sexes, but more common in females of all ages.

SIGNS & SYMPTOMS
- Fever and shaking chills.
- Burning, frequent urination.
- Cloudy urine or blood in the urine.
- Lower back (flank) pain (on one or both sides).
- Pain in the abdomen.
- Fatigue.
- Nausea and vomiting.

CAUSES—Most often, the infection is due to bacteria called *Escherichia coli*. Less often, other types of bacterial are the cause. The bacteria infection (called cystitis) begins in the bladder and the infected urine moves back up the tubes (ureters) that connect the bladder to the kidneys. This is called reflux.

RISK INCREASES WITH
- Sexual intercourse (for women). New sexual partner.
- Recent, or history of, urinary tract infection.
- Catheters, tubes, or some surgical procedures.
- Weak immune system due to illness or drugs.
- Diabetes.
- Recent incontinence.
- Recent spermicide use.
- Blockage or abnormality of the urinary system. This can be caused by stones, obstructions, nerve diseases, tumors, or prostate enlargement.
- Prolonged bed rest such as in nursing home.

HOW TO PREVENT
- Get treatment for any bladder infection.
- Women and girls always wipe from front to back (not back to front) after going to bathroom.
- Urinate within 15 minutes after sexual intercourse.
- Don't hold urine. If you have the urge to void, do so.

WHAT TO EXPECT

DIAGNOSTIC MEASURES
- Your own observation of symptoms.
- Your health care provider will do a physical exam along with a pelvic exam in females and a rectal exam (for prostate problems) in males. Questions will be asked about your symptoms.
- Medical tests may include urinalysis, urine culture, and blood studies. Other tests may be done to diagnose kidney stones or obstructions.

APPROPRIATE HEALTH CARE
- Treatment usually involves antibiotic drugs, or, in some cases, surgery or hospital care may be needed.
- Surgery may be needed for an obstruction or kidney stones, or for an abnormality diagnosed in a child.
- Hospital care may be needed for severe symptoms or if there are other medical problems.

POSSIBLE COMPLICATIONS
- Kidney infection recurs or becomes chronic.
- Kidney damage and chronic kidney disease.
- Blood infection (sepsis) or renal abscess.

PROBABLE OUTCOME—With early diagnosis and treatment, an uncomplicated kidney infection is usually curable in 10 to 14 days. Pregnant women, elderly, and people with other health problems are more at risk for complications.

HOW TO TREAT

GENERAL MEASURES
- Be sure to see your health care provider for follow-up urine tests to verify that the infection is cured.
- To learn more: National Kidney & Urologic Diseases Information Clearinghouse, 3 Information Way, Bethesda, MD 20892; (800) 891-5390; website: www.kidney.niddk.nih.gov.

MEDICATION
- Oral antibiotics. Take all the antibiotics prescribed, even if symptoms clear up.
- Antibiotics (intravenous or by injection), if oral antibiotics don't cure the infection.
- Take nonprescription drugs such as ibuprofen for pain symptoms.
- Urinary analgesics to relieve pain may be prescribed.

ACTIVITY—Rest in bed until any fever and discomfort are gone. Resume sexual relations when advised by your health care provider.

DIET—No special diet. Drink plenty of fluids. Drinking cranberry juice may be recommended.

CALL YOUR DOCTOR IF

- You or a family member has symptoms of a kidney infection.
- Symptoms and fever persist after 48 hours of antibiotic treatment.
- Symptoms return after treatment.

KIDNEY INFECTION, CHRONIC
(Pyelonephritis, Chronic)

 GENERAL INFORMATION

DEFINITION—Chronic kidney infection is a disorder of the kidneys that develops slowly and lasts for months or years. Over time, the kidneys become scarred or damaged. They begin to lose their ability to function as they normally would in removing waste products from the blood.

BODY PARTS INVOLVED—Kidneys.

SEX OR AGE MOST AFFECTED—It affects infants and young children more than it does adults. It is more common in females.

SIGNS & SYMPTOMS
- Usually there are no symptoms (unlike acute kidney infection). It may be diagnosed when medical tests are done for recurrent urinary tract infections.
- Symptoms that do occur may be vague, such as abdominal pain, fever, tiredness, nausea, and vomiting.
- Failure to thrive in infants or young children.

CAUSES—It results from recurrent or persistent kidney (renal) infection and inflammation. It occurs mostly in people who have a urinary tract abnormality (different from the normal).

RISK INCREASES WITH
- Acute kidney infection (acute pyelonephritis).
- Vesicoureteral reflux or VUR (backward flow of urine) in children.
- Diabetes.
- Urinary obstruction, such as from renal stones, tumors, or enlarged prostate.

HOW TO PREVENT
- There are no specific preventive measures.
- Controlling diabetes, getting treatment for urinary tract infections, or surgery for a urinary tract abnormality can help reduce risks.

 WHAT TO EXPECT

DIAGNOSTIC MEASURES
- Your health care provider will do a physical exam.
- Medical tests include blood and urine studies and urine culture. Other tests may include x-ray, ultrasound, kidney scan, cystoscopy, or a urine voiding study.

APPROPRIATE HEALTH CARE
- Treatment may include drugs or surgery.
- Surgery may be needed to relieve obstruction or correct any structural problem in the urinary tract.

POSSIBLE COMPLICATIONS
- Kidney failure.
- End-stage renal disease (ESRD).
- Need for a kidney transplant or kidney dialysis.
- Hypertension (high blood pressure).

PROBABLE OUTCOME
- The outcome depends on the extent of kidney damage. Early diagnosis and treatment can help delay disease progress.
- VUR in children may in time resolve on its own.

 HOW TO TREAT

GENERAL MEASURES
- Follow your treatment plan carefully. This may not be easy for an illness that causes few symptoms in the early stages.
- To learn more: National Kidney & Urologic Diseases information Clearinghouse, 3 information Way, Bethesda, MD 20892, (800) 891-5390; website: www.kidney.niddk.nih.gov.

MEDICATION
- Antibiotics may be prescribed. They are taken for months or years.
- Drugs may be prescribed to keep the urine slightly acidic.
- Drugs may be prescribed to lower blood pressure.

ACTIVITY—Usually, no limits. You will be advised of any temporary limits if surgery is performed.

DIET
- To help prevent urinary tract infections, drink plenty of fluids each day. Drinking cranberry juice may also help.
- A low-protein diet may be prescribed if kidney failure develops.

 CALL YOUR DOCTOR IF

- You or a family member has symptoms of chronic kidney infection.
- You or a family member has symptoms of an acute kidney infection, such as urgent, frequent, or burning urination; fever and chills; fatigue; and cloudy urine.

KIDNEY STONES
(Renal Calculi)

GENERAL INFORMATION

DEFINITION—Kidney stones are small, solid particles that form in one or both kidneys. They sometimes travel into the ureter (slender muscular tubes that carry urine from the kidneys to the urinary bladder). Stones vary from the size of a grain of sand to a golf ball, and there may be one or several.

BODY PARTS INVOLVED—Kidneys.

SEX OR AGE MOST AFFECTED—Adults of both sexes (more often in men); ages over 30.

SIGNS & SYMPTOMS
* Episodes of severe, off and on pain every few minutes. The pain usually appears first in the back, just below the ribs. Over several hours or days, the pain follows the stone's course through the ureter toward the groin. Pain stops when the stone passes.
* Frequent nausea.
* Cloudy or dark urine or blood in urine.

CAUSES—Stones are made up of crystals that form in the urine. Normally, the urine contains chemicals that stop crystals from forming. These chemicals do not seem to work for everyone, and some people form stones. Why this occurs is unknown. Kidney stones contain various chemicals. They may be made up of calcium (most common), struvite, uric acid, or cystine.

RISK INCREASES WITH
* Personal or family history of kidney stones.
* Men more than women.
* Obesity and weight gain.
* Caucasians and Asians more than other races.
* Hyperparathyroidism (excess parathyroid hormone).
* Urinary-tract infections (UTI) or blockage.
* Gout (uric-acid stones).
* Kidney disorders.
* Rarely, certain drugs may increase risk.
* Chronic bowel inflammation or bowel surgery.
* Bed rest for a long period of time.
* Diet factors (e.g., low fluid or high protein).

HOW TO PREVENT—No specific measures to prevent a first kidney stone. If you have had one kidney stone, you are more likely to have another and should take preventive measures. These will depend on the type of stone formed.

WHAT TO EXPECT

DIAGNOSTIC MEASURES
* Your health care provider will do a physical exam and ask about your symptoms and activities.

* Medical tests may include urinalysis, urine culture, x-rays, and other tests to confirm the diagnosis.

APPROPRIATE HEALTH CARE
* Small stones may need no specific treatment. They usually pass within 72 hours. Strain all urine and save the stone for analysis of the type of stone.
* Treatment may be done to remove larger stones if they don't pass on their own and are causing complications, infection, or severe pain. Options include chemical dissolution, endourologic stone extraction, percutaneous nephrolithotomy, extracorporeal shock wave lithotripsy, and rarely, open surgery. Other, new approaches are also being studied. Your health care provider will discuss these options with you.
* Stones due to excess calcium in the body may require surgical removal of abnormal parathyroid tissue.

POSSIBLE COMPLICATIONS
* Urinary-tract infection.
* Kidney damage or scarring.
* Kidney function may be lost or reduced.

PROBABLE OUTCOME—Most kidney stones will pass out of the body on their own. Stones that cause symptoms or complications can be treated successfully. Stones often recur.

HOW TO TREAT

GENERAL MEASURES—To learn more: National Kidney & Urologic Diseases Information Clearinghouse, 3 Information Way, Bethesda, MD 20892; (800) 891-5390; website: www.kidney.niddk.nih.gov.

MEDICATION
* Pain relievers may be prescribed.
* Antispasmodics to relax the ureter muscles and help the stone pass may be prescribed.
* Drugs may be prescribed that will stop the growth of new or existing stones.

ACTIVITY—During a kidney-stone episode, stay as active as possible. Activity may help the stone pass.

DIET—Drink lots of fluids (water is best). Eating less red meat may be helpful. You may be advised to make other diet changes to help prevent more stones.

CALL YOUR DOCTOR IF

* You or a family member has symptoms of a kidney stone.
* Kidney infection occurs (stinging, burning on urination, or a frequent urge to urinate).

LABYRINTHITIS

GENERAL INFORMATION

DEFINITION—Labyrinthitis is an inflammation of the labyrinth (fluid-filled canals and sacs) in the inner ear. The labyrinth contains the vestibular system, which controls a person's balance and eye movement. It also contains the cochlea, which controls hearing. Labyrinthitis may affect one or both ears.

BODY PARTS INVOLVED—Ears.

SEX OR AGE MOST AFFECTED—It can affect both sexes and all ages, including children.

SIGNS & SYMPTOMS
- Vertigo. A sensation that you or your surroundings are spinning around. Head movements make it worse.
- Hearing loss (one or both ears; may be mild or severe and may vary).
- Involuntary eye movement.
- Nausea and vomiting.
- Loss of balance (may fall toward affected side).
- Ringing in the ear (tinnitus).
- Feeling of fullness in the ears.

CAUSES—The cause is often a viral infection, but sometimes is unknown or unclear. It may result from other infection or trauma. The whole inner ear is about the size of a dime and the disorder often affects both hearing and balance.

RISK INCREASES WITH
- Upper respiratory viral infection (e.g., mumps).
- Bacterial infection in the middle ear.
- Head injury.
- Stress or fatigue.
- Allergies or family history of allergies.
- Smoking.
- Excess alcohol use.
- Some prescription or nonprescription drugs.
- Heart, brain, or blood-vessel disease.
- Cholesteatoma (cyst in middle ear) is rare.

HOW TO PREVENT
- Obtain prompt medical care for ear infections.
- Don't take drugs that have caused dizziness symptoms for you in the past.

WHAT TO EXPECT

DIAGNOSTIC MEASURES
- Your own observation of symptoms.
- Your health care provider will do an exam of the ears and your eye movements. Your head and body may be placed or moved in different positions to help determine what movements bring on the symptoms. You may be asked to walk so your balance can be checked.
- Medical tests may include hearing tests, CT, MRI, and others to determine any underlying disorder.

APPROPRIATE HEALTH CARE
- Treatment includes steps to treat any underlying disorder, rest, and drugs for symptoms if needed.
- Rarely, surgery is needed to drain pus or treat a cholesteatoma.

POSSIBLE COMPLICATIONS
- Injuries from falls that occur due to vertigo.
- Permanent hearing loss on the affected side (rare).

PROBABLE OUTCOME—The disorder usually resolves on its own in 1 to 6 weeks. Treatment can help relieve symptoms. Some mild vertigo symptoms may continue for several months.

HOW TO TREAT

GENERAL MEASURES—This disorder can be frightening and debilitating but complete recovery is usual.

MEDICATION
- Your health care provider may prescribe:
  - Antinausea drugs (oral or suppositories).
  - Tranquilizers to reduce dizziness.
  - Diuretics to decrease excess fluid in the inner ear.
  - Antibiotics for bacterial infection.
  - Antivirals for virus infection.
  - Antihistamines to relieve symptoms.

ACTIVITY—Keep the head as still as possible. Rest in bed until vertigo stops. Then resume your normal activities gradually. Avoid activities, such as driving, climbing, or working around dangerous machinery until symptoms clear up.

DIET—No special diet is needed. Nausea and vomiting symptoms may make eating difficult. Drink clear liquids and eat bland foods until symptoms improve.

CALL YOUR DOCTOR IF

- You or a family member has symptoms of labyrinthitis.
- The following occur during treatment:
  - Decreased hearing in either ear.
  - Persistent vomiting.
  - Convulsions or fainting.
  - Fever of 101°F (38.3°C) or higher.
  - New, unexplained symptoms develop.

LACTOSE INTOLERANCE
(Milk Intolerance; Lactase Deficiency)

 GENERAL INFORMATION

DEFINITION—Lactose intolerance is the inability to digest lactose, a sugar found in milk products. It is a common disorder. Lactose intolerance (a digestive problem) is different from a milk allergy (which involves the body's immune system).

BODY PARTS INVOLVED—Digestive system.

SEX OR AGE MOST AFFECTED—It usually develops in teens and adults of both sexes and continues for life. Some infants are born with it.

SIGNS & SYMPTOMS
* Symptoms will vary depending on the amount of lactose each person can tolerate. Symptoms occur about 30 minutes to 2 hours after eating or drinking foods that contain lactose. They may be mild to more severe.
* Rumbling stomach sounds.
* Stomach cramps and diarrhea.
* Gas and bloating.
* Nausea.
* Newborns may have foamy diarrhea, diaper rash, vomiting (maybe), and slow weight gain.

CAUSES
* Deficiency or absence of the enzyme lactase. Lactase is produced by the small intestine and is needed to digest all milk except mother's milk. Without it, sugars in milk absorb fluid and cause symptoms. Lactase production tends to decrease after childhood as the diet changes and is less dependent on milk.
* Secondary (or acquired) lactose intolerance occurs after an illness, surgery, injury, or along with certain diseases (e.g., Crohn's disease). This intolerance usually resolves on its own, but may be permanent.

RISK INCREASES WITH
* Family history of lactase enzyme deficiency.
* Genetic factors. It is more common in Blacks, Native Americans, Asians, Hispanics, and Ashkenazi Jews.

HOW TO PREVENT—Cannot be prevented at present.

 WHAT TO EXPECT

DIAGNOSTIC MEASURES
* Your own observation of symptoms.
* Your health care provider may do a physical exam. A trial period of no dairy products may be advised to see if symptoms stop.
* Medical tests may include blood studies, a hydrogen breath test, or lactose absorption test.

APPROPRIATE H
involves diet changes
person depending on th
people with lactose intolera
eat some amount of milk prod
Using lactase enzymes is also a

POSSIBLE COMPLICATIONS—Ca
deficiency and weak bones (rare).

PROBABLE OUTCOME—There is no cure
this disorder, but it does not cause a threat to
good health. Symptoms can be controlled with
diet changes. Symptoms may worsen at times
for unknown reasons.

 HOW TO TREAT

GENERAL MEASURES—To learn more: National Institute of Diabetes and Digestive and Kidney Disorders, 2 Information Way, Bethesda, MD 20892; (800) 891-5389; website: www.digestive.niddk.nih.gov.

MEDICATION
* The enzyme lactase is available without a prescription. It can be taken as a tablet or as a liquid that is added to milk and milk products. It acts in much the same way as the naturally occurring enzyme does.
* Some prescription and nonprescription drugs have lactose as an ingredient (e.g., some birth control pills and antacids). They may affect people who have severe lactose intolerance.

ACTIVITY—No limits.

DIET
* Reduce or restrict milk and milk products, such as cheese and ice cream. Lactose-free milk is available.
* Yogurt and fermented products such as hard cheese are often tolerated better than milk.
* Read food labels with care. Avoid products that contain milk, lactose, milk sugar, whey, curds, milk by-products, dry milk solids, and nonfat dry milk powder.
* Infants: If the condition is present at birth, an infant formula that contains little or no lactose, such as a soybean-based formula, will be recommended. If the lactose intolerance is short-term and caused by illness, a substitute formula is needed for a short time. Cow's milk can be introduced again later.
* Ask your health care provider about taking calcium supplements.

 CALL YOUR DOCTOR IF

* You or your child has lactose intolerance symptoms.
* Treatment is not helping symptoms.

WHAT TO EXPECT

DIAGNOSTIC MEASURES
- Your own observation of symptoms.
- Your health care provider can usually diagnose the problem by an exam of the affected skin area.
- Other medical tests may be done to confirm the diagnosis.

APPROPRIATE HEALTH CARE
- Self-care is usually all that is needed.
- Medical care may involve drug therapy.

POSSIBLE COMPLICATIONS
- If the blisters are scratched and opened, a bacterial infection may occur.
- Retreatment may be needed if the symptoms recur (larva may have been damaged, but not killed with original treatment).
- Very rarely, other complications may occur.

PROBABLE OUTCOME—The outcome is good. The infection may heal on its own over several weeks or months. Treatment with drugs can hasten the healing process.

HOW TO TREAT

GENERAL MEASURES—Apply cool, moist compresses to the affected area to help relieve itching.

MEDICATION
- Your health care provider may prescribe an antiparasitic drug to be taken by mouth (usually) or applied to the skin.
- Nonprescription oral antihistamines may be used to help relieve itching.

ACTIVITY—No limits.

DIET—No special diet.

CALL YOUR DOCTOR IF

- You or a family member has symptoms of larva migrans.
- Skin symptoms become worse or there are new symptoms.
- You take an oral anti-parasitic drug, and new, unexplained symptoms develop.

BODY PARTS ... that come in contact with the ground, usually feet, legs or buttocks.

SEX OR AGE MOST AFFECTED—Both sexes; all ages. It occurs more often in children.

SIGNS & SYMPTOMS—First, there may be a tingling or prickling of the skin area. Then it begins to itch. This is followed by a rash or small blisters on the skin. They often form thin, raised tracks (or lines) on the skin leading from the parasite's entry point. The tracks can get longer each day. There are usually several tracks at the same time, each of different length and pattern.

CAUSES—A hookworm-infested animal passes feces (stool) that contains the hookworm eggs into moist, sandy soil. The eggs hatch into larvae that infest the soil around the feces droppings. When a human comes in contact with the soil, the larvae are able to penetrate the skin and cause the symptoms. The infection cannot be spread from one person to another.

RISK INCREASES WITH
- Working or playing in warm, moist sand (such as a beach or a child's sandbox) in which cats or dogs have defecated.
- Walking barefoot in sand or dirt.
- Work that requires crawling in confined spaces and contact with infected soil (e.g., plumbers working under houses).

HOW TO PREVENT
- Wear shoes or sandals when walking on beaches that may be used by dogs or cats. Sit or lie on beach chairs or air mattress rather than towels on the sand.
- Don't work or play in soil used by cats and dogs for elimination.
- Have pets treated for worms.
- Clean up pet droppings.

LARYNGEAL CANCER
(Larynx Cancer)

 GENERAL INFORMATION

DEFINITION—Laryngeal cancer is cancer of the larynx (voice box). The larynx plays a role in helping a person breathe, swallow, and talk.

BODY PARTS INVOLVED—The larynx is about 2 inches long and 2 inches wide and located at the back of the throat.

SEX OR AGE MOST AFFECTED—Both sexes; (more common in men); adults over age 40.

SIGNS & SYMPTOMS
- Few or no symptoms in early stages.
- Hoarseness; scratchy, weak, or changed voice that does not go away.
- "Lump-in-the-throat" feeling.
- Painful or difficult swallowing.
- Trouble breathing.
- Hard, swollen lymph glands in the neck.
- Weight loss.
- Ear pain.
- Chronic cough.

CAUSES—Exact cause is unknown. Smoking or alcohol abuse are known major risk factors.

RISK INCREASES WITH
- Age over 55. Men more than women.
- African Americans more than whites.
- Smoking and/or excess alcohol use.
- Having had head or neck cancer.
- Exposure to certain chemicals, toxins, or asbestos.
- Gastroesophageal reflux disease (GERD).

HOW TO PREVENT
- Don't smoke. Don't drink more than 1 or 2 alcoholic drinks, if any, a day.
- Avoid exposure to known toxins.

 WHAT TO EXPECT

DIAGNOSTIC MEASURES
- Your own observation of symptoms. Be alert to hoarseness that persists beyond 2 weeks.
- Your health care provider will do a physical exam and ask questions about your symptoms.
- A variety of medical tests will be done to verify the exact type of cancer cells, the grade (fast or slow growing), and if the cancer has spread (called staging) to other places in the body.

APPROPRIATE HEALTH CARE
- Treatment will depend on the cancer type, grade and location, its stage, your health, age, and preferences. Preserving a good voice quality is a goal of treatment. Your health care provider will discuss your specific diagnosis and treatment options with you.

- Surgery, radiation, and/or chemotherapy (anticancer drugs) are the usual treatment steps. Other treatments are being studied.
- Advanced cancer often requires surgery. Part or all of the larynx may be removed (laryngectomy). A tracheostomy is performed. This is an opening (stoma) in the throat for breathing. It may be temporary or permanent. A "trach" tube or stoma button keeps it open.
- After larynx removal, therapy will help patients learn to breathe, swallow, eat, and talk. Talking will involve learning esophageal speech or use of a mechanical device.

POSSIBLE COMPLICATIONS
- Complications from treatments (chemotherapy, radiation, and surgery) that may affect the voice, breathing, swallowing, and eating.
- Spread of cancer in the body, which can be life-threatening.
- Cancer may recur after treatment.

PROBABLE OUTCOME—Early diagnosis and treatment offer the best outcome. Later diagnosis or spread of cancer has poorer outlook.

 HOW TO TREAT

GENERAL MEASURES
- Stop smoking. Find a way to quit that works.
- Use good mouth care on teeth and gums.
- Consider joining a cancer support group.
- To learn more: American Cancer Society; (800) ACS-2345; website: www.cancer.org or National Cancer Institute; (800) 4-CANCER; website: www.cancer.gov.

MEDICATION—Anticancer (chemotherapy) drugs may be prescribed.

ACTIVITY—Following larynx removal surgery, you should be able to do almost all the activities you did before. Straining and heavy lifting may be difficult since you cannot hold your breath. You can shower by using a shield over the stoma. Avoid swimming and water activities unless special instructions and equipment are used.

DIET
- Diet changes depend on the treatment. Surgery may require a liquid diet at first, then a soft diet. Learning to swallow again will take practice. Several small meals and snacks during the day may make eating easier.
- Avoid alcohol.

 CALL YOUR DOCTOR IF

- You or a family member has symptoms of laryngeal cancer.
- Symptoms worsen or new symptoms occur.

LARYNGITIS

GENERAL INFORMATION

DEFINITION—Laryngitis is an inflammation of the larynx (voice box) and surrounding tissues. Inflammation causes swelling and pain and is a reaction to infection, injury, or irritation. The disorder is common, affects all ages, and occurs more often in late fall, winter, and early spring. With acute laryngitis, the symptoms usually come on quickly and it heals on its own. With chronic laryngitis, the symptoms persist for 3 weeks or longer.

BODY PARTS INVOLVED—Larynx (voice box); the upper part of the neck, behind the Adam's apple.

SEX OR AGE MOST AFFECTED—Both sexes; all ages.

SIGNS & SYMPTOMS
• Hoarseness, weak voice, or loss of voice.
• Sore throat; tickling in the back of the throat.
• Feeling like you have a lump in your throat.
• Slight fever (sometimes).
• Swallowing difficulty (rare).

CAUSES—There are many factors that can lead to acute laryngitis. The most common is a viral infection. Chronic laryngitis may be caused by infection such as tuberculosis. Both types can be due to noninfectious causes such as voice abuse, smoking, and others.

RISK INCREASES WITH
• Viral infection from a recent cold or flu-like illness.
• Excessive use of the voice (such as singers, politicians, cheerleaders, or young children who cry or yell strenuously).
• Exposure to irritants such as mold, pollen and pollutants, or irritating chemicals.
• Allergies.
• Smoking or being around second-hand smoke.
• Gastroesophageal reflux disease (GERD).
• Rarely, it may be a bacterial infection, or be caused by disorders such as tuberculosis, syphilis, fungal infection, or tumor.
• Use of orally inhaled drugs (e.g., for asthma).

HOW TO PREVENT
• Most cases are caused by a virus. Taking steps to prevent viral infections such as hand washing may help.
• Take care to not overuse the voice.

WHAT TO EXPECT

DIAGNOSTIC MEASURES
• Your own observation of symptoms.
• Most people will self-treat this disorder. If symptoms persist, are severe, or cause concern, see your health care provider.
• An exam of the throat, ears, and nose, can usually confirm the diagnosis.
• Medical tests are normally not needed.

APPROPRIATE HEALTH CARE—Home care is the main form of treatment.

POSSIBLE COMPLICATIONS—Complications are rare.

PROBABLE OUTCOME—Acute laryngitis usually clears up on its own in about a week Voice rest and adequate fluid intake are important in healing. With chronic laryngitis, the outcome depends on the underlying condition.

HOW TO TREAT

GENERAL MEASURES
• Avoid using your voice as much as possible. Don't whisper (it can irritate the throat). Write notes to communicate. For most cases, resting the voice for a few days is all that is needed.
• Suck on throat lozenges, cough drops, or hard candy.
• To help relieve minor pain, gargle often with double-strength tea or warm salt water (one-half teaspoon of salt to 8 oz. of water).
• Hot, steamy showers may help.
• Avoid smoking and second-hand cigarette smoke.

MEDICATION
• If an underlying disorder is diagnosed, drugs may be prescribed for treatment.
• Since the cause is usually a viral infection, antibiotics are not helpful. They may be prescribed for suspected bacterial infection.

ACTIVITY—Usually no limits.

DIET—No special diet. Increased fluid intake may be helpful.

CALL YOUR DOCTOR IF

• You or a family member has hoarseness or other symptoms of laryngitis that last longer than 2 weeks.
• You feel very ill, are vomiting, have a high fever, or difficulty breathing. If these symptoms develop in a child, call immediately.

LATEX ALLERGY

GENERAL INFORMATION

DEFINITION—Latex allergy involves reactions of the body to natural rubber latex. Latex is a milky fluid produced by rubber trees. It is used in thousands of products (e.g., rubber gloves). Types of reactions are: irritant contact dermatitis, delayed (type IV) hypersensitivity (allergic contact dermatitis), and immediate (type I) hypersensitivity.

BODY PARTS INVOLVED—Skin.

SEX OR AGE MOST AFFECTED—Both sexes; all ages.

SIGNS & SYMPTOMS
- Irritant contact dermatitis:
  - Dry, crusty, itchy, sore areas on the skin.
  - Often affects the hands (e.g., rubber gloves).
- Delayed (type IV) hypersensitivity:
  - Rash that starts 6 to 48 hours after exposure. Usually starts on the skin area that has come into contact with latex. Rash may spread to other areas.
  - Skin is dry and crusty. May have blisters or sores.
- Immediate (type I) hypersensitivity:
  - Usually occurs right away, but can take hours.
  - Skin is red and itchy; may have hives.
  - Eyes are red and watery.
  - Runny nose, coughing, or sneezing.
  - Chest feels tight; may be short of breath.
  - Shock or a life-threatening reaction (rare).

CAUSES
- Irritant contact dermatitis is not an allergic reaction. It is due to the skin being irritated (e.g., sweating or rubbing under rubber gloves).
- Delayed (type IV) hypersensitivity is most often a reaction to the chemicals added to latex products.
- In immediate (type I) hypersensitivity, the body's immune system reacts to repeated exposure (e.g., over months or years) to latex. It may come from contact with latex or breathing in latex allergens (e.g., from the powder in gloves) that become airborne.

RISK INCREASES WITH
- Health care workers or others who use latex gloves often, or are exposed to them.
- Having had many operations (where you were exposed to latex gloves).
- Other allergies, such as hay fever or eczema.
- Food allergies, including avocado and banana.
- Rubber industry and latex manufacturing workers.
- Children born with spina bifida.

HOW TO PREVENT—For those diagnosed with the allergy, avoid latex.

WHAT TO EXPECT

DIAGNOSTIC MEASURES
- Your own observation of symptoms.
- Your health care provider will do a physical exam and may confirm the diagnosis with a blood test. Skin tests may be done (they carry a risk for serious allergic reactions).

APPROPRIATE HEALTH CARE—There is no treatment, except to avoid latex products.

POSSIBLE COMPLICATIONS
- Some people may need to change jobs due to latex exposure in their workplace.
- Rarely, anaphylaxis, a severe, life-threatening reaction occurs. Seek emergency help.

PROBABLE OUTCOME—There is no cure for latex allergy. Repeated exposure to latex can worsen the immune system response. Avoiding latex is the best action. Many products are made from latex, so this is not always easy to do.

HOW TO TREAT

GENERAL MEASURES
- Find out which products in your home and work contain latex. Thousands of items contain latex. Find substitutes you can use instead. Read labels, or ask, before buying a product.
- Health care workers and others should wear powder-free latex gloves or non-latex gloves. Powder can get in the air, and if breathed in can cause a reaction.
- Most male condoms, as well as diaphragms and cervical caps, are latex. If you use them, ask your health care provider about options for birth control and safe sex.
- Advise any health care provider you consult that you have a latex allergy. Wear or carry medical ID that shows you have this allergy.
- Discuss your latex allergy with your employer to find ways to avoid exposure at work.
- If your allergy is severe, carry a kit with a self-injecting device that contains the drug epinephrine. Instruct family and others on its use if you are unable to do so.
- To learn more: American Latex Allergy Assn., PO Box 198, Singer, WI, 53086; (888) 972-5378; website: www.latexallergyresources.org.

MEDICATION—Drugs may be prescribed for allergy symptoms.

ACTIVITY—No limits.

DIET—No special diet.

CALL YOUR DOCTOR IF

You or a family member has latex allergy symptoms.

LAXATIVE ABUSE

GENERAL INFORMATION

DEFINITION—Laxative abuse occurs when a person misuses or overuses laxatives. Laxative abuse is defined as (1) use of laxative for weight control, or (2) frequent use of laxatives over an extended period of time. It may result from a false belief that frequent bowel movements are necessary. Persons with eating disorders or binge eaters may abuse laxatives to get rid of large meals. Many individuals unintentionally develop the laxative habit.

BODY PARTS INVOLVED—Gastrointestinal system.

SEX OR AGE MOST AFFECTED—Both sexes; often occurs in adolescents or older adults.

SIGNS & SYMPTOMS
- Chronic constipation or chronic diarrhea.
- Gas and bloating.
- Laxative dependence (need laxatives to produce bowel movements).
- Dehydration due to excess loss of fluid.
- Electrolyte imbalance (minerals needed for body function), which causes tremors, muscle cramps, and spasms.
- Blood in the stools.
- Nausea or vomiting.
- Colon infection.

CAUSES—Short-term or long-term, laxatives create and continue the very problem they were trying to correct. Laxatives bring on constipation as the colon's tissues become dried out, muscles become weak, and the nerves lining the colon become damaged. Because of the damage that laxatives cause, ever-increasing dosages of laxatives may be required in order to achieve the desired effect. Where one laxative dose produced results, now two, then three doses a day are required. People who abuse laxatives for a long period of time may end up taking as many as 6 to 8 laxatives a day.

RISK INCREASES WITH
- Persons with eating disorders or binge eaters. They believe they are losing weight and that they are thinner. What is lost is water weight. It comes back on within 48 hours.
- False belief that you need a daily bowel movement.
- Preparing for competitions (sporting event, pageants, etc.).

HOW TO PREVENT
- Don't use laxatives on a routine basis.
- Avoid constipation. Read ideas under Diet. Go to the bathroom when you feel the urge.
- Exercise regularly to stimulate bowel activity.
- Get treatment for eating disorders (anorexia or bulimia) or disordered eating (abnormal change in eating patterns).

WHAT TO EXPECT

DIAGNOSTIC MEASURES
- Your own observation of symptoms.
- Ask your health care provider about how to recover normal bowel function and what steps to use to begin to reverse the laxative habit.

APPROPRIATE HEALTH CARE
- Self-care is usually all that is needed.
- Counseling may be useful for persons who are chronic laxative abusers. This type of therapy is important for people with eating disorders.

POSSIBLE COMPLICATIONS—It depends on the type of laxatives abused, the amount abused, and how long they have been abused. Can cause severe harm to the body and death.

PROBABLE OUTCOME—Will depend on the extent of the abuse and the motivation of the person. Withdrawal from laxatives can take days, weeks, or even months. Body functions should return to normal with no lasting damage.

HOW TO TREAT

GENERAL MEASURES
- Stopping laxatives may be done gradually or by going "cold turkey" (stopping in one day).
- Changing to products containing psyllium may help if you gradually withdraw from laxatives.
- Withdrawal symptoms may include nausea, constipation, bloating, and gas. They will stop as your body recovers and learns how to regulate itself again.

MEDICATION
- No drugs are usually needed. If a drug you take causes constipation, a change in drug or change in dosage amount may help.
- Your health care provider may suggest certain types of products to help ease constipation.

ACTIVITY—Exercise daily. It improves overall health and helps with digestion.

DIET
- Be sure to eat enough food to promote regular bowel movements. Eat high-fiber items like fruits, vegetables, and whole grains. Be careful, as some foods may cause intestinal gas, and if you already have discomfort, this may add to it.
- Drinking lots of water is important. Try to drink 8 to 10 glasses per day if possible. If you are constipated, warm/hot beverages can help.

CALL YOUR DOCTOR IF

You or a family member has a laxative abuse problem.

LEAD POISONING

GENERAL INFORMATION

DEFINITION—Lead poisoning occurs when there is a high level of lead in the body. Lead is all around us. It is found in older paint, batteries, drinking water, and pottery or other ceramic dishes. A little bit of lead finds its way into everyone and usually causes no problems. Too much lead in the body can cause serious problems, especially in infants and young children.

BODY PARTS INVOLVED—Gastrointestinal system; nervous system.

SEX OR AGE MOST AFFECTED—Both sexes; all ages, most common in young children.

SIGNS & SYMPTOMS
- Often no symptoms or they may be delayed.
- Pale skin, fatigue, feeling sluggish, sleeping problems.
- Behavior changes (such as being irritable).
- Child may be overly active.
- Stomach discomfort and poor appetite.
- Difficulty in concentrating.
- Headache; vomiting; weight loss; constipation.
- Higher lead levels: severe stomach cramps; rigid abdomen, muscle weakness, seizures, or coma.

CAUSES—Breathing in of lead dust or fumes, or taking lead in by mouth (ingestion). Lead in the body interferes with normal body functions. It affects red blood cells and the nerve cells in the brain.

RISK INCREASES WITH
- Children under 3. Their brain and nervous systems are still developing and are more affected by lead.
- Childhood behaviors such as hand-to-mouth activity and pica (repeated eating of nonfood products) increase the risk of taking in lead.
- Homes with lead-based paint (its use stopped in the mid-1970s). Children eat, chew, or suck on the paint. During remodeling, lead paint dust can get into the air.
- Lead plumbing (its use stopped in 1986).
- Using lead-glazed ceramics for food or drink.
- Some candies from Mexico have had high lead levels.
- Glazed pottery work, lead soldering, artists' paints, preparing lead shot, stained-glass work, some inks, car or boat repair, and others.
- Work or job exposure. Over 900 occupations have been connected with lead poisoning.
- Some cosmetics and folk remedies.
- Retained bullets or shrapnel.

HOW TO PREVENT
- Have children age 6 months to 6 years tested regularly for lead levels. Talk to your child's health care provider.
- Avoid risk factors where possible.
- Routine blood-lead tests for workers exposed to lead.
- Education about lead and ways to decrease lead exposure. Call (800) 424-LEAD; website: www.epa.gov/lead.

WHAT TO EXPECT

DIAGNOSTIC MEASURES
- Your health care provider may do a physical exam.
- Medical tests include blood studies to measure lead levels. Kidney and liver function testing and x-rays of the abdomen may be done.

APPROPRIATE HEALTH CARE
- Treatment involves avoiding any further exposure to the lead.
- Regular follow up blood testing is needed to be sure the blood lead levels are decreasing.
- For some patients, medical therapy will help the body excrete (get rid of) the lead. Hospital care may be needed for severe symptoms.

POSSIBLE COMPLICATIONS
- Damage to the nervous system, kidneys, liver, heart, and other body organ systems.
- Children may have mental retardation, behavior problems, learning disorders, aggressiveness, or delayed or slower growth. Seizures, coma, and death could occur.
- Adults may have loss of sex drive, impotence, or infertility. High lead levels in a pregnant woman can harm her unborn child.

PROBABLE OUTCOME—Lead poisoning without any apparent brain damage generally improves over time. Some problems may be long-lasting or permanent.

HOW TO TREAT

GENERAL MEASURES
- A report should be made to the local health department. An inspection of the home or workplace can be done to find the source of lead. Lead-level blood tests should be done for all family members.
- If the source is in the home, the patient needs to live elsewhere until lead source is removed.

MEDICATION—Chelating agents to excrete lead may be prescribed.

ACTIVITY—No limits.

DIET—No special diet unless advised.

CALL YOUR DOCTOR IF

You or a family member has symptoms of lead poisoning or you want blood lead levels tested.

LEGG-CALVÉ PERTHES DISEASE
(Coxa Plana)

 ## GENERAL INFORMATION

DEFINITION—Legg-Calve-Perthes disease is a hip disorder of childhood. It involves gradual weakening of the head of the thigh bone where it meets the pelvis.

BODY PARTS INVOLVED—Either leg at the hip joint (occasionally both).

SEX OR AGE MOST AFFECTED—It affects children ages 2 to 12 years (most often 4 to 8) of both sexes, but it is more common in boys (80% of the patients).

SIGNS & SYMPTOMS
- Pain and stiffness in the hip and thigh. Sometimes both sides are involved.
- Pain in the leg and often in the knee, even though the disorder is in the hip.
- Limping or other problems with walking.
- Symptoms usually begin slowly over time.

CAUSES—The bone becomes weak due to lack of a blood supply to the top of the bone. The weak bone is not able to handle weight. Why this occurs is unknown. It may involve growth factors in the body or blood clotting problems. Injury is usually not a factor.

RISK INCREASES WITH
- Boys more than girls. Ages 4 to 10.
- Whites, Eskimos, and Asians are more at risk.
- Possible risks: children who had low birth weight (less than 5 1/2 pounds) and are small for their age and very active; and secondhand smoke exposure.

HOW TO PREVENT—No specific preventive measures.

 ## WHAT TO EXPECT

DIAGNOSTIC MEASURES
- Your own observation of symptoms, especially a limp or knee pain in your child.
- Your child's health care provider will do a physical exam and ask questions about the symptoms.
- Medical tests usually include x-rays or other tests to find how far the problem has progressed.

APPROPRIATE HEALTH CARE
- Treatment depends on several factors: age and health of the child, extent of the disorder, child's tolerance for treatment procedures, and your preferences.

- Treatment may not be recommended for some patients with the disorder. These children will be watched to see if any problems develop. This can include children younger than 6 with no hip motion problems. Older children are usually treated.
- Treatment options are aimed at maintaining the range of motion and keeping the hip bone in the hip socket (called containment). Options include rest, limiting activities, drugs for inflammation, a cast, brace, physical therapy, traction, use of crutches (or wheelchair), or surgery.
- Surgery to reinforce the bone's attachment to the joint and prevent further problems may be needed.
- Traction therapy (involves equipment that places a steady pull on the leg) may be prescribed.

POSSIBLE COMPLICATIONS
- May cause permanent hip problem.
- Osteoarthritis may develop later in life.

PROBABLE OUTCOME—Often curable in 2 to 3 years with early treatment. The blood supply to the bone becomes normal, and new bone cells start growing to replace the old bone.

 ## HOW TO TREAT

GENERAL MEASURES
- Youngsters often have difficulty accepting the need for rest, casts, braces, or other treatment. Help your child find activities and interests that don't involve a lot of movement or athletics.
- Use heat to relieve pain. Warm compresses, heating pads, or other methods are effective.

MEDICATION—For minor discomfort, use nonprescription drugs, such as acetaminophen or ibuprofen. Don't give aspirin to children.

ACTIVITY
- A limited amount of bedrest may be prescribed. Certain activities may be limited, such as running. An activity such as swimming may be recommended.
- A child can and should attend school.
- A physical therapist can teach the child some simple exercises to do to maintain hip movement.

DIET—No special diet, unless the child is overweight.

 ## CALL YOUR DOCTOR IF

- Your child has hip or knee pain, stiffness, or a limp.
- After diagnosis, symptoms don't improve in 4 weeks, despite treatment or pain increases.

LEGIONNAIRE'S DISEASE
(Legionella Pneumophilia Bronchopneumonia)

 GENERAL INFORMATION

DEFINITION—Legionnaire's disease is a form of lung infection. It is named after an epidemic that affected people attending an American Legion convention in 1976. It occurs more often in the summer and early fall seasons.

BODY PARTS INVOLVED—Bronchial tubes; lungs.

SEX OR AGE MOST AFFECTED—It can affect both sexes and all ages, but is more common in older adults.

SIGNS & SYMPTOMS
- General ill feeling.
- Headache, muscle aches, and chest pain.
- Chills and fever up to 105°F (40.6°C).
- Cough without sputum that progresses to one with gray or blood-streaked sputum.
- Nausea, vomiting, diarrhea, and tiredness.
- Mental changes such as disorientation or confusion.

CAUSES
- Infection from *Legionella* bacteria. The bacteria are found in wet or moist environments. They have been found in hot water tanks, in water from shower-heads or faucets, cooling towers, air conditioners, whirlpool spas, soil, potting soil, and other locations.
- People become infected when they breathe in a mist or vapor (small droplets of water in the air) that is contaminated with the bacteria (germs). Symptoms begin 2 to 10 days after exposure. The germs are not spread from one person to another, or from drinking infected water. The risk of getting the infection is quite low, especially in healthy persons. The germs also cause a milder illness called Pontiac fever.
- Outbreaks are when two or more persons become ill in the same place at about the same time. This may happen in a hospital, on a cruise ship, or in a hotel.

RISK INCREASES WITH
- Certain people are more at risk of infection if exposed to *Legionella* bacteria:
  - Older adults.
  - Chronic illness (e.g., diabetes or emphysema).
  - Weak immune system due to illness or drugs.
  - Smokers.
- Working with cooling towers or air conditioners.

HOW TO PREVENT
- No specific preventive measures.
- Proper cleaning and maintenance of water systems, pools, and spas.
- Don't smoke (it increase your risk for infection if exposed to germs).

 WHAT TO EXPECT

DIAGNOSTIC MEASURES
- Your health care provider will do a physical exam and ask about your symptoms and activities.
- Medical tests may include blood and urine studies, sputum culture, and other testing to confirm the diagnosis.

APPROPRIATE HEALTH CARE
- Treatment is with antibiotics and supportive care.
- Hospital care may be needed.

POSSIBLE COMPLICATIONS
- Respiratory failure.
- Septic shock.
- Kidney failure.
- Can be fatal.

PROBABLE OUTCOME—Usually curable with prompt diagnosis and treatment.

 HOW TO TREAT

GENERAL MEASURES
- The following apply to mild cases or to care after a hospital stay:
  - Use a cool-mist humidifier to increase air moisture and thin lung secretions so that they can be coughed up more easily.
  - Use warm compresses or a heating pad on the chest to relieve chest pain.
  - Practice deep-breathing exercises as often as your strength allows.
  - Avoid talking loudly, laughing, or singing. They may trigger excessive coughing.
  - Don't smoke.

MEDICATION
- Antibiotics (finish all the dosage prescribed).
- If the cough is painful and doesn't produce sputum, you may use nonprescription drugs to suppress it. If the cough produces sputum, don't suppress it.
- You may take aspirin (not for children) or acetaminophen to reduce fever.

ACTIVITY—Rest in bed until symptoms improve. Allow 2 to 4 weeks for recovery.

DIET—No special diet. Drink plenty of fluids.

 CALL YOUR DOCTOR IF

- You or a family member has symptoms of Legionnaire's disease.
- During or after treatment you have higher fever; severe chest pain; shortness of breath; dark or bluish nails, lips, or skin; bloody sputum.

LEUKEMIA, ACUTE

GENERAL INFORMATION

DEFINITION
• Leukemia is cancer of the cells in the bone marrow. Bone marrow is the soft material in the center of bones and all blood cells are formed there. White blood cells fight infections, red blood cells carry oxygen, and platelets help control bleeding. With leukemia, the cancerous cells replace the normal bone marrow cells. As the amount of normal white blood cells, platelets, and red blood cells decrease, the body then develops infections, anemia, or bleeds easily. Acute leukemia usually has a sudden onset and symptoms progress rapidly. Acute leukemia has two types (each type has subtypes):
   - Acute lymphocytic leukemia (ALL). It affects all ages, but is more common in children.
   - Acute myeloid (myelogenous) leukemia (AML). It affects both children and adults (usually older adults).

BODY PARTS INVOLVED—Bone marrow and lymph tissue in early stages. The disease eventually affects all body tissues.

SEX OR AGE MOST AFFECTED—Both sexes and all ages depending on type of leukemia.

SIGNS & SYMPTOMS
• Low fever, chills, and sweating.
• Tiredness and weakness.
• Anemia (pale skin, fatigue).
• General ill feeling.
• Easy bruising or bleeding or cuts that heal slowly.
• Pin-head size spots on the skin.
• Repeated infections.
• Bone or joint pain.
• Loss of appetite and/or weight.
• Other symptoms may occur if cancer cells collect in organs such as brain, lungs, genitals, digestive tract, or kidneys.

CAUSES—It is unclear what causes the cancerous cells to develop in leukemia.

RISK INCREASES WITH
• ALL:
   - Children under age 6; having a brother or sister with ALL; adults over age 50.
   - Excess exposure to x-rays or radiation.
   - Genetic disorder, such as Down syndrome.
   - Being white or Hispanic.
   - Prior chemotherapy.
• AML:
   - Older ages; males.
   - Smoking.
   - History of blood disorder or previous cancer therapy with chemotherapy.
   - Exposure to radiation or chemical benzene.

HOW TO PREVENT—Cannot be prevented.

WHAT TO EXPECT

DIAGNOSTIC MEASURES
• Your health care provider will do a physical exam and ask questions about your symptoms.
• Medical tests include blood studies. Samples of bone marrow (liquid and solid) will be taken for viewing with a microscope. Further tests diagnose specific subtype of ALL or AML.

APPROPRIATE HEALTH CARE
• Treatment depends on the leukemia type, patient's age and health, and other factors. Treatment occurs in phases, such as initial treatment to remission to follow-up.
• Treatment may include anticancer drugs (chemotherapy), targeted or biologic therapy, stem cell transplant, or other newer treatments. Radiation or surgery are rarely used. Supportive care is treatment for infections, side-effects of therapy, pain, or other problems.
• Chemotherapy uses drugs to attack cancer.
• Biologic and targeted therapies fight cancer cells indifferent ways.
• Stem cell transplant replaces blood cells destroyed in treatment with stem cells.
• Blood and platelet transfusions may be given.
• Counseling may help you cope.

POSSIBLE COMPLICATIONS
• Hemorrhage or severe infection (can be fatal).
• Failure of leukemia to respond to treatment.
• Relapse (leukemia recurs after remission).

PROBABLE OUTCOME—Depends on the type of leukemia, stage of disease, the patient's health, and response to treatment. It is a potentially curable cancer.

HOW TO TREAT

GENERAL MEASURES
• Avoid crowds and people with infections.
• To learn more: American Cancer Society, 250 Williams St., NW, Atlanta, GA 30303; (800) ACS-2345; website: www.cancer.org.

MEDICATION
• You will be prescribed anticancer drugs; may be taken by mouth or given through a vein (IV).
• Antibiotics may be prescribed for infections.
• Other cancer-fighting agents/drugs may be used.

ACTIVITY—As tolerated.

DIET—No special diet.

☎ CALL YOUR DOCTOR IF

• You or your child has symptoms of leukemia.
• Any symptoms during or after treatment cause you concern.

LEUKEMIA, CHRONIC

GENERAL INFORMATION

DEFINITION
- Leukemia is cancer of the cells in the bone marrow. Bone marrow is the soft material in the center of bones and all blood cells are formed there. White blood cells fight infections, red blood cells carry oxygen, and platelets help control bleeding. With leukemia, the cancerous cells replace the normal bone marrow cells. As the amount of normal white blood cells, platelets, and red blood cells decrease, the body then develops infections, anemia, or bleeds easily. Chronic leukemia develops over a long period of time. Forms of chronic leukemia include:
  - Chronic lymphocytic leukemia (CLL). It often affects older adults; is twice as common as CML.
  - Chronic myeloid (myelogenous) leukemia (CML). It mostly affects adults (rare in children).

BODY PARTS INVOLVED—Blood-forming organs: bone marrow; lymph glands; liver; spleen.

SEX OR AGE MOST AFFECTED—Both sexes, usually adults and males more than females.

SIGNS & SYMPTOMS
- Sometimes, no symptoms occur.
- Low fever, chills, and sweating.
- Tiredness and weakness.
- Anemia (pale skin, fatigue).
- General ill feeling.
- Easy bruising or bleeding or cuts that heal slowly.
- Pin-head size spots on the skin.
- Repeated infections.
- Bone or joint pain.
- Appetite and/or weight loss. Fullness in the stomach.
- Other symptoms may occur if cancer cells collect in organs, such as brain, lungs, genitals, digestive tract, or kidneys.

CAUSES—It is unclear what causes the cancerous cells to develop in leukemia.

RISK INCREASES WITH
- CLL: males; age over 60; whites more than other races; family history of CLL or lymph system cancer.
- CML: males; middle age; excess exposure to radiation (e.g., for cancer treatment). Most people with CML have a genetic mutation called Philadelphia chromosome.

HOW TO PREVENT—No specific preventive measures.

WHAT TO EXPECT

DIAGNOSTIC MEASURES
- Your health care provider will do a physical exam and ask questions about your symptoms.
- Medical tests include blood studies. Samples of bone marrow (liquid and solid) will be taken for viewing with a microscope. Other tests are done to see if the cancer has spread.

APPROPRIATE HEALTH CARE
- Treatment depends on the leukemia type and other factors. The specific types of treatments available will be explained to you.
- CLL patients may not need any immediate treatment (watchful waiting). Follow-up exams are done. If disease progresses, then chemotherapy, radiation therapy, surgery, targeted or biologic therapy, stem cell transplant, or newer treatments may be options.
- CML treatment may include chemotherapy, surgery, targeted or biologic therapy, stem cell transplant (followed with donor lymphocyte infusion), or newer treatments.
- Blood and platelet transfusions may be given.
- Surgery may be done to remove the spleen.
- Counseling may help you cope.

POSSIBLE COMPLICATIONS
- Hemorrhage or severe infection (can be fatal).
- Failure of leukemia to respond to chemotherapy.
- Side effects of treatments.
- Relapse (leukemia recurs after remission).

PROBABLE OUTCOME—Depends on the type of leukemia, stage and grade of disease, the patient's health and age, response to treatment, and other factors. Overall, the outcome is improving due to quicker diagnosis and the different treatments available.

HOW TO TREAT

GENERAL MEASURES
- Avoid crowds and people with infections.
- To learn more: National Cancer Institute, 6116 Executive Blvd., MSC8322, Bethesda, MD 20892; (800) 422-6237; website: www.cancer.gov.

MEDICATION
- Chemotherapy, biologic, or targeted drugs/agents may be prescribed.
- Antibiotics may be prescribed for infections.
- Other drugs may be prescribed for specific complications.

ACTIVITY—As tolerated.

DIET—No special diet unless advised.

CALL YOUR DOCTOR IF

- You or a family member has symptoms of leukemia.
- Any symptoms occur during or after treatment that cause you concern.

LEUKOPLAKIA, ORAL

GENERAL INFORMATION

DEFINITION—Oral leukoplakia is a general term to describe a white patch on the mouth. Hairy leukoplakia is a different disorder, and it occurs in people who have a weak immune system due to drugs or illness. Another form of leukoplakia occurs in the genitals of women.

BODY PARTS INVOLVED—Inside of cheek; floor of mouth; tongue; palate; roof of mouth.

SEX OR AGE MOST AFFECTED—It affects all ages, but it is most common in adults over 60, and in men more than in women.

SIGNS & SYMPTOMS
• A white or off-white patch in the membranes of the mouth. The patch may be tiny or the size of a quarter. It can involve the lips, inside of the cheek, floor and roof of the mouth, tongue, or gums. It is not painful.
• The patch feels firm, rough, and stiff. It cannot be rubbed off.
• The area may be more sensitive when touched or when eating hot or spicy foods.
• It is sometimes first noticed by a dentist when doing a dental exam.

CAUSES—The exact cause is unknown. Chronic irritation of the mucous membranes appears to be involved. Certain risk factors, such as smoking, may lead to the disorder. It can not be spread from one person to another.

RISK INCREASES WITH
• Use of tobacco products, including cigarettes, chewing tobacco, snuff, pipes, or cigars.
• Poor oral hygiene. Repeated irritation to the mouth or tongue. This can be due to a sharp or broken tooth, ill-fitting dentures, cheek biting, or malocclusion (poor bite).
• Excess alcohol use.
• Candidiasis infection may be a risk factor.
• Other risk factors have been mentioned, but their involvement is unclear.

HOW TO PREVENT
• No specific preventive measures.
• For many health reasons, don't smoke or use tobacco products, and avoid or limit alcohol use.
• Use good oral hygiene. See your dentist on a regular basis to check for, and treat, any risk factors.

WHAT TO EXPECT

DIAGNOSTIC MEASURES
• Your own observation of symptoms.
• Your health care provider can diagnose the disorder with a physical exam of the mouth and tongue.
• A biopsy is usually done if a pre-cancerous risk is suspected. The biopsy involves the removal of a small amount of skin tissue to be viewed under a microscope.

APPROPRIATE HEALTH CARE
• Follow-up care may involve a wait-and-watch plan to see if any changes occur in the affected area.
• Drugs may be prescribed, or surgery may be recommended. Your health care provider will discuss the options with you.

POSSIBLE COMPLICATIONS
• In some cases, cancer may develop. Larger size of patch (lesion) has a greater risk.
• Leukoplakia may recur if the problem causing it (such as tobacco use) is not stopped.

PROBABLE OUTCOME—Leukoplakia by itself does not cause any problems and may not require treatment. The concern is that it may be pre-cancerous, and that makes it important to have it diagnosed. In the majority of cases, cancer will not develop.

HOW TO TREAT

GENERAL MEASURES
• Stop any tobacco use and/or alcohol use (including alcoholic mouthwashes).
• Get treatment for any tooth problems or have any denture problems fixed.
• Regular follow up visits with your health care provider are important to see if there are any changes.

MEDICATION
• Topical or oral forms of vitamin A may be prescribed.
• Other forms of treatment are currently undergoing study.

ACTIVITY—No limits.

DIET—No special diet.

CALL YOUR DOCTOR IF

You or a family member has symptoms of oral leukoplakia.

LICE
(Pediculosis; Head Lice)

GENERAL INFORMATION

DEFINITION—Lice are tiny parasites that live on the body or in clothing. Pediculosis (lice infestation) is the medical term. Three types of lice affect humans: head lice, pubic (crab) lice, and body lice (an uncommon type).

BODY PARTS INVOLVED—Head lice affect hair on scalp. Pubic lice usually affect hair in genital area and other areas (less often). Body lice affect skin in close contact with clothing.

SEX OR AGE MOST AFFECTED—Both sexes; all ages. Head lice are contagious and common in children in school or daycare.

SIGNS & SYMPTOMS
● Itching and scratching of the head or other body parts. It may take 2 to 3 weeks or longer after being infected before itching symptoms start. The itching is more common at night.
● You may see eggs ("nits") on hair shafts.

CAUSES—Tiny parasites that bite through skin to obtain nourishment (blood). The bites cause itching, redness, and soreness.

RISK INCREASES WITH
● Head lice:
 - Direct contact with head of infected person.
 - Contact with an infected object such as hair care item, hat, or bedding.
 - Crowded living conditions.
● Pubic lice: sexual contact with infected person; crowded living conditions; shared bed linens.
● Body lice: persons (e.g., homeless) who can't bathe or launder their clothes and bedding.

HOW TO PREVENT
● No specific prevention. Reduce risks if you can.
● Head lice:
 - Avoid head-to-head contact. Don't share combs, brushes, or hats with others.
 - If a child is at risk for lice, check their hair on a weekly basis.
 - If head lice or nits are found on your child, notify the child's school or daycare.
 - Check for lice in household members of an infected person.
● For pubic lice: avoid sexual contact with an infected person (condoms will not protect you).
● For body lice: launder clothing and bedding.

WHAT TO EXPECT

DIAGNOSTIC MEASURES
● Self-diagnosis and self-treatment are sometimes all that is needed.
● When unsure if head lice are the problem, or if pubic or body lice are suspected, see your health care provider. Lice are diagnosed with a physical exam of the affected area.

● A sample of the lice or nit may be removed for viewing under a microscope. Other medical tests may be done in some cases.

APPROPRIATE HEALTH CARE
● Self-care (usually) or medical care if needed.
● Head lice:
 - May be treated with an anti-lice (pediculicide) product (e.g., cream, lotion, or shampoo).
 - Manual removal can be done (e.g., nit picking or wet-combing) or using substances such as petroleum jelly to smother lice.
 - Other therapies, techniques, home remedies, "natural" products are options. Ask your health care provider for advice if unsure about using.
● Pubic lice: treat with anti-lice product. Sexual partners need to be advised about the lice.
● Body lice: destroy or wash infected clothing.

POSSIBLE COMPLICATIONS—Infection at the site of scratching.

PROBABLE OUTCOME—Curable with treatment. It will depend on the treatment used as to when a complete cure is achieved.

HOW TO TREAT

GENERAL MEASURES
● For head lice, you may want to clean items that have been in contact with infected person within the 2 day period before treatment. (Note: per CDC website [see below], this is not required to get rid of lice infestation.)
 - Wash articles such as combs, curlers, hairbrushes, and barrettes in hot water.
 - Machine-wash clothing and bedding in hot water. Dry in the dryer's hot-air cycle.
 - Vacuum floors, furniture, car seats, or other items to help remove any hairs with nits.
● To learn more: Centers for Disease Control & Prevention; (800) 232-4636; website: www.cdc.gov/parasites/lice/index.html

MEDICATION
● Use a nonprescription anti-lice product (e.g., permethrin or pyrethrin are often suggested). Follow label instructions for age group and proper use and follow-up care. You may use a special nit comb to help rid the hair of nits.
● Your health care provider may prescribe and give directions for using other anti-lice products.

ACTIVITY—No limits. A child should continue to attend school or daycare.

DIET—No special diet.

CALL YOUR DOCTOR IF

● You or a family member has symptoms of lice that you are concerned about.
● Self-treatment for lice has not worked.

LICHEN PLANUS

GENERAL INFORMATION

DEFINITION—Lichen planus (LP) is an inflammatory skin condition. It is not cancerous or contagious.

BODY PARTS INVOLVED—It may involve the skin of the legs, trunk, arms, wrists, scalp, or penis. Less often, the lining of the mouth or vagina, toenails, and fingernails (around or under the nailbed) may also be involved.

SEX OR AGE MOST AFFECTED—All ages, but most common in adults ages 30 to 60.

SIGNS & SYMPTOMS
- Small, slightly raised bumps that itch. The bumps are pinkish, purplish, or reddish-purple. They increase gradually and become more widespread.
- Irregular white lines (spider web-like) may be seen on the skin or in the mouth.
- Bumps in the mouth may be tender or cause burning sensation; may make it hard to eat.
- May have hair loss in patches on the head if scalp is affected.
- Affected nails may become thin and damaged with grooves along the nail.
- Pain with intercourse may occur if vagina is affected.

CAUSES—Unknown. It may be an immune or allergic reaction. Few risk factors are known.

RISK INCREASES WITH
- Hepatitis C infection.
- Hepatitis B vaccine or certain flu vaccines.
- Tattoo pigments.
- Very rarely, dental materials may cause a lichen planus-like allergic reaction.

HOW TO PREVENT—Cannot be prevented at present.

WHAT TO EXPECT

DIAGNOSTIC MEASURES
- Your own observation of symptoms.
- Your health care provider can usually diagnose the condition with an exam of the affected area.
- A biopsy may be done to confirm the diagnosis. This involves the removal of a small amount of skin tissue to be viewed under a microscope.

APPROPRIATE HEALTH CARE
- Treatment depends on the severity of symptoms and location on the body. No treatment may be needed in mild cases.
- Treatment helps relieve itching and inflammation and may include drug therapy, phototherapy, and self-care measures.
- Phototherapy called PUVA may be prescribed. It uses ultraviolet light combined with drugs.

POSSIBLE COMPLICATIONS
- Skin infection due to excessive scratching.
- Lichen planus may recur.
- Rarely, hair loss or nail loss may be permanent.
- Lichen planus in the mouth may increase risk for fungal infection and slightly increase the risk of oral cancer. Your health care provider will follow-up on a regular basis to watch for any problems.

PROBABLE OUTCOME—There is no specific cure. It often clears up in 6 to 18 months. Symptoms may come and go. Treatment can help relieve symptoms. Once the bumps are gone, a brown area may remain on the skin. It will fade in time. In some cases, the condition may last for up to 5 years (such as when mouth or genitals are affected).

HOW TO TREAT

GENERAL MEASURES
- Use cool-water soaks to relieve itching.
- Keep skin moisturized.
- Self-examine skin on a regular basis to find any new or changed skin symptoms.
- Manage stress in your life. It may worsen symptoms.
- Use good oral hygiene if mouth affected.
- To learn more: American Academy of Dermatology, PO Box 4014, Schaumburg, IL 60168; (888) 462-3376; website: www.aad.org.

MEDICATION
- You may use nonprescription antihistamines taken by mouth to help control itching.
- Nonprescription cortisone creams or ointments can help to reduce inflammation and itching. Follow directions on the label.
- Use medicated mouthwash for mouth discomfort.
- Topical, oral, or injected drugs may be prescribed for more severe symptoms.
- A lichenoid drug eruption clears up slowly once the drug causing it is stopped or changed.

ACTIVITY—No limits.

DIET—No special diet.

CALL YOUR DOCTOR IF

- You or a family member has symptoms of lichen planus.
- New, unexplained symptoms develop.

LIPOMAS

GENERAL INFORMATION

DEFINITION—Lipomas are benign (noncancerous), slow-growing tumors of fat cells. They grow under the skin (subcutaneous). In a few cases, lipomas may grow in deeper body tissues or in the body's organs.

BODY PARTS INVOLVED—They may involve the torso, neck, back, upper thighs, or arms.

SEX OR AGE MOST AFFECTED—They affect both sexes, and all ages, but are more common in adults.

SIGNS & SYMPTOMS
- Lumps are dome-shaped, and may be small or large.
- Lumps feel "doughy," smooth, and easily movable.
- One or many lipomas may occur on a person.
- Skin over the lump is normal in appearance.
- Most often, they cause no symptoms, such as itching or pain. However, a form of lipoma that contains blood vessels can cause pain.

CAUSES—Unknown. The tendency is probably inherited.

RISK INCREASES WITH—Family history of lipomas.

HOW TO PREVENT—Cannot be prevented at present.

WHAT TO EXPECT

DIAGNOSTIC MEASURES
- Your own observation of symptoms.
- Your health care provider can usually diagnose lipomas with an exam of the affected area.
- In a few cases, medical tests may be done to confirm the diagnosis or check for complications.

APPROPRIATE HEALTH CARE
- No treatment is needed for lumps that are stable in size.
- Surgical removal (if recommended) is usually done in a medical office. Lipomas can be removed with small incisions or removed by liposuction. Instructions for home care after surgery will be provided. (See Lipoma Removal in Surgery section.)
- Treatment with injections may be an option. Steroids are injected to shrink the lipoma. It will take 3 to 4 weeks for results. This treatment does not completely remove the lipoma.
- Your health care provider will discuss treatment for rare types or lipomas in unusual sites.

POSSIBLE COMPLICATIONS
- For the majority of people, there are no complications. In rare cases, certain forms of lipomas may cause complications.
- Rarely, lipomas that are removed may recur.
- Complications, such as wound infection, may develop after lipoma treatment.

PROBABLE OUTCOME—These lumps are benign and most often require no treatment. Treatment outcome is usually excellent.

HOW TO TREAT

GENERAL MEASURES—Follow medical advice about skin care after any surgical procedure.

MEDICATION—Drugs are not needed for this disorder.

ACTIVITY—No limits.

DIET—No special diet.

CALL YOUR DOCTOR IF

- You or a family member is concerned about skin growths.
- The following occur after lipoma surgery:
  - Bleeding that does not respond to moderate pressure.
  - Signs of infection (warmth, swelling or redness) at the surgical site.

LISTERIOSIS

GENERAL INFORMATION

DEFINITION—Listeriosis is a serious infection usually caused by consuming food or fluid contaminated with the bacterium *Listeria monocytogenes*. The risk of a person getting listeriosis after consumption of a contaminated product is very small. Healthy persons may consume contaminated foods without becoming ill.

BODY PARTS INVOLVED—Gastrointestinal system and sometimes, central nervous system.

SEX OR AGE MOST AFFECTED—Both sexes; all ages, but more common in older adults.

SIGNS & SYMPTOMS
* Diarrhea, nausea, fever, and muscle aches.
* If infection spreads to nervous system: headache, stiff neck, confusion, loss of balance, and convulsions.
* Pregnant women typically have only a mild, flu-like illness.
* Newborn may have loss of appetite, be lethargic, vomiting, and may be irritable.

CAUSES—Eating food contaminated with listeria. The bacteria is found in soil and water and infected animals. Babies can be born with listeriosis if their mothers eat contaminated food during pregnancy. Incubation period ranges from 3 to 70 days, but is usually about 3 weeks.

RISK INCREASES WITH
* Older adults.
* Pregnant women.
* People with weak immune system due to illness or drugs.
* Consuming contaminated food.

HOW TO PREVENT
* Do not drink raw (unpasteurized) milk or eat foods that contain raw milk.
* Wash hands and clean kitchen areas and utensils after preparing uncooked foods.
* Clean raw produce (including melons) with a brush and water.
* Thoroughly cook eggs and raw foods such as meat, poultry, or seafood.
* Eat perishable and ready-to-eat foods as soon as possible.
* People at risk—use caution in eating soft cheeses, hot dogs, luncheon meats, deli meats, meat spreads, or refrigerated smoked seafood.

WHAT TO EXPECT

DIAGNOSTIC MEASURES
* Your own observation of symptoms.
* Your health care provider may do a physical exam and ask questions about your symptoms and foods or beverages you have consumed.
* Medical tests may include blood test and urine and spinal fluid tests.

APPROPRIATE HEALTH CARE
* Treatment will depend on the severity of the symptoms, patient's age and immune status, and if pregnant. Drugs are normally prescribed.
* If you have eaten a contaminated product and do not have any symptoms or risk factors, no tests or treatment are usually recommended.
* Pregnant women are treated with drugs to help prevent the baby from being affected.
* Newborns with listeriosis are treated with drugs.

POSSIBLE COMPLICATIONS
* Blood infection, meningitis, or other complication may occur. They can be life-threatening.
* Infections during pregnancy can lead to miscarriage, stillbirth, premature delivery, or life-threatening infection of the newborn. Babies who survive may have long-term mental and physical health problems.

PROBABLE OUTCOME
* Mild symptoms may need no treatment and recovery takes 7 to 10 days. In others, the outcome often depends on the patient's symptoms, age, and health status.
* Pregnant women usually have a good outcome. Treatment can often prevent infection of the fetus.

HOW TO TREAT

GENERAL MEASURES—To learn more: Centers for Disease Control & Prevention; (800) 232-4636; website: www.cdc.gov.

MEDICATION—Antibiotics are prescribed if treatment is needed.

ACTIVITY—No limits except those caused by symptoms.

DIET
* May need liquid or soft diet if symptoms are severe. Drink plenty of fluids each day.
* See How to Prevent for other diet recommendations.

CALL YOUR DOCTOR IF

* You or a family member has symptoms of listeriosis.
* You are at risk for listeriosis and have consumed foods or fluids that may be contaminated.
* After treatment, any new symptoms occur.

LUNG ABSCESS

GENERAL INFORMATION

DEFINITION—A lung abscess is an infected area of lung tissue surrounded by lung inflammation. The infected lung tissue dies and is replaced with pus. The infection is not contagious from person to person.

BODY PARTS INVOLVED—Lung.

SEX OR AGE MOST AFFECTED—Both sexes; all ages. They occur more often in older adults and in men more than women.

SIGNS & SYMPTOMS
- Cough with sputum. The sputum is pus-like, often blood-streaked, and sometimes smells bad.
- Bad breath.
- Sweating.
- Fever up to 101°F (38.3°C) or higher.
- Chills.
- Weight loss.
- Chest pain (sometimes).

CAUSES—Lung abscesses are generally caused by a bacterial infection (less often by parasite or fungal infection). They are usually a result of aspiration (person inhales infected material from the upper-breathing passages). The patient may be unconscious from a head injury or heavily sedated.

RISK INCREASES WITH
- Alcoholism or substance abuse.
- Pneumonia.
- Recent general anesthesia or an injury that causes unconsciousness.
- Poor oral hygiene (e.g., dental or gum disease).
- Seizure disorder; cystic fibrosis.
- Esophageal disorder.
- Lung cancer.
- Diabetes
- There are other, more rare risk factors.

HOW TO PREVENT—No specific preventive measures. Be sure to seek prompt medical treatment for lung infections, especially pneumonia. Practice good dental hygiene.

WHAT TO EXPECT

DIAGNOSTIC MEASURES
- Your own observation of symptoms.
- Your health care provider will do a physical exam.
- Medical tests may include blood tests, a culture of pus from the abscess, and x-rays of the lung. A bronchoscopy may be done. This test uses an optical instrument with a lighted tip that is passed into the windpipe, and then into the bronchi.

APPROPRIATE HEALTH CARE
- Hospital care is usually required.
- Treatment is with antibiotic drugs. Surgery may be needed if antibiotics are not helping the abscess heal.
- Other care in the hospital may involve breathing support with oxygen and procedures to help loosen secretions. Physical therapy can help strengthen the breathing muscles.
- Surgery (sometimes) to remove pus from the abscess or to remove the abscess and part of the lung, if the abscess does not heal.

POSSIBLE COMPLICATIONS
- Abscess may not respond well to antibiotic treatment.
- Rupture of the abscess, causing empyema or massive bleeding in the lung.
- Spread of infection to other body parts, especially the brain.

PROBABLE OUTCOME—Usually curable with antibiotic treatment (may last for 4 to 6 weeks or for several months). In some cases, the underlying condition can affect the outcome.

HOW TO TREAT

GENERAL MEASURES
- Don't smoke. Find a way to quit that works.
- Practice deep-breathing exercises as often as possible.

MEDICATION—Antibiotics for prolonged periods to fight infection and prevent a recurrence. They are given through a vein (IV) at first, and then given by mouth.

ACTIVITY—Reduced activity until tests show a healed abscess.

DIET—No special diet. Increase your fluid intake. By drinking extra liquids, the body is forced to eliminate part of the fluid through the lungs. This makes thick lung secretions thinner, so they can be coughed up more easily.

CALL YOUR DOCTOR IF

- You or a family member has symptoms of a lung abscess.
- Symptoms of a lung infection recur after treatment, especially a sputum-producing cough, fever, or general ill feeling.

LUNG CANCER
(Bronchogenic Carcinoma)

GENERAL INFORMATION

DEFINITION—Lung cancer is cancer that begins in the lungs. There are two major types, non-small cell (more common) and small cell.

BODY PARTS INVOLVED—Bronchial tubes and lung tissues. Cancer spreads to the larynx, liver, brain, bones and kidneys.

SEX OR AGE MOST AFFECTED—Adults of both sexes between ages 40 and 70.

SIGNS & SYMPTOMS
- Usually no symptoms occur in early stages.
- Persistent cough.
- Wheezing or shortness of breath.
- Chest pain.
- Fatigue and weakness.
- Weight loss.
- Shoulder, arm, or bone pain.
- Coughing up blood.

CAUSES—Abnormal cells grow and destroy healthy lung tissue. Primary lung cancer is one that begins in the lungs. It can spread (metastasize) to other places in the body. Most lung cancers result from tobacco use, but it can occur in nonsmokers. Secondary lung cancer is when cancer from another place in the body spreads to the lungs.

RISK INCREASES WITH
- Adults over 65.
- Smoking. Cigarettes (highest risk and the risk increases with number smoked over time), pipes, and cigars.
- Secondhand smoke.
- Radon gas.
- Lung diseases.
- Personal or family history of lung cancer.
- Environmental exposure to asbestos, uranium ore, nickel, chromates, bischloromethyl ether, or air pollution.

HOW TO PREVENT
- Don't smoke. Because tumors don't develop for a long time, smokers can quit at any time and reduce risk of developing lung cancer.
- Obtain regular health check-ups that may include a chest x-ray or CT scan if you are a heavy smoker.
- Check your house for radon gas.

WHAT TO EXPECT

DIAGNOSTIC MEASURES
- Your health care provider will do a physical exam and ask questions about your symptoms. A number of medical tests will be done. The tests first help diagnose the cancer and then determine if it has spread (staging).

APPROPRIATE HEALTH CARE
- Treatment varies and depends on location and size of tumor, any spread of the cancer, your health, age, and preferences. Treatment may include surgery, anticancer drugs (chemotherapy), targeted therapy, and/or radiation therapy.
- Chemotherapy uses drugs and radiation therapy uses radiation to attack the cancer cells. Targeted therapy uses drugs/agents to fight cancer.
- Surgery to remove all of the lung (pneumonectomy) or part of the lung (lobectomy) may be recommended if cancer is at an early stage.
- Treatment may involve steps to relieve symptoms and make you comfortable, rather than treating the cancer.
- Counseling may help you cope.

POSSIBLE COMPLICATIONS
- Side effects of various treatments.
- Respiratory and heart problems or spread of cancer (all can be life-threatening).

PROBABLE OUTCOME—Outcome depends on the type of cancer, whether it has spread, patient's general health, and response to treatment. The outcome is more favorable with early diagnosis compared to diagnosis of advanced disease. Early diagnosis improves the success rate of treatment.

HOW TO TREAT

GENERAL MEASURES
- Stop smoking. Find a way to quit.
- To learn more: American Cancer Society; (800) ACS-2345; website: www.cancer.org or National Cancer Institute; (800) 4-CANCER; website: www.nci.nih.gov.

MEDICATION
- For minor pain, use nonprescription drugs such as acetaminophen, ibuprofen, or aspirin.
- Stronger pain drugs and nausea or anti-anxiety drugs may be prescribed.
- Chemotherapy or targeted therapy drugs/agents may be prescribed.

ACTIVITY—Be as active as possible. Follow medical advice about resuming activities.

DIET—No special diet.

CALL YOUR DOCTOR IF

- You or a family member has symptoms of lung cancer.
- Any symptoms occur during or after treatment that cause you concern.

LUPUS ERYTHEMATOSUS, DISCOID

GENERAL INFORMATION

DEFINITION—Discoid lupus erythematosus (DLE) is a chronic skin disorder. Localized DLE (the more common form) involves the skin on the face, scalp, ears, and neck. Generalized (or widespread) DLE involves other areas of skin. DLE is different from systemic lupus erythematosus (SLE), which affects many different internal organs.

BODY PARTS INVOLVED—Skin.

SEX OR AGE MOST AFFECTED—Both sexes, usually over age 10. The peak incidence occurs in women in their 30s.

SIGNS & SYMPTOMS
- Coin-shaped (discoid), red, raised, scaly skin patches (they may be referred to as rashes, plaques or lesions). Erythematosus means reddening of the skin.
- The centers are lighter in color than the outside ring.
- Patches may appear anywhere on the face. The cheeks and jawline are the most common sites. Some people describe them as "butterfly" rash when they appear on both sides of the nose.
- Sunlight can worsen rash.
- The patches may sometimes appear on the scalp with patches of hair loss.
- Mucous membranes of the mouth may be affected.
- Affected skin is usually not itchy or painful.
- Scarring occurs as the rash heals.

CAUSES—Unknown. It is thought to be an autoimmune disorder. In these disorders, the immune system by mistake attacks the body itself. It cannot be spread from one person to another. Genetic (hereditary), environmental, and hormonal factors may contribute.

RISK INCREASES WITH
- Family history of DLE.
- Females ages 15 to 44.
- Possible triggers for DLE include ultraviolet exposure (e.g., from the sun), smoking, or injury to the skin.

HOW TO PREVENT—No specific preventive measures.

WHAT TO EXPECT

DIAGNOSTIC MEASURES
- Your own observation of symptoms.
- Your health care provider will do an exam of the affected skin and may do a physical exam.
- Medical tests may include blood studies and a skin biopsy. A biopsy involves removal of a sample of the affected skin for viewing under a microscope.

APPROPRIATE HEALTH CARE—Treatment usually involves drug therapy. In some cases, laser therapy or surgery may be options.

POSSIBLE COMPLICATIONS
- Scarring.
- Bald areas can develop.
- Systemic lupus erythematosus (5 to 10% of patients). If it does occur, it is usually not severe.
- Rarely, skin cancer may develop.

PROBABLE OUTCOME—Outcome is generally good. Symptoms of the disorder may come and go over years, but they are not life-threatening. Treatment can help improve the cosmetic appearance of the rash.

HOW TO TREAT

GENERAL MEASURES
- Sun exposure is a trigger for a flare-up. If possible, don't go outdoors between 10 AM and 2 PM, when the sun's ultraviolet light is strongest. If you can't avoid exposure to bright sunlight, wear protective clothing and maximum-protection sunscreen products.
- Stop smoking and avoid secondhand smoke. Smoking can worsen symptoms and interfere with some drug treatments.
- Cosmetics may be used to improve the appearance of the skin.
- Regular checkups with your health care provider are important, even when in remission.
- To learn more: Lupus Foundation of America, 2000 L St., NW, Suite 710, Washington, DC 20036; (800) 558-0121; website: www.lupus.org.

MEDICATION
- Steroid skin creams or ointments are usually prescribed. Follow instructions carefully about their use.
- Injections of steroid into affected skin or oral steroids may be prescribed (with more severe symptoms).
- Antimalaria drugs may be prescribed. They are taken by mouth and often help the symptoms of this disorder.
- Other topical or oral drugs may be prescribed in some cases.
- Use sunscreens for sun protection.

ACTIVITY—No limit.

DIET—No special diet.

CALL YOUR DOCTOR IF

- You or a family member has symptoms of discoid lupus erythematosus.
- The following occur during treatment:
  - New skin symptoms.
  - Swelling, redness, or pain in joints.

LUPUS ERYTHEMATOSUS, SYSTEMIC

GENERAL INFORMATION

DEFINITION—Systemic lupus erythematosus (SLE) is an inflammatory disease that affects various parts of the body. Lupus symptoms often flare up and then subside.

BODY PARTS INVOLVED—Connective tissue (collagen). Many body systems are affected, including joints, skin, kidneys, brain, heart and lungs.

SEX OR AGE MOST AFFECTED—All ages and both sexes, but 90% of cases occur in women between ages 30 and 50.

SIGNS & SYMPTOMS
- Joint aches or pain, with redness and swelling.
- Fever and fatigue.
- Skin rash. Butterfly-like rash on the cheeks.
- Anemia (pale skin and feeling weak).
- Chest pain (with deep breathing).
- Increased sensitivity to the sun.
- Hair loss.
- Ulcers (sores) in the mouth or the nose.
- Seizures.

CAUSES—It is an autoimmune disorder. In these disorders, the immune system attacks the body itself by mistake. Why this occurs is unknown. The disease cannot be spread from one person to another. Genetic, environmental, and hormonal factors play roles.

RISK INCREASES WITH
- Females.
- Family history of lupus.
- Having other autoimmune disorders.
- Smoking.
- Genetic factors (occurs more in Blacks, Hispanics, Native Americans, Native Hawaiians, and Asians).
- Certain drugs can cause an SLE-like syndrome.

HOW TO PREVENT—Cannot be prevented.

WHAT TO EXPECT

DIAGNOSTIC MEASURES
- Your health care provider will do a physical exam and ask questions about your symptoms and activities.
- Medical tests include samples of blood to measure specific antibodies. Patients with vague, recurrent symptoms may require long-term observation and repeated testing before a final diagnosis can be made.

APPROPRIATE HEALTH CARE
- Treatment steps depend on the extent and severity of the disorder. There is no cure.
- Drugs are usually prescribed to treat the symptoms and any complications.

POSSIBLE COMPLICATIONS
- Anemia (often due to iron deficiency).
- Blood disorders and blood vessel disorders.
- Complications may occur in the heart, lung, gastrointestinal system, kidneys, nervous system, joint/muscle/bone, and eyes.
- Unable to continue regular job; changes are needed in working conditions.
- Pregnancies in SLE patients are high-risk.

PROBABLE OUTCOME—SLE is currently considered incurable. 20% to 30% of the cases are mild and may have only a skin rash. The majority of cases have continued remissions, flares, and relapses. The flares or relapses may occur 2 to 3 times a year. Many patients lead a normal lifestyle while in remission. Symptoms can often be relieved or controlled with treatment.

HOW TO TREAT

GENERAL MEASURES
- Obtain prompt medical treatment for any infection.
- Avoid sun exposure or use protection of hats, sunglasses, sunscreens, and long-sleeved clothing.
- Don't smoke. Find a way to quit.
- Apply heat or ice to relieve joint pain.
- Control the stress in your life. Learn relaxation techniques or obtain counseling if needed.
- Talk to your health care provider if you are thinking about becoming pregnant.
- Get regular medical and dental check-ups.
- To learn more: Lupus Foundation of America, 2000 L St., NW, Suite 710, Washington, DC 20036; (800) 558-0121; website: www.lupus.org.

MEDICATION—Drugs to suppress the immune system, steroid and nonsteroidal anti-inflammatory drugs, antimalarial drugs, or hormones may be prescribed. These may relieve symptoms but don't cure the disease. Other drugs may be prescribed depending on specific complications.

ACTIVITY
- Remain as active as possible. Extra rest may be needed. Exercises can help to retain range-of-motion an heart health. Exercise does not improve joint aches or fatigue.
- Physical therapy may be recommended.

DIET—Eat a healthy diet. Reduce salt intake.

CALL YOUR DOCTOR IF

- You or a family member has symptoms of systemic lupus erythematosus.
- New or worsening symptoms occur.

LYME DISEASE

 ## GENERAL INFORMATION

DEFINITION—Lyme disease is an infection caused by a tick bite. Most people who get Lyme disease do not become seriously ill. Symptoms vary as it can infect several parts of the body. It is named for Lyme, Connecticut, where it was first described.

BODY PARTS INVOLVED—Skin of the thighs, buttocks or underarms; central nervous system; heart and blood vessels; large joints, especially in the knee.

SEX OR AGE MOST AFFECTED—Both sexes; all ages.

SIGNS & SYMPTOMS
• Rash (called erythema migrans). It usually starts as a small red spot at the site of the tick bite. It slowly expands and becomes round or oval in shape with a clear center. It resembles a bulls-eye. Multiple rashes may appear elsewhere on the body in some cases.
• Mild flu-like symptoms (fever, chills, headache, fatigue, muscle/joint aches, and swollen lymph glands).
• More symptoms may develop if infection spreads to other parts of the body (e.g., facial palsy, stiff neck, severe headaches, joint pain and swelling [especially the knees], shooting pains, or heart palpitations).

CAUSES—Infection with the bacteria *Borrelia burgdorferi*. It is transmitted by the bite of an infected deer tick. The tick needs to be attached to the person for 2 to 3 days for infection to result. The tick bite may occur 3 to 30 days prior to the rash. Many people who get Lyme disease did not know they had a tick bite. The infection cannot be spread from one person to another.

RISK INCREASES WITH—Work, play, or recreational activities in states and locations at high risk for ticks. States include those in the northeast, mid-Atlantic, upper north-central United States, and some California counties. Ticks are often found in places that are grassy, brushy, or wooded.

HOW TO PREVENT
• Avoid tick-infested areas if possible. If in these areas, wear protective clothing with tight collars and cuffs. Use a permethrin spray to treat clothing and camping gear (such as tents). Use insect repellent (e.g., DEET).
• Have dogs and cats wear tick-repellent collars.
• Careful skin check and removal of any ticks. If the tick is removed from the skin within 36 to 48 hours, there is usually no infection. Remove any tick attached to you with tweezers. You may save tick in an air-tight container for possible medical exam.
• A drug may be prescribed to help prevent Lyme disease in certain cases of exposure.

 ## WHAT TO EXPECT

DIAGNOSTIC MEASURES
• Your own observation of symptoms.
• Your health care provider will do a physical exam and ask questions about your symptoms and activities.
• Medical tests may include blood studies and others to help confirm the diagnosis.

APPROPRIATE HEALTH CARE—Treatment is with antibiotic drugs. Early treatment helps prevent complications.

POSSIBLE COMPLICATIONS
• Late stages of untreated Lyme disease may occur months to years later. These include ongoing joint pain (Lyme arthritis), problems of the nervous system or heart, fatigue, memory problems, and other symptoms.
• In a few cases, non-specific symptoms continue after treatment (some call this post-Lyme disease syndrome). It has no specific treatment and symptoms gradually resolve.

PROBABLE OUTCOME—With early treatment, it is curable with antibiotics. Later disease stages can take weeks or months to respond to treatment. Untreated, it may clear up on its own or progress to other symptoms.

 ## HOW TO TREAT

GENERAL MEASURES
• Heat relieves joint pain or muscle aches. Take warm baths or showers, or use heating pads.
• To learn more: Lyme Disease Foundation, PO Box 332, Tolland, CT 06084; (800) 886-5963; website: www.lyme.org.

MEDICATION
• You may be prescribed:
  - An oral antibiotic (usually for 14 to 21 days) for early stage of the disease. The rash should begin to fade within a week.
  - Antibiotics given through a vein (IV) for later stages.
  - Nonsteroidal anti-inflammatory drugs.
  - Steroid drugs to reduce the inflammatory response in the heart or central nervous system.

ACTIVITY—Be as active as symptoms allow. Resume normal activities when able.

DIET—No special diet.

☎ CALL YOUR DOCTOR IF

• You or a family member has symptoms of Lyme disease.
• New, unexplained symptoms develop.

LYMPHEDEMA

GENERAL INFORMATION

DEFINITION—Lymphedema is a buildup of lymphatic fluid in the body's tissues that leads to swelling. It most often occurs in the arm(s) and/or leg(s), and sometimes other body parts. The lymphatic system is a part of the body's immune system that fights infections and diseases. Lymph vessels carry lymph fluid from body tissues back to the heart. Lymph nodes filter the fluid trapping bacteria and viruses and making antibodies to fight infection.

BODY PARTS INVOLVED—Lymphatic system, arms, legs, other parts of the body.

SEX OR AGE MOST AFFECTED—Adults of both sexes, but can occur in children.

SIGNS & SYMPTOMS
- Swelling of part of the arm or leg or entire arm or leg, including fingers or toes. The swelling can be mild, with little change in the size of the arm or leg. It can be extreme and make it impossible to use the affected limb.
- Feeling of heaviness or tightness in arm or leg.
- Restricted range of motion in arm or leg.
- Aching or discomfort in arm or leg.
- Recurring infections in affected limb.
- Skin on arm or leg may thicken or harden.

CAUSES
- Primary lymphedema (more rare) develops when lymphatic vessels are missing or impaired.
- Secondary lymphedema is more common and develops when lymph vessels are damaged or lymph nodes removed. It often occurs in patients treated for cancer. In many countries, the main cause is filiariasis (parasite infection).

RISK INCREASES WITH
- Primary type: certain rare inherited disorders or being born with lymph system abnormality.
- Secondary type:
  - Surgery, radiation, infection, injury, or tumors. (Lymphedema can develop right away, or weeks, months, even years later.)
  - Filariasis (a mosquito-borne illness found in many parts of the world).
  - Other, less common risk factors.

HOW TO PREVENT—No specific way to prevent. Early diagnosis may help prognosis.

WHAT TO EXPECT

DIAGNOSTIC MEASURES
- Your own observation of symptoms.
- Your health care provider will do a physical exam of the affected area and ask questions about your symptoms and medical history. Most cases are diagnosed in this way.
- Medical tests, if needed, may include MRI, CT, ultrasound, or other imaging study.

APPROPRIATE HEALTH CARE
- There is no cure for lymphedema. Treatment includes steps to reduce swelling, slow progression, and helping patients cope and continue with activities of daily living.
- Drugs may be prescribed for an infection.
- Treatment plan is usually based on the symptoms and may include skin care, compression garments, elevation, exercise, massage, bandaging, pneumatic compression, and counseling for emotional issues. The plan may be referred to as complete decongestive therapy (CDT). You and your health care provider will work together to format a treatment plan for your specific needs.
- In cases of severe lymphedema, your health care provider may suggest surgery to remove excess tissue in the arm or leg. This reduces severe swelling, but is not a cure.

POSSIBLE COMPLICATIONS
- Severe skin infection (cellulitis).
- Problems with function of arm or leg.
- Can affect almost all aspects of one's life (work, school, social life).
- Lymphangitis (infection of lymph vessels) or lymphangiosarcoma (a rare soft tissue cancer).

PROBABLE OUTCOME—It is a chronic and progressive condition. Adhering to a treatment plan can help symptoms and slow progression. Treatment is lifelong and requires daily involvement. New treatments are being researched.

HOW TO TREAT

GENERAL MEASURES
- Keep the swollen limb elevated as much as possible. Take steps to protect your skin from injury. Moisturize your skin daily. Don't use heating pads on the affected limb.
- Consider joining a support group.
- To lean more: National Lymphedema Network, 116 New Montgomery St., Suite 235, San Francisco, CA 94105; (800) 541-3259; website: www.lymphnet.org.

MEDICATION
- Drugs are not usually used in treatment.
- Antibiotics for infection or drugs for filariasis may be prescribed.

ACTIVITY—Exercise, and possibly physical therapy, will be part of the treatment plan and based on each individual's situation.

DIET—Eat a healthy diet.

CALL YOUR DOCTOR IF

- You or a family member has symptoms of lymphedema.
- Symptoms worsen despite treatment.

LYMPHOMA, NON-HODGKIN'S
(Lymphosarcoma; Reticulum Cell Sarcoma)

 GENERAL INFORMATION

DEFINITION—Non-Hodgkin's lymphomas are a group of closely related cancers that affect the lymphatic system. These cancers can be fast-growing or slow-growing. Hodgkin's disease is a related, yet different type of lymphoma. Lymphoma is a term that describes cancer of the body's lymphatic system. The lymphatic system is a part of the body's immune system that fights infections and diseases.

BODY PARTS INVOLVED
- Lymphocytes (white blood cells).
- Lymph glands (glands that fight infection and produce immune substances).
- Spleen (a large lymph gland).

SEX OR AGE MOST AFFECTED—Both sexes; all ages, but more common in older males.

SIGNS & SYMPTOMS
- May not have symptoms when first diagnosed.
- Swollen, non-tender, rubbery, distinct lymph nodes anywhere in the body, but most often in the armpit, neck, or groin.
- Fevers, night sweats, and weight loss.
- Loss of appetite and tiredness (may be severe).
- Cough or feeling breathless; itchiness.
- Other symptoms occur if cancer has spread.

CAUSES—The body produces too many lymphocytes (a type of white blood cell) that are abnormal. Why this occurs is unknown.

RISK INCREASES WITH
- Adults over 50. Males more than females.
- Weak immune system due to illness or drugs.
- Certain infections (e.g., human immuno-deficiency virus [HIV], Epstein-Barr virus, human T-cell lymphoma/leukemia virus type 1, Helicobacter pylori, and hepatitis C).
- Work that involves exposure to carcinogens (substances known to cause cancer).
- Radiation exposure, some autoimmune diseases, and chemotherapy.

HOW TO PREVENT—No specific preventive measures.

 WHAT TO EXPECT

DIAGNOSTIC MEASURES
- Your own observation of symptoms.
- Your health care provider will do a physical exam and ask questions about your symptoms.
- A variety of medical tests will be done to verify the exact type of cancer cells, the grade (fast or slow growing), and if the cancer has spread (called staging) to other places in the body.

APPROPRIATE HEALTH CARE
- Treatment will depend on the cancer type, grade and location, its stage, your health, age, and preferences. Your health care provider will discuss your specific diagnosis and treatment options with you.
- Treatment may include chemotherapy (anticancer drugs), biologic therapy (uses the immune system to treat cancer), radiation therapy, stem cell or bone marrow transplant, and possibly newer therapies. Hospital care may be needed for certain treatments or complications.
- In some cases, watchful waiting may be an option. This means monitoring the cancer cells for a period of time before deciding on treatment.
- Counseling may help you to cope.

POSSIBLE COMPLICATIONS
- Cancer spreads to other parts of the lymph system (spleen, tonsils, adenoids, thymus, and bone marrow). It may spread to other organs.
- Cancer treatments cause complications.
- Anemia.
- Recurrence of cancer after treatment.

PROBABLE OUTCOME—The outcome varies depending on the cancer cell type, if it is slow or fast growing, if it has spread, and the individual's age and response to treatment. If one treatment is not working, there may be other options that can be tried.

 HOW TO TREAT

GENERAL MEASURES—To learn more: American Cancer Society; (800) ACS-2345; website: www.cancer.org or National Cancer Institute; (800) 4-CANCER; website: www.cancer.gov.

MEDICATION
- Chemotherapy (anticancer drugs) and/or biologic drugs/agents are often prescribed.
- Steroid drugs may be prescribed.
- Antibiotics may be needed for an infection.

ACTIVITY
- Stay as active as you can. Walking and swimming are good ways to exercise.
- Avoid crowds and people with infections.

DIET—Eating a healthy diet can help you feel better and aid in healing. Consult a dietitian for help in meal planning if needed.

 CALL YOUR DOCTOR IF

- You or a family member has symptoms of non-Hodgkin's lymphoma.
- After diagnosis, any symptoms cause concern.

MALABSORPTION
(Malabsorptive Syndrome)

 GENERAL INFORMATION

DEFINITION—Malabsorption involves problems with digesting and absorbing nutrients (vitamins, minerals, proteins, sugars, fats, etc.) from foods. Most nutrients are absorbed through the small intestine. Malabsorption is not a disease in itself. It is a result of some other condition.

BODY PARTS INVOLVED—Intestinal tract; liver; pancreas.

SEX OR AGE MOST AFFECTED—Both sexes; all ages.

SIGNS & SYMPTOMS
- Diarrhea.
- Weakness.
- Weight loss.
- Gas with stomach discomfort and swelling.
- Bad-smelling, bulky stools, often with mucus.
- Mild anemia (pale skin and feeling weak and tired).
- Bone pain.
- Swollen hands and feet.

CAUSES—A variety of health problems can cause malabsorption. The small intestine can be affected by infections, inflammation, irritation, structural defects, injury, surgery, faults in the digestive process, congenital defects, and others.

RISK INCREASES WITH
- Lactose intolerance.
- Celiac disease.
- Crohn's disease; ulcerative colitis; chronic diarrhea.
- Chronic pancreatitis.
- Cystic fibrosis.
- Small intestine disorders such as diverticulosis, strictures, and partial obstruction.
- Bacteria or parasite infection.
- Short bowel syndrome (due to surgery that removed half or more of the small intestine).
- Stomach or bowel surgery or radiation.
- Liver disease.
- Excess use of laxatives or antacids.
- HIV infection.
- Imbalance of minerals in the body.

HOW TO PREVENT—No specific preventive measures. Get treatment for any risk factors.

 WHAT TO EXPECT

DIAGNOSTIC MEASURES
- Your own observation of symptoms.
- Your health care provider will do a physical exam and ask questions about your symptoms and activities.

- Medical tests may include blood, stool, and urine studies and x-rays of the intestinal tract. Other tests may be done to help diagnose the cause.

APPROPRIATE HEALTH CARE
- Treatment depends on the underlying cause and the needs of each patient. Steps may include special feeding methods, diet changes, or drugs.
- Some patients may need feeding through a vein (IV). This is called total parenteral nutrition (TPN).
- Some patients may need tube feeding. A tube is inserted into the stomach or the bowel for feeding.

POSSIBLE COMPLICATIONS
- Prolonged illness.
- Failure to thrive in infants.
- Additional illness caused by nutritional, vitamin, or mineral deficiency.
- Anemia.

PROBABLE OUTCOME—The degree to which symptoms can be controlled depends on the cause, but many things are common to all malabsorptive disorders. The onset is usually slow and sometimes difficult to diagnose. Disorders may be present for months or years before being recognized. Treatment can be long, complicated, and may need to be changed often.

 HOW TO TREAT

GENERAL MEASURES—Patience and a positive attitude are important in cure.

MEDICATION—You may be prescribed enzymes to aid digestion, antidiarrheals, antibiotics, anti-inflammatory drugs, intestinal hormones, medium chain triglycerides, vitamins and other supplements, and antacids.

ACTIVITY—As tolerated by symptoms and physical condition.

DIET—Diet changes may be prescribed. They may be milk-free, gluten-free, low-fat, no-fat, or have other restrictions. You will be provided specific diet instructions.

 CALL YOUR DOCTOR IF

- You or a family member has malabsorption symptoms.
- Any of the following occur during treatment:
  - Black, tarry bowel movements.
  - Fever of 101°F (38.3°C) or higher.
  - Severe abdominal pain.
  - Muscle cramps.

MALARIA

GENERAL INFORMATION

DEFINITION—Malaria is a serious infection caused by malarial parasites. It is transmitted by a mosquito bite. Most cases of malaria in the United States are in immigrants and travelers returning from malaria-risk areas. A few cases are transmitted by blood transfusion, from mother to fetus during pregnancy, or by mosquito bite that occurred in the United States.

BODY PARTS INVOLVED—Blood cells; blood vessels; liver; central nervous system.

SEX OR AGE MOST AFFECTED—Both sexes; all ages.

SIGNS & SYMPTOMS
• Symptoms usually occur about 7 to 30 days after infection (though it can be up to a year or more).
• Shaking chills, with a fever. This is followed by heavy sweating and temperature drops. These may repeat.
• Fatigue and general ill feeling.
• Muscle and joint pain.
• Symptoms may include headache, nausea, vomiting, and diarrhea.

CAUSES—The mosquito becomes infected with malaria after biting a person with the disease. The parasites multiply in the mosquito for a week, then enter the bloodstream of the next person the mosquito bites. Once in a person's bloodstream, the parasites travel to the liver, where they thrive and multiply rapidly. After several days, thousands re-enter the bloodstream and destroy red blood cells. Some parasites remain in the liver, continue to multiply, and are released again at intervals into the bloodstream.

RISK INCREASES WITH—Living in, or travel to, any country where malaria is a risk. It is most prevalent in rural tropical areas such as those found in Latin America, Asia, and Africa.

HOW TO PREVENT
• Take antimalaria drugs before visiting an area where malaria is a risk. Continue to take the drugs after you return. A travel health clinic or your health care provider can give you instructions. During your travels, you should have the name of a medical person or center to contact if symptoms develop.
• In mosquito-infested areas, wear long-sleeved shirts and pants, especially from dusk to dawn. Use a DEET insect repellent on exposed skin. Sleep under a bednet that has been dipped in permethrin insecticide.
• Contact Centers for Disease Control (CDC) traveler information about malaria risks and prevention: (877) 394-8747; website: www.cdc.gov/travel.

WHAT TO EXPECT

DIAGNOSTIC MEASURES
• Your own observation of symptoms.
• Your health care provider will do a physical exam and ask questions about your symptoms and recent travels.
• Medical tests will include special blood studies. Other tests may be done if complications are a concern.

APPROPRIATE HEALTH CARE
• Treatment is with drugs.
• Hospital care may be needed with severe symptoms.

POSSIBLE COMPLICATIONS
• Anemia, jaundice, or brain or kidney damage.
• Bleeding, seizures, or coma.
• Severe hypoglycemia (low blood sugar).
• Pulmonary edema (fluid in the lungs).
• Hemoglobinuria (hemoglobin in the urine).
• Enlarged spleen; rupture of the spleen (rare).

PROBABLE OUTCOME—Curable with treatment. Symptoms usually improve in about 48 hours and fever is gone in about 4 days. Children, persons with weak immune systems, and pregnant women are more at risk for complications.

HOW TO TREAT

GENERAL MEASURES
• Protect yourself from secondary bacterial infection while you are ill with malaria. Wash your hands often.
• All cases of malaria are reported to the local health department.

MEDICATION
• One or more antimalaria drugs to kill the parasite will be prescribed. It will depend on the type of malaria diagnosed.
• Take nonprescription acetaminophen for fever.

ACTIVITY—Rest in bed until fever and chills subside. Resume your normal activities gradually as symptoms improve.

DIET—No special diet.

CALL YOUR DOCTOR IF

• You or a family member has symptoms of malaria. Symptoms may begin up to one year after returning from travel in a malaria-risk area.
• After diagnosis, weakness lasts for a prolonged time. This may indicate anemia.
• Symptoms of malaria recur after treatment.
• New, unexplained symptoms develop.

...INFORMATION

...an syndrome is a rare, inhe...e tissue disorder. Connective tissue s... ...nd adds strength to other body tissue and b... parts such as tendons and ligaments and heart valves. The severity of the symptoms varies greatly among patients.

BODY PARTS INVOLVED—Musculoskeletal; endocrine system and metabolic system.

SEX OR AGE MOST AFFECTED—Newborns of both sexes.

SIGNS & SYMPTOMS
* Tall and thin body shape.
* Long arms and legs.
* Long, thin fingers (arachnodactyly).
* Chest deformity (may be sunken in or protrude out).
* Curved spine (scoliosis).
* High palate in the mouth; overcrowded teeth.
* "Double jointed;" joint weakness or looseness.
* Dislocation of eye lens, usually upward.
* Myopia (nearsighted).
* Symptoms of heart problems (e.g., shortness of breath, tiredness, irregular or rapid heartbeat).
* Stretch marks on the shoulders, hips, and lower back.
* Easy bruising or bleeding (uncommon).

CAUSES—Inherited disorder in about 75% of cases. Other cases occur with no known cause. The disorder is present from birth and diagnosis can sometimes be made in newborns. However, signs or symptoms are often not seen until adolescence or young adulthood.

RISK INCREASES WITH
* Advanced paternal age may be a risk in those cases that are not clearly inherited.
* Family history of Marfan syndrome.

HOW TO PREVENT
* No preventive measures.
* Each child has a 50% chance of inheriting the disorder from an affected parent. Children may be more or less severely affected.
* Get genetic counseling if you have Marfan syndrome or there is a family history of the disorder. Prenatal diagnosis is complicated and research is ongoing.

 WHAT TO EXPECT

DIAGNOSTIC MEASURES
* Your health care provider will do a physical exam and ask questions about family medical history. There is no one test to diagnose Marfan syndrome. Medical tests include echo-cardiogram (for diagnosing heart problems) and an eye exam. Genetic testing may be done.

APPROPRIATE HEALTH CARE
* Treatment will involve a team approach that involves eye, cardiac, orthopedic, and dental care. Drugs can help prevent complications.
* Annual screening echocardiograms are recommended beginning in adolescence in order to detect the start of any complications. During growth years, x-rays of spine are needed to detect scoliosis.
* Have annual eye exams. Special lenses and eye drops or surgery may be needed for lens dislocation.
* Surgery may be needed for cardiovascular problems.
* Scoliosis may require use of a brace or surgery.
* Surgery may be needed if chest bones are sunken in.
* Pregnant women with Marfan syndrome are managed as high-risk patients.

POSSIBLE COMPLICATIONS
* Cardiovascular (heart and blood vessels) problems.
* Lung problems (e.g., breathing difficulties).
* Eye problems (e.g., glaucoma, cataracts).

PROBABLE OUTCOME—Early diagnosis and steps to prevent and treat complications have improved the outlook for patients. Lifespan is about the same as an average person.

 HOW TO TREAT

GENERAL MEASURES—To learn more: National Marfan Foundation, 22 Manhasset Ave., Port Washington, NY 11050; (800) 862-7326; website: www.marfan.org.

MEDICATION
* Beta-blockers may be prescribed for heart problems.
* Hormone therapy may be given prior to puberty.
* Antibiotic therapy may be prescribed.

ACTIVITY
* Exercise is important, but follow medical advice. You may be advised to avoid certain sports, activities that risk head injury, rapid decompression (scuba diving), and isometric exercises (weightlifting, pull-ups, etc.).
* Get medical approval before starting any new sports activity or exercise routine.

DIET—No special diet.

 CALL YOUR DOCTOR IF

* You believe your child has signs or symptoms of Marfan syndrome.
* After diagnosis, symptoms change or worsen.

MASTITIS

GENERAL INFORMATION

DEFINITION—Mastitis is a breast disorder that usually occurs in a woman who has recently given birth. It develops in about 1% to 2% of new mothers and is more likely in women who are breastfeeding. However, it can occur even in women who are not breastfeeding or pregnant.

BODY PARTS INVOLVED—Breasts.

SEX OR AGE MOST AFFECTED—Females of childbearing age.

SIGNS & SYMPTOMS
- Symptoms may occur anytime while nursing, but usually begin 1 to 5 weeks after delivery.
- Tender or painful, swollen, hard, reddened, hot area of the breast(s).
- General feeling of weakness and lack of well-being.
- Fever and chills.

CAUSES—Infection from bacteria germs that enter the mother's breast. Most mastitis occurs only on one side. It is unknown exactly why some women get mastitis and others do not. Germs may gain access to the breast through a crack in the nipple, but women without sore nipples also get mastitis.

RISK INCREASES WITH
- Major risks are breastfeeding and cracked nipples.
- Women with a very abundant milk supply may be more prone to getting mastitis.
- Having mastitis previously.
- Tight-fitting bras.
- Women who are not breastfeeding but have diabetes, chronic illness, or weak immune system.

HOW TO PREVENT
- There are no specific preventive measures.
- Wash nipples before nursing. Wash hands before touching breasts.
- Regular emptying of the breasts. Breast-feed equally from both breasts. Change your body position for each feeding. Do not let baby use breast as a pacifier.

WHAT TO EXPECT

DIAGNOSTIC MEASURES
- Your own observation of symptoms.
- Your health care provider can usually diagnose mastitis by an exam of the breasts. Questions will be asked about your symptoms.
- Medical tests may be done, but are usually not needed.

APPROPRIATE HEALTH CARE—Treatment includes adequate breast emptying, rest, drinking plenty of fluids, and drug therapy, if needed.

POSSIBLE COMPLICATIONS
- Without proper treatment, or with incomplete treatment, mastitis may lead to breast abscess. This is a pus-filled infection in the breast.
- Mastitis may recur.
- Blockage of milk flow.

PROBABLE OUTCOME—Usually curable in 10 days with treatment. Symptoms will get better in 1 to 2 days.

HOW TO TREAT

GENERAL MEASURES
- Apply a warm compress or an ice pack (whichever feels better) to the engorged breast after feeding. Don't use ice packs within 1 hour of nursing; instead use warm compresses.
- Wear a good support bra during treatment.
- Most often, you can continue to breastfeed, even though breasts are infected. Offer the affected breast first to promote complete emptying. If needed, use a breast pump to completely empty the breast.
- Take your temperature 1 to 3 times a day at first, to check for any fever.

MEDICATION
- Pain relievers. For minor discomfort, you may use nonprescription drugs, such as acetaminophen or ibuprofen.
- Antibiotics for infection may be prescribed. Complete the entire dosage prescribed even if symptoms improve. Breast-feeding can usually be continued while taking the drug.

ACTIVITY—Get extra rest whenever you can.

DIET—No special diet. Eat regularly and drink extra fluids.

CALL YOUR DOCTOR IF

- You or a family member has symptoms of mastitis.
- During treatment, a fever occurs, you have nausea or vomiting, feel dizzy, or faint.
- You have signs of a breast abscess. An area with redness, pain, tenderness, and fluctuance (feels like pushing on an inflated inner tube).

MEASLES
(Red Measles; Rubeola)

 GENERAL INFORMATION

DEFINITION—Measles is a viral illness that infects the respiratory tract (lungs, throat, and nasal passages) and skin. It is one of the most easily spread diseases. Measles was once very common, but it is now rare in the United States due to immunization. It is still common in certain other countries in the world. Cases that occur in the United States are often in people who have become infected in other countries.

BODY PARTS INVOLVED—Skin; eyes; upper-respiratory tract.

SEX OR AGE MOST AFFECTED—All ages, but most common in children.

SIGNS & SYMPTOMS
- Measles symptoms usually occur in the following sequence:
  - Fever, often high.
  - Fatigue.
  - Appetite loss.
  - Sneezing and runny nose.
  - Harsh, hacking cough.
  - Red eyes and sensitivity to light.
  - Tiny white spots in the mouth and throat.
  - Rash on the forehead and around ears that spreads to the body.

CAUSES—Measles is caused by a virus. Germs are spread by contact with an infected person, breathing in germs in the air, or touching an object with germs on it. Symptoms first appear 7 to 14 days (may be longer in adults) after exposure. An infected person can spread the germs to others 4 to 5 days prior to the start of the rash and 4 to 5 days after it starts.

RISK INCREASES WITH
- People who are not immunized.
- Areas of the world that don't offer immunizations.
- Reduced protective affect of the vaccine over time. A teenager or young adult could become infected with measles if exposed.

HOW TO PREVENT
- Immunize children against measles. Prevention is important because measles can have rare, but serious, complications.
- Careful hand washing helps prevent spread of any type of germs.

 WHAT TO EXPECT

DIAGNOSTIC MEASURES
- Your health care provider will do a physical exam and ask questions about your symptoms and vaccine history. Measles is usually diagnosed by the symptoms.

- A blood test may be done to confirm the diagnosis.

APPROPRIATE HEALTH CARE—There is no specific treatment for measles. Home care involves rest, relief of symptoms, and keeping the patient away from other persons that are not immune to measles.

POSSIBLE COMPLICATIONS
- Ear and chest infections.
- Pneumonia.
- Encephalitis or meningitis.
- Complications can be life-threatening.

PROBABLE OUTCOME—Symptoms usually clear up after about 3 days.

 HOW TO TREAT

GENERAL MEASURES
- The eyes are more sensitive to light. Avoid reading books or watching TV for a few days.
- Use a cool-mist humidifier (if advised) to ease the cough and thin lung secretions so they can be coughed up more easily. Clean humidifier per instructions.
- Children who are old enough can suck on throat lozenges, cough drops, or hard candy to help ease throat discomfort.
- If fever is 101°F (38.3°C) or higher, take steps to lower it, if the child is uncomfortable, unable to sleep, or vomiting. Use drug therapy as advised by your child's health care provider. A lukewarm bath or sponge bath may help cool a febrile child.

MEDICATION
- Use acetaminophen or ibuprofen to relieve discomfort and reduce fever. Don't give aspirin if under age 18.
- An antihistamine or calamine lotion may help relieve the itchy rash. Follow instructions on label and be sure the product is approved for the age group.

ACTIVITY—Extra rest may help until the fever and rash get better. Children should not return to school or daycare until 4 to 5 days after the fever and rash disappear.

DIET—No special diet. Drink extra fluids, including water, tea, lemonade, and fruit juice.

 CALL YOUR DOCTOR IF

- You or your child has symptoms of measles.
- Breathing difficulty, wheezing, chest or stomach pain, earache, or vision problems occur.

MELANOMA

GENERAL INFORMATION

DEFINITION—Melanoma is a skin cancer that can occur on any skin or mucosal surface of the body. Melanoma can spread to other areas of the body, such as the lymph nodes, liver, lungs, and central nervous system.

BODY PARTS INVOLVED—Usually in skin of the head, neck, legs or back. It appears rarely in the eye, mouth, vagina or anus.

SEX OR AGE MOST AFFECTED—Both sexes and any age; usually occurs in adults, and is rare in children.

SIGNS & SYMPTOMS
- A changing mole is most common symptom.
- Flat or slightly raised skin lesion. It can be black, brown, blue, red, white, or a mixture of colors. Borders are often irregular. Some may bleed, itch, or cause pain.

CAUSES—Cells (melanocytes) that give skin its brownish color change into melanoma cells. It is unclear why this occurs. Melanomas may appear on normal skin or arise from a mole (nevus) or other abnormal skin area that has changed in appearance. They tend to occur at sites of sun exposure. When the cells grow down into deep skin layers, they invade blood vessels and lymph vessels and are spread to other body areas.

RISK INCREASES WITH
- Moles (more so with large numbers of moles).
- Occupations or activities involving excessive sun exposure, such as farming, athletics, or sunbathing.
- Excess sun exposure and sunburns in childhood (even one severe, blistering sunburn increases risk).
- Having atypical moles (dysplastic nevi).
- Increased age.
- Genetic factors. This is most common in fair-skinned, blond people. It is rare in African-Americans.
- Weak immune system due to illness or drugs.
- Personal or family history of melanoma.
- Sunny or high altitude climates.

HOW TO PREVENT
- Wear sunglasses, broad-rimmed hats, and protective clothing. Always use a sunscreen (15 SPF or higher). Avoid sun exposure between 10 AM and 4 PM.
- Examine your skin regularly for changes in pigmented areas (such as moles). Ask a family member to examine your back, scalp, and soles of the feet. Get medical advice about any skin lesion (especially brown or black) that becomes multicolored, develops irregular edges or surfaces, and bleeds or changes in any way.

WHAT TO EXPECT

DIAGNOSTIC MEASURES
- Your own observation of suspicious growths.
- Your health care provider will do an exam of the affected skin area.
- Biopsy (removal of a small amount of affected skin for viewing under a microscope) aids in diagnosis. Other tests may be done to see if the cancer has spread (staging).

APPROPRIATE HEALTH CARE
- Treatment varies and depends on location and size of affected area, stage of the cancer, your health, age, and preferences. Treatment may include surgery (most often), nonsurgical destruction or topical therapy, anticancer drugs (chemotherapy) and/or radiation therapy, biologic therapy, or other new therapies.
- Goal of surgery is to remove as much of the skin cancer as possible. Skin graft may be done if large areas of tissue are removed. Lymph nodes may also be removed. If surgery is not feasible, other modes of removal are options.
- Chemotherapy uses drugs, and radiation therapy uses radiation to attack the cancer cells. Biologic therapy uses the body's immune system to fight cancer.

POSSIBLE COMPLICATIONS
- Cancer spreads (metastasis) to other places in the body, which can be life-threatening.
- Melanoma recurs at same site or new site.

PROBABLE OUTCOME—Varies greatly. Early melanomas that have not spread are curable with surgical removal. Once the tumor has spread to distant organs, the prognosis is poor. Symptoms can be relieved or controlled.

HOW TO TREAT

GENERAL MEASURES
- Since there is a risk of melanoma recurring, be sure to have regular follow-up medical exams.
- To learn more: American Cancer Society, (800) ACS-2345; website: www.cancer.org or National Cancer Institute, (800) 4-CANCER; website: www.cancer.gov.

MEDICATION—Anticancer (chemotherapy) drugs or biologic therapy drugs may be prescribed.

ACTIVITY—No limits. Use sun protection.

DIET—No special diet.

CALL YOUR DOCTOR IF

- You or a family member has symptoms of melanoma.
- After diagnosis, any symptoms cause concern.

MÉNIÈRE'S DISEASE

GENERAL INFORMATION

DEFINITION—Ménière's disease is a disorder of the inner ear that causes a variety of symptoms. In most cases, only one ear is initially involved. Ménière's is named for the French doctor who described it in 1861.

BODY PARTS INVOLVED—Semicircular canals of the inner ear, usually on one side only (80% to 85%).

SEX OR AGE MOST AFFECTED—It usually affects adults between ages 30 and 60, and it is slightly more common in women than men.

SIGNS & SYMPTOMS
- Original symptoms often start suddenly, and recurrent attacks may come on with no warning. Attacks may occur daily, or in some persons, just once a year. Attacks may last 30 minutes to 2 hours, or longer. Symptoms may be mild to severe.
- Vertigo (feeling that you are spinning or everything around you is spinning).
- Noises in the affected ear (tinnitus), such as roaring, ringing, or buzzing.
- Low-frequency hearing loss that comes and goes and often increases over time.
- Feeling pressure or pain in the affected ear.
- Nausea, vomiting, and sweating may occur with the vertigo. Stomach discomfort, headache, and diarrhea may occur also.

CAUSES—The exact cause is unknown. There are a variety of suggested causes, and research continues.

RISK INCREASES WITH—Possible risks are viral infection, allergies, immune reaction, fluid in the ear, injury, and genetic factors.

HOW TO PREVENT—No specific preventive measures.

WHAT TO EXPECT

DIAGNOSTIC MEASURES
- Your own observation of symptoms.
- Your health care provider will do a physical exam and an exam of the ear.
- Medical tests may include blood studies, balance studies, hearing tests, and other tests to rule out disorders with similar symptoms.

APPROPRIATE HEALTH CARE
- Treatment can include lifestyle changes (such as diet), drugs, use of certain devices, or sometimes surgery to relieve the symptoms.
- Various treatments may be tried for tinnitus.
- Different types of surgery may be suggested for severe symptoms or to prevent further hearing loss.

POSSIBLE COMPLICATIONS
- Permanent hearing loss.
- Chronic tinnitus.
- The symptoms can affect all aspects of a person's life.

PROBABLE OUTCOME—There is no cure. Attacks of Ménière's disease recur and worsen over many years. Symptoms can often be relieved with one or more types of treatment. The disorder is frustrating, but not life-threatening.

HOW TO TREAT

GENERAL MEASURES
- You may find. certain triggers can set off your attacks (e.g., fatigue, overwork, stress, emotional upset, foods, salty diet, and others).
- During an attack, lie flat on a surface that does not move. Avoid bright lights. Focus eyes on an object that does not move. Don't eat or drink (to avoid nausea). Once the attack passes, get up slowly. You may feel sleepy and want to sleep for awhile.
- Learn techniques to control stress in your life. This helps some people with Ménière's.
- The Meniett device uses low pressure pulses to reduce symptoms. It may be an option for some.
- Quit smoking. Find a way to quit.
- To learn more: Vestibular Disorders Association; (800) 229-8064; PO Box 13305, Portland, OR 97213; website: www.vestibular.org.

MEDICATION
- Your health care provider may prescribe:
  - Antinausea drugs, to reduce nausea/vomiting.
  - Scopolamine patches, to treat nausea.
  - Tranquilizers, to reduce dizziness.
  - Antihistamines, to help lessen symptoms.
  - Diuretics, to decrease fluid in the inner ear.

ACTIVITY—Limit activities as needed during an attack, especially if it includes vertigo.

DIET
- Salt causes the body to retain fluid. By decreasing salt in your diet, it will help to reduce the amount of fluid in the inner ear.
- Limiting the use of caffeine and alcohol helps reduce attacks in some people.

CALL YOUR DOCTOR IF

- You or a family member has symptoms of Ménière's disease.
- The following occur during treatment: decreased hearing in either ear, persistent vomiting, fever of 101°F (38.3°C) or higher.
- New, unexplained symptoms develop. Drugs used in treatment may produce side effects.

MENINGITIS, ASEPTIC
(Viral Meningitis)

 GENERAL INFORMATION

DEFINITION—Aseptic meningitis is an inflammation of the thin membranes (meninges) and fluid surrounding the brain and spinal cord. It is more common in group settings such as young children in daycare, football team members, college students, and people who live in group care facilities. Aseptic meningitis is usually mild. Bacterial meningitis is different and much more serious.

BODY PARTS INVOLVED—Brain; spinal cord.

SEX OR AGE MOST AFFECTED—Both sexes; all ages.

SIGNS & SYMPTOMS
- Fever and/or chills.
- Headache, sometimes severe.
- Irritability.
- Eyes become more sensitive to light.
- Stiff neck.
- Vomiting.
- Confusion, lethargy, and drowsiness.
- Seizures may rarely occur.

CAUSES
- While this disorder is most often caused by a virus, other types of germs can be the cause. The most common cause is a group of viruses called enteroviruses. Less often, herpes virus, West Nile virus, mumps virus, HIV, and other viruses may be the cause. Germs are spread by contact with an infected person, or touching an object with germs on it and then touching the mouth, nose, or eyes.
- Other causes include tuberculosis, various fungi, certain diseases, parasites, exposure to certain chemicals, and some drugs.

RISK INCREASES WITH
- Weak immune system due to illness or drugs.
- Group homes, daycare, or schools where outbreaks may occur.
- Health care workers.

HOW TO PREVENT
- Keep immunizations up-to-date against viruses such as mumps, measles, and chickenpox. Currently, there is no vaccine for the enteroviruses.
- Wash hands carefully to prevent the spread of any type of germs.

 WHAT TO EXPECT

DIAGNOSTIC MEASURES
- Your health care provider will do a physical exam and ask about your symptoms and activities.
- Medical tests may include blood studies, cerebrospinal fluid studies, a stool culture, and others to confirm the diagnosis.

APPROPRIATE HEALTH CARE
- There is no specific drug therapy for most viruses. The body defenses will normally cure the disorder. Treatment involves getting extra bed rest, treating symptoms such as fever, and drinking fluids.
- If symptoms are severe, hospital care may be needed.

POSSIBLE COMPLICATIONS—Complications are rare. They may occur in those with weak immune systems or the very young.

PROBABLE OUTCOME—Most patients recover fully in 5 to 14 days. In some people, symptoms such as fatigue or lightheadedness may persist longer.

 HOW TO TREAT

GENERAL MEASURES—None specific.

MEDICATION
- Nonprescription drugs for fever, nausea, or minor pain may be used.
- Antibiotics may be given if there is a possibility the meningitis is caused by a bacterial infection.
- Drugs may be prescribed for other causes of the meningitis once they are identified.

ACTIVITY
- Rest in bed in a darkened room. Resume your normal activities as soon as symptoms improve.
- Children should stay home from school or daycare until symptoms improve.

DIET—No special diet. Drink plenty of fluids each day.

 CALL YOUR DOCTOR IF

- You or a family member has symptoms of aseptic meningitis.
- Symptoms don't improve in a week.

MENINGITIS, BACTERIAL

GENERAL INFORMATION

DEFINITION—Bacterial meningitis is an inflammation of the thin membranes (meninges) and fluid surrounding the brain and spinal cord. It is a rare, life-threatening disorder, and prompt treatment is vital.

BODY PARTS INVOLVED—Central nervous system.

SEX OR AGE MOST AFFECTED—Both sexes; all ages, but more severe in persons under age 2 or over age 60.

SIGNS & SYMPTOMS
- Fever, chills, and sweating.
- Headache.
- Irritability.
- Eyes sensitive to light; pupils may be of different sizes.
- Stiff neck.
- Vomiting.
- Red or purple skin rash (associated with one kind of bacteria).
- Confusion, lethargy, drowsiness, or unconsciousness.
- Sore throat or other signs of respiratory (nose, throat, and lungs) illness may occur before other symptoms.
- Poor feeding in infants.
- Seizures.

CAUSES—An infection usually caused by one of three types of bacteria. *Neisseria meningitidis*, *Streptococcus pneumoniae*, or *Haemophilus influenzae type b* (Hib). (Routine vaccines for children have lowered the risk of Hib infection.) Bacterial germs are spread by close contact with an infected person. The infection may start in another body part, such as the lung, ear, nose, throat, or sinus that spreads to the meninges.

RISK INCREASES WITH
- Newborns, infants, young people, and adults over 60.
- Ear, sinus, respiratory, or tooth infections.
- Weak immune system due to illness or drugs.
- Head injury.
- Close contact with a person with meningitis.
- People with cochlear implants (hearing device).

HOW TO PREVENT
- Get all the recommended vaccines for infants and adults. Other vaccines may be options depending on an individual's health condition.
- Vaccine against *Neisseria meningitidis* (meningococcal vaccine) may be recommended for students going to college and for travelers to certain areas of the world.
- Avoid contact with anyone who has meningitis. If contact occurs, ask your health care provider about possible preventive treatment.

WHAT TO EXPECT

DIAGNOSTIC MEASURES
- Your health care provider will do a physical exam and ask questions about the symptoms.
- Medical tests may include blood studies, culture of cerebrospinal fluid, x-rays, CT, and others to confirm the diagnosis.

APPROPRIATE HEALTH CARE
- Hospital care is usually needed, sometimes in an intensive care unit.
- Treatment involves antibiotics, supportive care for symptoms, and steps to prevent complications.

POSSIBLE COMPLICATIONS
- Brain damage, paralysis, speech difficulty, hearing loss, impaired vision or blindness, seizures, and mental impairment.
- Can be fatal.

PROBABLE OUTCOME—Full recovery is likely in 2 to 3 weeks with prompt treatment and if no complications arise.

HOW TO TREAT

GENERAL MEASURES—The family should stay in close contact with the patient's medical team.

MEDICATION
- Antibiotics will be give through a vein (IV).
- Steroids may be prescribed. They help prevent the risk of hearing loss.
- Anticonvulsants may be used to treat or prevent seizures.

ACTIVITY—After a 2- to 3-week period of recovery, you should be as active as your strength allows.

DIET—You may be given intravenous (IV) nutrients in the hospital. At home, eat a normal, well-balanced diet.

☎ CALL YOUR DOCTOR IF

- You or a family member has symptoms of bacterial meningitis. Get emergency help if needed.
- You have had contact with someone who has meningitis.

MENOPAUSE

GENERAL INFORMATION

DEFINITION—Menopause is the permanent cessation of menstruation. It can occur as early as age 40 or as late as early 60s. It usually spans 1 to 2 years. Menopause is only one event in the "climacteric." This is a biological change in all body tissue and body systems that occurs in both sexes between the mid-40s and mid-60s. Menopause that occurs before age 40 is termed premature. Menopause does not occur suddenly. Perimenopause usually begins a few years before the last menstrual cycle.

BODY PARTS INVOLVED—Female reproductive system, with effects in other body parts.

SEX OR AGE MOST AFFECTED—Women, especially between ages 45 and 50.

SIGNS & SYMPTOMS
- Some women may go through menopause without having symptoms. In most women, both physical and emotional symptoms usually occur.
- Irregular menstrual periods.
- Hot flashes or flushes and night sweats. These are sensations of heat spreading from the waist or chest toward the neck, face, and upper arms. The medical term is vasomotor symptoms.
- Headaches.
- Dizziness.
- Rapid or irregular heartbeat.
- Vaginal itching, burning; pain with intercourse.
- Bloating in the upper abdomen.
- Irritable bladder (urge to urinate).
- Tender breasts.
- Mood changes, including tension and anxiety.
- Sleeping difficulty.
- Changes in sex drive.
- Depression, feeling sad or down, and fatigue.

CAUSES
- A normal decline in ovary function. This results in decreased levels of the female hormones, estrogen and progesterone.
- Surgical removal of both ovaries.
- Medical treatment of endometriosis or cancer.

RISK INCREASES WITH—Menopause is a natural part of the aging process for women. Smoking and hysterectomy are risks for premature menopause.

HOW TO PREVENT—No prevention needed.

WHAT TO EXPECT

DIAGNOSTIC MEASURES—Your health care provider can determine if it is menopause by your age and symptoms. It is often diagnosed in females after 1 year of no menstrual periods.

APPROPRIATE HEALTH CARE—No specific medical treatment is usually needed.

POSSIBLE COMPLICATIONS
- Reduced skin elasticity and reduced vaginal moisture.
- Higher risk of hardening of the arteries, heart disease, stroke, and osteoporosis after menopause.
- Changes in feelings of self-worth.

PROBABLE OUTCOME—Menopause is a normal process, not an illness. Most women adapt without major problems or concerns.

HOW TO TREAT

GENERAL MEASURES
- Continue to use birth-control measures until 12 months after your last menstrual period.
- Reduce stress in your life as much as possible. Acupuncture, meditation, and relaxation techniques can be helpful ways to reduce any stress of menopause.
- Women who smoke start menopause about two years earlier than nonsmokers do. If you smoke, talk to your health care provider about programs to help you quit.
- Counseling may be helpful if emotional feelings interfere with personal relationships or work.
- To learn more: North American Menopause Society, PO Box 94527, Cleveland, OH 44101; (800) 774-5342; website: www.menopause.org.

MEDICATION
- Estrogen therapy alone or combination with progestogen are options for treating hot flashes. Hormone therapy has benefits as well as risks. The decision is made by a woman and her health care provider.
- Other drugs may be prescribed for hot flashes.
- Herbal (or those termed natural remedies) help some women. Discuss these with your health care provider.
- Drugs to prevent and/or treat loss of bone density may be prescribed.
- Take calcium supplements and vitamin D if needed.
- For vaginal dryness, use moisturizers and non-estrogen lubricants, such as KY Jelly or Replens.

ACTIVITY—No limits. Exercise helps your well-being. Weight-bearing activities (such as walking) help bone strength.

DIET—Eat a well-balanced diet.

CALL YOUR DOCTOR IF

- You or a family member has menopause symptoms that cause concern.
- Bleeding recurs 6 months or more after last period.

MENORRHAGIA

GENERAL INFORMATION

DEFINITION—Menorrhagia is a heavy blood loss during menstruation. The average amount of blood loss during a normal menstrual period is about two ounces. With menorrhagia, a woman may lose three ounces or more. Menorrhagia is more a symptom of a disease or condition rather than a disorder in itself. It can affect any woman who has begun menstruation.

BODY PARTS INVOLVED—Female reproductive system.

SEX OR AGE MOST AFFECTED—Females from age 12 to 55.

SIGNS & SYMPTOMS
* Menstrual periods at their regular cycle intervals have been extra heavy for several months in a row.
* Menstrual periods last for more than 7 days.
* Passing of large clots of blood.
* Paleness and fatigue (anemia).

CAUSES—The menstrual cycle is a process (series of events) that occurs in a woman's body each month. Different factors can disrupt the process and lead to menorrhagia.

RISK INCREASES WITH
* Women near menopause or young women who have not established a regular menstrual cycle.
* Hormone imbalance (estrogen/progesterone).
* Infections of the genitals or urinary tract. This includes sexually transmitted diseases.
* Kidney, liver, or thyroid disease.
* Pituitary tumors, polycystic ovarian syndrome, or blood vessel problems.
* Ectopic pregnancy or a miscarriage.
* Ovarian dysfunction (ovaries do not produce eggs).
* Fibroids (benign uterine tumors).
* Endometriosis or endometrial hyperplasia.
* Cervical or uterine polyps.
* Nonhormonal intrauterine device (IUD).
* Bleeding disorders.
* Drugs (steroids, blood thinners, or anticancer).
* Obesity or being overweight.
* Rarely, cancer of the uterus or cervix.

HOW TO PREVENT—No preventive measures.

WHAT TO EXPECT

DIAGNOSTIC MEASURES
* Your health care provider will do a physical exam and a pelvic exam and ask about your symptoms.
* Medical tests may include Pap smear, blood test, pregnancy test, ultrasound, and hysteroscopy (to see inside the uterus). Liver, kidney, and thyroid function tests, and endometrial biopsy may be done.

APPROPRIATE HEALTH CARE
* Treatment usually depends on the age of the woman, her desires for fertility, and any other medical disorder. Treatment steps may include drugs or surgery.
* A nonhormonal IUD may need to be removed.
* Surgery options may include endometrial ablation or endometrial resection, dilatation and curettage (D & C), uterine fibroid embolization, or hysterectomy. The options, risks, and benefits will be explained to you.

POSSIBLE COMPLICATIONS
* Anemia due to excess blood loss. Menorrhagia is a common cause of anemia in premenopausal women.
* Surgery may be required.
* Sometimes, bleeding is so severe that it interrupts normal daily routines like work, school, and social life.
* Other complications are related to the causes.

PROBABLE OUTCOME—Varies with cause of the bleeding. Treatment helps reduce the bleeding in most women.

HOW TO TREAT

GENERAL MEASURES—For self-care, wear extra sanitary pads during heavy flow. If a tampon is used, change tampon every 4 to 6 hours. Avoid scented pads and tampons. Don't douche.

MEDICATION
* Use nonsteroidal anti-inflammatory drugs, such as naproxen or ibuprofen, to relieve pain and possibly reduce bleeding. Avoid aspirin (may prolong bleeding).
* Hormones (oral, released via an IUD, or injected) may be prescribed to control the bleeding.
* If hormones cannot be taken for some reason, other drugs to control the bleeding may be recommended.
* Iron replacement may be prescribed for anemia.
* If a drug you take is the cause, a change in drug or a change in dosage amounts may be recommended.

ACTIVITY—Resting with feet up may help during heavy menstrual periods.

DIET—No special diet.

CALL YOUR DOCTOR IF

* You or a family member has signs or symptoms of menorrhagia.
* Symptoms worsen or new symptoms develop after treatment begins.

MENTAL RETARDATION
(Intellectual Disability)

GENERAL INFORMATION

DEFINITION—Mental retardation is below average, general intellectual functioning along with an inability to adapt to the normal aspects of daily life in a person under age 18. Intellectual functioning is typically measured by an intelligence quotient (IQ) test (if the person can take an IQ test). Those with mental retardation score 70 to 75 or below. The normal range is 80 to 130 (100 is average). Retardation is classified as mild (IQ 50 to 70), moderate (IQ 35 to 49), severe (20 to 34), or profound (IQ less than 20). Mild retardation is the most common form (over 80% of cases). Mildly retarded children may not be identified until they start school. Profoundly and severely retarded children are often diagnosed at birth.

BODY PARTS INVOLVED—All.

SEX OR AGE MOST AFFECTED—Both sexes; all ages. Males are affected more than females.

SIGNS & SYMPTOMS
• Failure to meet developmental milestones. These are the physical and behavioral signs of development or maturation of infants and children.
• Persistence of infantile behavior.
• Lack of curiosity; decreased learning ability.
• Unable to meet educational demands of school.
• Problems with communication and self-care.
• Behaviors may include: being aggressive, dependent, passive, stubborn; having low self-esteem, injures self; frustrates easily; mood disorders; attention difficulties.
• Physical traits may include: shortness in size, malformed ears and eyes, seizures, and birthmarks.

CAUSES
• Genetic: inborn errors of metabolism or chromosome disorders. Down syndrome is a genetic disorder that causes mental retardation.
• Intrauterine: congenital infections, placental-fetal malfunction, complications of pregnancy (infections, preeclampsia, eclampsia, maternal alcohol or drug abuse or poor diet).
• Perinatal (just before the birth): prematurity, postmaturity, birth injury, or metabolic disorders.
• Postnatal (after birth): endocrine or metabolic disorders, infection, trauma, toxic, and other causes of brain damage, or abuse.

RISK INCREASES WITH—Risk factors are related to the causes.

HOW TO PREVENT
• Genetic counseling and prenatal genetic tests for families with a history of mental retardation.
• During pregnancy, get good prenatal care; eat healthy; avoid smoking, alcohol, and drugs of abuse.
• Screening of newborns for metabolic disorders.
• Protect children from injury, poisoning, or abuse.

WHAT TO EXPECT

DIAGNOSTIC MEASURES
• Your own observation of symptoms.
• Your child's health care provider will do a physical exam and certain mental tests (if the child is old enough) to help with the diagnosis. You will be asked about your own observation of signs in your child.

APPROPRIATE HEALTH CARE—Goals are to develop the child's potential to the fullest. Retardation cannot be reversed, but much can be done to help the child function as normally as possible. Beginning in infancy, special education with social and behavioral training can enhance the child's skills.

POSSIBLE COMPLICATIONS
• Emotional and behavioral problems in child.
• Stresses placed on the family.

PROBABLE OUTCOME
• Mildly retarded people can learn to lead independent, productive lives.
• Moderately retarded people are trainable. They often require protective care (such as a group home).
• More severely and profoundly retarded people usually require continuous care.

HOW TO TREAT

GENERAL MEASURES
• The diagnosis has a profound effect on the family. It will affect every aspect of their lives. Counseling and/or spiritual support are both helpful for parents to learn to accept and cope. Joining a support group for families of children with mental retardation can help also.
• To learn more: The Arc of the United States, 1825 K St., Suite 1200, Washington, DC 20006; (800) 433-5255; website: www.thearc.org.

MEDICATION—Drugs for medical problems, such as seizures may be prescribed.

ACTIVITY—As fully active as child's physical condition permits.

DIET—No special diet.

CALL YOUR DOCTOR IF

You are concerned about your child's development.

METABOLIC SYNDROME
(Insulin Resistance Syndrome; Syndrome X)

GENERAL INFORMATION

DEFINITION
● Metabolic syndrome is not a specific disorder. Rather it is a group (or cluster) of health risks. Having any three of these five health risks would mean that you have the syndrome. A person with metabolic syndrome is more likely to develop heart disease, stroke, and diabetes. The health risks include:
- Large waistline (abdominal obesity).
- High triglyceride level (a type of fat).
- Low level of HDL("good" cholesterol).
- High fasting blood sugar (glucose).
- High blood pressure.
● Note: Not all medical experts agree on the definition of metabolic syndrome. In addition, some definitions include being prone to blood clots in blood vessels or low-grade inflammation throughout the body (as diagnosed with blood tests) as factors also.

BODY PARTS INVOLVED—Heart and blood vessels (cardiovascular system) and others.

SEX OR AGE MOST AFFECTED—Both sexes, children, adolescents, and adults.

SIGNS & SYMPTOMS—No symptoms usually. It is often found during routine medical exams.

CAUSES—The exact cause of the syndrome is unclear. It may be due to a combination of genetic makeup and lifestyle choices of diet and physical activity.

RISK INCREASES WITH
● Overweight/obesity, physical inactivity, insulin resistance (the body does not respond normally to insulin), aging, history of diabetes, and hormonal imbalance may be factors.
● Studies are ongoing to see who may be at specific risk for metabolic syndrome.

HOW TO PREVENT
● Eat a healthy diet.
● Exercise routinely.
● Don't use tobacco in any form.
● Maintain a healthy body weight.

WHAT TO EXPECT

DIAGNOSTIC MEASURES
● Your health care provider will order the medical tests and go over the results with you. Metabolic syndrome may be diagnosed with 3 or more of the following:
1. Waistline of 40 inches or more for men and 35 inches or more for women (measured across the belly).
2. Blood pressure of 130/85 mm Hg or higher.
3. Triglyceride level above 150 mg/dL.
4. Fasting blood glucose (sugar) level greater than 100 mg/dL.
5. HDL, the "good" cholesterol, less than 40 mg/dL (men) or under 50 mg/dL (women).

APPROPRIATE HEALTH CARE—You and your health care provider can decide on an action plan to reduce your risks of heart disease and stroke. This may include changes in diet, getting more exercise, weight loss, stopping smoking, and perhaps drug therapy.

POSSIBLE COMPLICATIONS—If not treated, the syndrome often leads to early heart disease, stroke, and other vascular (blood vessel) problems, as well as diabetes. The more risk factors you have, the more likely you are to have complications.

PROBABLE OUTCOME—Lifestyle changes involving your diet, weight loss, exercise, and drugs (if needed) can usually reverse the risk factors.

HOW TO TREAT

GENERAL MEASURES
● Diet and life-style changes do not mean you have to give up all the good things you enjoy. Even moderate changes can have a big impact on your risk factors.
● To learn more: American Heart Association, 7272 Greenville Ave., Dallas, TX 75231; (800) 242-8721; website: www.americanheart.org.

MEDICATION—Drugs may be prescribed to lower cholesterol, lower high blood pressure, or help with weight loss.

ACTIVITY—Increase physical activity. Get 30 to 60 minutes of aerobic exercise (such as brisk walking) every day. It does not need to be all at one time (e.g., take three 10 minute walks).

DIET
● Limit or avoid foods that contain saturated fats, trans fats, and high amounts of cholesterol. Read food labels carefully.
● Eat plenty of fresh fruits and vegetables and high-fiber foods.
● Begin a weight-reduction diet if you are overweight.

CALL YOUR DOCTOR IF

● You or a family member wants more information about the metabolic syndrome.
● You need help with diet and exercise planning.

METATARSALGIA

Toe

GENERAL INFORMATION

DEFINITION—Metatarsalgia is a general term for pain under the ball of the foot. The ball is the bottom, front part of the foot behind the toes. It is a common problem that can be very painful, but is usually not serious.

BODY PARTS INVOLVED—Muscles, ligaments, and bones of the foot.

SEX OR AGE MOST AFFECTED—Both sexes, usually adults ages 30 to 80.

SIGNS & SYMPTOMS
- Pain, dull ache, or burning feeling in the ball of one or both feet.
- It hurts when walking (especially on hard surfaces) and feels better when you rest.
- It is described as feeling like "have a stone in your shoe" or "walking on pebbles."
- Toes may be painful, or feel numb and tingly.
- Foot may be swollen.

CAUSES—There are five metatarsal bones in the foot that run from the arch to the toe joint. These bones take a lot of pressure when you walk, jump, or run. Anything that puts extra pressure on the front of the foot can cause metatarsalgia.

RISK INCREASES WITH
- High-impact sports that involve running or jumping.
- Wearing shoes that do not fit correctly, are poorly made, or are worn out.
- For women, wearing high heels and shoes that are too tight across the ball of the foot.
- Certain foot shapes (such as high arches) or other foot problems.
- With aging, the fat pad in the foot gets thinner.
- Certain medical problems, such as diabetes.
- Overweight or obesity.
- Walking barefoot on tile or concrete.

HOW TO PREVENT
- Wear shoes that fit well and are right for the activity.
- Start slowly with any new exercise or sports routines.
- Weight loss may help if overweight.

WHAT TO EXPECT

DIAGNOSTIC MEASURES
- Your own observation of symptoms.
- Consult your health care provider if self-treatment does not help to improve the symptoms. Your health care provider will examine the foot, and ask questions about symptoms, your activities, and the type of shoes you wear.
- An x-ray may be taken to make sure there is no bone fracture.

APPROPRIATE HEALTH CARE
- Self care is often all that is needed.
- Special shoes, or special shoe inserts (called orthotics), may be prescribed.
- Surgery may help if there is a problem such as bunions, hammertoes, or a pinched nerve.

POSSIBLE COMPLICATIONS—Without treatment, the foot joint may be less flexible and grow stiff. Pain may increase or occur elsewhere in the body (e.g., back) due to change in gait.

PROBABLE OUTCOME
- Treatment can often relieve symptoms in 10 to 14 days depending on what the cause is.
- In some cases, recovery may depend on treatment of any other medical disorder.

HOW TO TREAT

GENERAL MEASURES
- Rest with your feet elevated (raised up) after periods of standing or walking.
- Rub an ice pack over the painful area for about 15 minutes at a time, several times a day.
- Switch to heat after a day or two if it feels better. Use a heating pad or soak your feet in warm water.
- Do simple stretches while seated:
  - Place heels on floor, move toes in and out.
  - Lift one leg straight and flex ankle by pointing toes up and then toward the floor; repeat with other leg.
- Wear adhesive felt, gel, or foam padding around toe area. Cushioned insoles, metatarsal pads, or arch supports may help.
- Stop wearing the shoes that may cause the problem. Wear shoes that fit well and have plenty of toe room.

MEDICATION—For minor pain, you may use nonprescription pain drugs, such as ibuprofen.

ACTIVITY
- Limit activities until the symptoms improve.
- Try swimming or bicycling instead of running or walking while you have the symptoms.

DIET—No special diet. If overweight is a problem, begin a weight loss diet.

CALL YOUR DOCTOR IF

- You or a family member has metatarsalgia symptoms that have lasted several days or are very painful.
- Pain or discomfort gets worse despite treatment.

METHICILLIN-RESISTANT STAPHYLOCOCCUS AUREUS

 GENERAL INFORMATION

DEFINITION
- Methicillin-resistant *Staphylococcus aureus* (MRSA) is a type of bacteria infection. Usually, it is a mild type of skin infection. Its name comes from the fact that drugs such as methicillin and similar antibiotics are not effective in treating it.
- MRSA infections occur often in healthcare settings (e.g., a hospital), and are called healthcare-associated MRSA, or HA-MRSA. Community-associated MRSA, or CA-MRSA occurs in people in the wider community.

BODY PARTS INVOLVED—Skin, joints, heart, blood vessels, and lungs.

SEX OR AGE MOST AFFECTED—Both sexes; all ages.

SIGNS & SYMPTOMS
- Small bump(s) on the skin; may be red, swollen, painful, or warm to the touch; and look like a spider or insect bite. They may contain pus (e.g., boil or abscess).
- Rarely, infection may spread to other areas of skin or to other body parts. Serious symptoms can occur: fever, chills, low blood pressure, joint pain, severe headache, shortness of breath, and rash over most of the body.

CAUSES
- *Staphylococcus aureus* (*S. aureus* or staph). It is a common type of bacteria (or germ). The germs live on the skin or in the nose of many healthy people. They are called colonized or carriers. Most often, these germs cause no harm. If they enter the skin by way of a cut, scrape, or other skin flaw, an infection can develop.
- MRSA germs are spread by physical contact with someone who is either infected or is a carrier. Germs are also spread by physical contact of objects touched by an infected person or carrier. Objects may include towels, doorknobs, floors, athletic gear, or personal items. Germs can live on some surfaces for hours, days, or even months. Outbreaks of CA-MRSA can occur in places such as schools, gyms, military barracks, dorms, daycare centers, or prisons.

RISK INCREASES WITH
- HA-MRSA: older adults, hospital care, living in long-term care facility, recent antibiotic use, weak immune system, or invasive device (e.g., catheter).
- CA-MRSA: young age, skin injury, contact sports, sharing towels or athletic gear, weak immune system, close contact with health care workers, and living in crowded (e.g., barracks) or unclean home.

HOW TO PREVENT
- In health care settings—follow preventive guidelines.
- In community settings (these are basic steps)—always practice good hygiene. Wash your hands often or use a hand sanitizer. Don't share personal items or towels. Wash athletic clothes and gear after use. Keep your cuts or wounds covered. Avoid contact with other people's wounds or bandages.

 WHAT TO EXPECT

DIAGNOSTIC MEASURES
- Your health care provider will examine the infected area of skin.
- Lab culture studies are usually done (e.g., of pus). Studies can confirm the bacteria causing the infection is staph and if it is MRSA. Culture results take 48 to 72 hours. A rapid blood test (takes 2 hours) for MRSA is also being used.

APPROPRIATE HEALTH CARE
- Treatment will depend on the symptoms.
- Mild skin infections are often treated in a medical office. This is done by draining a boil or abscess. You will be advised about follow-up home care of the wound and how to prevent spreading an infection. In most cases, antibiotic drugs are prescribed.
- Patients with serious MRSA symptoms often require hospital care and extensive therapy.

POSSIBLE COMPLICATIONS—Severe MRSA can lead to pneumonia and other serious heart, blood, joint, and skin problems. It could be fatal.

PROBABLE OUTCOME
- A healthy person with a mild infection can be easily treated. MRSA infection may recur.
- With a severe infection, it depends on the health of the patient and the complications.

 HOW TO TREAT

GENERAL MEASURES—See How to Prevent.

MEDICATION—Oral antibiotics may be prescribed or given IV (with hospital care).

ACTIVITY
- Continue regular activities (unless advised).
- Athletes with MRSA should ask health care provider and coach about sports participation.

DIET—No special diet.

 CALL YOUR DOCTOR IF

- You or a family member has a skin infection that causes concern.
- After diagnosis, any symptoms cause concern.

MISCARRIAGE
(Spontaneous Abortion)

GENERAL INFORMATION

DEFINITION—Loss of a pregnancy prior to the 20th week is generally considered a miscarriage. It happens in about 20% to 30% of first pregnancies. It may occur so early that a woman is unaware of being pregnant. Sometimes, a miscarriage may be "threatened," but pregnancy continues to term.

BODY PARTS INVOLVED—Reproductive system.

SEX OR AGE MOST AFFECTED—Women of childbearing age.

SIGNS & SYMPTOMS
- Uterine cramps.
- Vaginal bleeding (from slight to heavy).
- Sudden decrease in signs of pregnancy.

CAUSES—There are many reasons a pregnancy ends in miscarriage. Most often, it is due to the pregnancy not developing normally. Sometimes, no cause is found.

RISK INCREASES WITH
- Genetic factors (problems with fetal chromosomes).
- Problems with a woman's uterus or cervix.
- Age over 30 years or under 15 years.
- Certain infections during pregnancy.
- Chronic maternal diseases.
- Alcohol use, drug or substance abuse.
- Cigarette smoking.
- Being very overweight or underweight.
- Caffeine use (heavy).
- Certain drugs.
- Conceiving after infertility.
- Conception within 3 to 6 months after prior birth.
- Exposure to environmental and workplace hazards.
- Intrauterine device use.
- Having two previous miscarriages.
- Radiation or severe malnutrition.
- Working, exercise, and having sex are not risk factors for normally healthy women.

HOW TO PREVENT
- May not be preventable. To reduce risk factors:
  - Obtain regular medical check-ups.
  - Eat a normal, well-balanced diet.
  - Avoid risk factors where possible.
  - Don't use nonprescription drugs or herbal products without medical advice.

WHAT TO EXPECT

DIAGNOSTIC MEASURES
- Your obstetric provider may do a pelvic exam. Questions will be asked about your symptoms.
- Tests can include blood studies, ultrasound, and tissue study (if you have passed tissue).

APPROPRIATE HEALTH CARE
- Types of miscarriage are: threatened, inevitable, incomplete, complete, missed, or septic. Treatment depends on type. Your obstetric provider will discuss options with you.
- For a threatened miscarriage, bed rest at home may help stabilize the pregnancy. Bleeding may be severe, requiring hospital care and blood transfusion.
- Surgery may be done to remove any remaining tissue or a dead fetus. D & C (dilatation and curettage) or D & E (dilatation and evacuation) may be needed.
- Counseling for patient and partner may be helpful.

POSSIBLE COMPLICATIONS
- Uterine infection (fever, chills, and aching).
- Hemorrhaging (bleeding).
- "Incomplete" abortion, in which some placenta or fetal tissue remains in the uterus, or missed abortion, in which the fetus dies but remains in the uterus.

PROBABLE OUTCOME—Complete recovery is expected. The majority of women will carry a healthy baby to term in the future. Feelings of loss and grief are common. Feelings of guilt may also be present.

HOW TO TREAT

GENERAL MEASURES
- Following a complete miscarriage:
  - Expect a small amount of vaginal bleeding or spotting for 8 to 10 days. Avoid tampons for 2 to 4 weeks.
  - Wait through 2 or 3 normal menstrual cycles (or as advised) before attempting to become pregnant again.

MEDICATION
- A drug to control bleeding may be given.
- Pain relievers may be prescribed.
- Antibiotics may be prescribed for an infection.
- RhoD (immune globulin) for Rh-negative female.

ACTIVITY
- For a threatened miscarriage, rest in bed until symptoms disappear. Avoid sexual intercourse.
- After a miscarriage, reduce activity and rest often during the next 48 hours.

DIET—Usually no special diet. Follow any medical advice.

CALL YOUR DOCTOR IF

- You or a family member has vaginal bleeding during pregnancy.
- Bleeding and cramps worsen, or you pass tissue, or fever and chills occur.

MITRAL VALVE PROLAPSE

GENERAL INFORMATION

DEFINITION—Mitral valve prolapse (MVP) is a heart valve disorder. The mitral valve is located in the left side of the heart. It is one of four heart valves that keep blood flowing in one direction. Prolapse means that openings (called leaflets) in the valve don't close as firmly as they should. This defect can allow a small amount of blood to leak backward (called mitral valve regurgitation). This leads to a heart "click" or murmur that may be heard through a stethoscope (an instrument used for listening to body sounds). MVP is common and it is often diagnosed in otherwise healthy teenagers and young adults.

BODY PARTS INVOLVED—Heart.

SEX OR AGE MOST AFFECTED—Both sexes; all ages.

SIGNS & SYMPTOMS
* Often no symptoms are present (about 60% of cases) and the condition may be discovered on a routine physical exam. When symptoms do occur, they may vary from a few that are mild to having many symptoms. The symptoms are sometimes referred to as mitral valve prolapse syndrome (MVPS).
* Chest pain (sharp, dull, or pressing).
* Fatigue, shortness of breath.
* Dizziness.
* Lightheadedness when rising up from a chair or bed.
* Heart palpitations.
* Anxiety and panic attacks.
* Migraines.

CAUSES—Why MVP occurs is unknown. The condition may be inherited or due to another disease.

RISK INCREASES WITH
* Family history of heart valve disorders.
* Connective tissue disorders (e.g., systemic lupus erythematosus, Marfan syndrome, and others).
* Other heart conditions and some muscle disorders.

HOW TO PREVENT—No preventive measures.

WHAT TO EXPECT

DIAGNOSTIC MEASURES
* Your own observation of symptoms.
* Your health care provider may do a physical exam and listen to the sounds of the heart.
* Medical tests may include an echocardiogram (heart function test) to confirm the diagnosis.

APPROPRIATE HEALTH CARE
* Treatment is usually not needed. A medical follow-up may be done every few years to check for proper heart function.
* In some cases where there is more blood leakage, drugs and lifestyle changes may be recommended for treatment.
* Surgery for valve replacement may be recommended in a few cases. New methods of repairing leaking valves are being researched.
* If other symptoms such as fatigue, anxiety, or panic attacks occur, your health care provider can discuss treatment options.

POSSIBLE COMPLICATIONS
* Excess blood may leak backward through the mitral valve.
* Endocarditis (inflammation of the heart valves and heart lining).
* Stroke.
* Sudden death.

PROBABLE OUTCOME—MVP is usually a benign disorder that needs no treatment and does not prevent a normal active life. Complications are rare.

HOW TO TREAT

GENERAL MEASURES—Be reassured that for most people, the condition is benign and requires no treatment except follow-up evaluation.

MEDICATION—Drugs may be prescribed depending on specific symptoms or to prevent complications.

ACTIVITY
* Daily exercise is helpful for most patients.
* Athletes with MVP who have many symptoms may be restricted from some types of sports.

DIET
* Weight-loss diet is suggested for overweight patients.
* Reducing intake of caffeine and alcohol may be recommended.

CALL YOUR DOCTOR IF

* You or a family member has signs or symptoms of mitral valve prolapse.
* Symptoms worsen or new symptoms occur after diagnosis.

MOLD ALLERGY

GENERAL INFORMATION

DEFINITION—An allergy is an abnormal reaction of the body's immune system to certain substances (or allergens) like mold. Mold is a fungus (fungi is plural) that can live indoors or outdoors. Mold spores (seeds) travel through the air. Spores are tiny, lightweight, and are basically everywhere. The spores are breathed in through the nose and mouth and travel to the lungs. Everyone is exposed to some mold every day with no bad effects. People with an allergy to mold can have a reaction that causes symptoms similar to hay fever or a cold.

BODY PARTS INVOLVED—Nose, eyes, lungs.

SEX OR AGE MOST AFFECTED—Both sexes; all ages.

SIGNS & SYMPTOMS
- Sneezing, coughing, and postnasal drip.
- Runny or stuffy nose. May have wheezing.
- Watery and itchy eyes.
- Itchy nose or throat.
- Sinusitis (sinus inflammation).
- Symptoms vary from person to person, and range from mild to severe.
- Symptoms may occur year-round. They may flare up during certain times of the year, in damp weather, or in indoor or outdoor spaces that have high levels of mold.

CAUSES—The body's immune system believes that the mold spores are harmful. It produces cells that release a chemical called histamine. Histamine in turn produces swelling and irritation in certain areas (e.g., nose, eyes, and sinuses). Future exposures to mold spores will then trigger that antibody response again.

RISK INCREASES WITH
- Personal or a family history of allergies.
- People who work in jobs involving high mold levels. These include baking, logging, dairy work, farming, etc.
- Workplace, home, or school has excess moisture, high humidity, or poor ventilation.

HOW TO PREVENT—There is no way to prevent having allergies. You can take measures to help prevent having the symptoms.

WHAT TO EXPECT

DIAGNOSTIC MEASURES
- Your own observation of symptoms.
- Your health care provider will ask questions about your symptoms, medical history, lifestyle, and allergies in family members. You will be asked about exposures to allergens. However, a person is unlikely to know they have been exposed to mold. An exam of the ears, eyes, nose, throat, and lungs is usually done.

- An allergy skin or blood test may be done to find out what allergens you are allergic to. For more severe symptoms, other medical tests may be done.

APPROPRIATE HEALTH CARE—Treatment usually involves drugs to help relieve the symptoms and avoiding exposure to molds. However, molds are common and can't be avoided completely.

POSSIBLE COMPLICATIONS
- Rarely, severe lung problems may develop. People with weak immune systems or who have asthma are more at risk.
- Anaphylaxis, a severe reaction, is very rare.
- Medical research is ongoing about the existence of other mold-related illnesses, such as the one called toxic mold syndrome.

PROBABLE OUTCOME—Treatment helps control the symptoms. Mold allergy continues over a lifetime.

HOW TO TREAT

GENERAL MEASURES
- Check your home for areas of mold growth, such as shower stalls, basements, and refrigerator drip trays. Watch for any water leaks.
- Make your home smoke-free.
- If your workplace or school is a possible source of mold, discuss the problem with the people in charge.
- If your job, such as in a bakery or greenhouse, is the problem, you may want to consider a career change.
- To learn more: American College of Allergy, Asthma & Immunology website: www.acaai.org/public or National Institute of Allergy and Infectious Diseases website: www3.niaid.nih.gov/topics/allergicdiseases.

MEDICATION
- Antihistamines, decongestants, eye drops, and nose sprays may be prescribed depending on the symptoms.
- A series of mold allergy shots may help in some cases, but not all.

ACTIVITY—Stay inside if it is windy or dusty outside. A dust mask may help if you go out.

DIET—An allergic reaction is unlikely to occur from eating food fungi such as mushrooms, dried fruits, and others. No one should eat food with mold growth on it.

CALL YOUR DOCTOR IF

- You or a family member has mold allergy symptoms.
- Symptoms worsen or don't improve with treatment.

MOLLUSCUM CONTAGIOSUM

GENERAL INFORMATION

DEFINITION—Molluscum contagiosum is a contagious, viral infection of the skin. It is usually a mild condition.

BODY PARTS INVOLVED—Skin anywhere on the body. The virus usually occurs on the face in children. In adults, it usually occurs on the inner thighs, abdomen and genitals.

SEX OR AGE MOST AFFECTED—Both sexes; all ages, but more common in children.

SIGNS & SYMPTOMS
- Small, raised bumps (papules) on the skin.
- Bumps are firm, smooth, domed with a central pit, and skin-colored or white. The skin over the bumps is transparent and thin.
- Bumps cause eye irritation if they are on the eyelids.
- They don't hurt or itch.

CAUSES—A virus of the pox group. The germs are usually spread by skin-to-skin contact in children and sexual contact in teens and adults. The time period from being exposed to having symptoms can range from 2 weeks to 6 months. It may also be spread by touching objects that have the germs on them, such as shared clothing, towels, wash cloths, and sports equipment.

RISK INCREASES WITH
- Close contact with an infected person.
- Weak immune system due to illness or drugs.
- Atopic dermatitis.
- Tropical climates.
- It is unclear if swimming pools are a risk.

HOW TO PREVENT
- Practice good personal hygiene. Wash hands often to avoid spreading any type of germs.
- Avoid sexual contact with infected people. It is unclear if condoms are effective in preventing spread.

WHAT TO EXPECT

DIAGNOSTIC MEASURES
- Your own observation of symptoms.
- Your health care provider can diagnose the disorder by a skin exam of the affected area.
- If needed, the diagnosis can be confirmed with a skin scraping and microscopic study.

APPROPRIATE HEALTH CARE
- Treatment is not always needed in healthy persons. It is important for those with weak immune systems to get treatment.
- Drugs may be applied to the skin.
- There are different options for removing the growths. They include cutting, burning (electrically or chemically), or freezing (cryotherapy). Treatments can be done in a medical office. There may be some discomfort with these treatments.

POSSIBLE COMPLICATIONS
- Some scarring can occur.
- The bumps can become irritated, inflamed, and infected by bacteria.
- The problem may recur.

PROBABLE OUTCOME—Outcome is good. They can heal on their own without treatment in otherwise healthy people. Healing can take a few months or up to a few years. Treatment helps to prevent their spread to other persons and to speed up the healing time.

HOW TO TREAT

GENERAL MEASURES
- An infected person is contagious until all the bumps are gone. Use care to avoid spreading the infection to other parts of your body and to other people.
  - Don't touch, pick or scratch a bump and then touch another part of your body or another person.
  - Keep bumps clean and covered with clothing or bandage if around other people.
  - Don't shave affected area.
  - Don't share clothing, towels, washcloths, personal items, toys, or sports gear.

MEDICATION
- Painless, medicated drops may be applied by your health care provider.
- Other drugs may be prescribed that you can apply to the bumps yourself.
- Ask your health care provider for advice before using any alternate forms of treatment.

ACTIVITY
- No limits for most activities. Avoid sexual relations until the bumps disappear.
- If using a swimming pool, cover the affected area with watertight bandages.

DIET—No special diet.

CALL YOUR DOCTOR IF

- You or a family member has symptoms of molluscum contagiosum.
- A reinfection occurs after treatment.

MONONUCLEOSIS, INFECTIOUS

GENERAL INFORMATION

DEFINITION—Infectious mononucleosis is a viral illness that affects the lungs, liver, and lymphatic system.

BODY PARTS INVOLVED—Lymph nodes; liver; spleen; throat; bronchial tubes.

SEX OR AGE MOST AFFECTED—It usually affects children and young adults (from 12 to 40 years of age) of both sexes.

SIGNS & SYMPTOMS
* Young children may have mild or no symptoms.
* Fever.
* Sore throat (sometimes severe).
* Appetite loss.
* Fatigue.
* Swollen lymph glands, usually in the neck, underarms, or groin.
* Enlarged spleen may cause pain in abdomen.
* Headache.
* General aching.

CAUSES
* Epstein-Barr virus (EBV) is the primary cause. The germs are spread in saliva and can be passed from person to person by close contact, such as kissing or sharing food. The incubation time can range from 2 to 6 weeks. Almost everyone will have been infected by EBV by adulthood, but not all infected persons will get infectious mononucleosis.
* Other causes are more rare and in some cases, no cause is found.

RISK INCREASES WITH—Close contact with saliva from an infected person.

HOW TO PREVENT—If you are in close contact with an infected person, don't kiss, don't share food or eating utensils or straws, don't share lip gloss or lipstick, don't share toothbrush.

WHAT TO EXPECT

DIAGNOSTIC MEASURES
* Your own observation of symptoms.
* Your health care provider will do a physical exam and ask questions about your symptoms.
* Medical tests may include blood studies.

APPROPRIATE HEALTH CARE—No specific cure or treatment is available. Extra rest and healthy diet are important.

POSSIBLE COMPLICATIONS
* Small risk for ruptured spleen, emergency surgery.
* In rare cases, the heart, lungs, or central nervous system could become involved. The disease can prove serious, even fatal.

PROBABLE OUTCOME—It usually clears up on its own in 10 days to 6 months. Fatigue usually lasts for 3 to 6 weeks after other symptoms get better. A few patients have a chronic form in which symptoms last for months or years.

HOW TO TREAT

GENERAL MEASURES
* There is no need to keep away from other people. Do not kiss or share any item that may have saliva on it.
* To relieve the sore throat, gargle frequently with warm or cold double-strength tea or warm salt water (mix one-half teaspoon of salt in one cup of water).

MEDICATION
* For minor pain, you may use nonprescription drugs such as acetaminophen. Don't use aspirin in children under age 18.
* If symptoms are severe, you may be prescribed a short course of cortisone drugs.
* Avoid penicillin, amoxicillin, or ampicillin as they can cause a rash in mononucleosis patients.

ACTIVITY
* Rest in bed while you have fever. Resume normal activities gradually. Rest when you are tired.
* Athletes involved in sports activity, especially contact sports, should ask their health care provider about returning to that activity.

DIET—No special diet. You may not feel like eating while you are ill. Eat soft foods or drink milk shakes. Drink plenty of fluids each day (especially with a fever).

CALL YOUR DOCTOR IF

* You or a family member has symptoms of infectious mononucleosis.
* The following occur during treatment:
  - Symptoms don't improve in a week or two.
  - Fever over 102°F (38.9°C).
  - Constipation, which may cause straining.
  - Severe pain in the upper left abdomen (rupture of the spleen is a medical emergency!).
  - Yellowing of the skin.
  - Difficulty swallowing or breathing due to severe sore throat.

...MA

...MATION

...oma is a thickening ...the foot. It typically ...and fourth metatarsal bone... ...rd and fourth toes. It may so... ...other toes as well. Most often, only ... ...is involved.

BODY PARTS INVOLVED—Muscles, ligaments, and nerves in the ball of the foot.

SEX OR AGE MOST AFFECTED—Usually adults of both sexes. It is more common in ages 40 to 50 and in women more than men.

SIGNS & SYMPTOMS
• Symptoms may begin gradually, they may come and go, and get worse over time.
• Pain, burning, tingling, or numbness in the ball of the foot, and sometimes, in the toes.
• Symptoms may increase when wearing shoes, walking, or when performing activities that put pressure on the foot.

CAUSES—The exact cause is unclear. It appears to result from pressure, injury, or irritation to the nerves in that part of the foot.

RISK INCREASES WITH
• People who have certain foot deformities (e.g., bunions, flatfeet, hammertoes, or more flexible feet).
• Activities that involve repetitive irritation to the ball of the foot, such as running or court sports.
• Ill-fitting or high-heel shoes.
• An injury or other type of trauma to the area.
• Obesity.

HOW TO PREVENT
• No specific way to prevent.
• Avoid poor-fitting shoes. Wear shoes with a wide toe box.
• Wear sports specific athletic shoes.

WHAT TO EXPECT

DIAGNOSTIC MEASURES
• Your own observation of symptoms.
• Your health care provider will do a physical exam of the foot and ask questions about your symptoms.
• A local anesthetic may be injected to see if it stops the pain. This helps confirm diagnosis.
• X-ray, ultrasound, or an MRI may be done.

APPROPRIATE HEALTH CARE
• Simple treatments are usually the first option. These may include footwear changes, shoe inserts, drugs for pain, physical therapy, and changes in activities.
• Custom orthotics (shoe inserts) may be prescribed.
• Options for patients who do not respond to simple treatments may include:
 - Surgery. See Morton's Neuroma Removal in the Surgery Section.
 - Cryogenic neuroablation. Extremely cold temperature is used to stop pain signals of nerve. It is not a permanent solution.

POSSIBLE COMPLICATIONS
• May develop an abnormal gait due to pain.
• Complications from surgery or symptoms recur after surgery.

PROBABLE OUTCOME—For some people, the simple treatment measures will control the symptoms. Surgery often helps in other cases. Surgery may leave some numbness in the area, but this is not a problem for most patients.

HOW TO TREAT

GENERAL MEASURES
• Use ice on the affected area to help ease symptoms. Apply 3 to 4 times a day for 10 minutes at a time. Stop if it worsens pain.
• Gently massage the area several times a day.
• Use nonprescription foot pads or arch supports in shoes to reduce nerve pressure.
• Wear comfortable, supportive, low-heeled shoes with plenty of toe room. Don't walk barefoot on hard surfaces.

MEDICATION
• Use nonprescription drugs such as aspirin or ibuprofen to reduce pain and swelling.
• One or more types of drugs injected into the affected area may be prescribed.

ACTIVITY
• You may want to temporarily limit activities that put pressure on the nerve (e.g., aerobics, running, or jogging).
• Stretching exercises or physical therapy may be recommended by your health care provider.

DIET—No special diet.

CALL YOUR DOCTOR IF

• You or a family member has symptoms of Morton's neuroma.
• Symptoms don't improve with treatment.
• The following occur after surgical treatment:
 - Bleeding at the surgical site.
 - Pain.

MOTION SICKNESS

GENERAL INFORMATION

DEFINITION—Motion sickness is an unpleasant, temporary condition that occurs as a response to certain kinds of movement.

BODY PARTS INVOLVED—The semicircular canals in the inner ear are affected. These fluid-filled canals normally maintain a person's sense of balance.

SEX OR AGE MOST AFFECTED—Both sexes; all ages.

SIGNS & SYMPTOMS
- Loss of appetite, nausea, and vomiting.
- Spinning sensation; weakness and being unsteady.
- Confusion; anxiety; sweating.
- Paleness.
- Yawning.

CAUSES—Motion that may be due to a plane, boat, car, train, amusement park ride, or swinging. The body, the inner ear, and the eyes send conflicting messages to the brain. The ears may sense motion that the eyes cannot see, or the eyes may see movement that the body does not feel. People who suffer from motion sickness may have the symptoms just thinking about movement (such as when sitting on a plane waiting for take-off).

RISK INCREASES WITH
- Certain persons: women more than men, children, being pregnant, migraine sufferers, and those who have ear disorders such as with allergies or infections.
- Certain situations: travel, smoky environment or poor ventilation, drinking too much alcohol, or visual stimuli (e.g., a moving horizon).

HOW TO PREVENT
- Avoid large meals and alcohol before and during trips.
- Sit in areas of the airplane (usually over the wings) or boat with the least motion. Sit in the front seat of the car.
- Recline in your seat, if possible.
- Breathe slowly and deeply. Don't read.
- In a car, airplane, or bus, turn on air vent to improve air flow. Focus eyes on the horizon.
- Avoid areas where others are smoking.
- Take preventive drugs before a trip.
- Mental and emotional factors can add to motion sickness. Try to resolve concerns about travel before leaving home.
- Acupressure may help. This is done by placing pressure on a point three finger-widths above the wrist on the inner arm. Elastic wristband products can be purchased to put pressure on this area.

- If your work or lifestyle requires travel and you suffer from motion sickness, consider preventive therapy. It may include behavior-modification techniques, biofeedback, controlled breathing, relaxation techniques, stress management, desensitization (repeated brief exposure therapy), and others undergoing research.

WHAT TO EXPECT

DIAGNOSTIC MEASURES
- Your own observation of symptoms.
- If your symptoms persist or cause concern, see your health care provider. A physical exam may be done and medical tests may be recommended to rule out other disorders.

APPROPRIATE HEALTH CARE—Self-care is usually all that is needed.

POSSIBLE COMPLICATIONS—None usually. Some people continue to suffer symptoms for a few days or longer after a trip (may be referred to as mal de debarquement syndrome).

PROBABLE OUTCOME—Usually resolves within an hour after the trip or other triggering event.

HOW TO TREAT

GENERAL MEASURES
- If symptoms occur, try to rest in a dark room with a cool cloth over the eyes and forehead.
  - Take sips of water until stomach calms.
  - Allowing yourself to vomit can help the nausea. However, don't make yourself vomit.

MEDICATION
- You may use nonprescription drugs. Try dimenhydrinate (Dramamine) or meclizine (Bonine) before and during travel, or for treatment. These can cause drowsiness.
- A scopolamine patch to control symptoms may be prescribed.
- Other drugs may be prescribed if simple treatment methods are not effective.

ACTIVITY—Limited only by the symptoms.

DIET
- Eat lightly or not at all before and during brief trips. For longer trips, sip liquids (tea and juices) to maintain your fluid intake. Avoid alcohol.
- Ginger helps some people. Take it on an empty stomach. It is available in a tea, capsules, or candied pieces.

CALL YOUR DOCTOR IF

You or a family member plans to travel and has had disabling motion sickness in the past.

MULTIPLE MYELOMA
(Plasma Cell Myeloma)

 GENERAL INFORMATION

DEFINITION—Multiple myeloma is a cancer of the plasma cells of the bone marrow. Plasma cells normally help the body destroy germs and protect against infection. It is called multiple because it occurs in many bones in the body.

BODY PARTS INVOLVED—Bone marrow of all bones, but most common in the thigh, back, pelvis or upper arms.

SEX OR AGE MOST AFFECTED—Older adults are more often affected and men more than women.

SIGNS & SYMPTOMS
- Pain in the affected bone. The pain is severe, boring, and deep. If the bone collapses, pain spreads to other parts of the body.
- Weight loss and/or infections or bleeding.
- Symptoms of anemia, such as weakness, paleness, tiredness, and breathlessness.

CAUSES—Unknown. The bone pain is caused by the cancerous plasma cells. The anemia is caused by damaged red blood cells and decreased platelets.

RISK INCREASES WITH
- Older adults.
- Other plasma cell disease (e.g., MGUS).
- Family history of myeloma.
- African Americans.
- Possibly—obesity, exposure to certain chemicals, or viruses.

HOW TO PREVENT—No specific preventive measures.

 WHAT TO EXPECT

DIAGNOSTIC MEASURES
- Your own observation of symptoms.
- Your health care provider will do a physical exam and ask questions about your symptoms and activities.
- Different medical tests are done to verify the diagnosis and to determine if the cancer has spread to other places in the body (called staging).

APPROPRIATE HEALTH CARE
- Treatment will depend on the stage of the disease, your health, age, and preferences. Your health care provider will discuss the options and their risks and benefits. All treatments have numerous side effects.
- Watchful waiting is usually recommended if there are no symptoms. This means monitoring the cancer cells for a period of time before deciding on treatment.

- Treatment may involve chemotherapy and other drug therapy, stem cell transplantation, radiation, treatment as needed for complications, and supportive care.
- Treatment may involve steps to relieve symptoms and make you comfortable, rather than treating the cancer.
- Counseling may help you cope with having cancer.

POSSIBLE COMPLICATIONS
- Recurrent infections, anemia, or hypercalcemia.
- Kidney failure or heart failure.
- Spontaneous bleeding.
- Bone fractures or paralysis.

PROBABLE OUTCOME—Treatment can help with the symptoms and improve quality of life. There is no cure. Some patients live up to 5 years or more after symptoms appear. Temporary remissions may occur with treatment. Research into causes and treatment continues, so there is hope for more effective treatment and cure.

 HOW TO TREAT

GENERAL MEASURES
- The more you can learn and understand about this disorder, the more you will be able to make informed decisions about treatments.
- To learn more: International Myeloma Foundation, 12650 Riverside Dr., Suite 206, North Hollywood, CA 91607; (800) 452-2873; website: www.myeloma.org.

MEDICATION
- Your health care provider may prescribe:
  - Anticancer (chemotherapy) and cortisone drugs.
  - Bisphosphonates for bone healing.
  - Pain relievers.
  - Antibiotics for infections.
  - Blood transfusions, if anemia is severe.
  - Drugs for hypercalcemia (too much calcium).
  - Other drugs may be prescribed depending on the response to initial therapy, for relapses, and to prevent or treat complications.

ACTIVITY
- Stay as active as pain or complications allow.
- Get medical advise about exercising.

DIET—No special diet.

 CALL YOUR DOCTOR IF

- You or a family member has symptoms of multiple myeloma.
- New or worsening symptoms occur.

MULTIPLE SCLEROSIS

GENERAL INFORMATION

DEFINITION
● Multiple sclerosis (MS) is a chronic disorder that affects the central nervous system (brain, spinal cord, and optic nerve). MS types include:
- Relapsing-remitting. Most common. Patients have flare ups followed by partial or complete recovery.
- Primary-progressive. Slow and continued worsening of symptoms. May be temporary minor improvements.
- Secondary-progressive. This type follows the relapsing-remitting type. Symptoms steadily worsen.
- Progressive-relapsing. Symptoms steadily worsen from the start. Has flare ups, with or without recovery.

BODY PARTS INVOLVED—Central nervous system.

SEX OR AGE MOST AFFECTED—It more often affects adults 20 to 50, and women twice as often as men.

SIGNS & SYMPTOMS
● Signs and symptoms may be mild, moderate, or severe. They vary from person to person and at times in the same person.
● Fatigue (called MS lassitude).
● Problems with walking. Lack of coordination.
● Bowel and bladder problems.
● Problems with vision or hearing (less often).
● Vague loss of sensation or numbness and tingling.
● Mood swings; depression; sexual problems.
● Difficulty with memory, concentration, attention, and problem solving.
● Speech or swallowing problems (sometimes).

CAUSES—It is believed to be an autoimmune disorder. In these disorders, the immune system attacks the body itself by mistake and in different ways. Genetic and environmental (such as a virus) factors may contribute.

RISK INCREASES WITH
● Females more than males.
● Family history of MS.
● Living in northern latitudes (e.g., northern United States or Canada).
● People of Northern European descent.
● Other possible factors are being studied.

HOW TO PREVENT—No preventive measures.

WHAT TO EXPECT

DIAGNOSTIC MEASURES
● Your health care provider will do a physical exam and ask questions about your symptoms, activities, and medical history. No specific test is available to diagnose MS.

● Medical tests may include blood, urine, and spinal fluid studies. An MRI scan of the brain and spinal cord may show typical changes that indicate MS. Often, a specialist called a neurologist is needed to make the diagnosis.

APPROPRIATE HEALTH CARE
● Treatment may include one or more drugs to treat symptoms, prevent complications, or slow progress of the disorder.
● Physical therapy and occupational therapy may be prescribed.
● Plasma exchange (a blood treatment) may be of help.
● Other treatments are undergoing research.
● Counseling may help you and your family cope.

POSSIBLE COMPLICATIONS—Numerous complications can occur. They often result from problems such as immobility, chronic urinary-tract infections, difficulty with swallowing and breathing, and mental and emotional disorders.

PROBABLE OUTCOME—There is no cure. The course of the disorder will be different for each person. Some will be favorable and others unfavorable. Symptoms can often be relieved or controlled.

HOW TO TREAT

GENERAL MEASURES
● Multiple sclerosis will affect every aspect of your life. You will want to educate yourself about your specific symptoms and what to expect and how to adjust to the disease.
● Joining a support group is a way to share feelings.
● To learn more: National Multiple Sclerosis Society, 733 Third Ave., New York, NY 10017; (800) 344-4867; website: www.nationalmssociety.org.

MEDICATION
● Drugs called disease-modifying agents are often prescribed. The options will be discussed with you.
● Oral or injected drugs for specific symptoms or complications will be prescribed as needed.

ACTIVITY—Get enough rest. Exercise to the extent possible. It helps physical and emotional well-being, keeps muscles limber and strong, and helps balance and coordination.

DIET—Eat a healthy diet that is low in fat and high in fiber (helps prevent constipation).

CALL YOUR DOCTOR IF

● You or a family member has symptoms of multiple sclerosis.
● After diagnosis, any symptoms cause concern.

MUMPS

GENERAL INFORMATION

DEFINITION—Mumps is a mild, contagious viral disease that causes painful swelling of the glands located between the ear and jaw. These are the parotid salivary glands. Mumps infections are now rare because of the routine vaccines given to infants. About 10% of adults are susceptible to mumps.

BODY PARTS INVOLVED—Parotid glands (salivary glands that lie between the ear and jaw). Other organs, including the testicles, ovaries, pancreas, breasts, brain and meninges (membranes that cover the brain) sometimes become involved.

SEX OR AGE MOST AFFECTED—All ages, but most common in children (2 to 12 years).

SIGNS & SYMPTOMS
- Mumps without complications:
  - Inflammation, swelling, tenderness, or pain of the glands. The glands feel firm. Discomfort increases with chewing or swallowing.
    - Fever.
    - Headache.
    - Sore throat.
    - Fatigue.
- Mumps symptoms with complications:
  - Painful, swollen testicles.
  - Abdominal pain.
  - Severe headache, if the brain or meninges (lining of the brain) are involved.

CAUSES—Person-to-person transmission of the mumps virus (*paramyxovirus*). The virus can be passed anytime from 48 hours before symptoms begin to 6 days after symptoms appear. Virus incubation is 14 to 24 days after contact; the average is 18 days.

RISK INCREASES WITH
- Lack of immunization.
- Travel to countries where mumps is still common.
- Outbreaks that may occur.

HOW TO PREVENT
- Obtain routine mumps vaccines for infants.
- If you have not had mumps or been vaccinated, and a close family member has mumps, seek advice from your health care provider.

WHAT TO EXPECT

DIAGNOSTIC MEASURES
- Your own observation of symptoms.
- Your health care provider can usually diagnose mumps by the signs and symptoms.
- Blood studies may be done to confirm the diagnosis.

APPROPRIATE HEALTH CARE
- Home care after diagnosis is usually all that is needed. Rarely, medical care may be needed for complications.
- Once the infection begins, it must run its natural course. There is no safe or effective drug that can treat mumps.

POSSIBLE COMPLICATIONS
- Complications are rare, and if they occur are usually in persons over age 19. Complications can involve the testicles, ovaries, thyroid, brain, spinal cord, prostate, pancreas, and the breasts. Testicle involvement may rarely lead to infertility in males.
- Mumps in the first trimester of pregnancy may lead to miscarriage.
- Hearing loss in children.

PROBABLE OUTCOME—Recovery in about 10–12 days. After having it once, a person almost always has lifetime immunity to mumps.

HOW TO TREAT

GENERAL MEASURES
- You do not need to keep the infected person away from the family. By the time symptoms appear, the disease has usually already spread.
- Apply heat or ice, whichever feels better, to the swollen, painful glands. Use a hot-water bottle, hot towel, or ice pack.

MEDICATION
- For minor pain, you may use nonprescription drugs such as acetaminophen or ibuprofen.
- If testicles are involved, stronger pain relievers and other drugs may be prescribed.

ACTIVITY—Allow as much activity as strength and feeling of well-being allow. Patients are no longer contagious when swelling disappears.

DIET—Soft food diet is helpful if chewing causes pain. Increase daily fluid intake to at least 6 to 8 glasses of liquid a day.

CALL YOUR DOCTOR IF

- You or a family member has symptoms of mumps.
- Fever rises above 101°F (38.3°C).
- The following occur during the illness:
  - Vomiting or abdominal pain.
  - Severe headache.
  - Drowsiness or inability to stay awake.
  - Swelling or pain in the testicles.
  - Twitching of the face muscles.
  - Convulsion.
  - Discomfort or redness in the eyes.

MUSCULAR DYSTROPHY

 GENERAL INFORMATION

DEFINITION—Muscular dystrophy is a group of inherited disorders that cause muscle weakness and wasting (decrease in size). There are nine major types of muscular dystrophy (and some subtypes within those types). Duchenne is one of the most common types.

BODY PARTS INVOLVED—Different types affect different areas of the body, such as shoulders, hips or face.

SEX OR AGE MOST AFFECTED—The disorders are usually diagnosed in children (most often boys), and less often in teens or adults.

SIGNS & SYMPTOMS
- Early symptoms:
  - Weakness.
  - Duck-like gait. Lack of coordination.
  - Falling, with difficulty getting up.
  - Muscles appear larger and stronger but are weaker than normal.
- Later symptoms:
  - Muscle loss severe enough to require use of a wheelchair by age 9 to 12.
  - Severe distortion of the body.
  - Recurrent respiratory infections.

CAUSES—Inherited. Muscular dystrophy is a genetic abnormality. It can be carried by a female who does not have symptoms, but passes it on to male children. In other cases, it may be passed on by one or both parents. In still other cases, there is no family history.

RISK INCREASES WITH—Family history of muscular dystrophy and males.

HOW TO PREVENT
- If there is family history of muscular dystrophy:
  - Obtain genetic counseling before pregnancy.
  - If pregnant, discuss option of prenatal testing with your obstetric provider.
  - Carriers can be detected with medical tests (blood contains high levels of a certain enzyme).

 WHAT TO EXPECT

DIAGNOSTIC MEASURES
- Your child's health care provider will do a physical exam and ask questions about the symptoms.
- Medical tests may include blood studies and muscle biopsy. A biopsy involves removal of a small amount of tissue for viewing under a microscope. An electromyogram (measures electrical impulses in muscles) and nerve conduction study may be done.

APPROPRIATE HEALTH CARE
- There is no cure for muscular dystrophy. Treatment can help improve the symptoms and help prevent complications. A child will need to be assisted in many ways to make the most of his abilities and keep his independence to the extent possible.
- Your child will need a health care team. This may include physical, occupational, speech, and respiratory therapists as well as routine medical care. Illnesses are more common and need to be watched for and treated.
- Surgery may be needed to release tight, painful muscles. If heart problems develop, a pacemaker may be surgically implanted to help the heart beat normally.
- Counseling can help parents cope with the diagnosis. It can help children if emotional problems develop.

POSSIBLE COMPLICATIONS
- Muscle weakness that leads to wheelchair use.
- Fractures or injuries from falls.
- Spinal curvature due to weak spine muscles.
- Pneumonia.
- Heart problems.
- Muscle shortening and tightening (contractures).

PROBABLE OUTCOME—Outcome varies depending on the type of muscular dystrophy. Some types are more mild, progress slowly, and patients may have a near normal lifespan. Other types progress more rapidly, leading to disability and a shortened lifespan. Research is ongoing for causes, prevention, effective treatments, and possible cures.

 HOW TO TREAT

GENERAL MEASURES
- Support groups are a good place to share.
- To learn more: Muscular Dystrophy Association, 3300 E. Sunrise Drive, Tucson, AZ 85718; (800) 572-1717; website: www.mdausa.org.

MEDICATION—Drugs may be prescribed to slow muscle loss, improve lung function, treat heart problems, for constipation, to treat infections, or for other complications.

ACTIVITY—The patient should be as physically and mentally active as possible. Many devices can help overcome handicaps caused by weakness. Braces may help.

DIET—Eat a healthy diet. Being overweight should be avoided (it adds more burden to already weak muscles).

 CALL YOUR DOCTOR IF

- Your child develops symptoms of muscular dystrophy.
- After diagnosis, symptoms develop that cause concern.

MYASTHENIA GRAVIS

GENERAL INFORMATION

DEFINITION—Myasthenia gravis is a disorder of the muscles that causes muscle weakness of varying degrees.

BODY PARTS INVOLVED—It often involves the muscles around the eyes, mouth, and throat, and the arms and legs. It can affect the breathing muscles also.

SEX OR AGE MOST AFFECTED—Both sexes; all ages; occurs more often in females under age 40 and men over age 60.

SIGNS & SYMPTOMS
- Drooping eyelids.
- Double vision.
- Loss of normal facial expression.
- Swallowing difficulty.
- Weakness of the arms and legs.
- Difficulty speaking clearly.
- Breathing difficulty.
- Most flare-ups appear after a period of normal muscle function and worsen as the muscle is used.

CAUSES—It is one of a group of autoimmune disorders. In these disorders, the immune system attacks the body itself by mistake. With myasthenia gravis, there is a miscommunication between the nerves and the muscles.

RISK INCREASES WITH
- Females under age 40 and men over age 60.
- Newborns of mothers with myasthenia gravis.
- Having other autoimmune disorders.
- Family history of myasthenia gravis.

HOW TO PREVENT—Cannot be prevented at present.

WHAT TO EXPECT

DIAGNOSTIC MEASURES
- Your own observation of symptoms.
- Your health care provider will do a physical exam and ask questions about your symptoms and activities.
- Medical tests may include studies of blood antibodies, electrical tests on muscle, and chest x-rays.

APPROPRIATE HEALTH CARE
- Some mild cases may not need treatment. In others, treatment will help control symptoms. It may involve extra rest, drug therapy, surgery, or plasmapheresis.
- Surgical removal (thymectomy) of the thymus gland may be recommended. It can improve symptoms in some patients, and even cure the disease in others.

- Plasmapheresis involves removal of blood from the patient, treating the blood, and reinjecting it. This therapy may be used when symptoms are severe.
- Acute flare-ups (myasthenia crises) may require emergency hospital care for breathing problems.

POSSIBLE COMPLICATIONS
- Swallowing difficulty.
- Long-term treatments may lead to various problems.
- Respiratory failure.
- Aspiration pneumonia.

PROBABLE OUTCOME—There is no known cure. Symptoms may get worse and then improve for a period of time. Symptoms can be helped with treatment. Patients with the disorder usually lead normal or near normal lives. Research into causes and treatment continues.

HOW TO TREAT

GENERAL MEASURES
- Avoid exposure to infections and try to avoid stress.
- To learn more: Myasthenia Gravis Foundation of America, 355 Lexington Ave., New York, NY 10017; (800) 541-5454; website: www.myasthenia.org.

MEDICATION
- Anticholinesterase drugs to help improve muscle function are usually prescribed.
- Immunosuppressive drugs may be prescribed at times when symptoms worsen.
- Intravenous immune globulin (IVIG) may be used for some patients to suppress the immune system.
- A number of drugs may worsen symptoms. Talk to your health care provider before taking any new drug.

ACTIVITY
- Plan activities to make the most of energy peaks. Frequent rest periods are important. Day-to-day changes in symptoms are common.
- Avoid strenuous activities and too much exposure to the sun or to cold weather.

DIET—Eat foods high in potassium. These include oranges, tomatoes, bananas, broccoli, and apricots. Soft diet may be helpful if chewing and swallowing are difficult.

CALL YOUR DOCTOR IF

- You or a family member has symptoms of myasthenia gravis.
- You develop swallowing or breathing difficulty.

MYOCARDITIS

 GENERAL INFORMATION

DEFINITION—Myocarditis is an inflammation of the heart muscle (myocardium). It can lead to poor heart function. Myocarditis usually occurs as a complication of another illness.

BODY PARTS INVOLVED—Heart muscle.

SEX OR AGE MOST AFFECTED—Both sexes; all ages; often affects adults under age 50.

SIGNS & SYMPTOMS
- No symptoms or symptoms may be mild and vague.
- Fatigue.
- Shortness of breath with physical activity.
- Irregular or rapid heartbeat.
- Fever.
- Chest discomfort or pain (sometimes severe).
- Muscle aches.
- If myocarditis causes heart failure, the following symptoms may also occur:
  - Swollen feet and ankles.
  - Distended (sticking out) neck veins.
  - Rapid heartbeat, even when at rest.
  - Breathing difficulty while resting or lying down.

CAUSES—The inflammation can result from numerous medical conditions. A viral infection is a common cause.

RISK INCREASES WITH
- Viral infection, such as Coxsackie, adenovirus, measles, influenza, herpes simplex, hepatitis, varicella, HIV, or others.
- Bacterial infections, such as tetanus, gonorrhea, typhoid fever, tuberculosis, or diphtheria.
- Immune system disorders (lupus, arthritis, and others).
- Parasitic or fungal infections.
- Certain drugs (e.g., sulfa, penicillin, or cocaine).
- Exposure to certain toxins or chemicals.

HOW TO PREVENT—No specific preventive measures. Avoid risk factors where possible.

 WHAT TO EXPECT

DIAGNOSTIC MEASURES
- Your own observation of symptoms.
- Your health care provider will do a physical exam.
- Medical tests may include blood studies, chest x-ray, and heart function tests. A biopsy may be done. This involves removal of a small amount of tissue for viewing under a microscope.

APPROPRIATE HEALTH CARE
- There is no specific treatment for myocarditis. Treatment usually involves rest, treating symptoms, and drugs for a diagnosed infection.
- Hospital care may be needed for more severe symptoms.

POSSIBLE COMPLICATIONS
- Heart failure.
- Heart rhythm problems.
- Weakened heart muscle (cardiomyopathy).
- Blood clots, heart attack, or stroke.
- Sudden death due to abnormal heart rhythm.

PROBABLE OUTCOME—Mild cases caused by a virus usually clear up on their own in about 2 weeks. Mild cases from other causes are usually treated successfully. In more severe cases, the outcome will depend on the underlying cause, patient's health status, and treatment.

 HOW TO TREAT

GENERAL MEASURES
- For home care, weigh daily and monitor your blood pressure. Tell your health care provider if unexpected changes occur.
- Stop smoking. Find a way to quit.
- To learn more: Myocarditis Foundation, 2201 River Rd, #3401, Point Pleasant, NJ 08742; (866) 846-1600; website: www.myocarditisfoundation.org.

MEDICATION
- Your health care provider may prescribe:
  - Antibiotics for a bacterial infection.
  - Steroid drugs to reduce inflammation.
  - Diuretics to reduce fluid build up.
  - Digitalis to stimulate a stronger heartbeat.
  - Anticoagulants to prevent clot formation.
  - Pain remedies.
  - Drugs to reduce the heart's workload (e.g., beta blockers or angiotensin-converting enzyme [ACE] inhibitors).

ACTIVITY
- Rest in bed until symptoms improve. Recovery time varies, depending on the underlying cause.
- After recovery, resume normal activities gradually.

DIET—A low-salt diet and limits on fluid intake may be recommended.

 CALL YOUR DOCTOR IF

- You or a family member has myocarditis symptoms.
- Symptoms get worse or don't improve with time or treatment.
- New, unexplained symptoms develop.

NARCOLEPSY

 GENERAL INFORMATION

DEFINITION—Narcolepsy is a sleep disorder that affects the control of sleep and wakefulness. Type and severity of symptoms can vary in people who have the disorder. Often, it goes undiagnosed for years.

BODY PARTS INVOLVED—Central nervous system.

SEX OR AGE MOST AFFECTED—Both sexes. It usually begins in the teen years or young adulthood. Young children and the elderly can also be affected.

SIGNS & SYMPTOMS
• Excessive daytime sleepiness (hypersomnia).
• Uncontrollable sleep attacks that may occur up to 10 times a day. They may last from 30 seconds up to 30 minutes or more. An attack leaves the person feeling refreshed, but another may occur again quickly. Attacks can occur while driving, talking, working, in warm environments, after large meals, or at social events.
• Hallucinations (seeing things that aren't there) when first going to sleep or waking up. This is called hypnagogic or hypnopompic.
• A short period of paralysis (sudden loss of muscle strength) when falling asleep or just before awakening.
• A few seconds of paralysis not related to sleep when feeling sudden emotion, such as anger, fear, or joy. This is called cataplexy.
• Nighttime sleep is disturbed by leg jerks, tossing and turning, nightmares, and frequent awakenings.

CAUSES—The exact cause is unknown. It is a neurologic (nervous system) disorder. Low levels of a brain chemical called hypocretin (that normally helps staying awake) play a role. It may also be linked to autoimmune disorders. In these disorders, the immune system by mistake attacks the body. There is also a genetic link.

RISK INCREASES WITH
• A family history of narcolepsy.
• Genetic factors.
• Brain injury (e.g., stroke or tumor), infections, contact with toxins (e.g., pesticides), or autoimmune disorders.

HOW TO PREVENT—Cannot be prevented.

 WHAT TO EXPECT

DIAGNOSTIC MEASURES
• Your own observation of symptoms.
• Your health care provider will do a physical exam and ask about your symptoms and activities. You may be asked to keep a 2-week diary about your sleep patterns.

• An overnight study in a sleep clinic followed by a daytime multiple sleep latency test (MSLT) may be done.

APPROPRIATE HEALTH CARE—Treatment usually involves lifestyle changes along with drugs to help control the drowsiness. It may take several weeks or months to achieve the best results.

POSSIBLE COMPLICATIONS
• Accidental injury during sudden sleep attack.
• The disorder may affect all aspects of one's life. This includes work, social life, personal relationships, and emotional health.

PROBABLE OUTCOME—The disorder appears to be lifelong. There is no cure. Drugs and lifestyle changes can help control the symptoms. Most people with the disorder can lead a near-normal lifestyle.

 HOW TO TREAT

GENERAL MEASURES
• Schedule a regular time for going to bed and getting up. Stick to the schedule. Get at least 8 hours of sleep.
• Take regular naps 2 to 3 times during the day. One 15-minute nap after lunch and another nap at around 5:30 PM may help symptoms.
• Avoid shift work, night work, or rotating hours.
• Avoid over-stimulating activities, if possible.
• Wear or carry medical ID to indicate you have this disorder.
• Talk to your employer or teachers about the disorder and ways to help you manage.
• To learn more: Narcolepsy Network, PO Box 294, Pleasantville, NY 10570; (888) 292-6522; website: www.narcolepsynetwork.org.

MEDICATION
• Stimulants to increase level of daytime alertness may be prescribed. It takes time to find best approach. Modafinil may be the first option.
• Antidepressants or sodium oxybate (Xyrem) for cataplexy or other symptoms may be prescribed.

ACTIVITY
• Use caution if doing an activity that carries the risk of injury from a sudden sleep attack. You may be advised to not drive or engage in dangerous activity at home or work.
• Exercise regularly, but not close to bedtime.

DIET—Diet changes may be recommended. Avoid stimulating drinks close to naps or bedtime.

 CALL YOUR DOCTOR IF

• You or a family member has symptoms of narcolepsy.
• New, unexplained symptoms develop.

NASAL POLYPS

GENERAL INFORMATION

DEFINITION—A nasal polyp is a benign (noncancerous) soft tissue growth that develops inside the nose or sinuses. Polyps look like small grapes and can grow alone, but usually occur in clusters. They often affect both sides of the nose.

BODY PARTS INVOLVED—Nasal mucous membranes.

SEX OR AGE MOST AFFECTED—Both sexes; all ages, but more common in adults.

SIGNS & SYMPTOMS
- Obstruction of air through the nose (chronic "stuffy-nose" feeling).
- Sense of smell is reduced.
- Nasal discharge.
- Sneezing.
- Facial pain or headaches.
- Feeling of fullness in the face.
- Itchy eyes.
- Snoring.
- Large polyps may cause the nose to be deformed.

CAUSES—Chronic inflammation of the lining of the nose and sinuses. Inflammation is normally a reaction to injury, infection, or irritation. Why it occurs in the nose and sinuses and causes polyps is not clearly understood.

RISK INCREASES WITH
- Chronic sinus, nasal, or lung disorders. This can include asthma, allergic rhinitis, cystic fibrosis, sinusitis, fungal infections, and others.
- Aspirin sensitivity. This is not a true allergy, but it may cause allergy-like reactions (such as hives, swelling, and asthma). People with this sensitivity need to avoid aspirin and other nonsteroidal anti-inflammatory drugs.

HOW TO PREVENT—No specific preventive measures. Getting treatment for risk factors may help. Use saline nasal spray or nasal lavage to help remove allergens and irritants.

WHAT TO EXPECT

DIAGNOSTIC MEASURES
- Your own observation of symptoms.
- Your health care provider will do an exam of the nasal passages.
- Medical tests may include a CT or endoscopy (small, lighted telescopic instrument) to see inside the nose. Allergy testing may be done in some cases.

APPROPRIATE HEALTH CARE
- Treatment may involve drugs to temporarily shrink the polyps and help relieve the symptoms.
- Surgery is often done to remove polyps. The type of surgery will depend on the location, size, and the number of polyps involved. Your health care provider will discuss the options, the risks, and the benefits with you. The use of a saltwater (saline) nasal rinse may be recommended before and/or after surgery. For information about surgery and postoperative care, see Nasal Polyp Removal in surgery section.

POSSIBLE COMPLICATIONS
- Polyps may recur after surgery.
- A number of different complications can occur due to blocked airflow and blocked mucus drainage.

PROBABLE OUTCOME—Treatment with drugs or surgery can help improve the symptoms.

HOW TO TREAT

GENERAL MEASURES—Try to avoid any substances that you know you are allergic to, such as dust mites, pollen, mold, and others.

MEDICATION
- For minor pain, you may use acetaminophen.
- Nonprescription antihistamines may help relieve symptoms, but they do not treat the polyps.
- Corticosteroid drugs in oral form may be prescribed for a short period to attempt to shrink the polyps.
- Corticosteroid drugs in nasal spray may be prescribed for treatment of smaller polyps. They are also prescribed following surgery to help prevent recurrence of polyps.
- Antibiotics or antifungal drugs may be prescribed for treatment of infection.

ACTIVITY—No limits.

DIET—No special diet. If you have food allergies, be sure to avoid those foods.

CALL YOUR DOCTOR IF

- You or a family member has symptoms of nasal polyps.
- Any new symptoms develop or other symptoms get worse after treatment is started.

NASAL SEPTUM, DEVIATED

GENERAL INFORMATION

DEFINITION—The septum is the structure that divides the nose into two parts. In some people it is significantly off-center, or deviated. This can result in the obstruction of normal airflow through the nasal passages. The septum is made up of cartilage (toward the tip) and bone (closer to the forehead). Ideally, the septum should divide the right and left side of the nose into two equal parts. It is estimated that 80% of all nasal septa are slightly off-center. These are usually not noticed and do not normally cause any problems.

BODY PARTS INVOLVED—Septum.

SEX OR AGE MOST AFFECTED—Both sexes; all ages.

SIGNS & SYMPTOMS
- An apparently crooked nose.
- Obstruction of air through one or both nostrils.
- Nasal congestion or discharge.
- Nosebleed, headache, or facial pain may occur.
- Sinus infections.
- Often, there are no symptoms.

CAUSES—Trauma to the nose, or it may be congenital (being born with a deviated septum).

RISK INCREASES WITH—None specific.

HOW TO PREVENT—Protect yourself from nose injury to reduce risk. Wear protective headgear for contact sports or cycling. Buckle your auto seatbelt.

WHAT TO EXPECT

DIAGNOSTIC MEASURES
- Your own observation of symptoms.
- Your health care provider can usually diagnose the problem by an exam of the nose. The exam involves the use of a bright light and nasal speculum (an instrument that spreads the nostril open).
- Medical tests may be done to confirm the diagnosis.

APPROPRIATE HEALTH CARE
- No treatment may be needed if there are no symptoms or if symptoms are mild.
- Surgery to correct the deviation may be recommended if the deviated septum is causing symptoms such as sinus infections or nosebleeds. Your health care provider will discuss the options with you. Surgery may involve:
    - Submucosal removal, which relieves obstruction.
    - Rhinoplasty, which corrects anatomical deformity.
    - Septoplasty, which relieves nasal obstruction and improves appearance.

POSSIBLE COMPLICATIONS
- Recurrent nosebleeds.
- Nasal obstruction.
- Recurrent nasal or sinus infections.

PROBABLE OUTCOME—Usually treatable with surgery. If symptoms are not troublesome, surgery is usually not needed.

HOW TO TREAT

GENERAL MEASURES—For an explanation of one type of corrective surgery and postoperative care, see Rhinoplasty in Surgery Section.

MEDICATION
- For minor discomfort, you may use nonprescription drugs temporarily, such as decongestants, to decrease nasal secretions.
- Antihistamines can help relieve symptoms.
- Antibiotics may be prescribed for infection.
- Inhaled nasal steroids may be prescribed.

ACTIVITY—No limits, unless surgery is needed. If so, resume your normal activities gradually.

DIET—No special diet.

CALL YOUR DOCTOR IF

- You or a family member has symptoms of a deviated nasal septum, especially recurrent nosebleeds, or nasal and sinus infections.
- New symptoms develop after surgery.

NAUSEA & VOMITING IN PREGNANCY
(Morning Sickness During Pregnancy)

 GENERAL INFORMATION

DEFINITION—50% to 80% of pregnant women suffer from nausea and vomiting in pregnancy. The symptoms often occur in the morning (from 6 to 9 AM), but they may occur at any time during the day.

BODY PARTS INVOLVED—Gastrointestinal system.

SEX OR AGE MOST AFFECTED—Females of childbearing age.

SIGNS & SYMPTOMS
- Mild to severe nausea with or without vomiting.
- It usually occurs during the first 12 to 14 weeks of pregnancy.
- It may continue longer, and for some women, last throughout pregnancy.
- By the end of the third month, most women stop having most of the symptoms.

CAUSES—Exact causes of nausea and vomiting during pregnancy are unknown. The hormonal changes due to pregnancy are thought to play a role.

RISK INCREASES WITH
- Being pregnant with twins, triplets, or more.
- You have history of morning sickness in previous pregnancy, have migraines, or past episodes of motion sickness.

HOW TO PREVENT—No specific preventive measures.

 WHAT TO EXPECT

DIAGNOSTIC MEASURES
- Usually self diagnosis and self-care are all that are needed.
- Talk to your obstetric provider if the symptoms are a concern.

APPROPRIATE HEALTH CARE
- Medical treatment is usually not needed. If symptoms are severe, hospital care may be needed.
- Acupuncture may be a helpful option for some women.

POSSIBLE COMPLICATIONS—Hyperemesis gravidarum. This is a rare condition of pregnancy that involves severe nausea, vomiting, dehydration, and weight loss.

PROBABLE OUTCOME—Morning sickness usually stops after the first 3 to 4 months of pregnancy. Your baby's well-being is not affected as long as you're able to keep food down, eat a well-balanced diet, and drink plenty of fluids.

 HOW TO TREAT

GENERAL MEASURES
- Try to identify odors or foods that are most upsetting, and avoid them. Many pregnant women figure out what they can and cannot eat, and how many times they need to eat each day.
- Keep rooms well aired out to rid your home of cooking smells or other odors.
- Don't smoke. Ask your family and friends not to smoke while you have morning sickness.
- Try to keep a positive attitude. If you have problems that you cannot resolve, ask for help from family, friends, or counselors.
- Keep a daily record of your weight.
- Ask your obstetric provider about using products that a woman can wear on her wrist to reduce symptoms.

MEDICATION
- Drugs are not usually prescribed for this disorder. If the symptoms are severe, your obstetric provider may prescribe certain drugs for the nausea.
- Nonprescription remedies (oral drugs or rectal suppositories) may ease the problem. Don't take or use any of these products without medical advice.
- A trial of vitamin B6 may be recommended, which appears safe at the present.
- If taking your pregnancy vitamin pill causes nausea, try taking it at night or take it with a snack or chew gum or suck hard candy right after you take it. If these ideas aren't helping with the nausea, ask your obstetric provider for advice.

ACTIVITY—No limits. Resting in a dark and quiet room provides some relief for most patients.

DIET
- The following may help lessen the nausea:
  - At night, place a small, quick-energy snack, such as soda crackers, at your bedside. Eat it before getting up.
  - Eat a small snack at bedtime and when you get up to go to the bathroom during the night.
  - Eat a snack every hour or two during the day. Avoid large meals.
  - Drink ginger ale or ginger tea.

 CALL YOUR DOCTOR IF

- You have morning sickness that does not improve, despite the self-help measures.
- You vomit blood or material that resembles coffee grounds.
- Abdominal pain, cramping, or fever occurs.
- You lose more than 1 or 2 pounds.

NEPHROTIC SYNDROME
(Nephrosis)

 GENERAL INFORMATION

DEFINITION—Nephrotic syndrome is a condition that results from damage to tiny blood vessels in the kidneys called glomeruli. Normally, the glomeruli filter the waste and excess water from blood and into urine. When they are damaged, they do not filter properly. This causes substances (proteins) to leak out of the blood and into the urine, which then leads to fluid building up in the tissues and swelling (edema).

BODY PARTS INVOLVED—Kidneys. Late or complicated stages involve all body cells.

SEX OR AGE MOST AFFECTED—It affects all age groups, and males more than females. In children, it is more common from ages 2 to 6.

SIGNS & SYMPTOMS
- Fluid retention (edema). At first, it causes puffy eyes and ankles, which is followed by general puffiness of the skin, and then, a swollen abdomen.
- Weight gain due to fluid retention.
- Reduced urine output (as low as 20% of normal).
- Frothy (foamy) urine.
- Appetite loss, weakness, and general ill feeling.

CAUSES—The cause of the kidney damage is often unknown. It may be due to numerous underlying disorders. In children, it is often due to a kidney disorder called minimal change disease.

RISK INCREASES WITH
- Disorders that affect kidney function. These include diabetes, lupus erythematosus, cancers, glomerulonephritis, autoimmune disorders, serum sickness and other severe allergic disorders, blood clot in the kidney, numerous types of infections, sickle cell anemia, congenital heart disease, severe high blood pressure, other disorders, and drugs that are toxic to the kidneys.
- Weak immune system due to illness or drugs.
- Family history of renal failure.
- Exposure to some chemical toxins or illegal drug use.

HOW TO PREVENT
- Getting treatment for any risk factor may help.
- Drugs may be prescribed to help prevent nephrotic disorder in persons at risk.

 WHAT TO EXPECT

DIAGNOSTIC MEASURES
- Your health care provider will do a physical exam and ask about your symptoms and activities.

- Medical tests may include urine and blood studies. A kidney biopsy may be done to diagnose any kidney disorder. A biopsy involves removal of a small amount of kidney tissue or fluid for viewing under a microscope.

APPROPRIATE HEALTH CARE
- Treatment will be prescribed for any underlying disorder diagnosed or to relieve the symptoms of nephrotic syndrome.
- Treatment is usually with drugs and sometimes with diet changes.

POSSIBLE COMPLICATIONS—Infections, kidney failure, blood clots, high blood pressure, failure to thrive in children, poor nutrition, high blood-fat levels, heart problems, or fluid overload.

PROBABLE OUTCOME—The outcome will depend on the underlying cause diagnosed. If it is treatable, such as an infection, the outcome is often good. In children with minimal disease, almost all patients respond to treatment. In other cases, the outcome may be less favorable and kidney failure and other complications may occur.

 HOW TO TREAT

GENERAL MEASURES—To learn more: National Kidney Foundation, 30 E. 33rd St., Suite 1100, New York, NY 10016; (800) 622-9010; website: www.kidney.org.

MEDICATION
- Your health care provider may prescribe:
  - Cortisone or immunosuppressive drugs.
  - Diuretics to reduce fluid retention.
  - Drugs to treat infections.
  - Angiotensin-converting enzyme (ACE) inhibitors to reduce protein loss.
  - Drugs for high blood pressure or high cholesterol.
  - Anticoagulants for blood clots.
  - Stopping the use of any drug that is the cause.

ACTIVITY—After the swelling decreases, be as active as your strength and condition allows.

DIET—You will be advised about any limits on fat, salt, protein, and fluid intake. A dietitian can help with diet changes.

 CALL YOUR DOCTOR IF

- You or a family member has symptoms of nephrotic syndrome.
- After diagnosis, any symptoms cause concern.

NOSE FRACTURE

GENERAL INFORMATION

DEFINITION—A nose fracture is a break in the bones or cartilage of the nose. It often happens when other facial bones are also fractured. The injury may be to the front or side of the nose.

BODY PARTS INVOLVED—Nose.

SEX OR AGE MOST AFFECTED—Older children (over age 8) and adults. Young children's noses have only cartilage. Males are more often affected than females.

SIGNS & SYMPTOMS
• Pain in the nose.
• Nosebleed.
• Swollen, discolored nose.
• Bruising around the eyes.
• Difficulty in breathing through the nose.

CAUSES—Injury or trauma to the nose. This may be from motor vehicle accident, being hit on the nose, running into a hard object, or from a fall.

RISK INCREASES WITH—Previous nose injury.

HOW TO PREVENT
• Wear protective headgear for contact sports or when riding motorcycles or bicycles.
• Use seatbelts in motor vehicles.

WHAT TO EXPECT

DIAGNOSTIC MEASURES
• Your own observation of symptoms.
• Your health care provider will do a physical exam of the face and nose.
• X-rays may or may not be needed depending on the injury. A CT scan may be done.

APPROPRIATE HEALTH CARE
• A minor nose fracture with no displacement may not require further medical treatment. It will heal on its own. Rest at home. Apply ice several times a day until the swelling is gone. Use two pillows when lying down to keep the head above the heart. This helps with pain.
• Treatment may involve reduction (correction) of the fracture. This can be done right after the injury, before any swelling occurs. It can also be done days later, when the swelling is gone. A local or general anesthetic is used.
• The reduction may be done by manipulating the nose into place with finger pressure. It may require the use of two probes inserted into the nose to move the bones back into place. More severe fractures may require surgery. An incision (cut) is made on the front of the nose. The bones are put back together with special tools. Wires, plates, or screws may be used to hold the bones in place. A splint may be needed.

• Plastic surgery can be done at a later date if there is a problem with the cosmetic appearance of the nose.

POSSIBLE COMPLICATIONS
• Infection of the nose and sinuses.
• Persistent breathing difficulty.
• Change in sense of smell.
• Permanent change in appearance.
• Deviated nasal septum. This occurs when the structure that divides the nose in half is off-center.
• Septal hematoma. Blood becomes trapped in the septum. This can lead to complications if it is not drained.

PROBABLE OUTCOME—Minor fractures with no deformity usually heal on their own. Major fractures can be repaired with treatment. Most of the swelling will be gone in 10 to 20 days, but some swelling may last for months. The nose may feel tender for about a month.

HOW TO TREAT

GENERAL MEASURES—First aid steps: Have the person sit down and lean forward to keep blood from going down the back of the throat. Have them breathe through the mouth. Apply cold compresses or an ice pack to the nose to reduce swelling. Do not try to move displaced bones in an attempt to straighten the nose. If a nosebleed is heavy or cannot be stopped, seek emergency medical care to get it under control.

MEDICATION
• For minor discomfort, you may use nonprescription drugs such as acetaminophen.
• Stronger pain relievers may be prescribed.
• Antibiotics may be prescribed to prevent or treat an infection.
• Decongestants may be prescribed, to reduce swelling.

ACTIVITY
• Rest until any bleeding stops.
• Most activities can be resumed right away.
• You can usually return to non-contact sports in two weeks, and contact sports in three weeks. Protective gear may need to be worn. Follow any medical advice.

DIET—No special diet.

CALL YOUR DOCTOR IF

• You or a family member has symptoms of a fractured nose.
• New symptoms develop after treatment.

NOSEBLEED
(Epistaxis)

GENERAL INFORMATION

DEFINITION—A nosebleed is sudden bleeding from one or both nostrils. Epistaxis is the medical term. The bleeding involves blood vessels in the nose. Nosebleeds may occur close to the nose opening or deeper in the nose.

BODY PARTS INVOLVED—Nose.

SEX OR AGE MOST AFFECTED—All ages, but twice as common in children as adults.

SIGNS & SYMPTOMS
- Blood oozing from the nostril. If the broken vessel is close to the nostril, the blood is bright red. If the broken vessel is deeper in the nose, the blood may be bright or dark red.
- Lightheadedness from a large amount of blood loss (rare).
- Rapid heartbeat, shortness of breath, and pallor (with significant blood loss only).
- Black stool from swallowed blood.

CAUSES—Injury to the nose, breathing dry air, allergies, illnesses, or for no apparent reason.

RISK INCREASES WITH
- Injury to the nose.
- Nasal or sinus infection.
- A foreign body in the nose.
- Dry mucous membranes in the nose from any cause, such as low humidity.
- Bleeding tendencies associated with some illnesses.
- Allergic rhinitis (hay fever) or nonallergic rhinitis.
- Use of certain drugs, such as anticoagulants, aspirin, or prolonged use of nose drops.
- Exposure to irritating chemicals.
- Excess alcohol use.
- High altitude or dry climate.

HOW TO PREVENT
- Avoid injury if possible.
- Get medical treatment for sinus or allergy problems.
- Humidify the air if you live in a dry climate or at high altitude.
- Avoid picking at nose or vigorous nose blowing.
- Use saline nasal spray to keep nose moist.
- Avoid aspirin or other nonsteroidal anti-inflammatories if you have frequent nosebleeds.

WHAT TO EXPECT

DIAGNOSTIC MEASURES
- Your own observation of symptoms.
- Exam by a health care provider (sometimes).

APPROPRIATE HEALTH CARE
- Seek emergency treatment if self-care is not successful. Gauze packing may be inserted to absorb blood, stop the dripping, and exert pressure on the ruptured blood vessels. Ongoing bleeding may require cauterization (use of heat to seal off blood vessels).
- Surgery (for severe bleeding only) to tie off the artery feeding the bleeding area.

POSSIBLE COMPLICATIONS—Bleeding may rarely be severe and require medical care.

PROBABLE OUTCOME—Most nosebleeds are harmless, even though it seems like a lot of blood is lost. They are usually controlled with self-care by applying pressure to the nose.

HOW TO TREAT

GENERAL MEASURES
- Sit up with your head bent forward.
- Clamp your nose closed with your fingers for 10 minutes. During this time, breathe through your mouth. Holding your nose tightly closed allows the blood to clot and seal the damaged blood vessels.
- If bleeding stops and recurs, repeat, but pinch your nose firmly on both sides for 8 to 10 minutes.
- You may apply cold compresses or an ice pack at the same time you are applying pressure.
- Don't blow your nose for several hours after bleeding stops to avoid dislodging the blood clot. Do not pack the nose with gauze.
- Don't swallow blood. It may upset your stomach or make you "gag," causing you to inhale blood. Spit out blood if it gets in mouth.
- Don't talk (also to avoid gagging).

MEDICATION
- A nonprescription nasal decongestant (e.g., oxymetazoline) may be used to help close off blood vessels if bleeding persists.
- Drugs may be prescribed to treat an underlying disorder.

ACTIVITY—Resume your normal activities as soon as symptoms improve.

DIET—No special diet.

CALL YOUR DOCTOR IF

- You or a family member has a nosebleed that won't stop with self-care steps.
- After the nosebleed, you become nauseous or vomit, or your temperature rises to 101°F (38.3°C) or higher.

OBESITY & OVERWEIGHT

 GENERAL INFORMATION

DEFINITION—Obesity is defined as having an excess amount of body fat. Overweight is defined as having extra body weight that includes muscle, bone, fat, and water. The common tool to measure obesity and overweight is the body mass index (BMI). It measures body weight in relation to height. Note: A BMI may indicate a person is overweight, but it could be due to lean muscle and not excess body fat (such as with an athlete).

BODY PARTS INVOLVED—Total body.

SEX OR AGE MOST AFFECTED—Both sexes; all ages.

SIGNS & SYMPTOMS
- Low energy levels.
- Breathing/snoring problems; sleep apnea.
- Appearance of large body size.
- Fatigue and joint pain due to excess weight.

CAUSES—Obesity and overweight occur when a person consumes more calories then he or she burns. There are a variety of risk factors (genetic, behavioral, environmental, and cultural) that play a role. It is a complex issue.

RISK INCREASES WITH
- Genetic—obesity runs in families.
- High fat and high calorie diet, lack of exercise, poverty, and lower education level.
- Certain underlying medical disorders.
- Use of some drugs (e.g., steroids, some antidepressants, and others).
- Older ages, pregnancy, shift work, lack of sleep, and people who stop smoking.

HOW TO PREVENT
- Proper diet and nutrition. Regular exercise.
- Behavior and lifestyle changes, as needed.

 WHAT TO EXPECT

DIAGNOSTIC MEASURES
- The body mass index (BMI) formula uses height and weight to measure weight status.
    - Adult BMI of 25 to 29.9 = overweight.
    - Adult BMI of 30 or more = obese.
    - BMI formula: *(weight, in pounds, times 703) divided by (height in inches squared).*
- Website to calculate BMI: www.cdc.gov/healthyweight/assessing/bmi/.
- Waist size (circumference) measures abdominal fat. Over 40 inches (102 cm) in men and over 35 inches (88 cm) in women indicates health and obesity risk factors.

APPROPRIATE HEALTH CARE
- Treatment steps depend on health status, age, degree of obesity or overweight, and motivation. Steps can include a combination of diet, exercise, behavior modification, and drugs.
- Gastrointestinal surgery may be recommended with severe obesity.
- You and your health care provider can develop a weight-loss plan based on your individual needs. Keep a food and activity diary to keep track of your progress.

POSSIBLE COMPLICATIONS
- High risk for many major physical health problems that can lead to disability and death.
- Emotional problems (e.g., depression; and feeling unattractive, rejected, and shameful).
- Prejudice or discrimination at work, school, social occasions, and travel.

PROBABLE OUTCOME—Obesity and overweight can be controlled if motivation is maintained for life.

 HOW TO TREAT

GENERAL MEASURES
- Books, websites, and weight loss programs are available to help with weight loss. Diet plans should provide proper nutrition, information on exercise and behavior changes, and maintaining the weight loss long-term.
- Behavior changes start with identifying the behaviors that lead a person to overeat and be inactive. Then learn how to change and maintain the new behaviors. Support groups or a weight-loss counselor can help.
- To learn more: Weight Control Information Network, 1 Win Way, Bethesda, MD 20892-3665; (877) 946-4627; website: www.win.niddk.nih.gov.

MEDICATION—Drugs for obesity may be prescribed on a trial basis to see if they help. Drugs are used along with diet, exercise, and behavior changes. Amphetamine compounds are not recommended for treating obesity.

ACTIVITY—Increase physical activity. Start with a daily 10 minute walk. Aim for 20 to 30 minutes of activity 3 to 5 days a week, plus muscle strengthening 2 to 3 times a week.

DIET
- Choose an eating plan that will work for you. Diets need to be healthy, help you lose weight, and maintain the new weight. A dietitian can help you choose a plan.
- A realistic weight-loss rate is 1 pound per week. It is normal to have periods when no weight is lost on your plan. Don't stop; weight loss will begin again.

 CALL YOUR DOCTOR IF

You or a family member wants to lose weight.

OBESITY, CHILDHOOD

GENERAL INFORMATION

DEFINITION—Childhood obesity means a child or teen has too much body fat. They weigh more than is healthy for their age, sex, and height. Obesity is a health risk as it can lead to many types of illnesses, disorders, and emotional and social problems.

BODY PARTS INVOLVED—Total body.

SEX OR AGE MOST AFFECTED—Both sexes; common in ages 2 to 19.

SIGNS & SYMPTOMS—A child may or may not appear overweight or obese.

CAUSES—Eating more calories than the body uses (or burns off) over a period of time. Excess calories are stored as fat. There are a number of risk factors (genetic, environmental, behavioral, and sometimes, cultural) that play a role. It is a complex issue.

RISK INCREASES WITH
- Obese parents.
- High fat and high calorie diet, too much sitting (e.g., computer use, television watching), lack of physical activity, or lack of enough sleep.
- Mother's weight gain in pregnancy, high birth weight, rapid weight gain as an infant, and weight gain in early childhood.
- Children raised in poorer families.
- Certain medical disorders.

HOW TO PREVENT
- Provide child with a healthy diet.
- Encourage healthy behaviors (e.g., exercise).
- Have medical well-child visits to check weight and discuss other risk factors.
- Parents should be watchful of their child's weight. The BMI (body mass index) can be used to help identify weight problems in a child. BMI is a tool to evaluate the weight based on height, age, and sex. Go online to: apps.nccd.cdc.gov/dnpabmi/.
- Support for healthy lifestyles from schools, communities, government, and industry.

WHAT TO EXPECT

DIAGNOSTIC MEASURES
- Your child's health care provider can check your child for weight problems such as obesity. This is done at well-child or other office visits and may include:
  - A physical exam and a review of the child's medical history. Other medical conditions will be ruled out.
  - Growth chart. This is used to keep track of changes in your child's weight and height as they grow.
  - Calculating the child's BMI (body mass index).
  - Finding out about the child's eating and physical activity habits, and sedentary (sitting) time (e.g., TV watching).
  - Finding out about the family's medical history and the family's history of obesity.
  - Lab tests (e.g., blood or urine) in some cases.

APPROPRIATE HEALTH CARE
- Treatment for childhood obesity involves behavior changes for the child and the family. The changes include eating a healthy diet, being more physically active, and a decrease in time spent on sitting activities. Treatment is based on each individual child's needs and the family's lifestyle. Rarely will treatment focus just on weight loss.
- You may be referred to other types of health care workers for special help. This could include family counseling or a dietitian for meal planning.
- Weight-loss surgery may be an option for certain obese adolescents.

POSSIBLE COMPLICATIONS
- Increased risk for being obese as an adult.
- Type 2 diabetes, high blood pressure, heart disease, and other disorders often develop.
- Child may have emotional problems, lose self-esteem, be depressed, and be teased by peers.

PROBABLE OUTCOME—Positive changes need to be made in eating and physical activity habits. This can result in a slow weight loss or help maintain healthy weight as a child grows. Praise and reward child (not with food). Child will have more self-esteem and fewer health risks.

HOW TO TREAT

GENERAL MEASURES—To learn more: website for Centers for Disease Control & Prevention: www.cdc.gov/healthyweight/children. Kids can find help at: kids.niehs.nih.gov.

MEDICATION—Weight loss drugs are not usually prescribed.

ACTIVITY—Work slowly toward a goal of 60 minutes (can be split up) of activity a day. Reduce sitting activities (e.g., TV) to 1–2 hours a day. Find activities the whole family can do (parents need to be active also).

DIET
- Prepare healthy meals, limit sugary foods and drinks, have healthy snacks on hand, eat together as a family, and limit fast-food meals.
- For help in planning meals, consult a dietitian or try the U.S. Dept. of Agriculture website: www.choosemyplate.gov.

CALL YOUR DOCTOR IF

You are concerned about your child's weight.

OBSESSIVE COMPULSIVE DISORDER

GENERAL INFORMATION

DEFINITION—Obsessive-compulsive disorder (OCD) involves having obsessions and/or compulsions that are unwanted and interfere with one's life. Obsessions are recurrent, intrusive thoughts or images. Compulsions are repetitive, ritualistic behaviors. Most people with OCD realize that these thoughts or behaviors are not rational, but are unable to stop them.

BODY PARTS INVOLVED—Nervous system.

SEX OR AGE MOST AFFECTED—Both sexes; symptoms often begin in ages 10 to 24; rarely starts after age 50.

SIGNS & SYMPTOMS
- Obsessions that recur. Trying to ignore or resist them is unsuccessful. Obsessions can include:
  - Fears of infection (from germs, dirt, etc.) and fear of serious illness.
  - Doubts (Is the door shut/locked? Is iron on?).
  - Excessive orderliness or symmetry.
  - Fear that one's actions hurt other people or cause bad thing to happen.
  - Inappropriate sexual and aggressive thoughts.
- Compulsions are repetitive, purposeful behaviors to try to suppress the anxiety caused by obsessions. Compulsions can include:
  - Asking for assurances.
  - Avoiding places or actions.
  - Doubts and rechecks (locks, lights, doors).
  - Excessive washing (hands or bathing).
  - Hoarding possessions.
  - Repeating behaviors such as dressing rituals.
  - Counting/cleaning/ordering/arranging.

CAUSES—The exact cause is unknown. Low levels of a brain chemical, serotonin, appear to play a role. Serotonin carries messages from one brain cell to another. Genetics or other factors may also play a role.

RISK INCREASES WITH
- Family history of OCD.
- Pregnancy and postpartum period.
- Certain strep infections in children.
- Certain neurological disorders.

HOW TO PREVENT—Cannot be prevented.

WHAT TO EXPECT

DIAGNOSTIC MEASURES
- Your health care provider may do a physical exam and will ask questions about the symptoms. No medical tests can diagnose OCD.
- A patient's description of the behavior offers the best clues to diagnosis. You may be asked if symptoms take up more than 1 hour a day; cause distress; and interfere with your work, personal relationships, or daily functioning.

APPROPRIATE HEALTH CARE
- Treatment may include psychotherapy (counseling), drugs, and education for both patient and family. Treatment can help relieve symptoms, improve functioning, reduce stress, and improve quality of life.
- Cognitive-behavioral therapy (CBT) is often used to help change thoughts and behaviors. One type of CBT is "exposure and response prevention." Combining CBT and drug therapy is effective treatment for some patients.
- Group therapy may help some patients.
- Other or new therapies may be options for those who do not respond to usual treatments.
- Hospital care or other inpatient care may be recommended for severe symptoms.

POSSIBLE COMPLICATIONS
- House-bound and limited lifestyle.
- Depression, anxiety, panic episodes, substance abuse problems, and suicidal feelings.

PROBABLE OUTCOME—Outcome varies for each person. The disorder is lifelong. Symptoms can be mild or moderate to severe and disabling. Symptoms may come and go or be chronic. Effective and specific therapy is available that can help control symptoms.

HOW TO TREAT

GENERAL MEASURES
- Family support is important during treatment.
- Be aware that stressful life events may worsen symptoms.
- To learn more: Obsessive-Compulsive Foundation, PO Box 961029, Boston, MA 02196; (617) 973-5801 (not toll free); website: www.ocfoundation.org.

MEDICATION
- Antidepressants are often prescribed. They are effective, but benefits may not be seen for 3 weeks or up to 12 weeks. Dosages may be adjusted or other drugs may be tried if one type is not effective, or a drug's side effects are not tolerable.
- Antianxiety or tranquilizer drugs may be prescribed.

ACTIVITY—No limits.

DIET—No special diet.

CALL YOUR DOCTOR IF

- You or a family member has symptoms of obsessive compulsive disorder.
- Symptoms continue or worsen during treatment.
- Drugs used in treatment produce side effects.

ORAL CANCER

GENERAL INFORMATION

DEFINITION—Oral cancer is cancer of the mouth or the part of the throat at the back of the mouth (oropharynx).

BODY PARTS INVOLVED—It can involve the lips, gums, palate (roof of the mouth), tongue, membranes inside the lip or cheek, floor of the mouth, and tonsils.

SEX OR AGE MOST AFFECTED—It is more common in adults over 40 and in males more than females.

SIGNS & SYMPTOMS
- In the early stages, there may be no symptoms. It may be found during a routine mouth or dental exam.
- Lump or bump in the mouth, throat, or on lip.
- Red, white, or speckled patch in the mouth or on the tongue.
- Sore throat or mouth sore that does not heal.
- Pain, bleeding, or numbness in the mouth.
- Difficulty in speaking, chewing, or swallowing.
- Feeling that something is caught in the throat.
- Hoarseness or a change in voice.
- Ear ache or pain.
- Lump in the neck if lymph nodes are involved.

CAUSES—The exact reason why cells become cancerous is unclear. Known risk factors exist.

RISK INCREASES WITH
- Use of tobacco in any form (including smokeless).
- Excess alcohol use.
- Having human papillomavirus (HPV) infection.
- Sun exposure (cancer on the lip).
- Family history of cancer.
- Possible risks: exposure to x-rays or certain toxins, poor oral hygiene, poorly-fitting dentures, previous head or neck cancer, poor nutrition (diet low in fruits and vegetables), or chewing betel nut.

HOW TO PREVENT
- Don't use tobacco in any form. Avoid alcohol or use in moderate amounts.
- Do use good oral hygiene. Have your dental care provider or health care provider perform routine exams of mouth and throat.
- Eat a healthy diet.

WHAT TO EXPECT

DIAGNOSTIC MEASURES
- Your own observation of symptoms.
- Your health care provider will do an exam of the mouth and throat area. Questions will be asked about risk factors (e.g., smoking and alcohol use). A number of medical tests will be done. The tests help diagnose the cancer and then determine if it has spread (staging).

APPROPRIATE HEALTH CARE
- Treatment will depend on location of the cancer, if the cancer has spread, and the patient's age and health.
- The main treatments are surgery, radiation, and/or chemotherapy. Additional options are targeted therapy (which uses drugs/agents to attack specific cancer cells) and experimental treatments. All options will be discussed with you. Treatment can affect your appearance and ability to eat, talk, and breathe.
- Surgery to remove the cancer is a common treatment. If needed, reconstructive surgery can be done on the oral cavity or facial features.
- Follow-up therapy may be needed to help adjust to new ways of eating and talking.
- Dental care before, during, and after treatment will be needed to maintain good oral health.

POSSIBLE COMPLICATIONS
- Treatments can lead to complications.
- Face, head, or neck may be disfigured by surgery.
- Speech and swallowing problems.
- Cancer may recur or spread.
- The five-year survival rate is about 60%.

PROBABLE OUTCOME—Recovery depends on where the cancer is located, if it has spread, and patient's general health. The outcome is more favorable with early diagnosis, as compared to diagnosis of advanced disease.

HOW TO TREAT

GENERAL MEASURES
- Patients need to stop smoking and avoid alcohol use.
- To learn more: Oral Cancer Foundation, 3419 Via Lido #205, Newport Beach, CA 92663; (949) 646-8000 (not toll-free); website: oralcancerfoundation.org.

MEDICATION
- Anticancer (chemotherapy) drugs or targeted therapy drugs/agents may be prescribed.
- Drugs may be prescribed for side effects of treatment.

ACTIVITY—Stay as physically active as you can. Ask your health care provider for advice.

DIET
- Weight loss is common with treatment. A dietitian can help you in maintaining nutrition.
- The ability to chew or swallow may be affected. Special therapy may be prescribed.

CALL YOUR DOCTOR IF

- You or a family member has any symptoms of oral cancer.
- New or worsening symptoms develop.

OSGOOD-SCHLATTER DISEASE
(Osteochondrosis)

GENERAL INFORMATION

DEFINITION—Osgood-Schlatter disease (OSD) is a common, temporary condition involving the knee and the shinbone (tibia). It occurs often in young athletes (boys more than girls) during the pre-teen or teenage growing years. One or both knees can be affected. Osgood-Schlatter disease is named for the two doctors who first described it.

BODY PARTS INVOLVED—Tibial tubercle, a prominence just below the knee cap attached to a large thigh muscle connecting the bone of the upper leg (femur) to the large bone in the lower leg (tibia). Usually, only one knee is affected.

SEX OR AGE MOST AFFECTED—It usually occurs during the pre-teen or teenage growing years. It is uncommon after age 16.

SIGNS & SYMPTOMS
- Swelling, pain, and tenderness below the knee joint and over the shinbone. The symptoms may be mild to severe.
- Pain worsens with activity and gets better with rest. Pain may occur with jumping, kneeling, running, climbing stairs, or anytime the knee is bent and extended.
- Bony bump may be felt just below the kneecap. It may feel tender, warm, and hurt when pressed.

CAUSES—It is thought to be a combination of rapid growth and stress on the knee joint due to overuse. The tendon that connects the kneecap to the shinbone becomes inflamed due to constant pulling by the quadriceps muscles. The tendon may stretch and tear away (avulsion) from the tibia and take a piece of bone with it.

RISK INCREASES WITH
- Sports and activities that involve running, jumping, cutting, or jogging.
- Boys.
- Ages 8 to 15.
- Rapid skeletal growth.

HOW TO PREVENT—No specific preventive measures. Regular stretching of leg muscles and gradual increase in intensity of any new sports or exercise may reduce risk.

WHAT TO EXPECT

DIAGNOSTIC MEASURES
- Your own observation of symptoms.
- Your health care provider will do a physical exam of the leg and ask questions about your symptoms and activities.
- Medical tests may include an x-ray or bone scan of the knee to confirm the diagnosis.

APPROPRIATE HEALTH CARE
- Treatment may involve ice or heat, drugs (if needed for pain), rest, and limits on sports activities.
- Stretching exercises may be prescribed.
- Occasionally, other treatments may be recommended depending on symptoms. These may include using crutches, having a leg cast or splint, or wearing an elastic knee brace.
- Surgery (rarely needed) if symptoms persist.

POSSIBLE COMPLICATIONS
- In a few cases, chronic pain may occur.
- Some adults who had OSD as a child have some pain when kneeling.

PROBABLE OUTCOME—Usually resolves on its own within one year. Some discomfort may persist for 2 to 3 years or until growth is completed. A permanent, painless bump may remain below the knee.

HOW TO TREAT

GENERAL MEASURES
- Apply ice to the affected area several times a day for the first 2 to 3 days to reduce swelling and pain.
- After a few days, heat may help discomfort. Use warm compresses, a heating pad, or take warm baths.

MEDICATION—For minor discomfort, use nonprescription drugs such as ibuprofen or naproxen.

ACTIVITY
- Your health care provider will advise you of the limits on sports and activities. Each patient is different. The usual recommendation is to stop any sports or activities that cause pain. Participation may be permitted when it does not cause pain. Resuming some activities too quickly could make the symptoms worse.
- When you return to normal sports activities, recommendations may include wearing a knee brace, special insoles in your shoes, using heat before and ice on your knee after your activity, and stretching and strengthening exercises.
- Physical therapy may be prescribed to help strengthen leg muscles. Exercises may be taught to do at home.

DIET—No special diet.

CALL YOUR DOCTOR IF

- Your child has symptoms of Osgood-Schlatter disease.
- After diagnosis, pain increases, fever, or other unexpected symptoms occur.

OSTEOARTHRITIS
(Degenerative Joint Disease)

 GENERAL INFORMATION

DEFINITION—Osteoarthritis (OA) is the gradual deterioration (degeneration) of cartilage in a joint. The cartilage normally forms a soft protective layer at the ends of bones at a joint. When the cartilage deteriorates, it allows the bones to rub together. This causes the pain and limited movement. It is the most common type of arthritis and can lead to disability.

BODY PARTS INVOLVED—Usually weight-bearing joints (feet, ankles, knees, hips). It also affects fingers, wrists, shoulders, and spine.

SEX OR AGE MOST AFFECTED—It can occur at any age in both sexes, but is more likely in adults over age 45.

SIGNS & SYMPTOMS
* Joint stiffness and pain, including backache. Weather changes, such as cold and damp, may increase aching.
* Joints have limited movement and less flexibility.
* No redness, heat, or fever in affected joints (usually).
* Swelling of affected joints, such as fingers.
* May have cracking or grating sounds in joints.

CAUSES—Why it occurs is unclear. There is no single cause. Biologic, mechanical, hereditary, trauma, or congenital factors are involved.

RISK INCREASES WITH
* Age over 50 and females more than males.
* Obesity; joint injury; muscle overuse or weakness.
* Family history of osteoarthritis.
* Having other bone or joint disorders.

HOW TO PREVENT—To reduce risks, maintain normal weight for height and body structure. Be physically active, but avoid activities that lead to joint injury, especially after age 40. A regular stretching routine or yoga classes may help.

 WHAT TO EXPECT

DIAGNOSTIC MEASURES
* Your health care provider will do a physical exam and ask questions about your symptoms and activities.
* Medical tests can include blood and joint fluid studies, x-rays, or MRI.

APPROPRIATE HEALTH CARE
* Treatment goals are to control pain, delay progress of the disorder, and improve mobility and function.
* Treatment may include lifestyle changes, self-care steps, drug therapy, physical and occupational therapies, and surgery.

* Lifestyle changes may involve diet (to achieve healthy weight) or exercises.
* Occupational therapy helps with problems of daily living.
* Mechanical aids can include: shock-absorbing or orthopedic shoes, canes, crutches, or walkers. They may include splints, braces, or elastic supports to help joints; neck brace, collar, or corset to help back pain.
* Other treatments (e.g., acupuncture) may help.
* Surgery for osteoarthritis may be an option for some patients. There are different types.

POSSIBLE COMPLICATIONS
* Symptoms can lead to limits in daily activities, affect ability to work, bring on depression or stress, and restrict social and other activities.
* Side effects of drug therapy.

PROBABLE OUTCOME—There is no cure and the disorder can slowly worsen with time. Treatment can help control pain symptoms and help maintain function.

 HOW TO TREAT

GENERAL MEASURES
* Heat can ease discomfort or pain. Use heating pads or warm soaks several times a day for 10 minutes at a time.
* Cold can help reduce swelling and inflammation. Use an ice pack several times a day for 20 to 30 minutes.
* To learn more: Arthritis Foundation, local chapter, or contact them at PO Box 7669, Atlanta, GA 30357-0669; (800) 283-7800; website: www.arthritis.org.

MEDICATION
* Self-care for pain:
  - Nonprescription topical pain creams/gels.
  - Acetaminophen for mild to moderate pain.
  - NSAIDs (nonsteroidal anti-inflammatory drugs) for pain and inflammation.
  - Get medical advice about any supplements.
* Stronger oral pain relievers or cortisone injections into joints may be prescribed.
* Artificial joint fluid injections may be an option.
* Other drugs may be prescribed as needed.

ACTIVITY
* Exercise is beneficial. Your health care provider can advise you about an exercise program. Swimming or water aerobics are good.
* Physical therapy may be prescribed.

DIET—If overweight, weight loss will help joints.

 CALL YOUR DOCTOR IF

* You or a family member has joint problems.
* Symptoms worsen after treatment starts.

OSTEOMYELITIS

GENERAL INFORMATION

DEFINITION—Osteomyelitis is an infection of the bone. It can involve any bone in the body. In a child, it usually affects the femur (upper leg bone), tibia (lower leg bone), or the humerus or radius (bones in the arm). In an adult, it usually affects the pelvis or spine.

BODY PARTS INVOLVED—Bones.

SEX OR AGE MOST AFFECTED—Both sexes and all ages (often children and the elderly).

SIGNS & SYMPTOMS
* High fever.
* Pain, swelling, redness, warmth, and tenderness in the area over the infected bone, especially when moving a nearby joint. Nearby joints, such as the knee, may also be red, warm, and swollen.
* May have limited use or not be able to use an infected extremity (arm or leg).
* Child may guard or protect area from being touched.
* General ill feeling.
* Excess sweating, chills, back pain may occur.

CAUSES—Bacterial infection (e.g., *Staphylococcus aureus*) is the most common cause. Other infections are more rare. Bones can be infected by: bacteria in the bloodstream from infection in another body part; bacteria in soft body tissue located next to the bone; and bacteria that directly infects the bone.

RISK INCREASES WITH
* Recent injury or surgery (especially orthopedic).
* Diabetes, sickle cell anemia, or chronic joint disease.
* Infection that occurs elsewhere the body.
* Periodontitis (gum inflammation).
* People on dialysis (hemodialysis).
* Weak immune system due to illness or drugs.
* Intravenous (IV) drug abuse.

HOW TO PREVENT—Not always preventable. Reduce your risk for infections where possible.

WHAT TO EXPECT

DIAGNOSTIC MEASURES
* Your own observation of symptoms.
* Your health care provider will do a physical exam of the affected area.
* Medical tests include blood studies and cultures to identify the bacteria. Samples of pus, joint fluid, and infected bone may be removed and used for tests to confirm the diagnosis.
* Imaging studies such as x-rays, bone scan, CT, or MRI may be done.

APPROPRIATE HEALTH CARE
* Treatment usually involves hospital care, drug therapy, rest, and other supportive measures.
* The affected bone and joint may be immobilized (not allowed to move). Bracing may be used for the spine.
* Surgery may be done to drain an abscess, remove dead bone tissue or infected bone, and to stabilize the spine. Bone or skin grafts may be required.
* An artificial joint that is infected may need to be removed and replaced.

POSSIBLE COMPLICATIONS
* Chronic osteomyelitis. It may last for months or years and be difficult to treat. It can cause periodic bone pain, tenderness, and abscess (area of pus) that may drain through the skin. Treatment may require more surgery and drugs for an extended period of time.
* Limited function of the affected limb and joint.
* Bone fractures.
* Serious blood infection (sepsis).
* Recurrence of the infection.
* Rarely, treatment is unsuccessful. Surgery may be done to fuse the joint or amputate the limb.

PROBABLE OUTCOME—Outcome will depend on severity of infection, the success of drug therapy, results of surgical procedures, and health of the patient. With early diagnosis and treatment, most patients recover with no complications.

HOW TO TREAT

GENERAL MEASURES—Follow medical advice about home care after treatment.

MEDICATION
* Antibiotics will be prescribed to treat the infection. They are sometimes given through a vein (IV) while in the hospital. The drugs usually need to be continued at home after the hospital stay. This may be done by continuing the IV drugs or with drugs that are taken by mouth.
* Pain relievers may be prescribed.

ACTIVITY
* Rest in bed until symptoms get better. Resume your normal activities gradually.
* Physical therapy can help affected limbs and joints regain function and flexibility.

DIET—No special diet.

CALL YOUR DOCTOR IF

* You or a family member has symptoms of osteomyelitis.
* Symptoms persist or recur despite treatment.

OSTEOPOROSIS

GENERAL INFORMATION

DEFINITION—Osteoporosis is the loss of normal bone density, bone mass, and bone strength. It is a progressive disease that leads to increased thinning of bones and risk of fractures (broken bones).

BODY PARTS INVOLVED—Bones.

SEX OR AGE MOST AFFECTED—It occurs in both sexes, but is most common in women after menopause due to a decrease in the hormone estrogen. Estrogen protects against bone loss.

SIGNS & SYMPTOMS
- It does not cause pain or other obvious symptoms. It is called a "silent" disease.
- People don't realize they have osteoporosis until they fall and suffer a fracture, or a spontaneous fracture occurs in a backbone. Pain from fractures may be mild to severe. The pain may stop when the fracture heals or it may be chronic due to permanent bone damage.

CAUSES—The body breaks down and rebuilds bones all through life and peak bone mass occurs in the 20s. When the bone loss occurs at a greater rate than the rebuilding, osteoporosis can develop. A number of factors are involved in the increased loss of bone.

RISK INCREASES WITH
- Females; older age; Asian or white persons.
- Early menopause (naturally or from surgery).
- Lack of exercise (sedentary lifestyle).
- A broad range of diseases and drugs.
- Poor nutrition.
- Women with small body frame or are quite thin.
- Eating disorders (bulimia or anorexia).
- Family history of osteoporosis or bone fractures.
- Smoking.
- Excess alcohol use.
- Men with low testosterone levels.

HOW TO PREVENT
- Prevention should start at a young age.
- Getting adequate calcium and vitamin D.
- Regular exercise such as walking (which is weight-bearing) and weightlifting.
- Avoid risk factors (e.g., alcohol and smoking).
- Get a bone mineral density test (if advised).
- Preventive drugs may be prescribed in high-risk cases.

WHAT TO EXPECT

DIAGNOSTIC MEASURES—Medical tests may include blood and urine studies, bone x-rays, ultrasound, and bone mineral density studies. The diagnosis may be osteopenia (an early stage of bone loss) or osteoporosis.

APPROPRIATE HEALTH CARE
- Treatment is aimed at stopping further bone loss, preventing fractures, relieving pain (if needed), and bone rebuilding. Treatment steps may include drugs, lifestyle changes, and medical care for any underlying disorder. A treatment plan will be based on each individual.
- Lifestyle changes may include diet changes, exercise, modifying behaviors, and home safety to prevent falls.
- If a drug you take is a risk factor for osteoporosis, the medical advice may be to stop the drug, reduce the dosage, or use an alternative drug.

POSSIBLE COMPLICATIONS
- Falls and bone fractures, such as hip, spine, and wrist.
- Severe, disabling pain.
- Deformed spinal column and bent back (sometimes called Dowager hump). Loss of height.

PROBABLE OUTCOME—There is no cure. Treatment (no matter what age) can help halt and may reverse some bone loss. Pain symptoms can usually be helped with drugs.

HOW TO TREAT

GENERAL MEASURES
- Stop smoking. Find a way to quit that works.
- Stop excess alcohol use.
- To learn more: National Osteoporosis Foundation, 1150 17th St NW, Suite 850, Washington, DC 20036; (800) 231-4222; website: www.nof.org.

MEDICATION
- Different prescription drugs are often used to prevent and treat bone loss. If one drug causes problems or is not effective, another drug can be prescribed.
- For minor pain, use nonprescription drugs such as acetaminophen or ibuprofen. Stronger pain drugs may be prescribed.
- Calcium and vitamin D supplements are usually recommended.

ACTIVITY—Exercise strengthens muscles and bones and improves balance. Aerobic and weight-bearing exercises should be part of a daily program. Ask you health care provider about a weightlifting routine to help build muscle strength.

DIET—Eat a healthy, well-balanced diet.

CALL YOUR DOCTOR IF

- You or a family member has concerns osteoporosis.
- Pain develops, especially after an injury.

OTOSCLEROSIS

GENERAL INFORMATION

DEFINITION—Otosclerosis is an abnormal growth of sponge-like bone in the middle ear. The growth prevents one of the small bones in the middle ear from transmitting sound waves. This can lead to hearing loss.

BODY PARTS INVOLVED—Middle-ear bones and nerves in the ear that allow us to hear. Otosclerosis usually affects both ears.

SEX OR AGE MOST AFFECTED—It occurs in all ages and both sexes, but is more common in middle-aged white women.

SIGNS & SYMPTOMS
- Slow, continuing hearing loss.
- Ringing or other types of noises in the ears (tinnitus).
- Dizziness or imbalance if the vestibular portion of the ear is affected.

CAUSES—The exact cause is unclear. It appears to be an inherited disorder. Sixty percent of those affected have a positive family history of the disorder. In other cases, the cause is unknown. A viral infection may be a factor.

RISK INCREASES WITH
- Family history of hearing loss.
- Genetics. Otosclerosis affects to some degree about 10% of all white persons.
- Pregnancy, which may trigger the onset.
- Osteogenesis imperfecta (a bone disease of the ear).

HOW TO PREVENT—Cannot be prevented at present. Obtain genetic counseling before starting a family if you or your spouse has otosclerosis.

WHAT TO EXPECT

DIAGNOSTIC MEASURES
- Your own observation of symptoms.
- Your health care provider will do a physical exam of the ears and ask questions about your symptoms and family history of hearing problems.
- Diagnosis is based on hearing tests such as an audiogram and Rinne test (study of bone conduction). A CT (an imaging study) of the head may be done to rule out other disorders.

APPROPRIATE HEALTH CARE
- Treatment will depend on the degree of hearing loss. It may involve surgery and/or hearing aids, and sometimes fluoride supplements.
- If the hearing loss is minor, no treatment is usually needed. Routine hearing tests will be given to check if hearing loss is getting worse.
- Treatment may involve surgery (stapedectomy) to remove a part or all of the stapes (a bone in the middle ear) and replace it with a prosthesis (artificial substitute). The hearing is improved in almost all cases.
- Hearing aids will benefit many patients. Different types are available. A hearing specialist can help you choose what will work best for your individual needs.

POSSIBLE COMPLICATIONS
- Without surgery, some hearing loss may progress for years. Total deafness is a rare complication.
- Hearing loss can cause problems with work, social events, and family relationships. Emotional distress may occur.
- Complications may result from surgery, such as infection or pain.

PROBABLE OUTCOME—Surgical treatment can help restore or improve hearing in most patients. In patients not needing or unable to have surgery, hearing aids can be of benefit.

HOW TO TREAT

GENERAL MEASURES—To learn more: National Institute on Deafness & Other Communication Disorders, 1 Communication Ave., Bethesda, MD 20892; (800) 241-1044; website: www.nidcd.nih.gov.

MEDICATION
- Antibiotics may be prescribed after surgery.
- Sodium fluoride may be prescribed to prevent further hearing loss by hardening the spongy bone. It won't, however, improve hearing.

ACTIVITY—After surgery, resume your normal activities gradually.

DIET—No special diet.

CALL YOUR DOCTOR IF

- You or a family member has symptoms of otosclerosis.
- Sudden hearing loss or dizziness occurs.
- New symptoms occur after surgery.

OVARIAN CANCER

 ## GENERAL INFORMATION

DEFINITION—Ovarian cancer is cancer that starts in one or both ovaries. The ovaries are female reproductive organs that store eggs and produce most of the female hormones.

BODY PARTS INVOLVED—One or both ovaries. It may spread to the lungs and bone.

SEX OR AGE MOST AFFECTED—It affects females of all ages, but is most common after age 40.

SIGNS & SYMPTOMS
- Early symptoms can be mild and vague or absent.
- Bloating.
- Pelvic or abdominal pressure or pain.
- Difficulty eating or feeling full quickly.
- A need to urinate often.
- Increase in size of waist or abdomen. May feel a firm swelling in lower abdomen.
- Nausea, gas, or indigestion.
- Changes in bowel habits (e.g., constipation).
- Menstrual period changes; irregular vaginal bleeding.
- Pain or discomfort with intercourse.
- Lack of energy, fatigue, weight loss or gain, or fever.

CAUSES
- The exact cause is unknown. There are different types of primary ovarian cancer. Epithelial tumors account for the majority, and they grow more rapidly. They can progress from an early to advanced stage within a year. Other types may be slow growing.
- Secondary ovarian cancer is due to spread of a primary cancer from elsewhere in the body.

RISK INCREASES WITH
- Having had breast, endometrial, or colon cancer.
- Family history of breast, ovarian, or hereditary colon cancer.
- Mutated genes such as BRCA1 and BRCA2.
- Advancing age.
- Never having had children.
- Obesity.
- Hormone replacement therapy (for 5 or more years).
- Infertility (with or without use of fertility drugs).

HOW TO PREVENT
- No specific preventive measures. Birth control pill use, giving birth at least once, and tubal ligation or hysterectomy can reduce risks.
- Women with high-risk factors should get medical advice about cancer preventive options. Surgical removal of the ovaries reduces, but does not entirely remove, the cancer risk.
- Routine pelvic exams are not a specific test for ovarian cancer, but are important for women's health care.

 ## WHAT TO EXPECT

DIAGNOSTIC MEASURES
- Your health care provider will do a physical exam and ask questions about your symptoms.
- A number of medical tests will be done. The tests help diagnose the cancer and also determine if it has spread (staging).

APPROPRIATE HEALTH CARE
- Treatment varies and depends on the location and size of a tumor, any spread of the cancer, health, age and preferences of the patient. Treatment includes surgery and/or chemotherapy (anticancer drugs). Other new therapies may be recommended.
- The goal of surgery is to remove as much of the cancer as possible. In patients who desire pregnancy, surgery may remove only the ovary and the fallopian tube (infertility may still result).
- Treatment may involve steps to relieve symptoms and make you comfortable, rather than treating the cancer.
- Counseling may help you cope.

POSSIBLE COMPLICATIONS
- Side effects occur from treatments.
- Infertility if both ovaries are removed.
- Bowel obstruction; fluid in lungs or abdomen.
- Cancer returns or persists after treatment.
- Spread of cancer to other organs (can lead to excess pain, complications, and can be fatal).

PROBABLE OUTCOME—The outcome depends on the stage of the disease when it is first diagnosed. Other factors that affect the outcome are a woman's age and her general health. Early diagnosis and treatment produce the best outcome.

 ## HOW TO TREAT

GENERAL MEASURES—To learn more: American Cancer Society; (800) ACS-2345; website: www.cancer.org or National Cancer Institute; (800) 4-CANCER; website: www.nci.nih.gov.

MEDICATION—Anticancer drugs (chemotherapy) and pain relievers, as needed, may be prescribed.

ACTIVITY—Be as active as symptoms and treatments permit.

DIET—Eat a healthy, well-balanced diet.

☎ CALL YOUR DOCTOR IF

- You or a family member has ovarian cancer symptoms.
- Symptoms cause concern during or after treatment.

OVARIAN CYST OR TUMOR, BENIGN

 GENERAL INFORMATION

DEFINITION
• A benign ovarian cyst or tumor is one that grows in or on the ovaries. The ovaries are the female reproductive organs that hold and release eggs and produce female hormones. Benign means noncancerous.
- Ovarian cysts are fluid-filled or semisolid-filled sacs. The most common type is called functional and occurs in premenopausal women. There are other, less common types. Rarely, a cyst may lead to cancer.
- Ovarian tumors are usually a solid mass, but can be cystic or mixed. One common type is a fibroma which can be quite large. It more often affects postmenopausal women. Another type, dermoid, occurs more often in younger women.

BODY PARTS INVOLVED—One or both ovaries.

SEX OR AGE MOST AFFECTED—Females.

SIGNS & SYMPTOMS
• Early symptoms can be mild and vague or absent.
• Bloating.
• Pelvic or abdominal pressure or pain.
• Loss of appetite or feeling full quickly.
• A need to urinate often.
• Increase in size of waist or abdomen. May feel a firm swelling in lower abdomen.
• Nausea, gas, or indigestion.
• Changes in bowel habits (e.g., constipation).
• Changes in menstrual periods.
• Pain or discomfort with intercourse.
• Lack of energy, fatigue, weight loss or gain, or fever.
• If a large ovarian cyst or tumor twists or ruptures, it can cause severe pain, rigid muscles, and swelling.

CAUSES—The exact causes for cysts and tumors are unclear. There are multiple factors that are likely to play a role.

RISK INCREASES WITH
• Obesity.
• Early menstruation.
• Infertility.
• Hypothyroidism.
• Tamoxifen drug therapy is a risk for cysts.
• Smoking may increase risk of benign tumors.

HOW TO PREVENT
• No specific preventive measures. Use of oral contraceptives may decrease risk.
• Have regular pelvic exams. They can help discover early changes in the reproductive organs.

 WHAT TO EXPECT

DIAGNOSTIC MEASURES
• Your own observation of symptoms.
• Your health care provider will do a physical and pelvic exam.
• Medical tests can include blood studies and an ultrasound. Laparoscopy (a telescope-like tool used to look inside the abdomen) may be used for diagnosis and treatment. A biopsy may be done.

APPROPRIATE HEALTH CARE
• Treatment will depend on the diagnostic results, symptoms, and a woman's age and health status.
• Treatment may not be needed for most cysts. Routine medical follow-up is done to verify the cyst goes away. A tumor may need surgery.
• Cyst treatment, if needed, may include removing the fluid in the cyst, drug therapy, or removal with surgery.
• A ruptured cyst usually does not require surgery. The fluid will be absorbed by the body. If bleeding continues, surgery may be required.
• Surgery may be done to remove a cyst or tumor. The ovary may be removed (oophorectomy) if it is damaged. Pregnancy can still occur with one ovary. Rarely, both ovaries are removed.
• A twisted cyst or tumor needs surgery right away to avoid damage to an ovary.

POSSIBLE COMPLICATIONS
• Complications from surgery may occur.
• Cyst or tumor may recur after treatment.
• Infertility.

PROBABLE OUTCOME—Most ovarian cysts require no treatment and disappear on their own within a few months. In other cases, treatment for a cyst or tumor usually provides a cure.

 HOW TO TREAT

GENERAL MEASURES—To learn more: try the library or do a web search. A good site to start with is www.womenshealth.gov.

MEDICATION—Female hormones may be prescribed. These help shrink or destroy some cysts. Oral contraceptives are often used as the first step in treatment.

ACTIVITY—No limits unless advised.

DIET—No special diet.

 CALL YOUR DOCTOR IF

• You or a family member has symptoms of an ovarian cyst or tumor.
• After diagnosis, any symptoms cause concern.

PAGET'S DISEASE OF BONE
(Osteitis Deformans)

 GENERAL INFORMATION

DEFINITION—Paget's disease of bone is a gradual, progressive bone disorder. It is named for an English doctor who first described the disease. Paget's disease of the breast is a different disorder.

BODY PARTS INVOLVED—It usually involves the bones of the skull, spine, legs, collar bone, and pelvis.

SEX OR AGE MOST AFFECTED—It can affect both sexes and is most common in older adults.

SIGNS & SYMPTOMS
- Most often, there are no early symptoms.
- Bone pain (especially at night).
- Skin over the bones is warm.
- Joint pain or stiffness.
- Headaches.
- Hearing loss and tinnitus (noises in the ear).
- Fractures (may occur from minor trauma).
- Bowing of long bones, such as of the legs.
- Nerve problems, from pressure on the nerves.

CAUSES—Unknown. It may involve genetics and/or a virus. The affected bone breaks down and then abnormal bone growth occurs. The new bone is weak, fragile, enlarged, and deformed.

RISK INCREASES WITH—Family history of Paget's disease.

HOW TO PREVENT
- No specific preventive measures.
- Those with a family history should consider a blood-screening test periodically to help with early diagnosis.

 WHAT TO EXPECT

DIAGNOSTIC MEASURES
- Your own observation of symptoms.
- Your health care provider will do a physical exam.
- Medical tests may include blood and urine studies, x-rays of affected bones, and a bone scan. Hearing and vision testing may be done if the skull is involved.

APPROPRIATE HEALTH CARE
- Treatment may include physical therapy, use of assistive devices, drugs, exercise, home care, and surgery.
- If there are no symptoms, treatment may not be needed. Follow-up exams will monitor the disease status.
- Physical therapy helps maintain and improve muscle strength, range of motion, flexibility, and endurance.

- Walkers, canes, crutches, special shoes, or shoe inserts may help if walking is a problem.
- Transcutaneous electrical nerve stimulation (TENS) or massage may help muscle pain and tightness.
- Hearing aid may be useful if hearing loss occurs.
- Rarely, splinting may be needed for severely affected areas to prevent fractures.
- Bone surgery may be needed to treat fractures, correct deformities, or treat arthritis.

POSSIBLE COMPLICATIONS—Many complications can occur that affect different organs and body parts. Complications include arthritis, heart disease, hearing loss, kidney stones, bone cancer, vision changes, spinal disease, enlarged head, loose teeth, and others.

PROBABLE OUTCOME—There is no cure, but treatment can control or reduce symptoms. With early treatment (before major bone changes occur), the outlook is generally good.

 HOW TO TREAT

GENERAL MEASURES
- Use heat to relieve pain (warm compresses, or soaks).
- Accident-proof your home. Avoid throw rugs and slippery floors. Install hand rails next to the tub. Other changes may be needed depending on patient's needs.
- To learn more: Paget Foundation, PO Box 24432, Brooklyn, NY 11202; (800) 237-2438; website: www.paget.org.

MEDICATION
- Drugs will usually be prescribed that help slow the rate of bone turnover. Several options are available and their risks and benefits will be discussed with you.
- Nonprescription drugs for pain can be used. Stronger ones may be prescribed (if needed).
- Calcium and vitamin D are often recommended.

ACTIVITY—Home exercises will help maintain mobility. Avoid stress on affected bones. Follow instructions provided by your physical therapist or health care provider.

DIET—Eat a healthy diet. Avoid weight gain.

 CALL YOUR DOCTOR IF

- You or family member has symptoms of Paget's disease of bone.
- New, unexplained symptoms develop.

PANCREAS CANCER

GENERAL INFORMATION

DEFINITION—Pancreas cancer is a type of cancer that affects the pancreas. The pancreas is an organ in the upper-middle part of the abdomen. It produces intestinal enzymes (juices) to help digest food, and insulin to control blood sugar.

BODY PARTS INVOLVED—Pancreas, an organ in the back of the upper abdomen.

SEX OR AGE MOST AFFECTED—It usually affects older adults, and men more than women.

SIGNS & SYMPTOMS
- Usually no symptoms occur in early stages of cancer.
- Weight loss. Loss of appetite.
- Pain in the back or upper abdomen.
- Fatigue.
- Jaundice (yellow skin and eyes). Intense itching may occur with jaundice.
- Nausea, vomiting, and digestion problems.
- Depression, though not caused by cancer, may occur.

CAUSES—Unknown. It may be a combination of hereditary, biologic, and environmental factors.

RISK INCREASES WITH
- Older adults and males more than females.
- Pancreatitis (inflammation of the pancreas).
- Family history of pancreatic, colon, or ovarian cancer.
- Diabetes.
- Jews and African Americans are more often affected.
- Smoking.
- Obesity and lack of physical activity.
- Heavy exposure to certain toxins in workplace.
- Certain hereditary conditions (or genetic syndromes).
- Prior surgery for peptic ulcers.
- Diet high in fats may play a role.

HOW TO PREVENT
- No specific preventive measures. To reduce cancer risks: get screening tests, maintain healthy weight, eat a healthy diet, exercise regularly, and don't smoke.
- Get genetic counseling if you have genetic risk.

WHAT TO EXPECT

DIAGNOSTIC MEASURES
- Your own observation of symptoms.
- Your health care provider will do a physical exam and ask questions about any symptoms. A number of medical tests will be done. The tests help to diagnose the cancer, and then determine if it has spread (staging).

APPROPRIATE HEALTH CARE
- Treatment varies and depends on location and size of tumor, any spread of the cancer, your health, age, and preferences. Treatment may include chemotherapy (anticancer drugs), radiation therapy, surgery, targeted therapy, or other new forms of treatment.
- Chemotherapy uses drugs and radiation therapy uses radiation to attack the cancer cells. Targeted therapy uses drugs/agents to attack specific cancer cells.
- Surgery may be performed to remove the tumor if the cancer has not spread to other places in the body.
- Treatment may involve steps to relieve symptoms and make you comfortable, rather than treating the cancer.
- Counseling may help you cope.

POSSIBLE COMPLICATIONS
- Spread (metastasis) of cancer to other organs (often occurred by the time of diagnosis).
- Surgical or drug therapy complications.
- Malnutrition (lack of nutrients for the body).
- Increased pain.

PROBABLE OUTCOME—Outcome depends on an individual patient's health, treatment response, and stage of the cancer at diagnosis. An early diagnosis provides a better outcome. The diagnosis often comes too late for effective treatment. Symptoms can be relieved or controlled to help improve quality of life.

HOW TO TREAT

GENERAL MEASURES—To learn more: American Cancer Society; (800) ACS-2345; website: www.cancer.org, or National Cancer Institute; (800) 4-CANCER; website: www.nci.nih.gov.

MEDICATION
- Your health care provider may prescribe:
  - Pain relievers.
  - Chemotherapy or targeted therapy.
  - Pancreatic enzymes to replace those that the pancreas cannot manufacture.
  - Sedatives for sleep if needed.
  - Vitamin supplements.

ACTIVITY—Remain as active as you can. It helps your quality of life.

DIET
- Low-fat diet may be recommended.
- Loss of appetite may make eating difficult. Try eating several small meals each day. Choose foods easy to digest.

CALL YOUR DOCTOR IF

- You have symptoms of pancreas cancer.
- New or changed symptoms occur.

PANCREATITIS

GENERAL INFORMATION

DEFINITION—Pancreatitis is an inflammation of the pancreas. The pancreas produces enzymes (juices) to help with digestion and hormones to help the body process sugar. Acute pancreatitis occurs suddenly and lasts for a short period. Chronic pancreatitis is inflammation that does not heal or improve with time.

BODY PARTS INVOLVED—Pancreas.

SEX OR AGE MOST AFFECTED—Children and adults of both sexes.

SIGNS & SYMPTOMS
- Upper abdominal pain that spreads to the back.
- Pain may worsen after eating or after drinking alcohol.
- Nausea and vomiting.
- Abdominal swelling and gas.
- Fever; rapid pulse.
- Diarrhea, oily stools, weight loss, and mild jaundice (yellow skin or eyes) with chronic pancreatitis.

CAUSES
- Inflammation is caused by digestive enzymes that become activated too soon and irritate the pancreas cells. This process can be brought on by a number of different risk factors. Sometimes the cause is unknown.
- Chronic pancreatitis develops when the pancreas has become damaged (scarred) from continued inflammation. These patients often have multiple risk factors (e.g., smoking and alcohol use).

RISK INCREASES WITH
- Chronic, heavy alcohol use.
- Gallstones.
- Infection, abdominal injury or surgery, or tumor.
- Use of certain drugs.
- Cigarette smoking.
- Some autoimmune or hereditary disorders.
- Family history of pancreatitis.
- High levels of calcium, triglycerides (fats), or parathyroid hormone in the blood.
- Endoscopic retrograde cholangio-pancreatography (ERCP), a medical procedure.

HOW TO PREVENT—No specific preventive measures. Avoid risk factors where possible.

WHAT TO EXPECT

DIAGNOSTIC MEASURES
- Your own observation of symptoms.
- Your health care provider will do a physical exam and ask questions about your symptoms and activities.
- Medical tests may include blood, stool, and urine studies; x-rays of the abdomen; CT scan or ultrasound of the pancreas; and others.

APPROPRIATE HEALTH CARE
- Acute pancreatitis normally requires hospital care for intravenous (IV) fluids and control of symptoms. Oxygen or breathing support with a machine may be needed. Surgery may be required for gallstones, perforated peptic ulcer, or to drain a source of infection.
- Chronic pancreatitis treatment may be in a hospital or as an outpatient. Treatment is with drugs, diet controls, and avoidance of alcohol. In some cases, surgery may be needed for a blockage or to control pain.

POSSIBLE COMPLICATIONS—They may occur from acute and chronic pancreatitis. They can affect the heart, lungs, kidneys, and other body organs, and could be fatal in a few cases.

PROBABLE OUTCOME—Most patients with acute pancreatitis improve in 3 to 7 days. Outcome sometimes depends on underlying cause. Chronic pancreatitis may have recurrent attacks for years. Drugs and diet changes can help symptoms.

HOW TO TREAT

GENERAL MEASURES
- Stop smoking. Find a way to quit.
- To learn more: National Digestive Diseases Information Clearinghouse, 2 Information Way, Bethesda, MD 20892; (800) 891-5389; website: www.digestive.niddk.nih.gov.

MEDICATION
- Your health care provider may prescribe:
  - Pain relievers.
  - Digestive enzymes that the damaged pancreas cannot manufacture.
  - Antibiotics, if bacterial infection develops.
  - Drugs to reduce stomach acid.
  - Drugs to lower fats in the blood.
  - Insulin, if diabetes is present.

ACTIVITY—Limits on activity will depend on symptoms and type of treatment. Follow your health care provider's advice about returning to work, school, or physical activities.

DIET
- In the hospital, the diet may progress from no foods to liquids to bland foods.
- At home, eat small, frequent, and low-fat meals.
- Avoid all alcohol.

CALL YOUR DOCTOR IF

- You or a family member has symptoms of pancreatitis.
- Symptoms worsen or don't improve.

PANIC DISORDER

GENERAL INFORMATION

DEFINITION—Panic disorder is a type of anxiety disorder. It involves repeated and unexpected episodes of irrational fear and panic. It occurs with attack-like symptoms (even during sleep). Most attacks last 2 to 10 minutes, but some may extend as long as an hour or two. The attacks may begin in the late teen years or early adulthood.

BODY PARTS INVOLVED—Central nervous system; heart; lungs; skin; hands; feet.

SEX OR AGE MOST AFFECTED—Females more than males; young adults, ages 25 to 44.

SIGNS & SYMPTOMS
- Physical symptoms:
  - Pounding, racing, or skipping heartbeat, chest pains, and shortness of breath.
  - Choking feeling, lump in the throat feeling, weakness, faintness, dizziness, lightheaded, and sweating.
  - Trembling, numbness, tingling, flushes, or chills.
  - Muscle spasms or contractions in the hands and feet.
  - Feeling of "butterflies" in the stomach or nausea.
- Emotional symptoms:
  - Intense fear of losing one's mind (fear of going crazy), an urge to flee, fear of dying.
  - Sense of terror, doom, or dread. Sense of unreality, loss of contact with people and objects, and fear of losing control. Fear of having another panic attack.

CAUSES—The brain's "alarm system" appears to be affected by a combination of biologic/genetic factors, illnesses, drugs, and one's personal history of traumatic events.

RISK INCREASES WITH
- Stress (emotional or physical); feelings of guilt, fatigue, or overwork; illness; alcohol or drug abuse.
- Personal history of emotional problems. A family history of panic disorder, alcoholism, or bipolar disorder.

HOW TO PREVENT—No specific measures to prevent a first panic attack. Treatment helps prevent repeated attacks.

WHAT TO EXPECT

DIAGNOSTIC MEASURES
- Your health care provider will do a physical exam and ask questions about your symptoms and activities.
- Medical tests may be done to rule out other disorders. A variety of physical disorders can mimic panic attacks.

APPROPRIATE HEALTH CARE
- Treatment may involve psychotherapy (treatment of emotional and mental problems), self-care, and drugs.
- Cognitive-behavioral therapy may help. Cognitive therapy teaches how to change thoughts, behaviors, or attitudes. Behavioral therapy teaches ways to reduce anxiety with deep breathing and muscle relaxation.

POSSIBLE COMPLICATIONS
- It can affect all aspects of life (work, family, friends, social, and recreational).
- Chronic anxiety or depression; phobias, including agoraphobia (fear of being alone or in public places).
- Some with this disorder feel there is a physical problem causing their symptoms and go from doctor to doctor for a diagnosis. Even if advised of their good health, they believe otherwise.
- Increased risk of drug or alcohol abuse.

PROBABLE OUTCOME—Outcome varies. Treatment can help reduce or completely prevent attacks. Most patients can lead normal lives. For some, the disorder gets better at times and worse at other times.

HOW TO TREAT

GENERAL MEASURES
- Self-care steps may include:
  - Talking to a friend or family member about your feelings. This may defuse your anxiety.
  - Keep a journal about your anxious thoughts or emotions. Consider causes and solutions.
  - Join a self-help group.
  - Reduce stress in your life, where possible.
  - Practice relaxation techniques.
- To learn more: National Institute of Mental Health; 6001 Executive Blvd., Bethesda, MD 20892-9663; (866) 615-6464; website: www.nimh.nih.gov.

MEDICATION
- Your health care provider may prescribe an antidepressant. It may be slowly reduced or stopped, after 6 months to a year, to determine if the panic attacks will return. If they do not return, the drug can be stopped.
- Get medical advice about use of supplements.

ACTIVITY—Exercise daily; get enough sleep.

DIET
- Consider giving up caffeine (coffee, tea, soft drinks). You may have withdrawal symptoms of headache or tiredness for a few days.
- Don't use alcohol as a way to numb feelings.

CALL YOUR DOCTOR IF

- You or a family member has panic attacks.
- Symptoms return after treatment.

PARALYSIS

GENERAL INFORMATION

DEFINITION—Paralysis is the loss of ability to move a part of the body caused by the inability to contract one or more muscles. The condition varies in degree and severity from paralysis of one small muscle to paralysis of almost the total body. The paralysis may be temporary or permanent. Types include: paraplegia (partial or complete paralysis of both legs), quadriplegia (partial or complete paralysis of both arms and legs), and hemiplegia (partial or complete paralysis of one side of the body).

BODY PARTS INVOLVED—Brain; spinal cord; nervous system; muscles.

SEX OR AGE MOST AFFECTED—Both sexes; all ages.

SIGNS & SYMPTOMS
- The following vary, depending on the site and extent of damage:
  - Loss of movement and sensation in affected arms or legs.
  - Loss of urinary and bowel control; impaired sexual function; loss of normal blood pressure; loss of body-temperature control; constipation.
  - Difficulty speaking, understanding or recognizing words.
  - Blurred, double or decreased vision.

CAUSES
- Normally, the brain originates the impulses for muscle movement. These impulses travel via the spinal cord and peripheral nerves to the muscles. Paralysis occurs when there is an injury or disruption in this nerve pathway. Causes include:
  - Stroke (most common). Stroke may be caused by bleeding in brain, or blood clot or obstruction of blood vessel to brain.
  - Brain: tumor, abscess, hemorrhage, infection (encephalitis).
  - Spinal cord: injury (from an accident); pressure on the spinal cord (disc prolapse, cervical osteoarthritis), decompression sickness.
  - Disease: multiple sclerosis, poliomyelitis, myelitis, Friedreich's ataxia, meningitis, motor neuron disease.
  - Nerve disorders (neuropathies): secondary to disorders such as diabetes mellitus, vitamin deficiency, liver disease, alcoholism, cancer and toxic effects of drugs or metals.
  - Muscle disorders such as muscular dystrophy and sometimes, myasthenia gravis.

RISK INCREASES WITH
- Any activity with a high risk of injury.
- Excess alcohol consumption or drug use.

HOW TO PREVENT
- Observe safety precautions; don't take risks.
- Don't dive into shallow water.
- Wear protective headgear during contact sports and while riding a bicycle or motorcycle.
- Obtain medical treatment to control any chronic medical condition.

WHAT TO EXPECT

DIAGNOSTIC MEASURES—Diagnosis with emergency care may be needed. Medical tests will be determined by the cause of the paralysis.

APPROPRIATE HEALTH CARE
- Treatment of any underlying cause.
- Hospital care in intensive unit if paralysis affects the breathing muscles.
- Surgery to limit further spinal-cord damage or to remove bones or a tumor.
- Time in an extended-care facility or special rehabilitation facility (sometimes).
- Physical and occupational rehabilitation.
- Psychotherapy or counseling for depression or for sexual problems.

POSSIBLE COMPLICATIONS—Kidney infections, especially if a urinary catheter is needed; lung infections; constipation; fecal impaction; pressure sores; deep-vein blood clot; depression; limb deformities.

PROBABLE OUTCOME—Depends on the extent of injury. Damaged spinal cord and nerves are limited in their ability to recover.

HOW TO TREAT

GENERAL MEASURES—To learn more: Christopher & Dana Reeve Foundation, 636 Morris Turnpike, Suite 3A, Short Hills, NJ 07078; (800) 225-0292; website: www.christopherreeve.org.

MEDICATION
- Your health care provider may prescribe:
  - Antibiotics to treat infection.
  - Drugs to control hypertension, diabetes, or other underlying disorders.
  - Anticoagulants to prevent blood clot.
  - Stool softeners and laxatives.

ACTIVITY—Resume activities gradually to the extent possible. With rehabilitation, many lost functions can be compensated for or restored. Use passive exercise for paralyzed or partially paralyzed muscles to prevent contractures.

DIET
- Eat a high-fiber diet to prevent constipation.
- If you have a urinary catheter, drink plenty of fluids a day to help prevent any problems.

CALL YOUR DOCTOR IF

After diagnosis, any symptoms cause concern.

PARKINSON'S DISEASE

 GENERAL INFORMATION

DEFINITION—Parkinson's disease is a chronic, progressive disorder of the central nervous system. It affects the movements of the body. The name comes from the doctor who first described it. Parkinsonism is a general term used for movement disorders, of which Parkinson's disease is the most common.

BODY PARTS INVOLVED—Area of the brain that regulates movement; muscles.

SEX OR AGE MOST AFFECTED—Parkinson's usually starts after age 50, but can occur in younger adults. It affects males more often.

SIGNS & SYMPTOMS
- Tremors (they get worse with rest and better with moving).
- General muscle stiffness (rigidity).
- Slowness of movement. Shuffling, wide-based walk, and balance problems.
- Stooped posture. Loss of facial expression.
- Voice changes. It becomes weak and high pitched.
- Swallowing difficulty; drooling.
- Mental functioning can slowly decease.
- Handwriting is small, cramped, and shaky.
- Depression and nervousness.
- "Freezing" (sudden, but a temporary inability to move).

CAUSES—Dopamine is a brain chemical that helps control normal muscle movement. With Parkinson's disease, less dopamine is produced due to a loss of nerve cell function. It is unknown why this loss of nerve cell function occurs. It is thought to be a combination of genetic and environmental factors.

RISK INCREASES WITH
- Family history of Parkinson's.
- Older age; males more than females.
- Toxin exposure.

HOW TO PREVENT—No preventive measures.

 WHAT TO EXPECT

DIAGNOSTIC MEASURES
- Your own observation of symptoms.
- Your health care provider will do a physical exam and ask questions about your symptoms and activities. You may be asked to walk or do other physical tasks.
- There is not a specific test to diagnose the disorder. Medical tests may be done to rule out other disorders. If symptoms get better after taking the drug levodopa, it usually means a person has Parkinson's disease.

APPROPRIATE HEALTH CARE
- Treatment will vary for each person. It is based on a person's age, stage of the disease, and symptoms. Treatment options can include exercise, drug therapy, other special therapies, self-care, or surgery.
- Physical therapy, occupational therapy (help with daily activities), and speech therapy may be helpful.
- Surgery may be an option for severe symptoms or when drugs are not helping. It is not a cure, but it may relieve symptoms.
- Counseling can help treat emotional problems (e.g., depression, anxiety, stress, or anger).

POSSIBLE COMPLICATIONS—Weakness and loss of strength, balance difficulty, depression, sleep problems, urinary problems, weight loss, constipation, sexual dysfunction, side effects of drug therapy, or dementia.

PROBABLE OUTCOME—There is no cure. It is progressive, but unpredictable. There may be good days and bad days. Symptoms can generally be relieved or controlled with treatment.

 HOW TO TREAT

GENERAL MEASURES
- Accident-proof your home to help prevent falls and injuries. Install handrails, remove area rugs, keep cords out of the way. Carry a cell phone.
- Getting dressed can be a problem. Choose clothes that are easy to slip on. Wear clothes and shoes that have Velcro fasteners.
- To learn more: National Parkinson Foundation, 1501 NW 9th Ave., Miami, FL 33136; (800) 473-4636; website: www.parkinson.org.

MEDICATION
- One or more of a variety of drugs can be prescribed to treat the symptoms. Your health care provider will discuss the options and the risks and benefits. If one does not help, stops being effective, or has side effects, others can be tried.
- Vitamins or supplements may be prescribed.

ACTIVITY—Exercises will help maintain mobility, balance, range of motion, and well-being. Follow instructions from your physical therapist or health care provider.

DIET—Eat a healthy diet. Add fiber to the diet and increase fluid intake to prevent constipation. If chewing is a problem, take small bites, eat slowly, and chop up food.

 CALL YOUR DOCTOR IF

- You or a family member has symptoms of Parkinson's disease.
- After diagnosis, any symptoms cause concern.

PARONYCHIA

GENERAL INFORMATION

DEFINITION—Paronychia is an inflammation of tissue folds that surround a nail. The inflammation is usually due to an infection, and is not contagious. It may be acute (rapid onset) or chronic (develops gradually).

BODY PARTS INVOLVED—It usually occurs on fingernails and less often on toenails.

SEX OR AGE MOST AFFECTED—Both sexes; all ages.

SIGNS & SYMPTOMS
- Acute paronychia:
  - Pain or tenderness, redness, warmth, and swelling of tissue along the edge of the nail.
  - Central whitish area produced by pus.
- Chronic paronychia:
  - Usually affects more than one nail.
  - Nail fold may be lifted off nailplate.
  - May be red, swollen, and have pus.
  - Nails may have ridges and be greenish.

CAUSES
- Acute type is preceded by injury, such as a torn hangnail. The infecting bacteria are usually *Staphylococcus.* Less often, it is caused by a fungus or yeast infection.
- Chronic type can be due to different infections or irritants.

RISK INCREASES WITH
- Injury around the fingernail.
- Hands are exposed to constant wetness (dishwashers, bartenders, housewives, or swimmers).
- Diabetes.
- Nail biting or finger sucking.
- Artificial nails.
- Ingrown toenail.
- Manicure procedures.
- Shoes that bind or pinch the toes.
- Certain drugs may lead to chronic paronychia.

HOW TO PREVENT
- Protect hands from wetness.
- Leave hangnails alone.
- Avoid fingertip injury.
- Avoid tight shoes.
- Do not trim or push back nail cuticles.
- Use care when trimming nails.

WHAT TO EXPECT

DIAGNOSTIC MEASURES
- Your own observation of symptoms.
- Your health care provider will do an exam of the affected nail.
- Medical studies, such as a culture of the discharge (pus), may be done to identify the germ.

APPROPRIATE HEALTH CARE
- Treatment involves avoiding factors that may be the cause, self-care, drug therapy, or surgery.
- If an abscess (pus-filled area) occurs, it may require incision (cutting) and drainage. Other surgery may be needed if acute paronychia does not heal with drug therapy.
- Treatment for chronic paronychia may include topical or oral drugs or surgery. It is somewhat difficult to treat and treatment can be prolonged.

POSSIBLE COMPLICATIONS
- If untreated, may permanently damage the fingernail and nail bed. Rarely, the infection may enter bone or bloodstream.
- Nail may separate from nailbed.

PROBABLE OUTCOME
- Acute paronychia is usually curable with treatment in a week to 10 days.
- Chronic paronychia is slow to heal and treatment can take weeks or months.

HOW TO TREAT

GENERAL MEASURES
- Wear vinyl gloves with cotton lining to prevent contact with water, irritating substances, or foods.
- Wear cotton, leather, or heavy-duty fabric gloves for housework or gardening.
- Use warm-water soaks several times a day for acute paronychia.
- Use mild soap or alcohol-based hand cleaner to clean hands. Use a cream, lotion, or gel for dry hands or feet.
- Avoid all nail products until healed.
- Protect hands from chapping in cold weather.

MEDICATION
- For minor pain, you may use nonprescription drugs, such as ibuprofen or acetaminophen.
- A topical antibiotic cream or lotion may be prescribed. An oral antibiotic may be needed for severe cases.
- Topical steroids may be prescribed.
- Topical antifungals may be prescribed for fungal infection. An oral antifungal may be needed for severe cases.

ACTIVITY—No limits.

DIET—No special diet.

CALL YOUR DOCTOR IF

- You or a family member has symptoms of paronychia.
- The disorder is not helped with treatment.

PATELLOFEMORAL PAIN SYNDROME

GENERAL INFORMATION

DEFINITION—Patellofemoral pain syndrome (PFPS) is a common cause of pain in the front (anterior) of the knee. The name refers to the knee joint that includes the patella (kneecap) and the femur (thigh bone). It can affect just about anyone. It occurs more often in physically active people (e.g., runners).

BODY PARTS INVOLVED—Knee.

SEX OR AGE MOST AFFECTED—It affects women more than men and ages under 40.

SIGNS & SYMPTOMS
- Pain that usually comes on gradually and may be under, behind, or around the kneecap. It can affect one or both knees. The pain may be described as aching, dull, sharp, shooting, or burning. It may last a few minutes, hours, or be chronic.
- Pain may occur during and after physical activity or when going up and down (more likely) steps or hills.
- Pain may occur with long periods of sitting with bent knees (e.g., watching a movie or airplane trip) or when kneeling or squatting.
- There may be a feeling that the knee might give out from under you or the knee may lock up.
- Other symptoms can include popping, clicking, or grinding sounds, or snapping sensation in the knee.

CAUSES—The exact cause is unclear. It is likely due to an imbalance in muscles, knee bones that are not aligned the right way, and overuse of the knee joint.

RISK INCREASES WITH
- Overtraining or overuse in a sports or fitness activity (too much, too soon, or too fast).
- Injury (such as from a fall).
- Prior knee surgery (such as for torn ligament).
- Some people are born with slightly misaligned bones or imbalanced muscles and may be more at risk. There is no simple and sure method to identify who may have these conditions.

HOW TO PREVENT
- In many cases, it cannot be prevented.
- You can reduce your risks. Stay in shape. Increase a new sport or fitness activity gradually. Use proper form for the activity and use or wear proper gear. Replace running shoes on a regular basis. Vary your workout intensity. Cross-train with a low impact activity.
- Arch supports or shoe inserts (foot orthotics) may be of help in some cases. Ask your health care provider.

WHAT TO EXPECT

DIAGNOSTIC MEASURES
- Your own observation of symptoms.
- Most often, your health care provider can diagnose PFPS during an office visit. Questions will be asked about your pain symptoms, physical activities, and your medical history. Your knee and the muscles of your leg will be examined. You may be asked to stand, sit, walk, jump, squat, lie down, or do other leg motions to see how the knee is functioning.
- In some cases, x-rays and other imaging studies are done to check for any knee damage or rule out other knee disorders.

APPROPRIATE HEALTH CARE
- There is no quick cure for the pain. Your health care provider will discuss a treatment plan with you. It depends on any physical problem found (such as weak muscles), severity of pain, your age and health, and your normal level and type of physical activity.
- A knee sleeve or brace, taping of the knee, or shoe inserts (orthotics) may be helpful.
- Rarely, surgery is an option if pain persists.

POSSIBLE COMPLICATIONS—Patellofemoral pain may recur or become chronic. It may lead to difficulty with daily activities.

PROBABLE OUTCOME—Most symptoms of patellofemoral pain clear up with time and treatment. It may take weeks or months.

HOW TO TREAT

GENERAL MEASURES—For self-care, icing the knee (for 10–15 minutes, 4–6 times a day) can help relieve pain.

MEDICATION—Nonprescription pain drugs may be used if needed.

ACTIVITY
- Avoid any activity that worsens the pain.
- You may be advised to stop or decrease your sports or fitness activities (such as running). Try low impact exercises (e.g., swimming or elliptical machine). Slowly resume your previous activity once pain eases up.
- Physical therapy may be prescribed. It can help improve muscle strength and flexibility.
- Exercises to do at home will be prescribed.

DIET—Eat a healthy diet.

☎ CALL YOUR DOCTOR IF

- You or a family member has symptoms of patellofemoral pain syndrome.
- Symptoms don't improve with treatment.

PELVIC INFLAMMATORY DISEASE

 GENERAL INFORMATION

DEFINITION—Pelvic inflammatory disease (PID) is an infection of the upper genital area (fallopian tubes, ovaries, and uterus). PID is one of the most common and serious complications of sexually transmitted diseases (STDs) in women. Up to 40% of untreated genital infections progress to PID. Salpingitis (fallopian tube inflammation) is another term for PID.

BODY PARTS INVOLVED—Fallopian tubes; cervix; uterus; ovaries; urinary bladder.

SEX OR AGE MOST AFFECTED—Sexually active females after puberty. The peak incidence occurs in late teens and early 20s.

SIGNS & SYMPTOMS
- Some women have no symptoms.
- Pain or cramps in the lower abdomen.
- Vaginal discharge (may have a foul odor).
- Painful intercourse or pain when urinating.
- Irregular menstrual bleeding.
- Fever, nausea, and vomiting.

CAUSES—Bacterial infection (usually chlamydial or gonorrheal). The bacteria infection starts in the vagina and cervix and then spreads to the upper genital area. PID usually develops from 2 days to 3 weeks after exposure to the bacteria, but can take months to develop. The infection may be transmitted by an infected sexual partner.

RISK INCREASES WITH
- Women who have a sexually transmitted disease.
- Teenagers (more at risk than older women).
- Multiple sexual partners, or exposure to a single partner who is infected.
- Use of an intrauterine contraceptive device (IUD).
- Prior episode of PID.
- Abortion.
- Pelvic surgery.
- Women who douche once or twice a month. This may push bacteria into the upper genital area.

HOW TO PREVENT
- Use latex (rubber) condoms to help prevent sexually transmitted infections.
- Oral contraceptives may help to decrease the risk.
- Get routine medical check-ups for sexually transmitted diseases if you have multiple sexual partners.
- Get medical care for abnormal vaginal discharge, unusual odor, fever, and bleeding between periods.
- Have your sexual partner tested and treated if needed. Don't resume sexual activity with your partner until tests show no infection, or it has been treated.

 WHAT TO EXPECT

DIAGNOSTIC MEASURES
- Your health care provider will do a physical and a pelvic exam.
- Medical tests may include blood studies, culture of the vaginal discharge, and a pregnancy test. Other tests may be done to confirm the diagnosis and rule out other disorders.

APPROPRIATE HEALTH CARE
- Treatment is with drugs.
- Most women can be treated as outpatients. It is important to follow your treatment schedule. Close medical follow-up care is needed.
- Hospital care may be needed for severe illness, more diagnostic tests, an abscess, pregnancy, if drugs are to be given in a vein (IV), and other reasons.
- Surgery to drain a pelvic abscess may be done.
- Surgery may help chronic PID or pelvic pain.
- Counseling can be helpful if infertility occurs.

POSSIBLE COMPLICATIONS
- Chronic pelvic pain.
- Infertility or ectopic pregnancy.
- Recurrent PID.
- Abscess (pus-filled pocket). It can be life threatening.

PROBABLE OUTCOME—With early diagnosis and treatment, most women recover with no complications. Late treatment or incomplete treatment can lead to serious complications.

 HOW TO TREAT

GENERAL MEASURES
- If you have a sexually transmitted disease (STD), your partner needs treatment (even if he has no symptoms).
- Use sanitary pads to absorb the discharge or menstrual flow. Don't douche during treatment.
- To learn more: Centers for Disease Control; (800) 232-4636; website: www.cdc.gov/std.

MEDICATION—Antibiotics (by injection or taken by mouth) for bacterial infection will be prescribed. Finish taking the entire drug course prescribed to be sure of a complete cure.

ACTIVITY—Avoid sexual intercourse until you and your sexual partner complete treatment.

DIET—No special diet.

☎ CALL YOUR DOCTOR IF

- You or a family member has symptoms of pelvic inflammatory disease.
- Fever, pelvic pain, or abnormal vaginal discharge occurs after treatment.

PENILE CANCER

GENERAL INFORMATION

DEFINITION—Penile cancer is cancer of the penis. It is a rare type of cancer.

BODY PARTS INVOLVED—Penis, including the glans (tip), corona (rounded border of the glans) or prepuce (foreskin covering the glans).

SEX OR AGE MOST AFFECTED—Men over age 50.

SIGNS & SYMPTOMS
- A small, circular lesion (resembles a pimple) or persistent, painless sore on the penis. The lesion is easily visible in a circumcised male, but it may go unnoticed in an uncircumcised male.
- Pain, bleeding, or discharge.
- Discomfort with urination.
- Enlarged lymph nodes in the groin.

CAUSES—Unknown. A human papillomavirus (HPV) may play a role in the cause. The virus can be sexually transmitted.

RISK INCREASES WITH
- Phimosis (inability to retract the foreskin over the glans).
- Smegma (thick, sometimes smelly substance that builds up under an intact foreskin).
- Lack of circumcision at birth.
- Cigarette smoking.
- HPV infection. Risk of infection increases with: starting sexual activity at early age, having many sexual partners, having sex with person who has many partners, or having unprotected sex.
- AIDS (acquired immunodeficiency syndrome).
- Psoriasis (skin disorder) treatment that uses drugs along with ultraviolet light.

HOW TO PREVENT
- No specific preventive measures. Avoid risk factors where possible. Practice good genital hygiene to reduce risks of infection or irritation. If uncircumcised, retract the foreskin and clean the entire penis when bathing.
- Do a self-exam of the penis and testicles monthly. This can help detect cancers early, when treatment is most successful. See your health care provider for any sign of infection or sores on the penis.
- Practice safe sex.
- Circumcision appears to reduce the risk if it is done shortly after birth. It offers little or no prevention when done in an adult.

WHAT TO EXPECT

DIAGNOSTIC MEASURES
- Your own observation of symptoms.
- Your health care provider will do a physical exam of the penis and ask questions about symptoms.
- A number of medical tests will be done. The tests help to diagnose the cancer and then determine if it has spread (staging).

APPROPRIATE HEALTH CARE
- Treatment varies and depends on the location and size of tumor, any spread of the cancer, health, age, and preferences. Treatment may include surgery, radiotherapy, or chemotherapy (anticancer drugs).
- Surgery is usually the main treatment.
  - With early diagnosis, it may involve just removing the tumor. Different surgical procedures are available.
  - Circumcision is done for cancer of the foreskin.
  - Invasive tumors may require part or total removal of the penis (penectomy). If needed, a new opening is created for urine to exit the body. Penis reconstruction may be an option.
  - Lymph nodes may be removed if cancer has spread.
- Radiation therapy may be used to kill cancer cells.
- Treatment may involve steps to relieve symptoms and make you comfortable, rather than treating the cancer.
- Counseling may help you cope with cancer.

POSSIBLE COMPLICATIONS—Men may delay treatment due to denial, embarrassment, fear of surgery, and loss of sexual function. A delay increases risk of the cancer spreading.

PROBABLE OUTCOME—Will depend on the extent of the cancer at diagnosis. Early diagnosis and treatment has a more favorable outcome. Recurrence is possible.

HOW TO TREAT

GENERAL MEASURES—To learn more: American Cancer Society; (800) ACS-2345; website: www.cancer.org or National Cancer Institute; (800) 4-CANCER; website: www.cancer.gov.

MEDICATION—Anticancer drugs may be prescribed. They may be used on the skin, taken by mouth, or given by injection.

ACTIVITY—Resume normal activities as soon as possible after treatment. Sexual relations are possible if enough penile tissue remains after surgery. If the total penis is removed, sexual pleasure is still possible using special techniques.

DIET—No special diet.

CALL YOUR DOCTOR IF

- You or a family member has penis symptoms.
- Symptoms after treatment cause concern.

PERICARDITIS

GENERAL INFORMATION

DEFINITION—Pericarditis is an inflammation of the pericardium. The pericardium is a sac (thin membrane) around the heart. It has two layers, with a small amount of "lubricating" fluid between them. The fluid lets the heart move around within the sac. With inflammation, the heart can become squeezed inside the sac.

BODY PARTS INVOLVED—Pericardium.

SEX OR AGE MOST AFFECTED—Both sexes; all ages (more often in men ages 20 to 50).

SIGNS & SYMPTOMS
- Usually a sharp, stabbing pain in the front of the chest. In some, the pain may be dull and achy. The pain moves to the neck, arm, and shoulder. The pain worsens with breathing and movement and eases when sitting up or leaning forward.
- Rapid breathing.
- Cough.
- Fever, sweating, and chills.
- Weakness.
- Anxiety.
- Pain with swallowing.

CAUSES—The inflammation is a reaction to injury, infection, or irritation of the heart lining. It can be caused by a number of different factors or the cause may be unknown.

RISK INCREASES WITH
- Males and ages 20 to 50.
- Autoimmune disorders, such as rheumatoid arthritis or lupus erythematosus.
- Complication of a heart attack.
- Complication following heart surgery.
- Complication of a chest injury.
- Viral, bacterial, tuberculous, amebic, toxoplasmotic, or fungal infection.
- Chronic kidney failure or dialysis.
- Spread of cancer to the pericardium.
- Radiation therapy.

HOW TO PREVENT—No specific preventive measures. To avoid risk factors, get treatment for disorders that may lead to pericarditis.

WHAT TO EXPECT

DIAGNOSTIC MEASURES
- Your own observation of symptoms.
- Your health care provider will do a physical exam and ask questions about your symptoms and activities.
- Medical tests may include blood studies, chest x-ray, heart tests (electrocardiogram and echocardiogram), and others.

APPROPRIATE HEALTH CARE
- Treatment is aimed at relieving symptoms and treating the underlying disorder. Treatment may include drugs and, sometimes, hospital care.
- Hospital care may be needed if there are complications. A needle may be used to draw off excess fluid if it is causing problems for heart function. Rarely, surgery may be needed on the pericardium.

POSSIBLE COMPLICATIONS
- Pericarditis becomes chronic if it lasts for 6 to 12 months following the initial (acute) episode.
- Excess fluid in the pericardium affects heart function.
- Pericardium becomes thick and scarred.
- Blood circulation problems.

PROBABLE OUTCOME—Usually curable with treatment. Allow 2 to 3 weeks for healing. It may recur in the next 6 to 12 months. In some cases, the outcome depends on underlying cause.

HOW TO TREAT

GENERAL MEASURES
- Apply a heating pad or warm compresses to the chest to relieve pain.
- To learn more: American Heart Association, 7272 Greenville Ave., Dallas, TX 75231; (800) 242-8721; website: www.americanheart.org.

MEDICATION
- Aspirin or other nonsteroidal anti-inflammatory drugs to reduce pain and inflammation are usually prescribed.
- Colchicine is often prescribed to reduce inflammation.
- Steroid drugs may be prescribed.
- Stronger pain drugs may be prescribed.
- Drugs to treat any infection (bacterial, fungal, etc.) will be prescribed.

ACTIVITY
- Get extra rest until fever and pain subside.
- Resume your normal activities gradually.
- Avoid strenuous exercise until advised.
- Athletes need to follow medical advice as to when to resume sports activities.
- Follow medical advice about when to resume sexual relations.

DIET—No special diet.

CALL YOUR DOCTOR IF

- You or a family member has symptoms of pericarditis.
- The following occur during treatment: fever, shortness of breath and rapid heartbeat, cough (with blood), unexplained weight loss, or increased pain.

PERIMENOPAUSE

Celina

GENERAL INFORMATION

DEFINITION—Perimenopause is the normal time in a woman's life that leads up to menopause. It may last 1 to 10 years (average about 4 to 5 years) and ends one year after your last period. Your body's hormone production starts to decrease and brings about changes (or symptoms). Symptoms will vary in each woman and may be mild to more severe. A woman can still become pregnant during perimenopause.

BODY PARTS INVOLVED—Female reproductive system and other body parts.

SEX OR AGE MOST AFFECTED—Females; average age of menopause is 51.

SIGNS & SYMPTOMS
- Hot flashes and night sweats.
- Tender breasts.
- Fatigue.
- Irregular periods. May have heavy bleeding.
- Trouble sleeping.
- Memory problems (fuzzy thinking) or forgetful.
- Mood swings, depressed, worried, or irritable.
- Hair loss or thinning. Skin dryness.
- Decreased libido (sex drive).
- Vaginal dryness; discomfort during sex.
- Weight gain (e.g., around the waist).
- Urinary tract infections.

CAUSES
- As a woman ages, hormone production begins to change. Ovaries produce less estrogen and progesterone. Eggs may not be released during a period. Estrogen levels can sharply rise and then quickly drop. Menstrual periods become shorter and more and more irregular until they stop.
- A woman who has a hysterectomy, but keeps her ovaries will have perimenopause. If the ovaries are removed surgically, menopause occurs right away. Other medical treatments may also lead to menopause.

RISK INCREASES WITH—Perimenopause may start early for some women (e.g., smokers, having a family history of early menopause, childhood cancer therapy, and possibly, others).

HOW TO PREVENT—It is a natural part of the aging process for women.

WHAT TO EXPECT

DIAGNOSTIC MEASURES
- Your own observation of symptoms.
- Your health care provider will ask questions about your medical and menstrual history and your symptoms and body changes. A diagnosis of perimenopause is often based on your age and your symptoms.
- Blood tests may be done to check hormone levels and thyroid function. Hormones go up and down during perimenopause so they may be tested at different times for comparison.

APPROPRIATE HEALTH CARE—Treatment may not be needed for mild symptoms. Drugs may be prescribed for problem symptoms.

POSSIBLE COMPLICATIONS
- Menstrual bleeding that may be abnormal (extremely heavy, lasting longer than 8 days, or occurs between periods).
- Decreasing fertility if you are trying to get pregnant.

PROBABLE OUTCOME—Most women will transition to menopause without any major problems. Uncomfortable symptoms can be relieved with treatment.

HOW TO TREAT

GENERAL MEASURES
- Make healthy lifestyle choices to help with symptoms of perimenopause. These include eating healthy, daily exercise, keeping a healthy weight, and reducing stress. If you smoke, stop. Avoid heavy alcohol use. Lifestyle changes can promote good health as you age.
- To learn more: North American Menopause Society, 5900 Landerbrook Dr., Ste 390, Mayfield Heights, OH 44124; (440) 442-7550 (not toll-free); website: www.menopause.org.

MEDICATION
- Low-dose birth control pills may be prescribed for some women to help relieve symptoms.
- Other drugs may be prescribed for certain symptoms.
- Calcium and vitamin D supplements may be recommended.
- Talk to your health care provider before using herbal supplements for symptom relief.

ACTIVITY
- Try to get 30 minutes a day (or most days) of aerobic exercise, such as walking. Start with a few minutes a day and increase gradually.
- Resistance exercise (weightlifting) will help build muscle and prevent bone loss as you get older.

DIET—Control your weight with a healthy diet. A weight-loss diet may be recommended if overweight is a problem.

CALL YOUR DOCTOR IF

- You or a family member has symptoms of perimenopause that cause concern.
- Symptoms don't improve with treatment.

PERIODONTITIS
(Gum Inflammation)

GENERAL INFORMATION

DEFINITION—Periodontitis is an inflammation and infection of the gums, causing loss of bone around the teeth. It is responsible for more tooth loss than tooth decay.

BODY PARTS INVOLVED—Gums; jaw bones.

SEX OR AGE MOST AFFECTED—Both sexes; usually adults over age 20.

SIGNS & SYMPTOMS
- There may be no symptoms.
- Gums may be swollen, red or purple, or tender.
- Gums may pull away from teeth.
- Unpleasant taste in the mouth and bad breath.
- Bleeding of the gums.
- Loosening of teeth in the sockets.
- Aching teeth and gums when eating hot, cold, or sweet food.

CAUSES—Plaque (a sticky deposit of food, bacteria, and mucus) builds up on the teeth. It turns hard and becomes tartar (calculus). Bacteria in the plaque and tartar can cause a gum inflammation called gingivitis. If untreated, gingivitis spreads to the bones that support the teeth causing periodontitis. Pockets of infection occur around the roots of the teeth.

RISK INCREASES WITH
- Poor dental hygiene.
- Weak immune system due to illness or drugs.
- Smoking.
- Certain drugs.
- Changes in hormones (e.g., with pregnancy).
- Diabetes and other diseases.
- Poor nutrition (not eating a healthy diet).
- Family history of gum disease.
- Clenching or grinding teeth.
- Older age.
- Substance abuse.

HOW TO PREVENT
- Maintain good oral hygiene.
  - Brush teeth twice a day or after each meal. Use a soft bristle toothbrush or a power toothbrush. A fluoride toothpaste is often recommended.
  - Floss teeth at least once a day with waxed or unwaxed dental floss or use an interdental cleaner. An oral irrigator may be used in addition to flossing.
  - A tongue scraper can be used to clean tongue.
  - Use an antiseptic mouthwash if desired.
  - Dental check-ups and cleaning every six months; more often if you are prone to plaque or gingivitis.
- Control chronic medical problems (e.g., diabetes).

- Do not smoke.
- Eat a healthy diet. Avoid snacks and junk foods packed with sugar.

WHAT TO EXPECT

DIAGNOSTIC MEASURES
- Your own observation of symptoms.
- Your dental care provider will do an exam of the teeth, gums, and supporting bones.
- X-rays may be done to check for bone loss.

APPROPRIATE HEALTH CARE
- Treatment may involve correcting dental problems, scaling, planing, and surgery. Your dental care provider will discuss a treatment plan with you.
- Dental work may be done for rough or jagged teeth.
- Dental appliances may need to be repaired.
- Scaling and root planing involves cleaning of deep pockets and smoothing roots of the teeth.
- Gum surgery may be needed. Pockets of infection may need to be cut open and cleaned. Loose teeth may need to be removed. Bone and tissue grafts may be needed to help support the teeth.
- Dental implants may be an option for lost teeth.

POSSIBLE COMPLICATIONS
- Without treatment, teeth loosen so much that they may fall out or need to be removed.
- Recurrence of periodontitis.
- Tooth abscess (pus-filled area).
- Mouth infections.

PROBABLE OUTCOME—Usually curable with a combination of dental treatment and maintaining a good oral hygiene program.

HOW TO TREAT

GENERAL MEASURES—To learn more: American Dental Association, 211 E. Chicago Ave., Chicago, IL 60611-2678; (312) 440-2500 (not toll-free); website: www.ada.org.

MEDICATION
- For minor pain, you may use nonprescription drugs such as acetaminophen.
- Antibiotics may be prescribed for infection.

ACTIVITY—No limits.

DIET—No special diet.

CALL YOUR DENTIST IF

You or a family member has symptoms of periodontitis.

PERIPHERAL NEUROPATHY

 GENERAL INFORMATION

DEFINITION
• Peripheral neuropathy is a term used for disorders (e.g., damaged nerves) of the peripheral nervous system (PNS). This system is made up of nerves that branch out of the spinal cord and go to all parts of the body. There are three types of PNS nerves with different functions:
- Sensory (feeling pain, temperature, and touch).
- Motor (voluntary movement as with the muscles).
- Autonomic (involuntary functions, such as breathing, blood pressure, sexual function, and digestion).

BODY PARTS INVOLVED—The symptoms
often affect fingers, toes, hands, feet, lower arms, or legs, and also bladder or bowel control.

SEX OR AGE MOST AFFECTED—Adults of both sexes.

SIGNS & SYMPTOMS
• Sensory nerve symptoms: Burning, tingling, numbness, or cold feeling in arm or leg. Painless injuries. Over-sensitive to touch. Loss of feeling.
• Motor nerve symptoms: Difficulty using hands to hold something or to write or button clothes. Tripping or problem lifting foot or toes. Problems using stairs or rising up from a chair. Knees give away and cause falls.
• Autonomic nerve symptoms: Unusual sweating, dizziness upon standing, urinary changes, or constipation. Men or women may have sexual problems.

CAUSES—Damage may be from nerve
destruction, pressure, or degeneration. The damage may be to one nerve or nerve group. Nerves become damaged due to a number of causes. Sometimes, no cause is found.

RISK INCREASES WITH
• Adults over 60.
• Diabetes or shingles (post-herpetic neuralgia).
• Exposure to certain chemicals or toxic substances.
• Certain drugs.
• Poor nutrition (not eating a healthy diet).
• Alcoholism.
• Family history of neuropathies.
• Nerve disorders or injury; pressure on nerves.
• Autoimmune disorder or connective tissue disease.
• Infections, kidney or liver failure, and some cancers.
• Bone fractures or herniated disc.
• Some hereditary disorders.

HOW TO PREVENT—No specific preventive
measures. Avoid risk factors where possible.

 WHAT TO EXPECT

DIAGNOSTIC MEASURES
• Your own observation of symptoms.
• Your health care provider will do a physical exam and ask questions about your symptoms and activities.
• Medical tests may be done to discover any underlying medical disorder.

APPROPRIATE HEALTH CARE
• The most important aspect of treatment is to identify and treat any underlying cause.
• Other treatments may include drugs, physical and occupational therapy, diet and exercise, assistive devices, relaxation techniques (such as biofeedback training), transcutaneous electrical nerve stimulation (TENS), surgery to relieve pressure, and others.
• Your health care provider will discuss your diagnosis and a specific treatment plan with you. No one treatment works for everyone.

POSSIBLE COMPLICATIONS—Complications
can cause chronic pain, disability, and may sometimes be life-threatening.

PROBABLE OUTCOME—It will depend on the
cause and treatment. Symptoms may improve come and go, stay the same, or worsen in time.

 HOW TO TREAT

GENERAL MEASURES—For self-care: Inspect
hands and feet daily for unnoticed wounds. Keep feet clean and toenails trimmed properly. Wear shoes that fit well. Take measures to make your home a safe place for you.

MEDICATION
• For minor pain, use nonprescription ibuprofen or acetaminophen. Other pain drugs may be prescribed.
• A variety of drugs can be used to treat the symptoms. Your health care provider will discuss the options and the risks and benefits.
• Drugs to treat underlying disorder may be prescribed.

ACTIVITY—Physical therapy and exercises to
do at home may be recommended. If you have difficulty maintaining balance, walk with a cane or other support.

DIET
• If poor nutrition is a cause, eat a healthy diet.
• Avoid or limit alcohol use.

 CALL YOUR DOCTOR IF

• You have symptoms of peripheral neuropathy.
• After diagnosis, any symptoms cause concern.

PERIPHERAL VASCULAR DISEASE
(Peripheral Artery Disease)

 GENERAL INFORMATION

DEFINITION—Peripheral vascular disease refers to disorders of the blood vessels outside the heart and brain. Most often, it involves the arteries and is called peripheral artery disease (PAD). In PAD, the arteries become clogged or blocked and normal blood flow is slowed or stopped. It typically affects the legs.

BODY PARTS INVOLVED—Arteries that carry oxygen- and nutrient-rich blood from the heart to the arms, legs, stomach, and kidneys.

SEX OR AGE MOST AFFECTED—Both sexes; men a little more than women; ages over 50.

SIGNS & SYMPTOMS
- In some cases, there will be no symptoms.
- Pain, cramping, ache, heaviness, or tired sensation in muscles of the affected area (usually legs). It may involve one or both calves, thighs, or hips.
- Early on, the symptoms occur while walking or climbing stairs and stop when resting.
- As disease worsens, symptoms may occur all the time (even at rest).
- Leg and foot may feel numb and cold.
- May have sores on legs that don't heal and may lose hair on legs and feet.
- Erectile dysfunction in males.

CAUSES—Atherosclerosis (hardening of the arteries). It develops when fatty material (called plaque) builds up inside the arteries. Other causes are rare.

RISK INCREASES WITH
- Ages over 50.
- Overweight or obesity; inactive (sedentary) lifestyle; smoking.
- Diabetes.
- High blood pressure.
- High LDL (bad cholesterol), plus high triglycerides, and low HDL (good cholesterol).
- Personal or family history of coronary heart disease, heart attack, or stroke.

HOW TO PREVENT
- Get medical treatment for any disorder that could lead to atherosclerosis.
- Don't smoke, do eat healthy, be active and exercise regularly, and maintain healthy weight.

 WHAT TO EXPECT

DIAGNOSTIC MEASURES
- Your health care provider will do a physical exam and ask questions about your symptoms and activities. Blood pressures in your ankles and arms may be taken and compared to find the ankle-brachial index, (ABI).
- Medical tests may include blood tests, angiography, arteriography, ultrasound, CT, MRA, and others if needed.

APPROPRIATE HEALTH CARE
- Treatment depends on the underlying cause, severity of your condition, and overall health. The goals are to improve symptoms and reduce risk of complications. Treatment options can include lifestyle changes, drugs, medical procedures, and/or surgery.
- Lifestyle changes will be prescribed (e.g., weight loss, no smoking, and regular exercise).
- Medical procedures or surgery may include: angioplasty (enlarges artery), stenting (for severely blocked artery), atherectomy (removal of plaque in artery), or bypass surgery.

POSSIBLE COMPLICATIONS
- Permanent numbness, weakness, and pain in legs or feet.
- Poor circulation makes infections hard to treat.
- Gangrene (tissues die due to lack of blood). Treatment is amputation of affected body part.
- Higher risk of heart attack and stroke.

PROBABLE OUTCOME—The outcome will vary depending on each individual's situation. PAD can't be cured, but it can often be controlled if your treatment plan is followed.

 HOW TO TREAT

GENERAL MEASURES
- Stop smoking. Find a way to quit.
- To learn more: American Heart Association, 7272 Greenville Ave., Dallas, TX 75231; (800) 242-8721; website: www.americanheart.org.

MEDICATION—Drugs may be prescribed to treat underlying causes, for pain, to prevent blood clots or clumping of platelets, to improve blood flow, or to dilate blood vessels. Get medical advice before taking any supplements.

ACTIVITY
- Regular physical activity will be prescribed. You and your health care provider will plan a program (e.g., walking and leg exercises). The program may be supervised at a special facility or done at home.
- A walking program may have you walk until pain occurs, then rest. You will slowly build up the time you can walk before pain occurs.

DIET—A low-fat diet may be recommended. A weight loss diet will be prescribed if overweight.

 CALL YOUR DOCTOR IF

You or a family member has symptoms of, or concerns about, peripheral vascular disease.

PERITONITIS

GENERAL INFORMATION

DEFINITION—Peritonitis is a serious inflammation of part or all of the lining of the abdominal cavity (peritoneum).

BODY PARTS INVOLVED—The abdominal cavity contains such organs as the stomach, intestines, spleen, gallbladder, liver, appendix, kidneys, and pancreas.

SEX OR AGE MOST AFFECTED—Both sexes; all ages.

SIGNS & SYMPTOMS
- Pain in one area of, or all through, the abdomen. Pain usually starts suddenly and becomes more severe with time. Pain may be cramp-like at first and then steady. The patient often prefers to lie quietly on the back because movement or pressure on the abdomen increases pain.
- Shoulder pain (sometimes).
- Chills and fever (often high).
- Dizziness and weakness.
- Rapid heartbeat and rapid breathing.
- Low blood pressure.
- Nausea and vomiting.

CAUSES—The inflammation is a reaction to infection (most often), injury, or irritation of the abdominal lining. Primary (or spontaneous) peritonitis is rare. Secondary peritonitis is caused by other medical conditions.

RISK INCREASES WITH
- Infection inside the abdomen (e.g., appendicitis or bowel infection).
- Inflammation of the stomach, gallbladder, or pancreas.
- Penetrating injury to the abdominal wall, such as from a knife or bullet wound.
- Peptic ulcer.
- Pelvic inflammatory disease.
- Rupture of an ectopic pregnancy.
- Recent abdominal surgery.
- Bowel obstruction.
- Advanced liver disease.
- Hernia.
- Tuberculosis.
- Ovarian cyst or abscess.

HOW TO PREVENT—No specific preventive measures. Get medical treatment for any disorder that could lead to peritonitis.

WHAT TO EXPECT

DIAGNOSTIC MEASURES
- Your health care provider will do a physical exam and ask questions about your symptoms.
- Blood tests, x-rays, and other medical tests are usually done to help diagnose the underlying disorder.

APPROPRIATE HEALTH CARE
- Hospital care is needed to treat this condition and any underlying disorder. You may require treatment for dehydration, breathing support, drugs injected into a vein (IV), blood transfusions, and surgery.
- Surgery may be needed to help diagnose the cause of the inflammation, and repair organ damage or injury.

POSSIBLE COMPLICATIONS
- Shock.
- Blood poisoning (septicemia).
- Intestinal obstruction caused by adhesions (bands of scar tissue).
- Kidney or liver failure.

PROBABLE OUTCOME—Usually curable with early diagnosis and treatment. Treatment delay and complications can be fatal. Outcome depends on age, length of illness, cause, and any pre-existing condition(s).

HOW TO TREAT

GENERAL MEASURES—Early diagnosis and treatment of the underlying disorder, such as appendicitis, ulcer or ectopic pregnancy, are essential. If abdominal pain develops, don't waste valuable time with home treatments—especially laxative use. Laxatives may cause inflamed abdominal organs to rupture.

MEDICATION
- Antibiotics to fight infection are usually prescribed.
- Pain relievers (sometimes) after diagnosis or surgery.

ACTIVITY—Rest in bed, after treatment, until symptoms disappear. If surgery is needed, resume your activities gradually after surgery.

DIET—While in the hospital, fluids and nutrients may be given through a vein. Oral feedings will resume when your gastrointestinal system can tolerate them.

CALL YOUR DOCTOR IF

- You or a family member has symptoms of peritonitis. This is an emergency! Early diagnosis and treatment of the underlying disorder are essential.
- Any new symptoms occur after treatment.

PERSONALITY DISORDERS

GENERAL INFORMATION

DEFINITION—Personality disorders are a group of conditions that are not illnesses, but ways of behaving. Each condition is defined by its main symptoms. Persons with these conditions have patterns of abnormal behavior, thought, and emotion. These patterns interfere with daily activity, personal relationships, and social and work functioning. The person feels their behavior patterns are "normal" and "right."

SEX OR AGE MOST AFFECTED—Both sexes; all ages.

SIGNS & SYMPTOMS
- Paranoid: shows unwarranted suspiciousness and distrust of others; is defensive, oversensitive, angers easily.
- Schizoid and schizotypal: cold (emotionally); has difficulty forming relationships; is withdrawn, shy, superstitious, or socially isolated.
- Compulsive—perfectionist, rigid in habits, indecisive; needs control.
- Histrionic—dependent, immature, excitable, vain; constantly craves stimulation and attention; communicates by appearances or behavior (not verbally).
- Narcissistic: has an exaggerated sense of one's own importance; is preoccupied with power; lacks interest in others; demands attention; feels entitled to special consideration.
- Avoidant: fears and overreacts to rejection; has low self-esteem; is socially withdrawn; dependent.
- Dependent: passive, over-accepting, unable to make decisions; lacks confidence.
- Passive-aggressive—stubborn, sulking; fears authority; procrastinates; is chronically late, argumentative, helpless, clinging.
- Antisocial: selfish, callous, promiscuous, impulsive, reckless; unable to learn from experience; fails at school and work.
- Borderline: impulsive; has unstable and intense interpersonal relationships; displays inappropriate anger, fear, and guilt; lacks self-control; has identity problems; may self-mutilate (cut or burn oneself to relieve tension); may be suicidal; views world as good or evil.

CAUSES—Unknown. May be multiple factors, including genetics, type of parenting in childhood, one's own personality traits, and early social experiences (such as abuse).

RISK INCREASES WITH
- History of abuse as a child.
- Family history of mood disorders.

HOW TO PREVENT—No specific preventive measures.

WHAT TO EXPECT

DIAGNOSTIC MEASURES
- Diagnostic measures may include observation of symptoms by other people.
- Diagnosis may include medical history, behavioral history, physical exam, and psychological evaluation by your health care provider.

APPROPRIATE HEALTH CARE
- Treatment requires a trusting relationship between the therapist and patient. This can be difficult, as motivation for treatment often comes from someone other than the person with the disorder.
- Psychotherapy provides help with thoughts, feelings, and behavior. It may include:
  - Family and group therapy, group living situations, and self-help groups.
  - Behavior-changing techniques involve the learning of social skills, reinforcement of appropriate behavior, setting limits on inappropriate behavior, learning to express feelings, self-analysis of behavior, and accepting accountability for actions.

POSSIBLE COMPLICATIONS
- Difficulty maintaining personal relationships and jobs; anxiety and depression. Risk of suicide.
- Drug and alcohol abuse. Behaviors may lead to trouble with the law.
- Noncompliance with treatment.

PROBABLE OUTCOME—Treatment can be effective for some patients, bringing about a gradual change in behavior. For others, prognosis is guarded; and for some, the outcome is poor.

HOW TO TREAT

GENERAL MEASURES—To learn more: Visit a library or do an Internet search.

MEDICATION—No drugs will cure a personality disorder. They may be prescribed for treatment of specific symptoms (e.g., antidepressants, antianxiety drugs, or antipsychotic drugs).

ACTIVITY—No limits.

DIET—No special diet.

CALL YOUR DOCTOR IF

- You or a family member has symptoms of a personality disorder.
- Symptoms don't improve with treatment.

PHARYNGITIS

 GENERAL INFORMATION

DEFINITION—Pharyngitis is an inflammation or infection of the pharynx. The pharynx is the hollow passage at the back of the throat. It is made up of the nasopharynx (which leads to the nose) and oropharynx (which leads to the mouth). The larynx (voice box) is located below the pharynx.

BODY PARTS INVOLVED—Throat area.

SEX OR AGE MOST AFFECTED—It occurs in both sexes and all age groups, but most often affects children.

SIGNS & SYMPTOMS
- Sore throat.
- Swallowing difficulty.
- Tickle or "lump" in the throat.
- Fever and/or chills.
- Swollen glands in the neck (sometimes).
- Throat may be red or covered with a white or grayish membrane (sometimes).
- Body aches (sometimes).

CAUSES—Viral infection (most common cause) or bacterial infection (such as *Streptococcus*). The germs are spread by person-to-person contact. Rarely, there may be other causes.

RISK INCREASES WITH
- Common cold, flu, or seasonal allergies.
- Weak immune system due to illness or drugs.
- Smoking or secondhand smoke.
- Chronic illness, such as diabetes.
- Close quarters, such as with military recruits, in schools, and daycare centers.
- Young age.

HOW TO PREVENT
- No sure way to prevent. Avoid close contact with anyone with a sore throat.
- Avoid germs. Wash hands often, especially children.

 WHAT TO EXPECT

DIAGNOSTIC MEASURES
- Your own observation of symptoms.
- Your health care provider will do an exam of the throat, ears, nose, neck, and lungs.
- Medical tests may include blood study and throat culture (from a swab of the throat), or rapid strep test to diagnose the type of infection.

APPROPRIATE HEALTH CARE—Treatment will include self-care measures and antibiotic drugs for bacterial infections. Antibiotics will not help viral infections.

POSSIBLE COMPLICATIONS
- Airways may become blocked.
- Abscess (pus-filled area of infection).
- Rheumatic fever, scarlet fever, or glomerulonephritis, if pharyngitis is caused by streptococcal bacteria and does not receive adequate antibiotic treatment.

PROBABLE OUTCOME—Most cases of viral infection clear up on their own in a week. Antibiotic drugs can successfully treat bacterial infections. Complications are rare.

 HOW TO TREAT

GENERAL MEASURES
- To relieve the sore throat, gargle frequently with warm or cold double-strength tea or warm salt water (mix one-half teaspoon of salt in one cup of water).
- Wash hands often to help prevent the spread of germs to other family members. Avoid kissing or sharing cups or other utensils.

MEDICATION
- For minor discomfort, you may use nonprescription drugs such as ibuprofen. Don't give aspirin to a child under age 18.
- Nonprescription throat lozenges (for patients over age 3) may help ease discomfort.
- Antibiotic drugs are usually prescribed for bacterial infection. Finish entire course of drugs even if symptoms improve.

ACTIVITY—Return to normal activities as symptoms improve.

DIET—Drink plenty of fluids. If swallowing solid food is painful, try a liquid or soft diet for a few days.

 CALL YOUR DOCTOR IF

- You or a family member has symptoms of pharyngitis.
- The following occur during treatment:
  - Breathing/swallowing difficulty or chest pain.
  - Fever worsens or severe headache develops.
  - Thick mucus drainage from the nose.
  - Cough that produces colored or bloody sputum.
  - Skin rash.
  - Dark urine.

PHEOCHROMOCYTOMA

GENERAL INFORMATION

DEFINITION—Pheochromocytoma is a rare type of tumor of the adrenal glands. There are two adrenal glands, each located above a kidney. They produce hormones for important body functions. The tumor usually affects one adrenal gland. In some cases, it may develop outside the glands. This type of tumor is most often benign (90%), but can be cancerous.

BODY PARTS INVOLVED—Adrenal glands.

SEX OR AGE MOST AFFECTED—Adults of both sexes between ages 30 and 50.

SIGNS & SYMPTOMS
- Episodes of at least some of these symptoms may occur several times a day or may occur less often (up to 2 months apart). Symptoms increase as tumor grows.
- High blood pressure episodes.
- Severe headaches; abdominal or chest pain.
- Rapid heartbeat following exercise, emotional upset, or exposure to cold.
- Tremors and nervousness.
- Feelings of doom.
- Feelings of hunger.
- Episodes of flushing.
- Sweating, paleness.
- Weakness and fatigue.
- Unexplained weight loss.
- Nausea and vomiting.

CAUSES—Hormones produced by adrenal glands work with the central nervous system to control heart rate, blood pressure, and other vital body functions. When a tumor (the pheochromocytoma) exists, even though it is benign, excess hormones are produced. The excess hormones cause symptoms. Cause of the tumor is unknown.

RISK INCREASES WITH
- Unknown for most cases.
- Certain inherited disorders (e.g., multiple endocrine neoplasia [MEN] syndrome, Von Hippel-Lindau disease, and neurofibromatosis type 1).

HOW TO PREVENT—No specific preventive measures. Screening tests are recommended for people at risk for pheochromocytoma. Consult your health care provider.

WHAT TO EXPECT

DIAGNOSTIC MEASURES
- Your own observation of symptoms.
- Your health care provider will do a physical exam.
- Medical tests may include studies of urine and blood to measure hormone production, x-ray, CT, MRI, and other tests. These help to diagnose the tumor, determine if it is benign or cancerous, and determine any spread of the cancer.

APPROPRIATE HEALTH CARE
- Treatment will depend on the diagnosis. It may include surgery, drug therapy, chemotherapy (anticancer drugs), and radiation.
- Surgery is usually done to remove the tumor.

POSSIBLE COMPLICATIONS
- Hypertensive crisis (severe blood pressure increase).
- Tumor may recur.
- Stroke, caused by very high blood pressure.
- High blood pressure may continue after surgery. It can be treated with drugs.
- Kidney, brain, heart damage, and death caused by unrecognized and untreated pheochromocytoma.

PROBABLE OUTCOME—The outlook is generally good for those with benign tumors removed by surgery. For those tumors that are cancerous, the outlook is more guarded.

HOW TO TREAT

GENERAL MEASURES—For a description of abdominal surgery and postoperative care, see Laparotomy in Surgery section.

MEDICATION
- Drugs are sometimes prescribed before surgery to suppress the effect of hormones.
- Drugs to treat high blood pressure may be needed.
- Anticancer drugs may be prescribed.

ACTIVITY—Usually, no limits after recovery from surgery.

DIET—Prior to surgery, a high-salt diet may be recommended to increase blood volume.

CALL YOUR DOCTOR IF

- You or a family member has symptoms of pheochromocytoma.
- Symptoms recur after treatment.

PHOBIAS

GENERAL INFORMATION

DEFINITION
• Phobias are a type of anxiety disorder involving intense and/or unrealistic fears. The fears may involve an object, situation, activity, event, or even a bodily function. The fear leads to avoidance of the stimulus. Phobias can cause minor or major problems for a person. Most people with phobias realize the fear is not appropriate to the situation. Phobias are classified as:
- Social—fear of embarrassment in social situations, such as public speaking or using a public bathroom.
- Agoraphobia—fear of being in crowds or fear of public places.
- Specific (simple)—fear of a specific object or situation, such as animals, insects, heights, flying, or closed places.

BODY PARTS INVOLVED—Nervous system.

SEX OR AGE MOST AFFECTED—Females more than males; onset often in ages 7 to 10.

SIGNS & SYMPTOMS
• The following anxiety symptoms occur when exposed to, or thinking of the phobic stimulus:
- Palpitations (irregular and rapid heartbeat).
- Desire to flee.
- Sweating, tremors, shortness of breath, or dizziness.
- Flushing.
- Nausea.
- Negative thoughts and scary images.

CAUSES—When fears are real (due to danger or a threat to life), the body's alarm system switches on and is ready to help protect us. With phobias, this alarm system switches on when there is no real threat or danger. The exact cause for this is unknown. It may involve genetics, family influence, traumatic events, medical conditions, or imbalance of certain brain chemicals.

RISK INCREASES WITH
• Family history of anxiety.
• Having other anxiety disorders.
• Women more than men.

HOW TO PREVENT—No specific preventive measures to prevent the phobia. After diagnosis, treatment can help symptoms.

WHAT TO EXPECT

DIAGNOSTIC MEASURES
• Your own observation of symptoms.
• Your health care provider will usually do a physical exam and ask about your symptoms and activities.
• Medical tests may be done to rule out other disorders.

APPROPRIATE HEALTH CARE
• Treatment may involve psychotherapy, drug therapy, and self-help methods. No treatment may be needed if the phobia is not interfering with daily life.
• Cognitive-behavioral therapy may help. Cognitive therapy teaches how to change thoughts, behaviors, or attitudes. Behavioral therapy teaches ways to reduce anxiety with deep breathing and muscle relaxation.

POSSIBLE COMPLICATIONS
• Limits in lifestyle due to avoiding the phobic stimulus. Agoraphobia, especially, restricts a person's activities and is severely disabling.
• Overuse of drugs or alcohol to relieve anxiety.

PROBABLE OUTCOME
• Specific phobias—some stop on their own as the person ages. Others do not cause any problems if the object can be avoided (such as snakes). Some get better as people go through their fearful situations (such as flying). Others can be cured or helped with treatment.
• Social phobias—usually can be resolved with treatment. Drugs are often helpful.
• Agoraphobia—is more difficult to treat because the person has so many fears, but treatment can help.

HOW TO TREAT

GENERAL MEASURES
• Simple self-help ideas if you feel your fear taking hold:
- Shift a thought from a negative ("The dog will bite") to a real and positive one ("The dog is on a leash").
- Do something you can control—count backward from 1000, read a book, talk aloud, or take deep, measured breaths.
- Shift your thoughts to pleasant ones.
- Practice relaxation techniques.
• Joining a support group is helpful for some patients.
• To learn more: Anxiety Disorders Association of America, 8730 Georgia Ave., Suite 600, Silver Spring, MD 20910; (240) 485-1001 (not toll free); website: www.adaa.org.

MEDICATION—Drugs may be helpful. Your health care provider will discuss the options, the risks, and the benefits.

ACTIVITY—No limits.

DIET—No special diet. Avoid caffeine and alcohol.

CALL YOUR DOCTOR IF

• You or a family member has symptoms of a phobia.
• Symptoms of the phobia return after treatment.

PHOTOSENSITIVITY
(Polymorphous Light Eruption; Solar Urticaria)

 GENERAL INFORMATION

DEFINITION
• Photosensitivity is a skin reaction to sunlight. There are several types, including:
  - Polymorphous light eruption (PMLE; sun poisoning) is a common, recurrent, abnormal, delayed reaction.
  - Chemical (drug) photosensitivity occurs from use of certain oral drugs or topical drugs and skin products. This reaction can be an irritant (toxic) or immune.
  - Solar urticaria is a rare reaction that causes hives within a few minutes of exposure to sunlight.

BODY PARTS INVOLVED—Skin.

SEX OR AGE MOST AFFECTED—Both sexes; all ages.

SIGNS & SYMPTOMS
• Red or pink skin rash (called photodermatosis), sometimes with small blisters, in areas exposed to sunlight.
• Rash may itch or burn.
• Large hives with solar urticaria. May also have faintness or nausea.

CAUSES—Symptoms are triggered by exposure to sun (ultraviolet light). It is not known why the body develops this reaction. Sunlight exposure may come through glass (e.g., in an automobile) or thin clothing. Some people react to winter-daylight as well. Tanning booths are a source of ultraviolet light. Fluorescent lights affect some.

RISK INCREASES WITH
• Use of drugs, products, or herbs that cause increased sensitivity to ultraviolet light:
  - Common drugs include tetracycline antibiotics, thiazide diuretics, sulfa drugs, nonsteroidal anti-inflammatory drugs, birth control pills, the herb St. John's Wort, and others.
  - Some sunscreens and some cosmetics, including lipstick, perfume, and soaps.
  - Certain plants (either eaten or skin contact).
• Certain skin disorders such as porphyria.
• Previous episodes of photosensitivity.
• Systemic lupus erythematosus.
• Family history of polymorphous light eruption.

HOW TO PREVENT
• Stay out of the sun when possible if you have a history of photosensitivity. The hours of strongest ultraviolet light are 10 am to 2 pm. Avoid tanning booths.
• Wear dark colored clothing that is tightly woven when in sunlight. Wear wide brim hat.
• Sunscreen can help. Use with care. Some sunscreens cause a reaction in photosensitive persons.
• Avoid the drugs or products known to cause photosensitivity. Not all persons who use these drugs will have a photosensitive reaction. Also, a reaction differs in different people. A person may have a one time reaction and not again.

 WHAT TO EXPECT

DIAGNOSTIC MEASURES
• Many people with mild symptoms self-treat.
• See your health care provider if you have concerns about the symptoms or they are severe. A physical exam of the affected skin area will be done. Questions will be asked about your sun exposure, products you use, and drugs that you take.
• A medical test may be done to check your skin's reaction to ultraviolet light.

APPROPRIATE HEALTH CARE
• Treatment depends on the cause. Changing drugs or skin care products may be advised.
• Phototherapy (a controlled light exposure) or PUVA (uses a drug and light) may be an option.

POSSIBLE COMPLICATIONS
• Skin may be hyperpigmented (darker).
• Chronic rash.

PROBABLE OUTCOME
• PMLE rash usually clears up within 5 to 10 days (if sun is avoided). A person becomes less sensitive with gradual sun exposure over time. This is called hardening.
• If a drug or other product is the cause, avoiding it or using sun protection improves symptoms. Healing may take weeks to months.
• In other photosensitivity cases, symptoms may come and go depending on sun exposure.

 HOW TO TREAT

GENERAL MEASURES—Apply cool, moist compresses to the skin. For sun protection, see Preventive Measures.

MEDICATION
• Use aspirin (if over age 18), acetaminophen, or an antihistamine for mild pain or itching.
• Beta-carotene taken orally may help some.
• Steroid drugs for severe cases, or other drugs to reduce photosensitivity may be prescribed.

ACTIVITY—Avoid prolonged sun exposure.

DIET—No special diet.

 CALL YOUR DOCTOR IF

You or a family member has symptoms of photosensitivity and self-care does not help.

PICA

GENERAL INFORMATION

DEFINITION—Pica is a craving, eating, or mouthing items that are not food. Pica can occur in adults, but usually affects children between ages 2 and 6, and persons with developmental disorders. Pica does not apply to infants 18 months to 2 years old who "put everything" in the mouth. That is normal.

BODY PARTS INVOLVED—Brain; gastrointestinal tract.

SEX OR AGE MOST AFFECTED—Both sexes; adults and children.

SIGNS & SYMPTOMS
- Eating non-food substances, such as starch, clay, ice, plaster, paint, cigarette ashes, hair, gravel, chalk, needles, string, pencil erasers, and others.
- Stomach pain (sometimes).

CAUSES—The exact cause is unknown. Factors that may contribute to the cause include physical, emotional, nutritional, family, social, economic, and cultural.

RISK INCREASES WITH
- Family history of pica.
- Poor nutrition or a vitamin deficiency.
- Poverty.
- Developmental disorders.
- Anemia.
- Pregnancy.
- Cultures where clay eating is a common practice.
- People on diets who try to ease hunger with non-food items.

HOW TO PREVENT—There are no specific preventive measures. To reduce risks, provide a well-balanced diet for yourself and your children.

WHAT TO EXPECT

DIAGNOSTIC MEASURES
- Your own observation of symptoms.
- Your health care provider will usually do a physical exam.
- Medical tests may include x-rays, blood studies, and other tests to rule out medical disorders. There is no diagnostic test for pica.

APPROPRIATE HEALTH CARE
- Treatment usually includes behavior and diet changes, if needed.
- Several different types of behavioral training are used to treat pica. Your health care provider will discuss the options with you depending on your individual situation.

POSSIBLE COMPLICATIONS
- Lead poisoning from paint or plaster.
- Intestinal infections from parasites in soil.
- Anemia.
- Malnutrition (not getting enough nutrients).
- Intestinal obstruction.

PROBABLE OUTCOME
- It may go on for years with no harmful effects.
- It may stop on its own in a few months.
- In some cases, it can be helped with treatment.
- For others, it may continue (even with treatment) into the teenage years. This occurs more often with developmental disorders.
- Pica during pregnancy usually ends with childbirth.

HOW TO TREAT

GENERAL MEASURES—Childproof your home by removing nonfood substances the child is eating. Repaint homes in which lead-base paints have been used. Don't use older baby cribs painted with lead-base paint.

MEDICATION—Drugs are usually not needed for this disorder.

ACTIVITY—No limits.

DIET—A well-balanced diet will be prescribed. A dietitian may help plan meals if any nutritional deficiency is diagnosed.

CALL YOUR DOCTOR IF

- You or a family member has symptoms of pica.
- You are pregnant and have symptoms of pica.
- Pica does not improve in 2 weeks, despite treatment.

PILONIDAL DISEASE

GENERAL INFORMATION

DEFINITION—Pilonidal disease is an infection in the skin—almost always located just above the crease of the buttocks. It starts with a pilonidal cyst (a sac) under the skin. The cyst can become infected and form an abscess (pus-filled area). An opening (sinus tract) may also develop that goes from the abscess to the outside skin.

BODY PARTS INVOLVED—Skin.

SEX OR AGE MOST AFFECTED—The disease affects both sexes, but is more common in males, from teenagers to age 40.

SIGNS & SYMPTOMS
• Symptoms may go unnoticed in mild cases.
• Pain, redness, tenderness, and swelling in the area.
• Fever and chills.
• Discharge of pus.
• Sitting or walking may be difficult.

CAUSES—The exact cause is unclear. It was thought for many years that people were born with the cysts. Now the theory is that they are acquired and caused by problems within a hair follicle.

RISK INCREASES WITH
• Obesity.
• Men more than women.
• Family history of pilonidal disease.
• Sedentary lifestyle (lack of exercise).
• Repeated trauma (injury) to the tailbone area.
• Work that requires a lot of sitting.
• Activities, such as biking or motorcycle riding, that can cause sweating and friction to the tailbone area.
• Heavy growth of body hair.
• Hair that is stiff or course.
• White persons are affected more often than African American or Asian persons.

HOW TO PREVENT
• Bathe or shower daily to keep the area clean. Warm tub baths seem more effective in preventing infection of the cyst than showers.
• Avoid risk factors where possible.

WHAT TO EXPECT

DIAGNOSTIC MEASURES
• Your own observation of symptoms.
• Your health care provider will do a physical exam of the cyst.
• Medical tests may include blood studies and a culture of the discharge from the cyst.

APPROPRIATE HEALTH CARE
• Treatment may not be needed for mild disease. Use extra care in keeping that area of the body clean. You may be advised to shave or use a hair remover product to keep the area free of hair.
• Incision and drainage may be recommended. This involves opening the cyst so that any hair or pus can be removed. The opening is then packed with gauze. Healing may take several weeks. Recurrence may be somewhat more common than with surgery.
• Surgical removal (excision) of the cyst or sinus may be recommended. Several different surgical methods can be used. Healing time will depend on the procedure. You will be advised about follow-up home care. See Pilonidal Cyst Removal in Surgery Section.

POSSIBLE COMPLICATIONS
• The disease recurs in about 40% of the patients after the initial treatment. It may clear up on its own after age 40.
• Without proper treatment, there may be an increased risk of skin cancer.

PROBABLE OUTCOME—Mild cases may need no treatment. In cases of abscess or recurrence of the disease, treatment can help. Healing time may take weeks to months, depending on treatment procedure.

HOW TO TREAT

GENERAL MEASURES—If the cyst is infected, take warm baths to relieve pain. Sit in a tub of warm water for 10 to 15 minutes as often as it feels good.

MEDICATION—Antibiotics may be prescribed for infection.

ACTIVITY—No limits, unless the cyst becomes infected. Then, limit activities until the infection is cured. Use a special doughnut cushion if sitting is uncomfortable.

DIET—No special diet. A weight-loss diet may be recommended if overweight is a problem.

CALL YOUR DOCTOR IF

• You or a family member has symptoms of a pilonidal disease.
• Symptoms recur after treatment.

PINWORMS

GENERAL INFORMATION

DEFINITION—Pinworms are small parasitic worms that infect the intestines (colon and rectum) of humans. Pinworms are a type of roundworm called *Enterobius vermicularis*. Pinworm infections are common and are not a serious medical problem.

BODY PARTS INVOLVED—Cecum (pouchlike beginning of the large intestine on the right side to which the appendix is attached); large intestine; anus; skin around the anus.

SEX OR AGE MOST AFFECTED—Both sexes; all ages, but most common in children.

SIGNS & SYMPTOMS
- A person may be infected and have no symptoms.
- Skin irritation and painful itching around the anus, especially during sleep.
- Restless sleep.
- Vaginal discharge, itching and discomfort if pinworms migrate into the vaginal opening.

CAUSES
- Infestation of the intestine by a very small worm about 1/4 to 1/2 inch long. Pinworms travel from the intestine to the rectum to lay eggs around the anus and buttocks. If a person scratches the area, the eggs can get under the fingernails and be passed to anything or anyone that person touches.
- Pinworms are easy to catch from someone who is infected. Eggs are passed to others on toilet seats or by hand-to-hand or hand-to-mouth contact. They may drift in the air, where they are inhaled or swallowed. Eggs hatch and the larvae travel to the large intestine, where they mature, mate, and repeat the cycle.

RISK INCREASES WITH—Groups of children, as in daycare, school, or at camps.

HOW TO PREVENT
- Wash hands carefully before meals and after using the toilet.
- Keep the nails short and clean.
- Bathe daily, right after waking up. This helps rid the body of any eggs before they can be spread.
- Have children wear clean underwear and pajamas daily.
- Don't scratch the anus or put fingers near the nose or mouth.
- Vacuum children's play area frequently.
- Wash bedding and pajamas regularly.

WHAT TO EXPECT

DIAGNOSTIC MEASURES
- You may help diagnose the pinworms yourself.

- They look like small pieces of white or yellow thread.
- They may sometimes be seen on a child's stool.
- Since they are active at night, check your child a few hours after bedtime. Shine a flashlight on the rectal area and you may see the worms in action.
- Perform a tape test for the eggs:
  - Your health care provider may give you a tongue depressor with clear tape on it and a glass slide. If you do not have this, use your own clear (scotch) tape. This procedure may need to be done three times for accurate diagnosis.
  - Place tape against your child's anal skin first thing in the morning (before getting up) to collect eggs.
  - Then place the sticky side of the tongue depressor tape on the glass slide. If your own tape was used, put it in a plastic bag and seal it.
  - Take slide or bag to the medical office for viewing under a microscope to check for pinworm eggs.

APPROPRIATE HEALTH CARE—Once the pinworm diagnosis is confirmed, the infection is usually treated with a drug to kill the worms. All family members should be treated even if they have no symptoms.

POSSIBLE COMPLICATIONS—No serious complications expected.

PROBABLE OUTCOME—The infection is curable in two weeks with treatment. If worms reappear soon after treatment, it usually means a new infection, not treatment failure. A second treatment can be effective.

HOW TO TREAT

GENERAL MEASURES—On the day of treatment, wash sheets, towels, and clothing, especially bedclothes, in hot water. Cut and clean fingernails.

MEDICATION
- A two-dose course of an antiworm drug is usually prescribed. The second dose is taken 2 weeks after first dose.
- Nonprescription creams or lotions to relieve itching may be helpful.

ACTIVITY—No limits.

DIET—No special diet.

CALL YOUR DOCTOR IF

- Anyone in your family has symptoms of pinworms.
- Pinworms reappear after treatment.

PITUITARY GLAND, UNDERACTIVE
(Hypopituitarism)

GENERAL INFORMATION

DEFINITION
- An underactive pituitary gland fails to release enough of one or more of its hormones. The pituitary is a small, dime-sized gland located just below the brain. It works with the hypothalamus in the brain to regulate body functions. Hormones released by the pituitary are used in many of these functions. If all hormones are absent, it is called panhypopituitarism. Hormones include:
  - Growth hormone—for growth of tissue and bones.
  - Prolactin hormone—for female breast development and milk production.
  - Thyroid-stimulating hormone—used by the thyroid gland for metabolism functions.
  - Adrenocorticotropic hormone—used by the adrenal gland to control blood pressure.
  - Luteinizing hormone and follicle stimulating hormones—control sexual function in males and females.
  - Antidiuretic hormone—affects the kidneys in the production of urine.
  - Oxytocin—for contractions of the uterus during childbirth and the release of milk during breast-feeding.

BODY PARTS INVOLVED—Pituitary gland and body parts mentioned above.

SEX OR AGE MOST AFFECTED—Both sexes; all ages.

SIGNS & SYMPTOMS
- Decrease in appetite and weight loss.
- Unusual tiredness or fatigue.
- Abdominal pain; nausea.
- More sensitive to cold or heat.
- Persistent headaches.
- Mental changes.
- Changes in vision.
- Women may have menstrual period changes, failure to produce milk, hot flashes, and infertility.
- Men may have decreased sexual interest.
- Severe thirst and lack of urination.
- Failure of growth (seen after age 6 months).
- Lack of secondary sexual features that develop in puberty. These include voice changes, breast development, and growth of pubic hair.

CAUSES—Usually caused by disorders that affect the pituitary, the hypothalamus, or surrounding structures. Sometimes the cause is unknown.

RISK INCREASES WITH
- Tumors.
- Head injury.
- Infection (tuberculosis, syphilis, or meningitis).
- Blocked blood supply to the pituitary.
- Immune system problem.
- Pregnancy and delivery.
- Radiation or surgery.
- Congenital defect (present since birth).

HOW TO PREVENT—None specific. Obtain medical care for any risk factors.

WHAT TO EXPECT

DIAGNOSTIC MEASURES
- Your own observation of symptoms.
- Your health care provider will do a physical exam and ask about your symptoms and activities.
- Medical tests may include blood studies of hormone levels and hormone function. CT or MRI scans may be done.

APPROPRIATE HEALTH CARE
- Treatment is aimed at treating the cause of the pituitary failure. It may include drugs or surgery and hormone replacement as needed.
- Surgery may be needed to remove underlying tumors or blood clots.

POSSIBLE COMPLICATIONS—Hormonal failure and possible death without treatment. Other complications depend on the underlying cause.

PROBABLE OUTCOME—It is usually a lifelong disorder. Outcome is generally favorable if an underlying disorder is successfully treated and hormone-replacement therapy is continued.

HOW TO TREAT

GENERAL MEASURES
- This disorder requires close medical supervision and continuing treatment.
- Wear or carry medical ID indicating your hormone deficiencies and the proper treatment.

MEDICATION
- Hormones are usually prescribed to replace those the pituitary is not producing.
- Drugs may be prescribed for treatment of an underlying disorder.

ACTIVITY—Stay as active as your condition allows.

DIET—No special diet.

CALL YOUR DOCTOR IF

- You or a family member has symptoms of an underactive pituitary gland.
- Symptoms occur with treatment that cause concern.

PITUITARY TUMOR

GENERAL INFORMATION

DEFINITION
- Pituitary tumors are usually benign (noncancerous) tumors called adenomas. Other, less-common types may be cancerous. Tumors are also classed as functioning (producing hormones) or nonfunctioning (not producing hormones).
- The pituitary is a small, dime-sized gland located just below the brain. It works with the hypothalamus to regulate body functions from within the brain. Hormones released by the pituitary are used in many of these functions. Hormones released by the pituitary include:
  - Growth hormone—for growth of tissue and bones.
  - Prolactin hormone—for female breast development and milk production.
  - Thyroid-stimulating hormone—used by the thyroid gland for metabolism functions.
  - Adrenocorticotropic hormone—used by the adrenal gland to control blood pressure.
  - Luteinizing hormone and follicle stimulating hormones—control sexual function in males and females.
  - Antidiuretic hormone—affects the kidneys in the production of urine.
  - Oxytocin—for contractions of the uterus during childbirth and the release of milk during breast-feeding.

BODY PARTS INVOLVED—Pituitary gland.

SEX OR AGE MOST AFFECTED—Both sexes and all ages; more common in ages 30 to 60.

SIGNS & SYMPTOMS
- Symptoms may occur due to tumor growth. It can put pressure on eye nerves causing vision problems, headaches, and other symptoms.
- Numerous symptoms may occur due to an over-production or under-production of any of the hormones listed above. No symptoms are specific for diagnosing a tumor. Often, symptoms may go unnoticed, fail to cause alarm, or be attributed to another illness.

CAUSES—Unknown.

RISK INCREASES WITH—Certain hereditary disorders (for some types of tumors).

HOW TO PREVENT—No preventive measures.

WHAT TO EXPECT

DIAGNOSTIC MEASURES
- Your own observation of symptoms.
- Your health care provider will do a physical exam and ask about your symptoms. Medical tests may include cerebrospinal fluid and blood studies, x-rays of the skull, CT scan or MRI of the brain, and vision tests.

APPROPRIATE HEALTH CARE
- Treatment may involve a combination of surgery to remove the tumor, radiation treatment, hormone therapy, or other drugs.
- Different types of surgery are used to treat the tumors. The procedure depends on the type of tumor, its location, and its size. Your health care provider will explain the options to you.
- Radiation therapy may be used in combination with surgery. It may also be used for people who, for medical reasons, are not able to have surgery.

POSSIBLE COMPLICATIONS
- Spread of the tumor to other parts of the brain.
- Blindness due to pressure from tumor.
- Recurrence of tumor after treatment.

PROBABLE OUTCOME—Outcome will depend on the type of tumor, and the patient's age and general health status. Early diagnosis and treatment offer the most favorable outcome.

HOW TO TREAT

GENERAL MEASURES
- Wear or carry medical ID indicating your hormone deficiencies and the proper treatment.
- To learn more: Pituitary Network Association, PO Box 1958, Thousand Oaks, CA 91358; (805) 499-9973 (not toll free); website: www.pituitary.org.

MEDICATION
- Pain relievers may be prescribed.
- Hormone-replacement drugs may be prescribed. They may require frequent dosage adjustments.
- Drugs to reduce hormone production may be prescribed.
- Anticancer drugs may be prescribed.

ACTIVITY—Resume your normal activities gradually after treatment.

DIET—No special diet unless advised.

CALL YOUR DOCTOR IF
- You or a family member has symptoms of a pituitary tumor.
- The following occur after surgery:
  - Bleeding at the surgical site or general signs of infection, such as fever, chills, headache, and muscle aches.
  - Clear discharge from the nose or nosebleeds.

PITYRIASIS ALBA

GENERAL INFORMATION

DEFINITION—Pityriasis alba is a common disorder of the skin. It causes a temporary loss of pigmentation (coloring) in patches found usually on the cheeks and, sometimes, the neck and shoulders. Pityriasis means "scaly" and alba means "white" in Latin.

BODY PARTS INVOLVED—Skin.

SEX OR AGE MOST AFFECTED—It occurs mostly in children of both sexes, but may appear in adults up to ages 20 to 30.

SIGNS & SYMPTOMS
- Small white or light-pink patches with vague borders. They sometimes have pinpoint-sized white papules (small, raised bumps). Patches feel smooth.
- Patches are most apparent in summer because the areas do not tan. Tanning will increase the contrast. A scaly appearance may be visible in winter when air in the home is dry.
- There may be 1 to 20 patches at a time. They may range in size from 1/4 to 2 inches.
- Patches may itch occasionally, but they are not painful.

CAUSES—Unknown. The tendency may be inherited.

RISK INCREASES WITH
- Family history of allergies of any kind.
- Skin that is extra dry and sun exposure may be risk factors.

HOW TO PREVENT—No specific preventive measures.

WHAT TO EXPECT

DIAGNOSTIC MEASURES
- Your own observation of symptoms.
- Your health care provider can usually diagnose the disorder by an exam of the affected skin.
- Medical tests are generally not needed.

APPROPRIATE HEALTH CARE—No truly effective therapy is available. Some skin-care products may help the dry skin.

POSSIBLE COMPLICATIONS—None expected.

PROBABLE OUTCOME—Patches may come and go for years. Between ages 20 and 30, they disappear completely.

HOW TO TREAT

GENERAL MEASURES—Use sunscreen or protective clothing to prevent sunburn in affected areas.

MEDICATION
- Moisturizers may improve roughness or dryness, but do not improve the color.
- Prescription or nonprescription topical steroid drug(s) to control itching may be recommended.

ACTIVITY—No limits.

DIET—No special diet.

CALL YOUR DOCTOR IF

You or a family member has symptoms of pityriasis alba.

PITYRIASIS ROSEA

 GENERAL INFORMATION

DEFINITION—Pityriasis rosea is a common skin disorder with a faint rash that lasts weeks to months. Pityriasis means "scaly" and rosea means "pink" in Latin.

BODY PARTS INVOLVED—Skin, especially of the chest and abdomen.

SEX OR AGE MOST AFFECTED—It affects all ages, but is most common in adolescents and young adults. Women are affected more often than men are.

SIGNS & SYMPTOMS
- A faint rash (often found in skin creases) of oval or round, pale-pink or light-brown areas. One larger patch (the "herald patch") may appear first. They may evolve into a "Christmas tree" pattern on the chest or back.
- Mild fatigue.
- Itching, usually mild, but worsens in hot weather.
- Slight fever, headache, and stuffy nose occasionally occur before rash appears.

CAUSES—Unknown, but may be caused by a virus or autoimmune disorder. It does not appear to be contagious (easily spread from one person to another).

RISK INCREASES WITH
- Fall and spring seasons.
- Weak immune system due to illness or drugs.

HOW TO PREVENT—Cannot be prevented at present.

 WHAT TO EXPECT

DIAGNOSTIC MEASURES
- Your own observation of symptoms.
- Your health care provider can usually diagnose the disorder by an exam of the affected skin.
- Medical tests may include blood studies. A scraping of the skin or a sample of the skin may be removed for viewing under a microscope.

APPROPRIATE HEALTH CARE
- No specific treatment will cure the disorder.
- Treatment can help relieve the itching. In more severe cases, treatment with ultraviolet light or moderate exposure to sunlight may be recommended.

POSSIBLE COMPLICATIONS
- Affected skin areas may have color changes in darker-skinned persons.
- Rarely, bacterial infection may occur in affected skin.

PROBABLE OUTCOME—Pityriasis rosea usually runs its natural course in 5 weeks to 4 months. No drug or treatment is available to shorten its course, but itching and discomfort can be relieved. New rash areas continue to break out for several weeks. Once over, it is unlikely to recur.

 HOW TO TREAT

GENERAL MEASURES—Bathe as usual with a mild soap. Use warm water, as hot water may increase the itching. Oatmeal baths may help.

MEDICATION
- For minor discomfort, you may use nonprescription drugs, such as:
  - Calamine lotion, to decrease itching.
  - Steroid cream, to control more severe itching.
  - Acetaminophen, to reduce fever.
- Other topical or oral steroids and antihistamines may be prescribed.

ACTIVITY—Avoid activities that cause excess sweating. This can make the rash worse.

DIET—No special diet.

 CALL YOUR DOCTOR IF

You or a family member has symptoms of pityriasis rosea.

PLACENTA PREVIA

GENERAL INFORMATION

DEFINITION
● In placenta previa, the placenta is covering or near the cervical opening (called the os). The placenta normally attaches high on the uterus wall, away from the cervix. With placenta previa, it can block the cervical opening to the vagina (birth canal). Placenta previa carries a risk of excessive bleeding, which can threaten the well-being of the mother and the baby. A low-lying placenta diagnosed in early pregnancy usually self-corrects as the uterus enlarges. Types of placenta previa include:
   - Total placenta previa: The placenta completely covers the opening of the cervix. This type presents the most serious risk to the mother.
   - Partial placenta previa: The placenta partially covers the opening of the cervix.
   - Marginal placenta previa: The placenta just reaches the margin of the cervix.
   - Low-lying placenta previa: The placenta is near the cervix.

BODY PARTS INVOLVED—Uterus; placenta (the organ that transfers nourishment and oxygen from mother to fetus); cervix (opening to the uterus).

SEX OR AGE MOST AFFECTED—Pregnant women.

SIGNS & SYMPTOMS
● Sudden, painless bleeding during the second or third trimester of pregnancy. Bleeding may be mild at the start and become severe. Bleeding may not occur until after labor begins in some cases.
● Cramping may occur in some patients.

CAUSES—The exact cause is unknown. There may be a number of factors involved.

RISK INCREASES WITH
● Previous uterine surgery involving the lining of the uterus. This includes dilation and curettage (D & C) and cesarean section.
● Smoking.
● Prior induced abortion.
● Multiple previous pregnancies and births.
● Pregnancy with twins or other multiples.
● Mothers over age 35.
● Previous placenta previa.

HOW TO PREVENT—It cannot be prevented. Good prenatal care during pregnancy can help identify it early.

WHAT TO EXPECT

DIAGNOSTIC MEASURES
● Your own observation of symptoms, especially of vaginal bleeding during pregnancy.

● If bleeding occurs, medical tests may include blood studies and ultrasound to determine the exact location of the placenta. Rarely, a vaginal exam may be done.

APPROPRIATE HEALTH CARE
● Treatment depends on type of previa, amount of bleeding, fetal age, presentation and condition, and presence or absence of labor.
● Hospital care that includes blood transfusions, intravenous (IV) fluids, and oxygen may be needed with severe bleeding.
● If the bleeding is heavy or the pregnancy is at term, delivery is usually done. There may be a trial of labor for vaginal delivery or a cesarean delivery.
● If the pregnancy is between 34 and 37 weeks and the mother and fetus are stable, amniocentesis may be done to check fetal lung maturity. With mature lungs, the newborn will not need breathing support.
● If the baby's lungs are immature or the pregnancy is less than 34 weeks, the treatment may involve medical observation for a period. You may be placed on bed rest at home. Follow your obstetric provider's instructions carefully.

POSSIBLE COMPLICATIONS
● Poor fetal growth, due to an abnormal placenta providing a decrease in blood flow and oxygen delivery.
● Premature delivery, or (possibly) fetal death.
● Risk of clotting disorder (disseminated intravascular coagulopathy or DIC).
● Rarely, blood loss could lead to maternal shock and death.

PROBABLE OUTCOME—With prompt care, the outcome for mothers and term infants is good. Outcome for premature baby will depend on number of weeks of gestation and the baby's condition at birth.

HOW TO TREAT

GENERAL MEASURES—Follow medical advice.

MEDICATION
● Steroids may be prescribed to help fetal lungs mature.
● Drugs to delay labor may be used.

ACTIVITY—Rest in bed until bleeding stops or you deliver your child. Avoid sexual intercourse or douching.

DIET—No special diet.

CALL YOUR DOCTOR IF

You or a family member has symptoms of placenta previa. Report any bleeding immediately. This is an emergency!

PLANTAR FASCIITIS

Joe P.

GENERAL INFORMATION

DEFINITION—Plantar fasciitis is an inflammation (red, sore, swollen) of the plantar fascia. The plantar fascia is a thick band of tissue on the bottom of the foot. It extends from the heel bone to the base of the toes. Plantar refers to the sole of the foot. Fascia describes thin, fibrous, supportive tissue. It is a common foot problem, and is different from heel spurs. But, a person may have both of these foot problems at the same time.

BODY PARTS INVOLVED—Foot.

SEX OR AGE MOST AFFECTED—It can affect anyone, of any age, no matter their fitness level.

SIGNS & SYMPTOMS
• Pain and tenderness in the heel and sole of the foot under the heel bone.
• Pain often occurs after resting or after rising in the morning. There may be no pain when sitting.
• One or both feet can be affected.
• It hurts worse when running faster or when weight is on the ball of the foot.

CAUSES—The exact cause is unknown. It may be a combination of factors, such as inflammation, mini tears, and chronic changes in the fascia.

RISK INCREASES WITH
• People over age 40; women more than men.
• Athletes who overtrain, wear improper shoes, or fail to warm up.
• Running, jumping, or walking on hard surface.
• Having flat feet, high arches, or tight calf muscles.
• Previous foot or ankle injury.
• High-heels; poor-fitting or worn-out shoes.
• Being on the feet for many hours a day.
• Overweight.

HOW TO PREVENT
• Wear proper footwear for sports, exercise, and work. Consult a podiatrist (foot specialist) if needed.
• Do stretching exercises for the Achilles tendon (tendon from the heel to the calf).
• With any new exercise or sport, build up your pace gradually. Warm up before exercise.
• Maintain a healthy weight for your height.
• Avoid running or walking on hard surface.

WHAT TO EXPECT

DIAGNOSTIC MEASURES
• Your own observation of symptoms.
• Your health care provider will examine your foot and ankle and ask about your symptoms. The bottom of your foot will be touched and pressed to identify the cause of the pain.

• X-rays and other tests may be done to check for other disorders.

APPROPRIATE HEALTH CARE
• There are a variety of treatment options. Follow your health care provider's advice. Basic ideas are listed under General Measures.
• If other treatments fail after 6 months, shock wave therapy (nonsurgical) or surgery may be options.

POSSIBLE COMPLICATIONS—Pain may become chronic which can lead to limping and other walking problems. This can limit everyday activities as well as sports and fitness activities.

PROBABLE OUTCOME—Different types of treatment work for different people. Complete healing may take months and up to a year or more. Other methods of treatment are being studied and may be available in the future.

HOW TO TREAT

GENERAL MEASURES
• Massage an ice pack over the painful area. Do this for 15 minutes, 3 or 4 times a day, and after activities.
• Before getting out of bed, use a towel to pull toes back toward the ankle. Count to 10, and do it 10 times.
• While sitting, grab a towel with your toes or roll your foot back and forth over a can of frozen juice. Stand on the ball of your foot on the edge of a step and raise and lower leg.
• Try heel cushions or arch supports. Use them in both shoes so other problems don't develop. Custom orthotics (special shoe inserts) may be prescribed.
• Taping helps some people. Apply athletic tape as directed on the product's instructions.
• Night splints may help. They are products that keep the muscles stretched while sleeping.
• Buy shoes that fit well. Sandals help some people.

MEDICATION
• For minor pain and inflammation, use nonprescription drugs, such as ibuprofen or aspirin (if over age 18).
• Steroids may be injected into the foot.

ACTIVITY—Stay off your feet as much as possible until symptoms are better. Try swimming or cycling for exercising.

DIET—If overweight is a problem, begin a weight-loss diet.

CALL YOUR DOCTOR IF

• You or a family member has symptoms of plantar fasciitis.
• Symptoms don't improve despite treatment.

PLEURAL EFFUSION
(Hemothorax)

GENERAL INFORMATION

DEFINITION—Pleural effusion is an abnormal accumulation of fluid in the pleural space. It is not a disease in itself, but a complication of some disorder or injury. Pleura are the thin membranes that line the lungs and chest cavity. Normally the fluid in this area provides lubrication and allows smooth, uniform contractions of the lungs during breathing. The fluid may be termed exudate (often cloudy) or transudate (watery). Special types of pleural effusion include: empyema, (pus is present), hemothorax (blood is present), pneumothorax (air is present), and chylothorax (milky fluid made up of lymph and fat is present).

BODY PARTS INVOLVED—Lung; pleura.

SEX OR AGE MOST AFFECTED—Both sexes; all ages.

SIGNS & SYMPTOMS
* No symptoms sometimes (with small effusion). It may be discovered on a routine health exam.
* Chest pain. Pain varies from vague discomfort to stabbing pain. It is often worse with coughing or breathing. Pain may extend to the lower chest wall or abdomen.
* Shortness of breath.
* Dry cough.
* Other symptoms may be associated with an underlying disease. Symptoms can include edema (e.g., swollen feet and ankles), night sweats, fever, weight loss, bloody sputum.

CAUSES—Many conditions can cause pleural effusion, and sometimes, no cause is found. The effusion results from too much fluid being produced, too little fluid draining out, or an excess accumulation of fluid.

RISK INCREASES WITH
* Congestive heart failure.
* Lung or chest infections, such as pneumonia, tuberculosis or lung abscess.
* Cancer.
* Collapsed lung or chest injury (trauma).
* Pulmonary embolism (blood clot in the lung).
* Viral or fungal infection.
* Pleurisy (lung inflammation).
* Benign (noncancerous) tumor.
* Kidney or liver disorders.
* Adverse drug reaction.
* Vascular disease (e.g., rheumatoid arthritis).
* Surgery complication.

HOW TO PREVENT—Not usually preventable. To reduce risk, get medical care for any problem that may lead to pleural effusion.

WHAT TO EXPECT

DIAGNOSTIC MEASURES
* Your own observation of symptoms.
* Your health care provider will do a physical exam.
* Medical tests may include culture of pleural fluid obtained by thoracentesis (needle inserted into the chest to withdraw fluid), x-ray, MRI, CT, ultrasound (see Glossary for all), or biopsy (removal of tissue sample for viewing under a microscope).

APPROPRIATE HEALTH CARE
* Small effusions may need treatment only for the cause.
* With larger effusions, the fluid may be removed via a needle or a tube placed in the chest. A fibrinolytic drug may be added to the space to help prevent fluid accumulation.
* Surgery may be needed to remove fibrous material from the lung.
* Treatment will be provided for any disorder that caused pleural effusion.

POSSIBLE COMPLICATIONS—Will depend on the underlying cause.

PROBABLE OUTCOME—A pleural effusion can be treated successfully, but the outcome of the underlying disorder depends on diagnosis and treatment. If a drug is the cause, stopping the drug usually resolves the problem.

HOW TO TREAT

GENERAL MEASURES—Follow medical instructions for any home care.

MEDICATION
* You may be prescribed antibiotic or antifungal drugs.
* Different drugs including anticancer drugs (chemotherapy) may be prescribed once an underlying disorder is diagnosed.

ACTIVITY—Reduce activity until treatment is complete. Gradually return to normal activity.

DIET—No special diet.

CALL YOUR DOCTOR IF

* You or a family member has symptoms of pleural effusion.
* Symptoms recur after treatment.
* New symptoms develop. They may be due to the underlying disorder.

PLEURISY
(Pleuritis)

GENERAL INFORMATION

DEFINITION—Pleurisy is an inflammation of the pleura. The pleura is a thin, two-layered membrane that surrounds the lungs and lines the chest wall. When inflamed, the normally smooth membranes rub against each other which leads to the symptoms. In some cases, fluid may build up in the space between the two membrane layers. This is called pleural effusion.

BODY PARTS INVOLVED—Pleura.

SEX OR AGE MOST AFFECTED—Both sexes; all ages.

SIGNS & SYMPTOMS
- Sudden chest pain that worsens with breathing and coughing. The pain varies from vague discomfort that occurs only with deep breathing or coughing to intense, stabbing pain. Pain is usually over the area of pleural inflammation, but it may also occur in the lower chest or abdomen.
- Fever (sometimes).
- Discomfort on moving the affected side.
- Rapid, shallow breathing.
- Breathing difficulty if pleural effusion develops.

CAUSES—Pleurisy can be caused by infection (e.g., bacterial, fungal, or viral), injury, irritation, blood clot, or disease. Sometimes, no cause is found.

RISK INCREASES WITH
- Lung or chest infection (e.g., pneumonia, bronchitis, tuberculosis).
- Blood clot in the lung.
- Injury to the chest or rib fracture.
- Cancer in other parts of the body.
- Collagen vascular disease, such as systemic lupus erythematosus or rheumatoid arthritis.
- Collapse of a part of the lung.
- Kidney, liver, or pancreas disorders.
- Weak immune system due to illness or drugs.
- Smoking.
- Sickle cell disease.

HOW TO PREVENT—No specific preventive measures. Obtain medical treatment for any risk factors listed above to reduce the risk of pleurisy.

WHAT TO EXPECT

DIAGNOSTIC MEASURES
- Your own observation of symptoms.
- Your health care provider will do a physical exam and ask about your symptoms and activities.
- Medical tests may include blood and pleural fluid studies, x-rays of the chest, and others to diagnose the cause.

APPROPRIATE HEALTH CARE
- The main treatment is aimed at the underlying cause. Other treatment may help the symptoms of pleurisy.
- Excess fluid in the pleura may need to be removed. This is done with a needle inserted into the pleura to draw out the fluid.

POSSIBLE COMPLICATIONS
- Fluid build-up (pleural effusion).
- Pneumonia.
- Scar tissue (adhesions) may form that cause pain and shortness of breath.

PROBABLE OUTCOME—Outcome depends on successful treatment of the disorder causing it. Sometimes, pleurisy symptoms clear completely on their own in 1 to 2 weeks.

HOW TO TREAT

GENERAL MEASURES
- Lie with the sore side down, on a firm surface. This will help ease the pain.
- Holding a pillow firmly against the chest wall helps ease the pain when coughing.
- Quit smoking. Find a way to stop that works.

MEDICATION
- You may take nonsteroidal anti-inflammatory drugs, such as aspirin (if over age 18) or ibuprofen, to relieve pain and inflammation.
- Antibiotics, bronchodilators, or stronger pain relievers may be prescribed.

ACTIVITY—Reduce activity until pain and cough get better. Then resume normal activities gradually.

DIET—No special diet.

CALL YOUR DOCTOR IF

- You or a family member has symptoms of pleurisy.
- The following occur during treatment:
  - Fever.
  - Increased pain.
  - Increased breathlessness.
  - Cough that is dry and non-productive.
  - Blue or dark fingernails, toenails, or lips.
  - Blood in the sputum.

PNEUMOCONIOSIS

GENERAL INFORMATION

DEFINITION—Pneumoconiosis is a lung inflammation caused by breathing in certain dusts. The dusts most often come from work-place exposure. It usually takes at least 10 years of exposure and up to 25 years for pneumoconiosis to develop. Only a few persons exposed to the dusts actually become ill.

BODY PARTS INVOLVED—Lungs.

SEX OR AGE MOST AFFECTED—Men over age 40.

SIGNS & SYMPTOMS
- Early symptoms:
  - Shortness of breath.
  - Cough that produces little or no sputum.
  - General ill feeling.
- Late symptoms:
  - Restless sleep.
  - Appetite and weight loss.
  - Chest pain.
  - Hoarseness; coughing up blood.
  - Bluish nails.

CAUSES
- Inhaling certain dusts for many years may cause little patches of irritation to form in one or both lungs. The scar tissue (called fibrosis) formed by the irritation may make the lungs less flexible and porous. There are several forms of pneumoconiosis:
  - Coal dust causes black-lung disease (coal miner's pneumoconiosis, anthracosis).
  - Beryllium and its compounds (once used in manufacturing fluorescent lamp bulbs, ceramics, and chemicals) cause berylliosis.
  - Talc, iron, cotton, synthetic fiber, and aluminum dusts cause a rare form of pneumoconiosis.
  - Asbestos and silica cause asbestosis and silicosis.

RISK INCREASES WITH—Amounts of dust inhaled over the years.

HOW TO PREVENT
- Practice safety during exposure to work-place dusts. Wear a protective mask or external-air-supplied hood. Get an x-ray once a year.
- Don't smoke. Smoking is not a risk factor in itself, but can worsen symptoms and increase complications.

WHAT TO EXPECT

DIAGNOSTIC MEASURES
- Your health care provider will do a physical exam and ask questions about your symptoms and activities. Be sure to tell your provider about your work history and any exposure to work-place dusts.
- Medical tests may include a chest x-ray, pulmonary function tests, and others to confirm diagnosis and check for complications.

APPROPRIATE HEALTH CARE
- Drugs and lung therapy may help the symptoms and treat complications.
- Chest physical therapy (such as controlled coughing) and bronchial drainage help clear secretions. Get special training about the use of these procedures.
- Supplemental oxygen may be needed.
- Lung transplantation may be an option for some patients.

POSSIBLE COMPLICATIONS
- Congestive heart failure.
- Lung collapse, pleurisy, or other lung disease.
- Tuberculosis (in the late stages).
- Lung cancer.

PROBABLE OUTCOME—This condition is currently considered incurable. Symptoms can be relieved or controlled. It reduces life span, but many patients live into their 60s and 70s.

HOW TO TREAT

GENERAL MEASURES
- Avoid any further exposure to industrial dusts.
- Quit smoking. Find a way to stop that works.
- Get medical care for any respiratory infection (such as a cold). Get pneumococcal and annual influenza vaccines.
- To learn more: American Lung Association, 61 Broadway, 6th Floor, New York, NY 10006; (800) 586-4872; website: www.lungusa.org.

MEDICATION
- Bronchodilators (inhaled or oral) with inhalation therapy may be prescribed. This is supervised at first by an inhalation therapist.
- Corticosteroids may be prescribed for certain types of pneumoconiosis.
- For minor discomfort, use nonprescription drugs, such as acetaminophen or aspirin.
- Antibiotics may be prescribed for infections.

ACTIVITY—No limits, except those caused by symptoms. An exercise program is usually recommended.

DIET—No special diet.

CALL YOUR DOCTOR IF

- You or a family member has pneumoconiosis symptoms.
- The following occur during treatment:
  - Temperature of 101°F (38.3°C) or more.
  - Increased chest pain or shortness of breath.
  - Blood in sputum.
  - Continuing weight loss.
  - Unexplained symptoms develop.

PNEUMOCYSTIS JIROVECI PNEUMONIA
(Pneumonia Pneumocystis Carinii)

GENERAL INFORMATION

DEFINITION—*Pneumocystis* penumonia (PCP) is an inflammation of the lungs caused by infection with *Pneumocystis jiroveci* germs. It occurs in children (including infants) and adults with a weakened immune system. They are usually AIDS patients. Most people have been exposed to these germs by age four, but their immune systems are able to fight off any infection.

BODY PARTS INVOLVED—Lower-respiratory system (bronchial tubes and lungs).

SEX OR AGE MOST AFFECTED—All ages, both sexes, but most common in adult men.

SIGNS & SYMPTOMS
- Dry, nonproductive cough.
- Fever.
- Difficulty in breathing (more so with exertion).
- Fatigue.
- Weight loss.
- Night sweats.
- Tightness in the chest.
- Lips, fingernails, or skin may turn blue or gray.

CAUSES—*Pneumocystis jiroveci*, a fungus. It is most likely transmitted through the air. It is unknown if it lives in soil or other places. It is also unknown how long it takes symptoms to start after exposure. Person-to-person spread is a possibility, but is not yet proven.

RISK INCREASES WITH
- HIV (human immunodeficiency virus) and AIDS (acquired immunodeficiency syndrome).
- People with weak immune systems due to illness or drugs.
- Cancer chemotherapy (anticancer drugs).
- Long-term steroid drug use.
- Severe malnutrition (any disorder of nutrition).
- History of *Pneumocystis jiroveci* pneumonia.

HOW TO PREVENT—It is almost entirely preventable with drugs. Preventive drugs can be prescribed for those at risk.

WHAT TO EXPECT

DIAGNOSTIC MEASURES
- Your own observation of symptoms.
- Your health care provider will do a physical exam and ask questions about the symptoms.
- Medical tests may include x-rays, a study of a specimen of sputum, and high-resolution CT scan. A bronchoscopy may be done. This involves inserting a tube down the throat to view the lungs and to get a sample of tissue for diagnosis.

APPROPRIATE HEALTH CARE
- Treatment is with drugs given by mouth or given through a vein (IV).
- Treatment may be done at home for mild cases. For more severe infection, hospital care may be needed.

POSSIBLE COMPLICATIONS
- Prolonged illness, sometimes fatal.
- Side effects of drugs, especially skin rash and low white blood cell count.

PROBABLE OUTCOME—With prompt diagnosis and treatment, the outlook is generally good for mild cases. In more severe cases, the risk of complications is higher.

HOW TO TREAT

GENERAL MEASURES—To learn more: American Lung Association, 61 Broadway, 6th Floor, New York, NY 10006, (800) 586-4872; website: www.lungusa.org.

MEDICATION
- Antibiotics, such as trimethoprim-sulfamethoxazole or pentamidine (oral or aerosol) will be prescribed. (The infection does not respond to antifungal drugs.)
- Corticosteroids may be prescribed.
- Cough medicine may be recommended.

ACTIVITY—Bed rest is recommended until fever subsides. Normal activities should be resumed gradually.

DIET—No special diet. Extra fluid helps to thin lung secretions so they can be coughed up more easily.

CALL YOUR DOCTOR IF

- You or a family member has symptoms of *Pneumocystis jiroveci* pneumonia.
- The following occur during treatment:
  - Higher fever.
  - Pain becomes worse.
  - Increased shortness of breath.
  - Dark or bluish fingernails, toenails, or skin.
  - Blood in the sputum.
  - Nausea, vomiting, or diarrhea.

PNEUMONIA, BACTERIAL

GENERAL INFORMATION

DEFINITION—Bacterial pneumonia is an inflammation of the lungs caused by bacterial infection. The inflammation causes fluid to build up in the air sacs (alveoli), making it difficult to breathe. Bacterial pneumonia is not usually contagious.

BODY PARTS INVOLVED—Lungs; bronchial tubes.

SEX OR AGE MOST AFFECTED—Both sexes; all ages, but most severe in young children and adults over age 60.

SIGNS & SYMPTOMS
- High fever (over 102°F or 38.9°C) and chills.
- Shortness of breath.
- Cough with sputum that may contain blood or blood streaks.
- Rapid breathing.
- Chest pain that worsens with inhalations.
- Abdominal pain.
- Fatigue.
- Bluish lips and nails (rare).
- Loss of appetite and weight loss.

CAUSES—Infection with bacteria, such as *Streptococci, Haemophilus, Klebsiella, Staphylococci*, and others. The germs are usually breathed in, but may be spread in other ways.

RISK INCREASES WITH
- Age (newborns, infants, and adults over 60).
- Use of anticancer drugs.
- Smoking.
- Chronic diseases.
- Recent surgery.
- Poor general health from any cause.
- Weak immune system due to illness or drugs.
- Hospital care, for any reason.
- Persons who have had their spleen removed.

HOW TO PREVENT
- Obtain medical care for respiratory infections.
- Ask your health care provide about pneumococcal and influenza vaccines.
- Avoid risk factors where possible.

WHAT TO EXPECT

DIAGNOSTIC MEASURES
- Your own observation of symptoms.
- Your health care provider will do a physical exam and ask questions about your symptoms.
- Medical tests may include a sputum culture, blood studies, and x-rays.

APPROPRIATE HEALTH CARE
- Hospital care is often needed for more severe cases. Treatment may include breathing support, fluids and/or drugs injected into a vein (IV), and removal of excess fluids from the lung.
- Some cases may be treated at home.

POSSIBLE COMPLICATIONS
- Pleurisy and pleural effusion (problems of the membrane layers that cover the lung).
- Bronchiectasis (damaged airways in the lungs).
- Spread of infection.
- Pulmonary abscess (pus-filled area).
- Complications are more likely in older persons who have other respiratory disorders or serious diseases. They can be life-threatening.

PROBABLE OUTCOME—Usually curable, in otherwise healthy persons, in 1 to 2 weeks with treatment. It may take longer for the very young, elderly, or those with other disorders.

HOW TO TREAT

GENERAL MEASURES
- Don't suppress the cough with a drug if the cough produces sputum or mucus. It is useful in ridding the body of lung secretions.
- Use a heating pad on low heat or warm compresses to relieve chest pain.
- Use a humidifier (if advised) to increase air moisture and loosen lung secretions. Follow instructions for its use.
- Stop smoking. Find a way to quit.
- To learn more: American Lung Association, 61 Broadway, 6th Floor, New York, NY 10006; (800) 586-4872; website: www.lungusa.org.

MEDICATION
- Antibiotics for infection will be prescribed.
- You may use nonprescription drugs, such as acetaminophen, to relieve minor discomfort.

ACTIVITY—Rest in bed until fever declines and pain and shortness of breath disappear. Then resume normal activities gradually.

DIET—No special diet. Increase fluid intake. Extra fluid helps thin the lung secretions so they are easier to cough up.

CALL YOUR DOCTOR IF

- You or a family member has symptoms of bacterial pneumonia.
- Symptoms worsen or new symptoms occur during treatment.

PNEUMONIA, MYCOPLASMA
(Atypical Pneumonia; Walking Pneumonia)

 GENERAL INFORMATION

DEFINITION—Mycoplasma pneumonia is a lung inflammation caused by infection with *Mycoplasma pneumoniae,* an organism (germ) that is similar to bacteria. The disorder is also called walking pneumonia, because a patient is usually not confined to bed or in need of hospital care. Some people may not even realize they have pneumonia, as the symptoms are often mild.

BODY PARTS INVOLVED—Upper-respiratory system.

SEX OR AGE MOST AFFECTED—Can affect all ages, but is more common in ages 5 to 20.

SIGNS & SYMPTOMS
* Cough that is dry. May have some sputum.
* Fever.
* Sore throat.
* Stuffy nose.
* Chest or ear pain may occur.
* Headache.
* Wheezing.
* Muscle aches and fatigue.

CAUSES—Mycoplasma pneumonia is infectious and is spread through close contact with an infected person. Germs are spread into the air when the infected person coughs or sneezes. Symptoms may begin 15 to 25 days after being exposed to the germs.

RISK INCREASES WITH
* Close living conditions (military barracks, college dorms, and families).
* Weak immune system due to illness or drugs.

HOW TO PREVENT—No specific preventive measures. Avoid exposure to persons who are ill with respiratory infections. Wash hands often to prevent spread of any type of germs.

 WHAT TO EXPECT

DIAGNOSTIC MEASURES
* Your own observation of symptoms.
* Your health care provider will do a physical exam and ask questions about your symptoms.
* Medical tests may include blood studies, sputum culture, and chest x-rays.

APPROPRIATE HEALTH CARE
* Treatment may include extra rest, treatment of symptoms, and antibiotics. For most patients, treatment can be done at home.
* Hospital care may be needed for someone with severe symptoms or complications.

POSSIBLE COMPLICATIONS
* Skin rash.
* Ear infection or sinus inflammation.
* Asthma.
* Hemolytic anemia (lack of red blood cells).
* Severe pneumonia.
* Other, less common complications may occur.

PROBABLE OUTCOME—Symptoms usually clear up in about two weeks. Some symptoms, such as cough or fatigue, may persist for 4 to 6 weeks. The disorder will heal on its own, but treatment with antibiotics can help speed recovery. Once a person has had the infection, there is some immunity, but it is not life-long.

 HOW TO TREAT

GENERAL MEASURES
* Use a heating pad on low heat or warm compresses to relieve chest pain.
* To learn more: American Lung Association, 61 Broadway, 6th Floor, New York, NY 10006; (800) 586-4872; website: www.lungusa.org.

MEDICATION
* Antibiotics, such as erythromycin, clarithromycin, azithromycin, or tetracycline (for ages over 8), may be prescribed. They will shorten the duration of fever and other symptoms, but you can carry the germs for weeks in spite of treatment.
* Cough medicine, nose drops, sprays, or oral decongestants may be recommended.
* You may use acetaminophen or ibuprofen for fever or minor pain.

ACTIVITY—Get extra rest until symptoms improve. Normal activities should be resumed gradually. Children may return to school once symptoms improve.

DIET—No special diet. Extra fluid helps thin lung secretions so they can be coughed up more easily.

 CALL YOUR DOCTOR IF

* You or a family member has symptoms of mycoplasma pneumonia.
* The following occur during treatment:
  - High fever, increased pain, or shortness of breath.
  - Dark or bluish fingernails, toenails, or skin.
  - Blood in the sputum, nausea, vomiting, or diarrhea.
  - Rash or earache.
  - Severe headache.

PNEUMONIA, VIRAL

GENERAL INFORMATION

DEFINITION—Viral pneumonia is a lung inflammation caused by a virus infection. Inflammation causes fluid to collect in the air sacs (alveoli) making it difficult to breathe.

BODY PARTS INVOLVED
* Lower respiratory tract (bronchial tubes, bronchioles and lungs).
* Upper respiratory tract (nose, throat, tonsils, sinuses, trachea and larynx).

SEX OR AGE MOST AFFECTED—Both sexes; all ages, but can be more severe in young children and adults over age 60.

SIGNS & SYMPTOMS
* Fever, chills, and sweating.
* Muscle aches and fatigue.
* Cough, with or without sputum, or "croup."
* Rapid, difficult (sometimes) breathing.
* Sore throat.
* Loss of appetite.
* Enlarged lymph glands in the neck.

CAUSES—Viral infection. These include influenza, chickenpox, and respiratory syncytial virus (especially in adults); respiratory viruses, measles, and cytomegalovirus (especially in infants).

RISK INCREASES WITH
* Newborns and infants.
* Adults over 60.
* Weak immune system due to illness or drugs.
* Persons with chronic diseases.
* Smoking.
* Crowded living conditions.
* Recent upper respiratory infection.

HOW TO PREVENT
* No specific preventive measures.
* Measles vaccines for children, chickenpox vaccine, and annual flu vaccines can help prevent infections that can lead to pneumonia.
* Wash hands often to prevent spread of any germs.

WHAT TO EXPECT

DIAGNOSTIC MEASURES
* Your own observation of symptoms.
* Your health care provider will do a physical exam and ask questions about your symptoms.
* Medical tests may include a sputum culture, blood studies, and x-rays.

APPROPRIATE HEALTH CARE
* Treatment may involve providing relief for the symptoms and drug therapy.
* Most patients can be treated at home.
* Hospital care may be needed for more severe cases.

POSSIBLE COMPLICATIONS
* Bacterial infection of the lungs.
* Other lung disorders such as bronchitis.

PROBABLE OUTCOME—Usually clears up on its own in 1 to 3 weeks. In more severe cases, recovery may take longer. Some people are fatigued and weak for up to 6 weeks after recovery.

HOW TO TREAT

GENERAL MEASURES
* Coughing and deep breathing are helpful to clear secretions. Dispose of tissues carefully.
* Use a heating pad on low heat or warm compresses to relieve chest pain.
* Use a humidifier (if advised) to increase air moisture and loosen lung secretions. Follow instructions for its use.
* Stop smoking. Find a way to quit.
* To learn more: American Lung Association, 61 Broadway, 6th Floor, New York, NY 10006, (800) 586-4872; website: www.lungusa.org.

MEDICATION
* Antiviral drugs may be prescribed depending on the virus and how long it's been since symptoms started.
* For minor pain, fever, and congestion, you may use nonprescription drugs, such as acetaminophen or decongestant nose drops, nasal sprays, or tablets.
* Antibiotics do not cure viral infections. They may be prescribed to prevent or treat a complicating bacterial infection.

ACTIVITY—Bed rest is helpful until fever, pain, and shortness of breath have been gone at least 48 hours. Then normal activity may be resumed slowly.

DIET—No special diet. Drink plenty of fluids. This helps to thin lung secretions so they are easier to cough up.

CALL YOUR DOCTOR IF

* You or a family member has symptoms of viral pneumonia.
* The following occur during treatment:
  - Temperature rises over 102°F (38.9°C).
  - Pain gets worse.
  - Nausea, vomiting, or diarrhea.
  - Increasing shortness of breath.
  - Blood in the sputum.
  - Increasingly bluish nails and skin.

PNEUMOTHORAX

GENERAL INFORMATION

DEFINITION
• A pneumothorax (collapsed lung) occurs when there is air between the two layers of the pleura. The pleura are thin membranes that cover the lung and line the chest wall. Pneumothorax types include:
- Spontaneous—it occurs without a cause. It is common in young men age 20 to 40.
- Secondary spontaneous—complication of lung disease.
- Traumatic—caused by an injury to the chest.
- Tension—excessive pressure builds up around lung. Air gets in, but cannot get out. It can be life-threatening.

BODY PARTS INVOLVED—Lung; pleura.

SEX OR AGE MOST AFFECTED—Both sexes; all ages; most common in active young men (ages 20 to 40).

SIGNS & SYMPTOMS
• The symptoms vary according to the degree of lung collapse and extent of other lung disease. Symptoms may be less acute if the pneumothorax develops slowly.
• Sharp chest pain. Pain may extend to a shoulder or across the chest or abdomen.
• Shortness of breath and rapid breathing.
• Anxiety.
• Dry, hacking cough (sometimes).
• Bluish nails.
• Coughing bloody sputum (sometimes).
• Rapid pulse.
• Fainting and shock (in tension pneumothorax).

CAUSES
• When air gets into the pleural space, it increases the pressure against the lung. This causes a partial or a complete collapse of the lung. Air may get into the pleural space as a result of:
- Rupture of the small air or fluid sacs in lungs.
- Air enters the chest from the outside, such as with a chest wound.
- Air results from a medical procedure on chest cavity.
- Air results from damaged lungs due to chronic lung disease, other diseases, or injury.

RISK INCREASES WITH
• Body build that is tall and slender.
• Males ages 20 to 40.
• Asthma, emphysema, chronic bronchitis, empyema, lung abscess, lung cancer, cystic fibrosis, or other lung disease.
• A wound to the chest area, which permits outside air to rush into the pleural space.
• Removing fluid from the lung (thoracentesis).
• Smoking.
• Personal or family history of pneumothorax.
• Marfan syndrome.

HOW TO PREVENT—No specific preventive measures. Get medical care for chronic lung disorders. Don't smoke.

WHAT TO EXPECT

DIAGNOSTIC MEASURES
• Your own observation of symptoms.
• Your health care provider will do a physical exam and ask about your symptoms and activities.
• X-rays of the chest help to confirm the diagnosis, determine the size of the pneumothorax, and track progress of treatment.

APPROPRIATE HEALTH CARE
• Treatment depends on the size of the pneumothorax and the condition of the lungs.
• No treatment may be needed in some cases. Small amounts of air are reabsorbed naturally and the lung will re-expand on its own.
• Hospital care may be needed for treatment.
- A small needle may be inserted into the chest cavity to relieve excess pressure.
- A tube may be placed in the chest and attached to a special vacuum bottle. This allows the air to be slowly removed and the lung to reexpand.
- Surgery may be needed if the pneumothorax has recurred or if the lung does not reexpand after 5 days.

POSSIBLE COMPLICATIONS
• Critical illness and death with tension pneumothorax.
• Repeated pneumothorax.

PROBABLE OUTCOME—Most patients recover fully in 2 to 4 weeks.

HOW TO TREAT

GENERAL MEASURES
• Don't smoke; try not to cough; avoid loud talking, laughing, or singing.
• Rest in a sitting position. It may be more comfortable.

MEDICATION—You may use nonprescription drugs, such as acetaminophen, for minor pain. Stronger pain relievers may be prescribed if needed.

ACTIVITY—Rest often. Allow two or more weeks for recovery.

DIET—No special diet.

CALL YOUR DOCTOR IF

• You or a family member has pneumothorax symptoms.
• New symptoms develop during recovery.

POISON IVY, OAK, SUMAC

GENERAL INFORMATION

DEFINITION—Poison ivy, oak, and sumac are three types of plants that cause a skin reaction (contact dermatitis). The reaction results from contact with an oily substance (or resin) produced by these plants. This particular type of allergic reaction is the most common one in the United States. 60% to 80% of the population has developed an allergy to these plants.

BODY PARTS INVOLVED—Skin.

SEX OR AGE MOST AFFECTED—Both sexes; all ages.

SIGNS & SYMPTOMS
- Skin rash with the following signs:
  - Bright red spots that develop 24 to 48 hours (sometimes may take several days) after contact.
    - Weeping, crusting, and swelling.
    - Intense itching and burning.
    - Blisters (the fluid in blisters is not contagious).
    - Enough of the oily resin remains on hands or clothing so that the rash is carried to other body parts, such as the face or genitals.

CAUSES—Contact with any part of the poison ivy, poison oak, or poison sumac plants. They grow as vines or bushes and have three leaves (poison ivy and poison oak), or a row of paired leaves (poison sumac). They produce a potent oil (urushiol) that is the cause of the problem. A reaction may also occur from touching the poison substance when it is on clothing, equipment (e.g., hunting, golfing, or athletic), or animals, such as pets. It can also come from any smoke these plants give off if they are burned. This may affect the face, eyelids, throat, and lungs.

RISK INCREASES WITH
- Spring and summer (though plants are dangerous year round).
- Not wearing protective clothing.

HOW TO PREVENT
- Learn to identify and avoid contact with these plants.
- When walking in areas where these plants grow, wear shoes, socks, long pants, long-sleeved shirts, and, sometimes, gloves. Wash this clothing right after you return if possible. Use a product that prevents the poison from getting on your skin.
- If you are exposed, washing the skin immediately (within 30 minutes) with soap and water and sponging with rubbing alcohol may prevent the rash.

WHAT TO EXPECT

DIAGNOSTIC MEASURES
- Your own observation of symptoms.
- Consult your health care provider if rash is severe or does not improve. The diagnosis can be confirmed.

APPROPRIATE HEALTH CARE
- Self-care at home.
- If needed, drugs may be prescribed.

POSSIBLE COMPLICATIONS—A skin infection may develop.

PROBABLE OUTCOME—Itching, redness, and swelling are often improved by the second day, and complete healing usually occurs within 7 to 14 days. Some cases may persist for 6 weeks.

HOW TO TREAT

GENERAL MEASURES
- Sweating and heat make the itching worse, so try to stay cool.
- Apply cool compresses to the affected area.
- A soothing bath helps. Use Aveeno (a product made of oatmeal) or baking soda (about a half cup per bath).
- Wash all clothing and shoes, and any equipment that came in contact with the plant oils, with soap and water.
- Give pets a warm, soapy bath to remove any oil from the fur.
- To learn more: CDC-National Institute for Occupational Safety & Health; (800) 232-4636; website: www.cdc.gov/niosh/topics/plants.

MEDICATION
- Nonprescription topical steroid creams may be used for itching and swelling.
- You may use calamine lotion to relieve the itching.
- Oral antihistamines may be helpful also.
- Your health care provider may prescribe oral or stronger topical steroid drugs for severe symptoms.

ACTIVITY—No limits. Avoid activities that can cause sweating. This can worsen itching.

DIET—No special diet.

CALL YOUR DOCTOR IF

- You or a family member has a severe rash.
- Swelling or pain develops around the eyes, nose, or genitals.
- Rash gets worse or doesn't improve with self-care methods.

POLYARTERITIS NODOSA
(Necrotizing Angiitis)

GENERAL INFORMATION

DEFINITION—Polyarteritis nodosa is an inflammation of the small and medium size arteries in the body. This results in a decrease in blood supply to the body's organs and tissues supplied by the affected arteries.

BODY PARTS INVOLVED—Can affect the muscles, joints, skin, heart, brain, intestinal tract, nerves, liver, kidneys, and genitals.

SEX OR AGE MOST AFFECTED—It is more common in middle-age adults, and occurs in men slightly more often than women.

SIGNS & SYMPTOMS
- General symptoms include weight loss, fever, fatigue, general ill feeling, muscle and joint aches, weakness, high blood pressure, and headache.
- Other symptoms may be due to the affected organ:
  - Blood in the urine (kidney involved).
  - Chest pain (heart involved).
  - Abdominal pain (intestinal tract and liver involved).
  - Numbness and tingling of the hands and feet (nerves involved).
  - Purplish rash and other skin disorders (skin involved).
  - Testicle pain (testicles involved).

CAUSES—It is considered an autoimmune disease, although the cause is unknown. Hepatitis B appears to be a factor in some cases.

RISK INCREASES WITH
- Hepatitis B and sometimes hepatitis C.
- Other autoimmune diseases.
- Methamphetamine abuse.
- Smoking.
- Use of certain drugs, including penicillin, antithyroid drugs, thiazide diuretics, and some vaccines.

HOW TO PREVENT—No specific preventive measures.

WHAT TO EXPECT

DIAGNOSTIC MEASURES
- Your own observation of symptoms.
- Your health care provider will do a physical exam and ask questions about your symptoms.
- No single test can diagnose the disorder. Medical tests may include blood and urine studies, x-ray, biopsy, and MRI. Angiography may be done—a dye is injected into the arteries to highlight the affected areas and x-rays taken.

APPROPRIATE HEALT
- Treatment is with drugs t[...] inflammation.
- Hospital care may be needed [...] cases and complications.
- Surgery may be needed if there a[...] complications involving the intestinal tr[...]

POSSIBLE COMPLICATIONS
- Kidney failure.
- Heart attack, heart failure, or stroke.
- Nervous system disorders.
- Intestinal perforation.
- Aneurysm rupture.
- Side effects of drugs used in treatment.
- Blood clots.

PROBABLE OUTCOME—With early diagnosis and treatment, the disorder can be controlled and, sometimes patients recover completely. Without treatment, few patients live beyond 5 years.

HOW TO TREAT

GENERAL MEASURES
- Wear or carry medical ID to show that you have this disorder.
- Avoid close contact with people who have infections.

MEDICATION
- Cortisone drugs and immunosuppressive drugs are usually prescribed. They need to be continued even after symptoms improve. The dosage may be adjusted once the symptoms are controlled. Some patients want to stop the drugs because of side effects. Without drugs, however, the disorder will progress and cause complications.
- Drugs to treat other disorders such as hepatitis B, heart drugs, or drugs for high blood pressure may be prescribed.

ACTIVITY—Resume your normal activities gradually as symptoms improve.

DIET—No special diet unless advised by your health care provider.

CALL YOUR DOCTOR IF

- You or a family member has symptoms of polyarteritis nodosa.
- New, unexplained symptoms develop.

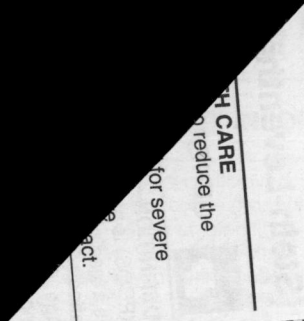

...RY SYNDROME
(...drome)

...TION

...ne
...dition. It
... PCOS
...bearing
...come
...in
...y ... older and is rare after
menopause.

BODY PARTS INVOLVED—Ovaries, but can affect the entire body.

SEX OR AGE MOST AFFECTED—Women of childbearing age.

SIGNS & SYMPTOMS
* Irregular menstrual bleeding. This results in periods of light flow along with heavy flow. There is increased time between periods, often up to several months.
* Hirsutism—increased hair growth on the face, arms, legs, and from pubic area to navel.
* Thinning of the scalp hair (alopecia).
* Overweight or obesity.
* Trouble getting pregnant; miscarriages.
* Acne and oily skin.
* Dark patches of skin or skin tags (small skin growths).
* Polycystic ovaries. These are fairly common and involve enlarged ovaries from many small cysts.
* Anovulation (absence of ovulation). The monthly release of the egg from the ovary fails to take place.
* High cholesterol level; high blood pressure.

CAUSES—The exact cause is unclear. Hormone imbalances, insulin production, and hereditary factors all seem to play a role.

RISK INCREASES WITH
* Obesity or overweight.
* Family history of PCOS or diabetes.
* Ages 20 to 30.
* Having diabetes or insulin resistance.

HOW TO PREVENT—No known way to prevent.

WHAT TO EXPECT

DIAGNOSTIC MEASURES
* Your own observation of symptoms.
* Your health care provider will usually do a physical exam and a pelvic exam. Questions will be asked about your symptoms, menstrual cycle, and pregnancies.
* Blood studies will be done. These measure levels of hormones, glucose, insulin, and fats (cholesterol and triglyceride). An ultrasound may be done to rule out other disorders. There is no one test to diagnose PCOS.

APPROPRIATE HEALTH CARE
* Treatment goals: regulate menstrual cycle, reduce hair growth and acne problems, help with fertility (if pregnancy desired), and prevent long-term problems.
* A diet and exercise program for overweight or obese women will help improve physical and mental health.
* Infertility can be treated successfully with diet, exercise, weight loss, and drug therapy. If these steps are not helpful, surgery (ovarian drilling) may be an option.
* Counseling may help you cope with diagnosis.

POSSIBLE COMPLICATIONS
* Infertility or miscarriages.
* Depression and anxiety.
* A decrease in HDL (the good) cholesterol.
* High triglyceride levels.
* Heart and blood vessel disease; high blood pressure.
* Diabetes or metabolic syndrome.
* Uterine bleeding.
* Endometrial cancer. There may be an increased risk of ovarian or breast cancer.

PROBABLE OUTCOME—There is no cure. Treatment, along with weight control and exercise, can often relieve or eliminate symptoms. Pregnancy (if desired) can be achieved in many patients.

HOW TO TREAT

GENERAL MEASURES
* Options for removing excess hair from your face, arms, and legs include drugs, bleaching, electrolysis, laser therapy, plucking, waxing, and depilation.
* Quit smoking. Find a way to stop that works.

MEDICATION
* Diabetic drugs (such as metformin), birth-control pills, or other drugs may be prescribed.
* Drugs to help with fertility may be prescribed.
* Vaniqa (eflornithine cream) for excess facial hair or spironolactone for excess body hair may be prescribed.

ACTIVITY—No limits on activity, including sexual intercourse. Physical activity is important. Exercise daily.

DIET—A weight-loss program is often prescribed for overweight women. A dietitian can help you plan a diet.

☎ CALL YOUR DOCTOR IF

* You or a family member has symptoms of polycystic ovary syndrome.
* New symptoms occur with treatment.

POLYCYTHEMIA

GENERAL INFORMATION

DEFINITION
• Polycythemia is an increase of red blood cells in the body. The different types are:
- Primary polycythemia (polycythemia vera) involves an overproduction of red blood cells, white blood cells, and platelets, by an abnormality of the bone marrow.
- Secondary polycythemia (reactive polycythemia) involves an overproduction of red blood cells caused by a disease (rather than the bone marrow).
- Relative polycythemia (sometimes called pseudo-polycythemia) involves an increase in red blood cells that is due to decreased blood plasma.

BODY PARTS INVOLVED—Blood-forming organs: bone marrow; spleen; lymph glands; lymph channels.

SEX OR AGE MOST AFFECTED—It usually affects adults over age 50 and is rare in children.

SIGNS & SYMPTOMS
• Some patients have no symptoms. It may be diagnosed when a routine blood test is done.
• Fatigue, headache, drowsiness, dizziness, weight loss, or weakness.
• Itching or flushed skin.
• Enlarged spleen.
• Unexplained bleeding or bruising.
• Vision changes, shortness of breath, or bone pain.

CAUSES
• Polycythemia vera—a genetic mutation (change in the body's genes) is involved, but exact cause is unknown.
• Secondary polycythemia—congenital heart disease, chronic lung disease, living at high altitude, and others.
• Relative polycythemia—dehydration or use of diuretic drugs.

RISK INCREASES WITH
• Adults over age 50 and males more than females.
• Ashkenazi Jewish ancestry.
• Family member has polycythemia.

HOW TO PREVENT—Cannot be prevented.

WHAT TO EXPECT

DIAGNOSTIC MEASURES
• Your health care provider will do a physical exam and ask questions about your symptoms.
• Medical tests may include studies of bone marrow and blood (red blood cell count, hematocrit), x-ray of the kidneys, and others.

APPROPRIATE HEALTH CARE
• Treatment steps will depend on the age of patient, disease duration, type of polycythemia, complications, disease activity, and response to treatment.
• Treatment steps to keep the red blood cell range near normal and prevent clotting or hemorrhage include phlebotomy (withdrawal of excess blood) and drug therapy. Other therapies are usually prescribed for high risk patients.
• For secondary or relative polycythemia, proper treatment of the underlying cause is important. Drug therapy or surgery may be recommended.

POSSIBLE COMPLICATIONS
• Blood clots in veins or arteries. Clots can lead to strokes or heart attack.
• Gout, heart failure, peptic ulcer, or kidney stones.
• Leukemia.
• Hemorrhage.
• Bone marrow scarring.

PROBABLE OUTCOME
• There is no cure for polycythemia vera. Treatment can help manage symptoms and reduce complication risks. Life expectancy varies. Ongoing research may help find the cause and a cure.
• Outcome of other types of polycythemia will depend on treatment of the underlying cause.

HOW TO TREAT

GENERAL MEASURES
• Stop smoking. Find a way to quit.
• Adherence to your treatment plan brings about improved survival and well-being.

MEDICATION
• Your health care provider may prescribe:
- Drugs to suppress production of red blood cells and platelets.
- Allopurinol if uric acid levels are high.
- Low-dose aspirin for ages over 18.
- Anti-itching drugs, such as antihistamines.
- Drugs for stomach acidity.
- Other drugs as needed for complications.

ACTIVITY—Your health care provider may recommend an exercise program. Moderate exercise, such as walking improves blood flow.

DIET—No special diet. Drink enough fluids to help maintain adequate body fluid.

CALL YOUR DOCTOR IF

• You or a family member has symptoms of polycythemia.
• Symptoms recur after treatment.
• New, unexplained symptoms develop.

POLYMYALGIA RHEUMATICA & GIANT CELL ARTERITIS

 GENERAL INFORMATION

DEFINITION—Polymyalgia rheumatica (PMR) and giant cell arteritis (GCA) are related inflammatory disorders. They often occur together. In PMR, inflammation affects the whole body. In GCA, certain arteries, such as those in the head and neck, are inflamed.

BODY PARTS INVOLVED—Muscles; temporal arteries; eyes; connective tissue.

SEX OR AGE MOST AFFECTED—Adults over 50. The disease occurs more often in women than men.

SIGNS & SYMPTOMS
- The symptoms may resemble those of an infection such as influenza. Symptoms can come on suddenly.
- Low fever and weakness.
- Muscle stiffness or aches and pains, especially in the morning. The muscles involved are usually those of the shoulders, upper arms, and legs.
- Headache (usually in one temple).
- Pain in the temples or scalp, and sometimes, the jaw and tongue.
- Blurred or double vision; vision loss in one eye.
- Appetite loss and weight loss.

CAUSES—Exact cause of the inflammation is unknown. It may involve the immune system, or be due to viral, genetic, or environmental factors.

RISK INCREASES WITH—Adults over age 50, especially women.

HOW TO PREVENT—No specific preventive measures.

 WHAT TO EXPECT

DIAGNOSTIC MEASURES
- Your own observation of symptoms.
- Your health care provider will do a physical exam and ask questions about your symptoms.
- There is no specific diagnostic test for either disorder. Medical tests may include blood studies, tests for anemia, a CT or MRI, and a biopsy. Biopsy involves the removal of a small amount of tissue or fluid for viewing under a microscope.

APPROPRIATE HEALTH CARE—Treatment involves drug therapy and exercise.

POSSIBLE COMPLICATIONS
- PMR may recur. It can be successfully treated again with drugs. GCA rarely recurs after treatment.

- Without treatment for GCA, there is a risk for loss of vision, stroke, heart failure, chest pain, and aneurysm.
- Adverse effects of steroid treatment (osteoporosis, high blood pressure, cataracts, and others).

PROBABLE OUTCOME—With treatment, the symptoms can clear up quickly and complications are unlikely. Treatment with drugs needs to continue for months to years depending on each individual patient. An active lifestyle is expected.

 HOW TO TREAT

GENERAL MEASURES
- For headache relief, apply heat to the painful side of the head. For muscle stiffness, apply heat directly to the affected area or take warm baths.
- To learn more: National Institute of Arthritis & Musculoskeletal & Skin disorders, 1 AMS Circle, Bethesda, MD 20892; (877) 226-4267; website: www.niams.nih.gov.

MEDICATION
- Cortisone drugs are usually prescribed until the acute phase ends. These relieve symptoms by reducing inflammation. Adverse effects may occur. For ongoing treatment with cortisone, the dosage will be reduced as low as possible to keep symptoms under control.
- Nonsteroidal anti-inflammatory drugs may be prescribed for polymyalgia rheumatica. They may not completely control symptoms.

ACTIVITY
- Physical therapy may be prescribed.
- Exercise regularly. Swimming, walking, biking, and stretching exercises will help keep muscles strong, flexible, and functional. Avoid straining the muscles (such as doing heavy lifting). Adequate rest is also important. Don't overdo physical activities.

DIET—No special diet.

 CALL YOUR DOCTOR IF

- You or a family member has symptoms of polymyalgia rheumatica or giant cell arteritis.
- The following occur during or after treatment:
  - Any changes in vision. Call immediately!
  - Temperature of 101°F (38.3°C).
  - Blood in the urine.
  - Shortness of breath and/or chest pain.
  - Bloody bowel movements.
  - Severe abdominal pain.
- New, unexplained symptoms develop. Drugs used in treatment may produce side effects.

POLYMYOSITIS & DERMATOM[...]

GENERAL INFORMATION

DEFINITION—Polymyositis is muscle inflammation that leads to a gradual weakening of the muscles. When the disorder involves the skin, it is called dermatomyositis.

BODY PARTS INVOLVED—Muscles, including large muscles of the skeleton and tiny muscles that control small arteries; skin; connective tissue.

SEX OR AGE MOST AFFECTED—Women are affected more often than men. It usually begins after age 20. It may also occur in children.

SIGNS & SYMPTOMS
- Symptoms vary from person to person and may be mild to severe. Their onset may be sudden or slow.
- Muscle weakness that often begins in the hip, thighs, and shoulder muscles. Other muscles may be affected.
- Frequent falls and difficulty in getting up.
- Difficulty in climbing stairs and getting up from a chair or bed.
- Muscle pain, stiffness, or swelling.
- Skin rash (may itch) on the face, shoulders, arms, and over joints. The rash may be red or violet.
- Cold hands and feet.
- Speaking or swallowing difficulty.

CAUSES—Exact cause is unknown. They may be autoimmune disorders. In these disorders, the immune system by mistake attacks the body. Other factors may be involved such as viral, genetic, or environmental.

RISK INCREASES WITH
- Females over age 30.
- Family history of autoimmune disorders.

HOW TO PREVENT—No known preventive measures.

WHAT TO EXPECT

DIAGNOSTIC MEASURES
- Your health care provider will do a physical exam and an exam of any affected skin.
- Medical tests may include blood studies, heart tests, x-ray, and MRI. A biopsy may be done, which involves removal of a small amount of muscle tissue for viewing under a microscope. An electromyogram may be done. This test studies the electrical activity of muscles.

APPROPRIATE HE[...]
usually involves drugs, [...]
other therapy to help you [...]
daily living.

POSSIBLE COMPLICATIONS
- Progressive muscle weakness.
- Heart, gastrointestinal, and lung prob[...]
- Adverse effects of drugs.
- Skin ulcers (open sores), infections, and scarring.
- Polymyositis has been associated with an increased risk of certain cancers (e.g., colon, lung, ovarian, and breast).

PROBABLE OUTCOME—The outcome varies. Symptoms can improve at times and get worse at other times. Earlier diagnosis and treatment improves the outcome. Some patients recover completely. Others have persistent symptoms, such as weakness. Others may have complications that can lead to disability and be life-threatening.

HOW TO TREAT

GENERAL MEASURES
- Cool-water compresses may relieve itching.
- To learn more: The Myositis Association, 1737 King St., Suite 600, Alexandria, VA 22314; (800) 821 7356; website: www.myositis.org.

MEDICATION
- Your health care provider may prescribe:
  - Cortisone drugs, in high doses until acute symptoms diminish, then in lower doses.
  - Drugs to suppress the immune system.
  - Drugs to help control itching.
  - Drugs for pain.
  - Drugs for bone building.

ACTIVITY—Physical therapy may be prescribed. It helps keep muscles flexible, strong, and functional. Follow instructions for exercises to do at home. Swimming is a good exercise. Don't overdo any activity. Rest as needed.

DIET—Chewing and swallowing may become more difficult for some patients. A dietitian can help with meal planning and easy-to-eat foods.

CALL YOUR DOCTOR IF

- You or a family member has symptoms of polymyositis or dermatomyositis.
- Symptoms don't improve or recur despite treatment.
- New, unexplained symptoms develop.

...YOSITIS

...ALTH CARE—T...physical thera...with the activities of...

...TION

...which the ...yrin is a ...the body ...of blood that ...n. Types include:
...yria (AIP).
...P).
- Hereditary coproporphyria (HCP).
- Porphyria cutanea tarda (PCT).
- Erythropoietic porphyria (EPP).
- Congenital erythropoietic porphyria (CEP).
- Hepatoerythropoietic porphyria (HEP).
- Aminolevulinic dehydratase deficiency porphyria (ALAD).

BODY PARTS INVOLVED—Blood, nervous system, skin, liver, and digestive system.

SEX OR AGE MOST AFFECTED—The sex and age affected varies depending on type.

SIGNS & SYMPTOMS
- Symptoms vary and can appear over hours or days. Symptoms often affect the nervous system or the skin. A variety of factors can trigger an attack.
- Chest, abdominal, or leg pain.
- Muscle cramps and weakness.
- Numbness and tingling in the feet and hands.
- Emotional and mental changes including depression, mania, anxiety, agitation, confusion, and others.
- Skin changes, including itching, blistering, and sensitivity to the sun.
- Excessive hair growth.
- Urine turns color (dark-red, purplish, or brown).

CAUSES—Porphyrin builds up in the body due to enzyme deficiencies. Enzymes are required to complete the porphyrin-heme process. There are several different types of enzyme deficiencies. Most types are inherited. Others develop during a person's life.

RISK INCREASES WITH—Family history of porphyria.

HOW TO PREVENT
- Cannot be prevented at present.
- Porphyria attacks may result from drugs, alcohol, smoking, infection, reduced calorie intake, stress (physical and emotional), sun exposure, fasting, excess iron, hepatitis C, pregnancy, and before a menstrual period. Ask your health care provider about avoiding attacks.

 WHAT TO EXPECT

DIAGNOSTIC MEASURES
- Your own observation of symptoms.

- Your health care provider will do a physical exam and ask questions about your symptoms and activities and family medical history.
- Medical tests are done to measure porphyrins in the urine, blood, and stool.

APPROPRIATE HEALTH CARE
- Treatment involves medical care during attacks, preventing attacks, and counseling if needed. Specific treatment will depend on the type of porphyria.
- Phlebotomy may be done. A unit of blood is removed on a regular basis to get rid of excess iron in the body.
- Hospital care may be required for severe symptoms.

POSSIBLE COMPLICATIONS—Physical problems as well as psychological problems.

PROBABLE OUTCOME—There is no cure. Some people with porphyria never have symptoms. In others, the symptoms may be mild to severe. Symptoms can usually be relieved with treatment. A few patients may have complications.

 HOW TO TREAT

GENERAL MEASURES
- Don't take any drugs, herbs, or supplements without medical advice.
- Avoid bright sunlight. If you must be in bright sun, use a hat and protective clothing.
- Wear or carry medical ID to show you have this disorder.
- Genetic counseling before starting a family is advised.
- To learn more: American Porphyria Foundation, 4900 Woodway, Suite 780, Houston, TX 77056; (866) 273-3635; website: www.porphyriafoundation.com.

MEDICATION
- Your health care provider may prescribe:
  - Intravenous (IV) glucose or heme to help prevent or treat acute attacks.
  - Drugs for depression or anxiety.
  - Drugs to reduce nausea and vomiting.
  - Drugs to reduce the excess porphyrin in the body.
  - Drugs to help reduce premenstrual attacks.
  - Drugs for anemia (if needed).
  - Beta carotene for skin symptoms.

ACTIVITY—No limits except for sun avoidance.

DIET—No special diet.

 CALL YOUR DOCTOR IF

- You or a family member has symptoms of porphyria.
- Any symptoms develop that cause concern.

POSTMENOPAUSAL BLEEDING

 GENERAL INFORMATION

DEFINITION—Postmenopausal bleeding is unexpected vaginal bleeding that begins 6 or more months after menstrual periods stop due to menopause. This is not a normal condition and can be a symptom of a serious medical problem.

BODY PARTS INVOLVED—Reproductive system.

SEX OR AGE MOST AFFECTED—Females after menopause.

SIGNS & SYMPTOMS
- Vaginal bleeding. It may be a light-brown discharge or heavy, red bleeding (with or without clots).
- Mucus may be a part of the bleeding.
- Bleeding episodes vary in length.
- Pelvic pain (sometimes).

CAUSES
- Most common cause is atrophy of the lining of the uterus (endometrium) or the vagina. Atrophy means shrinking, drying or wasting away of tissue.
- Hormone therapy. Using estrogens (female hormones).
- Cancer.
- Endometrial hyperplasia (the uterine lining becomes overgrown).
- Endometrial or cervical polyps (benign growths).
- Myoma (benign fibroid tumor in the uterus).
- Trauma (injury) to the vagina.

RISK INCREASES WITH
- Women over 60, due to fragile blood vessels and thin vaginal or uterine lining.
- Obesity.
- Hormone therapy. Women are likely to have some bleeding the first year.

HOW TO PREVENT—No specific preventive measures.

 WHAT TO EXPECT

DIAGNOSTIC MEASURES
- Your own observation of symptoms.
- Your health care provider will usually do a physical exam, including a pelvic exam. (Be sure to tell your health care provider about nonprescribed substances that you take, such as soy protein.) Unexplained postmenopausal bleeding requires further medical testing. Tests start with blood studies and a Pap smear.

- Additional tests may include:
  - Biopsy of a small amount of tissue removed from the uterine lining. This is done with a thin suction device.
  - Ultrasound of the pelvic area.
  - Sonohystogram, an ultrasound with a saline (salt-water solution) injected into the uterus.
  - A hysteroscopy. A telescopic instrument with a special light is used to look inside the uterus.
  - A dilatation and curettage, referred to as D & C (dilatation of the cervix and a scraping out of the uterus with a curette). It may be both diagnostic and treatment to relieve the bleeding.

APPROPRIATE HEALTH CARE
- Specific therapy, usually drugs or surgery depends on the cause. Sometimes, even after testing, no clear-cut reason for the bleeding is found.
- Surgery (hysterectomy) to remove the uterus may be needed.

POSSIBLE COMPLICATIONS If cancer is the cause, the outcome will depend on the type of cancer and the stage at which it is diagnosed. Many of these cancers are caught early, when treatment is more effective.

PROBABLE OUTCOME—The outcome will depend on the cause of the bleeding. In the majority of cases, the cause is not cancer. Benign conditions can usually be treated and bleeding symptoms should clear up.

 HOW TO TREAT

GENERAL MEASURES—Follow medical advice about home care after any treatment.

MEDICATION
- If hormone drugs are currently being taken, the dose may need to be adjusted. In other cases, hormones may be prescribed.
- Drugs may be prescribed to treat any underlying disorder diagnosed.

ACTIVITY
- No limits unless advised by your health care provider.
- Sexual relations may be resumed as soon as desired after diagnosis and treatment.

DIET—No special diet.

 CALL YOUR DOCTOR IF

You or a family member has unexplained vaginal bleeding after menopause or bleeding persists, despite treatment.

POSTPARTUM INFECTION
(Puerperal Infection)

GENERAL INFORMATION

DEFINITION—Postpartum infection is a bacterial infection in the genital tract following delivery of a baby.

BODY PARTS INVOLVED—The infection most often occurs in the uterus and causes inflammation (endometritis). It can also affect the vagina, vulva, perineum (area between the vagina and rectum), cervix, or peritoneum (membrane that covers abdominal organs).

SEX OR AGE MOST AFFECTED—Females of childbearing age.

SIGNS & SYMPTOMS
- Fever and chills for two or more days after the first postpartum day (first day after delivery).
- Headache and muscle aches.
- Appetite loss.
- Vaginal discharge with a foul odor.
- Stomach (abdominal) pain.
- General ill feeling.

CAUSES—Infection by bacteria germs during childbirth.

RISK INCREASES WITH
- Cesarean delivery.
- Genital or urinary tract infection prior to delivery.
- Use of a fetal scalp electrode during labor.
- Anemia, either before pregnancy, or from loss of blood during delivery.
- Poor nutrition during pregnancy.
- Long delay between water break (rupture of the placental membranes) and delivery (more than 24 hours).
- A small part of the placenta is left in the uterus.
- Extra-long labor.
- Multiple vaginal exams.
- Obesity.
- Diabetes.

HOW TO PREVENT
- No specific preventive steps. To reduce risk factors:
  - Avoid anyone with an active infection for the last 2 weeks of pregnancy.
  - Notify your obstetric provider as soon as your water breaks. Don't have sexual intercourse after this occurs.
  - Wash the genital area often during the first week after delivery.

WHAT TO EXPECT

DIAGNOSTIC MEASURES
- Your health care provider will do a physical exam including a pelvic exam.

- Medical tests may include blood and urine studies and studies of the vaginal discharge. Other tests may be done if drug treatment fails.

APPROPRIATE HEALTH CARE
- Treatment usually involves antibiotics for the infection. Hospital care may be needed for severe infection.
- Surgery may be done to remove fragments of placenta or to treat an abscess or blood clot. An infected episiotomy (incision made during delivery) may need to be opened and drained.

POSSIBLE COMPLICATIONS
- Deep-vein blood clot in pelvis; pelvic abscess.
- Shock.
- Scarring.
- Infertility.
- Blood poisoning (although rare, could be life-threatening).

PROBABLE OUTCOME—Usually curable in 7 to 10 days with treatment.

HOW TO TREAT

GENERAL MEASURES
- To relieve pain, place a heating pad or hot-water bottle on the abdomen or back. Take frequent, warm baths to relax muscles and help relieve pain.
- Use sanitary pads, rather than tampons, for the vaginal discharge.
- If you breastfeed, ask your health care provider about continuing to do so during treatment.

MEDICATION
- One or more antibiotics for infection will be prescribed. They may be taken by mouth or given through a vein (IV).
- Drugs to reduce fever and relieve pain may be prescribed.
- Anticoagulants may be prescribed to prevent blood clots from forming.

ACTIVITY—Rest in bed, except to use the bathroom, until fever and other signs of infection clear up. You may be more comfortable lying on your left side.

DIET—Drink plenty of fluids.

CALL YOUR DOCTOR IF

- You or a family member has symptoms of a postpartum infection after delivery.
- Symptoms of infection recur after treatment.

POSTPARTUM MOOD DISORDE
(Postpartum Blues, Depression, & Psyc

 GENERAL INFORMATION

DEFINITION
- Mood disorders following the birth of a baby affect nearly half of all new mothers. The symptoms are most common 3 to 10 days following delivery, but can occur anytime in the first 6 months. Types include:
  - Postpartum blues (baby blues), which involves mild symptoms that last a short time.
  - Postpartum depression symptoms are sometimes described as baby blues that deepen and last longer.
  - Postpartum psychosis is a rare, severe depression.

BODY PARTS INVOLVED—Brain.

SEX OR AGE MOST AFFECTED—Females of childbearing age.

SIGNS & SYMPTOMS
- Symptoms vary for different women.
- Mild sadness, crying spells, and mood swings.
- Appetite loss and weight loss, or weight gain.
- Sleep problems; unable to sleep when baby sleeps, or waking up and having trouble returning to sleep.
- Loss of energy; fatigue.
- Irritability; anxiety, or feelings of tension or anger.
- Slow speech and thought, unable to make decisions.
- Frequent headaches, and other physical discomfort.
- Confusion about one's ability to improve life.
- Feelings of hopelessness, worthlessness, gloom, or guilt. Fears about personal health and infant's health.
- Poor personal hygiene.

CAUSES—Exact cause is unknown. It may involve physical, emotional, social, genetic, and hormone factors.

RISK INCREASES WITH
- Personal or family history of depression or bipolar disorder or postpartum depression in previous pregnancy.
- Physical and emotional stress, lack of sleep; poor nutrition, or problems with the baby's health.
- Severe pregnancy problem (e.g., preterm birth).
- Lack of support from one's partner, family, or friends.

HOW TO PREVENT
- No specific way to prevent . Screening tests may help identify women at risk.
- If you have had postpartum blues or depression before, ask your obstetric provider about ways to help guard against a recurrence.

 WHAT TO EXPE

DIAGNOSTIC MEASURES
- Your own or other's observation of sympto
- Your health care provider will ask questions about your symptoms and medical history.
- A depression-screening test may be given. Urine and blood tests may be done.

APPROPRIATE HEALTH CARE—Treatment
may involve counseling (psychotherapy) and/or group therapy, drugs, self-help, and education. Treatment depends on the type and degree of the symptoms. Rarely, hospital care is needed.

POSSIBLE COMPLICATIONS
- Lack of bonding between mother and baby.
- Children of depressed mothers are more at risk for behavioral or developmental problems.
- Relationship problems with partner.
- Depression may become chronic or recurrent.
- Postpartum psychosis. A mother may harm herself or her baby.

PROBABLE OUTCOME
- It's common for mothers to have some degree of baby blues. It clears up on its own in days.
- For most women, postpartum depression is treatable. It may last a few weeks to months.

 HOW TO TREAT

GENERAL MEASURES
- Don't feel guilty if you have mixed feelings the baby. Adjustment and bonding take time.
- Schedule outings, such as walks and short visits with friends or family so you don't feel alone.
- Ask for daytime help from family or friends (shop for you or care for baby while you rest).
- Find time for you and your partner to be alone.
- Share your feelings with your partner, friends, other mothers, or a support group.
- To learn more: Postpartum Support, PO Box 60931, Santa Barbara, CA 93160; (800) 944-4773; website: www.postpartum.net.

MEDICATION—Antidepressant drugs may be
prescribed. These are effective when used for 3 to 4 weeks. If you are breastfeeding, your health care provider will discuss your options.

ACTIVITY—Try to get some exercise each day.

DIET—Eat a well-balanced diet. Avoid alcohol.

 CALL YOUR DOCTOR IF

- You or a family member has symptoms of a postpartum mood disorder.
- You have thoughts of hurting yourself or the baby. Seek help promptly!

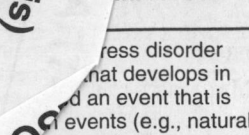

BASIC INFORMATION

...ress disorder ...hat develops in ...d an event that is ...l events (e.g., natural ...ar, imprisonment, torture, a... ...uce psychological (emotional) stress... everyone. PTSD involves a persistent re-experiencing of the trauma and other symptoms. The symptoms may begin right after the event or develop months or years later.

BODY PARTS INVOLVED—Nervous.

SEX OR AGE MOST AFFECTED—Both sexes; all ages (more common in women than men).

SIGNS & SYMPTOMS
- Recurrent, intrusive, and distressing memories of the event. A sense of reliving the event (flashbacks).
- Recurrent dreams or nightmares relating to the event.
- Chronic anxiety; insomnia; easily startled.
- Difficulty in concentrating; memory problems.
- A sense of personal isolation (feeling alone).
- Lack of interest in activities previously enjoyed.
- Phobic (fearful) reactions to situations or avoiding activities that recall memories of the event.
- Emotional effects (irritability, restlessness, tearfulness, explosive outbursts of behavior including violence, a numbness of feelings, or painful guilt feelings).

CAUSES—Exact cause is unknown. Exposure to an overwhelming, distressing event is a main factor. Other factors may involve a person's personality type, chemical imbalance in the brain, environmental stresses, and genetics.

RISK INCREASES WITH
- Event:
  - The type, severity, and duration of the event.
  - Being directly involved or witness to the event.
- Personal:
  - Emotional problems (e.g., low self-esteem).
  - Lack of support from family, friends, or community.
  - Childhood history of alcoholic parents, neglect, abuse, separation of parents, poverty, or violence.
  - Previous experience with trauma.
  - Personal or family history of mental disorders.
  - Alcohol or drug abuse.

HOW TO PREVENT
- Counseling and crisis intervention right after a traumatic event may help prevent PTSD.
- Debriefing soon after an event. Persons involved discuss the event, their emotions, and their reactions.

WHAT TO EXPECT

DIAGNOSTIC MEASURES
- Your own or other's observation of symptoms.
- Your health care provider will do a physical exam and ask questions about your symptoms and exposure to a traumatic event.
- Medical tests may be done to rule out physical disorders. Mental health tests may be done.

APPROPRIATE HEALTH CARE
- Treatment may include medical care (if needed for injuries or substance abuse), counseling (psychotherapy), drugs, education, self-help, and support groups. Treatment depends on each person's situation (safety from harm), the symptoms, and health status.
- Cognitive-behavioral therapy is often helpful. Cognitive therapy teaches how to change thoughts, behaviors or attitudes. Behavioral therapy teaches ways to reduce anxiety with deep breathing and muscle relaxation. Other types of therapies can be effective.

POSSIBLE COMPLICATIONS
- Marriage and family conflicts, difficulty in parenting children effectively, loss of friends, and unemployment.
- Depression, anxiety, phobias, drug abuse, or alcohol abuse.
- Self-inflicted violence and suicide.

PROBABLE OUTCOME—For some patients, the symptoms go away on their own after 6 months. Most patients are helped with therapy. In others, the disorder may become chronic.

HOW TO TREAT

GENERAL MEASURES
- Learn relaxation techniques.
- Talking about the event may help. Talk to family, friends, clergy, or join a support group.
- To learn more: National Institute of Mental Health; 6001 Executive Blvd., Bethesda, MD 20892-9663; (866) 615-6464; website: www.nimh.nih.gov.

MEDICATION—Drugs for depression, anxiety, or insomnia may be prescribed.

ACTIVITY—Try to exercise each day (helps mental and physical health). Get enough sleep.

DIET—No special diet.

CALL YOUR DOCTOR IF

- You or a family member has symptoms of post-traumatic stress disorder.
- Symptoms don't improve or become worse.

POTASSIUM IMBALANCE

 GENERAL INFORMATION

DEFINITION—A potassium imbalance is a higher- or lower-than-normal level of potassium in the blood, body fluids, and body cells. Important electrolytes, including potassium, sodium, and calcium, maintain normal heart rhythm and regulate the body's water balance. They also help control muscle contractions and nerve impulses. Electrolytes need to be in a certain balance. A high or low potassium level results in an electrolyte imbalance and can cause heart and muscle symptoms.

BODY PARTS INVOLVED—Blood, which affects all body cells and body fluids.

SEX OR AGE MOST AFFECTED—Both sexes; all ages.

SIGNS & SYMPTOMS
- For higher-than-normal levels (hyperkalemia):
  - Tingling in hands and feet.
  - Extreme weakness and paralysis.
  - Dangerously rapid, irregular heartbeat.
- For lower-than-normal levels (hypokalemia):
  - Mild weakness and muscle cramps, often following or during exercise.
  - Discomfort in the legs while sitting.
  - Confusion and disorientation.
  - Extreme weakness and paralysis.
  - Life-threatening rapid, irregular heartbeat.

CAUSES—Usually, the imbalance is due to the body either excreting too little or too much potassium. This can be due to different medical disorders usually involving the kidneys. Less often, an imbalance is caused by a lack or an excess of potassium in the diet.

RISK INCREASES WITH
- Hyperkalemia:
  - Kidney or renal disease.
  - Severe burns, infections, or muscle injuries.
  - Acidosis (high acid concentration in the blood).
  - Rhabdomyolysis (muscle and kidney injury).
  - Chemotherapy (anticancer drugs).
  - Adrenal gland disorders.
  - Certain drugs that decrease potassium excretion.
  - Rarely, strenuous exercise.
- Hypokalemia:
  - Use of diuretic drugs for medical or other purposes. Athletes may use diuretics to meet certain weight limits before competing (e.g., jockeys, boxers, wrestlers).
  - Excessive sweating, vomiting, or diarrhea.
  - Eating disorders; laxative abuse, prolonged fasting or starvation, or alcoholism (can lead to poor diet).
  - Hyperaldosteronism, Cushing's syndrome, inherited kidney defects, chronic kidney disease, and eating too much black licorice.

HOW TO PREVENT—If you take diuretics or have renal or kidney disease, have frequent blood studies to check potassium levels.

 WHAT TO EXPECT

DIAGNOSTIC MEASURES
- Your own observation of symptoms.
- Your health care provider may do a physical exam.
- Medical tests may include blood and urine studies of potassium and other electrolytes. An ECG (electrocardiogram) may be done. It measures the electrical activity of the heart.

APPROPRIATE HEALTH CARE
- Treatment usually involves drugs to correct the potassium imbalance.
- Most cases are treatable at home. Hospital care and intravenous (IV) therapy may be needed for severe cases of hypokalemia or hyperkalemia. Dialysis (a way to clean the blood) may be required if kidneys fail.

POSSIBLE COMPLICATIONS
- Treatment of hypokalemia may result in hyperkalemia and vice versa.
- Life-threatening cardiac arrest.

PROBABLE OUTCOME—Treatment can help correct the potassium imbalance, but In most cases, the outcome will depend on the underlying cause.

 HOW TO TREAT

GENERAL MEASURES—If you take diuretics and digitalis, your family members should learn cardiopulmonary resuscitation (CPR). Learn to count your own pulse at the wrist or neck.

MEDICATION
- Your health care provider may prescribe:
  - Oral or intravenous (IV) potassium supplements to raise low levels.
  - Diuretics to increase urination and decrease high potassium levels.
  - Intravenous (IV) fluids (electrolytes) to correct a serious imbalance.
  - Drugs to treat an underlying disorder.
  - Changes in your current drugs if they are causing the potassium imbalance.

ACTIVITY—Resume normal activities once symptoms improve.

DIET—You may be advised to eat more or less high-potassium foods.

 CALL YOUR DOCTOR IF

You or a family member has symptoms of a potassium imbalance.

PREECLAMPSIA & ECLAMPSIA
(Pregnancy-Induced Hypertension; Toxemia)

 GENERAL INFORMATION

DEFINITION—Preeclampsia and eclampsia are serious problems of pregnancy. They may develop from the 20th week of pregnancy up to 6 weeks after delivery. Preeclampsia is high blood pressure and protein in the urine. Eclampsia includes seizures and possibly coma. Eclampsia may follow preeclampsia or occur on its own.

BODY PARTS INVOLVED—It involves blood pressure, kidney function, and the central nervous system.

SEX OR AGE MOST AFFECTED—Pregnant females.

SIGNS & SYMPTOMS
- Mild preeclampsia usually has no symptoms. It can be diagnosed on a routine pregnancy check-up.
- More severe preeclampsia symptoms may include:
  - Swelling (edema) of the hands and face.
  - Rapid weight gain.
  - Changes in vision.
  - Headache.
  - Changes in mental status.
  - Nausea or vomiting and abdominal pain.
  - Low urine output.
- Eclampsia symptoms can include seizures or coma.

CAUSES—Exact cause is unknown. A dysfunction of the placenta may start the process that leads to other problems.

RISK INCREASES WITH
- First pregnancy or first pregnancy with new partner.
- Preeclampsia in a previous pregnancy.
- Family history of preeclampsia or eclampsia.
- Obesity.
- Multiple gestation (twins, triplets, etc.).
- Mother's age over 40 or less than 20.
- Prolonged time between pregnancies.
- African American women.
- Diabetes prior to pregnancy or gestational diabetes.
- Chronic medical problems before pregnancy (e.g., high blood pressure, kidney disease, vascular or connective tissue disorders, or thrombophilic diseases).
- Medical problems during pregnancy, such as urinary tract infection, and others.
- Complications of pregnancy, such as chromosome abnormalities, and others.

HOW TO PREVENT—None specific. Reduce risk factors where possible. Low dose aspirin may be prescribed for pregnant women at risk.

 WHAT TO EXPECT

DIAGNOSTIC MEASURES—Diagnosis may include blood pressure tests, blood studies, 24-hour urine study (to check the protein levels), and ultrasound (to assess fetal development). Other tests may be done if complications occur.

APPROPRIATE HEALTH CARE
- Treatment will depend on results of medical tests, the severity of the symptoms, and how far along you are in the pregnancy. In some cases, mild preeclampsia may be treated as an outpatient. Hospital care is needed if the condition worsens or for early delivery. Eclampsia, because of seizure activity, requires hospital care.
- The decision to have a vaginal delivery or cesarean section is based on each individual's situation.

POSSIBLE COMPLICATIONS
- Mother—placenta abruption, stroke, kidney failure, seizures, high blood pressure, HELLP syndrome (a severe preeclampsia), pulmonary edema, hemorrhage, heart failure, and death.
- Baby—premature birth, low birth weight, intrauterine growth restriction, and stillbirth.

PROBABLE OUTCOME—The cure is to deliver the baby. Complications for mother and baby can often be prevented with prompt diagnosis and treatment. The high blood pressure and other symptoms usually resolve within days to weeks after delivery. If premature labor occurs, the newborn's survival depends on its maturity.

 HOW TO TREAT

GENERAL MEASURES—To learn more: Preeclampsia Foundation, 6767 N. Wickham Rd., Ste 400; Melbourne, FL 32940; (800) 665-9341; website: www.preeclampsia.org.

MEDICATION
- Drugs may be given for high blood pressure, to prevent or control seizures, or induce labor.
- Corticosteroids may be given for complications or to help mature the baby's lungs before delivery.

ACTIVITY—You will be advised of any limits. Bedrest at home may be recommended.

DIET—No special diet (unless advised).

 CALL YOUR DOCTOR IF

- You or a family member has symptoms of preeclampsia at any stage of pregnancy.
- After diagnosis, any symptoms cause concern.

PREMATURE EJACULATION

GENERAL INFORMATION

DEFINITION—Premature ejaculation (PE) involves ejaculating shortly before intercourse begins or shortly afterward, lack of control of ejaculation, and concern or distress about the situation. PE is a common problem in males ages 18 to 59. PE may be lifelong (called primary). It may be acquired (called secondary) if a male was previously able to have ejaculatory control. If acquired, it may occur with specific partners or situations or it may occur in all situations and partners.

BODY PARTS INVOLVED—Brain and central nervous system; reproductive system.

SEX OR AGE MOST AFFECTED—Male adolescents and adults.

SIGNS & SYMPTOMS
- Difficulty in delaying ejaculation.
- Ejaculating before you or your partner wishes or with little stimulation. It is sometimes described as taking place 1 to 2 minutes before or after vaginal penetration.
- Frustration about the premature ejaculation.
- Concerns about partner being sexually unfulfilled.

CAUSES—The exact cause is unknown. In most cases, the male is healthy. PE involves psychological (mental or emotional) factors. Biologic factors may play a role (e.g., an oversensitive glans penis [head of the penis]).

RISK INCREASES WITH
- Erectile dysfunction.
- Lack of sexual experience, infrequent sexual intercourse, stress, fear, anxiety, sexual performance pressure, social phobia, and lack of sexual education have all been mentioned as risk factors.

HOW TO PREVENT—No specific preventive measures.

WHAT TO EXPECT

DIAGNOSTIC MEASURES
- Your own observation of signs.
- Your health care provider may do a physical exam and ask questions about your symptoms and sexual history. You may be asked to fill out a questionnaire.
- Medical tests may be done, but they are usually normal.

APPROPRIATE HEALTH CARE
- Treatment may include sexual therapy or behavior therapy for patient and partner, and/or drug therapy. Most often, the couple (not just the man) needs to work on the problem together.

- Sexual therapy techniques may be recommended. These can include:
  - Sensate-focus exercises, in which each partner caresses the other's body without intercourse to learn relaxed, pleasurable aspects of touching.
  - Start and stop technique, which delays ejaculation by withdrawing the penis or stopping the thrusts.
  - Masturbating 1 or 2 hours before intercourse so you can delay ejaculation during sex.
  - Squeeze technique, in which the woman squeezes her partner's penis with her thumb and forefinger when he feels an impending ejaculation.
- Counseling from a mental health provider or qualified sex therapist may be recommended if other methods are not successful.

POSSIBLE COMPLICATIONS
- Problem can recur after successful treatment.
- Relationship difficulties with sexual partner. PE may cause stress, feelings of guilt, and resentment.
- Can cause difficulty in achieving a pregnancy.

PROBABLE OUTCOME—Treatment can help in many cases and the man is able to learn ejaculatory control.

HOW TO TREAT

GENERAL MEASURES—Work on ways to improve communication with your partner and try to reduce your performance anxiety.

MEDICATION
- There is no specific drug to treat the problem. Antidepressants or other drugs help some men and may be prescribed. The drug may be used as a single dose prior to sexual intercourse or taken on a daily basis.
- A topical anesthetic agent (e.g., cream) may be recommended. It may help to reduce penile sensitivity and delay ejaculation. An example is lidocaine. It can be applied to the penis under a condom about 30 minutes before intercourse. Follow instructions provided with the product.

ACTIVITY—No limits.

DIET—No special diet.

CALL YOUR DOCTOR IF

- You or a family member has repeated episodes of premature ejaculation.
- Problem continues despite treatment.

PREMATURE LABOR & PREMATURE BIRTH

GENERAL INFORMATION

DEFINITION—Premature labor is labor that begins before the 37th week of pregnancy. Full-term pregnancy is about 40 weeks. Premature birth may follow premature labor.

BODY PARTS INVOLVED—Female reproductive system.

SEX OR AGE MOST AFFECTED—Pregnant females.

SIGNS & SYMPTOMS
- Uterine contractions at regular intervals that begin before the 37th week of gestation.
- Passage of mucus (may be bloody).
- A feeling of pelvic pressure; low back pain; cramping.
- May have flow of fluid (amniotic fluid) from the uterus (can be a gush or a steady watery discharge).
- Some degree of vaginal bleeding or spotting.

CAUSES—The cause is not clearly understood. Multiple factors are usually involved.

RISK INCREASES WITH
- Premature rupture of membranes (water breaks).
- Pregnant with twins, triplets, or more.
- Illness of the mother, including preeclampsia, high blood pressure, or diabetes.
- Abnormal shape or size of the uterus; weak cervix.
- Placenta problems (e.g., placenta previa).
- Excessive amniotic fluid (polyhydramnios).
- Poor nutrition (more so if weight loss occurs).
- Previous premature labor or premature birth.
- Smoking, excess alcohol use, or drug abuse.
- Infection (e.g., in urinary tract or amniotic fluid).
- Mother-to-be is under age 18 or older than 35.
- Underweight or overweight before pregnancy. Too little or too much weight gain during pregnancy.
- Poor prenatal care or none at all.
- Low income, nonwhite racial groups, emotional stress, or certain work (e.g., standing for hours).
- Less than 6 months between pregnancies.
- In vitro fertilization (IVF).

HOW TO PREVENT
- Obtain good prenatal care throughout pregnancy.
- Don't smoke, abuse drugs, or drink alcohol.
- Eat a well-balanced diet during pregnancy. Take prescribed prenatal vitamins. Use good dental hygiene.
- Don't use drugs of any kind, including nonprescription drugs, without medical advice.
- Follow medical advice about physical activity levels and sexual activity during pregnancy.
- Keep control of any chronic health conditions such as diabetes or high blood pressure. Try to control stress.
- Premature contractions can sometimes be stopped by drinking extra fluids (e.g., 16 ounces of water or juice) and then lying down for an hour on your left side.

WHAT TO EXPECT

DIAGNOSTIC MEASURES
- Your own observation of watery vaginal drainage or regular uterine contractions.
- Medical tests usually include a pelvic exam. Lab tests of blood, urine, and fetal fibronectin (a protein secreted by the cervix) are often done. Ultrasound can be used to determine fetal weight, age, growth, and position. An amniocentesis can help determine baby's maturity or diagnose infection. Fetal monitoring may be done.

APPROPRIATE HEALTH CARE
- Treatment depends on the number of weeks of pregnancy, any health problems diagnosed, fetal maturity, and if the cervix has opened (dilated) or begun to thin (efface). Hospital care may be needed. You may be sent home if labor stops or you are not really in labor.
- Labor is usually allowed to continue if near term or there is a serious medical problem for mother or baby. Delivery may be cesarean.
- Labor can often be stopped with treatment. This allows the fetus to mature until the 36th or 37th week of pregnancy when there is less risk.

POSSIBLE COMPLICATIONS
- Premature infant.
- Uterine infection after delivery.
- Fetal death.

PROBABLE OUTCOME
- In about 50% of cases, the premature labor ceases, either on its own or with treatment.
- In some cases delivery must proceed; outcome depends on fetal maturity.

HOW TO TREAT

GENERAL MEASURES—Follow medical advice.

MEDICATION
- Drugs to stop the labor may be given.
- Antibiotics may be used to treat or prevent infection.
- Corticosteroids may be used to aid fetal lung maturity.

ACTIVITY—Activity limits and extra rest may be recommended.

DIET—Diet limits will depend on treatment.

CALL YOUR DOCTOR IF

You or a family member has symptoms of premature labor. Get emergency help if needed.

PREMENSTRUAL DYSPHORIC DISORDER

 GENERAL INFORMATION

DEFINITION—Premenstrual dysphoric disorder (PMDD) is a severe form of premenstrual syndrome (PMS). Symptoms of PMDD interfere with daily activities, and can cause problems with personal relationships. PMDD is also called late-luteal dysphoric disorder.

BODY PARTS INVOLVED—Gastrointestinal system; central nervous system; skin; reproductive system; breasts.

SEX OR AGE MOST AFFECTED—Females who have menstrual periods.

SIGNS & SYMPTOMS
- The symptoms occur 5 to 14 days before, and go away a few days after, the start of menstruation.
- Symptoms vary for every woman, and vary at times in the same woman. Most of the symptoms involve emotional or behavioral factors. Symptoms may include:
  - Being irritable or angry.
  - Feeling depressed, sad, and hopeless.
  - Feelings of tension, anxiety, or panic.
  - Mood swings marked by periods of crying.
  - Lack of interest in daily activities and relationships.
  - Trouble paying attention and unable to concentrate.
  - Fatigue or lack of energy.
  - Food cravings or overeating.
  - Trouble sleeping.
  - Feeling out of control.
  - Physical symptoms, such as bloating, breast tenderness, headaches, diarrhea, and joint or muscle pain.

CAUSES—No single cause has been found. Some studies suggest it may be an abnormal response to normal hormonal changes. Genetic factors are likely involved. Research into the cause is ongoing.

RISK INCREASES WITH
- Women with a personal or family history of mood disorders, such as depression or postpartum depression.
- Stressful life events.

HOW TO PREVENT—No preventive measures for the first episode.

 WHAT TO EXPECT

DIAGNOSTIC MEASURES
- Your own observation of the symptoms.
- Your health care provider will do a physical exam (including a pelvic exam). Questions will be asked about your symptoms and lifestyle.

- To aid in the diagnosis, you may be asked to keep a symptom diary for two or more months. List the dates of your period and which symptoms you have (and their severity) on the days before and after your period.

APPROPRIATE HEALTH CARE
- Treatment options for PMDD include lifestyle changes, counseling, drugs, and use of alternative therapies. No single treatment works for every woman.
- Lifestyle changes include diet changes, stopping smoking, aerobic exercise, and steps to reduce stress.
- Counseling may help a woman find ways to cope with the PMDD symptoms.
- Biofeedback, acupuncture, and massage may help some women. Relaxation techniques may be used as treatment for stress. Phototherapy (treatment with light) may help in some cases.

POSSIBLE COMPLICATIONS—The symptoms may get worse over time and last until menopause (when menses ceases).

PROBABLE OUTCOME—Treatment can help reduce some PMDD symptoms. Treatment may be needed for at least a year. There are a variety of treatment options. It is important to find what works for you.

 HOW TO TREAT

GENERAL MEASURES—Consider joining a support group. Talking about your PMDD symptoms with others can help.

MEDICATION
- Antidepressant drugs may be prescribed. These help the symptoms of PMDD.
- Other drugs may be prescribed for specific symptoms such as headaches, anxiety, pain, and bloating.
- Vitamins and supplements may be prescribed.

ACTIVITY
- Do aerobic exercise (20 to 30 minutes) daily, or at least three times per week.
- Be sure to get enough sleep.

DIET
- Eat a healthy diet. Try eating frequent, small meals.
- Reduction of salt, caffeine, sugar, and alcohol helps some patients.

 CALL YOUR DOCTOR IF

- You or a family member has PMDD symptoms.
- Symptoms get worse or new symptoms develop despite treatment.

PREMENSTRUAL SYNDROME

GENERAL INFORMATION

DEFINITION—Premenstrual syndrome (PMS) involves symptoms that begin 7 to 14 days prior to a menstrual period and usually stop when menstruation begins. About half of all women experience PMS at some time, some very frequently.

BODY PARTS INVOLVED—Gastrointestinal system; central nervous system; skin; reproductive system; breasts.

SEX OR AGE MOST AFFECTED—It most often affects women ages 25 to 40.

SIGNS & SYMPTOMS
- Depressed mood.
- Nervousness and irritability.
- Dizziness or fainting.
- Fatigue.
- Emotional instability; mood swings.
- Increased or decreased sex drive.
- Headaches.
- Tender, swollen breasts.
- Bloating, constipation, or diarrhea.
- Other digestive disturbances.
- Fluid retained (edema) in ankles, hands, or face.
- Having more minor infections such as colds.
- Acne outbreaks.
- Decreased urination.
- Many other symptoms (over 150) have been attributed to PMS.

CAUSES—Unknown, but may be due to changes in the level of hormones (especially estrogen and progesterone). These changes cause retention of sodium in the bloodstream, resulting in edema in body tissues including the brain. Increased levels of prostaglandin (a chemical) in the bloodstream may be a factor. More theories about the basis of PMS include emotional, stress, diet, changes in brain chemicals, and other factors.

RISK INCREASES WITH
- Younger women (often begins in mid-20s).
- Family history of PMS.
- Personal history of depression or mood disorder.
- Stress, smoking, or painful menstrual periods may increase PMS risk or worsen its symptoms.

HOW TO PREVENT—Cannot be prevented. After diagnosis, you can plan ahead to reduce, control, and better cope with symptoms. Let people close to you know about the PMS.

WHAT TO EXPECT

DIAGNOSTIC MEASURES
- Your own observation of symptoms.

- Your health care provider may do a physical exam, pelvic exam, and blood tests to rule out other disorders. Diagnosis is usually based on the symptom history. Keep a menstrual diary for 2 months. Write down your symptoms, dates, and other details.

APPROPRIATE HEALTH CARE
- Treatment can include lifestyle changes, drug therapy, psychotherapy, and other therapies. No single treatment works for everyone. Several may be needed.
- Healthy lifestyle changes can include regular exercise, diet changes, good sleep habits, and quitting smoking.
- Psychotherapy includes cognitive-behavioral therapy (CBT), learning relaxation techniques, or biofeedback.
- Other therapies may include chiropractic care, massage, acupuncture, or phototherapy.

POSSIBLE COMPLICATIONS
- Severe symptoms that disrupt a woman's life.
- Premenstrual dysphoric disorder.

PROBABLE OUTCOME—There is no cure. Different treatments can relieve the symptoms for different women. PMS symptoms often decrease after age 35 and stop at menopause.

HOW TO TREAT

GENERAL MEASURES—Consider joining a support group. Talking about your PMS symptoms with others can help.

MEDICATION
- These are used with varying success:
  - Nonsteroidal anti-inflammatory drugs (NSAIDs) or acetaminophen for pain, cramping, and headaches.
  - Antidepressants or antianxiety drugs.
  - Diuretics to reduce fluid retention.
  - Vitamins B-6 and E, magnesium, or calcium.
  - Hormones to suppress ovarian function.
  - Herbal products (e.g., evening primrose oil).
  - Oral contraceptives.

ACTIVITY
- Begin a regular exercise program. It can help relieve or reduce PMS symptoms.
- Try to get enough sleep at night.

DIET—Eat a low-fat, low-salt, high complex carbohydrate diet with frequent small meals. Limit use of caffeine.

CALL YOUR DOCTOR IF

- You or a family member has symptoms of PMS that interfere with normal activities.
- Symptoms don't improve, despite treatment.

PRIAPISM

GENERAL INFORMATION

DEFINITION—Priapism is a persistent erection of the penis without sexual arousal or desire. It is an emergency condition that requires medical care to prevent complications.

BODY PARTS INVOLVED—Penis.

SEX OR AGE MOST AFFECTED—Males; all ages (including children).

SIGNS & SYMPTOMS—A prolonged, usually painful erection. The erection may last hours to days.

CAUSES
- It may be associated with certain diseases or use of drugs. Sometimes, no cause is found. Types include:
  - Low-flow—blood becomes trapped in the penis causing its engorgement.
  - High-flow (rarer)—occurs when the blood in the penis does not circulate properly. It is usually due to an injury.

RISK INCREASES WITH
- Drugs that are used to treat impotence.
- Blood disease (sickle-cell disease or thalassemia).
- Cancer (leukemia or multiple myeloma).
- Certain drugs used to treat other disorders (such as chlorpromazine, prazosin, trazodone, some corticosteroids, anticoagulants, and antihypertensives).
- Spinal tumor, injury, or anesthesia.
- Carbon monoxide poisoning.
- Black widow spider bite.
- Malaria.
- Cocaine, marijuana, ecstasy, and alcohol abuse.
- Use of anabolic steroids.
- Prolonged sexual activity.
- Tumors or blood clots in the pelvis.
- Nervous system disorders (e.g., multiple sclerosis).

HOW TO PREVENT—No specific preventive measures. Avoid risk factors where possible.

WHAT TO EXPECT

DIAGNOSTIC MEASURES
- Your own observation of symptoms.
- Emergency treatment is necessary because of the risk of permanent damage to the penis. Your health care provider will do a physical exam and an exam of the penis. Questions will be asked about your symptoms, activities, and drug use.
- Medical tests may include a small amount of blood taken from the penis for study. Ultrasound or angiogram (special type of x-ray) tests may be done.

APPROPRIATE HEALTH CARE
- Treatment may include drug therapy, aspiration of the blood, or surgery. Any underlying cause will also need treatment. Patients with sickle-cell disease may need a blood transfusion. Spinal anesthesia is sometimes helpful.
- As a temporary measure, ice packs may be applied to the penis and perineum to help reduce swelling. Walking up a flight of stairs may help divert blood flow.
- Aspiration involves using a needle to remove blood from the penis. This will reduce pressure and swelling.
- Surgery may be needed if other treatment measures are not effective. A shunt (passageway) may be inserted to divert the blood flow. In high-flow priapism, surgery may be done to tie off an injured artery to restore normal blood flow.

POSSIBLE COMPLICATIONS
- Impotence.
- Recurrence of priapism.
- Infection.
- Complications from surgical procedures may occur.

PROBABLE OUTCOME—With prompt medical care, the outcome is good. Delayed treatment can lead to increased risk of erectile dysfunction.

HOW TO TREAT

GENERAL MEASURES—No measures other than medical care.

MEDICATION
- One or more drugs may be used in the treatment of priapism.
- If a drug you take is the cause of priapism, it may be discontinued. An alternative drug may be prescribed.

ACTIVITY—Rest until erection is relieved.

DIET—No special diet.

CALL YOUR DOCTOR IF

You or a family member has an erection that persists for no apparent reason. Do not waste time trying to get it down with cold compresses. Go immediately to an emergency room.

PRICKLY HEAT
(Miliaria Rubra)

GENERAL INFORMATION

DEFINITION—Prickly heat is a skin disorder caused by blocked sweat-gland ducts. Miliaria rubra is the medical name.

BODY PARTS INVOLVED—Skin.

SEX OR AGE MOST AFFECTED—Both sexes; all ages. It is common in infants and children.

SIGNS & SYMPTOMS
- Clusters of vesicles (small, fluid-filled skin blisters that may come and go within a matter of hours) or red rash without vesicles in areas of heavy sweating.
- In adults, it occurs more often in the skin fold areas or where clothes cause friction. In infants, it can occur on the chest, back, neck, head, and, sometimes, the groin or armpits.
- May have itching, burning, tingling, prickling, or stinging.

CAUSES—Blockage of sweat-gland ducts (such as with dead skin cells or bacteria). The trapped sweat causes an inflammatory response. There are different type of miliaria depending on the skin level that is blocked. When it occurs in the upper skin level (epidermis), it results in prickly heat (miliaria rubra). Other types of miliaria are less common.

RISK INCREASES WITH
- Heavy sweating.
- Hot, humid weather.
- Clothing that keeps in heat and moisture.
- Infants and young children (sweat glands are not mature).
- Infants that are bundled up.
- High fever.
- Use of certain drugs.

HOW TO PREVENT
- Avoid risk factors where possible.
- Use anhydrous lanolin to help prevent blockage of sweat ducts. Apply to affected skin areas prior to activity in hot weather.
- Bathe regularly, especially in hot, humid situations. This helps get rid of salt and bacteria on the skin.
- Use water-based product for moisturizing skin.
- Use sunscreens, but avoid those that are oily/cocoa butter types.

WHAT TO EXPECT

DIAGNOSTIC MEASURES
- Your own observation of symptoms.
- See your health care provider if skin symptoms cause concern.

APPROPRIATE HEALTH CARE—Self-care is usually all that is needed.

POSSIBLE COMPLICATIONS
- A bacterial skin infection may develop.
- Some people never adapt to hot climates and may end up moving to milder weather location.

PROBABLE OUTCOME—Prickly heat is not a serious condition. Most rashes heal on their own within days to weeks. Symptoms can often be relieved with treatment.

HOW TO TREAT

GENERAL MEASURES
- Avoid further sweating. Provide a cool, dry environment. Spend time in an air-conditioned room or office.
- Avoid clothing that irritates the skin or clothing that is too tight.
- Use cool-water soaks to relieve itching. Pat skin dry and dust with cornstarch after soaks.
- Wear cotton socks and leather-soled footwear rather than shoes made of synthetic materials.
- Expose the affected skin to air as much as possible.
- Don't use binding materials, such as adhesive tape.
- Change diapers on infants as soon as they are wet.
- Avoid sunburn once you have had prickly heat. The body's inflammatory reaction to sunburn may trigger a new outbreak of prickly heat.

MEDICATION
- Use lotions that contain menthol or pramoxine, or use calamine lotion to relieve symptoms.
- Nonprescription cortisone cream may be recommended by your health care provider. Follow product instructions carefully.
- Oral antibiotics may be prescribed if there is a secondary bacterial infection.
- Drugs may be prescribed for a fever or illness.

ACTIVITY—Decrease activity during hot, humid weather or until skin heals.

DIET—No special diet.

CALL YOUR DOCTOR IF

Prickly heat doesn't improve in 10 days, despite home care.

PROCTITIS

GENERAL INFORMATION

DEFINITION—Proctitis is an inflammation of the lining of the rectum. It may be acute (short-term) or chronic (long-term).

BODY PARTS INVOLVED—Anus; rectum.

SEX OR AGE MOST AFFECTED—It affects teens and adults of both sexes, but it is more common in adult males.

SIGNS & SYMPTOMS
- Rectal and anal pain.
- Constant urge to have a bowel movement, often when little or no stool is present.
- Blood or mucus discharge from the rectum.
- Cramping pain in the left lower abdomen.
- Diarrhea.

CAUSES—The inflammation can be due many conditions that cause infection, irritation, or injury to the rectum. Sexually transmitted diseases (STDs) are the most common cause.

RISK INCREASES WITH
- STD (e.g., gonorrhea, syphilis, herpes simplex virus, chlamydia, anal warts, and others).
- Anal or oral-anal intercourse (more so with multiple partners).
- Weak immune system due to illness or drugs.
- Radiation therapy.
- Bacterial infection not sexually transmitted (e.g., streptococcus, Campylobacter, salmonella, and others).
- Rectal injury, rectal drug, or chemical enemas.
- Inflammatory bowel disease (Crohn's disease or ulcerative colitis), or vasculitis.
- Antibiotic use.

HOW TO PREVENT
- Practice safe sex methods to help prevent an STD. Use condoms. Have sex with only one partner.
- Avoid risk factors where possible.

WHAT TO EXPECT

DIAGNOSTIC MEASURES
- Your own observation of symptoms.
- Your health care provider will do a physical exam.
- Medical tests may include blood studies, stool cultures, and tests for sexually transmitted diseases. Diagnostic tests often include use of a telescope-like instrument (e.g., proctoscope or sigmoidoscope) to look inside the rectum and colon.

APPROPRIATE HEALTH CARE
- Infectious proctitis is usually treated with drug therapy for the underlying cause.
- Radiation proctitis may be treated with ablation therapy. This will destroy abnormal, bleeding tissue.
- Proctitis due to inflammatory bowel disease is treated along with the underlying disorder. This can include drugs, diet changes, and/or surgery.
- Proctitis due to use of an antibiotic drug is treated with drug therapy that destroys the harmful bacteria.

POSSIBLE COMPLICATIONS
- Tears or constrictions in rectal tissue.
- Fistula (abnormal passageway).
- Rectal ulcer (open sore) or abscess.
- Anemia from chronic bleeding.
- Chronic ulcerative colitis.
- Treatment failure.

PROBABLE OUTCOME—The outcome of proctitis depends on the treatment of the underlying cause. Infections can usually be cured with antibiotics. Symptoms of other disorders can be relieved or controlled with treatment.

HOW TO TREAT

GENERAL MEASURES
- Keep the anal area clean with frequent bathing.
- Take sitz baths often to relieve pain. Sit in a tub of warm water for 10 to 15 minutes as often as necessary.

MEDICATION
- Your health care provider may prescribe:
  - Antibiotics for sexually transmitted infections, other bacterial infections, or for destroying harmful bacteria
  - Antivirals for virus infection.
  - Steroids (oral, suppositories, or rectal foam) to reduce inflammation
  - Iron supplements for anemia.
  - Antidiarrheals for diarrhea.
- You may use nonprescription topical anesthetics to relieve discomfort.

ACTIVITY—No limits.

DIET
- You may be advised to eat a high-fiber diet.
- Drink plenty of fluids each day.

☎ CALL YOUR DOCTOR IF

- You or a family member has symptoms of proctitis.
- Symptoms recur after treatment or new, unexplained symptoms develop.

PROSTATE CANCER

GENERAL INFORMATION

DEFINITION—Prostate cancer is a growth of malignant (cancerous) cells in the prostate gland. The prostate is about the size of a walnut and is located just below the urinary bladder in men. It helps form semen. This cancer often grows very slowly and may never cause symptoms. In some cases, it grows more rapidly, such as in younger men.

BODY PARTS INVOLVED—Prostate gland.

SEX OR AGE MOST AFFECTED—Men over age 50.

SIGNS & SYMPTOMS
- No symptoms (usually). Most prostate cancers are found with routine blood work or routine rectal exam.
- Difficult, frequent, weak, or painful urination.
- Low back or pelvic pain (if cancer spreads).
- Painful ejaculation.

CAUSES—Unknown. Hormonal, environmental, genetic, and dietary factors may play a role.

RISK INCREASES WITH
- Age over 50.
- Family history of prostate cancer.
- African American more than whites or others.
- High-fat diet; lack of exercise; obesity.

HOW TO PREVENT—No specific preventive measures. A yearly rectal exam after age 40 and PSA testing may help detect early prostate cancer. Lifestyle changes (e.g., diet and exercise) may have some preventive benefits.

WHAT TO EXPECT

DIAGNOSTIC MEASURES
- Your own observation of symptoms, especially urinary obstruction.
- Your health care provider will do a digital rectal exam (DRE). During a DRE, a gloved, lubricated finger is inserted into the rectum to check the prostate gland for lumps.
- Blood levels of prostate-specific antigen (PSA) will be checked. PSA, a protein produced by the prostate, is higher than normal in prostate diseases.
- Ultrasound, biopsy, CT, and other tests may be done to confirm the cancer diagnosis and to see if it has spread to other places in the body (staging).

APPROPRIATE HEALTH CARE
- Treatment depends on the cancer stage, age, health status, and personal preferences of the patient.
- Treatment may include watchful waiting, surgery, radiation, hormone therapy, chemotherapy, ultrasound, or newer therapies being tested. It helps to discuss your options

with family and friends and/or support groups.
- With watchful waiting, the cancer is monitored for a time before deciding on treatment. Prostate cancer may grow slowly and never cause symptoms or problems.
- Surgery to remove the prostate gland and surrounding tissues, if the cancer has not spread. Your health care provider will discuss options, risks, and benefits.
- Cryosurgery may be used. It treats cancer (that has not spread) by freezing cancer cells.
- Radiation or hormone treatment if the cancer has spread.
- Tiny, radioactive "seeds" may be inserted into the prostate to deliver a radiation dose over 3 to 6 months.
- High-intensity focused ultrasound may be an option.
- Counseling, if sexual difficulties occur.

POSSIBLE COMPLICATIONS
- Cancer may recur after treatment.
- Urinary incontinence.
- Sexual impotence after treatment.
- Life-threatening spread of cancer to bone, bladder, and other organs.

PROBABLE OUTCOME—Often curable if treated before cancer spreads. If the cancer has spread, treatment can relieve symptoms and prolong life.

HOW TO TREAT

GENERAL MEASURES—To learn more: American Cancer Society; (800) 227-2345; website: www.cancer.org or Prostate Cancer Foundation; website: www.prostatecancerfoundation.org.

MEDICATION
- Your health care provider may prescribe:
  - Hormones (e.g., estrogens or luteinizing hormone-releasing hormone) to slow cancer growth.
  - Chemotherapy (anticancer drugs).
  - Drugs for pain.

ACTIVITY
- Resume normal activities after treatment.
- Follow medical advice on resuming sexual relations.
- Exercise daily.

DIET—Eat a healthy diet. One that is high in fiber and fruits and vegetables, and low in fat is often recommended.

CALL YOUR DOCTOR IF

- You or a family member has symptoms of prostate cancer.
- After diagnosis, any symptoms cause concern.

PROSTATIC HYPERPLASIA, BENIGN
(Prostate Hypertrophy)

GENERAL INFORMATION

DEFINITION—Benign prostatic hyperplasia (BPH) is an enlargement of the prostate gland. The prostate is about the size of a walnut and is located just below the urinary bladder in men. An enlarged prostate presses against the urethra (tube that carries urine outside) making it narrower. The bladder muscle becomes thicker and more sensitive, causing urinary tract symptoms.

BODY PARTS INVOLVED—Prostate gland; bladder; urethra.

SEX OR AGE MOST AFFECTED—Men over age 50.

SIGNS & SYMPTOMS
* Increased urinary urgency and frequency, especially at night.
* Weak urinary stream.
* Stopping and starting again while urinating.
* Straining and dribbling during urination.
* Feeling that the bladder cannot be emptied completely.
* Leaking of urine and sometimes blood in the urine.

CAUSES—Exact cause unknown. It is common for the prostate to enlarge as a man ages. Changes in male hormones may be a factor.

RISK INCREASES WITH
* Aging; white and African American men.
* Family history of prostate problems.

HOW TO PREVENT—No specific prevention measures are known.

WHAT TO EXPECT

DIAGNOSTIC MEASURES
* Your own observation of symptoms.
* Your health care provider will do a digital rectal exam (DRE). During a DRE, a gloved, lubricated finger is inserted into the rectum to feel the prostate gland's size and check for lumps.
* Blood levels of prostate-specific antigen (PSA) will be checked. Other medical tests may include urine flow rate study, urinalysis, urine culture, x-ray of the urinary tract, and ultrasound.
* A question and answer interview is done about your symptoms. This can help in making treatment decisions. After treatment, it can help show how much the symptoms have changed.

APPROPRIATE HEALTH CARE
* Treatment may include watchful waiting, nonsurgical treatment, surgery, or drug therapy. Emergency treatment may be needed if all urine output is blocked.

* Watchful waiting is an option. This means monitoring the symptoms for a time before deciding on treatment. For home care—urinate when you get the urge, use bathrooms when you get the chance, avoid drinking large amounts of fluid at one time, and reduce stress.
* Several types of nonsurgical procedures are available. They include balloon dilation, prostatic stents, microwave therapy, needle ablation using radiofrequency, laser therapy, or electrovaporization. Your health care provider will explain and discuss these options.
* Surgery may be recommended if there are more severe symptoms, if complications occur, or there is a health risk. Several surgical options are available. The choice usually depends upon the size of the enlarged prostate.

POSSIBLE COMPLICATIONS
* Urinary retention, urinary stones, or urinary-tract infections.
* Reduced kidney function.
* Sexual dysfunction.

PROBABLE OUTCOME—Symptoms may improve, worsen, or stay the same. Treatment can help to relieve the symptoms.

HOW TO TREAT

GENERAL MEASURES—To relieve discomfort—sit in a tub with 6 to 8 inches of warm water for 15 minutes 3 times a day. Use an inflatable donut cushion for sitting.

MEDICATION
* 5-alpha-reductase inhibitors may be prescribed. They cause the prostate to shrink.
* Alpha-adrenergic blockers may be prescribed. They help relax the muscles in the prostate.
* Antibiotics if urinary-tract infection occurs.
* Get medical advice before using herbal remedies or other dietary supplements for BPH.
* Read labels on nonprescription drugs. Avoid those that state "not recommended if you have prostatic hypertrophy," such as antidiarrheals or antihistamines.

ACTIVITY—Stay active. Exercise can help reduce urinary problems. Walking is a good exercise.

DIET—Avoid alcohol, coffee, and spicy foods. These irritate the urethra. Drink plenty of fluids, but not within 2 hours of bedtime.

CALL YOUR DOCTOR IF

* You or a family member has BPH symptoms.
* Symptoms recur, worsen, or change.

PROSTATITS

GENERAL INFORMATION

DEFINITION
• Prostatitis is an inflammation of the prostate gland. The prostate is about the size of a walnut and is located just below the urinary bladder in men. Inflammation causes swelling of the prostate. The swelling can occur gradually or come on suddenly. Symptoms occur when the swollen prostate presses against the urethra. This is the tube that carries urine from the bladder to the outside. Types include:
   - Acute bacterial prostatitis.
   - Chronic bacterial prostatitis.
   - Chronic nonbacterial prostatitis/chronic pelvic pain syndrome. This is the most common type.
   - Asymptomatic prostatitis.

BODY PARTS INVOLVED—Prostate gland; bladder; urethra.

SEX OR AGE MOST AFFECTED—Men over age 50.

SIGNS & SYMPTOMS
• Urgency to urinate. Burning or pain with urination.
• Frequent urination. Waking at night to urinate.
• Difficulty starting urination and emptying the bladder completely.
• Fever, chills (acute bacterial prostatitis).
• Tiredness and muscle and joint aches.
• Pain between the scrotum and anus.
• May have blood in the urine or in the semen.
• Low back pain.
• Not enjoying sex; unable to get and keep an erection.

CAUSES
• Acute and chronic bacterial types are caused by bacteria infection.
• In nonbacterial types, the causes are unclear. It is not contagious, nor infectious, and does not cause cancer.

RISK INCREASES WITH—Aging.

HOW TO PREVENT—No specific prevention measures are known.

WHAT TO EXPECT

DIAGNOSTIC MEASURES
• Your own observation of symptoms.
• Your health care provider may do a physical exam and a digital rectal exam (DRE). With DRE, a gloved, lubricated finger is inserted into the rectum to feel the prostate gland.
• Medical tests may include blood, urine, and prostate secretion studies. Urodynamic tests can check bladder function. Other tests may be done.

APPROPRIATE HEALTH CARE
• Treatment depends on the type of prostatitis.
• Bacterial infections are treated with drugs. In some cases, hospital care and IV drugs may be needed.
• Treatment for nonbacterial types of prostatitis may include drugs, other therapies, lifestyle changes, counseling, and, rarely, surgery. There is no specific cure. More than one type of treatment is often needed. Your health care provider will discuss treatment options with you.
• Lifestyle changes may involve diet and exercise.
• Counseling may help with stress or sexual dysfunction problems. Support groups may help some patients.
• Rarely, surgery is needed for complications.

POSSIBLE COMPLICATIONS
• Recurrence or chronic prostatitis.
• Abscess (pus-filled infection).
• Bladder obstruction and urinary retention.
• Urinary-tract infection.
• Infertility.
• Blood poisoning.

PROBABLE OUTCOME—Outcome is generally good for bacterial prostatitis. Treatment may take 2 weeks to 6 months or longer and different drugs may be tried. Other types can be more difficult to treat, and the outcomes will vary.

HOW TO TREAT

GENERAL MEASURES—For home care to relieve discomfort—sit in a tub with 6 to 8 inches of warm water for 15 minutes 3 times a day. Use an inflatable donut cushion for sitting.

MEDICATION
• Your health care provider may prescribe:
   - Antibiotics for bacterial infection.
   - Anti-inflammatory drugs for pain.
   - Drugs to help improve bladder or prostate function.
   - Other agents (e.g., herbal or plant-based).
   - Stool softeners.

ACTIVITY
• Stay active. Walking is a good exercise.
• Pelvic floor exercises (called Kegel) may be recommended.

DIET—Avoid alcohol, coffee, and spicy foods. These irritate the urethra. Drink plenty of fluids.

CALL YOUR DOCTOR IF

• You or a family member has symptoms of prostatitis.
• Symptoms recur, worsen, or change.

PRURITUS ANI
(Anal Itching)

GENERAL INFORMATION

DEFINITION—Pruritus ani is chronic itching around the anus (opening of the rectum). It results in a compelling need to scratch the area.

BODY PARTS INVOLVED—Anus.

SEX OR AGE MOST AFFECTED—Both sexes; all ages; more common in men than in women.

SIGNS & SYMPTOMS
- Itching, which can be intense. It often occurs at night or after a bowel movement.
- Scratching makes the itch worse (scratch-itch cycle).
- May have burning and soreness.
- Itching may worsen with heat, moisture, leaking, wearing certain clothing, stress, or anxiety.

CAUSES
- The itching can be a symptom of many conditions. Often the cause is not clear (called idiopathic pruritus ani). The skin can become sensitized from a variety of causes that can't readily be pinpointed.
- Certain cycles can develop. For example, a person has a mild anal itch and cleans the area with a scented soap (which can sensitize the skin). A worse itch occurs, so you clean again which makes itching even more severe.

RISK INCREASES WITH
- Contact dermatitis caused by soaps, contraceptive foam or jelly, perfumed toilet paper, deodorant sprays, douches, or underwear made of synthetic fabric.
- Skin disorders (e.g., psoriasis, seborrheic dermatitis, atopic dermatitis, neurodermatitis, and others).
- Fissures, fistulas, proctitis, prolapsing hemorrhoids, skin tags, and dysfunction of the sphincter muscle.
- Chronic diarrhea or constipation.
- Fecal incontinence.
- Chronic disorders (e.g., diabetes or thyroid disease).
- Food irritants (e.g., caffeine, tomatoes, beer or wine, citrus, carbonated drinks, spices, hot peppers, milk, chocolate, cheese, or nuts).
- Pinworms, scabies, lice, or yeast infections.
- Excess sweating.
- Excessive or harsh cleaning of the anal area.
- Use of certain drugs.

HOW TO PREVENT—No specific preventive measures. Avoid risk factors if possible.

WHAT TO EXPECT

DIAGNOSTIC MEASURES
- Your own observation of symptoms.
- Your health care provider will do an exam of the affected area.
- Medical tests may include blood, urine, stool studies, and others.

APPROPRIATE HEALTH CARE—Treatment will be provided for any specific infection or problem that is diagnosed and for the itching.

POSSIBLE COMPLICATIONS
- Skin damage or secondary bacterial infection.
- Recurrence is common.
- Some may occur from an underlying cause.

PROBABLE OUTCOME—Treating the cause may provide a cure. Symptoms can be helped with treatment, even if the cause cannot be found. It may take weeks for the itching to stop.

HOW TO TREAT

GENERAL MEASURES
- Keep showers or baths brief to reduce dryness and soap irritation. Don't overclean the anal area by rubbing. Use plain soap or no soap.
- Keep the rectal area clean, dry, and cool. Clean carefully after bowel movements. Use moist wipes or moistened toilet paper. Dry toilet paper can be irritating.
- Avoid contact with substances to which you may be sensitive (colored toilet tissue, soaps, or skin products).
- Wear loose clothing and underclothing. Wear underwear with a cotton crotch or made of cotton, rather than nylon or other synthetics.
- Try not to scratch. Wear mittens or cotton gloves on your hands at night, if you are scratching while asleep.
- Get medical advice if stress or anxiety are problems.

MEDICATION
- Use a bland, soothing ointment on the area.
- You may use nonprescription cortisone ointment or cream. Apply as directed.
- Antihistamines for itching or stronger topical cortisone drugs may be prescribed.
- Drugs to treat an infection or other medical problem may be prescribed.

ACTIVITY—Avoid excessive sweating.

DIET—Avoid spicy or highly-seasoned foods and coffee. These irritate mucous membranes of the anus. Eat plenty of high-fiber foods to help avoid constipation.

CALL YOUR DOCTOR IF

- You or a family member has symptoms of pruritus ani that persist despite self-care.
- Symptoms don't improve with treatment.

PRURITUS VULVAE

GENERAL INFORMATION

DEFINITION—Pruritus vulvae is an acute or chronic itching of the skin around the vulva (the vaginal lips) and anus. It is not contagious.

BODY PARTS INVOLVED—Vulva and skin surrounding the vulva and anus.

SEX OR AGE MOST AFFECTED—Female adolescents and adults, especially after menopause.

SIGNS & SYMPTOMS
- Itching that may be severe and burning. The itching may be continuous or come and go.
- Sensitivity and irritation in the genital area.
- The skin may be dry.
- Thin, white vaginal discharge (sometimes).
- Discomfort during sexual intercourse.

CAUSES—It may be a symptom of an infection or other health problem. It may develop without any known cause.

RISK INCREASES WITH
- Skin disorder such as psoriasis or lichen planus.
- Systemic disease, such as diabetes.
- Atrophy and dryness due to lack of estrogen.
- Skin reaction to irritants such as toilet tissue, sanitary pads, soap, douches, deodorants, powders, perfume, and fabric.
- Systemic allergies, including food allergies.
- Disorder of the vagina or rectum, such as vaginitis or hemorrhoids.
- Genital warts (human papilloma virus).
- Vulvar cancer (rare).
- Days prior to menstruation.
- Hot, humid weather.
- Obesity.
- Lack of urinary or bowel control (incontinence).

HOW TO PREVENT—No specific preventive measures. Obtain medical care for any underlying disorders to reduce risk.

WHAT TO EXPECT

DIAGNOSTIC MEASURES
- Your own observation of symptoms.
- Your health care provider will do an exam of the affected area and ask questions about your symptoms and activities.
- Medical tests may include study of vaginal discharge and, if needed, a biopsy of the vulva (removal of a small amount of tissue for viewing under a microscope). In some cases, the exact cause is not found.

APPROPRIATE HEALTH CARE—Treatment for the underlying cause and topical skin-care products are usually recommended.

POSSIBLE COMPLICATIONS
- Secondary bacterial infection of inflamed skin.
- Chronic itch can lead to emotional problems (e.g., embarrassment) and/or insomnia.
- Complications occur from underlying cause.

PROBABLE OUTCOME—Treatment can help symptoms, but it may be long term.

HOW TO TREAT

GENERAL MEASURES
- Avoid the irritants listed among the risk factors.
- Wear cotton underpants rather than nylon or other synthetic material.
- Keep the area as dry and cool as possible. Wear loose clothing. Don't douche.
- Don't scratch the itchy area. Scratching will aggravate soreness and cause more irritation.
- Wash the genital area with water and plain soap or soap-free cleanser once a day.
- Use a lubricant, such as K-Y Lubricating Jelly or petroleum jelly, during intercourse. Avoid intercourse if it is painful.
- After urinating or having a bowel movement, clean the genital area gently with moist cotton or antiseptic wipes. Wipe from front to back (vagina to anus).
- During menstruation, insert tampons carefully. Change sanitary napkins frequently.
- Sit in bathtub of warm (tepid, not hot) water several times a day to help relieve itching.

MEDICATION
- Drugs may be prescribed for any infection.
- Use nonprescription steroid creams or ointments. Follow instructions on the label.
- Stronger steroid creams or lotions, or hormone ointment may be prescribed.
- Hormone therapy or topical application of estrogen is sometimes recommended for postmenopausal women.
- Sedating antihistamines may be recommended to help in sleeping at night.

ACTIVITY—Avoid excess sweating.

DIET—Avoid foods that produce allergic reactions.

CALL YOUR DOCTOR IF

- You or a family member has symptoms of pruritus vulvae.
- Symptoms don't improve in 2 weeks, despite treatment or if scratching leads to skin infection.

PSEUDOGOUT

GENERAL INFORMATION

DEFINITION—Pseudogout is an acute (sudden), inflammatory form of arthritis that usually involves the large joints of the body. It usually occurs in acute attacks, but often the disease may progress without the attacks.

BODY PARTS INVOLVED—Large joints (most often, the knee, wrist, ankle).

SEX OR AGE MOST AFFECTED—Elderly; more common in men than women.

SIGNS & SYMPTOMS
- Acute attacks of swelling, pain, and warmth in one or more of the joints.
- Joints involved most often are the knee (50% of the time), ankle, wrist, and shoulder.
- Attacks may last for 2 or more days (up to 2 weeks).
- Freedom from pain or less severe pain between attacks.
- Limited range of motion of the joints.
- Fever.

CAUSES—Pseudogout involves deposits of calcium crystals in and around the joints. The medical term is calcium pyrophosphate dihydrate (CPPD). Why the crystals form is unknown. The joint becomes inflamed leading to problems with cartilage, tendons, ligaments, and muscles that all connect to the joint. It is similar to gout, which is caused by a different type of crystal deposit.

RISK INCREASES WITH
- Trauma (injury).
- Aging.
- Metabolic diseases (e.g., hypothyroidism, hyperparathyroidism, or hemochromatosis).
- Family history of pseudogout.
- Eating too much calcium is not a risk factor.

HOW TO PREVENT—None known.

WHAT TO EXPECT

DIAGNOSTIC MEASURES
- Your own observation of symptoms.
- Your health care provider will do a physical exam of the affected area and ask questions about your symptoms and activities.
- Medical tests may include blood studies, a microscopic exam of a sample of joint fluid, and x-rays.

APPROPRIATE HEALTH CARE
- Treatment may include drugs, physical therapy, exercise, and self-care.
- Drainage of joint fluid from the inflamed joint may be done to relieve pain and pressure.
- Rarely, joint surgery (e.g., joint replacement) may be recommended.

POSSIBLE COMPLICATIONS
- Recurrences of the attacks.
- Permanent joint damage.
- Depression or other emotional problems.

PROBABLE OUTCOME—There is no cure. Treatment can usually help relieve the symptoms.

HOW TO TREAT

GENERAL MEASURES
- Apply ice to the affected area several times a day for the first 2 to 3 days to reduce swelling and pain.
- After a few days, heat may help discomfort. Use warm, moist compresses or heating pad, or take warm baths.
- To learn more, do an Internet search or visit a library.

MEDICATION
- Use acetaminophen for pain.
- Nonsteroidal anti-inflammatory drugs (NSAIDs) may be prescribed for pain and inflammation.
- Stronger pain medicine may be prescribed.
- A corticosteroid injection into the joint may be given to help relieve symptoms. An oral corticosteroid may be prescribed if other treatments fail to help.
- Colchicine, an antigout drug, may be prescribed.

ACTIVITY
- Rest as needed during an acute attack.
- Physical therapy may be prescribed to help maintain range of motion. You may be taught exercises to do at home. These will help keep joints and muscles flexible, strong, and functioning as well as possible.
- If an affected joint causes pain when walking, use a cane, crutches, or a walker temporarily.
- Swimming, water aerobics, or riding an exercise bike are good forms of exercise.
- Avoid heavy lifting or other tasks that put too much stress on your joints.

DIET—Avoid gaining weight. If your weight is a problem, a weight-loss diet may be recommended.

CALL YOUR DOCTOR IF

- If you or a family member has symptoms of pseudogout.
- Symptoms worsen after treatment begins.
- New or unexplained symptoms develop.

PSEUDOMEMBRANOUS COLITIS

GENERAL INFORMATION

DEFINITION—Pseudomembranous colitis is a severe illness that involves the colon (large intestine). It affects the lining and deeper layers of the colon. It usually occurs after a person has taken antibiotics.

BODY PARTS INVOLVED—Large intestine.

SEX OR AGE MOST AFFECTED—More often affects the elderly and women more than men.

SIGNS & SYMPTOMS
- Symptoms may be mild to severe.
- Watery diarrhea (sometimes bloody) with stomach cramps or pain.
- Fever.
- Drop in blood pressure, sometimes to shock levels, with weak pulse and rapid heartbeat.
- Nausea and vomiting.
- Disorientation.
- Symptoms usually begin 3 to 9 days after starting antibiotic treatment. In some cases, they may appear days to weeks after treatment has stopped.

CAUSES—Usually caused by the bacterial germ, *Clostridium difficile*. This germ is found in about 5% of healthy persons and normally causes no problems. It lives in a delicate balance in the colon with other bacteria. When antibiotics are used for treating bacterial infections, they can upset this bacterial balance of the intestinal tract. This allows *Clostridium difficile* to grow rapidly and produce a toxin that damages the intestinal wall.

RISK INCREASES WITH
- Use of antibiotics, especially lincomycin, clindamycin, ampicillin, chloramphenicol, cephalosporins, penicillin, or sulfa drugs. Multiple antibiotics and longer use increase risk.
- Adults over age 60.
- Recent surgery and/or a stay in a hospital.
- Cancer treatment.
- Poor general health.

HOW TO PREVENT—No specific preventive measures. Maintaining good health can help prevent the need for treatment with antibiotics.

WHAT TO EXPECT

DIAGNOSTIC MEASURES
- Your own observation of symptoms.
- Your health care provider will do a physical exam.
- Medical tests may include blood studies, stool cultures, and x-rays. An colonoscopy with biopsy may be done. This involves using a lighted, tube-like instrument to see inside the intestine. It is also used to remove a small bit of tissue for viewing under a microscope.

APPROPRIATE HEALTH CARE
- Treatment usually involves drug therapy, supportive care, hospital care if needed, and discontinuing or changing the antibiotic causing the problem.
- Mild cases can be treated at home.
- Hospital care for moderate to severe cases. Fluids given through a vein (IV) may be required to prevent dehydration.
- In rare cases, surgery may be needed due to complications of the bowels and to prevent or treat a perforation (a tear in the wall of the intestine).

POSSIBLE COMPLICATIONS
- Shock and severe dehydration.
- Peritonitis caused by perforation of the intestine.
- In people who are elderly and have a serious illness, it can sometimes be fatal.

PROBABLE OUTCOME—Almost all patients recover. Symptoms will usually disappear in 1 to 2 weeks with treatment. Some may have a relapse, which can be treated successfully.

HOW TO TREAT

GENERAL MEASURES—Follow medical advice for any home care.

MEDICATION
- Vancomycin, metronidazole, or other drugs may be prescribed to treat the *Clostridium difficile* infection. They may be taken by mouth or given by injection. Sometimes, repeat treatments may be needed.
- Don't take drugs for the diarrhea unless prescribed. They can prolong the infection.
- Supplements (e.g., probiotics) that help healthy bacteria grow in the intestines may be recommended.

ACTIVITY—Limit activities until symptoms of the illness get better. Move legs often while in bed to reduce the risk of deep-vein blood clots. Resume normal activities gradually.

DIET
- Patients in the hospital may need nutrition given through a vein (IV) for a few days. Then a soft diet may be prescribed until intestinal tract is back to normal.
- Patients at home need to drink plenty of fluids.

CALL YOUR DOCTOR IF

- You or a family member has symptoms of pseudomembranous colitis.
- Symptoms return after treatment.

PSITTACOSIS
(Parrot Fever; Ornithosis)

GENERAL INFORMATION

DEFINITION—Psittacosis is a rare infection transmitted by birds. The infection may be mild to severe. It is primarily a lung disease, but it may affect other organs.

BODY PARTS INVOLVED—Lungs.

SEX OR AGE MOST AFFECTED—Both sexes; all ages.

SIGNS & SYMPTOMS
- Fever and chills.
- General ill feeling.
- Appetite loss.
- Cough without sputum that progresses to a cough with occasional discolored sputum.
- Shortness of breath.
- Headache (may be severe).

CAUSES—Infection by the germ, *Chlamydia psittaci*, a special type of bacteria. Psittacosis is found in psittacine birds (parrots, parakeets, and lovebirds), poultry, pigeons, canaries, and some sea birds. Birds may not appear to be sick. Germs enter the human body by breathing in air that contains the germ or by a bite from an infected bird. Symptoms may begin 5 days to 4 weeks after exposure. Human-to-human transmission is rare but possible.

RISK INCREASES WITH
- Bird owners.
- Pet shop employees.
- Veterinary clinic employees.
- Poultry farmers or ranchers.
- Zoo workers.
- Working in poultry processing plants.

HOW TO PREVENT
- Avoid dust from bird feathers and cage contents.
- Don't handle any sick bird. Imported psittacine birds must be treated for 45 days with feed that contains chlortetracycline. This eliminates the germs from the birds' blood and feces.

WHAT TO EXPECT

DIAGNOSTIC MEASURES
- Your own observation of symptoms.
- Your health care provider will usually do a physical exam and ask questions about your exposure to birds.
- Medical tests may include blood studies or a sputum culture. X-rays of the lungs may be done.

APPROPRIATE HEALTH CARE
- Treatment usually involves drugs and supportive care for symptoms.
- Hospital care may be needed in severe cases. Breathing support may be required and fluids may be given through a vein (IV).
- Public health agencies will be notified about cases of psittacosis.

POSSIBLE COMPLICATIONS
- Hepatitis.
- Heart inflammation.
- Nervous system complications.
- Infection may recur.
- Kidney failure.
- Severe or fatal pneumonia (rare).

PROBABLE OUTCOME—Usually curable in 10 to 21 days with treatment.

HOW TO TREAT

GENERAL MEASURES
- Use a heating pad or warm, moist compresses on the chest to relieve pain.
- Don't smoke.

MEDICATION
- Doxycycline, tetracycline, or another antibiotic drug will be prescribed. They may be taken by mouth or given through a vein (IV). Take the full course of drugs prescribed, even if symptoms improve in a day or two.
- For minor pain, take nonprescription drugs such as acetaminophen or ibuprofen.

ACTIVITY—Usually no limits unless hospital care is needed. Fatigue and weakness may persist for several weeks for some patients.

DIET—No special diet. Increase fluid intake to at least one glass of fluid every hour. This helps to thin lung secretions so they can be coughed up more easily.

CALL YOUR DOCTOR IF

- You or a family member has symptoms of psittacosis.
- Symptoms get worse or do not improve with treatment.

PSORIASIS

GENERAL INFORMATION

DEFINITION—Psoriasis is a chronic, scaly skin disorder. There are several types. The most common is plaque (discoid) psoriasis.

BODY PARTS INVOLVED—It affects the skin of the scalp, elbows, knees, chest, back, arms, legs, toenails, fingernails, and the fold between the buttocks.

SEX OR AGE MOST AFFECTED—Begins in late childhood or young adulthood and continues throughout life.

SIGNS & SYMPTOMS
- Skin areas that are slightly raised, have sharp red borders, and are covered with large white or silver-white scales. The areas crack and become painful. Psoriasis often goes through cycles with flares and remissions.
- May have itching, burning, or joint pain.

CAUSES—The exact cause is unclear. The body's immune system and genetics appear to be factors. With psoriasis, new skin cells mature too rapidly and the dead skin cells build up on the skin's surface.

RISK INCREASES WITH
- Family history of psoriasis.
- Genetic factors. People with psoriasis have HLA antigens, and the incidence is highest among white people.
- Certain trigger factors may induce psoriasis or worsen its symptoms for different people. These can include stress, skin injury, infection, certain drugs, cold weather, excess alcohol use, smoking, or hormonal changes.

HOW TO PREVENT—Cannot be prevented at present. After diagnosis, try to identify and avoid any trigger factors to help prevent flare-ups.

WHAT TO EXPECT

DIAGNOSTIC MEASURES
- Your own observation of symptoms.
- Your health care provider can diagnose the disorder with an exam of the affected skin.
- A biopsy may sometimes be done. It involves removing a small amount of skin tissue for viewing under a microscope.

APPROPRIATE HEALTH CARE
- No permanent cure exists. Steps in treatment depend on the type of psoriasis, extent of the disorder, your response to it, and the effect on your lifestyle.
- Treatment steps include drugs to be used on the skin or taken by mouth, phototherapy, and self-care.
- Phototherapy may be prescribed. It involves use of sunlight or artificial light. Expose skin to moderate amounts of sunlight as often as possible. Artificial light may be used. This can be done at a medical office, or, in some cases, patients may have a unit they use at home.
- Get counseling if needed for emotional problems.

POSSIBLE COMPLICATIONS
- It can cause embarrassment, self-consciousness, and depression about one's appearance.
- Drugs used in treatment cause side effects.
- Pustular psoriasis (skin has pus-filled blisters).
- Psoriatic arthritis (inflammation in the joints).

PROBABLE OUTCOME—Symptoms can be controlled, but not cured. There may be long periods of inactivity of the disorder.

HOW TO TREAT

GENERAL MEASURES
- Maintain good skin hygiene with daily baths or showers. Avoid skin injury, including harsh scrubbing, which can trigger new outbreaks.
- Avoid skin dryness to decrease the risk of recurrences. To reduce scaling, use nonprescription, waterless cleansers and hair products that contain coal tar or cortisone. Use a moisturizer after bathing.
- Oatmeal baths may loosen scales. Use one cup of oatmeal to a tub of warm water.
- To learn more: National Psoriasis Foundation, 6600 SW 92nd Ave., Suite 300, Portland, OR 97223; (800) 723-9166; website: www.psoriasis.org.

MEDICATION
- No one drug therapy works for everyone. You may be prescribed one or more of the following:
  - Topical drugs including corticosteroids, forms of vitamin D-3, coal tar, anthralin, retinoids, or salicylic acid. Some of these may be combined into one product.
  - Oral retinoids, methotrexate, cyclosporine, and biologic therapies may be prescribed in more severe cases.
  - PUVA (combines use of a psoralen drug and exposure to ultraviolet light–wavelength A).
  - Combination of tar baths with UVB (ultraviolet therapy wavelength B).
  - Antihistamines may help relieve itching.

ACTIVITY—No limits. Your health care provider may suggest small amounts of sun exposure.

DIET—No special diet.

CALL YOUR DOCTOR IF

- You or a family member has symptoms of psoriasis.
- Symptoms do not improve with treatment.
- New, unexplained symptoms develop.

PSORIATIC ARTHRITIS

GENERAL INFORMATION

DEFINITION—Psoriatic arthritis is joint inflammation that occurs along with psoriasis (a skin disorder). Rarely, it may occur without obvious psoriasis.

BODY PARTS INVOLVED
- Joints in any part of the body, but most likely in finger joints and low-back and neck joints in the spine.
- Skin or nails that have psoriasis lesions and are close to the affected joint. Sometimes additional skin sites include the scalp, navel, underarm and groin.

SEX OR AGE MOST AFFECTED—Both sexes; usually begins between ages 30 and 35 and continues intermittently throughout life.

SIGNS & SYMPTOMS
- Pain, swelling, limited movement, tenderness, and warmth in the affected joints.
- Psoriasis. Skin areas that are slightly raised, have red borders, and are covered with large white or silver-white scales. The areas crack and become painful. (Rarely, a person may have psoriatic arthritis without obvious signs of psoriasis.)
- Tiredness and fever (sometimes).

CAUSES—Unknown. It is thought to be one of a group of autoimmune disorders. In these disorders, the immune system by mistake attacks the body itself. Genetic (family) factors may be involved. In some cases, it may be linked to an infection or injury to joint or tendon.

RISK INCREASES WITH
- Psoriasis.
- Family history of psoriasis or psoriatic arthritis.
- Human immunodeficiency virus (HIV) infection.
- Joint or tendon injury.

HOW TO PREVENT—No specific preventive measures.

WHAT TO EXPECT

DIAGNOSTIC MEASURES
- Your own observation of symptoms.
- Your health care provider will do a physical exam and ask about your symptoms.
- There is no one test that will diagnose the disorder. Medical tests may include blood studies, joint fluid studies, x-rays, CT, or MRI.

APPROPRIATE HEALTH CARE
- Treatment may include drugs, physical therapy, exercise, and self-care. Psoriasis therapy will continue also.
- Ultrasound or diathermy (heat therapy) may be prescribed.
- Splints for the affected joints may be recommended.
- In some cases, surgery may be recommended for severe joint problems or for joint replacement.

POSSIBLE COMPLICATIONS
- May progress to chronic arthritis and severe crippling may occur.
- Drugs used in treatment may have adverse effects.

PROBABLE OUTCOME—There is no cure for this disorder. The symptoms often go away and then return. Symptoms can be relieved or controlled with treatment.

HOW TO TREAT

GENERAL MEASURES
- Use heat to relieve joint pain. Warm soaks, heating pads, or warm compresses may help. If heat does not help, try cold compresses.
- Protect your joints where possible (e.g., use bottle and jar opener, special gloves, or cane for walking).
- To learn more: National Psoriasis Foundation, 6600 SW 92nd Ave., Suite 300, Portland, OR 97223; (800) 723-9166; website: www.psoriasis.org.

MEDICATION
- Nonsteroidal anti-inflammatory drugs, other anti-inflammatory drugs, cortisone injections into inflamed joints, drugs to suppress the immune system, or tumor necrosis factor (TNF) inhibitors may be prescribed.
- Drugs will be prescribed for psoriasis at the same time as treatment for the arthritis symptoms.

ACTIVITY
- Rest during flare-ups, then resume your normal activities gradually. Exercise regularly to help keep your strength and flexibility. Swimming is a good exercise.
- Physical therapy can help with joint range of motion, flexibility, stretching, and muscle strength.

DIET—No special diet. Maintain a healthy weight.

CALL YOUR DOCTOR IF

- You or a family member has symptoms of psoriatic arthritis.
- Symptoms do not improve with treatment.

PTOSIS
(Blepharoptosis)

GENERAL INFORMATION

DEFINITION—Ptosis is a drooping of the upper eyelid, partially or completely covering the eye. It is pronounced as TOE-sis. The disorder may be acquired (most common type) or present at birth (congenital).

BODY PARTS INVOLVED—Upper eyelid; eye.

SEX OR AGE MOST AFFECTED—Both sexes; all ages (usually occurs in adults over age 30).

SIGNS & SYMPTOMS—Drooping of one or both eyelids, along with poor blinking reflexes. The extent of droop may vary at different times of the day.

CAUSES
- The acquired type is usually due to the muscles that elevate the eyelid becoming weak, thin, or stretched. This is often due to aging, but may be caused by disease, injury, or other medical problem.
- The congenital type is usually due to lack of development in the eyelid muscles (levators).

RISK INCREASES WITH
- Aging.
- Family history of ptosis.
- Paralysis of nerve fibers to the eyelids.
- Myasthenia gravis.
- Muscular dystrophy.
- Diabetes.
- Stroke.
- Brain tumor.
- Horner's syndrome.
- Birth injury.
- Head or eyelid injury.
- Tumor in the upper lobe of a lung.
- Eye surgery (such as cataract).

HOW TO PREVENT—No specific preventive measures.

WHAT TO EXPECT

DIAGNOSTIC MEASURES
- Your own observation of symptoms.
- Your health care provider can diagnose the disorder by an exam of the affected eyelid.
- Medical tests may be done to determine the cause of acquired ptosis.

APPROPRIATE HEALTH CARE
- No treatment may be needed if the symptoms are mild and no cause is found.
- Specific treatment will be directed toward any underlying disease that is diagnosed.
- Surgery to tighten the muscles of the eyelid may be done to prevent interference with vision or to improve appearance.
- Special glasses with a crutch attachment to hold up the eyelid may be an option.

POSSIBLE COMPLICATIONS
- If uncorrected in a child, it can lead to amblyopia (lazy eye).
- In some uncorrected cases, there may be decreased field of vision and headaches.
- Complications may occur from surgery. Ptosis may recur after surgery or the muscle can be overtightened.

PROBABLE OUTCOME—If surgery is performed, it is usually successful in improving appearance and eyelid function. The outcome may depend on treatment of the cause.

HOW TO TREAT

GENERAL MEASURES—Follow medical advice about home care after surgery or other treatments.

MEDICATION—Drugs are usually not needed for ptosis, but it may be prescribed for the underlying disorder.

ACTIVITY—No limits (unless advised).

DIET—No special diet.

CALL YOUR DOCTOR IF

- You or a family member has symptoms of ptosis.
- Ptosis worsens or vision is affected.

PULMONARY EDEMA

GENERAL INFORMATION

DEFINITION—Pulmonary edema is a condition of excess fluid (edema) in the lungs. Symptoms may begin suddenly or develop more slowly over weeks or months.

BODY PARTS INVOLVED—Lungs and heart.

SEX OR AGE MOST AFFECTED—Both sexes; it more often affects middle-aged and elderly adults.

SIGNS & SYMPTOMS
- Shortness of breath. Rapid breathing. May have wheezing. Symptoms may be worse when lying down.
- Restlessness and anxiety.
- Paleness and sweating.
- Weakness and fatigue.
- Swollen feet and ankles.
- Cough. This may be unproductive at first, but later it can produce frothy, blood-stained sputum.
- Fever (sometimes).

CAUSES—Lungs are normally air-filled. They take in oxygen and pass it on to the blood for transport to all cells in the body. When fluid builds up in the lungs, it interferes with oxygen intake. This can affect all body functions. Pulmonary edema can be caused by a number of different disorders, but heart disorders are the most likely.

RISK INCREASES WITH
- Heart disorders (e.g., heart failure or heart attack) can cause fluid to build up in veins in the lungs. Pressure causes the veins to leak excess fluid into the lungs.
- Acute respiratory distress syndrome (ARDS).
- Pulmonary embolism (blood clot).
- Drug overdose (such as from heroin or narcotics).
- High altitude illness.
- Pneumothorax or pleural effusion.
- Brain injury.
- Near drowning.
- Kidney failure.
- Inhaled toxins (e.g., ammonia, chlorine, or smoke from a fire).
- Eclampsia in pregnant women.
- Aspirin overdose or chronic high dose use.

HOW TO PREVENT—Get treatment for any illness or disease that could be a risk factor for pulmonary edema.

WHAT TO EXPECT

DIAGNOSTIC MEASURES
- Your own observation of symptoms.
- Your health care provider will do a physical exam and ask questions about your symptoms.

- Medical tests may include blood studies, blood-oxygen levels, chest x-ray, pulmonary function studies, and heart function studies.

APPROPRIATE HEALTH CARE
- Treatment will help reduce the excess fluid, improve lung and heart function, and treat any underlying disorder.
- Hospital care is almost always needed. Emergency treatment is often required.
- Hospital treatment may include supplemental oxygen, breathing support with a ventilator (breathing machine), fluids given through a vein (IV), drugs, and special diet. Patients are sometimes more comfortable sitting with legs dangling over the side of the bed.

POSSIBLE COMPLICATIONS—Heart attack, heart rhythm problems, shock, adverse effect of drugs, or death (if treatment is delayed or unsuccessful).

PROBABLE OUTCOME—In most cases, symptoms can be controlled with treatment. The underlying disease causing pulmonary edema may require lifelong treatment.

HOW TO TREAT

GENERAL MEASURES—Self-care is not appropriate for pulmonary edema.

MEDICATION
- Your health care provider may prescribe:
  - Diuretics to help remove excess fluid from the bloodstream and the lungs.
  - Drugs such as beta-blockers, ACE inhibitors, nitrates, calcium-channel blockers, digoxin, and others to reduce workload on the heart.
  - Drugs to treat any underlying disorder.

ACTIVITY
- Rest in bed until symptoms get better. After treatment, resume your normal activities gradually. Walking is a good activity to help increase strength. Resume sexual relations when you have medical approval.
- Check weight daily to be aware of any fluid buildup.

DIET—In the hospital, sodium and fluids are usually restricted. After recovery, a low-salt, low-fat diet and reduced fluid intake may be recommended.

CALL YOUR DOCTOR IF

- You or a family member has symptoms of pulmonary edema that appear suddenly. This is an emergency! Call 911 first.
- Weight goes up 2 to 3 pounds in one day.

PULMONARY EMBOLISM

 GENERAL INFORMATION

DEFINITION—A pulmonary embolism occurs when a blood clot blocks the flow of blood through an artery in the lungs. The clot prevents blood from flowing to a portion of the lung which results in a decrease of oxygen to the body.

BODY PARTS INVOLVED—Veins, especially veins in the legs; pulmonary artery and smaller artery branches that nourish the lungs.

SEX OR AGE MOST AFFECTED—Both sexes; all ages, but most common in adults.

SIGNS & SYMPTOMS
- Sudden shortness of breath.
- Faintness or fainting.
- Pain in the chest.
- Cough (sometimes with bloody sputum).
- Rapid heartbeat.
- Low fever.
- These symptoms are often preceded by swelling and pain in the leg.

CAUSES—In almost all cases, the blood clot begins in a deep vein of the leg (deep vein thrombosis or DVT), and rarely, another place in the body. The clot moves through the bloodstream, passing through the heart, and into an artery in the lungs. The blockage reduces breathing ability and can destroy lung tissue. Rarely, other types of clots form that are made up of fat, air bubbles, tissue from a tumor, or bacteria.

RISK INCREASES WITH
- Previous embolism or deep vein thrombosis.
- Any injury or illness that requires prolonged bed rest.
- Sitting for long periods, as on car or plane trip.
- Recent surgery.
- Heart disease, high blood pressure, or lung disorders.
- Bone fractures, such as hip fracture.
- Overweight.
- Pregnancy.
- Use of birth-control pills or hormone replacement therapy (risk increases if you smoke or are overweight).
- Cancer, severe burns, or inflammatory bowel disease.
- Smoking.
- Inherited blood clotting conditions.

HOW TO PREVENT
- Avoid prolonged bed rest during illnesses. Wear compressive stockings during recovery (in or out of bed).
- Start moving legs and walking as soon as possible after surgery.
- Don't smoke, especially if you are a woman age 35 or older who takes birth-control pills.
- If traveling, stand, stretch, and walk as often as possible.

 WHAT TO EXPECT

DIAGNOSTIC MEASURES
- Your own observation of symptoms.
- Your health care provider will do a physical exam and ask questions about your symptoms and activities.
- Medical tests may include chest x-ray, lung scan, pulmonary angiogram (a special x-ray study of blood flow), CT, blood studies, and other tests as needed.

APPROPRIATE HEALTH CARE
- Treatment is aimed at maintaining heart, blood vessel, and lung functions and preventing clot recurrence.
- Hospital care is necessary. Supplemental oxygen will be provided. Drugs will be given through a vein (IV).
- Rarely, surgery (embolectomy) is used to remove clot.
- A filter may be placed (using a catheter) into the main vein (vena cava) leading to the heart and lungs to trap recurrent clots.

POSSIBLE COMPLICATIONS
- High blood pressure in the lungs (pulmonary hypertension).
- Heart damage (a condition called cor pulmonale).
- Death (from a large clot that blocks artery).

PROBABLE OUTCOME—Usually curable with treatment. Embolism may recur.

 HOW TO TREAT

GENERAL MEASURES—To learn more: National Heart Lung Blood Institute, PO Box 30105, Bethesda, MD 20824; (301) 592-8573 (not toll free); website: www.nhlbi.nih.gov.

MEDICATION
- Anticoagulant drugs to treat the clots will be prescribed. You may need indefinite treatment with these drugs to prevent a recurrence.
- Clot-dissolving (clot buster) drugs may be prescribed. They break down the blood clots.
- Drugs to treat other disorders may be prescribed.

ACTIVITY—Rest in bed until all symptoms of the clot improve. While in bed, move legs often.

DIET—No special diet. Drink plenty of fluids.

 CALL YOUR DOCTOR IF

- You or a family member has symptoms of pulmonary embolism. This is an emergency! Call 911.
- After treatment, any symptoms cause concern.

PURPURA, HENOCH-SCHONLEIN
(Anaphylactoid Purpura)

 GENERAL INFORMATION

DEFINITION—Henoch-Schönlein purpura (HSP) is a disease that causes small blood vessels in the skin to leak because of inflammation.

BODY PARTS INVOLVED—Skin, joints, and gastrointestinal system (sometimes).

SEX OR AGE MOST AFFECTED—It usually affects children ages 2 to 11, most often boys. Adults are rarely affected.

SIGNS & SYMPTOMS
- Headache, fever, and loss of appetite may occur first.
- Itching, red skin rash that seems to be just beneath the skin surface. The rash usually consists of large hives with small bruises or blood spots in the centers. The rash is most often on the legs, thighs, and lower abdomen, but it may be scattered over the body. The rash turns a bruised, purple color. (That is why the name purpura is given to the disorder.)
- Joint pain and swelling at the knees, ankles, hips, wrists, or elbows.
- Cramping stomach (abdominal) pain and vomiting.
- Blood in urine or stools.

CAUSES—The cause is unclear. It may develop as an immune response to an infection. The immune system continues to attack cells after the infecting germs are gone. HSP has also been associated with insect bites and exposure to cold weather. Other cases have developed after a person received vaccination for typhoid, measles, cholera, hepatitis B, or yellow fever. Some foods, drugs, or other chemical toxins may trigger HSP as well. Often no cause can be found.

RISK INCREASES WITH
- Children between ages 2 and 11; boys more than girls.
- White and Asian children.
- Autumn, winter and spring seasons, and rarely in summer.
- Recent illness such as cold or flu. Both viral and bacterial infections are risks.
- Use of certain drugs. These include antibiotics such as penicillin and ampicillin, and some vaccines, such as typhoid, measles, yellow fever, and cholera.
- Bee stings, some chemical toxins, cold exposure, and food allergies have also preceded HSP.

HOW TO PREVENT—No specific preventive measures. Avoid any of the risk factors where possible.

 WHAT TO EXPECT

DIAGNOSTIC MEASURES
- Your own observation of symptoms.
- Your health care provider will do an exam of the skin and ask questions about the symptoms.
- No one test can diagnosis HSP. Medical tests may include blood and urine studies, skin biopsy, kidney biopsy, or ultrasound of abdomen.

APPROPRIATE HEALTH CARE
- There is no specific treatment for HSP. The main goals of treatment are to relieve symptoms such as joint pain, abdominal pain, or swelling.
- Hospital care may be needed for some cases.
- Treatment involves discontinuing any drugs or trigger factors that could be the cause.

POSSIBLE COMPLICATIONS
- Kidney damage. It may occur years later.
- The disorder can cause complications in almost every organ system. These include gastrointestinal, cardiovascular (heart and blood vessels), and the lungs.
- Women who had HSP during childhood may be at increased risk of high blood pressure during pregnancy.

PROBABLE OUTCOME—Most children recover completely. Mild cases may last a few days. Usually, recovery takes 1 to 4 weeks. In about 30% of cases, the disorder will recur. Recurrences usually occur within a few months and are usually less severe than first episode.

 HOW TO TREAT

GENERAL MEASURES—At home, use warm soaks to relieve joint pain.

MEDICATION
- There is no specific drug to treat the disorder. Drugs to reduce inflammation (such as ibuprofen or naproxen), or to treat an infection may be prescribed.
- In some cases, corticosteroids may be prescribed.

ACTIVITY—Get extra rest. When fever and pain are gone, the patient may gradually resume normal activities.

DIET—A bland diet may help if stomach pain occurs with eating.

 CALL YOUR DOCTOR IF

- Your child has symptoms of Henoch-Schönlein purpura.
- New symptoms occur or others worsen or recur.

PYLORIC STENOSIS
(Hypertrophic Pyloric Stenosis)

 GENERAL INFORMATION

DEFINITION—Pyloric stenosis is a condition of infancy in which encircling muscles at the end of the stomach enlarge and cause obstruction.

BODY PARTS INVOLVED—It affects the pylorus (a muscular tube that carries food from the stomach to the small intestine).

SEX OR AGE MOST AFFECTED—It is more common in firstborn males and usually begins between 2 and 5 weeks of age, but can occur as late as 4 months.

SIGNS & SYMPTOMS
- Recurrent vomiting episodes that become more forceful (projectile vomiting). It usually occurs after feeding.
- Muscular, olive-sized mass in the upper abdomen (sometimes).
- No pain or fever. Infant seems happy, but hungry, after vomiting.
- Gradual weight loss and dehydration.

CAUSES—The muscular band that encircles the pylorus thickens and eventually closes off the outlet from the stomach. Why this occurs is unknown.

RISK INCREASES WITH—Family history of pyloric stenosis.

HOW TO PREVENT—Cannot be prevented at present.

 WHAT TO EXPECT

DIAGNOSTIC MEASURES
- Your child's health care provider will do a physical exam.
- An ultrasound may be done to confirm the diagnosis.

APPROPRIATE HEALTH CARE
- Treatment is surgery to cut the thickened muscle (pyloromyotomy). In rare cases, treatment may involve a nonsurgical method.
- Fluids and electrolytes will be given through a vein (IV) until the baby is ready for surgery.

POSSIBLE COMPLICATIONS
- Without treatment, it can cause dehydration, weight loss, stomach irritation, and possibly jaundice (yellow skin and eyes).
- Rarely, complications from surgery may occur such as bleeding or infection.

PROBABLE OUTCOME—Curable with surgery. The child typically recovers quickly with no long-lasting ef fects.

 HOW TO TREAT

GENERAL MEASURES—Following surgery, you will be advised as to how to care for the incision and when you can give the baby a bath.

MEDICATION—Acetaminophen may be recommended after surgery if the baby appears to have pain or discomfort.

ACTIVITY—You will be advised of any limits.

DIET
- The baby will start being fed liquids about 4 to 6 hours after surgery. Feedings are gradually increased until a normal feeding schedule is resumed. This may take 1 to 2 days and then you can take the baby home.
- Your baby may still vomit a small amount for a day or two after surgery.

 CALL YOUR DOCTOR IF

- Your baby vomits repeatedly.
- The following occur after surgery:
  - Pain, swelling, redness, bleeding, or drainage at the surgical site.
  - Temperature rises to 101°F (38.3°C).

RABIES
(Hydrophobia)

GENERAL INFORMATION

DEFINITION—Rabies is a serious viral infection of the central nervous system, transmitted by an infected animal. In two-thirds of patients, symptoms may appear 1 to 3 months after the bite. Sometimes they may appear in as short as 5 days or as long as 7 years.

BODY PARTS INVOLVED—Brain and central nervous system; body parts bitten by the rabid animal.

SEX OR AGE MOST AFFECTED—Both sexes; all ages.

SIGNS & SYMPTOMS
• The first symptoms may be nonspecific and flu-like (e.g., fatigue, fever, or headache) and may last for days.
• Discomfort, numbness, or tingling at the site of exposure (e.g., bite or scratch).
• Symptoms progress within days to brain dysfunction (e.g., anxiety, confusion, agitation).
• Worsening symptoms—delirium, abnormal behavior, hallucinations, insomnia, violent movements, and inability to swallow.

CAUSES
• The infection is caused by the rabies virus. It is spread from the saliva of an infected animal. The transmission may come from a bite or nonbite exposure (e.g., scratch, being licked over an open wound or mucus membrane, or exposure to infected brain tissue).
• Animals that are commonly infected include dogs (especially wild dogs), bats, skunks, foxes, coyotes, and raccoons. Other animals can also be infected, so consult your local health department after any animal bite.

RISK INCREASES WITH—Professions or activities that may involve exposure to wild animals (cave exploration, hunting, farm or ranch workers, forest rangers, some laboratory workers, and veterinarians).

HOW TO PREVENT
• Vaccinate your dog or cat against rabies.
• Report stray animals in the neighborhood, and teach children to avoid them.
• Get rabies vaccine if work involves animals.
• Keep tetanus immunizations current.
• Avoid wild animals. In the United States, bats, skunks, and raccoons are the most likely to be infected, but any carnivore can carry rabies.

WHAT TO EXPECT

DIAGNOSTIC MEASURES
• Your health care provider will examine the wound.

• Medical tests may include blood tests and fluid and electrolyte studies.
• An exam of the animal's tissue (if available) will be done. Your own observation of the animal's behavior is important. Determine if the animal was provoked. Animals that attack without reason are more likely to be infected.

APPROPRIATE HEALTH CARE
• Treatment will be determined by type of exposure (bite or nonbite), the risk of rabies in the type of animal, circumstances of the biting incident, and vaccination status of animal.
• Hospital care is needed for serious wounds. Surgery may be done to clean and repair the bite wound.

POSSIBLE COMPLICATIONS—Acute period of rabies typically ends after 2 to 10 days. Once symptoms of rabies appear, the disease is nearly always fatal.

PROBABLE OUTCOME—Rabies can be prevented with early treatment following exposure to animal bites.

HOW TO TREAT

GENERAL MEASURES
• For animal bites or scratches:
  - Wash hands first. Wash the bite area for 3 to 5 minutes with mild soap and water to remove all saliva.
  - Cover the wound with a clean bandage or dry cloth.
  - Immediately call your health care provider's office or emergency room for advice.
  - Call your local animal control center to catch the animal, if possible.
  - Seek medical help if you have been exposed to a bat (such as waking up and finding one in the room) even if you have no bite or scratch marks.
  - Don't panic. The incubation period allows time for diagnosis and treatment.

MEDICATION
• Injections of rabies-immune globulin. (Painful injections in the abdomen are no longer used.)
• Injections of human-diploid-cell-strain vaccine, if the animal is proven rabid.
• Tetanus booster will be prescribed if needed.

ACTIVITY—No limits.

DIET—No special diet.

CALL YOUR DOCTOR IF

Anyone is bitten by an animal or has other exposure to an animal that may have rabies.

RADIATION SICKNESS

GENERAL INFORMATION

DEFINITION—Radiation sickness can develop from radiation therapy for medical reasons or after accidental exposure to radiation. Symptoms vary widely and are often temporary, depending on the radiation dosage and area radiated.

BODY PARTS INVOLVED—Depends on the location of treatment or exposure. See Signs & Symptoms below.

SEX OR AGE MOST AFFECTED—Both sexes; all ages.

SIGNS & SYMPTOMS
- Symptoms may start in 30 minutes after severe exposure and in 24 to 48 hours after mild exposure.
- Nausea, vomiting and diarrhea.
- Headache.
- Fatigue and shortness of breath.
- Rapid heartbeat.
- Yeast infection in the mouth.
- Dry mouth and loss of taste.
- Swallowing difficulty.
- Worsening of tooth or gum disease.
- Hair loss; dry cough.
- Heart inflammation with chest pain.
- Burning, inflammation, or scarring of the skin.
- Permanent skin darkening.
- Bleeding spots anywhere under the skin.
- Anemia; sexual impotence.

CAUSES
- Damage to the immune system and to healthy body tissues from high-dose radiation exposure.
- Exposure to low-dose radiation (e.g., x-ray exams) does not cause radiation sickness.

RISK INCREASES WITH
- Dose and rate of radiation treatment exposure.
- Amount of body area exposed to radiation treatment.

HOW TO PREVENT
- If you work with radiation, learn and adhere to all safety procedures for yourself and for patients.
- Avoid unnecessary radiation exposure.

WHAT TO EXPECT

DIAGNOSTIC MEASURES
- Your health care provider will do a physical exam and ask about radiation exposure.
- Medical tests may include blood studies of hemoglobin, platelet counts and white blood cell counts, x-rays of treated areas, and dosimetry (test to detect and measure radiation exposure).

APPROPRIATE HEALTH CARE
- Hospital care is usually needed. Treatment is aimed at controlling symptoms and preventing infections. Treatment may include drugs, fluids given through a vein (IV), blood transfusions, and surgery.
- Surgery to treat wounds or bone-marrow transplant may be needed for severe exposure.

POSSIBLE COMPLICATIONS
- Increased risk of infections due to poor immune system function.
- Sterility or birth defects may occur.
- Increased risk of cancer especially bone marrow cancer or leukemia.
- With radiation treatment, other complications depend upon the area involved. Modern radiation equipment makes serious complications unlikely.
- Death is likely with severe radiation sickness.

PROBABLE OUTCOME
- If from radiation treatment, most side effects or complications disappear gradually afterward.
- If from radiation accidents not severe enough to cause immediate death, radiation sickness may not appear for years.

HOW TO TREAT

GENERAL MEASURES—Use effective birth control measures to prevent pregnancy until it is determined that it is safe to have children. Genetic counseling may be recommended.

MEDICATION
- Your health care provider may prescribe:
  - Antinausea drugs and/or pain relievers.
  - Drugs to promote the growth of blood cells.
  - Blood transfusions for anemia.
  - Antibiotics to fight infections.
  - Antidiarrheal drugs.
  - Sedatives if sleeping is a problem.
  - Drugs to counter the effects of radiation.

ACTIVITY—Be as active as your strength allows. Rest often.

DIET—Eat a balanced diet. You may need a liquid diet for a short time or you may want to prepare food in a blender if you have trouble swallowing. Intravenous (IV) feeding or use of a small stomach tube is also possible until you can resume normal eating.

CALL YOUR DOCTOR IF

- You or a family member is accidentally exposed to radiation.
- Feelings of illness occur during radiation treatment or unexpected symptoms occur.
- Signs of infection develop, such as fever and chills, muscle aches, headache, and dizziness, during or after exposure or treatment.

RAPE TRAUMA SYNDROME

GENERAL INFORMATION

DEFINITION—Rape trauma syndrome involves the physical and emotional aftereffects of rape. The term rape refers to forcible sexual intercourse with an unwilling partner. In most cases, the rapist is a man and the victim is a woman.

BODY PARTS INVOLVED—Genitals; rectum; mouth; brain.

SEX OR AGE MOST AFFECTED—All ages and both sexes, but most common in females.

SIGNS & SYMPTOMS
- Right after the rape:
  - Physical injuries such as cuts, bruises, or other injuries, including vaginal and rectal tears.
  - Fear, anger, crying, or unusual behavior such as laughter.
  - No outward emotional signs (sometimes).
- Later effects (may be weeks to months):
  - Feelings of self-blame and guilt.
  - Depression and withdrawal, even from family and friends.
  - Mood swings; feelings of grief, shame, and revenge.
  - Loss of appetite.
  - Fear of intercourse; fear of men.
  - Nightmares and sleep disorders.
  - Fear of being alone.
  - Anxiety.

CAUSES—Rape is extremely traumatizing. All rape victims will suffer physical and emotional effects.

RISK INCREASES WITH—Any victim of rape or attempted rape.

HOW TO PREVENT
- There is no prevention for rape trauma syndrome.
- The scope of rape prevention is complex. It involves individuals, society, communities, and the government.

WHAT TO EXPECT

DIAGNOSTIC MEASURES—See Appropriate Health Care below.

APPROPRIATE HEALTH CARE
- Immediate care:
  - Emergency medical care will be provided for your physical injuries. A general physical exam and pelvic exam will be done according to specific medical guidelines. A report is normally made to local law agencies.
  - Ask for help from a rape crisis center (or similar agency). They help you through the medical, emotional, and legal necessities.
  - You will be advised about the risks of pregnancy, sexually transmitted diseases, HIV/AIDS, hepatitis B, and other infections, and what can be done to prevent the risks, and the need for any follow-up tests.

POSSIBLE COMPLICATIONS
- Sexually transmitted diseases.
- Emotional trauma that may last years.
- Pelvic injury.
- Pregnancy.

PROBABLE OUTCOME
- It takes most rape victims a long time to feel like they've returned to a normal existence. Some never do, and some say that they are completely changed people.
- Length of recovery time will be different for every person. Recovery may involve stages:
  - Acute. This involves dealing with the immediate physical and emotional effects.
  - Outward adjustment. Individual appears to be resuming "normal life," but still suffers from turmoil.
  - Reorganization. The assault, though not forgotten, is no longer the central focus. Person begins to accept the rape as part of their life, but chooses to move on.

HOW TO TREAT

GENERAL MEASURES
- After the medical care:
  - Get counseling help. This is important for your emotional recovery. Don't just try to put the matter out of your mind, and don't try to "go it alone." Hiding feelings can increase distress.
  - Keeping a journal or diary about your feelings, thoughts, and reactions may be helpful. Talk over your feelings with trusted friends and family.
  - Prepare yourself as much as possible for legal proceedings that force you to relive the trauma.
- To learn more: National Sexual Assault Hotline (800) 656-4673, which connects callers to a nearby rape crisis center; website: www.rainn.org.

MEDICATION
- Your health care provider may prescribe:
  - Antibiotics, if infection is suspected or diagnosed.
  - Emergency contraception.
  - Sedatives or tranquilizers to reduce anxiety.
  - Tetanus prevention.

ACTIVITY—No limits.

DIET—No special diet.

CALL YOUR DOCTOR IF

- You or someone you know has been raped.
- Emotional and/or physical symptoms worsen.

RAYNAUD DISEASE & PHENOMENON

 GENERAL INFORMATION

DEFINITION
• Raynaud disease (primary Raynaud) and Raynaud phenomenon (secondary Raynaud) are disorders of the circulatory system. Both types involve small blood vessels in the body. They usually affect blood circulation to the fingers, but may affect other areas.
- Primary Raynaud is not associated with an underlying cause.
- Secondary Raynaud is associated with an underlying cause.

BODY PARTS INVOLVED—Both types involve small blood vessels and fingers, may affect the toes; rarely, nose, lips, nipples, knees, or ears.

SEX OR AGE MOST AFFECTED—Primary Raynaud is more common in females under 40; secondary is more common in adults over 40.

SIGNS & SYMPTOMS
• Symptoms may develop over a period of years. In secondary Raynaud, they may begin suddenly.
• When exposed to cold or after emotional stress, fingers turn pale followed by a bluish tinge, then redness.
• Numbness and tingling occur along with the color changes. Pain is not common, but can occur.
• Symptoms may last from several minutes to a few hours. This is often called an attack.
• Warmth helps relieves these symptoms. Hands may become swollen and painful when warmed.

CAUSES—The exact cause is unknown. The blood vessels may constrict (narrow) due to cold or emotional stress, or there may be increased thickness to the blood.

RISK INCREASES WITH
• Females and under age 30 (for primary type).
• Family history of Raynaud.
• Living in a cold climate.
• Personal history or family history of autoimmune disorders, such as scleroderma, lupus erythematosus, rheumatoid arthritis, or others.
• Environmental factors, such as use of vibrating tools or exposure to certain chemicals or toxins.
• Smoking (it affects blood circulation).
• Certain drugs.

HOW TO PREVENT
• None specific. Avoid risk factors where possible. Don't smoke. It triggers symptoms. Avoid secondhand smoke.
• If attack occurs, take action to warm hands or feet or affected area of skin.

 WHAT TO EXPECT

DIAGNOSTIC MEASURES
• Your own observation of symptoms.
• Your health care provider will do a physical exam of the affected areas and ask questions about your symptoms and activities.
• Medical tests may include blood studies and a cold challenge test (putting hands in cold water). A nailfold capillary test may be done to check tiny blood vessels at base of fingernail.

APPROPRIATE HEALTH CARE
• Treatment involves treating any underlying cause, lifestyle changes, and drug therapy.
• Biofeedback training to teach you how to raise skin temperature may be helpful.
• Surgery to sever (cut) sympathetic nerves to the involved hands or feet (rare).

POSSIBLE COMPLICATIONS
• Fingertip or toe ulcers (open sores).
• Smooth skin on fingertips or toes.
• Development of an autoimmune disorder.
• Gangrene and amputation (rare, severe cases).

PROBABLE OUTCOME—Self-care and other treatments can help prevent symptoms. Symptoms may stop as person gets older. Secondary Raynaud may be curable if underlying cause can be resolved.

 HOW TO TREAT

GENERAL MEASURES
• Stop smoking. Symptoms will improve.
• Avoid exposure to cold if possible. Wear mittens or gloves outdoors and when handling ice or frozen foods. Wear comfortable, roomy shoes and wool socks.
• Avoid drugs that can worsen symptoms.
• Use caution in handling iced drinks or being in air-conditioned rooms.
• Avoid stress. Learn relaxation techniques.
• To learn more: Raynaud's Association, 94 Mercier Ave., Hartsdale, NY 10530; (800) 280-8055; website: www.raynauds.org.

MEDICATION
• Vasodilator drugs may be prescribed to dilate (widen) blood vessels which helps circulation.
• Topical drugs for the fingertips may be prescribed to protect them from skin ulcers.

ACTIVITY—Exercise daily. It helps circulation.

DIET—No special diet. Avoid caffeine.

☎ **CALL YOUR DOCTOR IF**

• You or a family member has Raynaud symptoms.
• Symptoms worsen or don't improve.

REACTIVE ARTHRITIS
(Reiter's Syndrome)

GENERAL INFORMATION

DEFINITION—Reactive arthritis is a joint inflammation that develops as a reaction to an infection in the body. It can cause swelling, redness, heat, and pain. Reactive arthritis can have two other symptoms—red and inflamed eyes and an inflamed urinary tract. Reactive arthritis is also known as Reiter's syndrome. It is not contagious.

BODY PARTS INVOLVED—Joints; eyes, including white eye covering; urethra and head of the penis; skin.

SEX OR AGE MOST AFFECTED—Both sexes; males ages 20 to 40.

SIGNS & SYMPTOMS
- Symptoms vary from person to person.
- Inflammation of the urethra (tube that takes urine from the bladder to the outside).
- Discharge from the penis or vagina. It often occurs 1 to 2 weeks after sexual contact.
- Pain or discomfort when urinating.
- Painful, swollen joints, especially in the knees, ankles, feet, and wrists.
- Stiffness and pain in the back and neck due to inflammation of the spine.
- Small ulcers (sores) inside the mouth, tongue, and on the penis tip.
- Red, itchy, burning and tearing of the eyes.
- Skin rash similar to psoriasis on the soles, palms, and around fingernails and toenails.
- Diarrhea may occur before other symptoms.
- General ill feeling.

CAUSES—The cause is unknown. It tends to occur after a person has had an intestinal infection or sexually transmitted disease. Genetic factors appear to play a role.

RISK INCREASES WITH
- Men ages 20 to 40.
- Certain genetic factors.

HOW TO PREVENT—To reduce risk, men can use rubber (latex) condoms during sexual intercourse or abstain from sex.

WHAT TO EXPECT

DIAGNOSTIC MEASURES
- Your own observation of symptoms.
- Your health care provider will do a physical exam and ask questions about your symptoms and activities.
- Medical tests may include blood studies and a culture of the urethral discharge. X-rays may be done. There is no specific test to diagnose reactive arthritis.

APPROPRIATE HEALTH CARE
- There is no treatment to cure reactive arthritis. Symptoms are managed with drug therapy and physical therapy.
- Physical therapy is often recommended to help maintain range of motion of the joints.
- Usually, no treatment is needed for eye symptoms, unless they are severe or chronic.

POSSIBLE COMPLICATIONS
- Chronic or recurrent symptoms that lead to disability.
- Iritis/uveitis (eye inflammation).
- Osteoarthritis.

PROBABLE OUTCOME—Symptoms may range from mild to severe. Arthritis symptoms may continue for a few weeks or up to 6 months. Many patients have recurrences over the years.

HOW TO TREAT

GENERAL MEASURES—Follow medical advice.

MEDICATION
- Your health care provider may prescribe:
  - Nonsteroidal anti-inflammatory drugs for arthritis symptoms.
  - Antibiotics for infection.
  - Corticosteroid injections for painful joints.
  - Corticosteroid eye drops for eye symptoms.
  - Topical corticosteroids for skin problems.
  - Drugs that suppress the immune system.
  - Drugs called tumor-necrosis factor inhibitors that are used for other forms of arthritis.

ACTIVITY
- After inflammation improves, exercise the affected joints daily with stretching and strengthening routines. Follow medical instructions. Maintain good posture.
- To relieve foot pain, wear cushion pads and arch supports in your shoes.

DIET—No special diet. Drink plenty of fluids.

CALL YOUR DOCTOR IF

- You or a family member has symptoms of reactive arthritis.
- Symptoms recur or new symptoms develop.

RECTAL PROLAPSE
(Procidentia)

GENERAL INFORMATION

DEFINITION—Rectal prolapse is a protrusion (bulging) of rectal tissues outside the anus. Partial prolapse is protrusion of the mucosa (inner lining) alone. Complete prolapse (procidentia) is protrusion of the entire thickness of the rectum.

BODY PARTS INVOLVED—Anus and rectum.

SEX OR AGE MOST AFFECTED—It can affect adults of both sexes, usually over age 60, and children ages 1 to 3. Rectal prolapse in infants can be a sign of cystic fibrosis.

SIGNS & SYMPTOMS
- Sense of fullness in the lower abdomen or rectal area.
- Mucus discharge sometimes tinged with blood from the rectum.
- Firm mass of tissue that can be felt at the anus. It may worsen after a bowel movement.
- Pain when having bowel movements.
- Bowel incontinence. Stool may leak from anus.

CAUSES—Weakness of muscles and ligaments holding the rectum in place. Why the weakness occurs is unknown.

RISK INCREASES WITH
- Aging.
- Previous surgery on the rectum or vagina.
- Constipation and straining to have bowel movements.
- Chronic diarrhea.
- Weak anal sphincter.
- Multiple sclerosis.
- Stroke, paralysis, or spinal tumor.
- Anal or pelvic injury.
- Chronic obstructive pulmonary disease.
- Multiple pregnancies.
- Malnutrition.
- Parasitic infections.
- Cystic fibrosis (children).

HOW TO PREVENT—No specific measures. Don't strain when having bowel movements. Avoid constipation and diarrhea. Eat a high-fiber diet.

WHAT TO EXPECT

DIAGNOSTIC MEASURES
- Your own observation of symptoms.
- Your health care provider will do an exam of the rectal area.
- Medical tests may include a defecogram (a special x-ray), anal muscle function tests, and others if needed. Cystic fibrosis tests may be done in children.

APPROPRIATE HEALTH CARE
- Treatment varies according to underlying cause. Causes of straining need to be corrected.
- In children, prolapse is usually temporary.
- Occasionally, minor prolapse can be reversed by gently pushing the protruding tissue back into the rectum.
- For most patients, surgery is needed to repair the prolapse. There are several different options available. Your health care provider will explain them to you and discuss the risks and benefits. Surgery is usually done under a general anesthetic.

POSSIBLE COMPLICATIONS
- Ulceration (sores) and bleeding in tissue that protrudes.
- Rectal prolapse may occur with another prolapse, such as the uterus or the bladder.
- Rectal prolapse may recur.
- Complications can occur from underlying condition or from surgery.

PROBABLE OUTCOME—Good prognosis with treatment. In children, there is usually complete recovery.

HOW TO TREAT

GENERAL MEASURES—Use sanitary napkins or absorbent pads to absorb the mucus discharge.

MEDICATION—To prevent constipation, bulk-formers, stool softeners, enemas, or suppositories may be prescribed.

ACTIVITY—Recovery from surgery may take 4 to 6 weeks. Then resume normal activities gradually.

DIET—Drink plenty of fluids each day and eat a diet high in fiber to help prevent constipation.

CALL YOUR DOCTOR IF

- You or a family member has symptoms of rectal prolapse.
- Rectal pain or bleeding occur.
- Fever or chills develop, indicating infection.
- Symptoms return after treatment.

REGIONAL PAIN SYNDROME, COMPLEX
(Reflex Sympathetic Dystrophy)

GENERAL INFORMATION

DEFINITION
• Complex regional pain syndrome (CRPS) is a chronic pain condition. The main symptom is continuous, intense pain which typically gets worse rather than better over time. Symptoms vary in severity and length. It most often affects one of the arms, legs, hands, or feet. Types:
  - CRPS 1 is frequently triggered by tissue injury with no underlying nerve injury.
  - CRPS 2 is associated with a nerve injury (this type previously known as causalgia).

BODY PARTS INVOLVED—The nerves, skin, muscles, blood vessels, and bones.

SEX OR AGE MOST AFFECTED—It occurs in both sexes at any age, but is more common in ages 30 to 60, and in women more than men.

SIGNS & SYMPTOMS
• Pain (may be burning or aching) and swelling. These symptoms may increase over time.
• Skin changes color from pale to purple/blue or gray. Affected skin may be tender, thin, and shiny.
• Hair and nail growth is increased. These symptoms may slow with time.
• Stiff joints and muscle spasms.
• Excessive sweating.
• Extreme sensitivity to touch.

CAUSES—The exact cause is unknown. It most often develops after an injury, sprain, or fracture. The pain that occurs is more severe and lasts longer than would be expected after the event. The sympathetic nervous system that controls blood flow and sweat glands appears to play a role. The immune system and other factors may be involved.

RISK INCREASES WITH
• Certain genetic factors may increase the risk.
• A tendency toward increased sympathetic activity. This includes cold hands, excessive sweating, or a history of fainting.
• Major or minor injury to an arm or leg.
• Heart attack, stroke, pancreatic cancer, herpes zoster, arthritis, nerve disorder, and others.
• Chest, neck, or shoulder injury.
• The period following surgery.
• Prolonged time in a cast or splint.

HOW TO PREVENT—No known way to prevent.

WHAT TO EXPECT

DIAGNOSTIC MEASURES
• Your own observation of symptoms.
• Your health care provider will do a physical exam and ask questions about your symptoms, activities, and medical history. This is often enough for diagnosis.

• A stimulus test (such as touch, pinprick, heat, or cold) to the area to see if it causes pain, x-ray, bone scan, and other tests may be done.

APPROPRIATE HEALTH CARE
• There is no cure, but there are treatment options. These include drugs, counseling, physical therapy, splinting, surgery, spinal cord stimulation, implanted drug pumps, and others. Your health care provider will devise a treatment plan based on your symptoms.
• TENS (transcutaneous electrical stimulation) may be prescribed. Brief pulses of electricity applied to nerve endings help relieve pain.
• Massage therapy will help some people.
• Biofeedback may help. It is a technique that involves learning to become more aware of your body to help you relax and control the pain.
• Counseling may help you learn ways to cope.

POSSIBLE COMPLICATIONS
• Disabling pain can affect an entire arm or leg.
• Muscle wasting (atrophy) and joint damage.
• Skin damage that cannot be reversed.
• Tightening of the muscles as they lose their tone. Hand and fingers or foot and toes may contract into a fixed position.
• Depression and anxiety due to chronic pain.

PROBABLE OUTCOME—Outcome will vary in different people. Some may be helped with treatment, some cases clear up on their own, and others have ongoing pain despite treatment.

HOW TO TREAT

GENERAL MEASURES
• Applying cold may help swelling and sweating. If the affected area is cool, heat may offer relief.
• Consider joining a support group.
• To learn more: Reflex Sympathetic Dystrophy Syndrome Association; website: www.rsds.org.

MEDICATION
• Take nonprescription drugs for pain and inflammation such as ibuprofen or naproxen.
• Steroids to reduce swelling and inflammation, drugs that widen blood vessels, injections of local anesthetic, stronger pain drugs, or other drugs may be prescribed.

ACTIVITY
• Maintain normal daily activities as best you can.
• Physical therapy and/or occupational therapy may be prescribed.

DIET—Eat a healthy diet.

☎ CALL YOUR DOCTOR IF

• You or a family member has symptoms of complex regional pain syndrome.
• Symptoms don't improve with treatment.

RENAL FAILURE, ACUTE
(Kidney Injury, Acute)

 GENERAL INFORMATION

DEFINITION—Acute renal failure is a sudden failure of the kidneys to function. Kidneys produce certain hormones, regulate electrolytes, and help rid the body of waste products. When kidneys fail, the waste products build up and cause symptoms. This disorder usually has a short, sometimes severe course.

BODY PARTS INVOLVED—Kidneys.

SEX OR AGE MOST AFFECTED—Both sexes; all ages.

SIGNS & SYMPTOMS
- Reduced urine output and increased thirst.
- Fluid build-up causing swelling in legs, ankles, or feet.
- Fatigue, drowsiness, or shortness of breath.
- Nausea, vomiting, diarrhea, or appetite loss.
- Mental (e.g., confusion) or mood changes.
- Bruising.
- Convulsions or coma in severe cases.
- The symptoms of the underlying cause will also be present.

CAUSES
- Conditions in the kidney, or in other areas of the body, that cause the kidneys to stop functioning. This leads to a buildup of waste products in the blood and tissues. Underlying conditions include:
  - Shock with very low blood pressure.
  - Blood poisoning (septicemia).
  - Congestive heart failure.
  - Fluid and electrolyte imbalance.
  - Blood-transfusion reaction.
  - Severe accident with severe muscle injury.
  - Acute glomerulonephritis (kidney inflammation).
  - Multiple myeloma (bone cancer).
  - Blockage of blood vessels to the kidney.
  - Kidney stones obstruct the ureters or urethra.
  - Prostate enlargement.
  - Use of certain drugs.
  - Overdose of poisons or drugs (e.g., drugs of abuse).

RISK INCREASES WITH
- Person with one kidney.
- Recent surgery.
- Being in the hospital.
- Accidents with severe injuries.
- Medical history of conditions that affect the kidney, such as diabetes, gout, multiple myeloma, high blood pressure, or congestive heart failure.

HOW TO PREVENT—No specific preventive measures. Seek medical care for causes and risk factors when possible.

 WHAT TO EXPECT

DIAGNOSTIC MEASURES
- Your health care provider will do a physical exam and ask questions about your symptoms and activities.
- Medical tests may include blood and urine studies that measure kidney function and fluid and electrolyte balance. Ultrasound, x-ray, heart studies, and other tests may be done to diagnose any complications.

APPROPRIATE HEALTH CARE
- Hospital care is usually needed.
- Treatment will depend on the cause. It may involve drug therapy, discontinuing a drug, surgery, or other type of treatment.
- Food and water intake is controlled to stop fluid and electrolyte imbalance and to reduce buildup of body wastes.
- Dialysis (artificial method of removing waste products from the blood) may be required until the kidneys recover their function.

POSSIBLE COMPLICATIONS—Shock, uremia, infections, seizures, heart or lung problems, chronic kidney failure, coma, or death.

PROBABLE OUTCOME—If the underlying cause can be treated, the kidneys usually start working again (may take days or weeks). Some patients may have only partial recovery. Older adults and those with serious medical problems are more at risk for complications.

 HOW TO TREAT

GENERAL MEASURES—To learn more: National Kidney Foundation, 30 E. 33rd St., New York, NY 10016; (800) 622-9010; website: www.kidney.org.

MEDICATION
- Diuretics (to remove excess fluid) and drugs to treat the underlying condition may be prescribed.
- Antibiotics may be given to treat or prevent infection.
- Other drugs will be prescribed as needed.

ACTIVITY—Follow medical instructions.

DIET—A diet high in carbohydrates and low in protein, potassium, and salt to reduce kidneys' work load may be a part of the treatment.

 CALL YOUR DOCTOR IF

- You or a family member has acute renal failure symptoms.
- Symptoms recur after treatment.

RENAL FAILURE, CHRONIC
(Kidney Disease, Chronic)

GENERAL INFORMATION

DEFINITION—Chronic renal failure is a gradual failure (over months to years) of the kidneys to function. Kidneys produce certain hormones, regulate electrolytes, and help rid the body of waste products. When kidneys fail, the waste products build up and cause symptoms.

BODY PARTS INVOLVED—Kidneys, which eventually affect all body systems.

SEX OR AGE MOST AFFECTED—Both sexes; all ages (often the elderly).

SIGNS & SYMPTOMS
- None or few symptoms until 60% to 75% of the kidney function fails. The symptoms listed may then occur.
- Listlessness, mental confusion, and drowsiness.
- Mild shortness of breath. Swelling of feet and ankles.
- Sudden weight change or nausea and vomiting.
- Itching, dry skin, and easy bruising.
- Headaches.
- Frequent hiccups.
- Changes in urine flow.
- Muscle cramps, twitches, or pain. Bone or joint pain.
- Numbness or tingling in hands or feet.
- Anemia with paleness and fatigue.
- Unusual bleeding.
- High blood pressure.

CAUSES—The kidneys are damaged as a complication of other medical conditions.

RISK INCREASES WITH
- Diabetes types 1 and 2.
- High blood pressure.
- Autoimmune disorders (e.g., systemic lupus erythematosus).
- Glomerulonephritis (kidney inflammation).
- Polycystic kidney disease; other hereditary disorders.
- Chronic kidney stones and infections.
- Use of certain drugs that are toxic to kidneys.
- Blood vessel diseases and various cancers.

HOW TO PREVENT—None specific. Get treatment for any condition that is a risk factor.

WHAT TO EXPECT

DIAGNOSTIC MEASURES
- Your health care provider will do a physical exam and ask questions about your symptoms and activities.
- Medical tests may include blood and urine tests that measure kidney function and fluid and electrolytes. Ultrasound, x-ray, heart studies, and other tests may be done to diagnose underlying disorder or complications.

APPROPRIATE HEALTH CARE
- Treatment is aimed at slowing the progress of the disease, treating the underlying disorder, treating complications, and replacing kidney function.
- Treatment steps may include hospital care, drugs, diet changes, dialysis, and kidney transplant.
- Hospital care may be needed for severe symptoms.
- Dialysis to filter and remove waste products from the blood may be needed for advanced kidney failure. Hemodialysis uses a machine. Peritoneal dialysis uses the body's abdominal lining as a filter.
- A kidney transplant may be recommended.

POSSIBLE COMPLICATIONS
- Kidney failure can affect almost any body function.
- End stage renal disease (ESRD).

PROBABLE OUTCOME—Kidney failure is a condition that worsens gradually. Treatment can help slow the progress. Kidney dialysis or kidney transplant will eventually be needed.

HOW TO TREAT

GENERAL MEASURES—To learn more: National Kidney Foundation, 30 E. 33rd St., New York, NY 10016; (800) 622-9010; website: www.kidney.org.

MEDICATION
- Your health care provider may prescribe:
  - Diuretics to reduce fluid build-up in the body.
  - Drugs to lower high blood pressure, treat anemia, treat an underlying disorder, prevent bone loss, treat symptoms (such as itchy skin), or treat complications.
  - Changes in drugs you now take that may be toxic to the kidneys.

ACTIVITY—Reduce activity as needed. Get adequate sleep.

DIET—Limits on protein, salt, and fluids are usually needed. A dietitian can be helpful in providing instructions.

CALL YOUR DOCTOR IF

- You or a family member has symptoms of chronic renal failure.
- Chest pain, fainting, difficulty breathing, severe vomiting, bleeding, weakness, or a change in alertness occur.

RESPIRATORY SYNCYTIAL VIRUS

 ## GENERAL INFORMATION

DEFINITION—Respiratory syncytial virus (RSV) is a viral infection of the nose, throat, and lungs. It is easily spread from one person to another. It occurs mainly in winter and spring months. RSV is common and most children have had an infection by age three. Symptoms are usually mild, but can be serious, especially in infants. A person can get it more than once, but the symptoms tend to be milder.

BODY PARTS INVOLVED—Upper and lower respiratory tracts.

SEX OR AGE MOST AFFECTED—Both sexes; all ages; most common in infants and children (it is the major cause of respiratory tract infections in this age group).

SIGNS & SYMPTOMS
- Mild symptoms (are like a common cold):
  - Runny nose, low-grade fever, headache, sore throat.
  - Feeling tired and loss of appetite.
  - Dry cough.
- More severe symptoms:
  - Infant or child refuses to eat. High fever.
  - Increase in coughing. Wheezing can occur.
  - Less active and sleeping more than usual.
  - Breathing problems. Skin color may be bluish. Spells of apnea (breathing stops for 10 to 15 seconds).

CAUSES—The virus is spread by close contact with an infected person. The viral germs enter the body through the eyes, nose, or mouth. The germs can be inhaled (from coughing) or passed by direct contact (e.g., holding hands). Germs are also spread by touching a surface or object, such as a toy, that an infected person has handled. The germs can live on an object, a hard surface, or on used facial tissues for several hours and on hands for 30 minutes or longer.

RISK INCREASES WITH
- Under age 2. Children with weak immune system or have a chronic medical disorder or born prematurely.
- Daycare centers. Both children and teachers.
- Living, working, or being in crowded places.

HOW TO PREVENT
- Wash hands often. Clean surfaces such as doorknobs. Wash toys that are shared.
- Take care to throw away used facial tissues.
- Cover your mouth when coughing or sneezing.
- Avoid crowds during seasonal outbreaks.
- Avoid close contact with people with cold symptoms.
- Preventive injections may be prescribed for young children at risk of a severe RSV illness.

 ## WHAT TO EXPECT

DIAGNOSTIC MEASURES
- If there are any concerns about the symptoms, call your health care provider.
- Your health care provider may confirm an RSV diagnosis with a physical exam. Often, they know if there is an RSV outbreak in the area.
- Medical tests are normally not required for healthy patients. They may be done for people who have a risk of complications.

APPROPRIATE HEALTH CARE
- Home care is usually all that is needed.
- Hospital care may rarely be needed for more severe symptoms. Oxygen, special drugs, and fluids to prevent dehydration may be required.

POSSIBLE COMPLICATIONS
- Ear infection.
- Serious lung disorders. More likely in premature infants, or people who have heart or lung problems. Most everyone will recover, but may be life threatening.

PROBABLE OUTCOME—Most cases are mild, need no special treatment, and last 7 to 14 days.

 ## HOW TO TREAT

GENERAL MEASURES
- Treatment of mild symptoms in otherwise healthy people is the same as for a cold. Get extra rest and drink plenty of fluids until the symptoms are better. Be alert for any serious problems that might develop.
- Avoid being around cigarette smoke.
- Use salt (saline) nose drops for a stuffy nose.

MEDICATION
- Children may be given acetaminophen. Other drugs should be approved by their health care provider.
- A child in a hospital may be given bronchodilators, antivirals, or other drugs for severe symptoms.
- Adults may take nonprescription drugs for pain or cold remedies.
- Antibiotics won't help a virus infection. They may be prescribed if bacterial infection develops.

ACTIVITY—Reduce daily activity while ill.

DIET—No special diet. Drink plenty of fluids.

CALL YOUR DOCTOR IF

You or your child has symptoms of respiratory syncytial virus that cause you concern.

RESTLESS LEGS SYNDROME
(Willis-Ekbom Disease)

 GENERAL INFORMATION

DEFINITION
- Restless legs syndrome (RLS) is a disorder that causes an urge to move the legs and other sensations.
- More than 80% of people with RLS also have a more common condition known as periodic limb movement disorder (PLMD). PLMD involves involuntary leg twitching or jerking movements during sleep. They typically occur every 10 to 60 seconds, sometimes throughout the night. People have no control over them.

BODY PARTS INVOLVED—Legs.

SEX OR AGE MOST AFFECTED—RLS occurs more often in women than in men. It may begin at any age, even infancy. Patients with severe symptoms are usually middle-aged or older.

SIGNS & SYMPTOMS
- A compulsive urge to move the legs. Lying down and trying to relax worsens symptoms.
- Sensations in the legs are described as burning, creeping, tugging, or like insects crawling inside the legs.
  - They usually occur deep inside the leg, between the knee and ankle. More rarely, they occur in the feet, thighs, arms, and hands. The sensations usually affect both sides of the body.
  - The sensations range from uncomfortable, to irritating, to painful. They may come and go.
- Symptoms may be mild during the day and more severe in the evening or at night. They cause difficulty in falling, and staying, asleep.
- Long car or plane trip, sitting in a movie theater, or relaxation exercises can trigger symptoms.

CAUSES—In most cases, the cause is unknown (primary RLS). In others (secondary RLS), there are certain factors or conditions that may be related to RLS.

RISK INCREASES WITH
- Family history of RLS.
- Low iron levels or anemia.
- Chronic diseases such as diabetes, kidney failure, Parkinson's disease, or peripheral neuropathy.
- Obesity.
- Pregnancy.
- Certain drugs.
- Caffeine, alcohol, and tobacco may aggravate or trigger symptoms in some patients.

HOW TO PREVENT—No preventive measures.

 WHAT TO EXPECT

DIAGNOSTIC MEASURES
- Your own observation of symptoms.

- Your health care provider will do a physical exam and ask questions about your symptoms and activities.
- Medical tests (including a sleep study) may be done to identify any medical disorder that may be a factor in the symptoms.

APPROPRIATE HEALTH CARE
- Treatment options for RLS may include lifestyle changes and drugs or supplements.
- Treatment will be given for underlying disorder.

POSSIBLE COMPLICATIONS
- Left untreated, the condition causes exhaustion and daytime fatigue.
- Symptoms may gradually worsen with age.

PROBABLE OUTCOME
- There is no cure for primary RLS. Symptoms may disappear for weeks or months, but usually return. Treatment can reduce the symptoms and increase periods of restful sleep.
- Secondary RLS can be cured if the cause is managed.

 HOW TO TREAT

GENERAL MEASURES
- Don't smoke. Find a way to quit.
- A regular sleep pattern can help reduce symptoms. Try to go to bed and get up at the same times each day.
- Taking a hot bath, massaging the legs, or using a heating pad or ice pack can help.
- To learn more: Restless Legs Syndrome Foundation, 1610 14th St., Suite 300, Rochester, MN 55901; (507) 287-6312 (not toll free); website: www.rls.org.

MEDICATION
- No one drug works for everyone with RLS. There are several options and your health care provider will discuss the options. If one type doesn't help, another can be tried.
- Iron supplements may be prescribed.
- Diet supplements may be recommended.
- If a drug you take could be a cause of RLS, you may be advised to change the dose or take a different drug.

ACTIVITY—A program of regular, moderate exercise may help you sleep better. Excessive exercise may worsen symptoms.

DIET—Avoid caffeine and alcohol. They may trigger symptoms.

 CALL YOUR DOCTOR IF

- You or a family member has symptoms of restless legs syndrome.
- Symptoms continue despite treatment.

RETINAL DETACHMENT

GENERAL INFORMATION

DEFINITION—A retinal detachment is a separation or tear of the retina (the light-receptive tissue at the back of the eye) from the remainder of the eye. It usually affects one eye, but sometimes both are affected. Retinal detachment is a medical emergency.

BODY PARTS INVOLVED—Eye.

SEX OR AGE MOST AFFECTED—All ages (most often ages 40 to 70) and both sexes.

SIGNS & SYMPTOMS
- Light flashes in the field of vision.
- Floating spots in the field of vision.
- Blurred vision.
- A shadow or curtain over the field of vision.
- Gradual loss of vision. This may not be noticed because it is so gradual.
- No pain.

CAUSES—Retinal detachments may develop in eyes with retinas weakened by a hole or a tear. This allows fluid to seep underneath and weaken the attachment so that the retina then becomes detached.

RISK INCREASES WITH
- Aging.
- Eye injury.
- Diabetes (which can lead to diabetic retinopathy).
- Previous retinal detachment.
- Family history of retinal detachment.
- Extreme nearsightedness (myopia).
- Cataract surgery.
- Other eye diseases.

HOW TO PREVENT
- No specific preventive measures.
- Use safety precautions to prevent eye injury (e.g., eye protection in contact sports).
- People at risk should have regular eye exams.
- Following cataract surgery, call your eye care provider about any new or unexpected symptoms.

WHAT TO EXPECT

DIAGNOSTIC MEASURES
- Your own observation of symptoms.
- Your eye doctor (ophthalmologist) can diagnose the detachment by an exam of the eye using special equipment. Vision testing will usually be done.
- An ultrasound, CT, or MRI may be done in some cases.

APPROPRIATE HEALTH CARE
- Treatment will depend on location and severity of the detachment. There are several procedures available. Sometimes, a combination of one or more procedures is used. The procedures are most often done as an outpatient, but hospital care may be needed for surgery. A local or general anesthetic may be used. Your eye doctor will explain the procedures to you.
- The retina may be reattached using special lasers or cryotherapy (using below-freezing temperatures).
- A gas bubble may be injected into the eye. It holds the retina in place while, over a period of days, the fluid that seeped in is resolved. The gas bubble is eventually absorbed by the body. This procedure may require the head to remain in a certain position for days to weeks.
- More advanced detachments may require surgery. Scleral buckle or vitrectomy are two types of surgery that may be recommended.

POSSIBLE COMPLICATIONS
- With delayed or no treatment—partial or complete blindness may occur in affected eye.
- Cataracts and/or glaucoma.
- Detachment may recur. This can occur within a few months of surgery. Treatment will need to be repeated. Detachment occurs in other eye.

PROBABLE OUTCOME—Usually curable with prompt treatment. Recovery of vision may take weeks to months. If vision was good before the detachment, good vision should return. If vision was poor prior to the detachment, the return may be slow and remain poor.

HOW TO TREAT

GENERAL MEASURES—Follow medical advice about home care after any eye surgery.

MEDICATION—After surgery, one or more types of eye drops are usually prescribed for short time period.

ACTIVITY—You will be advised about limits on activity depending on the type of procedure used. Follow all instructions carefully.

DIET—No special diet.

CALL YOUR DOCTOR IF

- You or a family member has flashes or floating spots in your field of vision. Do not delay in getting medical help. This can be an emergency.
- Any sign of infection occurs (bleeding, redness, pain, swelling, or fever) or vision worsens after surgery.

REYE'S SYNDROME

GENERAL INFORMATION

DEFINITION—Reye's syndrome is a rare disease that causes swelling of the brain, liver, and other major organs.

BODY PARTS INVOLVED—Can affect all body organs.

SEX OR AGE MOST AFFECTED—It can occur at any age, but most often affects children and young teenagers.

SIGNS & SYMPTOMS
- Vomiting.
- Lethargy.
- Drowsiness.
- Confusion.
- Delirium.
- Personality changes (such as irritability).
- Seizures.
- Arm or leg weakness, or unable to move them.
- Double vision.
- Speech problems.
- Coma.

CAUSES—Unknown. Reye's syndrome usually occurs after a virus infection. Studies link most cases to the use of salicylate drugs, such as aspirin, during a viral illness (e.g., chickenpox and influenza). Genetics may play a role.

RISK INCREASES WITH
- Recent illness, such as chickenpox, influenza, or other respiratory illness.
- Use of aspirin with the viral illness.
- Having fatty acid oxidation disorder (a genetic metabolic deficiency).

HOW TO PREVENT—Don't give a child under the age of 18 aspirin for fever until it has been diagnosed. If the illness is diagnosed as viral, never use aspirin.

WHAT TO EXPECT

DIAGNOSTIC MEASURES
- Your own observation of symptoms.
- Your health care provider will do a physical exam.
- Medical tests may include blood studies of liver function and a study of cerebrospinal fluid (CSF). An EEG (electroencephalogram) may be done. It measures electrical activity of the brain

APPROPRIATE HEALTH CARE
- There is no specific treatment that will cure the disorder. Hospital intensive care is needed.
- Treatment steps are aimed at preventing complications such as swelling of the brain. This may involve inserting a feeding tube, intravenous (IV) fluids, urinary catheter, mechanical breathing support, kidney dialysis, blood transfusion, cardiovascular (heart and blood vessel) monitoring, and therapies to reduce pressure on the brain.

POSSIBLE COMPLICATIONS
- Pneumonia.
- Respiratory failure.
- Heart rhythm problems or heart attack.
- Seizures.
- Permanent brain damage, coma, or death caused by pressure on the brain.

PROBABLE OUTCOME—Some patients will have a mild illness with complete recovery. Others may have more severe symptoms and develop varying degrees of brain damage. Early diagnosis is important to help prevent complications.

HOW TO TREAT

GENERAL MEASURES—To learn more: National Reye's Syndrome Foundation, 426 N. Lewis, P.O. Box 829, Bryan, OH 43506, (800) 233-7393; website: www.reyessyndrome.org.

MEDICATION
- Your health care provider may prescribe:
  - Steroids or other drugs to reduce pressure and swelling of the brain.
  - Diuretics to help remove excess fluid from the body.
  - Glucose solutions to maintain normal levels of glucose.

ACTIVITY—Bed rest is needed until the symptoms improve. Normal activities may then be resumed gradually.

DIET—Nothing by mouth initially. After recovery, no special diet required.

CALL YOUR DOCTOR IF

- Your child has symptoms of Reye's syndrome. Call at the first sign of confusion, lethargy, or other mental changes!
- After hospital care, any symptoms of Reye's syndrome recur or the child develops a fever.
- New, unexplained symptoms develop. Drugs used in treatment may produce side effects.

RH INCOMPATIBILITY

 GENERAL INFORMATION

DEFINITION—Rh incompatibility is a difference between an infant's blood type and that of its mother. This results in the destruction of the infant's red blood cells during pregnancy and after birth by antibodies from its mother's blood.

BODY PARTS INVOLVED—Blood of pregnant mother and fetus.

SEX OR AGE MOST AFFECTED—Newborn infants only.

SIGNS & SYMPTOMS
- Symptoms affect the fetus or newborn.
- Excessive amniotic fluid around the fetus.
- Jaundice (yellow skin and eyes) that begins within 24 hours after delivery.
- Infant has floppy or decreased muscle tone.

CAUSES—The baby of an Rh-negative (blood type) mother and an Rh-positive father may be Rh-positive. (If the father is known to be Rh negative, there is no concern.) During pregnancy, but more commonly during delivery, a small amount of the infant's blood is absorbed by the mother through the placenta, stimulating her body to produce antibodies against Rh-positive blood. The antibodies are produced after delivery, so the first infant is not affected (unless mother had prior miscarriage or abortion). With each subsequent pregnancy, anti-Rh antibodies cross the placenta and may destroy fetal blood cells. The resulting anemia can be severe enough to cause fetal death. If the fetus survives, antibodies can cross to the baby during birth, causing jaundice and other symptoms shortly after birth.

RISK INCREASES WITH—Each pregnancy after the first one that involved different blood types. This includes ectopic pregnancies and spontaneous (miscarriage) and elective abortions.

HOW TO PREVENT—Medical care early in pregnancy is important to determine the risk of Rh incompatibility and provide treatment if needed.

 WHAT TO EXPECT

DIAGNOSTIC MEASURES
- Blood tests are done to type the mother's, father's, and infant's blood, measure the mother's Rh-positive antibodies, and to detect anemia in the infant's blood.
- Amniocentesis may be done. A small amount of amniotic fluid is withdrawn from the amniotic sac that surrounds the unborn child in the uterus for a diagnostic procedure. It can be used sometimes to determine the fetal blood type.

- Cordocentesis (percutaneous umbilical blood sampling [PUBS]) may be recommended. It is done to determine fetal blood type and the degree of anemia.

APPROPRIATE HEALTH CARE
- Intrauterine blood transfusions (sometimes).
- Transfusion to completely exchange the infant's blood after birth.
- Hospital care. The newborn child will remain in the hospital up to 2 weeks after an exchange transfusion.

POSSIBLE COMPLICATIONS
- Complications may develop from procedures such as amniocentesis or cordocentesis.
- Emergency delivery of the baby may be required.
- Hydrops fetalis in the newborn. This involves severe edema (swelling), heart, lung, and liver problems.
- Mental deficiency, movement disorders, seizures, or hearing or speech problems.

PROBABLE OUTCOME—With prompt diagnosis, monitoring, and treatment, the outcome is generally good. Complications are rare.

 HOW TO TREAT

GENERAL MEASURES
- If you have an Rh-negative blood type, tell any health care provider who treats you. Be sure this information is in your medical records.
- Wear or carry medical ID to identify your medical problem.

MEDICATION—If you are pregnant and have Rh-negative blood type, you will be prescribed an anti-Rh gamma globulin injection (RhoGAM) at 28 weeks and again within 72 hours after delivery or at the end of a pregnancy for any reason. You may have an antibody titer drawn during pregnancy to see if you are producing anti-Rh antibodies. You do not need RhoGAM if your fetus is Rh-negative.

ACTIVITY—No limits after treatment.

DIET—No special diet.

 CALL YOUR DOCTOR IF

You have further questions about RH incompatibility.

RHEUMATIC FEVER

GENERAL INFORMATION

DEFINITION—Rheumatic fever is an inflammatory disorder that affects many parts of the body, especially the joints and heart. It is a complication of a throat infection caused by group A streptococcus. Strep throat infections are contagious, but rheumatic fever is not.

BODY PARTS INVOLVED—Joints; heart and heart valves; skin and brain (sometimes).

SEX OR AGE MOST AFFECTED—Children and adults of both sexes. It is most common in ages 5 to 15.

SIGNS & SYMPTOMS
- Joint inflammation that causes pain, redness, swelling, and warmth. Wrists, elbows, knees, or ankles are most often affected. The symptoms may move from one joint to another.
- Fever; fatigue; paleness.
- Appetite loss, general ill feeling.
- Stomach (abdominal) pain; chest pain.
- Mild skin rash on the chest, back, and abdomen.
- Small, painless bumps just under the skin in bony areas such as the elbows or knees.
- Uncontrolled arm and leg movement (chorea).
- If the heart is involved:
  - Shortness of breath.
  - Fluid build-up that causes swelling of legs and back.
  - Rapid heartbeat, especially when lying down.

CAUSES—Rheumatic fever is caused by a preceding strep infection that occurs 1 to 6 weeks prior to the start of symptoms. It is an autoimmune disorder in which antibodies produced by the body to attack the strep bacteria also attack tissues of the joints or heart. Why this occurs is unknown.

RISK INCREASES WITH
- Family history of rheumatic fever.
- Crowded or unclean living conditions. poverty.

HOW TO PREVENT—Obtain prompt antibiotic treatment of any strep infection, including those of the skin. Strep infections must be treated with antibiotics.

WHAT TO EXPECT

DIAGNOSTIC MEASURES
- Your own observation of symptoms.
- Your health care provider will do a physical exam and ask questions about your symptoms and previous illnesses.
- Medical tests may include blood studies, a throat culture, and x-rays of the chest and heart. An ECG (electrocardiogram) may be done. This test measures electrical activity of the heart. No test is specific to diagnose rheumatic fever.

APPROPRIATE HEALTH CARE
- Treatment includes rest and drugs to treat the symptoms and to prevent rheumatic fever from recurring.
- Home care is recommended for some cases. Hospital care may be required for more severe cases.

POSSIBLE COMPLICATIONS
- Rheumatic heart disease. In some cases, rheumatic fever may permanently damage the heart valves. It may take 10 to 30 years for symptoms of valve damage to appear. A damaged valve can usually be replaced with surgery.
- Relapse of rheumatic fever.

PROBABLE OUTCOME—Rheumatic fever usually resolves in 2 to 12 weeks. Some cases may take 15 weeks or more.

HOW TO TREAT

GENERAL MEASURES
- Good oral hygiene is important. See your dentist for regular exams.
- To learn more: American Heart Association, 7272 Greenville Ave., Dallas, TX 75231; (800) 242-8721 website: www.americanheart.org.

MEDICATION
- Your health care provider may prescribe:
  - Drugs to reduce inflammation.
  - Diuretics to reduce fluid build-up in the body.
  - Drugs for congestive heart failure if it occurs.
  - Antibiotics for strep bacteria. Once rheumatic fever reaches the inactive stage, low-dose antibiotics may be continued indefinitely to prevent recurrence. They may be taken by mouth or given as an injection.

ACTIVITY—Bed rest normally (or very limited activity) until studies show the disease has subsided. Then return to normal activities gradually. Your health care provider will advise when to return to school.

DIET
- A liquid or soft diet in the early stages. Then provide a normal diet high in protein, calories, and vitamins.
- A low-salt diet may be recommended if patient has carditis (inflammation of the heart).

CALL YOUR DOCTOR IF

- You or your child has symptoms of rheumatic fever.
- Symptoms recur or new symptoms develop.

RINGWORM
(Tinea)

GENERAL INFORMATION

DEFINITION—Ringworm is a fungal (tinea) infection of the skin. It can involve the scalp (tinea capitis), skin (tinea corporis), groin skin (tinea cruris), nails (tinea unguium), feet (tinea pedis), and skin with beard (tinea barbae).

BODY PARTS INVOLVED—Skin.

SEX OR AGE MOST AFFECTED—It affects children and adults and is more common in males than females.

SIGNS & SYMPTOMS
* Lesions (sores) that itch (sometimes).
* On the scalp—lesions cause patchy hair loss and scaling scalp.
* On body skin—lesions are red, circular, flat, scaling, and have well-defined borders.
* On the bearded area of the face—lesions cause an itchy, scaling rash under the beard.
* On the feet—in the skin between the toes, a soft scaling (may be blistered), itchy rash.
* Of the nails—thickened, yellow, dull nails with crusting at the free edge.

CAUSES—Fungal infection with one or more of 5 different fungi. They are found almost everywhere. Transmission is by person-to-person contact, by touching infected surfaces (e.g., towels, shoes, or shower stalls), or contact with infected pet (cats are common carriers). (Worms have nothing to do with the infection.)

RISK INCREASES WITH
* Crowded living conditions.
* Contact with infected persons or animals.
* Daycare centers or schools.
* Weak immune system due to illness or drugs.
* Chronic moisture and irritation of the skin.
* Warm, humid climates.

HOW TO PREVENT
* The fungi are so prevalent that total prevention is impossible. To reduce risk:
  - Get treatment for pets that have skin problems.
  - Carefully dry feet after bathing in a tub or shower or after swimming. Apply antiperspirant to your feet if they perspire excessively.
  - Good personal hygiene.
  - Don't share headgear (hats, combs, brushes).
  - Avoid tight shoes or underwear that may rub or irritate the skin. Wear cotton underwear and socks.

WHAT TO EXPECT

DIAGNOSTIC MEASURES
* Your own observation of symptoms.

* In most cases, self-care is all that is needed. See your health care provider if self-care does not help.
* Your health care provider can usually diagnose the disorder by a skin exam.
* Medical tests may include microscopic exam of skin scrapings and exam with ultraviolet light (Wood's lamp) for ringworm on the scalp.

APPROPRIATE HEALTH CARE—Treatment is usually with topical drugs. Other specific care depends on location of infection.

POSSIBLE COMPLICATIONS
* Bacterial infection of ringworm lesions.
* Recurrence is common and ringworm becomes chronic in 20% of cases.

PROBABLE OUTCOME—Usually curable with treatment. It may take weeks to months depending on the location.

HOW TO TREAT

GENERAL MEASURES
* For infection on the body—wash clothing, towels, or bed linens that have touched lesions.
* Keep the skin dry. If the area is red, swollen, and weeping, use compresses made of 1 teaspoon salt to 1 pint water. Apply 4 times a day for 2 to 3 days before starting the local antifungal medication.
* For infection of the scalp, shampoo hair daily.
* For infected feet, expose feet to air whenever possible. Wear sandals or leather shoes; wear cotton socks. Wash and dry your feet daily.
* For an infected beard, let the beard grow. If necessary to shave, use an electric shaver and not a blade.
* For nail infection, keep nails short.

MEDICATION
* Use topical antifungal drugs in the form of creams, lotions, or ointments. Treatment may continue after symptoms clear up to help prevent a recurrence.
* In widespread infections or nail infections, an oral antifungal may be prescribed.
* Topical steroids may be prescribed for itching or inflammation.
* Antibiotics may be prescribed for a bacteria infection.

ACTIVITY—No limits.

DIET—No special diet.

CALL YOUR DOCTOR IF

You or a family member has symptoms of ringworm that do not improve in 4 weeks or skin symptoms cause concern.

ROCKY MOUNTAIN SPOTTED FEVER
(Tick Typhus)

GENERAL INFORMATION

DEFINITION—Rocky Mountain spotted fever is an acute illness caused by a germ transmitted by infected ticks. The disorder gets its name from the area where it was first identified.

BODY PARTS INVOLVED—Skin; central nervous system; gastrointestinal tract; muscles.

SEX OR AGE MOST AFFECTED—Both sexes; all ages, more likely to occur in children and young adults.

SIGNS & SYMPTOMS
- Symptoms can begin 3 to 12 days after tick bite.
- Fever, often high, with chills.
- Red skin rash that begins on hands and feet and spreads to ankles, wrists, legs, trunk, and abdomen.
- Headache that may be severe.
- Muscle aches and weakness; stiff back.
- Nausea and vomiting.
- Mental confusion; coma.

CAUSES—*Rickettsia* germs that live inside ticks. People are infected through tick bites, usually in the spring or summer. *Rickettsia* also infect rodents, squirrels, and chipmunks. The disease occurs in all states of the United States, especially on the East Coast from Georgia to Maryland, and in heavy brush areas, such as Long Island. It is not contagious from person to person.

RISK INCREASES WITH
- Outdoor activities in tick-infested areas.
- Contact with dogs.

HOW TO PREVENT
- Wear protective clothing in tick-infested areas, and use insect repellent.
- During outdoor activity, carefully inspect the body frequently to remove ticks. If ticks are removed within 4 hours, it will reduce the risk of infection. Use tweezers to remove a tick. Wear latex gloves or cover fingers with paper towel. Grasp tick as close to the skin as possible and pull upward. Disinfect the bite site and wash hands with soap and water. Do not remove ticks by squeezing, using petroleum jelly (Vaseline), or burning them with a match. Save the tick in a plastic bag in a freezer. If illness occurs, it may be used to help with diagnosis.

WHAT TO EXPECT

DIAGNOSTIC MEASURES
- Your own observation of symptoms.
- Your health care provider will do a physical exam and ask questions about your symptoms and activities.

- Medical tests may include blood studies and skin biopsy (small piece of skin is removed to view under a microscope). The history of a tick bite or travel to a tick-infested area helps confirm diagnosis.

APPROPRIATE HEALTH CARE
- Treatment is with drugs and supportive care.
- Patients with mild disease may be treated at home. Moderate to severe infections require hospital care. Treatment may include mechanical breathing support, blood transfusions, and close watch for complications such as kidney failure.
- Treatment is with drugs and supportive care.
- Patients with mild disease may be treated at home. Moderate to severe infections require hospital care. Treatment may include mechanical breathing support, blood transfusions, and close watch for complications such as kidney failure.

POSSIBLE COMPLICATIONS—They rarely can develop in the skin, heart, lungs, joints, kidneys, brain, and central nervous system. Very rarely, it can be fatal.

PROBABLE OUTCOME—With treatment, most patients recover completely. Symptoms usually being to improve within 72 hours of start of treatment. Complications can occur with delayed or no treatment.

HOW TO TREAT

GENERAL MEASURES
- Good mouth care is important.
- To learn more: Centers for Disease Control & Prevention, 1600 Clifton Rd, Atlanta, GA 30333; (800) 232-4636; website: www.cdc.gov/ticks.

MEDICATION—Antibiotics, such as doxycycline, tetracycline, or chloramphenicol will be prescribed.

ACTIVITY—Rest in bed until fever and other symptoms improve.

DIET—No special diet. Very ill patients may require intravenous (IV) feedings. For others, small frequent meals may be needed.

CALL YOUR DOCTOR IF

- You or a family member has symptoms of Rocky Mountain spotted fever.
- New, unexplained symptoms develop. Drugs used in treatment may produce side effects.

ROSEOLA INFANTUM
(Exanthem Subitum)

GENERAL INFORMATION

DEFINITION—Roseola infantum is a common, mild childhood illness.

BODY PARTS INVOLVED—Skin; central nervous system.

SEX OR AGE MOST AFFECTED—It usually affects infants and young children (ages 6 months to 3 years). Most children have had the infection by the time they start school. Older children and adults are rarely infected.

SIGNS & SYMPTOMS
- Fever, often high, for several days. It may be the only symptoms until the rash appears.
- Flat, reddish skin rash after 3 to 5 days of high fever. The rash usually starts on the trunk and spreads to neck and arms. In some cases, it may reach the face or legs. When the rash appears, the fever subsides. Some children may never develop the rash.
- Irritability.
- Drowsiness.
- Loss of appetite.

CAUSES—It is caused by herpes virus types (HHV)-6 (most often) or (HHV)-7. The fever begins 5 to 15 days (usually 9 days) after exposure. A child is infectious during the fever phase of the illness. The infection is probably spread by contact with an infected person's saliva or respiratory secretions. The infected person may have no symptoms.

RISK INCREASES WITH—Children ages 6 months to 3 years.

HOW TO PREVENT—There is no specific way to prevent the infection. Take general precautions such as frequent hand washing and not exposing your child to someone who is sick.

WHAT TO EXPECT

DIAGNOSTIC MEASURES
- Your own observation of symptoms.
- Call your child's health care provider if you have any concern about the symptoms. The disorder can usually be diagnosed without any medical tests, but a blood or urine study may be done.

APPROPRIATE HEALTH CARE
- There is no specific treatment for roseola.
- Rest at home, drink extra fluids, and drug therapy to reduce the fever if needed.

POSSIBLE COMPLICATIONS
- Rarely, seizures caused by high fever. They will not cause brain damage and will stop after the fever subsides.
- Person with weak immune system may have more severe infection or other complications.

PROBABLE OUTCOME—The illness heals on its own in about 1 week. The rash will fade and clear up without leaving scars.

HOW TO TREAT

GENERAL MEASURES
- It is usually unnecessary to keep the patient away from other people in the family. Everyone should wash their hands often to help prevent spreading germs.
- Lukewarm water bath or a warm sponge bath may be used to help reduce fever. Don't use ice or cold water or a fan (they can cause chills).

MEDICATION
- For relief from minor discomfort and to reduce fever, you may use nonprescription drugs such as acetaminophen or ibuprofen. Don't give aspirin to children under age 18.
- Antibiotics will not help a virus infection.
- Anticonvulsant drugs (if child has seizure) may be prescribed.
- Antiviral drugs may be prescribed for persons with weak immune systems.

ACTIVITY—The child should get extra rest until the fever disappears. Return to day care or school once temperature is normal.

DIET—The child should eat a normal, well-balanced diet. Encourage extra fluid intake. Continue baby-vitamin supplements if the child is accustomed to taking them.

CALL YOUR DOCTOR IF

- Your child has symptoms of roseola infantum.
- High fever occurs.
- Twitching or other signs of a convulsion begin.
- The child refuses liquids.
- The child cries loudly and persistently, and does not stop when picked up.
- The child is listless and has a stiff neck.

ROUNDWORMS
(Ascariasis)

GENERAL INFORMATION

DEFINITION—Roundworms thrive in the gastrointestinal tract (and sometimes in the lungs). They are contagious.

BODY PARTS INVOLVED—Gastrointestinal tract; lungs (sometimes).

SEX OR AGE MOST AFFECTED—Both sexes; all ages, but most common in children.

SIGNS & SYMPTOMS
- Often, there may be no symptoms.
- Irritability.
- Restlessness at night.
- Erratic or poor appetite.
- Frequent fatigue.
- Weight loss or lack of weight gain.
- Stomach (abdominal) discomfort.
- Diarrhea (sometimes).
- Cough and wheezing (rare).
- Worms may sometimes be seen in bowel movements or in the child's bed. Rarely, one may be vomited.
- Fever.

CAUSES—There are several types of roundworms (or nematodes). Some can be seen by the human eye, and others can only be seen with a microscope. Their eggs can enter the human body through contaminated water, food, or soil-contaminated hands. In some types, the larvae (young worms) enter through the skin.

RISK INCREASES WITH
- Crowded or unclean living conditions.
- Warm climate.
- Young children.
- Lack of clean water supply.
- Contact with animal feces.

HOW TO PREVENT
- Wash hands often, and always before eating and after using the bathroom.
- Keep fingers away from the mouth.
- Have pets treated for worms. Avoid strange animals.

WHAT TO EXPECT

DIAGNOSTIC MEASURES
- Your own observation of symptoms.
- Your health care provider may do a physical exam.
- Medical tests may include studies of the stool or a study of an adult worm, if passed, to identify the worm. X-ray of the lungs or an ultrasound may be done in some cases.

APPROPRIATE HEALTH CARE
- Treatment can be given at home and involves anti-worm drug therapy.
- In rare cases, surgery may be needed for complications, such as a bowel perforation (tear).

POSSIBLE COMPLICATIONS—Intestinal obstruction (rare).

PROBABLE OUTCOME—Usually curable in one week with treatment.

HOW TO TREAT

GENERAL MEASURES—Wash hands carefully after using the toilet or before meals. Keep fingers away from the mouth. Keep nails short and clean.

MEDICATION—Drugs called anthelmintics that kill roundworms may be prescribed. Follow the instructions provided for taking the drug.

ACTIVITY—No limits.

DIET—No special diet.

CALL YOUR DOCTOR IF

- You or a family member has symptoms of roundworms.
- Roundworms reappear after treatment.
- Drugs used for treatment cause side effects.

RUBELLA
(German Measles)

 GENERAL INFORMATION

DEFINITION—Rubella is a mild, contagious, viral illness. Use of the rubella vaccine has reduced the number of cases in the United States by 99%. Rubella is likely to cause serious birth defects in the unborn baby of a pregnant woman who develops the disease in the first 3 or 4 months of pregnancy.

BODY PARTS INVOLVED—Skin; lymph glands behind the ears and in the neck.

SEX OR AGE MOST AFFECTED—Both sexes; all ages, but most common in children.

SIGNS & SYMPTOMS
- Fever.
- Muscle aches and stiffness (often in the neck).
- Fatigue and headache.
- Reddish rash on the head and body after the 2nd or 3rd day. May have tiny purple spots in the throat. May have eye redness or irritation. The rash lasts 1 or 2 days.
- Swollen lymph glands, especially behind the ears and at the back and sides of the neck.
- Joint pain (adults).

CAUSES—The rubella virus is spread by person-to-person contact. It takes 14 to 23 days after exposure before symptoms appear. Patients are contagious from one week before the rash appears until one week after it started.

RISK INCREASES WITH
- People who remain unvaccinated.
- Incomplete immunization.
- Foreign-born immigrants.

HOW TO PREVENT
- Vaccination:
  - For children, rubella vaccine is usually given with the measles and mumps vaccine (MMR).
  - Nonpregnant women of childbearing age should be vaccinated if they have not had rubella or have not been vaccinated before. Pregnancy should be prevented for one month after vaccination. A blood test can be done if a woman is unsure about her rubella immunity.
  - Health care workers and daycare workers should get vaccinated if they have not been, or if their vaccination history is unknown. Young adults, such as college students should get two doses of MMR if not previously vaccinated.
- A person should talk to their health care provider before being vaccinated if he or she has a weak immune system.
- Persons, such as pregnant women, who are exposed to rubella and have not had it, or been vaccinated for it, should consult a health care provider right away.

 WHAT TO EXPECT

DIAGNOSTIC MEASURES
- Your own observation of symptoms.
- Your health care provider can usually diagnose the disorder with a physical exam.
- Medical tests are normally not done for rubella. If needed, cultures of the throat, blood, urine, or cerebrospinal fluid can confirm the presence of the virus.

APPROPRIATE HEALTH CARE—Home care is usually all that is needed. Get extra rest and drink plenty of fluids.

POSSIBLE COMPLICATIONS
- Encephalitis (brain inflammation).
- Thrombocytopenia (a blood disorder).
- Agranulocytosis (reduced white blood cells).
- Rubella infection in a pregnant woman may cause miscarriage or birth defects. The baby may have growth restriction; mental retardation; deafness; blindness; or liver, spleen, and bone marrow problems.

PROBABLE OUTCOME—No specific treatment is needed. The illness will heal on its own in one week in children, sometimes longer in adults. Complications are rare.

 HOW TO TREAT

GENERAL MEASURES—Be sure to contact any pregnant woman who has been exposed to the patient. Exposure includes contact with the infected person 1 week prior to, during or 1 week after the infection. This woman should consult her obstetric provider immediately.

MEDICATION—For minor discomfort, you may use nonprescription drugs such as acetaminophen or ibuprofen. Don't give aspirin to children under age 18.

ACTIVITY—Get extra rest until the symptoms get better.

DIET—No special diet.

 CALL YOUR DOCTOR IF

- You or a family member has symptoms of rubella.
- The following occur during treatment: high fever, red eyes, cough, shortness of breath, severe headache, drowsiness, lethargy, or convulsion.
- Unusual bleeding occurs 1 to 4 weeks after the illness (from gums, nose, uterus, or blood specks on the skin).

SALIVARY GLAND INFECTION

GENERAL INFORMATION

DEFINITION
• Salivary gland infection is an infection of a saliva-producing gland. Saliva is the moisture in the mouth that helps with chewing and swallowing.
• There are three pairs of major salivary glands:
  - Parotids are the largest. They are located in each cheek, over the jaws, in front of the ears.
  - Submandibulars are located at the back of the mouth on both sides of the jaw.
  - Sublinguals are located under the floor of the mouth.

BODY PARTS INVOLVED—Salivary glands and ducts.

SEX OR AGE MOST AFFECTED—Adults of both sexes.

SIGNS & SYMPTOMS
• Pain, tenderness, and swelling of the face or mouth.
• Dry mouth.
• May be hard to open mouth wide.
• Foul taste or food may taste strange.
• There may be a bitter tasting pus, which is a creamy fluid, in the mouth caused by the infection.
• Fever, chills.
• Facial redness.

CAUSES—There are a wide variety of causes of salivary gland infections. They can be due to bacteria (e.g., staph infection), viruses (e.g., mumps), autoimmune diseases, or result from other medical conditions. A gland can also become blocked by tiny, stone-like substances.

RISK INCREASES WITH
• Poor oral hygiene.
• Adults over age 60.
• Not vaccinated against mumps.
• Certain medical conditions (e.g., diabetes, Sjögren's syndrome, dehydration, malnutrition, HIV/AIDS, alcoholism, or bulimia).
• Radiation therapy of the head or neck.
• Use of certain drugs.

HOW TO PREVENT
• No specific preventive measures.
• Brush and floss teeth often and use germ-killing mouthwash, especially when ill.
• Visit your dentist regularly for checkups.
• Eat a healthy diet.

WHAT TO EXPECT

DIAGNOSTIC MEASURES
• Your own observation of symptoms.
• Your health care provider will do a physical exam of the head, neck, mouth, and throat.
• Tests may be done on a sample of the fluid from the infected gland. An x-ray, ultrasound, CT, or MRI may be done.

APPROPRIATE HEALTH CARE
• Treatment may involve self-care, drug therapy if needed, and, rarely, surgery.
• If the gland becomes blocked with a stone or scar tissue, surgery may be needed before the infection can heal. This is rare.

POSSIBLE COMPLICATIONS
• Infection may recur or bacterial infection may spread.
• Abscess (pus-filled sore).

PROBABLE OUTCOME—Symptoms usually improve within a week with self-care or drug therapy. In some cases, the outcome depends on the underlying cause.

HOW TO TREAT

GENERAL MEASURES
• For pain control, apply warm soaks or a heating pad on low setting.
• Rinse the mouth with warm salt water a few times a day. Use one-half teaspoon of salt in one cup of warm water. This may help ease the pain.
• Suck on hard candy, such as lemon drops to increase moisture in the mouth.
• Don't smoke. Smoking can delay healing.

MEDICATION
• Antibiotics may be prescribed for bacterial infection.
• For minor pain, you may use nonprescription drugs such as acetaminophen.
• If a drug you take is a risk factor, you may be advised to discontinue its use.
• Drugs may be prescribed for an underlying condition.

ACTIVITY—No limits.

DIET—No special diet. Drink plenty of fluids each day.

CALL YOUR DOCTOR IF

• You or a family member has symptoms of a salivary gland infection.
• The infection does not improve in four days or symptoms get worse despite treatment.
• Fever persists or recurs after treatment.

SALIVARY GLAND TUMOR

GENERAL INFORMATION

DEFINITION
• A salivary gland tumor is a rare type of growth in the saliva-producing glands. Saliva is the moisture in the mouth that helps with chewing and swallowing. These tumors can be benign and slow growing (most often) or cancerous.
• There are three pairs of major salivary glands:
- Parotids are the largest. They are located in each cheek, over the jaws, in front of the ears. These glands have the most tumors and the majority are benign.
- Submandibulars are located at the back of the mouth on both sides of the jaw. They have fewer tumors and about half of them are benign.
- Sublinguals are located under the floor of the mouth. Tumors are rare in these glands.
• There are also hundreds of minor salivary glands that are microscopic in size. Tumors in these glands are uncommon, but they are less often benign.

BODY PARTS INVOLVED—Salivary glands and ducts.

SEX OR AGE MOST AFFECTED—Older adults of both sexes.

SIGNS & SYMPTOMS
• There may be no symptoms. It may be found during a routine exam.
• A soft or firm mass that gradually increases in size in the jaw or in the floor of the mouth. There may be pain, tenderness, or swelling.
• Trouble swallowing or opening mouth widely.
• Face may have numbness or weakness.

CAUSES—Unknown. Environmental and genetic factors may play a role.

RISK INCREASES WITH
• Older adults.
• Radiation therapy to the head or neck.
• Exposure to certain substances in workplace.
• Tobacco use may be a risk factor.

HOW TO PREVENT—Most can't be prevented. To reduce your risks—avoid smoking, limit radiation therapy when possible, and have your health care or dental care provider check your salivary glands during routine checkups.

WHAT TO EXPECT

DIAGNOSTIC MEASURES
• Your own observation of symptoms.
• Your health care provider will do a physical exam of the head, neck, mouth, and throat.
• Medical tests may include blood studies, CT, or MRI. A fine needle aspiration biopsy removes tumor cells that are then examined under a microscope. If cancer is found, other tests help determine the cancer type, grade, and stage.

APPROPRIATE HEALTH CARE
• Surgery is the usual treatment for a benign or cancerous tumor. Your health care provider will discuss your options with you. It often involves removing the salivary gland in which the tumor is located. Sometimes, the surrounding bone and tissue or lymph nodes are removed also. Reconstruction surgery may be needed.
• Radiation therapy may be used to kill cancer cells or keep them from growing.

POSSIBLE COMPLICATIONS
• Infection or bleeding at the surgical site.
• Rarely, surgery may injure the facial nerve causing loss of control of facial muscles. Other nerve injury may affect your speech or swallowing.
• Cancer may recur or spread in the body.

PROBABLE OUTCOME
• Tumors with cancer cells are often cured with surgery and radiation treatment. Outcome depends on the stage and type of cancer and the patient's health.
• Tumors that are not cancerous are usually cured with surgery alone.

HOW TO TREAT

GENERAL MEASURES
• After surgery, keep the mouth clean with salt water mouthwashes. At least three or four times a day, rinse the mouth with a solution of one-half teaspoon salt in one cup of warm water.
• Suck on hard candy, such as lemon drops to increase moisture in the mouth.
• Stop smoking. This will help in recovery.

MEDICATION
• Anticancer drugs (chemotherapy) are not standard treatment for salivary gland cancer, but may be used if cancer has spread.
• Your health care provider may prescribe pain medicine or drugs for any infection.

ACTIVITY
• Resume your normal activities gradually after surgery.
• Physical therapy or speech therapy may be needed after extensive surgery.

DIET—After surgery, a liquid diet may be needed for a short time until your mouth heals.

CALL YOUR DOCTOR IF

• You or a family member has symptoms of a salivary gland tumor.
• After surgery, signs of infection occur in your mouth, such as feeling warmer or tender, redness, pain, and swelling.
• Symptoms recur after treatment.

SALMONELLA INFECTIONS

 GENERAL INFORMATION

DEFINITION—Salmonella infection is an illness caused by a bacteria named *Salmonella*. This is a type of germ sometimes found in food or drinks. The illness can cause symptoms that affect the stomach and the intestines (digestive tract). A group of people may get sick at the same time if they all eat the same infected food at a picnic, a party, or at a restaurant. A mild *Salmonella* illness may feel like a simple upset stomach for some people.

BODY PARTS INVOLVED—Gastrointestinal tract; lymphatic system.

SEX OR AGE MOST AFFECTED—Both sexes; all ages.

SIGNS & SYMPTOMS
- Diarrhea, often with stomach cramps.
- Nausea, vomiting, and fever.
- Blood in the stool (sometimes).
- Headache.
- Some people may have a rash.

CAUSES
- Symptoms can start 6 to 72 hours after eating food, such as meat, chicken, or eggs, or drinking raw (unpasteurized) milk or water that contains the *Salmonella* germs. The germs can stay alive even in frozen foods, but careful cooking will kill them.
- The illness can also be passed from person to person.
- Pet turtles, lizards, and other pets or animals can carry the germ and cause illness in humans.

RISK INCREASES WITH
- Living in a place with many other people, such as a school dorm, or living in a place that is not kept clean.
- Age over 60; young children; infants.
- Weak immune system due to illness or drugs.
- Certain stomach or bowel disorders.

HOW TO PREVENT
- Keep the kitchen area where you prepare meals very clean. Kill germs on knives and other items you use for cooking by washing them with hot water and soap.
- Stay away from pets or animals that might be sick.
- Drink only milk that is pasteurized. Avoid raw eggs.
- Always wash your hands after you go to the bathroom, before you handle any food, and if you have touched an animal or pet.
- Avoid being around someone who has this illness.

 WHAT TO EXPECT

DIAGNOSTIC MEASURES
- Your own observation of symptoms.
- Your health care provider may do a physical exam and may want to have a medical test done on a sample of the stool (bowel movement).

APPROPRIATE HEALTH CARE
- Most patients recover by getting some extra rest and replacing the fluids the body loses (due to the diarrhea).
- People who have a severe case of this illness or have complications may need treatment in a hospital.

POSSIBLE COMPLICATIONS
- Dehydration from diarrhea and vomiting. This can be serious for infants and older persons.
- Arthritis can occur weeks after an infection.

PROBABLE OUTCOME—In most cases, the illness is mild and over in 2 to 7 days.

 HOW TO TREAT

GENERAL MEASURES
- Keep the ill person away from other people in the house, if possible.
- Use a heating pad or hot-water bottle to relieve abdominal cramps.
- If diarrhea is severe, use a bedside commode.

MEDICATION
- Drugs are not needed for mild cases, but may be prescribed for severe cases and for patients who have other health problems.
- Do not use any drugs for the diarrhea unless your health care provider tells you to do so. The diarrhea is the way your body gets rid of the germs.

ACTIVITY—Rest in bed, except for trips to the bathroom, until the symptoms get better. Then begin your normal routine slowly, day by day.

DIET—Replace the fluids lost from the body due to diarrhea with sports drinks such as Gatorade or a special children's product such as Pedialyte. Begin to eat regular food within 12 to 24 hours or when you feel better.

☎ **CALL YOUR DOCTOR IF**

- You or a family member has symptoms of a *Salmonella* illness.
- An infant has signs of dehydration (e.g., dry, wrinkled skin, less urine output, or dark urine).
- A patient has a fever 102°F (38.9°C) or higher, yellow skin or eyes, cough with blood, or diarrhea gets worse.

SARCOPENIA
(Muscle Loss, Age-related)

 GENERAL INFORMATION

DEFINITION—Sarcopenia is defined as the age-related loss of muscle mass, strength, and function. It is not considered a disease, but it can contribute to medical disorders and disability. Sarcopenia affects everyone, but people who are physically inactive will have a greater and faster loss of muscle. Sarcopenia and osteoporosis (loss of bone) are related conditions and often occur together or one follows the other.

BODY PARTS INVOLVED—Muscles.

SEX OR AGE MOST AFFECTED—Both sexes; (women more than men); older adults.

SIGNS & SYMPTOMS
• Usually, there are no specific symptoms. The muscle loss occurs over time and symptoms may not be apparent or are accepted as a sign of getting older.
• Loss of strength and increased weakness that can affect the ability to perform basic tasks of daily living. A person may not be able to rise out of a chair on their own or put groceries away on a shelf. They may have trouble walking or climbing stairs, have stooped posture, or slow, unsteady movements.
• Decrease in the size of the muscles. This may not be noticed as the muscle loss is often replaced by fat.

CAUSES—The exact cause is unclear. Muscle strength begins to decline after age 40 and 25% of muscle mass can be lost by age 65. There are a number of factors that may be involved. These include decreasing hormone levels, inadequate nutrition, lack of exercise, changes in muscle cells and muscle fibers, impaired protein synthesis, and inflammation in the body.

RISK INCREASES WITH
• Aging.
• Women. They have less muscle than men and those with less muscle to begin with can have a greater loss.
• Inactive lifestyle.
• Poor nutrition (e.g., decreased protein intake).
• Prolonged bedrest.

HOW TO PREVENT—An ongoing program of physical activity (particularly resistance training) and eating a healthy diet can reduce the risks for muscle loss.

 WHAT TO EXPECT

DIAGNOSTIC MEASURES—There is no specific exam or test to diagnose sarcopenia or the degree of muscle loss in an individual. Your health care provider may discuss sarcopenia prevention as a part of a routine recommendation for a healthy aging lifestyle.

APPROPRIATE HEALTH CARE
• Your health care provider can help develop an overall exercise plan depending on your age, health status, and fitness level. It will normally include resistance (weight) training to maintain or gain muscle strength and aerobic activity to maintain or improve cardiovascular fitness.
• Diet changes may be helpful in some cases.

POSSIBLE COMPLICATIONS
• Loss of ability to perform daily living tasks. This leads to a cycle of more inactivity and then, more weakness.
• Sarcopenic obesity (sarcopenia along with obesity).
• Frailty, risk for falls or other injures, risk of cardiovascular disease or diabetes, or other health problems.
• Unable to care for oneself. Loss of independent living.

PROBABLE OUTCOME
• An individual can make the necessary lifestyle changes to preserve muscle mass.
• Preventing and treating sarcopenia can improve the health and quality of life for older adults.

 HOW TO TREAT

GENERAL MEASURES—Follow medical advice about treating sarcopenia.

MEDICATION—Drugs are not used to treat sarcopenia. Hormone replacements may be prescribed if levels are low.

ACTIVITY
• Begin a resistance training (e.g., weight-lifting or strength training) program. Start low and slowly increase the weights. A personal trainer or physical therapist can help plan and monitor your workout.
• Balance training can help reduce the risk of falls.
• To maintain cardiovascular fitness, get 30 minutes a day (or most days) of aerobic exercise, such as walking. Start with a few minutes a day and increase gradually.

DIET—Eat a healthy diet. An increase in protein intake may be recommended.

 CALL YOUR DOCTOR IF

• You or a family member has symptoms of muscle weakness or loss of strength.
• You want to begin a fitness program.

SCABIES

GENERAL INFORMATION

DEFINITION—Scabies is a skin disorder caused by little bugs called mites (the "itch" mite). Scabies is very contagious and can be spread from person to person or less often, by sharing clothing, towels, or bedding. It can be spread by sexual contact. It may take as long as two to ten weeks after being exposed for the rash to first appear. Scabies can still be spread during this time (even though there are no symptoms).

BODY PARTS INVOLVED—Skin of the finger webs and folds under the arms, breasts, elbows, genitals, and buttocks.

SEX OR AGE MOST AFFECTED—Both sexes; all ages.

SIGNS & SYMPTOMS
- A rash with small, very itchy, red bumps or blisters. They may look like pimples. Scabies usually infects the skin of the finger webs, and folds under the arms, breasts, elbows, genitals, and buttocks.
- Sores can form on the skin where it has been scratched.

CAUSES—A mite (*Sarcoptes scabiei* var. *hominis*) that burrows into deep skin layers, where the female mite lays her eggs. Eggs grow into adult mites in three weeks. If you scratch the skin area, the mites and eggs get under the fingernails and then get spread to other places in the body that you touch.

RISK INCREASES WITH
- Living in a place with many other people, such as a school dorm, or living in a place that is not kept clean.
- Children in daycare.
- Contact with a person who has scabies.
- Sexual contact with new or multiple partners.
- Weak immune system due to illness or drugs.

HOW TO PREVENT—It is difficult to prevent scabies. Avoid skin-to-skin contact with persons or bedding and clothing that you suspect may be infected with scabies.

WHAT TO EXPECT

DIAGNOSTIC MEASURES
- Your own observation of symptoms.
- Your health care provider can diagnose scabies by looking at the affected skin area.
- Sometimes the skin may be scraped to gather the mites so they can be viewed under a microscope.

APPROPRIATE HEALTH CARE—Treatment is with a drug to be used on the skin. Patients and their close contacts in the preceding month should be treated (even when they have no symptoms).

POSSIBLE COMPLICATIONS
- Sores from scratching the itchy skin may become infected with bacteria.
- Severe form of scabies called crusted (or Norwegian) scabies. Person will have thick crusts of skin that contain large number of mites.
- You can be reinfected with scabies.

PROBABLE OUTCOME—The skin will usually heal in about two weeks with treatment. The itching can last for up to four weeks even after treatment.

HOW TO TREAT

GENERAL MEASURES—Use hot water to wash all clothes, towels, bedding and washable toys used two days before and during treatment. You don't need to clean furniture or floors with special care. Put items you can't wash in plastic bags for one week to kill the mites.

MEDICATION
- Several different creams or lotions (called scabicides) can be prescribed for treatment. Infants and pregnant women may need a milder product than that used for other family members. These are general directions (follow your health care provider's instructions or read the directions that come with the product):
  - Take a bath or shower before applying the product.
  - Apply from the neck down, and cover the entire body. Wait 15 minutes before dressing.
  - Leave product on the skin for 8 to 12 hours, then take a bath or shower to remove it.
  - Your family or other close contacts should be treated at the same time.
  - You may need to repeat the treatment if the rash does not go away in a few weeks or if it gets worse after being treated.
- An oral drug may be prescribed for difficult or severe cases.
- In some cases, an anti-itching drug may be prescribed.

ACTIVITY—Until the disorder is resolved, avoid sports or recreational activities that involve skin-to-skin contact with other persons.

DIET—No special diet.

CALL YOUR DOCTOR IF

- You or a family member has symptoms of scabies.
- After treatment, the skin shows signs of infection (redness, pus, swelling, or pain).

SCARLET FEVER

GENERAL INFORMATION

DEFINITION—Scarlet fever is an illness caused by group A streptococcus (strep) bacteria. It begins with a strep throat infection, or rarely, a strep infection elsewhere such as the skin. About 10% of strep throat infections lead to scarlet fever.

BODY PARTS INVOLVED—Throat; tonsils; skin.

SEX OR AGE MOST AFFECTED—Both sexes; children and adolescents ages 5 and 15 are most often affected. It is less common in adults.

SIGNS & SYMPTOMS
• Symptoms may vary in different children. The following is the usual course of the disease:
• Day 1
 - Fever as high as 104°F (40°C); a red sore throat, swollen tonsils (tonsils may have a whitish coating), enlarged lymph glands in the neck, cough, vomiting.
• Day 2
 - Bright red rash on the face, except around the mouth.
• Day 3
 - Reddened tongue ("strawberry tongue") and rash in body creases, which spreads to the neck, chest, back, and then the entire body. The rash looks like a sunburn with bumps.
• Day 6
 - The rash fades and skin may begin peeling, which can go on for 10 to 14 days.

CAUSES
• Scarlet fever is caused by a toxin that is produced by the streptococcal bacteria. The toxin causes the rash and reddened tongue. Not everyone is susceptible to the toxin. In a family, one child may get scarlet fever and a second may have only the strep throat.
• Strep germs are spread by contact with an infected person, breathing in germs in the air, or touching an object with germs on it. It usually takes 2 to 4 days for symptoms to appear after exposure. Sometimes, a person can be a carrier of the strep germs, but have no symptoms. They can still spread the infection to others.

RISK INCREASES WITH
• Children ages 5 to 15.
• History of strep throat or scarlet fever in the community, school, or neighborhood.

HOW TO PREVENT—Cannot be prevented completely. Avoid contact with infected persons when possible. Wash hands frequently.

WHAT TO EXPECT

DIAGNOSTIC MEASURES
• Your own observation of symptoms.
• Your health care provider will do a physical exam.
• Tests will include throat culture for strep bacteria. Testing may be done on other family members if they have symptoms.

APPROPRIATE HEALTH CARE—Treatment is with drug therapy for the bacteria infection and supportive care for symptoms. Precautions help reduce the spread of infection to other persons.

POSSIBLE COMPLICATIONS—Without treatment, the infection may spread to other body parts. Rarely, it can lead to rheumatic fever or other serious conditions.

PROBABLE OUTCOME—With treatment, it is typically cured in about 10 days.

HOW TO TREAT

GENERAL MEASURES
• Keep the ill person away from other family members as much as possible to avoid spread of germs.
• Keep the ill person's dishes and utensils separate from others and wash them carefully.
• Keep fingernails short to avoid excessive scratching of the rash.
• Use a cool-mist humidifier to help relieve the sore throat. Clean the humidifier as directed.

MEDICATION
• Antibiotics will be prescribed. Be sure to take all the doses even if the symptoms improve.
• Use acetaminophen for pain relief and fever. Do not give aspirin for fever in children under age 18.

ACTIVITY—Person can return to school, daycare, or work after being on an antibiotic for 24 hours and there is no fever.

DIET—Soft food, warm food (e.g., soup), or cold foods (e.g., milkshake) may be easier to swallow. Drink plenty of fluids.

CALL YOUR DOCTOR IF

• You or your child has symptoms of strep throat or scarlet fever.
• The following occur during treatment:
 - Fever goes away and then returns.
 - New symptoms begin, such as nausea; vomiting; earache; cough; headache; thick, colored nasal drainage; chest pain; dark urine; or difficulty breathing.

SCHIZOPHRENIC DISORDERS

GENERAL INFORMATION

DEFINITION—Schizophrenic disorders are severe mental illnesses. Schizo means "split," and phrenia refers to the mind. A person with schizophrenia can't tell fact from fantasy, and therefore does not behave rationally. Symptoms may begin in early teen years or early adulthood. It may take months or years for the symptoms to be apparent.

BODY PARTS INVOLVED—Brain.

SEX OR AGE MOST AFFECTED—Both sexes; all ages.

SIGNS & SYMPTOMS
- Delusions (fixed false, unreal beliefs).
- Hallucinations (hearing voices or seeing things that are not there).
- Becomes more withdrawn; wants to be alone.
- Lack of energy and desire to do things.
- Showing few emotions, or showing emotions that are not appropriate.
- Disordered thoughts that are shown in disorganized or disjointed speech.
- A belief that other people hear and "steal" one's thoughts or that one is being controlled by others.
- Suspicious and paranoid behavior (in paranoid schizophrenia).

CAUSES—Exact cause is unknown. An imbalance in brain chemicals, genetics, biologic, and environmental factors play roles.

RISK INCREASES WITH
- Family history of schizophrenia; older age of father.
- Many environmental risk factors have been suggested.

HOW TO PREVENT—No specific preventive measures are known.

WHAT TO EXPECT

DIAGNOSTIC MEASURES
- Other's observation of symptoms.
- Your health care provider will do a physical exam and ask questions about the symptoms and activities.
- Medical tests are often done to rule out other problems. There is no specific test to diagnose schizophrenia. A psychological evaluation will be done. Family members may help provide information about the symptoms. Diagnosis depends on having the symptoms for at least 6 months, the impairment they cause, and being sure that no other mental disorder is involved.

APPROPRIATE HEALTH CARE
- The goal of therapy is to help the person get back in touch with reality. Treatment often begins with drugs to reduce the symptoms.

- Once symptoms are improved, treatment continues to help the person learn to cope with daily aspects of life. Treatment depends on the patient's needs and the severity of their symptoms. It may include social and work skills training, self-help groups, and counseling.

POSSIBLE COMPLICATIONS
- Life-long disability. Physical illnesses are common.
- Alcohol and substance abuse.
- Drugs may not be effective in treatment.
- Patients stop taking the drugs because of side effects, impaired thinking, or they feel they don't need them.
- Self-inflicted injuries; suicide.
- Hostile behavior or violence toward others.
- Relapse, neglect, homeless, or in prison.

PROBABLE OUTCOME—Outcome will vary. There is no known cure. Treatment can help some patients lead independent lives. Others will improve, but still need a support network. Some patients fail to improve and may need care in a treatment facility.

HOW TO TREAT

GENERAL MEASURES
- The family or other important persons in the patient's life should also be involved in the therapy. This will help them understand the problem and what they can do to help the patient. Schizophrenia patients are sometimes difficult to live with.
- To learn more: National Alliance for the Mentally Ill; (800) 950-6264; website: www.nami.org or National Institute of Mental Health; (866) 615-6464; website: www.nimh.nih.gov.

MEDICATION—Antipsychotic drugs are usually prescribed. Some are taken by mouth. Others may be injected. If side effects are too severe with one drug or the symptoms are not controlled, a different drug is prescribed. The dose is reduced as symptoms improve. For most patients, the drugs may need to be taken for life.

ACTIVITY—Normally no limits, unless advised by your health care provider. Daily exercise is often recommended.

DIET—Eat a regular healthy diet.

CALL YOUR DOCTOR IF

- You or a family member has schizophrenia symptoms.
- Symptoms continue or worsen with treatment.
- Drugs prescribed cause unwanted side effects.

SCLERODERMA

GENERAL INFORMATION

DEFINITION—Scleroderma is a disease in which the skin and other body parts change gradually, becoming thick, stiff, and hardened. Scleroderma has two main classes, localized and systemic. Localized affects only certain parts of the body such as the skin. Systemic affects the whole body, including blood vessels and major organs. There are subgroups defined within these two classes.

BODY PARTS INVOLVED—Skin, joints, digestive system, heart, kidneys, lungs, blood vessels, fingers; and toes.

SEX OR AGE MOST AFFECTED—It affects all age groups and females more than males. Localized form is more common in children and systemic form more often affects adults.

SIGNS & SYMPTOMS
- Patches on the skin that start in one place and spread.
- Fingers, toes, cheeks, nose, and ears may have numbness, pain, and color changes. Symptoms may be brought on by cold weather or emotional upset. This is called Raynaud phenomenon.
- Skin changes—thickened patches, especially on the fingers. Tight skin around the hands, face, or mouth.
- Digestive system problems—swallowing difficulty, poor food absorption, bloating after eating, weight loss, heartburn, and a feeling that food sticks in the chest.
- Feet and hands may be swollen.
- Feeling weak and tired.
- Joint pain, stiffness, and swelling.

CAUSES—The exact cause is unknown. It is an autoimmune disorders. In these disorders, the immune system by mistake attacks the body itself. With scleroderma, it produces too much collagen, a fibrous type of protein found in connective tissues. Genetic and environmental factors may play a role also.

RISK INCREASES WITH—Family history of scleroderma.

HOW TO PREVENT—Cannot be prevented.

WHAT TO EXPECT

DIAGNOSTIC MEASURES
- Your own observation of symptoms.
- Your health care provider will do a physical exam and check the affected skin. Questions will be asked about your symptoms.
- Medical tests may include blood and urine studies, heart and lung function tests, x-rays, CT, and others. A biopsy may be done.

APPROPRIATE HEALTH CARE
- There is no cure for the disorder. The goals of treatment are to help with the symptoms and prevent complications. Drug therapy is used.
- Physical therapy and occupational therapy (to help with day-to-day living activities) may be prescribed.

POSSIBLE COMPLICATIONS—Complications can cause severe symptoms in the skin, heart, lungs, gastrointestinal system, and kidneys. Dental problems and sexual problems may occur.

PROBABLE OUTCOME—Outcome will depend on each individual patient and their symptoms. Many treatments are available.

HOW TO TREAT

GENERAL MEASURES
- Wear warm clothing, such as heavy socks and gloves, if going out in the cold. Cover your head and face.
- Sleep on 2 or 3 pillows, or raise the head of your bed 5 to 8 inches to help prevent digestion problems.
- Stop smoking. Find a way to quit that works for you.
- Use heat to relieve joint stiffness.
- Seek counseling to help adjust to living with the disease. Joining a support group may help.
- To learn more: Scleroderma Foundation, 300 Rosewood Dr., Suite 105, Danvers, MA 01923; (800) 722-4673; website: www.scleroderma.org.

MEDICATION
- Different drugs may be prescribed, depending on your symptoms. Drugs can improve circulation, help joint stiffness and pain, aid digestive problems, improve the immune system, and lower high blood pressure.
- Use skin lotions, lubricants, and bath oils to soften skin. Other topical drugs may be prescribed.

ACTIVITY
- Be as active as your strength permits; avoid fatigue.
- Regular exercise (or movement) helps keep skin flexible, helps blood circulation, and prevents fixed joints.

DIET—Eat frequent, small meals to minimize bloating, heartburn, and stomach discomfort. A soft diet is sometimes helpful. Drink extra fluids to help with swallowing. A dietitian can help plan a nutritious diet.

CALL YOUR DOCTOR IF

- You or a family member has symptoms of scleroderma.
- Any symptoms of infection occur.
- Symptoms get worse or new ones develop.

SCOLIOSIS
(Curvature of the Spine)

GENERAL INFORMATION

DEFINITION—Scoliosis is an abnormal, side-to-side curve of the spinal column.

BODY PARTS INVOLVED—It can involve the thoracic (middle) spine, the lumbar (lower) spine, or the thoracolumbar (between the two areas).

SEX OR AGE MOST AFFECTED—It most often affects children during their growth spurt just before puberty. It is more common in girls than in boys. Adults can also be diagnosed with scoliosis.

SIGNS & SYMPTOMS
- No obvious symptoms or signs in the early stage. It comes on gradually. Scoliosis can be detected by a health care provider with a simple screening test. Schools sometimes have scoliosis screening programs.
- Entire body may lean to one side.
- The hip, shoulder, or rib cage on one side of the body is higher than the other side.
- Head may be off center.
- One shoulder blade is more prominent.
- Waist is uneven.
- May walk with a rolling gait.
- May have back pain or tire easily.

CAUSES
- Most often the cause is unknown (called idiopathic scoliosis).
- Scoliosis is sometimes a result of:
  - A disease of the central nervous system, such as cerebral palsy or muscular dystrophy.
  - Congenital (being born with) spinal defects.
  - Uneven leg length.

RISK INCREASES WITH—Family history of scoliosis.

HOW TO PREVENT—Cannot be prevented at present.

WHAT TO EXPECT

DIAGNOSTIC MEASURES
- Your own observation of symptoms.
- Your child's health care provider can diagnose scoliosis with a physical exam.
- An x-ray may be done to confirm the diagnosis. The amount of curve in the spine is measured by degrees.

APPROPRIATE HEALTH CARE
- Treatment will depend on the age of the child, how severe the curve is, and how much it is progressing.
- Many cases of scoliosis are minor (less than 20 degrees) and require no treatment. Follow up medical exams will be done to see if the problem is progressing.
- For children with more of a curve (usually 25 to 40 degrees), treatment often involves wearing an orthopedic back brace. Sometimes this is needed for several years. Some braces are less visible and permit the person to wear regular clothes.
- Surgery to correct scoliosis is typically advised if the curve is more than 40 to 50 degrees or bracing is not helping. Surgery can help improve posture and back function.
- For adults with scoliosis, physical therapy or exercises to strengthen back muscles are sometimes helpful. Talk to your health care provider.

POSSIBLE COMPLICATIONS
- Severe curving of the spine and ribs.
- Social embarrassment, due to wearing a brace.
- Complications such as lung and heart damage, loss of bone strength, and back pain may occur. These are more likely when scoliosis is more severe and goes untreated.
- Complications can occur with scoliosis surgery.

PROBABLE OUTCOME—Mild curves may not require treatment. If treatment is done, the outcome is usually successful.

HOW TO TREAT

GENERAL MEASURES—To learn more: National Scoliosis Foundation, 5 Cabot Place, Stoughton, MA 02072; (800) 673-6922; website: www.scoliosis.org.

MEDICATION—Drugs will not correct this disorder.

ACTIVITY
- Limits on sports activities are generally not needed. Follow medical advice.
- Special exercises may be part of therapy.
- Some activities, such as swimming, may help. They can tone and strengthen the back.
- If surgery is done, activities will be limited for a time to allow for healing.

DIET—No special diet.

CALL YOUR DOCTOR IF

You suspect your child is developing scoliosis.

SEASONAL AFFECTIVE DISORDER

GENERAL INFORMATION

DEFINITION—Seasonal affective disorder (SAD) is a type of depression. It usually recurs each year during the winter months and stops when spring begins. Light plays a major part in its origin and in its treatment. In rarer instances, the seasonal disorder symptoms occur in the summer months and may be caused by intolerance to heat.

BODY PARTS INVOLVED—Nervous system.

SEX OR AGE MOST AFFECTED—Adults and children and is more common in women.

SIGNS & SYMPTOMS
- Symptoms usually begin in September when days get shorter, and last through the winter into March when the days get longer again.
- Depression.
- Feeling tired, sluggish, and needing more sleep.
- Increased appetite (craves sweet or starchy foods).
- Weight gain.
- Irritability and feeling less cheerful.
- Being less social.
- Decreased interest in sex and physical contact.
- Joint aches, stomach problems, and more infections.

CAUSES—Exact cause is unknown. Decreased amounts of sunlight may lead to chemical changes in the brain or interfere in the body's natural clock (circadian rhythms). The disorder can run in some families.

RISK INCREASES WITH
- Living far from the equator.
- Females more than males.
- Family history of SAD.

HOW TO PREVENT—No prevention for first episode. Treatment may be provided to prevent recurrence of symptoms.

WHAT TO EXPECT

DIAGNOSTIC MEASURES
- Your own observation of symptoms.
- Your health care provider will do a physical exam and ask questions about your symptoms and activities. Diagnosing SAD can be difficult. The same symptoms can arise from other types of depression.
- Blood tests may be done to rule out other medical disorders. Diagnosis usually requires a two-year pattern of mood changes that begin in the autumn and stop in the spring.

APPROPRIATE HEALTH CARE
- Treatment may involve light therapy (phototherapy). Duration and intensities of this therapy will vary for each person. (It is recommended that light therapy not be used without medical advice.) Types include:
  - Sitting in a very bright light (equal to 10 or more 100-watt bulbs) for a period in the morning and, sometimes, in the evening. The term lux (Latin for light) is the unit of measure for the light therapy.
  - Installing a computerized system of lighting in a patient's bedroom that creates an artificial dawn. The light goes from very dim to bright like a sunrise.
  - Avoid tanning beds for therapy. The ultraviolet (UV) rays are harmful to skin and eyes.
- Other forms of treatment include drugs or counseling to help the person cope with the symptoms.

POSSIBLE COMPLICATIONS
- Problems in coping with life because of symptoms.
- May progress to more severe depression.
- Substance abuse.

PROBABLE OUTCOME—With correct diagnosis and treatment, symptoms can be helped. The symptoms may recur the following year.

HOW TO TREAT

GENERAL MEASURES
- Mild symptoms may be helped with simple measures. Keep drapes and blinds open in your house and sit near windows and gaze outside often. Turn on bright lights on cloudy days. Keep a diary or journal of your mood changes so that any changes or patterns can be tracked.
- Stay social, visit friends, and stay busy with activities.
- To learn more, search the internet or visit a library.

MEDICATION—Antidepressants may be prescribed.

ACTIVITY
- Stay as active as your energy permits. Physical activity is almost always good for mood disorders.
- Get outside as much as possible, especially in the early morning light.
- Take vacations in the winter months to places that are sunny and warm.

DIET—Eat a normal well-balanced diet to maintain good health.

CALL YOUR DOCTOR IF

- You or a family member has symptoms of seasonal affective disorder.
- Symptoms continue or worsen, despite treatment.

SEVERE ACUTE RESPIRATORY SYNDROME

GENERAL INFORMATION

DEFINITION—Severe acute respiratory syndrome (SARS) is a type of respiratory illness. Respiratory refers to the lungs and breathing. In 2003, SARS was first diagnosed in Asia and then spread to other countries, including the United States.

BODY PARTS INVOLVED—Respiratory system.

SEX OR AGE MOST AFFECTED—Adults and children of both sexes.

SIGNS & SYMPTOMS
- Fever higher than 100.4°F (38.0°C). The fever starts 2 to 7 days after being infected.
- May include headache, an overall feeling of discomfort, and body aches.
- Some people also have mild breathing problems.
- After 2 to 7 days, patients may develop a dry cough and have more trouble breathing.

CAUSES
- The cause is a form of the coronavirus. It is one of a family of viruses that in humans usually cause mild infections like common colds. How the new type came into being is unknown.
- SARS germs spread by close, person-to-person contact. A cough or sneeze can spread the germs into the nearby air and be breathed in by someone. They are also spread if you touch the skin of an infected person or objects that have the germs on them, and then touch your eyes, nose, or mouth. SARS may spread more broadly in the air or by other ways that are not now known. Also unknown is the time period that an infected person can spread germs to others.

RISK INCREASES WITH
- Travel to an area where the infection is present.
- Close contact with an infected person.

HOW TO PREVENT
- Check for any travel precautions for the area you plan to visit. The Centers for Disease Control & Prevention has updated information about travelers' health; website: www.cdc.gov or toll free hotline (877) 394-8747.
- If you are in an area where this infection is present, wash your hands often or use alcohol-based hand wipes. Avoid crowds if possible.
- Wearing a facemask or other protective device may be helpful.

WHAT TO EXPECT

DIAGNOSTIC MEASURES
- The symptoms for SARS are like those for other viral illnesses, such as cold and flu. If you have been exposed to SARS or have recently been traveling, and symptoms occur, seek medical help right away. Advise any health care provider in advance of your visit about the SARS exposure. Arrangements can be made, as needed, to prevent the spread of germs to others.
- Your health care provider will do a physical exam and have blood and urine studies done.
- An x-ray and other medical tests may be needed.

APPROPRIATE HEALTH CARE
- Once a SARS infection is diagnosed, hospital treatment is needed. This may be in an intensive care unit.
- Treatment is aimed at assistance with the breathing problems. Oxygen is provided through a facemask. Some patients require breathing support with a ventilator (a device to help the lungs).

POSSIBLE COMPLICATIONS
- Severe breathing problems that may lead to death.
- Survivors may have long term medical and psychological problems. These include bone problems (such as osteoporosis) and depression.

PROBABLE OUTCOME—Outcome varies depending on the severity of the symptoms. Most people will recover from the infection.

HOW TO TREAT

GENERAL MEASURES—None specific.

MEDICATION—Drugs are not available to cure the infection. Drugs to treat the symptoms will be given while in the hospital.

ACTIVITY—Resume normal activities slowly once symptoms improve.

DIET—May require feeding through a vein (IV) while in the hospital. Then return to a regular diet with recovery.

☎ CALL YOUR DOCTOR IF

You or a family member has symptoms of SARS. You should seek emergency care. Be sure to advise any health care providers in advance of your visit about the SARS exposure.

SEXUAL DYSFUNCTION, FEMALE

GENERAL INFORMATION

DEFINITION—Female sexual dysfunction is not a disease. It is a term used to describe problems with sexual desire, arousal, orgasm, and sexual pain in women. Over 40% of women have sexual problems at some time in their lives.

BODY PARTS INVOLVED—Brain and central nervous system; autonomic nervous system.

SEX OR AGE MOST AFFECTED—Sexually active women.

SIGNS & SYMPTOMS
- Lack of sexual desire or no interest in sex.
- Not able to feel aroused. There may be no sexual response in the body, or it may start, and then stop.
- Failure to achieve orgasm (climax), even when sexually aroused.
- Pain with sexual intercourse.

CAUSES—Sexual dysfunction is usually due to a variety of factors involving a woman's mind, body, and sexual partner.

RISK INCREASES WITH
- Depression, stress, or anxiety. Worries about family problems, finances, career, childcare, marital problems.
- Previous sexual abuse or trauma.
- Feelings of shame or guilt about sex.
- Pregnancy (during and after), or a fear of pregnancy.
- Lack of experience or knowledge about sex on the part of either partner.
- Male sexual partner is having sexual problems.
- Not enough or ineffective foreplay. Feeling boredom with the same sexual routine.
- Couples differ in what they expect from sex, and their attitude toward sex.
- Other people close by in the home (e.g., children or mother-in-law).
- Fatigue (e.g., working and caring for small children).
- Medical conditions such as cancer, diabetes, heart disease, thyroid disorders, arthritis, and others.
- Drug abuse, including alcohol.
- Heavy smoking.
- Gynecology factors (e.g., infection or other disorders).
- Side effects of some drugs.
- Intercourse causes pain.
- Hysterectomy with removal of ovaries.
- Menopause (reduced estrogen levels affect sexual function).

HOW TO PREVENT
- Avoid the risk factors where possible.
- Get counseling for any anxieties or fears about sex.
- Good communication with sexual partner.

WHAT TO EXPECT

DIAGNOSTIC MEASURES
- Your health care provider will do a physical exam and ask questions about your symptoms and sexual history. It may be difficult to discuss your sexual concerns, but it is important to be open and honest.
- Medical tests may be done to check for any health problems.

APPROPRIATE HEALTH CARE
- Treatment depends on the type(s) of problem and the causes. Your health care provider will discuss the options regarding treatment steps.
- Treatment will be provided for any medical disorder. This includes vaginal dryness or other physical problems that may be causing painful intercourse.
- Counseling can help with emotional problems (e.g., stress, anxiety, depression, or sexual fears).
- Sex education may be needed for the woman and her partner. Learn about the female anatomy, sexual response, and arousal.
- Treatment with a sex therapist may be helpful. Partners can learn techniques to help stimulate each other, perform self-stimulation, use sexual aids, new sexual routines, and communicate about sexual desires.
- A small vacuum device to improve blood flow to the clitoris may help sexual arousal.

POSSIBLE COMPLICATIONS
- Ongoing inability to enjoy sex.
- Relationship problems with partner.

PROBABLE OUTCOME—Some sexual problems go away on their own. Others are helped with treatment and the support of a caring partner. Some problems are more difficult to resolve.

HOW TO TREAT

GENERAL MEASURES—None specific.

MEDICATION—Nonprescription vaginal lubricants may help. Hormone therapy may be prescribed.

ACTIVITY
- Exercise daily. It can reduce stress, improve physical well-being, and may lead to better sexual health.
- Pelvic floor exercises (Kegel) may be recommended.

DIET—Eat a well-balanced diet.

CALL YOUR DOCTOR IF

You or a family member has sexual dysfunction problems and wants help in resolving them.

SEXUALLY TRANSMITTED DISEASES

GENERAL INFORMATION

DEFINITION—Sexually transmitted diseases (STDs) are infections spread from person to person through any type of sexual contact. They include HIV, chancroid, chlamydial infections, trichomoniasis, genital herpes, pubic lice, genital warts, gonorrhea, lymphogranuloma venereum, syphilis, viral hepatitis, scabies, candidiasis, molluscum contagiosum, and others. STDs affect more than 12 million men and women in the United States each year. Many are teenagers or young adults.

BODY PARTS INVOLVED—Whole body.

SEX OR AGE MOST AFFECTED—Sexually active males and females.

SIGNS & SYMPTOMS
- Sometimes, early in an infection, there may be no symptoms or they may be confused with other illness.
- Discharge from the vagina, penis, or rectum.
- Pain or burning during urination or intercourse.
- Pain in the abdomen (women), testicles (men), and buttocks and legs (both men and women).
- Blisters, open sores, warts, rash, or swelling in the genital or anal area or the mouth.
- Persistent, flu-like symptoms. These include fever, headache, aching muscles, or swollen glands.

CAUSES—STDs are spread by sexual activity. They are usually caused by viruses or bacteria, and less often by parasites or fungi.

RISK INCREASES WITH
- High-risk behaviors include having sex—vaginal, anal, or oral—with:
  - A person who has an STD.
  - Someone who has shared needles to inject drugs with an infected person.
  - Someone with a past partner(s) who was/were infected. Your partner may seem perfectly healthy.
- The more sexual partners you have, the higher your chance of being exposed to STDs.
- Using drugs or alcohol increases your chances of getting STDs. They can interfere with your judgment and your ability to use a condom correctly.
- Intravenous (IV) drug use puts a person at higher risk for human immunodeficiency virus (HIV) and hepatitis B, because IV drug users usually share needles.

HOW TO PREVENT
- Abstinence (no sexual activity) or sex with only one partner (neither partner has an STD).
- Avoid risk factors. If you know your partner is infected, avoid intercourse (including oral sex).
- People who take part in risky sexual behavior should always use a condom. Be sure to use a new condom from start to finish, every time.
- Use of a condom for an uninfected pregnant woman. It helps protect her and her unborn child from STDs.

WHAT TO EXPECT

DIAGNOSTIC MEASURES
- Your health care provider may do a physical and genital area exam. Questions will be asked about the symptoms and sexual activity history.
- Medical tests may include blood studies or a study of fluid discharge from vagina or penis.

APPROPRIATE HEALTH CARE
- Treatment may include drugs for the STD diagnosed or for symptoms of the STD.
- Your sexual partner(s) should be checked for STDs.

POSSIBLE COMPLICATIONS
- Pelvic inflammatory disease (PID). It can damage a woman's fallopian tubes and cause pelvic pain and infertility.
- Tubal pregnancies (where pregnancy grows in the fallopian tube instead of the womb). It is sometimes fatal to the mother and always fatal to the fetus.
- Infertility in both men and women.
- Cancer of the cervix in women.
- Damage to major organs, such as the heart, kidney, and brain, if STDs go untreated.

PROBABLE OUTCOME—Some STDs can be treated and cured with drugs. Some cannot be cured, but symptoms can be treated and the risk of transmission lowered.

HOW TO TREAT

GENERAL MEASURES—To learn more: Centers for Disease Control & Prevention, 1600 Clifton Rd., Atlanta, GA 30333; (800) 232-4636; website: www.cdc.gov/std.

MEDICATION—Oral, intravenous (IV), or topical drugs may be prescribed. Take or use all of the prescribed drug.

ACTIVITY—Avoid sexual activity while being treated.

DIET—Eat a well-balanced diet.

CALL YOUR DOCTOR IF

- You or a family member has symptoms of a sexually transmitted disease (STD).
- You think you have been exposed to an STD.
- Symptoms worsen or don't improve.

SHIN SPLINTS
(Medial Tibia Stress Syndrome)

 GENERAL INFORMATION

DEFINITION—Shin splints is a common term that has been used to describe a variety of different leg injuries. It is generally being replaced by more specific diagnostic terms. The most common shin pain is caused by medial tibia stress syndrome (MTSS). The tibia (shin bone) is the larger of the two bones between the knee and the ankle. Medial refers to the inside part of the tibia (the most common injury site).

BODY PARTS INVOLVED—Legs.

SEX OR AGE MOST AFFECTED—Both sexes and almost all ages.

SIGNS & SYMPTOMS—Pain, dull ache, or tenderness, and, sometimes, swelling, redness, and warmth in inner side (medial), back side (posterior), or outer side (anterior) of the lower leg. At first, the pain decreases with exercise and increases with rest. Later, it becomes continuous.

CAUSES—It is an overuse condition that can be caused by several factors. This shin problem usually develops gradually over weeks to months or could occur after a single excessive or intense training session. The problem is exercise-induced, but the specific cause of the pain is difficult to pinpoint. It may be periostitis (inflammation of the outer layer of the bone), myositis (muscle inflammation), tendinitis (inflammation of the muscle-tendon complex), or a combination of two of these. Faulty foot mechanics contribute to the injury.

RISK INCREASES WITH
- Sports involving running or jumping activities.
- Running on uneven surfaces. Climbing hills.
- Training too quickly, too hard, and for too long.
- Training that involves switching from one type of sport to another (e.g., a triathlon).
- High impact aerobics or aerobic dancing.
- Poorly fitting or worn-out running shoes.
- Foot arches that are flat (pronated) or high (supinated), or imbalance in leg muscles.

HOW TO PREVENT
- Stretch and strengthen the muscles in the lower leg.
- Stretch before and after running.
- Slowly increase intensity/duration of a new exercise.
- Avoid hard and uneven surfaces. Use soft surfaces, such as dirt or grass, for jogging, running, and walking.
- Warm up before activity; avoid overtraining.
- Shoes with good fit, cushioning, and arch support.
- Try sports activities, such as swimming or biking, that have less impact on the shins.

 WHAT TO EXPECT

DIAGNOSTIC MEASURES
- Your own observation of symptoms.
- See your health care provider if self-care does not help. A physical exam and x-ray or bone scan may be done to rule out a stress fracture.
- Physical therapy may be recommended.

APPROPRIATE HEALTH CARE
- Self-care is all that is usually needed.
- Medical care (if needed) may involve drug therapy, physical therapy, and other treatments.

POSSIBLE COMPLICATIONS
- May progress to stress fracture.
- Shin splints may recur.

PROBABLE OUTCOME—Healing time may range from a few days to two weeks to two months.

 HOW TO TREAT

GENERAL MEASURES
- Use ice massage over the painful area (in a circle about the size of a softball). Do this for 15 minutes at a time 3 or 4 times a day.
- After a few days, apply heat if you want. Use hot soaks, hot showers, or heating pads.
- Massage area gently and often to provide comfort and decrease swelling. Stretch the calf and foot frequently.

MEDICATION
- For minor pain, use nonprescription anti-inflammatory drugs (e.g., aspirin or ibuprofen).
- Nonsteroidal anti-inflammatory drugs may be prescribed.

ACTIVITY
- Discontinue sports or exercise until the pain is gone. Return to pre-injury activity level slowly.
- In some cases, severe pain may require the use of crutches for a short period of time.
- If foot mechanics are a problem, such as excessive pronation, special shoes, heel lifts, or orthotics (inserts for the shoes) may be prescribed. Orthotics can be nonprescription products. In some cases, custom-made orthotics are recommended.
- Try different exercises (cross-training) such as swimming or walking in water, bicycle riding, or regular walking.

DIET—No special diet.

 CALL YOUR DOCTOR IF

You or a family member has shin splints and the symptoms cause concern.

SHOCK

GENERAL INFORMATION

DEFINITION—Shock occurs when the heart and blood vessels are unable to supply enough blood and oxygen to meet the demands of the body. Shock can be caused by several different conditions and is a medical emergency.

BODY PARTS INVOLVED—Whole body.

SEX OR AGE MOST AFFECTED—Both sexes; all ages.

SIGNS & SYMPTOMS
- Fast, weak pulse.
- Not knowing where you are or confusion.
- Anxiety with feelings of impending doom.
- Skin that is cold, pale, moist, and sweaty.
- Shortness of breath and rapid breathing.
- Lack of urination.
- Low blood pressure.
- Dizziness or fainting.
- Chest pain or bluish lips or nails.

CAUSES
- Hypovolemic shock is a sudden loss of blood or body fluids. The bleeding may be visible, or bleeding may occur inside the body. Sudden fluid loss occurs with severe burns, severe vomiting, and/or diarrhea.
- Cardiogenic shock is due to damaged heart function (e.g., heart attack or heart failure).
- Anaphylactic shock is an adverse reaction to a substance to which the body is sensitive. These can include drugs such as penicillin, insect bites, or food allergies.
- Septic shock is caused by blood poisoning or major infections in the body.
- Neurogenic shock is caused by damage to the nervous system, such as a spinal cord injury.
- Shock can be caused by exposure to extreme heat or cold for too long.

RISK INCREASES WITH
- Serious injury, illness, or surgery.
- Heart disorders.
- Contact with a substance you are allergic to.
- Overdose of mind-altering drugs.
- Excess alcohol consumption.

HOW TO PREVENT
- You can't prevent shock. You can avoid the risk factors where possible.
- You may be able to help someone in shock, or prevent shock, until emergency help is available if you are prepared. To prepare yourself:
    - Take a first aid course.
    - If you or a family member has a severe allergy, be sure an emergency kit is available and that you know how to give the injection.
    - Carry emergency supplies, such as a first aid kit, in your car or truck.
- Wear or carry medical ID if you have a serious medical or allergy problem.

WHAT TO EXPECT

DIAGNOSTIC MEASURES—A careful physical exam will be done.

APPROPRIATE HEALTH CARE
- Emergency care in the hospital will include fluids given through a vein, oxygen for breathing support, and drugs. A careful physical exam will be done.
- Treatment will be provided for the injuries or other causes of the shock. The patient will be watched closely for any complications until the risk is over.

POSSIBLE COMPLICATIONS
- Heart or lungs are unable to function.
- Permanent brain damage.
- Death.

PROBABLE OUTCOME—The outcome will depend on how severe the symptoms are and receiving prompt treatment.

HOW TO TREAT

GENERAL MEASURES
- Call for emergency help right away. Shock requires immediate medical care.
- While waiting for emergency help:
    - Do not move person if spinal injury is suspected.
    - Have person lie down on his or her back.
    - Keep person warm and comfortable.
    - Take direction from the 911 operator. They can advise you on what to do to help the patient.

MEDICATION
- If shock is from blood or fluid loss, treatment includes blood transfusion or fluids given through a vein.
- If blood pressure is at a dangerous low level, drugs to raise blood pressure may be given.
- If infection is present, antibiotics may be used.

ACTIVITY—Rest in bed until completely recovered. Move legs actively while in bed to decrease the risk of blood clots.

DIET—Diet will depend on your medical condition.

CALL YOUR DOCTOR IF

You or a family member has symptoms of shock or observe them in someone else. Call 911 immediately. This is a life-threatening emergency!

SHOULDER, FROZEN
(Adhesive Capsulitis)

GENERAL INFORMATION

DEFINITION—Frozen shoulder is a general term used to describe pain and stiffness in the shoulder joint that leads to loss of shoulder movement. Adhesive capsulitis is the medical term.

BODY PARTS INVOLVED—It affects the shoulder capsule (tissues surrounding the ball and socket joint) and the ligaments that attach the shoulder bones to each other. Sometimes both shoulders are affected.

SEX OR AGE MOST AFFECTED—It occurs more often in people over age 40, and in women more than men.

SIGNS & SYMPTOMS
- Stage 1 (painful)—ache or pain in the shoulder, often mild. It progresses to severe pain that interferes with sleep and normal activities. Pain gets worse with shoulder movement. This stage may last for 2 to 9 months.
- Stage 2 (adhesive)—pain gradually lessens, but stiffness increases in the shoulder. This prevents normal range of motion movement. Reduced movement increases stiffness. This stage may last 4 to 12 months.
- Stage 3 (recovery)—healing starts. For most patients, the range of motion begins to increase. This stage may last for 12 months or up to several years.

CAUSES—The cause is unknown. It may be due to an inflammatory process. In some cases, it may result from an injury that leads to lack of use due to pain. Adhesions (a type of scar tissue) grow between the joint surfaces, causing restricted motion. There is less synovial fluid that lubricates the shoulder joint to help it move.

RISK INCREASES WITH
- Shoulder surgery, injury, or fracture.
- Previous frozen shoulder.
- Diabetes or thyroid disorder.
- Being immobile (prolonged inactivity) due to trauma, overuse injuries, or surgery.

HOW TO PREVENT
- Can't always be prevented. Obtain medical care for any shoulder injury, pain, or stiffness.
- Do regular stretching exercises.

WHAT TO EXPECT

DIAGNOSTIC MEASURES
- Your own observation of symptoms.
- Your health care provider will do an exam of the affected shoulder and ask questions about your symptoms and activities.
- X-rays or other tests may be done to confirm the diagnosis.

APPROPRIATE HEALTH CARE
- Exercises, and drugs are used in treatment to restore joint movement and reduce the pain.
- Physical therapy and stretching exercises will help improve joint movement. They may be uncomfortable to do, but should not cause excess pain. You will be instructed about exercises to do at home.
- Other treatments may include acupuncture, ultrasound therapy, and electrical stimulation.
- Manipulation may help some patients. This procedure can be done under a local or general anesthesia. The shoulder joint capsule is stretched to break up scar tissue. It helps right away, but exercise is still needed.
- If other treatment does not help the symptoms after several months, your health care provider may recommend shoulder surgery. This is usually done with an arthroscope (small instrument) through tiny incisions.

POSSIBLE COMPLICATIONS—Some permanent shoulder disability and pain may occur despite treatment.

PROBABLE OUTCOME—Most patients will have increased shoulder mobility and function with time and treatment. Full recovery usually takes 18 to 24 months. You may need help with daily activities that require lifting your arms.

HOW TO TREAT

GENERAL MEASURES—Apply heat (warm compresses or heating pad) to the affected area or apply ice packs if it feels better.

MEDICATION
- Nonsteroidal anti-inflammatory drugs or muscle relaxers may be prescribed. An injection of cortisone or local anesthesia into joints may help to reduce severe pain. Repeated injections are generally not recommended.
- For minor pain, you may use nonprescription drugs such as ibuprofen or aspirin.

ACTIVITY
- Follow instructions for home exercises.
- Resume athletic or fitness activities as your symptoms ease and you have medical approval.

DIET—No special diet.

CALL YOUR DOCTOR IF

- You or a family member has symptoms of a frozen shoulder.
- Symptoms don't improve with treatment.

SICKLE CELL ANEMIA & SICKLE CELL TRAIT

GENERAL INFORMATION

DEFINITION—Sickle cell anemia is an inherited blood disorder. It causes chronic anemia, periods of severe pain, high risk of infections, and general poor health. People with the sickle cell trait usually have no symptoms of the disorder, but may pass it onto their children.

BODY PARTS INVOLVED—Bone marrow; lymph glands; spleen; liver; thymus.

SEX OR AGE MOST AFFECTED—Symptoms usually begins around 6 months of age and last a lifetime.

SIGNS & SYMPTOMS
- Swollen hands or feet, fever, and paleness.
- Shortness of breath; rapid heartbeat; fatigue.
- Painful episodes (crises) in a joint or an organ that can last hours or days.
- Frequent infections (e.g., pneumonia).
- Eye problems.
- Delayed growth and development in children.
- Jaundice (yellow skin and/or eyes).

CAUSES—A gene that causes defective hemoglobin (blood cells). The gene occurs mostly in African Americans (about 8% are carriers) and some Hispanics. Defective hemoglobin changes blood cells from smooth and round to a stiff, sickle shape. These abnormal cells cause a blockage of blood flow in blood vessels. This leads to the symptoms and sickle crisis. A chronic short supply of red blood cells causes anemia.

RISK INCREASES WITH—Family history of sickle cell anemia. If both parents have the gene, their child may have sickle cell anemia. If one parent has the gene, the child will not get the disorder, but may carry the sickle cell trait.

HOW TO PREVENT
- If you have a family history of sickle cell anemia, ask for testing. If the condition is present, obtain genetic counseling before starting a family.
- Early pregnancy test to see if the baby has inherited the double-dose gene (both parents are carriers).

WHAT TO EXPECT

DIAGNOSTIC MEASURES
- Prenatal testing during pregnancy.
- Screening tests are done on newborns in most states. Older children and adults can also be tested. If this test shows sickle hemoglobin, more tests are done to confirm the diagnosis.

APPROPRIATE HEALTH CARE
- A health care provider with special knowledge of this disorder can help with ongoing health care.

- Education and counseling are helpful in adapting to this condition, especially for children as they get older. Support groups may help.
- Hospital care may be required at times of severe attacks for intravenous (IV) therapy and oxygen therapy, and blood transfusions.
- Bone marrow transplant may be an option. It is a cure, but risks and lack of donors limits use.

POSSIBLE COMPLICATIONS—Infections, other medical problems, stroke, and death.

PROBABLE OUTCOME—Life span is reduced, but has gradually increased to over 40 years. More effective treatments are helping.

HOW TO TREAT

GENERAL MEASURES
- Home treatment involves good nutrition and hygiene, rest as needed, and steps to avoid infection and stress. Encourage a child to lead as normal a life as possible.
- Some things may worsen symptoms. These include an injury or infection, pregnancy, surgery, dehydration, traveling to high altitudes (as in driving up a mountain, or an airplane trip).
- See your health care and dental care providers on a regular basis. Keep all vaccines and flu shots up to date.
- Wear or carry medical ID that shows you have this disorder.
- To learn more: Sickle Cell Disease Association of America, 231 East Baltimore St., Ste. 800, Baltimore, MD 21202; (800) 421-8453; website: www.sicklecelldisease.org.

MEDICATION
- No drug is effective for the disorder. Drugs are used for symptoms and to prevent complications.
- Use nonsteroidal anti-inflammatory drugs or acetaminophen for pain.
- Penicillin started in infancy helps prevent infections.
- Adults need prompt treatment for infections.
- Hydroxyurea may be prescribed. It helps to reduce the frequency of painful crisis.
- Vitamin supplements are often recommended.

ACTIVITY
- Avoid strenuous exercise. Avoid being out in very hot or cold temperatures. Rest in bed during acute attacks.
- Activity may be somewhat limited due to chronic anemia and poor muscle development.

DIET—Eat a healthy diet. Drink plenty of fluids.

CALL YOUR DOCTOR IF

After diagnosis of sickle cell anemia in a child, any signs of infection occur, pain increases, or symptoms develop that cause concern.

SILICOSIS

GENERAL INFORMATION

DEFINITION—Silicosis is a chronic lung condition caused by breathing silica (quartz) dust. Silicosis is world-wide and is the most common form of pneumoconiosis. This is a group of lung diseases caused by inhaling certain mineral dusts.

BODY PARTS INVOLVED—Lungs.

SEX OR AGE MOST AFFECTED—It usually affects men (due to work exposure).

SIGNS & SYMPTOMS
- Early symptoms:
  - Shortness of breath.
  - Cough that produces little or no sputum.
  - General ill feeling.
- Later symptoms:
  - Fitful sleep and appetite loss.
  - Chest pain, hoarseness, and coughing blood.
  - Symptoms of heart failure.
  - Bluish nails.

CAUSES—Chronic breathing in of small particles of free crystalline silica dust. The dust may be invisible to the naked eye. It is so light that it can remain in the air for a long time. The disorder causes lung inflammation and then scarring of lung tissues. It usually takes 20 to 30 years of exposure to develop silicosis. If exposure is extremely high, it may take less than 10 years. An acute form may occur following massive exposure to dusts.

RISK INCREASES WITH
- Work such as mining, granite-cutting, concrete mixing and drilling, manufacturing pottery, metal-grinding, tunneling, sand-blasting, and others.
- Smoking adds to possible lung damage.

HOW TO PREVENT
- Be aware of the risks and follow all training and preventive instructions provided for your work. Get health screenings on a regular basis.
- Employers are required to take preventive measures to reduce exposure for workers.
- Don't smoke.

WHAT TO EXPECT

DIAGNOSTIC MEASURES
- Your health care provider will do a physical exam and ask questions about your symptoms and activities. Be sure to tell your provider about your work history and any exposure to silica.
- Medical tests may include x-ray of the chest, pulmonary function tests, CT, and others to confirm the diagnosis and check for complications.

APPROPRIATE HEALTH CARE
- No specific treatment is known for silicosis. Drugs and lung therapy may help the symptoms and treat complications.
- Chest physical therapy (such as controlled coughing) and bronchial drainage help clear secretions. Get medical training about these procedures.

POSSIBLE COMPLICATIONS
- Pulmonary tuberculosis (late stages of silicosis).
- Chronic obstructive pulmonary disease (COPD).
- Lung fibrosis (scar tissue).
- Heart failure.

PROBABLE OUTCOME—There is no cure. Outcome will vary for each individual depending on amount of lung damage. Symptoms can sometimes be relieved or controlled.

HOW TO TREAT

GENERAL MEASURES
- Avoid any further exposure to silica dust.
- Quit smoking. Find a way to stop.
- Obtain medical treatment for any respiratory infection, including the common cold.
- Get influenza and pneumococcal vaccines.
- Consider moving to a warm, dry climate if you have advanced disease.
- To learn more: American Lung Association, 61 Broadway, 6th Floor, New York, NY 10006; (800) 586-4872; website: www.lungusa.org.

MEDICATION
- Bronchodilators (inhaled or oral) with inhalation therapy may be prescribed. This is supervised at first by an inhalation therapist.
- Antibiotics may be prescribed for infections.
- For minor discomfort, you may use nonprescription drugs, such as acetaminophen or aspirin.

ACTIVITY—No limits, except those caused by symptoms.

DIET—No special diet. Maintain high fluid intake.

CALL YOUR DOCTOR IF

- You or a family member has symptoms of silicosis.
- Fever, increased chest pain or breathing problems, blood in the sputum, or other new symptoms develop.

SINUSITIS

GENERAL INFORMATION

DEFINITION—Sinusitis is an infection or inflammation (redness and soreness) of the sinuses. Sinuses are air-filled spaces that make mucus to help clean the air we breathe. Sinuses open into the nose for mucus and air exchange. Sinusitis can be acute (short illness), or chronic if it continues for several weeks or recurs often.

BODY PARTS INVOLVED—The 8 sinuses (mucosa-lined air pockets) located within the facial bone structure and connected to the nose. Usually involved are the ethmoidal sinuses, located between the eyes; and the maxillary sinuses, located in the cheekbone.

SEX OR AGE MOST AFFECTED—Both sexes; all ages.

SIGNS & SYMPTOMS
* Nasal congestion with white or greenish-yellow (sometimes blood-tinged) discharge.
* Feeling of pressure inside the head.
* Eye pain.
* Headache that is worse in the morning or when bending forward.
* Cheek pain that may resemble a toothache.
* Post-nasal drip.
* Cough (sometimes) that is usually non-productive.
* Disturbed sleep (sometimes).
* Fever (sometimes).
* Swelling of the sinus openings, blocking the discharge, and increasing pain.
* Bad breath.

CAUSES
* Viral or bacterial infection. A common cold can cause the sinuses to swell and increase the amount of mucus they produce. In some cases, bacteria begins to grow in the excess mucus in the swollen sinuses.
* Fungal infection, such as aspergillosis, may occur in people who have a weakened immune system.

RISK INCREASES WITH
* Common cold or other viral illness.
* Weak immune system due to illness or drugs.
* Swimming or diving.
* Using nasal decongestant sprays too often.
* Growths (polyps) in the nose or a deviated septum.
* People with asthma or an allergic disease.
* Smoking.
* People with cystic fibrosis.
* Dental problems.

HOW TO PREVENT—None specific. Wash hands often to avoid germs. Prompt treatment of any cold or other viral infection may reduce the risk. Avoid irritants such as smoking.

WHAT TO EXPECT

DIAGNOSTIC MEASURES
* Your own observation of symptoms.
* Your health care provider will do a physical exam and ask questions about your symptoms and recent illnesses, such as a cold. Diagnosis can usually be made based on this information.
* Medical tests (such as blood tests or CT scan) may be done in certain cases, such as repeated infections.

APPROPRIATE HEALTH CARE
* Drug treatment is aimed at improving symptoms and curing the Infection.
* Sinusitis not responding to drug treatment may require surgery to drain blocked sinuses.
* Surgery may be done for polyps or a deviated septum.
* Sinusitis due to a fungus may require surgery.

POSSIBLE COMPLICATIONS
* Sinusitis may become chronic.
* Rarely, infection may spread into bones, eyes, or brain.

PROBABLE OUTCOME—Most cases clear up on their own within 10 days. Some patients may require drug therapy or, rarely, surgery.

HOW TO TREAT

GENERAL MEASURES—Apply moist heat to relieve pain in the sinuses and nose. Take a warm shower once or twice a day.

MEDICATION
* For stuffy nose, use nonprescription nasal decongestants. Limit use to 3 days in a row. Saline nasal sprays may be used several times a day. Nonprescription antihistamines are sometimes helpful.
* For minor pain, you may use drugs such as acetaminophen or ibuprofen.
* Drugs to reduce congestion may be prescribed.
* Antibiotics for bacterial infection may be prescribed.
* Nasal or oral steroid drugs may be prescribed.

ACTIVITY—Resume your normal activities gradually. Exercise can help to clear your head.

DIET—No special diet, but drink extra fluids to help thin secretions.

CALL YOUR DOCTOR IF

* You or a family member has symptoms of sinusitis.
* The following occur during treatment: fever; bleeding from the nose; severe headache, or swelling of the face.

SJÖGREN'S SYNDROME

GENERAL INFORMATION

DEFINITION—Sjögren's (pronounced show-grun) syndrome is one of a group of autoimmune disorders. In these disorders, the immune system by mistake attacks the body itself. Sjögren's syndrome mainly affects the glands that produce moisture, but it can affect the body as a whole. Symptoms may be mild or severe.

BODY PARTS INVOLVED—May involve only the exocrine (mucus secreting) glands or involve other organs, such as the lung or kidneys.

SEX OR AGE MOST AFFECTED—It occurs mostly in women (about 90% of cases) with an average age of 50.

SIGNS & SYMPTOMS
- Dry eyes. It may cause foreign body sensation, gritty feeling, redness, burning, sensitivity to light, itching, feeling that there is a "film" across the field of vision, and eye discharge.
- Dry mouth, nose, and throat. This can cause problems in swallowing and talking, changes in taste, thirst, ulcers (sores), or dental cavities. Nosebleeds, hoarseness, chronic nonproductive cough, ear infection, or other infections may occur.
- Vaginal dryness can cause painful intercourse.
- Dry skin.
- Severe fatigue.
- Parotid glands become enlarged (referred to as "chipmunk face" or "chipmunk cheeks").
- Joint pain and stiffness.
- Other symptoms include hair loss, low-grade fever, itching skin, and muscle aches or pain.

CAUSES—Unknown. Genetic, immunologic, hormonal, and environmental factors may play roles. Viral infection may trigger the disorder in some people. It may occur alone or along with other autoimmune disorders such as rheumatoid arthritis, scleroderma, systemic lupus erythematosus, or polymyositis.

RISK INCREASES WITH
- Females over age 50.
- Family history of autoimmune disorders.
- Having other autoimmune disorders.

HOW TO PREVENT—No specific measures.

WHAT TO EXPECT

DIAGNOSTIC MEASURES
- Your health care provider will do a physical exam and ask questions about your symptoms.
- Medical tests of blood, tear production, saliva production, an eye exam, and others may be done to confirm the diagnosis.

APPROPRIATE HEALTH CARE
- Treatment is directed to relieving the dryness symptoms and preventing complications.
- Self-care is usually all that is needed.

POSSIBLE COMPLICATIONS
- Damage to the kidneys, blood vessels, lungs, liver, eyes, pancreas, and brain may occur.
- Children born to some younger women with the disorder may be at risk for heart defects.
- Small risk of cancer of lymph nodes.

PROBABLE OUTCOME—Sjögren's syndrome is a chronic disorder. Symptoms sometimes stay the same, worsen, or sometimes disappear for a period. Treatment can relieve symptoms and help prevent complications.

HOW TO TREAT

GENERAL MEASURES
- Brush and floss teeth daily. Use a fluoride mouthwash. See a dentist for checkups.
- Wear sunglasses when outside to help protect eyes from dust, wind, and strong light. See your eye care provider for regular exams.
- Warm compresses or heating pad may help ease joint pain or swollen gland discomfort.
- To learn more: Sjögren's Syndrome Foundation, 6707 Democracy Blvd., Suite 325, Bethesda, MD 20817; (800) 475-6473; website: www.sjogrens.org.

MEDICATION
- Use artificial tears for dry eyes. Use an eye ointment at night. Other drugs for dry eyes may be prescribed.
- Use nonprescription saliva substitutes and mouth-coating products for dry mouth.
- Vaginal moisturizers and lubricants (not petroleum jelly) will help vaginal dryness.
- Use nonsteroidal anti-inflammatory drugs (e.g., ibuprofen, naproxen) for joint pain and muscle aches.
- Avoid decongestants and antihistamines. They can cause dry mouth or eyes.
- Steroids and other drugs may be prescribed.

ACTIVITY—Mild exercise daily helps keep joints flexible.

DIET
- Chew sugarless gum or suck on sugarless candies.
- Drink or sip fluids all during the day.
- If mouth soreness prevents eating regular foods, drink high-calorie, high-protein liquid supplements.

CALL YOUR DOCTOR IF

- You or a family member has symptoms of Sjögren's syndrome.
- Symptoms don't improve with treatment.

SKIN GROWTHS, BENIGN

GENERAL INFORMATION

DEFINITION—Benign skin growths are noncancerous growths or areas of pigment or color change on the skin.

BODY PARTS INVOLVED—Skin.

SEX OR AGE MOST AFFECTED—Both sexes; all ages.

SIGNS & SYMPTOMS
- Tags—soft, flesh-colored buds, often on stalks, found on the neck, armpits or groin.
- Moles—flat or raised lesions with clearly defined borders. Moles may be black, blue, red, yellow or brown.
- Cherry spots—pinhead-sized, bright-red lesions on the chest or back.
- Strawberry marks—bright-red raised areas in infants that grow until they are removed.
- Keloids—thick, pale, irregular growths that begin at the site of a scar and gradually increase in size.
- Dermatofibromas—rounded nodules, usually brownish and usually on the legs.
- Freckles—flat, brownish spots of pinhead-size or larger.

CAUSES—Unknown, but most people have a few benign skin growths.

RISK INCREASES WITH
- Family history of benign skin lesions.
- Pregnancy or use of oral contraceptives (brownish, freckle-like patches only).

HOW TO PREVENT—To decrease freckles, avoid excessive sun exposure. Other forms cannot be prevented.

WHAT TO EXPECT

DIAGNOSTIC MEASURES
- Your own observation of symptoms.
- If needed, your health care provider will examine the skin growth for any abnormal appearance.
- Rarely, all, or part, of the skin tissue may be removed for biopsy. The tissue is viewed under a microscope to see if it is cancerous.

APPROPRIATE HEALTH CARE
- Usually, no treatment is needed.
- Surgery to remove lesions that enlarge, bleed, change color, are slow to heal or are unsightly. (See Skin Lesion Removal in Surgery section.)

POSSIBLE COMPLICATIONS—None expected for benign lesions.

PROBABLE OUTCOME—Treatment is usually unnecessary because most skin lesions are harmless. Suspicious or unsightly lesions can be removed surgically. If the affected area is large or in a prominent place, plastic surgery may be necessary after removal.

HOW TO TREAT

GENERAL MEASURES
- Examine skin growth—especially those that are constantly rubbed or irritated by clothing—regularly for signs of growth, color change, pain, infection or bleeding.
- Makeup may be helpful in covering unsightly blemishes.
- If a growth is removed, cover the area with a clean dressing and protect against injury. Ointments are rarely needed.

MEDICATION—Drugs are usually not needed.

ACTIVITY—No limits.

DIET—No special diet.

CALL YOUR DOCTOR IF

You or a family member has a skin growth that enlarges, bleeds, changes color, is painful or doesn't heal.

SLEEP APNEA

GENERAL INFORMATION

DEFINITION—Sleep apnea is a disorder in which a person's breathing stops briefly and repeatedly during sleep. In most cases, the person is unaware of these episodes.

BODY PARTS INVOLVED—Central nervous system, upper airways (soft palate and tongue).

SEX OR AGE MOST AFFECTED—All ages, but is more common in adults over 60 and men.

SIGNS & SYMPTOMS
- Periods of 10 seconds or longer of not breathing while asleep. They may occur hundreds of time a night. It causes less oxygen to get to the lungs and eventually triggers the lungs to suck in air. The person may make a gasping or snorting sound, but is usually not fully awake. A bed partner may notice symptoms first.
- Loud snoring and restless sleep.
- Daytime sleepiness and fatigue.
- Sexual dysfunction.
- Morning headaches, dry mouth, or sore throat.
- Mental or emotional problems (e.g., memory loss, feeling irritable, poor judgment, or depression).

CAUSES
- Obstructive apnea (most common type). Breathing stops because the airway collapses and prevents air from getting into the lungs. Airway collapse may be due to several factors. There may be excess tissue at the back of the throat (large tonsils). The tongue may fall back and close off the airway. The muscles controlling the airway have become weakened.
- Central sleep apnea (less common type). It is caused by a central nervous system problem.
- Mixed apnea. The two types occur together.

RISK INCREASES WITH
- Overweight.
- Older adults and males.
- Family history of sleep apnea.
- Persons having a large neck, recessed chin, or abnormal structure of the upper airway.
- Smoking; use of alcohol or sedative drugs; diabetes.
- African Americans, Hispanics, and Pacific Islanders.

HOW TO PREVENT—No specific preventive measures. Avoid risk factors where possible.

WHAT TO EXPECT

DIAGNOSTIC MEASURES
- A bed partner may be the first to notice the symptoms.
- Your health care provider may do a physical exam and ask questions about your symptoms and lifestyle.

- Tests to check your airways may be done. An overnight study at a sleep center may be prescribed. Diagnostic devices to be used at home may be an option.

APPROPRIATE HEALTH CARE
- Treatment depends on severity of apnea, other health problems, and daytime sleepiness. It may involve lifestyle changes (e.g., weight loss), drug therapy, use of certain devices, or surgery.
- Oral appliances may be suggested. They keep airway open by moving lower jaw forward.
- Devices to keep the airway open may help. Continuous positive airway pressure (CPAP) is often prescribed. A mask is worn over the nose and mouth during sleep. A small air compressor forces air into the nasal passages to keep airway open. Other devices are being researched.
- For severe apnea, surgery may be an option.

POSSIBLE COMPLICATIONS
- High blood pressure, heart problems, or stroke.
- Other health and emotional problems, motor vehicle accidents, or impaired work or school functioning.
- Sleep quality of bed partner is affected. This can cause sleepiness and fatigue for that person.

PROBABLE OUTCOME—Outcome depends on the individual and how severe the symptoms are. Treatment can help improve apnea.

HOW TO TREAT

GENERAL MEASURES
- Try sleeping on your side, not your back. Pillows may help. Or put a tennis ball in a sock and pin sock to back of pajamas.
- Quit smoking. Find a way to stop that works.
- To learn more: American Sleep Apnea Assn., 6856 Eastern Ave., Ste. 203, Washington, DC 20012; (202) 293-3650 (not toll free); website: www.sleepapnea.org.

MEDICATION
- Drugs may be prescribed for daytime sleepiness, depression, acid reflux, or other health problems.
- Avoid drugs like sedatives, barbiturates, hypnotics, or narcotics. Nasal strips do not treat apnea.

ACTIVITY—Exercise daily, but not right before bedtime.

DIET—Lose weight, if you are overweight. Avoid alcohol.

CALL YOUR DOCTOR IF

- You suspect you have sleep apnea or observe signs of sleep apnea in another family member.
- Symptoms don't improve with treatment.

SLEEP PROBLEMS, TEMPORARY

GENERAL INFORMATION

DEFINITION—Temporary sleep problems can involve difficulty falling asleep or remaining asleep, being awake off and on, early-morning awakening, or a combination of these. Everyone has occasional sleep problems. They are usually temporary. *Sleep disorders* are different and more specific (e.g., insomnia or sleep apnea) and can be chronic.

BODY PARTS INVOLVED—Brain; may affect whole body.

SEX OR AGE MOST AFFECTED—Both sexes; all ages; more common in older adults.

SIGNS & SYMPTOMS
- Feeling restless when trying to fall asleep.
- Brief sleep followed by wakefulness.
- Normal sleep until very early in the morning (such as 3 am to 4 am), then being wide awake (often with frightening thoughts).
- Periods of no sleep that alternate with periods of excess sleep.
- Feeling sleepy, tired, and irritable in daytime.

CAUSES—Sleep is a normal and natural function of the human body. Nerve cells in the brain control whether you are asleep or awake. When something affects the balance or normal rhythm of those nerve cells, changes in sleep patterns can occur.

RISK INCREASES WITH
- Emotional problems:
  - Depression or anxiety.
  - Stress.
- Physical problems:
  - Allergies and early-morning wheezing. Other health problems that cause shortness of breath.
  - Heartburn/gastroesophageal reflux disease (GERD).
  - Painful disorders, such as fibromyalgia or arthritis.
  - Medical problems that require urination or bowel movements during the night.
  - Alcoholism.
  - Use of certain drugs, such as decongestants.
  - Drug abuse, including overuse of sleep inducers.
  - Use of stimulants (e.g., caffeine drinks or chocolate).
  - Withdrawal from addictive substances.
  - Obesity.
  - Sleep disorders (e.g., apnea, restless leg syndrome, or narcolepsy).
- Lifestyle problems:
  - Erratic work hours.
  - New environment or location.
  - Jet lag after travel.
  - Noisy environment (including a snoring partner).
  - Lack of physical exercise.

HOW TO PREVENT—Maintain a healthy lifestyle that includes good sleep habits. Avoid or treat risk factors where possible.

WHAT TO EXPECT

DIAGNOSTIC MEASURES
- Your own observation of symptoms.
- If self-help fails, see your health care provider. A physical exam and medical tests may be done to help find the cause. An overnight sleep study may be prescribed.

APPROPRIATE HEALTH CARE—A medical treatment plan may include lifestyle changes, drug therapy, or other treatments.

POSSIBLE COMPLICATIONS
- Short-term sleep problems become chronic.
- Excess daytime sleepiness can affect all aspects of life.

PROBABLE OUTCOME—The problem usually clears up on its own. Most people can establish good sleep patterns.

HOW TO TREAT

GENERAL MEASURES
- Self-care steps can often resolve problem.
- Have routine bedtime and wake up times.
- Try to find ways to reduce stress in your life.
- Relax in a warm bath before bedtime.
- Create a comfortable bedroom (dark, cool, and quiet). Don't use the bedroom as an office.
- Turn off your mind. Think peaceful and relaxing thoughts. Listen to soft music or relaxation audios.
- Use ear plugs or eye shades.
- To learn more: National Sleep Foundation, 1522 K St., Ste. 500, Washington, DC 20005; (202) 347-3471 (not toll-free); website: www.sleepfoundation.org.

MEDICATION
- Melatonin, a nonprescription product, may help some people. Ask your health care provider's advice.
- Your health care provider may prescribe sleep-inducing drugs for a short period of time.

ACTIVITY—Exercise regularly, but not within 2 hours of bedtime.

DIET—Don't eat within 3 hours of bedtime if indigestion is a problem. A glass of warm milk before bedtime may help. Avoid caffeine.

CALL YOUR DOCTOR IF

- You or a family member has sleep problems that cause concern.
- Sleep problems don't improve with treatment.

SMOKING ADDICTION

 GENERAL INFORMATION

DEFINITION—Cigarette smoking is an addiction (uncontrollable dependence) disorder and the cause of many serious health problems. There are many chemicals in cigarette smoke. Among them are tar, nicotine, and carbon monoxide (a poisonous gas). These three substances are a health risk to the person smoking and to those who breathe in the secondhand smoke. Tar condenses into a sticky substance in the lungs. Nicotine is the addictive component of tobacco smoke. Carbon monoxide decreases the oxygen carried by the red blood cells in the body.

BODY PARTS INVOLVED—Brain, nervous system, and other body systems.

SEX OR AGE MOST AFFECTED—Both sexes; smoking often starts in adolescence.

SIGNS & SYMPTOMS
- An average smoker smokes 15 to 20 cigarettes a day. The more one smokes, the greater the health risks. Someone who smokes even 1 to 4 cigarettes a day has more risks for health problems than nonsmokers.
- Certain activities also become linked with smoking. These include smoking after a meal, when drinking coffee, while on the phone, relaxing, or if stressed.

CAUSES—The inhaled nicotine travels to the brain in 8 seconds. It activates a certain area of the brain involved with pleasure and reward. Over time, the brain develops a resistance to nicotine and a smoker has to increase the number of cigarettes to get the same pleasure.

RISK INCREASES WITH
- Teenagers. Smoking often begins as a social behavior and an adventure. Teens feel pressure from friends; they want to be socially accepted in certain groups, and to appear more mature.
- People who are under stress or feel nervous.
- Less education (high school dropouts are more likely to smoke than college graduates).
- Lower economic group.
- Ages 25 to 44 have highest smoking rates.
- Blue-collar occupations.
- Risk-taking and outgoing personality types.
- Family history of smoking.
- Alcoholics.

HOW TO PREVENT
- Education about health risks.
- Prohibiting smoking in public places.

 WHAT TO EXPECT

DIAGNOSTIC MEASURES—None needed usually.

APPROPRIATE HEALTH CARE
- Smokers can quit on their own or be helped by a variety of methods. No one method works for everyone.
- See your health care provider for help.

POSSIBLE COMPLICATIONS
- Cancer; heart, blood vessel, or lung diseases.
- Problems with infertility.
- Problems in pregnancy and risks to the baby's health.
- Earlier menopause and possible osteoporosis.
- Skin is rougher, thicker, and more wrinkled.
- Secondhand smoke is harmful to others.
- Home fire deaths (most are due to smoking).

PROBABLE OUTCOME—It is never too late to quit. Anyone who smokes should make every attempt to stop. If you do, it can reverse many health risks and bring a better quality of life.

 HOW TO TREAT

GENERAL MEASURES
- Self-help steps in quitting: 1) Think about your smoking habits and when and why you smoke. 2) Make up your mind to quit. 3) Choose the day and quit on that day. 4) Use any kind of substitute (gum, hard candy). Give up those activities, for now, that you link with smoking. 5) Reward yourself for not smoking (e.g., a fun activity). 6) During the first few weeks, eat plenty of low-calorie snacks; drink lots of water.
- Call local office of the American Cancer Society or American Lung Association for help.
- Ask family and friends for help. Join a support group or a smoking-cessation program.
- Try other ideas (e.g., hypnosis or acupuncture).
- Concerns about quitting: 1) *Weight gain.* Average amount is 5–8 pounds over 5 years (for some, there is no weight gain). 2) *Stress.* It may occur. Get counseling or help with managing stress. 3) *Withdrawal.* Physical symptoms stop in about 10 to 14 days. Psychologic symptoms may go on for months or longer. 4) *Fear of failure.* Relapse is common. Many people have had to try more than once, and by more than one method.

MEDICATION
- Drugs to reduce cravings may be prescribed.
- Stop smoking aids include nicotine gum, skin patch, nasal spray, or inhaler. They can help reduce withdrawal symptoms. They are used with counseling or smoking-cessation program.

ACTIVITY—Exercise daily. It helps lower stress, control weight, and reduce craving for cigarette.

DIET—Eat a healthy diet.

 CALL YOUR DOCTOR IF

You or family member wants to quit smoking.

SNAKEBITE

GENERAL INFORMATION

DEFINITION—A snakebite is a skin wound caused by the fangs of a snake. Venomous snakes (e.g., rattlesnake, copperhead, water moccasin, or coral snake) can cause severe reactions. Nonvenomous snake bites are rarely serious. Bites on the legs and feet are more common. Bites on the head and trunk are more dangerous. Snakes are more likely to bite runners, joggers, walkers, hikers, backpackers, fishers, boaters, and campers, or anyone playing or working where snakes live.

BODY PARTS INVOLVED—Exposed skin; blood; lymphatic system.

SEX OR AGE MOST AFFECTED—Both sexes; all ages.

SIGNS & SYMPTOMS
- If the bite is from a coral snake, it will have multiple fang marks and small cuts; symptoms may not appear for 3 to 4 hours. If the bite is from another snake, it will have deep single or double fang marks, and symptoms will begin quickly.
- Severe pain and swelling around the bite.
- Skin color around the bite looks bruised.
- Bleeding spots under the skin, all over the body.
- Numbness and tingling around the mouth and in the hands and feet.
- Excessive sweating; fever.
- Low blood pressure and life-threatening shock.
- Breathing difficulty; blurred vision; headache.
- Seizures; coma.

CAUSES—Snakes use their fangs to bite a person. Venomous snakes inject a venom through the fangs.

RISK INCREASES WITH—Bites from venomous snakes occur during outdoor activities in warm months in areas where snakes are known to live. People handling snakes or trying to capture snakes put themselves at risk.

HOW TO PREVENT
- Wear protective shoes, boots, and clothing for hiking, camping, fishing, and hunting. Consider taking a snakebite kit with instructions with you.
- Don't try to pick up or handle snakes.

WHAT TO EXPECT

DIAGNOSTIC MEASURES—Emergency care will include a physical exam, blood studies, urinalysis and other tests as needed to monitor vital signs.

APPROPRIATE HEALTH CARE
- In the hospital, the treatment may include:
  - Breathing support with a machine if needed.
  - Treatment to prevent any complications.

- Surgical debridement (removal of dead or infected tissue) after 3 or 4 days. Skin grafts may be needed. Affected skin may take weeks to months to heal.

POSSIBLE COMPLICATIONS
- Wound infection and skin loss.
- Heart, lung, blood, or kidney complications.
- Compartment syndrome (swelling of muscles and tissue in a closed space, which cuts off the blood supply).
- Reaction to the antivenin includes anaphylaxis (severe allergic) and delayed serum sickness.
- Death from snakebite is rare.

PROBABLE OUTCOME—Venomous bites are usually curable with rapid medical care. Other snakebites usually heal on their own, but may need medical care.

HOW TO TREAT

GENERAL MEASURES
- If possible, identify the snake, but don't waste time looking for it. If unsure about the snake, treat all bites as poisonous.
- Don't panic! Venom will spread more quickly in the body if the victim runs or gets excited.
- Call 911 for emergency help. If help cannot get there right away, go to the nearest emergency center.
- Follow snakebite kit instructions if one is handy.
- Some basic first aid steps include: remain calm. Keep bitten area below or at heart level, if possible. Remove jewelry and tight clothing. Do not cut or suction the bite. Cover area with a clean, dry pad. Do not use a tourniquet. If elastic bandage is available, wrap firmly around the area. Don't use ice on the area (cool compresses may be used). Cover victim with a blanket. Don't give victim food or drink, especially alcohol.

MEDICATION
- Your health care provider may prescribe:
  - Antivenin to counter the snake poison.
  - Tetanus booster injection.
  - Antibiotics to prevent infection.
  - Pain relievers. Narcotics cannot be used for coral snake bites. They may cause shock.

ACTIVITY—Resume normal activities as soon as symptoms improve.

DIET—No special diet.

CALL YOUR DOCTOR IF

- You or someone you are with receives a snakebite.
- New, unexplained symptoms develop after snakebite treatment.

SODIUM IMBALANCE
(Hypernatremia; Hyponatremia)

 GENERAL INFORMATION

DEFINITION—Sodium imbalance is an above-normal sodium level (hypernatremia) or a below-normal sodium level (hyponatremia) in the blood. Sodium, an electrolyte, helps regulate the body's water balance and maintain normal heart rhythm. It is responsible for the conduction of nerve impulses, and the contraction of muscles.

BODY PARTS INVOLVED—All body cells.

SEX OR AGE MOST AFFECTED—Both sexes; all ages.

SIGNS & SYMPTOMS
• Confusion.
• Restlessness and anxiety.
• Weakness.
• Muscle cramps (usually in the legs).
• Changes in pulse rate and blood pressure.
• Tissue swelling (edema).
• Stupor or coma (if severe imbalance).
• Sodium imbalance may be part of a disease with other symptoms, such as fever, vomiting, diarrhea, or excessive sweating.

CAUSES—The sodium and water levels in the body are normally kept in balance by different body functions. There are many disorders that can disrupt these functions.

RISK INCREASES WITH
• Hyponatremia (below-normal sodium):
 - Excess loss of body fluids from vomiting or diarrhea.
  - Addison's disease.
  - Congestive heart failure.
  - Prolonged, excess drinking of water or fluids.
  - Some cancers of the adrenal glands.
  - Infections with high fever.
  - Certain drugs (e.g., diuretics).
  - Poor kidney function.
  - Prolonged exercise with sweat loss and excessive water intake.
• Hypernatremia (above-normal sodium):
  - Inability to drink water, as with stroke or gastrointestinal diseases.
  - Use of cortisone drugs.
  - Excess intake of salty food or liquid, as in near drowning in salt water.
  - Inappropriate secretion of antidiuretic hormone.
  - Diabetes, kidney disease, or heart disease.
  - Aldosteronism.

HOW TO PREVENT—Sodium imbalance is the result of an underlying disorder. Medical treatment for that disorder will help prevent sodium imbalance.

 WHAT TO EXPECT

DIAGNOSTIC MEASURES
• Your own observation of symptoms.
• Your health care provider may do a physical exam.
• Medical tests may include blood and urine studies of sodium and other electrolytes.

APPROPRIATE HEALTH CARE
• Treatment will depend on the underlying cause.
• If a drug is the cause for sodium imbalance (above or below normal), it may be stopped or the dose lowered.
• For below-normal sodium levels, water restriction is usually the therapy. This will increase the sodium levels in the body. It is important that the treatment not overcorrect the sodium levels, as that can be dangerous.
• For above-normal levels of sodium, providing fluids (such as dextrose in water) to return sodium levels to normal is the usual therapy.

POSSIBLE COMPLICATIONS
• Shock, which can be life threatening.
• Problems may occur from an underlying disorder.

PROBABLE OUTCOME—Usually, the imbalance can be corrected and the underlying disorder treated to prevent a recurrence.

 HOW TO TREAT

GENERAL MEASURES—None specific.

MEDICATION
• Your health care provider may prescribe:
 - Intravenous (IV) sodium, if sodium levels are low.
  - Diuretics to decrease high sodium levels.
  - Drugs to correct underlying disorders.

ACTIVITY—Get extra rest until stable, or underlying condition resolved or controlled. Resume normal activities after recovery.

DIET—Usually, no special diet for low sodium levels. Most persons with high sodium levels benefit from a low-salt diet. Low-salt diets contain enough sodium to prevent hyponatremia. However, sodium levels are not influenced by diet alone.

 CALL YOUR DOCTOR IF

• You or a family member has symptoms of a sodium imbalance.
• Symptoms recur after treatment.

SORES, PRESSURE
(Bed Sores; Decubitus Ulcers)

 GENERAL INFORMATION

DEFINITION—Pressure sores are areas of damaged skin caused by pressure. The most common places for the sores are over bony areas. These include the lower back, buttocks, elbows, knees, shoulders, heels, or ankles.

BODY PARTS INVOLVED—Skin; body tissue.

SEX OR AGE MOST AFFECTED—Both sexes; all ages, but most likely in the elderly.

SIGNS & SYMPTOMS—Spots of the skin that are red and shiny. Spots progress to blisters, then ulcers (deep sores), leading to a breakdown of tissue under the ulcer.

CAUSES—Constant pressure on the skin, especially over the bony areas. Pressure reduces the blood supply, causing death in the tissue layers. Pressure sores usually develop in persons who cannot move because of chronic illness or disability that confines them to bed.

RISK INCREASES WITH
* Elderly.
* People who are frail, disabled, ill, or immobile.
* Being confined to bed or a chair for long, or even short periods of time. Sores can start within 24 hours.
* Poor nutrition, impaired blood circulation, or poor mental or sensory function.
* Surgery, cast or splint, anemia, weak immune system, urinary or stool incontinence, and others.

HOW TO PREVENT
* Provide good nursing care for the disabled.
* Daily skin inspection in good light. Frequent changes of position in bed or wheelchair (may need hourly).
* Keep skin clean. Clean the skin of any urine or fecal matter as soon as possible. Apply moisturizers.
* Maintain good nutrition (e.g., vitamins and protein).

 WHAT TO EXPECT

DIAGNOSTIC MEASURES—Your health care provider can diagnose a pressure sore by an exam of the affected area. The diagnosis includes a stage (1 to 4) depending on the severity.

APPROPRIATE HEALTH CARE
* Treatment involves relieving the pressure, treating the sores, and improving nutrition, or other conditions. Your health care provider will discuss the steps to take.

* A water mattress, an egg-crate rubber mattress, an alternating-pressure mattress, or special airbed may be recommended.
* Special dressings for pressure sores may be prescribed.
* Dead skin and tissue may need to be removed. This can be done in different ways and can be painful to the patient.

POSSIBLE COMPLICATIONS—Serious infections of bone (osteomyelitis), skin (cellulitis), or whole body (sepsis).

PROBABLE OUTCOME—Usually curable with treatment. Sores heal in 2 to 4 weeks, or sometimes longer. Healing time varies with the site and size of the ulcer and the patient's health.

 HOW TO TREAT

GENERAL MEASURES
* Relieve pressure by not lying on the sores. Other options include protective, soft padding, such as gel flotation pads or sheepskin, over the affected area.
* Clean the area with mild soap and warm water and pat dry. Avoid harsh soaps, tincture of benzoin, or hexachlorophene. Cover the sore with bandage or dressing.
* Apply a skin product if prescribed. Apply a thin layer of the cream, ointment, or lotion 3 or 4 times daily. Rub in gently for several minutes, until it disappears.

MEDICATION
* Antibiotics will be prescribed if infection develops.
* Ointments, dressings, and drying agents may be recommended.
* Drugs for pain may be needed when dead skin tissue is removed.
* Vitamin and mineral supplements may be needed.

ACTIVITY
* Change the position of an immobilized patient every 1 to 2 hours. A wheelchair patient should change position every hour.
* Passive or active exercises (if the patient is able). Instructions will be provided by your health care provider or physical therapist.

DIET—Normal, well-balanced diet that includes extra protein. Good nutrition is important in prevention and healing.

 CALL YOUR DOCTOR IF

* You or a family member has symptoms of pressure sores.
* Sores don't improve with treatment.

SPINAL CORD TUMOR

GENERAL INFORMATION

DEFINITION—A spinal cord tumor is an abnormal growth that presses on the spinal cord or its nerve roots. The growth may be benign (noncancerous) or malignant (cancerous). A benign tumor may be as damaging as a malignant tumor if it is not treated.

BODY PARTS INVOLVED—Spinal cord; nerves below the level of the spinal-cord tumor.

SEX OR AGE MOST AFFECTED—Both sexes; all ages, but most common in adults.

SIGNS & SYMPTOMS
- Symptoms may come on gradually and then suddenly be more severe.
- Dull, burning, or aching pain due to tumor putting pressure on the spinal cord. Pain may be constant and, sometimes, severe. It may feel like it's coming from various parts of the body.
- Pain may be located near the level of the tumor on the spinal cord. Midway affects the chest, higher affects arms and neck, and lower affects the back and legs. The pain may also occur in other areas of the spine or body.
- A loss of sensation that may include a feeling of numbness and skin being less sensitive to heat and cold.
- Muscle weakness or stiffness.
- Urination problems or incontinence (unable to control urination or bowel movements).
- If not treated, muscle wasting (loss of tissue) and paralysis may occur.

CAUSES
- A spinal cord tumor usually comes from cancer that has spread from another part of the body. The cancer may have started in the lung, breast, intestinal tract, prostate, kidney, thyroid, or lymphatic system.
- Tumors that start first (primary tumors) in the spinal cord are more rare, especially in childhood or old age. Their cause is often unknown. A few may result from a genetic disease or radiation exposure.

RISK INCREASES WITH—Cancer in other parts of the body.

HOW TO PREVENT—Take steps to help reduce your cancer risk or diagnose the cancer early. Don't smoke. Eat a healthy diet. Maintain a healthy weight. Get recommended cancer screening exams. Learn the warning signs and symptoms of cancer.

WHAT TO EXPECT

DIAGNOSTIC MEASURES
- Your own observation of symptoms.
- Your health care provider will do a physical exam and ask questions about your symptoms.

This exam may include checking: your eye movement, reflexes, hearing, sense of touch, and balance.
- Medical tests may include x-ray, CT, or MRI. A biopsy (tumor tissue is viewed under a microscope) can check for cancer cells.

APPROPRIATE HEALTH CARE
- Treatment depends on the tumor type, your health, other cancer treatment, and your preferences. Options include monitoring (no treatment right away), surgery, radiation, and/or chemotherapy (anticancer drugs).
- A slow-growing, benign tumor may be monitored for a period of time. It may have been found on a routine exam and not be causing symptoms, or the symptoms are mild.
- Surgery is often the first option if the tumor can be removed without damage to the spinal cord or nerves. Several different types of surgery are available. If the tumor is benign, surgery can provide a cure.
- Radiation therapy is usually done after surgery for a cancerous tumor. Radiation may also be done if the tumor cannot be removed with surgery.

POSSIBLE COMPLICATIONS—Paralysis, spread of cancer in the body, treatment complications, infections, and other medical problems.

PROBABLE OUTCOME—Early diagnosis and early treatment offer the most favorable outcome for cancerous tumors. Many benign tumors are cured with surgery.

HOW TO TREAT

GENERAL MEASURES—To learn more: American Cancer Society; (800) ACS-2345; website: www.cancer.org or National Cancer Institute; (800) 4-CANCER; website: www.cancer.gov.

MEDICATION
- Pain relievers may be prescribed.
- Cortisone drugs may be given to decrease swelling around the tumor and reduce spinal cord pressure.
- Anticancer drugs may be prescribed.

ACTIVITY—Activity levels will depend on your condition. Be as active as your energy permits.

DIET—Eat a normal, well-balanced diet.

CALL YOUR DOCTOR IF

- You or a family member has any symptoms of a spinal cord tumor.
- new or unexpected symptoms occur during or after treatment.

SPINAL STENOSIS

GENERAL INFORMATION

DEFINITION—Spinal stenosis occurs when the space around the spinal cord narrows. This puts pressure on the spinal cord and the spinal nerve roots. The narrowing can occur in the space at the center of the spine, the canals where nerves branch out from the spine, or the space between vertebrae (the bones of the spine).

BODY PARTS INVOLVED—It usually affects the upper spine (cervical spinal stenosis) or lower spine (lumbar spinal stenosis).

SEX OR AGE MOST AFFECTED—Both sexes; most common in adults over age 50.

SIGNS & SYMPTOMS
- May not cause symptoms or they may start gradually and worsen over time. Symptoms may come and go. Symptoms are usually worse with standing or walking.
- Back pain. It lessens with leaning forward or sitting.
- Numbness, weakness, cramping, or pain in the arms or legs.
- Burning pain in buttocks or legs (sciatica).
- Pain in the neck or shoulders.
- Foot drop (problem with lifting front part of foot).
- Loss of balance.
- Loss of bowel or bladder function (cauda equina syndrome). In severe cases, nerves to your bladder or bowel may be affected.

CAUSES—Spinal stenosis is either acquired or primary. Acquired spinal stenosis is the most common type and is usually a result of arthritic changes in the spine that occur with aging. Primary spinal stenosis is less common and is present at birth.

RISK INCREASES WITH
- Age over 50.
- Osteoarthritis or rheumatoid arthritis.
- Rarer risks include herniated disc, spinal tumors, injury, Paget's disease (a bone disease), or inherited disorders.

HOW TO PREVENT—No specific preventive measures. To reduce risk, exercise regularly and maintain a healthy weight.

WHAT TO EXPECT

DIAGNOSTIC MEASURES
- Your own observation of symptoms.
- Your health care provider will do a physical exam and ask questions about your symptoms and activities.
- Medical tests may include x-ray, CT, MRI, bone scan, nerve study, or myelogram (a special x-ray).

APPROPRIATE HEALTH CARE
- Treatment depends on the severity of the symptoms. Nonsurgical options are drug therapy, physical therapy, lifestyle changes, or use of a back support device.
- Lifestyle changes can include extra rest, limits on activities, and home exercises.
- A neck brace, back brace, or corset device may be recommended for supporting the back.
- Surgery is an option if other treatments do not help or if symptoms are severe. There are different surgical procedures and the choices will be explained. Surgery can relieve the pressure, lessen pain, and improve function. It does not stop the degenerative process.
- Alternative therapies (e.g., massage, chiropractor therapy, acupuncture, acupressure, or others) may be of help.

POSSIBLE COMPLICATIONS
- Loss of feeling in the arms, hands, feet, or legs. May not feel the effects of an injury or infection.
- Limited activities of daily living; disability.
- Loss of bladder or bowel control.
- Surgery complications or symptoms recur a few years after surgical treatment.
- Dependence on pain medication.

PROBABLE OUTCOME—Conservative treatment helps improve symptoms in many cases. Others can be helped with surgery.

HOW TO TREAT

GENERAL MEASURES—Use heat (to relax muscles) or cold therapy (reduce pain) on back.

MEDICATION
- Your health care provider may prescribe:
  - Nonsteroidal anti-inflammatory drugs (NSAIDs) to reduce inflammation and pain.
  - Other drugs for pain.
  - Epidural injections to relieve pain and inflammation (can be done more than once).

ACTIVITY
- Limited activity is recommended. Avoid activities that worsen symptoms (e.g., excess standing). Bed rest is not usually recommended.
- Leaning forward helps reduce pain symptoms. A walking stick or walker can help with walking.
- Physical therapy can help to maintain strength and flexibility. Biking or pool exercises are other options.

DIET—Eat a normal, well-balanced diet. Being overweight can worsen symptoms. A weight-loss diet may be recommended.

CALL YOUR DOCTOR IF

- You or a family member has symptoms of spinal stenosis.
- Symptoms don't improve with treatment.

SPONDYLITIS, ANKYLOSING
(Marie-Strümpell Disease)

 GENERAL INFORMATION

DEFINITION—Ankylosing spondylitis is a chronic, progressive, rheumatic disease of the joints. Ankylosing means "fusing together." Spondylitis means "inflammation of the vertebrae" (bones in the spine). It often starts where the lowest part of the spine (sacrum) joins the ilium bone of the pelvis.

BODY PARTS INVOLVED—Joints.

SEX OR AGE MOST AFFECTED—Males are affected more often than females. The onset is usually in the late teens or early twenties.

SIGNS & SYMPTOMS
- Early stages:
  - Recurrent episodes of low back ache. Pain can also occur along the sciatic nerve (along the leg).
  - Stiffness in the spine (especially in the morning).
  - The symptoms can be mild and a person may think it is just a common back ache.
- Later stages:
  - Symptoms gradually become worse. Pain often spreads from the lower back to the middle back, or higher in the neck. Joints in the arms, legs, feet, and hands may be affected.
  - It can bring about a "bent forward" posture caused by stiffening of the spine and support structures.
  - Muscle stiffness.
  - Fatigue; weight loss.
  - Iritis (eye redness and soreness).

CAUSES—Unknown. Genetic factors appear to play a role. The disorder causes some or all the bones of the spine to fuse together.

RISK INCREASES WITH
- Family history of ankylosing spondylitis.
- Having a certain gene called HLA-B27.

HOW TO PREVENT—No specific preventive measures. Consult your health care provider if you have a family history of the disorder and have ongoing back or joint pain.

 WHAT TO EXPECT

DIAGNOSTIC MEASURES
- Your own observation of symptoms.
- Your health care provider will do a physical exam and ask questions about your symptoms.
- Medical tests may include blood studies and x-rays of the spine.

APPROPRIATE HEALTH CARE
- Physical therapy, exercise, and drugs can help delay or prevent deformity, ease pain, and maintain function.

- Physical therapy includes exercises for breathing techniques, to maintain proper posture, and to build up muscle groups (to oppose the direction of possible deformities).
- Surgery to replace a damaged hip or to insert bone grafts in the spine (advanced stages only).

POSSIBLE COMPLICATIONS
- Heart and lung problems.
- Eye inflammation.
- Difficulty walking and standing.
- Osteoporosis and fractures of the spine.
- Anemia.
- Permanent disability.

PROBABLE OUTCOME—There is no cure for this disorder. Symptoms change with mild or moderate flare-ups and they may stop for periods of time. With treatment, symptoms can be relieved or controlled. Most patients can lead normal, productive lives. For some, the disease is severe and incapacitating due to deformities.

 HOW TO TREAT

GENERAL MEASURES
- Sleep on your back on a firm mattress. Use a small pillow or none at all.
- Take hot baths or use heat compresses before exercising or to relieve pain. Get regular massages, if possible.
- Quit smoking. Find a way to stop that works.
- See your eye care provider for regular exams.
- To learn more: Spondylitis Association of America, PO Box 5872, Sherman Oaks, CA 91413; (800) 777-8189; website: www.spondylitis.org.

MEDICATION
- Use nonprescription, nonsteroidal anti-inflammatory drugs to help ease discomfort.
- Drugs to treat arthritis symptoms, stronger pain drugs, and muscle relaxants may be prescribed.

ACTIVITY
- Exercise to maintain good posture and retain as much upright carriage as possible.
- Swim regularly, if possible. Your buoyancy in water lets you move stiff, painful areas.
- Avoid activity that puts stress on the back. Avoid contact sports (risk of spinal injury).

DIET—No special diet. Maintain a healthy body weight.

 CALL YOUR DOCTOR IF

- You or a family member has symptoms of ankylosing spondylitis.
- Increasing back pain or stiffness, or eye pain occur.

SPOROTRICHOSIS

GENERAL INFORMATION

DEFINITION—Sporotrichosis is a fungal infection that affects the skin. It is not contagious from person to person.

BODY PARTS INVOLVED—Skin; lymph system; lungs; joints; bones (rare).

SEX OR AGE MOST AFFECTED—Adults of both sexes.

SIGNS & SYMPTOMS
- A small, movable, non-tender bump (nodule) usually on the fingers, hands, or arms. It starts at the place where the fungus entered the skin. The color may be pink, red, or purple.
- More bumps occur around the same area.
- The bumps may ulcerate (become open sores).
- The skin infection can spread in a line-like formation up the fingers, hands, or arms. They spread along what is called lymphatic channels.

CAUSES
- Infection by a fungus, *Sporotrichum schenckii*, that lives in soil, sphagnum moss, weeds, baled hay, and decaying organic vegetation. It enters the skin through small cuts or punctures, such as from thorns. The infection may appear on the skin 1 to 12 weeks after exposure. Very rarely, an inhaled form may occur.
- Research has shown that a pet cat may have the infection and pass it to a human through a bite or scratch. Rarely, other animals may be a source.

RISK INCREASES WITH
- Farm laborers, plant nursery workers, gardeners, and others who handle rosebushes, sphagnum moss, hay bales, or barberry bushes.
- Kids playing among hay bales.
- Those with weak immune system due to illness or drugs are more at risk for complications.

HOW TO PREVENT
- Wear gloves and long sleeves when working with plants with thorns, hay bales, pine seedlings, or other materials that could cause minor skin breaks.
- Avoid skin contact with sphagnum moss. It has been the cause of some outbreaks.

WHAT TO EXPECT

DIAGNOSTIC MEASURES
- Your own observation of symptoms.
- Your health care provider will do a physical exam of the affected skin.
- Medical tests may include a culture of fluid from the sores or a small bit of tissue is removed for viewing under a microscope.

APPROPRIATE HEALTH CARE
- The disorder is treated with antifungal drugs.
- Rarely, hospital care may be needed if complications occur.

POSSIBLE COMPLICATIONS—Spread of the fungal infection to joints, lungs, and central nervous system. This is rare, but may occur in those who have diabetes or weak immune systems.

PROBABLE OUTCOME—Curable with treatment, but it can take several months to heal completely.

HOW TO TREAT

GENERAL MEASURES
- You may be advised to apply warm compresses or a heating pad to the affected skin for 40 to 60 minutes a day. This can help control the skin symptoms.
- Cover lesions with loose-fitting bandages to prevent secondary infection with bacteria.

MEDICATION—Oral (taken by mouth) antifungal drugs are usually prescribed. Drugs may be continued for 1 to 2 months or more after the skin symptoms have cleared up.

ACTIVITY—No limits.

DIET—No special diet.

CALL YOUR DOCTOR IF

- You or a family member has symptoms of sporotrichosis.
- Any new sores occur after treatment starts.
- New, unexplained symptoms develop. Antifungal drugs used in treatment may produce side effects.

SPRAINS & STRAINS

 GENERAL INFORMATION

DEFINITION—A sprain is a stretched or torn ligament. A strain is a stretched or torn muscle or tendon. Sprains occur most often in ankles, knees, or fingers, although any joint can be sprained. Strains often occur in the back or hamstring muscles (at the back of the thigh). It is sometimes difficult to know if the injury is a sprain or strain. Sprain and strain grades are:
1 (mild)—some stretching or minor tear,
2 (moderate)—partial tear, but intact,
3 (severe)—complete tear.

BODY PARTS INVOLVED—Muscles, tendons and any ligament attached to any joint. Ligaments are the fibrous, elastic connective bands that attach bone to bone (tendons connect muscle to bone).

SEX OR AGE MOST AFFECTED—Both sexes; all ages.

SIGNS & SYMPTOMS
• Pain or tenderness in the area of injury; severity varies with the extent of injury.
• Swelling of the affected joint. Area feels warm.
• Redness or bruising in the area of injury (sometimes), either right away, or several hours after injury.
• Loss of normal mobility in the injured joint.

CAUSES
• Sprains usually occur as a result of trauma (fall, twisting injury, or automobile accident). The ankle is injured most often because of its normal weakness, its exposed position, and the stress it sustains in sports and other activities.
• Strains (also called a pulled muscle) are often caused by abrupt twisting, pulling, or contraction. A chronic strain is often due to overuse or repetitive movement.

RISK INCREASES WITH
• Sports requiring running, jumping, and change of direction.
• High-risk activities such as skateboarding, contact sports, ice and roller skating, mountain biking, skiing, and rock climbing.
• Overweight.
• Trauma.
• Excessive exercise.
• Fatigue and tired muscles.
• Poor conditioning.
• Poor fitting shoes and high-heeled shoes.

HOW TO PREVENT
• Maintain good level of physical fitness.
• Maintain a healthy weight.
• To avoid injury:
  - Wear proper shoes and other protective gear for the sport or activity.
  - Stretch muscles before and after exercise.
  - Strengthen weak muscles with exercises.
  - Accident-proof your home.

 WHAT TO EXPECT

DIAGNOSTIC MEASURES
• Your health care provider will do an exam of the injured area. Questions will be asked about your symptoms and activities that led to injury.
• Medical tests may include x-rays or other test of the injured area.

APPROPRIATE HEALTH CARE
• Treatment for a sprain or strain will depend on how mild or severe the injury is. It may range from simple self-care, to wearing a cast or brace, to having surgery.
• Special boots, cast, brace, or splint may be prescribed.
• Rehabilitation for a sprain or strain starts after the pain and swelling improve. The goals are to restore complete joint function and a return to full activity levels.

POSSIBLE COMPLICATIONS
• Joint may remain unstable.
• Arthritis may develop later on in the joint.

PROBABLE OUTCOME—Mild sprains or strains heal on their own in a few weeks. More severe injuries may take several months to heal.

 HOW TO TREAT

GENERAL MEASURES
• Use RICE therapy—Rest, Ice, Compression, Elevation.
  - Rest and reduce activities as needed. A cane or crutches or may be required to get around.
  - Apply ice. Place ice in a plastic bag and separate it from the skin with a thin towel. Continue the ice treatment for 20 minutes at a time at 2-hour intervals. After 24 hours, continue ice treatment or switch to heat.
  - Compression may be done with elastic wrap.
  - Elevate the injured area on a pillow, above the heart level if possible, to reduce swelling.

MEDICATION—Use nonprescription pain relievers such as acetaminophen, ibuprofen, or naproxen. If the sprain is severe, a stronger pain reliever may be prescribed.

ACTIVITY
• You may be taught exercises to do at home.
• Physical therapy may be needed.
• Consider a return to previous activity levels—once the pain is gone, you have full range of motion, and normal strength in injured joint.

DIET—No special diet.

📞 CALL YOUR DOCTOR IF

• You or a family member has a joint injury.
• Pain, swelling or bruising, increases.

STOMACH CANCER
(Gastric Carcinoma)

 GENERAL INFORMATION

DEFINITION—Stomach cancer is a growth of cancer cells in the stomach. Most people do not have symptoms until the disease is advanced.

BODY PARTS INVOLVED—Stomach.

SEX OR AGE MOST AFFECTED—It most often affects adults over age 50 and is more common in men than in women.

SIGNS & SYMPTOMS
- Early stages:
  - Vague symptoms of indigestion, such as fullness, burping, nausea, and poor appetite.
- Later stages:
  - Unexplained weight loss.
  - Loss of appetite.
  - Vomiting blood.
  - Black stools.
  - Fullness after eating small amounts.
  - Pain in the stomach.
  - Mass in the stomach that can be felt (sometimes).

CAUSES—Exact cause is unknown. Genetic and environmental factors are likely involved. *Helicobacter pylori* infection, a bacteria infection of the stomach and dietary factors are believed to play a role.

RISK INCREASES WITH
- Age over 50; men more than women.
- Tobacco use.
- *Helicobacter pylori* infection (a bacterial infection of the stomach).
- Diet that includes high amounts of smoked, pickled, and salted foods; and low amounts of protein, green, leafy vegetables, and fresh fruit.
- Pernicious anemia (unable to absorb vitamin B-12).
- Family history of stomach cancer.
- Gastritis (chronic stomach inflammation).
- Stomach polyps or stomach surgery.
- Certain racial groups (Asian, Pacific Islander, Hispanic, and African American).

HOW TO PREVENT
- There are no specific preventive measures. Changing some lifestyle behaviors may help lower the risks.
  - Eat a nutritious, well-balanced diet with plenty of fresh fruits and vegetables. Lose weight if overweight.
  - Don't smoke. If you do smoke, try to quit.
- To help find stomach cancer early, don't ignore symptoms of indigestion that last more than a few days. Ask your health care provider about a yearly home test for blood in the stool.
- Get treatment for any medical disorder that increases your risk for stomach cancer.

 WHAT TO EXPECT

DIAGNOSTIC MEASURES
- Your health care provider will do a physical exam and ask questions about your symptoms.
- Medical tests may include blood studies, CT, x-rays, and endoscopy of the stomach.

APPROPRIATE HEALTH CARE
- Treatment varies and depends on location and size of tumor, any spread of the cancer, your health, age, and preferences. Treatment may include surgery, radiation, chemotherapy, and/or other drug therapy. More than one type of treatment may be recommended.
- Surgery to remove part or all of the stomach is the primary treatment for stomach cancer.
- Drugs to treat the cancer and/or radiation therapy may be used alone or with surgery.
- Treatment may involve steps to relieve symptoms and make you comfortable, rather than treating the cancer.

POSSIBLE COMPLICATIONS
- Spread of cancer to other parts of the body.
- Treatment complications often occur.
- Cancer is diagnosed too late for effective treatment.

PROBABLE OUTCOME—Early diagnosis and treatment offer the best outcome. A complete cure is possible. The outcome will vary for patients with a more advanced stage of cancer.

 HOW TO TREAT

GENERAL MEASURES—To learn more: American Cancer Society; (800) ACS-2345; website: www.cancer.org or National Cancer Institute; (800) 4-CANCER; website: www.cancer.gov.

MEDICATION
- Anticancer (chemotherapy) drugs or other drugs for cancer treatment (e.g., biologics) may be prescribed.
- Pain relievers may be prescribed.

ACTIVITY—As tolerated by your energy level.

DIET—Treatments for stomach cancer will affect your eating and drinking habits. Problems can occur right after surgery or weeks to months later. Maintaining a healthy diet can be hard. A dietitian can help you with meal plans.

 CALL YOUR DOCTOR IF

- You or a family member has symptoms of stomach cancer.
- New symptoms occur during treatment.

STOMATITIS, HERPETIC

GENERAL INFORMATION

DEFINITION—Herpetic stomatitis is a contagious, viral infection of the mouth that causes blisters, ulcers (open sores), and inflammation. It is a common and usually mild condition. This infection is not the same as canker sores (aphthous stomatitis).

BODY PARTS INVOLVED—It may involve the cheeks, gums, lips, tongue, roof, and floor of the mouth.

SEX OR AGE MOST AFFECTED—Both sexes; occurs most often in young children who have never had the virus before.

SIGNS & SYMPTOMS
- Burning, tingling, or pain in the mouth.
- Fever.
- Blisters in the mouth, often on the tongue or cheeks.
- Ulcers form after the blisters pop.
- Swollen gums.
- Drooling.
- Difficulty swallowing (dysphagia) and eating.
- Irritability.
- May have bad breath, sore throat, or swollen glands in the neck.

CAUSES—Herpes simplex virus type 1 (HSV-1). This is the same herpes virus that causes cold sores. Less often, the cause is HSV-2. The virus enters the body when the mouth comes in contact with saliva from someone who is infected by the virus. Usually, no source for the infection will be discovered. Once the first infection occurs, the virus remains inside the body for life.

RISK INCREASES WITH
- Exposure to someone who has herpetic stomatitis.
- Physical contact with someone who has blisters or ulcers around the mouth.

HOW TO PREVENT
- It is difficult to prevent children from exposure to the virus at some time during their childhood.
- Children should avoid close contact with anyone who has cold sores (e.g., don't kiss a parent who has a cold sore).
- Children should also avoid other children with herpetic stomatitis. They should not share silverware, cups or glasses, or food.

WHAT TO EXPECT

DIAGNOSTIC MEASURES
- Your own observation of symptoms.
- See your health care provider if sores persist, cause excess pain, or cause concern. An exam of the mouth is usually all that is needed for diagnosis.
- Medical tests such as smears or cultures of the sores may be done.

APPROPRIATE HEALTH CARE
- Most people will let the sores heal on their own or use self-treatment methods.
- Treatment may include temporary diet changes, extra rest, drugs for pain and fever, or antiviral drugs.

POSSIBLE COMPLICATIONS
- High fever.
- Dehydration (if a child refuses to eat or drink enough because of a sore mouth).
- Infection recurs (will appear as cold sores).
- Herpes eye infection (rare).

PROBABLE OUTCOME—It will clear up on its own. Ulcers and other symptoms are generally healed within 10 to 14 days.

HOW TO TREAT

GENERAL MEASURES
- Wash your hands and the child's hands often, and especially before eating.
- Avoid touching the mouth sores and then touching the eyes. It can lead to a serious herpes eye infection.

MEDICATION
- Antiviral drugs (e.g., acyclovir) may be prescribed.
- Use ibuprofen or acetaminophen for minor pain. Don't give aspirin to children under age 18.
- Nonprescription topical anesthetics may relieve more severe pain. Follow product instructions carefully.

ACTIVITY—Activity limits will depend on severity of symptoms. Extra rest is usually recommended when a child has a fever.

DIET
- Give a child cool liquids. They can be soothing to the mouth and help numb the pain. Choices include milk, milkshakes, and clear liquids. Use a straw if there are blisters on the lips or tongue.
- Avoid citrus or carbonated drinks. These can make the sores hurt more.
- Feed the child soft foods to make chewing and swallowing easier. Choices include soft fruits, mashed potatoes, applesauce, yogurt, pudding, or strained baby foods. Avoid spicy, salty, or hard foods.

CALL YOUR DOCTOR IF

- You or a family member has symptoms of herpetic stomatitis that cause concern.
- Your child will not drink and cannot swallow, has a high temperature, becomes more fussy, or won't stop crying, or isn't better in a few days.

STRABISMUS

GENERAL INFORMATION

DEFINITION
- With strabismus, the eyes do not line up in the same direction when focusing. One or both eyes may turn inward, outward, upward, or downward. Normally, eye movements are controlled by brain signals to six muscles around each eye. Loss of this coordinated movement results in an unequal focusing ability. Strabismus (also called crossed eyes) usually affects children, but can develop in adults.
  - In young children, when the two eyes fail to focus on the same image, the brain can ignore the input from one eye. If this continues, that ignored eye will never see well (called amblyopia or lazy eye). Children do not outgrow strabismus.
  - Adults who develop strabismus often have double vision. This happens because the brain has been trained to receive images from both eyes and will not ignore the image from the affected eye.

BODY PARTS INVOLVED—Eyes; brain area that controls vision.

SEX OR AGE MOST AFFECTED—A true eye problem shows up from 3 or 4 months of age. It also may occur in childhood or later.

SIGNS & SYMPTOMS
- Eyes of infants may appear to be crossed, though they are not (this is called pseudostrabismus).
- An eye that is not straight.
- Eye movement that is not coordinated. This may be constant, or it may come and go.
- Child may look at you with one eye closed, squint, or with the head turned to one side.
- Adults have double vision, eyestrain, headaches, or abnormal head position (from trying to see properly).

CAUSES   For most children, the cause of strabismus is unknown. It is often present at, or shortly after, birth (congenital strabismus). In adults, there are known risk factors.

RISK INCREASES WITH
- Children:
  - Family history of strabismus.
  - Down syndrome, cerebral palsy, or hydrocephalus.
  - Brain tumor, prematurity, cataract, or eye injury.
- Adults:
  - Eye disease, eye injury, stroke, head injury, certain surgeries, thyroid disease, myasthenia gravis, diabetes, or having had childhood strabismus.

HOW TO PREVENT—No preventive measures. Ask your child's health care provider about routine visual exams to detect any problems.

WHAT TO EXPECT

DIAGNOSTIC MEASURES
- Your own observation of symptoms. If a young child covers one eye—this may indicate the eyes are not focusing together.
- Your health care provider will do an exam of the eyes.
- Medical tests may include a visual acuity test, a retina exam, and others.

APPROPRIATE HEALTH CARE
- Treatment depends on the patient's age, the cause of the problem, and the type and degree of the eye turn.
- The goals of treatment are to straighten the eyes and preserve binocular (both eyes) vision.
- Treatments may include:
  - Eyeglasses to correct vision in weaker eye (child).
  - Wearing a patch over the good eye or using eye drops to temporarily blur the vision of the good eye will force a child to use the weaker eye.
  - Eye exercises to strengthen eye muscles.
  - Surgery to tighten, loosen, or reinforce eye muscles is often an option to realign the eyes.
  - Eyeglasses with prisms to correct mild double vision in adult strabismus.

POSSIBLE COMPLICATIONS
- Without treatment in children, vision weakness or vision loss in one eye may become permanent. In adults, the symptoms will continue or worsen.
- In adults and children, surgery complications may occur. Symptoms may recur after treatment.

PROBABLE OUTCOME
- With early diagnosis and treatment for children, the outcome is usually excellent.
- Strabismus symptoms in adults can be improved with treatment.

HOW TO TREAT

GENERAL MEASURES—To learn more: American Academy of Ophthalmology, PO Box 429098, San Francisco, CA 94142; (877) 887-6327; website: www.eyecareamerica.com.

MEDICATION—Botulinum toxin (Botox) injection may be prescribed to relax an overactive eye muscle.

ACTIVITY—No limits.

DIET—No special diet.

☎ CALL YOUR DOCTOR IF

- You or a family member has symptoms of strabismus.
- Symptoms recur after treatment.

STREP THROAT
(Streptococcal Sore Throat)

GENERAL INFORMATION

DEFINITION—Strep throat is a streptococcal bacterial infection of the throat (the pharynx). It can spread from person to person and is most common in children over age 2. An infection can be present in someone with no symptoms, but who can still spread the germs (carrier state).

BODY PARTS INVOLVED—Throat; tonsils.

SEX OR AGE MOST AFFECTED—Both sexes; all ages, but most common in children.

SIGNS & SYMPTOMS
- Rapid onset of throat pain.
- Throat pain that is worse when you swallow.
- Headache, fever, general ill feeling.
- Children may have nausea and vomiting.
- Tender, swollen glands in the neck.
- Bright-red tonsils that may have spots of pus.

CAUSES—Group A streptococcus (GAS) bacteria. Germs are spread by contact with an infected person, breathing in germs in the air, or touching an object with germs on it. A person usually has symptoms within 2 to 5 days of exposure. Strep throat is one of the most common types of infection caused by group A streptococcus. It can also cause skin infections and other health problems.

RISK INCREASES WITH
- Recent strep infection in a family member.
- Crowded living conditions such as a dorm.
- Being in a daycare center or attending school.

HOW TO PREVENT
- There are no specific preventive measures.
- Avoid close contact with anyone with strep throat.
- Avoid germs. Wash hands often, especially children.

WHAT TO EXPECT

DIAGNOSTIC MEASURES
- Your own observation of symptoms.
- Your health care provider will examine the throat. A sore throat (pharyngitis) can also be caused by virus infection, allergies, or other problems. Further tests are usually needed.
- A throat culture or rapid strep test can confirm a strep infection.

APPROPRIATE HEALTH CARE—Treatment for strep infection is with antibiotic drugs and self-care.

POSSIBLE COMPLICATIONS
- Ear infection.
- Sinusitis.
- Rheumatic fever or scarlet fever.
- Glomerulonephritis (kidney disorder).

PROBABLE OUTCOME—A strep throat infection will normally clear up in 3 to 7 days. Antibiotic therapy will shorten the time you can spread the germs to others (be contagious). Antibiotics also reduce the risk of complications and the risk of spreading the infection to other parts of your body. Without antibiotics, a person may be contagious for 2 to 3 weeks after symptoms are gone. Complications are rare.

HOW TO TREAT

GENERAL MEASURES—To relieve the sore throat, gargle frequently with warm or cold double-strength tea or warm salt water (mix one-half teaspoon of salt in one cup of water).

MEDICATION
- Penicillin, amoxicillin, or another antibiotic is usually prescribed. Be sure to take the full course of the drug even if symptoms are better.
- Use a nonprescription pain drug, such as acetaminophen or ibuprofen, if needed. Don't give aspirin to children under age 18.
- Throat lozenges or anesthetic sprays for sore throats may be used to help with pain relief.

ACTIVITY—Get extra rest. Return to normal activities as symptoms improve. A person can no longer spread the germs if they have taken the antibiotic drug for at least 24 hours.

DIET—A liquid diet may be helpful while the throat is sore. Drink plenty of fluids, including milkshakes, soups, tea, carbonated drinks, or iced coffee. Any type and amount of solid food is fine as long as you can swallow it without too much pain.

CALL YOUR DOCTOR IF

- You or a family member has symptoms of strep throat.
- The following occur during treatment:
  - Fever recurs after being normal for a few days.
  - New symptoms appear, such as nausea, vomiting, earache, cough, swollen glands, skin rash, severe headache, nasal drainage, or shortness of breath.
  - Joints become red or painful.
  - Symptoms don't improve in 3 or 4 days.

STRESS

GENERAL INFORMATION

DEFINITION—Stress is a general term that described the physical, mental, and emotional reactions you experience due to changes and demands in your life. The changes and demands can be small to large and each person will respond to them differently. Some people are more prone than others to stress. Positive stress can be a motivator. Negative stress occurs when these changes and demands are overwhelming to you.

BODY PARTS INVOLVED—Almost all.

SEX OR AGE MOST AFFECTED—Both sexes; all ages.

SIGNS & SYMPTOMS
- Physical symptoms include muscle tension, headache, chest pain, upset stomach, diarrhea or constipation, racing heartbeat, cold clammy hands, fatigue, profuse sweating, rashes, rapid breathing, shaking, tics, jumpiness, changes in appetite, weakness, tiredness, and dizziness.
- Emotional reactions include anger, low self-esteem, depression, lack of interest, irritability, fear and phobic responses, guilt, worry, difficulty concentrating, agitation, anxiety, and panic.
- Behavioral reactions may lead to alcohol or drug abuse, an increase in smoking, overeating, memory loss, confusion, sleep disorders, or nervous habits such as nail biting or pacing.

CAUSES—In stressful times, the body increases the production of certain hormones. These cause changes in the heart rate, blood pressure, metabolism, and physical activity.

RISK INCREASES WITH
- Recent loss of loved one (spouse, child, friend).
- Holidays, such as Christmas.
- Injuries or severe illnesses.
- Problems with work or school.
- Recent move to a new city or state.
- Sexual difficulties between you and partner.
- Business or financial problems.
- Buying a new home.
- Conflict between you and a spouse or family member, business associate, or close friend.
- Constant fatigue.
- Demands on your time and energy by other family members leaving little time for self-care.
- World or national events (e.g., war or disaster).
- Women; people with certain personality traits or genetic factors.

HOW TO PREVENT
- Stress can't be entirely prevented. Avoid or reduce the impact of your stressors where possible. It helps if you get enough sleep, eat healthy, avoid excess caffeine, exercise daily, and take time to relax.
- Avoid use of pain drugs, alcohol, smoking, or eating in dealing with stress.

WHAT TO EXPECT

DIAGNOSTIC MEASURES—Diagnosis is often by your own or others' observation of symptoms. Sometimes medical tests may be needed to rule out medical problems that could cause the symptoms. A person may not realize they are stressed.

APPROPRIATE HEALTH CARE
- Counseling may be helpful. Talking about your problems is one way of relieving stress.
- Drug therapy may be recommended.

POSSIBLE COMPLICATIONS—Chronic stress can cause problems with your personal relationships and job. Stress is a risk factor for many types of medical problems and illnesses.

PROBABLE OUTCOME—Varies for each person. Many people can learn to recognize when they are stressed and find ways to manage their symptoms. This improves their well-being.

HOW TO TREAT

GENERAL MEASURES
- Here are some tips to help reduce stress:
  - Learn a meditation or relaxation technique and practice it regularly, daily if possible.
  - Share your feelings with a friend.
  - Arrange daily schedules to make them less stressful.
  - Decide what is important and has to get done and what can be put off, left undone, or passed on to others.
  - Take a short time away from any stressful situation you encounter during a day. A short walk can help.
  - Learn and practice a muscle-tensing and muscle-relaxing technique. Take warm bath.
  - Make lists of what needs to be done each day. Cross items off as they are completed.
  - Take time for some enjoyable recreation.
  - Avoid taking problems home or to bed with you. At the end of the day, take a few minutes and review the day. Let go of negative emotions. Decide about undone activities. Release mental or muscular tension.
- To learn more: Mental Health America; (800) 969-6642; website: www.nmha.org.

MEDICATION—If symptoms are severe, drug therapy may be recommended.

ACTIVITY—Exercise 20 to 30 minutes daily. It helps relieve stress.

DIET—Eat a healthy diet. Don't skip meals.

CALL YOUR DOCTOR IF

You or a family member has stress symptoms.

STROKE
(Brain Attack)

GENERAL INFORMATION

DEFINITION—A stroke is a sudden decrease or block in the blood supply to part of the brain. This causes damage to the brain so it cannot function normally.

BODY PARTS INVOLVED—Central nervous system; musculoskeletal system.

SEX OR AGE MOST AFFECTED—Both sexes (men more than women); adults over 55 are most often affected.

SIGNS & SYMPTOMS
- The symptoms can vary in different people.
- Inability to speak.
- Inability to move part of the body.
- Loss of consciousness.
- Sudden heavy feeling in an arm or leg, or feeling numb and unable to control muscles.
- Headache.
- Vision changes.
- Confusion.
- Dizziness.
- Loss of bowel and bladder control.

CAUSES
- Ischemic stroke—blood flow to the brain is blocked by a blood clot. A clot can form in the brain itself due to narrowed arteries. A clot can form elsewhere in the bloodstream and travel to the brain.
- Hemorrhagic stroke—bleeding due to ruptured blood vessel. The bleeding may occur in the brain or in the space between the brain and the skull.

RISK INCREASES WITH
- Age over 55.
- Personal or family history of stroke, heart attack, or transient ischemic attack (TIA).
- Cigarette smoking.
- High blood pressure.
- High cholesterol.
- Heart disease, irregular heartbeat, diabetes, sickle cell anemia, and carotid or other artery disease.
- Obesity and/or sedentary lifestyle (lack of exercise).
- Use of birth control pills.
- Excess alcohol use and certain types of drug abuse.

HOW TO PREVENT
- Exercise regularly.
- Eat a healthy diet.
- Don't smoke.
- Get treatment for diabetes, heart disease, or other chronic disorders.
- Have your blood pressure checked regularly. If it is high, see your health care provider.
- Get medical advice about taking aspirin daily.

WHAT TO EXPECT

DIAGNOSTIC MEASURES
- Call 911 if you think you might be having a stroke or have someone take you to an emergency center. The first few hours are critical for effective treatment.
- Emergency care will include a physical exam and medical tests to check heart, brain, and other body functions.

APPROPRIATE HEALTH CARE
- Treatment may include drugs, oxygen to help with breathing, and sometimes surgery. You will stay in the hospital until symptoms improve. Long-term care may be needed in some cases.
- Early rehabilitation after a stroke will help improve physical abilities. Outcome will depend on the extent of the brain injury. Physical therapy, occupational therapy, and speech therapy may be needed. Patient attitude and family support are important in the success.

POSSIBLE COMPLICATIONS
- Serious physical and mental health problems. Major lifestyle changes that affect work, family, and social life.
- Recurrence of stroke.
- Stroke can be fatal.

PROBABLE OUTCOME—Depends on severity of the stroke. Recovery is a lifelong process.

HOW TO TREAT

GENERAL MEASURES—To learn more: American Stroke Association, 7272 Greenville Ave., Dallas, TX 75231; (888) 478-7653; website: www.strokeassociation.org.

MEDICATION
- Drugs to break up clots, control brain swelling, and prevent complications may be given.
- Drugs for high blood pressure, clot prevention, and other preventive drugs may be prescribed.

ACTIVITY—If you have lost muscle control, therapy will help you learn to use affected limbs. You can often regain basic skills, such as eating, dressing, and toilet functions.

DIET—At first, you may require feeding tube, then progress to a pureed, soft, and then to a regular diet.

CALL YOUR DOCTOR IF

- You or a family member has symptoms of a stroke or observe them in someone else. This is an emergency!
- After diagnosis, any symptoms cause concern.

STROKE, SILENT

GENERAL INFORMATION

DEFINITION—A silent stroke can occur when small blood vessels in the brain become blocked. It is called "silent" because there are none of the usual stroke symptoms (e.g., trouble walking, talking, or seeing, or paralysis or weakness on one side). Minor symptoms may not be noticeable. A person is not aware of having had a stroke. A silent stroke is detected only with a medical imaging test. However, silent strokes can cause real brain damage. They affect the brain areas involving mood, thinking, and personality. They are more common than strokes with symptoms.

BODY PARTS INVOLVED—Brain.

SEX OR AGE MOST AFFECTED—Both sexes; older adults.

SIGNS & SYMPTOMS
- Over time, subtle changes may develop in memory, thinking, concentration, or other cognitive effects.
- Depression. It is more a feeling of apathy and a loss of interest in usual activities, rather than sadness.

CAUSES—Silent stroke is a brain injury usually caused by a blood clot interrupting blood flow in the brain. A person still feels fine and doesn't even know it happened. Over time, the blood and oxygen supply to the brain decreases and cells die. This causes damage in the brain that can be seen on imaging tests.

RISK INCREASES WITH
- Age 55 or older.
- High blood pressure (hypertension).
- Diabetes.
- High cholesterol.
- Heart disease (especially atrial fibrillation), or carotid and/or coronary artery disease, or previous transient ischemic attack (TIA or mini-stroke).
- Smoking and/or excess alcohol use.
- Obesity and/or sedentary (inactive) lifestyle.
- Personal or family history of stroke or heart attack.
- Use of birth control pills or other hormone therapy.

HOW TO PREVENT
- Get medical care for any treatable risk factors, such as high blood pressure.
- Your health care provider can help determine your risk factors for a stroke and counsel you on ways to reduce your risks.
- Reducing risks may include stopping smoking, diet changes, losing weight, exercising more, and limiting alcohol use. Be sure to follow any prescribed treatment for high blood pressure, high cholesterol, and diabetes. See your health care provider on a regular basis.

WHAT TO EXPECT

DIAGNOSTIC MEASURES
- Brain damage due to a silent stroke is detected by an MRI of the brain. It is often an incidental finding. Incidental finding means the MRI was performed for another reason. There is no way to know from the MRI results just when a silent stroke occurred. Patients who have had a silent stroke typically have no memory of any specific stroke symptoms at any time in their lives. Very few patients will have a silent stroke detected.
- The MRI is not a routine screening test.

APPROPRIATE HEALTH CARE—If you have a silent stroke detected, your health care provider will discuss the MRI test with you. Additional tests, medical follow up, and treatment will depend on your individual situation and your risk factors.

POSSIBLE COMPLICATIONS
- Vascular dementia (mental decline due to disease of blood vessels in the brain).
- Higher risk of having another stroke and/or dementia.

PROBABLE OUTCOME—Many risk factors can be controlled to reduce the risk of stroke.

HOW TO TREAT

GENERAL MEASURES—None specific.

MEDICATION
- Drugs may be prescribed to lower blood pressure, reduce cholesterol level, control diabetes, manage heart rhythm problems, or treat other medical disorders.
- Blood thinners or drugs to help prevent blood clots (e.g., aspirin) may be prescribed for some patients.

ACTIVITY—Try to get 30 minutes a day (or most days) of aerobic exercise, such as walking. Start with a few minutes a day and increase gradually.

DIET
- Eat a healthy diet. Avoid excess fat and sodium (salt).
- A weight-loss diet may be advised for some patients.
- Limit or avoid alcohol use.

CALL YOUR DOCTOR IF

You or a family member has questions or concerns about stroke prevention.

STYE
(Hordeolum)

GENERAL INFORMATION

DEFINITION—A stye is an infection or inflammation (red, sore, swollen) of one of the glands of the upper or lower eyelids. It is typically harmless. The medical term for stye is hordeolum.

BODY PARTS INVOLVED—Eyelid; eyelashes; conjunctiva (white of the eye).

SEX OR AGE MOST AFFECTED—Both sexes; all ages.

SIGNS & SYMPTOMS
* A bump on the edge of the eyelid.
* The eyelid area is red, swollen, painful, or tender. The head of the stye is usually on the outside, but it may be on the underside of the lid.
* Eye may be sensitive to bright light.
* A gritty feeling in the eye.
* Eye may water.

CAUSES—Bacterial infection (most often, staphylococcal) in a hair follicle or a gland in the corner of the eye. The infection may be limited to the eyelid or may have spread from somewhere else in the body.

RISK INCREASES WITH
* Having diabetes or other health problem.
* Blepharitis (infection of eyelid margin).
* High cholesterol.
* History of styes.
* Certain chronic skin problems.

HOW TO PREVENT—There are no specific preventive measures. Use a mild shampoo on eyelashes when bathing or washing face. Don't share eye makeup with anyone.

WHAT TO EXPECT

DIAGNOSTIC MEASURES
* Your own observation of symptoms.
* Consult your health care provider if the stye does not drain or is spreading. Your eye will be examined to make sure there is not another eye problem.

APPROPRIATE HEALTH CARE
* Self-care and time is usually all that is needed.
* Drug therapy may be prescribed.
* Sometimes minor surgery to drain the stye or drugs may be needed to help heal the infection.

POSSIBLE COMPLICATIONS
* Spread of infection to other glands in the eyelid.
* Ongoing infection that may not respond to treatment.

PROBABLE OUTCOME—The infection usually heals on its own. It will drain in about two days. Styes often recur, even with treatment.

HOW TO TREAT

GENERAL MEASURES
* Use warm-water pressure to relieve pain and inflammation and hasten healing. Apply soaks for 10 minutes, then rest at least 1 hour. Repeat as often as needed.
* Don't squeeze the stye. It will soon open and release the pus, bringing relief from the pain.
* Do not wear contact lenses until the infection is resolved.

MEDICATION—Antibiotic ointments or creams may be prescribed. Apply according to package instructions.

ACTIVITY—No limits.

DIET—No special diet.

CALL YOUR DOCTOR IF

* You or a family member has a stye that does not drain on its own.
* Pain occurs in the eye.
* Vision changes.

SUBCONJUNCTIVAL HEMORRHAGE

 GENERAL INFORMATION

DEFINITION—Subconjunctival hemorrhage is the sudden appearance of blood in the white area of the eye. Although the bleeding may seem alarming, it is not serious. The bleeding is from tiny blood vessels under the thin, clear membrane (conjunctiva) that covers the white of the eye (the sclera). Often, a person discovers the problem after waking up in the morning.

BODY PARTS INVOLVED—Eye.

SEX OR AGE MOST AFFECTED—Both sexes; all ages, including newborns.

SIGNS & SYMPTOMS
• A small, usually painless spot of bright red blood in the white of the eye. It may first appear as a patch, but may spread to cover the entire white area of the eye.
• Swelling may occur in that part of the eye.
• There are no vision problems.

CAUSES—When one of the tiny, unseen blood vessels in the conjunctiva breaks, it can bleed and cause the problem. There is often no obvious reason why the vessel breaks. It may follow coughing, sneezing, vomiting, heavy lifting, diving under water, or rubbing of the eyes.

RISK INCREASES WITH—Certain disorders such as high blood pressure, diabetes, or use of blood thinner drugs can be risk factors.

HOW TO PREVENT—No specific preventive measures.

 WHAT TO EXPECT

DIAGNOSTIC MEASURES—Your own observation of symptoms.

APPROPRIATE HEALTH CARE—No treatment is necessary, except time.

POSSIBLE COMPLICATIONS—None expected.

PROBABLE OUTCOME—The blood will go away by itself. It should be absorbed in 1 to 3 weeks. The blood may change color from red to yellow before disappearing.

 HOW TO TREAT

GENERAL MEASURES—Cool compresses may be applied at first. After 24 hours, you may use warm compresses applied to the eye to help hasten the removal of the blood.

MEDICATION
• Drugs are usually not needed for this disorder.
• Nonprescription artificial tears may help if there is any irritation.

ACTIVITY—No rest is needed and you may continue with your regular activities.

DIET—No special diet.

 CALL YOUR DOCTOR IF

• You or a family member has symptoms of subconjunctival hemorrhage with eye pain, your vision changes, or both eyes are affected.
• Your subconjunctival hemorrhage does not get better within 3 weeks, or it recurs often.

SUBDURAL HEMORRHAGE & HEMATOMA

 GENERAL INFORMATION

DEFINITION—Subdural hemorrhage is bleeding that causes blood to collect and clot (hematoma) beneath the outermost of 3 membranes that cover the brain (meninges). There are 2 types of subdural hematomas. An acute subdural hematoma occurs soon after a severe head injury. A chronic subdural hematoma is a complication that may develop days or weeks after a head injury. The injury may have been so minor that the patient does not remember it.

BODY PARTS INVOLVED—Brain; meninges; blood vessels to the brain.

SEX OR AGE MOST AFFECTED—Both sexes; all ages.

SIGNS & SYMPTOMS
- Recurrent headaches that worsen each day.
- Drowsiness or tiredness, dizziness, mental changes, or confusion.
- Weakness or numbness on one side.
- Slurred speech.
- Vision disturbances.
- Nausea and vomiting.
- Pupils of different size.
- Loss of consciousness after original injury.
- Seizures (convulsions).
- An infant may have increased head size, bulging fontanelles (soft spots in the skull), irritability, high-pitched cry, or seizures. Skull fracture can occur with child abuse.

CAUSES—Injury causes the blood vessels (located between the surface of the brain and its outer covering) to tear and spill blood into the subdural space.

RISK INCREASES WITH
- Head injury.
- Excess alcohol use.
- Drugs that thin the blood (anticoagulants).
- Very young or the elderly.
- Child abuse, such as shaken baby syndrome.

HOW TO PREVENT
- Use seat belts in motor vehicles. Don't drink alcohol or use mind-altering drugs and drive.
- Wear protective head gear during contact sports, or while riding a bicycle or motorcycle.
- Use of safety gear at work, such as hard hats.
- Safety measures at home to prevent falls.
- Report any suspected child abuse.
- Get medical care for illnesses that affect consciousness or balance.

 WHAT TO EXPECT

DIAGNOSTIC MEASURES
- Your own or other's observation of symptoms.
- Your health care provider will do a physical exam and ask questions about the symptoms and any recent head injury.
- Medical tests may include studies of blood and cerebrospinal fluid. X-ray, arteriography, CT, and/or MRI are different tests that may help determine the extent of injury.

APPROPRIATE HEALTH CARE
- Hospital care for emergency treatment.
- Treatment steps include lifesaving therapy, controlling symptoms, and preventing permanent brain damage.
- Emergency surgery may be needed to reduce pressure within the brain. This can involve drilling a hole in the skull to let the hematoma drain. Solid clots may be removed through a larger hole (craniotomy).
- Drug therapy may be required.
- In some cases, the hematoma may be small and not as serious. Blood will be absorbed in a few weeks.

POSSIBLE COMPLICATIONS—Death or permanent brain damage, including partial or complete paralysis, behavioral and personality changes, and speech problems.

PROBABLE OUTCOME—The degree of recovery depends upon general health, age, severity of the injury, rapidity of the treatment, and severity of the bleeding or clot. After the clot is removed, brain tissue that has been compressed usually expands slowly to fill its original space. The outlook is good under the best circumstances.

 HOW TO TREAT

GENERAL MEASURES—Follow medical advice.

MEDICATION
- You may be prescribed:
  - Drugs to reduce swelling inside the skull.
  - Anticonvulsant drugs for seizures.
  - Other drugs for specific symptoms.

ACTIVITY—During recovery stay as active as your strength allows. Work and exercise moderately. Rest when you tire. If your speech or muscle control has been damaged, you may need physical therapy or speech therapy.

DIET—Most likely will require intravenous or tube feeding during acute phase and then shift to regular food as tolerated.

 CALL YOUR DOCTOR IF

- You or someone else has a head injury (even if it seems minor) and develops any symptoms of subdural hemorrhage. This is an emergency!
- Fever, surgical wound becomes infected (red, swollen, or tender), headache recurs, or other symptoms occur during or after treatment.

SUBSTANCE ABUSE

 GENERAL INFORMATION

DEFINITION
• Substance abuse is the continuing misuse of any mind altering substances or chemicals. There is a loss of self-control and a compulsion to continue despite adverse personal, physical, mental, and social outcomes that may result. Common substances of abuse include:
- Nicotine and alcohol.
- Marijuana.
- Amphetamines; barbiturates; cocaine.
- Opiates. These include codeine, heroin, opium, morphine, methadone, hydrocodone, and oxycodone.
- Anabolic steroids.
- Psychedelic or hallucinogenic drugs (club drugs), including PCP ("angel dust"), mescaline, GHB, and LSD.
- Volatile substances, such as glue, solvents, and paints that are inhaled.
- Misuse of cough remedy dextromethorphan.

BODY PARTS INVOLVED—Whole body.

SEX OR AGE MOST AFFECTED—Males more than females; adolescents and young adults.

SIGNS & SYMPTOMS
• Symptoms vary depending on substance.
• A temporary pleasant mood.
• Relief from anxiety.
• False feelings of self-confidence and being in control.
• Increased sensitivity to sights and sounds (including hallucinations).
• Altered activity levels (lethargy and sleep-like states, or frenzied states [being very active]).
• Unpleasant or painful symptoms when abused substance is no longer used (withdrawal).
• Tolerance (need more of the substance to get "high").
• Other persons may observe new and odd behavior changes.

CAUSES—For most people, the first time use of a substance of abuse is voluntary. Repeated use causes changes in the brain and leads to addiction. It is a disease, not just a matter of willpower.

RISK INCREASES WITH
• Family history of drug or alcohol abuse.
• Family problems (conflict, stress, lack of closeness, poor parenting, loss of job, physical or sexual abuse).
• Genetic factors (more prone to addiction).
• Peer pressure, especially in teenagers.
• Fatigue or overwork; problems at work or school.
• Ease of obtaining the substances of abuse.
• Emotional problems, including depression, dependency, poor self-esteem, anxiety, and stress.

HOW TO PREVENT
• Don't socialize with persons who abuse drugs.
• Medical care for emotional or mental problems.
• Parents who are involved in a child's life.
• Drug education and prevention programs.

 WHAT TO EXPECT

DIAGNOSTIC MEASURES
• Your own or other's observation of symptoms.
• Your health care provider may do a physical exam.
• Medical tests may include blood studies and substance abuse screening studies.

APPROPRIATE HEALTH CARE
• Treatment can be voluntary or involuntary. Family, legal, or job factors may lead a person into treatment.
• No single treatment works for everyone. A plan needs to address the person's type of abuse, their physical and emotional health, and job, social, and legal aspects. A person is rarely able to quit without some help.
• The plan may require a combination of counseling, drug therapy, other medical services, family therapy, parenting instruction, job training, and social and legal services. Treatment may take 3 months, or up to a year.
• Counseling (group or alone) helps in recovery.
• Symptoms of withdrawal will be treated.

POSSIBLE COMPLICATIONS
• Accidents, infections, other health problems.
• Relapse after treatment.
• Loss of job or family. Involvement in crime and violence. Legal problems. Death from overdose.

PROBABLE OUTCOME—Successful recovery from substance abuse can improve all aspects of one's life. It is not easy, but it can be done.

 HOW TO TREAT

GENERAL MEASURES
• Join a local support group.
• To learn more: Substance Abuse & Mental Health Services Administration; (800) 726-4727; website: www.samhsa.gov.

MEDICATION—Your health care provider may prescribe drugs to help you through withdrawal symptoms. Other drugs may be prescribed to treat emotional or mental problems.

ACTIVITY—Exercise on a regular basis.

DIET—No special diet.

☎ **CALL YOUR DOCTOR IF**

You or a family member has a problem with, or has symptoms of, substance abuse.

SUNBURN

GENERAL INFORMATION

DEFINITION—Sunburn is redness and soreness of the skin that follows excess exposure to the sun or tanning devices.

BODY PARTS INVOLVED—Exposed skin.

SEX OR AGE MOST AFFECTED—Both sexes; all ages.

SIGNS & SYMPTOMS
• Sunburn symptoms develop 2 to 4 hours after exposure.
• Red, swollen, hot, and (sometimes) blistered skin. Pain occurs and is worse in the first 6 to 48 hours.
• Fever, nausea, and feeling faint (sometimes).

CAUSES—Melanin, a pigment, in the skin helps to protect the skin from exposure to the ultraviolet light from the sun. When there is overexposure, the melanin is unable to keep up the protection, and sunburn occurs.

RISK INCREASES WITH
• People who have fair skin, blue eyes, and red or blonde hair.
• Sun exposure from 10:00 am to 4:00 pm.
• Certain drugs, soaps, or cosmetics may cause a photosensitive reaction. This causes the skin to be even more sensitive to the sun.
• Living close to the equator or at high altitudes.

HOW TO PREVENT
• Avoid the sun from 10:00 am to 4:00 pm when possible. Sunburn can occur even on cloudy days. Ultraviolet light is not blocked by thin clouds on overcast days. It is partially screened by smoke and smog. A great deal of ultraviolet light can reflect from snow, water, sand, and sidewalks.
• Use sunscreen daily. Use products with a sun-protective factor (SPF) of 15 or more (an SPF of 30 or more is recommended by some experts). Some of these resist water and perspiration. Reapply them every 2 hours or after swimming. Baby oil, mineral oil, and cocoa butter offer no protection from the sun.
• For the best protection, use a physical barrier agent such as zinc oxide or titanium oxide ointment. Reapply after swimming and at frequent intervals during exposure. Barrier agents are helpful on skin areas that are more likely to burn. These include the nose, ears, backs of the legs, and back of the neck.
• Wear clothing that covers your whole body. Protect your face with a wide-brimmed hat. Wear sunglasses.
• If you feel you must get a tan, do it very gradually. A "base" tan is not proven to offer protection from sunburn.

WHAT TO EXPECT

DIAGNOSTIC MEASURES—See your health care provider for severe sunburn or if you have other symptoms such as nausea, vomiting, or swelling. An exam of the affected area will be done and treatment prescribed for any complications.

APPROPRIATE HEALTH CARE—Self-care is usually all that is needed. Medical care may rarely be required for severe symptoms.

POSSIBLE COMPLICATIONS
• Blisters may become infected.
• Years of overexposure to the sun can lead to wrinkled, saggy, and leathery skin. The risk of skin cancer is greatly increased.

PROBABLE OUTCOME—Recovery in 3 days to 3 weeks. Tanning or peeling of the skin usually occurs, depending on severity of the sunburn.

HOW TO TREAT

GENERAL MEASURES
• To reduce heat and pain, dip gauze or towels in cool water and lay these on the burned areas. Take cool showers.
• Soak in a tub of cool water to which an oatmeal product (Aveeno) or baking soda has been added. Pat skin dry, do not rub. Use a moisturizer to keep the skin from feeling dry.
• If blisters occur, do not break them. They aid in the healing process.

MEDICATION
• Use nonprescription drugs, such as antihistamines, aspirin (not for children), or acetaminophen to help relieve discomfort.
• Ask your health care provider about using nonprescription burn remedies that contain local anesthetics such as benzocaine or lidocaine. They can produce allergic reactions in some persons.
• Drugs for pain or cortisone drugs to use briefly may be prescribed.

ACTIVITY—Rest in any comfortable position until symptoms get better. Cover yourself with an upside-down "cradle" or tent of cardboard or other material. This will keep bed linens off the burned skin.

DIET—No special diet. Increase fluid intake.

CALL YOUR DOCTOR IF

You or a family member has sunburn that seems severe or there are other symptoms from sun exposure.

SURGICAL WOUND INFECTION

 GENERAL INFORMATION

DEFINITION—A surgical wound infection is one that develops after a surgical procedure. Infections after surgery occur in 1.5% to 30% of cases, depending on the type of procedure. The medical term is surgical site infections (SSIs).

BODY PARTS INVOLVED—Surgery site.

SEX OR AGE MOST AFFECTED—Both sexes; all ages.

SIGNS & SYMPTOMS
- Symptoms usually begin within 5 to 10 days after surgery, but in some cases, they begin weeks later.
- Pain, redness, and heat around the surgical wound.
- Pus and other collections of fluid around the incision.
- Red streaks in the skin around the wound.
- Fever, chills (sometimes).

CAUSES—Infection with bacteria. These include *streptococcus*, *staphylococcus*, or other germs. These sometimes cause infection, in spite of careful preventive measures. Germs get into wounds by direct contact (e.g., from instruments or surgical team), being airborne, or self-contamination.

RISK INCREASES WITH
- Very young and very old persons.
- Poor nutrition (weakness from not being able to eat).
- A pre-existing illness, such as diabetes.
- Weak immune system due to illness or drugs.
- Obese patients.
- Smoking.
- Other infection at the time of surgery.
- Type of surgery being performed.
- Type of surgery wound. It may range from clean to contaminated, depending on several medical factors.
- Increased length of time for the surgery.
- Emergency surgery.

HOW TO PREVENT
- Surgery team members need to follow all medical guidelines for preventing wound infections.
- In some cases, antibiotic drugs may be given to help prevent infections.

 WHAT TO EXPECT

DIAGNOSTIC MEASURES
- Your own or other's observation of symptoms.
- Your health care provider will do a physical exam of the surgical wound area.
- Medical tests may include blood tests and a culture of pus or blood from the infection site.

APPROPRIATE HEALTH CARE
- Treatment may include antibiotic drugs and wound-cleaning procedures.
- Surgery to open the wound and remove infected or damaged tissue or treat an abscess may be required.
- Negative pressure wound therapy may be an option.

POSSIBLE COMPLICATIONS
- Delayed healing.
- Sepsis (also called blood poisoning) is a bloodstream infection.
- Chronic infection in some patients.

PROBABLE OUTCOME—In most patients, surgical wound infections heal in about 2 weeks.

 HOW TO TREAT

GENERAL MEASURES
- After treatment, relieve pain with heat. Use a heating pad or warm compress 3 or 4 times a day for 30 to 40 minutes.
- Change wound dressings as directed.

MEDICATION
- Antibiotics may be prescribed for an infection. They may be taken by mouth or given intravenously (into a vein).
- Vitamin and mineral supplements may be prescribed to hasten healing.
- You may use nonprescription drugs, such as acetaminophen, to relieve minor pain.

ACTIVITY—Limits will depend on the severity of the symptoms. Follow your health care provider's instructions.

DIET—Usually, no special diet required.

 CALL YOUR DOCTOR IF

- You or a family member has symptoms of a surgical-wound infection.
- High fever occurs and a general ill feeling, or infection seems to worsen after treatment.
- New, unexplained symptoms develop.

SYPHILIS

GENERAL INFORMATION

DEFINITION—Syphilis is a sexually transmitted disease. It is known as the "great mimic," because its symptoms are like those of many other diseases. There are two types. Congenital form occurs in babies (age 0 to 2 weeks) born to mothers with syphilis. Contagious form is the type that affects persons of all ages and both sexes who get it by sexual contact. There may be no symptoms or very mild ones. A person may not know they are infected.

BODY PARTS INVOLVED—Genitals; skin; central nervous system.

SEX OR AGE MOST AFFECTED
• Newborns born to mothers with syphilis.
• Persons of all ages and both sexes who have sexual contact.

SIGNS & SYMPTOMS
• Primary stage (contagious; begins 9 to 90 days after exposure; usually at about 3 weeks):
  - A painless, red sore (chancre) on the genitals, mouth, or rectum. The sore usually affects the penis in males and vagina or cervix in females.
• Secondary stage (occurs if not treated; contagious; begins 2 to 8 weeks after the chancre appears):
  - Enlarged lymph glands in the neck, armpit, or groin.
  - Headache, sore throat, and feeling tired.
  - Rash on skin and mucous membranes of the penis, vagina, or mouth. The rash has small, red, scaly bumps.
  - Fever (sometimes).
• Latent stage or hidden stage (can be 2 to 30 years after second stage; may be contagious):
  - There are no signs or symptoms.
• Tertiary stage (rare; not contagious; may appear 2 to 30 years after other stages):
  - The infection can seriously damage the heart, brain, nervous system, eyes, skin, bones, and joints.

CAUSES
• A germ (bacteria) called *Treponema pallidum*.
• Contagious form is spread by sexual contact (vaginal, anal, or oral sex) with someone who has the sores or rash. Germs cannot be spread from toilet seats, towels, or other objects.
• Congenital form passes to a baby by an infected mother.

RISK INCREASES WITH—Unsafe sex.

HOW TO PREVENT
• Latex male condoms used during sexual contact help stop the risk, but do not provide 100% protection.
• Avoid sexual contact with an infected person or a person whose health history you don't know.

• Obtain blood test for syphilis early in pregnancy. If infected, get treatment right away.

WHAT TO EXPECT

DIAGNOSTIC MEASURES
• Your own observation of symptoms.
• Your health care provider will do a physical exam.
• Blood tests and microscope studies of material from a sore are usually done to confirm the diagnosis. Tests for other sexually transmitted diseases are often done.

APPROPRIATE HEALTH CARE
• Syphilis is treated with drugs.
• Be sure that all your sexual partners obtain treatment. The public health department will help you if needed.
• After drug treatment, blood tests will be done at regular intervals to verify that you are no longer infectious.
• The tertiary stage of syphilis generally requires treatment in a hospital.

POSSIBLE COMPLICATIONS
• After penicillin treatment, you may have a Jarisch-Herxheimer reaction. A fever, headache, muscle aches, and other symptoms may last for about 24 hours.
• Treatment in a few patients may need to be repeated.
• Syphilis sores makes it easier to get an HIV infection.
• Without treatment, the disease may progress to the next stage. A number of medical problems and death may occur with tertiary syphilis.

PROBABLE OUTCOME—Curable with antibiotic treatment.

HOW TO TREAT

GENERAL MEASURES—To learn more: Centers for Disease Control & Prevention (CDC); 800232-4636; website: www.cdc.gov.

MEDICATION—Penicillin will be given by injection for all stages. If someone is allergic to penicillin, other antibiotics are equally effective.

ACTIVITY—Avoid sexual activity until cured.

DIET—No special diet.

CALL YOUR DOCTOR IF

• You or a family member has symptoms of syphilis.
• Symptoms recur after treatment.
• You had sexual contact with person who has syphilis.

TAPEWORM

GENERAL INFORMATION

DEFINITION—Tapeworm is a parasitic infection of the digestive tract or other organs. Tapeworms are typically acquired from eating undercooked meat or fish.

BODY PARTS INVOLVED—Intestinal tract.

SEX OR AGE MOST AFFECTED—Both sexes; all ages.

SIGNS & SYMPTOMS
* Most people with this problem have no symptoms.
* Pain in the upper abdomen.
* Diarrhea.
* Unexplained weight loss.
* Symptoms of anemia (weakness, fatigue, and shortness of breath).
* Bowel movements containing worm eggs and worm body parts.

CAUSES
* Parasites: *Taenia saginata* from beef, *Taenia solium* from pork, and *Diphyllobothrium* from fish. People become infected by eating improperly cooked or raw food infected with the parasite.
* *Echinococcus* tapeworm is found in dogs and some livestock (often in sheep). Humans can get an infection (echinococcosis) from this tapeworm. Infected dogs leave feces in soil or water. Humans are infected by eating food grown in the soil or drinking the water. It can also be spread by handling an infected dog or livestock. The infection causes cysts (sores), usually in the liver. Symptoms may not develop for 10 to 20 years after exposure.

RISK INCREASES WITH—Travel to places such as Asia, Africa, or Latin America. This disorder is uncommon in the United States.

HOW TO PREVENT
* Cook beef, pork, and fish thoroughly. Additional information available from the National Center for Nutrition (800) 366-1655 or the Department of Agriculture Meat and Poultry Hotline (800) 535-4555.
* Buy only meat that has been inspected.
* Wash your hands after handling any raw meat or fish.
* Keep pet dogs clean and dewormed. Wash hands after handling pets or livestock.

WHAT TO EXPECT

DIAGNOSTIC MEASURES
* Your own observation of symptoms.
* Your health care provider may do a physical exam.
* Medical tests usually include a study of a stool sample to check for eggs or worms. If echinococcosis is suspected, an x-ray or blood study may be done.

APPROPRIATE HEALTH CARE
* The usual treatment is with drug therapy.
* Cysts from echinococcosis infection may need to be removed surgically.
* Have all family members examined for possible infection.

POSSIBLE COMPLICATIONS
* Cysticercosis, a more widespread infection from tapeworm larvae (rare).
* Obstruction of intestine (rare).
* Echinococcosis can cause severe health problems including death.

PROBABLE OUTCOME—Usually curable with appropriate treatment.

HOW TO TREAT

GENERAL MEASURES—Follow medical advice.

MEDICATION—Anthelmintic (antiparasitic) drug to kill the parasite will be prescribed. The drug can cure with a single dose. Medical tests should be repeated in 3 to 6 weeks to make sure the disorder is cured.

ACTIVITY—No limits.

DIET—No special diet.

CALL YOUR DOCTOR IF

* You or a family member has symptoms of a tapeworm.
* New, unexplained symptoms develop. Drugs used in treatment may produce side effects.

TASTE & SMELL DISORDERS

 GENERAL INFORMATION

DEFINITION
- A taste disorder may involve a distorted sense of taste (dysgeusia) or decrease in taste (hypogeusia) or a rare total loss of taste (ageusia). Taste buds on the tongue can detect sweet, sour, salty, bitter, and umami (savory) tastes. Often, what one perceives as "taste" is actually smell. People with taste problems often have a smell disorder that makes it hard to identify a food's flavor. Flavor is a combination of taste and smell. The sense of smell contributes to 75% of flavor sensations.
- A smell disorder may involve a distorted sense of smell (dysosmia) or decreased ability to detect odors (hyposmia) or complete loss of sense of smell (anosmia).

BODY PARTS INVOLVED—Olfactory nerve cells in the nose and gustatory nerve cells in mouth and throat that send messages to brain.

SEX OR AGE MOST AFFECTED—Both sexes; usually older adults.

SIGNS & SYMPTOMS
- Phantom taste perception (tasting something that isn't there); a reduced ability to taste sweet, sour, bitter, and salty; or a distorted taste.
- Familiar odors become distorted. An odor that usually smells pleasant may smell foul. May perceive an odor that isn't present.
- May not feel satisfied after eating. Person may eat too much and gain weight or may eat too little and lose weight. May use too much sugar and/or salt in an effort to make food taste better.

CAUSES—Taste and smell disorders can be caused by numerous medical disorders, injuries, surgeries, oral health problems, environmental factors, certain drugs, aging, or congenital conditions. Sometimes, no cause is found (idiopathic).

RISK INCREASES WITH
- Upper respiratory infections (colds and flu).
- Breathing allergies.
- Nasal congestion from irritants, such as pollutants and cigarette smoke.
- Sinus infections.
- Nasal polyps.
- Head injury.
- Aging (taste and smell senses decrease after age 60).
- Exposure to certain chemicals, such as insecticides and solvents.
- Certain drugs, such as antibiotics and blood pressure pills.
- Radiation therapy for head and neck cancers.
- Poor oral hygiene or dental problems.
- Some surgeries to ear, nose, or throat.
- Smoking or cocaine use.
- A number of other health problems.

HOW TO PREVENT—No specific preventive measures. Avoid risk factors where possible. Get medical care for treatable risk factors.

 WHAT TO EXPECT

DIAGNOSTIC MEASURES
- Your own observation of symptoms.
- Your health care provider will do an oral and nasal exam and ask questions about the symptoms and your medical history.
- Medical tests can include smell and taste tests. Other tests depend on suspected causes. They may include blood studies, CT, or MRI.

APPROPRIATE HEALTH CARE
- Some taste and smell disorders can be treated, but others cannot (e.g., aging).
- Treatment may include treating an underlying medical condition, changing or adjusting drugs, surgery (e.g., for polyps), and lifestyle changes (e.g., modify diet).
- Counseling may help you cope with the loss.

POSSIBLE COMPLICATIONS
- Taste or smell loss becomes permanent.
- Can affect everyday enjoyment of food.
- Impairs ability to smell odors such as smoke, natural gas leaks, and spoiled food.
- Anxiety, depression, or poor nutrition.

PROBABLE OUTCOME—Often, the sense of taste or smell returns when underlying cause resolves. Treatment of other causes can help, but recovery of taste and smell can take weeks or months. Changes in lifestyle may help.

 HOW TO TREAT

GENERAL MEASURES
- Stop smoking. It impairs both taste and smell.
- For home safety, install smoke alarms and natural gas detectors.
- Get regular dental care.

MEDICATION—Drugs for an underlying cause or its symptoms may be prescribed. No specific drug is available to treat loss of taste or smell.

ACTIVITY—No limits.

DIET
- Eat warm food, flavor-enhanced foods, or stronger flavored foods. Be careful not to add too much salt or sugar. Increase flavor with herbs. Prepare foods with a variety of colors and textures.
- Write dates on stored foods to avoid eating food that is spoiled.
- A dietitian can help with recipes.

 CALL YOUR DOCTOR IF

You or a family member has taste or smell loss.

TAY-SACHS DISEASE

 GENERAL INFORMATION

DEFINITION—Tay-Sachs disease is a rare, inherited disorder in which harmful quantities of a fatty substance build up in the central nervous system. The classic form causes progressive impairment and early death. Less than 100 children are born with the disease each year in the United States.

BODY PARTS INVOLVED—Brain and central nervous system.

SEX OR AGE MOST AFFECTED—Infants and young children (up to age 5).

SIGNS & SYMPTOMS
- The child seems normal at birth. Symptoms begin to appear before 6 months.
- Loss of alertness and retarded mental development.
- Loss of muscle strength, such as difficulty sitting up or turning over.
- Unable to swallow.
- Deafness.
- Blindness.
- Severe constipation caused by an impaired nerve supply to the colon.
- Seizures.

CAUSES
- An inherited disease resulting from a recessive gene that causes enzyme deficiency. If both parents have the gene, they have a 25% chance of having a child with Tay-Sachs disease. If only one parent is a carrier, the children will not have the disease. The gene occurs in 1 out of 60 people of Ashkenazi Jewish or French Canadian ancestry.
- Other forms of Tay-Sachs include:
  - Juvenile form which appears about ages 2 to 5. Symptoms are like the classic form and death occurs by age 15.
  - Chronic form may appear at age 5. Symptoms are like classic form but are milder.
  - Adult form, which appears between teens and 30s. Symptoms are like the chronic form.

RISK INCREASES WITH—Genetic factors. Many parents who carry the recessive gene are of Eastern European Jewish (Ashkenazi) or French Canadian origin.

HOW TO PREVENT
- A simple blood test can identify Tay-Sachs carriers. It can't be used in pregnant women. For pregnant women, an amniocentesis or chorionic villus testing can be done.
- Obtain genetic counseling if you or your spouse have a family history of Tay-Sachs or are of Ashkenazi or French Canadian background.
- Assisted reproductive technologies can be used to help at-risk couples have a non-affected baby.

 WHAT TO EXPECT

DIAGNOSTIC MEASURES
- Your own observation of symptoms.
- To make the diagnosis, your baby's health care provider will do a physical exam and an eye exam. A cherry-red spot at the back of the eye occurs in a baby with Tay-Sachs disease.
- A blood test will be done to confirm the diagnosis.

APPROPRIATE HEALTH CARE
- Treatment consists of providing comfort and support for the baby.
- Counseling may help parents and siblings to learn to cope with the distress produced by this condition.

POSSIBLE COMPLICATIONS—Symptoms progress to loss of all voluntary movement, which eventually causes death.

PROBABLE OUTCOME—There is no cure or treatment. Death usually occurs before age 5 with the classic form. Research is ongoing.

 HOW TO TREAT

GENERAL MEASURES
- Join support groups for families of Tay-Sachs victims.
- To learn more: National Tay-Sachs and Allied Disease Association, 2001 Beacon St., Suite 204, Brookline, MA 02146; (800) 906-8723; website: www.ntsad.org.

MEDICATION
- Anticonvulsants to control seizures.
- Stool softeners and laxatives to relieve constipation.
- Other drugs to help with complications as they arise.

ACTIVITY—In the early stages, encourage the child to be as active as possible. Increasing loss of mental, nervous, and muscular functions will eventually confine the child to bed much of the time.

DIET—Provide plenty of fluids and a normal, high-fiber diet to reduce constipation. Feeding by tube usually becomes necessary as the disease progresses.

 CALL YOUR DOCTOR IF

- You are concerned about your infant's mental and physical development.
- You think you or any member of your family carries the abnormal gene. A genetic counselor can advise you on how to prevent having children with this disease.

TEAR DUCT INFECTION OR BLOCKAGE
(Dacryocystitis; Dacryostenosis)

 GENERAL INFORMATION

DEFINITION—An infected or blocked tear duct causes tears to gather or pool in the eyes and then run down the cheeks even though the person is not crying. Infection of the tear duct is called dacryocystitis. It is most common in children. A blocked tear duct is called dacryostenosis. It may occur in infants ages 3 to 12 weeks or in older children and adults.

BODY PARTS INVOLVED—Eye; tear (nasolacrimal) gland, sac or duct.

SEX OR AGE MOST AFFECTED—Both sexes; all ages.

SIGNS & SYMPTOMS
- Increased tearing of one or both eyes.
- Mucus and pus drains out of the tear duct. It may drain on its own or come out when pressure is put on the area.
- Pain, redness, or swelling of the eye area.
- Fever (sometimes).

CAUSES—Tears are stored in a sac (lacrimal sac) and are released into the eyes to help keep them clean, for protection, and to provide lubrication. The tears drain out of the eyes through small pinpoint openings in the corner of the eyes. They then flow through a duct or tube into the nose. The duct is called the nasolacrimal duct. When infection or blockage occurs in the duct, the tears cannot drain normally and they back up.

RISK INCREASES WITH
- Tear duct that is not fully developed or formed properly in a newborn.
- Bacterial infection of the duct.
- Sinus or nasal infection, or abnormal growths or tumors.
- Surgery on the face, nose, or sinuses.
- Eye injury.
- Conjunctivitis (pink eye).
- Fracture of the nose or facial bones.
- Thickening of the tear duct lining as a person ages.

HOW TO PREVENT—No specific preventive measures. Get prompt medical treatment for eye, nose, or sinus infections. For contact sports, wear helmets and facemasks to protect the face from injury.

 WHAT TO EXPECT

DIAGNOSTIC MEASURES
- Your own observation of symptoms.
- Your health care provider will do a physical exam of the eye area.

- A sample of the discharge may be tested to check for the germs causing the infection. To confirm the diagnosis, a harmless dye may be placed in the eye. This helps determine if tears are flowing normally. Other tests may be needed in adults.

APPROPRIATE HEALTH CARE
- Treatment may involve drugs for infection, massaging the area, and, for some, surgery to open the duct. In some cases, no treatment is needed.
- If there is excessive tearing, surgery may be recommended to probe the tear duct. A thin wire is passed through the duct to open any obstruction.
- Other surgery options involve placing tubes in the tear duct that stay in for about 6 months or inserting a balloon that stretches the tear duct and then is removed.
- In adults, tear ducts damaged by chronic infection may need to be surgically replaced by creating a new passage or inserting an artificial duct. Tumors or nasal polyps may need to be removed with surgery.

POSSIBLE COMPLICATIONS—A blocked tear duct may cause chronic infection. Infection may spread to other areas of the face.

PROBABLE OUTCOME—Infected or blocked tear ducts are usually cured with treatment. Blocked tear ducts in an infant are usually outgrown when they are 9 to 12 months of age.

 HOW TO TREAT

GENERAL MEASURES
- Clean any drainage from the eye with a cotton ball or washcloth moistened with warm water. Gently wipe away any pus or crusted areas.
- For a child with a blocked duct, massage can help. Do it several times a day for 2 months, or as directed. Wash your hands carefully. Place your index finger alongside the nose and firmly massage down toward the corner of the nose. Use a warm compress on the eye area to provide comfort and promote drainage.

MEDICATION—Antibiotics for infection may be prescribed. These may be eyedrops, eye ointment, or drugs taken by mouth.

ACTIVITY—No limits unless advised.

DIET—No special diet.

 CALL YOUR DOCTOR IF

- You or a family member has symptoms of a tear duct infection or blockage.
- Symptoms don't improve or vision changes.

TEETHING
(Cutting Teeth; Tooth Eruption)

GENERAL INFORMATION

DEFINITION
• Teething is a normal process that occurs when a baby's teeth grow and break (erupt) through the gums. New teeth erupt continually from around age 6 months to 3 years.
• The timing of teeth eruption is highly variable. However, the sequence of normal tooth eruption in children is:
   - First teeth (lower front teeth) at about 6 months, sooner in girls than boys. Teething may start as early as one month or as late as one year. Rarely, a baby is born with one or more teeth visible.
   - Complete set of baby teeth by about age two and a half.
   - First adult teeth at about age 6.
   - Bicuspids (side teeth) between ages 10 and 12.
   - Permanent molars at about age 12.

BODY PARTS INVOLVED—Mouth; teeth.

SEX OR AGE MOST AFFECTED—Both sexes of children from ages 6 months to 3 years and 6 to 12 years.

SIGNS & SYMPTOMS
• Excess saliva production, drooling, and chewing on anything the baby can hold.
• Pain. (This symptom cannot be proven, but probably does occur.)
• Gums may become red or swollen.
• Irritability.
• Fretful and clinging.
• Difficulty in sleeping.
• Crying more than usual.
• Teething should never be considered the cause of fever, vomiting, diarrhea, prolonged loss of appetite, earache, convulsions, cough, or diaper rash. These are symptoms of an illness.

CAUSES—Teething is normal. There are 20 baby (or primary) teeth and 32 permanent teeth.

RISK INCREASES WITH—Teething problems are not related to any known risk factor.

HOW TO PREVENT—Teething problems cannot be prevented, but the symptoms can be relieved.

WHAT TO EXPECT

DIAGNOSTIC MEASURES
• Your own observation of teething symptoms.
• Your baby's health care provider will examine the baby's mouth and gums and any new teeth at well-baby check ups.

APPROPRIATE HEALTH CARE—Home care is all that is needed. Follow any special medical instructions if advised.

POSSIBLE COMPLICATIONS—None expected.

PROBABLE OUTCOME—Teething discomfort can be partially relieved.

HOW TO TREAT

GENERAL MEASURES
• Rub the child's gums with a clean finger; this is very comforting.
• Freeze a wet washcloth for the baby to chew on.
• Offer the child a safe, one-piece teething ring. It can be cooled in the refrigerator (don't freeze the ring).
• Don't put anything into the baby's mouth that might cause choking. Don't tie anything around the neck.
• Sucking a thumb, finger, or pacifier will not harm the baby's teeth. If sucking continues after age 3, talk to your child's dentist to see if there are any concerns.
• Clean new teeth and gums with your finger using a soft washcloth. When the teeth are bigger, start brushing them with a baby's toothbrush.
• Wipe baby's face often using a soft cloth to remove drool to help prevent rashes.
• At age five, explain to the child that losing baby teeth is normal. This prevents the child from becoming concerned when tooth loss begins.

MEDICATION—Medicine is not usually needed for teething. In some cases, the baby's health care provider may suggest an oral or topical pain reliever.

ACTIVITY—No limits.

DIET
• Don't let your baby go to bed or walk around with a bottle with milk in it. Milk that stays in contact with the teeth for a long time can cause decay.
• Start your baby or toddler off to a healthy diet that will promote healthy teeth. Avoid too many sweets, sticky foods, or constant snacks during the day.

CALL YOUR DOCTOR IF

• Your child's temperature rises above normal.
• Signs of infection such as pain, pus, a lot of swelling, or very red gums occur.

TELOGEN EFFLUVIUM

GENERAL INFORMATION

DEFINITION—Telogen effluvium is a common hair loss disorder in which numerous, scattered hair follicles simultaneously change from the growth phase (called anagen) to the resting phase (called telogen) of the hair-growth cycle. The disorder can be acute (short term) or chronic (long term). Persons with telogen effluvium rarely progress to significant baldness and it is not contagious.

BODY PARTS INVOLVED—Scalp hair usually. It can cause hair loss on all parts of the body.

SEX OR AGE MOST AFFECTED—Both sexes (somewhat more common in females) and all ages; even infants can be affected.

SIGNS & SYMPTOMS
- Hair loss at much more than the normal rate. Normal hair loss is about 100 hairs a day (on a comb or brush, on a pillow, or in the sink).
- No itching or pain.

CAUSES—Major stresses that affect the body's systems. The hair loss may begin several months after the event (such as childbirth) occurred.

RISK INCREASES WITH
- Illness (acute or chronic).
- Major surgery.
- Severe trauma.
- Severe emotional stress or chronic stress.
- High fever.
- Thyroid gland problems.
- Changes in diet (such as crash dieting, low protein intake, anorexia, and iron deficiency).
- Hormonal changes (such as those that occur during adolescence, following childbirth or starting or discontinuing use of oral contraceptives).
- Certain drugs (such as beta blockers, anticoagulants, and others, and immunizations).

HOW TO PREVENT—No specific preventive measures.

WHAT TO EXPECT

DIAGNOSTIC MEASURES
- Your own observation of symptoms.
- Your health care provider will do a physical exam of the scalp and ask questions about your symptoms and activities.
- Medical tests may be done to check for any underlying medical disorder.
- You may be asked to collect all hairs that are shed for a 24 hour period. This test may be repeated 3 to 4 times over several weeks. If the number shed decreases, then the disorder is resolving itself.

APPROPRIATE HEALTH CARE—No specific treatment is usually needed.

POSSIBLE COMPLICATIONS—None expected.

PROBABLE OUTCOME—Spontaneous recovery in 6 to 12 months.

HOW TO TREAT

GENERAL MEASURES
- Continue to wash and brush your hair as usual. A change of hair style may disguise the hair loss and improve cosmetic appearance.
- To learn more: American Hair Loss Association, 23679 Calabasas Rd #682, Calabasas, CA 91301; website: www.americanhairloss.org.

MEDICATION
- Drugs are usually not necessary for this disorder. They may be prescribed if an underlying disorder is diagnosed.
- Nonprescription hair growth products for the scalp may be tried if desired.
- If a drug you take is the cause, your health care provider will discuss other options.

ACTIVITY—No limits. Engage in a regular exercise program at 3 or more times a week to reduce stress and maintain good overall fitness.

DIET—If diet problems are involved, consult a dietitian. Steps can be taken to be sure a healthy diet is a part of your lifestyle.

CALL YOUR DOCTOR IF

- Hair loss doesn't improve in 4 months.
- Signs of infection (pain, redness, tenderness, swelling) begin at the site of hair loss.

TEMPOROMANDIBULAR JOINT DISORDERS

 GENERAL INFORMATION

DEFINITION—Temporomandibular joint (TMJ) disorders are conditions that affect the temporomandibular joint. This is the joint on either side of the lower jaw that opens and closes the mouth. Normally the jaw, the skull, the muscles that attach to and move the jaw, and the involved nerves work together in a smooth relationship. The symptoms develop when an imbalance occurs in the way one or more of these parts function.

BODY PARTS INVOLVED—Temporomandibular joint; facial muscles; nerves.

SEX OR AGE MOST AFFECTED—Adults of both sexes, but more common in women.

SIGNS & SYMPTOMS
* Symptoms may come on slowly or they may begin suddenly if there is an injury to the area.
* Dull, aching pain on one side of the jaw. It occurs below or in front of the ear, in the temples, in back of the head, and along the jaw line.
* It may hurt to chew.
* "Clicking" or "popping" joint sounds.
* Unable to open the jaw all the way or, rarely, jaw may "lock" in open position.
* Headache, dizziness, and toothache.
* Ears feel pressured, clogged, aching, or you may hear ringing.
* Tired facial muscles from yawning, speaking, or when waking up. Head, shoulder, and neck muscles may ache.

CAUSES—The cause is often unknown. There are known contributing factors. Genetic, hormone, and environmental factors may play roles.

RISK INCREASES WITH
* Physical and emotional stress.
* Joint is affected by jaw, head, or neck injuries.
* Grinding or clenching teeth (e.g., during sleep).
* Chewing gum or biting nails.
* Tension of the masticatory (chewing) muscles.
* Faulty alignment ("bite") between the upper and lower jaws (disc derangement).
* Osteoarthritis, rheumatoid arthritis, or gout.
* Work habits such as holding a phone between shoulder and ear.

HOW TO PREVENT—No specific preventive measures. Avoid risk factors where possible.

 WHAT TO EXPECT

DIAGNOSTIC MEASURES
* Your own observation of symptoms.
* Your health care provider will do a physical exam of the jaw area and ask questions about your symptoms and habits.
* Medical tests may include jaw range-of-motion studies, x-rays, and others.

APPROPRIATE HEALTH CARE
* Treatment plans may include lifestyle changes, drugs for pain, diet changes, and simple jaw exercises. For tooth or denture problems, see a dental care provider.
* Counseling may be helpful for stress problems.
* Simple jaw exercises may help. You will be instructed on how to do stretching and relaxing exercises.
* You may be fitted with a special splint or biteplate that will help reduce clenching or teeth grinding.
* A procedure to wash out the joint or inject pain drugs may be done in a medical office with local anesthesia.
* Severe cases that do not respond to simpler measures may need surgery to reconstruct the joint (rare).

POSSIBLE COMPLICATIONS
* Arthritis of the joint.
* Chronic pain of the face.

PROBABLE OUTCOME—The symptoms often clear up on their own in about 2 weeks. In most other cases, time and simple treatment measures can relieve symptoms.

 HOW TO TREAT

GENERAL MEASURES
* Try to limit jaw movements and learn to relax the jaw. Don't open it wide. Block a yawn by putting your fist under your chin. Don't chew gum.
* Ice and/or heat may be of benefit in relieving discomfort. Try one and then the other to see what works best for you. Massage the TMJ muscle area.
* To learn more: TMJ Association, PO Box 26770, Milwaukee, WI 53226; (262) 432-0350 (not toll free); website: www.tmj.org.

MEDICATION
* For pain and inflammation, use nonprescription drugs such as aspirin (not for children) or ibuprofen.
* Muscle relaxants, drugs for pain, steroids, antidepressants, or botulism toxin injections may be prescribed.

ACTIVITY—No limits.

DIET—Eat a soft diet until symptoms subside. Avoid hard or chewy foods (such as bagels).

 CALL YOUR DOCTOR IF

* You or a family member has symptoms of a temporomandibular joint disorder.
* Symptoms don't improve with treatment.

TENDINITIS & TENOSYNOVITIS

GENERAL INFORMATION

DEFINITION—Tendinitis is an inflammation of a tendon. Tenosynovitis is an inflammation of the protective covering (tendon sheath) around a tendon. They often occur at the same time. Tendons are made up of tough, fibrous, cord-like tissue. They connect muscles to bones.

BODY PARTS INVOLVED—Common sites are the shoulder (rotator cuff), elbow, heel (Achilles' tendon), knee or hamstring.

SEX OR AGE MOST AFFECTED—Both sexes; adolescents and adults.

SIGNS & SYMPTOMS
● Limited movement, tenderness, pain, and swelling around the inflamed tendon. Common sites are the shoulder, elbow, Achilles' tendon (heel), or hamstring.
● Weakness in the tendon caused by calcium deposits that often accompany tendinitis.

CAUSES—Inflammation or a small tear in a tendon. The tendons become inflamed for a variety of reasons. Inflammation is a reaction of the body's tissues to injury, infection, or irritation. Inflammation symptoms include redness, swelling, heat, and pain.

RISK INCREASES WITH
● Injury or overuse, usually from an athletic activity, exercising, or during work.
● Incorrect movement and strain during activity. For example, repeatedly holding and swinging a tennis racket incorrectly may cause tendinitis at the elbow (tennis elbow).
● Certain joint diseases (rheumatoid arthritis, scleroderma, gout, and Reiter's disease).
● Aging (tendons are more prone to injury).

HOW TO PREVENT
● Gradually build up the intensity and frequency of an activity.
● Avoid overuse of muscles and tendons. Maintain strength and flexibility. Warm up before each workout and stretch afterwards.
● Learn the proper techniques for any exercise or sport you intend to do regularly.
● Wear proper gear for any sport or exercise activity including well-fitting shoes.

WHAT TO EXPECT

DIAGNOSTIC MEASURES
● Your own observation of symptoms.
● See your health care provider if symptoms persist or are more severe. A physical exam of the affected area will be done and questions asked about your symptoms and activities.
● X-rays do not show tendon problems, but they may be done to rule out a fracture, if an injury occurred.

APPROPRIATE HEALTH CARE
● Treatment usually involves self-care.
● Treatment may involve rest, ice or heat, drugs, range-of-motion exercises, and steps to prevent recurrence.
● Surgery may be recommended in chronic tendinitis.
● Physical therapy may be needed to help regain strength and flexibility.

POSSIBLE COMPLICATIONS
● Chronic disability.
● Tendon rupture.
● Frozen shoulder.

PROBABLE OUTCOME—Usually curable with treatment and rest of the affected tendon area. Pain and swelling usually decrease in a few days. Allow 6 weeks for complete healing.

HOW TO TREAT

GENERAL MEASURES
● When resting, sleeping, or sitting, place the injured area on a pillow—at or above heart level.
● Wrap the area in a compressive (Ace) bandage to reduce swelling.
● Apply ice packs to the affected area. Do this several times a day for the first 24 to 48 hours. Then apply them twice a day until pain is gone. You can apply heat if it feels good. Take hot showers, soak in a warm bath, apply warm compresses, or use a heating pad.
● You may want to use a sling or splint for an arm or shoulder to limit movement. Use crutches, a cane, or a brace for affected leg, knee, or heel, if needed.

MEDICATION
● Use nonprescription nonsteroidal anti-inflammatory drugs and pain relievers such as ibuprofen.
● Steroid injection for painful tendons may be prescribed. This reduces pain and inflammation and allows movement. Injections are done just a few times because steroids can weaken the tendon.

ACTIVITY
● Resume normal activities as symptoms ease.
● After a few days, begin range-of-motion exercises to prevent stiffness in the area. Do them 3 to 4 times a day.
● Physical therapy may be recommended.

DIET—No special diet.

CALL YOUR DOCTOR IF

● You or a family member has symptoms of tendinitis that are severe or the symptoms don't improve with self-care.
● Pain and swelling increase despite treatment.

TENNIS ELBOW
(Epicondylitis, Lateral)

 GENERAL INFORMATION

DEFINITION—Tennis elbow is an inflammation of the tendons on the outside of the elbow at the epicondyle. The epicondyle is the bony area on the outside of the elbow. This is where the muscles of the forearm attach to the bone of the upper arm.

BODY PARTS INVOLVED—Elbow muscles, tendons, and epicondyle.

SEX OR AGE MOST AFFECTED—Both sexes; adults (20 to 40 years).

SIGNS & SYMPTOMS
- Pain and tenderness over bony part of elbow.
- Unable to straighten the arm completely.
- Stiffness in elbow in the morning.
- Pain when bending or twisting hand and arm.
- Weak grip (even when grabbing a light object such as a coffee cup).

CAUSES—The tendon becomes inflamed due to a variety of reasons. Most often, it is a result of overuse or repetition. Small tears in the tendon may lead to the problem. Inflammation is a reaction of the body's tissues to injury, infection, or irritation.

RISK INCREASES WITH
- Work or activity that requires repetitive forearm movement (e.g., hedge clipping, racket sports, or golf).
- Work or activity that requires excessive, constant gripping or squeezing.
- Poor physical condition.
- Sudden strain on the forearm.

HOW TO PREVENT
- Don't play sports, such as tennis, for long periods until you are in good condition. Learn proper playing techniques. Tennis racquets can worsen tennis elbow. Trying a different size or type (larger, more flexible, larger grip) may help.
- For work or sports activity requiring elbow movement, warm up the arm for 5 to 10 minutes. Take frequent breaks. Use ice pack on elbow if pain develops.
- Do flexibility and strength exercises for the arm and elbow.

 WHAT TO EXPECT

DIAGNOSTIC MEASURES
- Your own observation of symptoms.
- See your health care provider if symptoms persist or are more severe. A physical exam of the affected area will be done and questions asked about your symptoms and activities.
- X-rays do not show tendon problems, but they may be done if an injury occurred.

APPROPRIATE HEALTH CARE
- Mild cases may be self-treated if desired.
- Treatment may involve rest, ice or heat, massage, drugs, exercises, and steps to prevent recurrence.
- Surgery possibly (if other methods of treatment fail).

POSSIBLE COMPLICATIONS
- Recurrence of tennis elbow.
- Chronic pain if left untreated.

PROBABLE OUTCOME—Usually curable, but it takes time. Healing may require 3 to 6 months or longer.

 HOW TO TREAT

GENERAL MEASURES
- When resting, sleeping, or sitting, place the injured area on a pillow—at or above heart level.
- Wrap the thickest portion of the forearm in a compressive (Ace) bandage to reduce swelling. Massage the area several times a day.
- Apply ice packs to the affected area (several times a day) for the first 24 to 48 hours. Then apply heat if it feels good. Take hot showers, soak in a bath, apply hot compresses, or a heating pad.
- You may need to wear a forearm brace or splint to immobilize the elbow. Do the following exercise 3 or 4 times a day while wearing the splint. Stretch your arm, flex your wrist, and then press the back of your hand against a wall. Hold for 1 minute.

MEDICATION
- Use nonprescription nonsteroidal anti-inflammatory drugs and pain relievers such as ibuprofen or aspirin (not for children).
- Steroid injection for painful tendons may be recommended. This reduces pain and inflammation and allows movement. Injections are done just a few times as steroids can weaken the tendon.

ACTIVITY
- Don't repeat the activity that caused tennis elbow until symptoms clear up. Stretching and strength exercises are often prescribed to do at home. Do them daily or as directed.
- Physical therapy may be prescribed.

DIET—No special diet.

 CALL YOUR DOCTOR IF

- You or a family member has symptoms of tennis elbow.
- Symptoms don't improve in 2 weeks with treatment.

TESTICLE, UNDESCENDED
(Cryptorchidism)

GENERAL INFORMATION

DEFINITION—Undescended testicle occurs when one or both testicles fail to descend (move down) into the scrotum before birth. While in the uterus, a baby boy's testicles grow in his abdomen and then descend into his scrotum. Over 3% of full-term newborn males and 30% of premature newborn males are affected. The medical term for the condition is cryptorchidism.

BODY PARTS INVOLVED—One or both testes (testicles); scrotum; spermatic cord.

SEX OR AGE MOST AFFECTED—Male infants and children.

SIGNS & SYMPTOMS—One or both testicles can't be felt in the normal position in the scrotum. "Testes" is another name for testicles.

CAUSES—Unknown. It may be related to a hormone deficiency in the mother or fetus. Genetic, environmental, and other factors may also be involved.

RISK INCREASES WITH
- Family history of undescended testicle.
- Premature birth.
- Low birth weight.

HOW TO PREVENT—No specific preventive measures.

WHAT TO EXPECT

DIAGNOSTIC MEASURES
- Your own observation of symptoms.
- Your child's health care provider will do a physical exam. One or both testicles will not be in the scrotum, but they can often be felt above it. If they cannot be located, medical testing may be needed. Follow-up exams are done to check if they have descended.

APPROPRIATE HEALTH CARE
- If the testicle lies in the scrotum at times and then occasionally retracts, the problem normally resolves itself by puberty. No treatment is needed.
- Surgery (called orchiopexy) to move the testicles into the scrotum is usually recommended. Surgery is normally performed between 6 and 24 months of age and is successful in most cases. Your child may have the surgery, which takes about one hour, and go home the same day. Follow-up care instructions will be provided.
- In cases where a testicle is missing or cannot be moved surgically, artificial ones (implants) are available.
- Adult men with undescended testicles may have them removed or left in place. Your health care provider will discuss the options with you.

POSSIBLE COMPLICATIONS
- Inguinal hernia (weak area in wall of abdomen where intestines may protrude).
- Increased risk of testicular cancer as an adult.
- Sterility or reduced fertility rate.
- Emotional problems, about the physical appearance of an empty scrotum, may develop as a boy gets older.
- Testicular torsion (twisting).

PROBABLE OUTCOME—Most testicles will descend without treatment by 3 to 6 months of age. If they remain undescended, treatment can usually correct the problem.

HOW TO TREAT

GENERAL MEASURES—None specific.

MEDICATION
- Hormone therapy may be prescribed in some cases. It helps increase male hormones, which may cause the testicles to descend.
- Pain relief drugs may be prescribed following surgery.

ACTIVITY—No limits, except those following surgery.

DIET—No special diet.

CALL YOUR DOCTOR IF

- Your child has an undescended testicle that has not been diagnosed.
- An undescended testicle has not descended within 3 to 4 months.

TESTICULAR CANCER

GENERAL INFORMATION

DEFINITION—Testicular cancer is a growth of malignant cells in the testicle. Testicles are the male sex glands and are located in the scrotum. It is the most common cancer in young men.

BODY PARTS INVOLVED—Testicles (usually one only).

SEX OR AGE MOST AFFECTED—It can affect all ages, but occurs more often in ages 18 to 32.

SIGNS & SYMPTOMS
- A firm swelling in one testicle discovered by accident or by self-examination.
- No pain (90% of cases).
- Sense of fullness in the scrotum.
- A rarer type of the cancer may cause breast tenderness or swelling and loss of sexual desire.
- If cancer has spread, there may be back or chest pain, cough, and shortness of breath.

CAUSES—Unknown. There are several types of testicular cancer depending on the cells where it develops. The most common type is called germ cell. It develops in cells that produce sperm. Rarely are both testicles affected.

RISK INCREASES WITH
- Undescended testicles in infancy. (Surgery to bring the testicle down may reduce the risk. Research is ongoing.)
- White males, especially of Scandinavian descent.
- Being a younger male. Men over age 40 are less likely to get this form of cancer.
- Personal or family history of testicular cancer.
- Testicles that did not develop normally.

HOW TO PREVENT—Males should examine their testicles routinely at least once a month. This will not prevent the cancer, but the self-exam may detect a tumor early enough for effective treatment. Your health care provider can give you instructions on how to do a self-exam.

WHAT TO EXPECT

DIAGNOSTIC MEASURES
- Your own observation of symptoms. Testicular self-examination is an important diagnostic measure.
- Your health care provider will do a physical exam of the genital area.
- Different medical tests are usually done to verify the diagnosis and to determine if cancer has spread (called staging). These can include blood tests, ultrasound, CT, MRI, x-ray, and biopsy.

APPROPRIATE HEALTH CARE
- Treatment often involves surgery (called orchidectomy) to remove the cancerous testicle. Radiation therapy and/or chemotherapy (anticancer drugs) may be prescribed depending on the type and stage of the cancer.
- Some patients may want to arrange to have their sperm frozen in a sperm bank before treatment. This will allow them to produce children (if fertility is lost).
- Testicular prosthesis (implants) may be a choice of some patients after surgery. They are made of saline and are implanted in the scrotum to look and feel natural.

POSSIBLE COMPLICATIONS
- Without treatment, cancer may spread to other places in the body.
- Cancer recurs or develops in the other testicle.
- Patient is more at risk for other forms of cancer.
- Treatment-related complications (e.g., infertility due to chemotherapy or radiation).

PROBABLE OUTCOME—Most types of testicular tumors are curable with early diagnosis and treatment. Surgical removal of one testicle does not interfere with normal sexual function or the ability to have children.

HOW TO TREAT

GENERAL MEASURES—To learn more: American Cancer Society, (800) ACS-2345; website: www.cancer.org or National Cancer Institute, (800) 4-CANCER; website: www.nci.nih.gov.

MEDICATION
- Chemotherapy (anticancer drugs) may be prescribed.
- Pain medicine may be prescribed if needed.

ACTIVITY
- Resume your normal activities as soon as possible. Radiation and chemotherapy may cause temporary fatigue requiring extra rest.
- Resume sexual relations when you are able. Men often wait a few weeks until healing is complete and the groin area is no longer tender.

DIET—No special diet.

CALL YOUR DOCTOR IF

- You or a family member has a firm swelling or mass in the scrotum.
- New, unexplained symptoms develop due to a treatment procedure.

TESTICULAR TORSION

GENERAL INFORMATION

DEFINITION—Testicular torsion is a twisting of the spermatic cord of the testicle. This may damage the testicle. Testicular torsion usually occurs on one side only. Prompt treatment is necessary to save the affected testicle.

BODY PARTS INVOLVED—Testicle; spermatic cord; blood supply to each.

SEX OR AGE MOST AFFECTED—Males of all ages, but most common in ages 12 to 20 years.

SIGNS & SYMPTOMS
- Sudden pain in one testicle. It often starts in the night. Some prior pain may have been felt off and on, but went away on its own.
- Swelling, redness, and tenderness of the scrotum.
- Nausea and vomiting.
- Sweating.
- Fever (sometimes).

CAUSES
- In some males, the testicles are not attached firmly within the scrotum. The testicle is more movable and more likely to become twisted.
- Injury or exercise may cause torsion. There may be no obvious cause.

RISK INCREASES WITH
- Age under 20.
- Undescended testicles.
- Trauma to the scrotum.
- Physical activity.
- Previous testicular torsion.
- Cold weather.

HOW TO PREVENT—No specific preventive measures. Wear an athletic supporter or cup when participating in contact sports to prevent genital injury.

WHAT TO EXPECT

DIAGNOSTIC MEASURES
- Your own observation of symptoms.
- Your health care provider will do a physical exam of the scrotum area and ask questions about your symptoms and activities.
- Medical tests such as ultrasound may be done to confirm the diagnosis.

APPROPRIATE HEALTH CARE
- Immediate surgery is the usual treatment.
- In some cases, gentle manipulation by hand may undo the twisting. This is a temporary measure and is usually followed up with surgery to stop recurrence.
- Surgery is done to untangle the twisted spermatic cord. The affected testicle is attached to the inside scrotal wall, which prevents recurrence. The surgery will probably also include treatment on the unaffected testicle to prevent torsion.

POSSIBLE COMPLICATIONS
- The testicle is usually injured beyond repair unless surgery is done within about 6 hours after symptoms begin. If one testicle must be removed, the remaining healthy testicle should provide enough hormones for normal male growth, sex life, and fertility. A prosthetic testicle may be inserted in some cases.
- Infection in the scrotum and testicle.
- Recurrent torsion.

PROBABLE OUTCOME—Curable with prompt diagnosis and treatment.

HOW TO TREAT

GENERAL MEASURES—After surgery, use ice packs to relieve pain and swelling. Wrap the ice in plastic. Apply it to the affected side, separating the ice from the skin with a cloth towel. Apply ice 5 to 10 minutes at a time. Repeat as often as necessary.

MEDICATION—Pain relievers are usually given.

ACTIVITY—Resume your normal activities gradually after surgery.

DIET—No special diet.

CALL YOUR DOCTOR IF

- You or a family member has symptoms of testicular torsion. This is an emergency!
- Signs of infection begin after surgery. These include fever, chills, muscle aches, headache, dizziness, and a general ill feeling.
- Excessive bleeding occurs at the surgical site.

TETANUS

GENERAL INFORMATION

DEFINITION—Tetanus is an infection in a wound that causes severe muscle spasms and can lead to death. Tetanus cannot be spread from person to person. It is now rare, due to tetanus immunization.

BODY PARTS INVOLVED—Injured tissue; muscles throughout the body, especially the jaw, neck, back and abdomen.

SEX OR AGE MOST AFFECTED—Both sexes; all ages.

SIGNS & SYMPTOMS
- Stiffness and spasms of the jaw.
- Muscle pain and frequent, severe spasms.
- Stiff neck, arms, and legs.
- Headache.
- Sore throat and difficulty in swallowing.
- Difficulty using chest muscles to breathe.
- Fast pulse.
- Profuse sweating.

CAUSES—Bacteria (*Clostridium tetani*) that are present almost everywhere, especially in soil, manure, or dust. Bacteria may enter through any break in the skin, including burns or puncture wounds. The wound can be tiny such as with a splinter. Toxins produced by the bacteria travel to nerves that control muscle contraction, producing muscle spasms and seizures.

RISK INCREASES WITH
- Lack of up-to-date tetanus immunization.
- Newborn infants born to non-immunized mothers.
- Use of street drugs with unclean needles and syringes.
- Burns, surgical wounds, puncture wounds, bites, skin ulcers, crush injuries, ear infections, and others.

HOW TO PREVENT
- Obtain tetanus vaccination. It is given in a series of shots in combination with a diphtheria and pertussis vaccine in children. Booster shots are recommended every 10 years thereafter.
- An additional booster shot may be needed at the time of an injury.
- Take proper care of any wound.

WHAT TO EXPECT

DIAGNOSTIC MEASURES
- Your own observation of symptoms.
- Your health care provider will do a physical exam and ask questions about your symptoms and activities.
- Medical tests may include blood tests and culture studies of wound.

APPROPRIATE HEALTH CARE
- Hospital care is required. A quiet, dark room may be recommended. Treatment may include the use of breathing tubes, a respirator (machine to help breathing), intravenous (IV) fluid support, and drugs.
- Surgery to remove infected tissue may be needed.

POSSIBLE COMPLICATIONS
- Pneumonia or other infections.
- High blood pressure.
- Severe pain with muscle spasms.
- Irregular heartbeat.
- Bone fractures.
- Brain damage.
- Coma, respiratory paralysis, and death.

PROBABLE OUTCOME—With early diagnosis and treatment, full recovery is likely in mild or moderate tetanus. Allow 4 weeks for recovery. The death rate for severe tetanus is about 50%.

HOW TO TREAT

GENERAL MEASURES—Provide the patient with reassurance and emotional support. Despite the seriousness of tetanus, patients are usually conscious.

MEDICATION
- You may be given:
  - Antitoxins to neutralize the nerve toxin.
  - Muscle relaxants to control spasms.
  - Sedatives to relieve anxiety.
  - Anticonvulsants.
  - Antibiotics.
  - Tetanus combination vaccine.

ACTIVITY—During hospital time, bed rest is needed with as little disturbance as possible. During recovery, activities should be resumed gradually.

DIET—During treatment, intravenous (IV) fluids will be needed because of difficulty in swallowing.

CALL YOUR DOCTOR IF

- You or a family member has symptoms of tetanus or observes them in someone else. Call immediately. This is an emergency!
- You or someone in your family needs basic or booster tetanus immunizations.
- You have a puncture wound or injury that breaks the skin, and you have not had an immunization or booster in 5 years.

THALASSEMIA
(Mediterranean Anemia)

 GENERAL INFORMATION

DEFINITION
- Thalassemia is an inherited blood disorder in which red blood cells contain less hemoglobin than normal. Types are:
  - Alpha-thalassemia—found in populations from the Chinese subcontinent (Malaysia, Indochina, Africa). It is less common than the beta type.
  - Beta-thalassemia—found in Mediterranean area and Africa. If a person inherits one defective gene, it is called beta thalassemia minor (or trait); with two defective genes (one from each parent), it is called beta thalassemia major (or Cooley's anemia) and is a more serious disorder; a milder form also exists, beta-thalassemia intermedia.

BODY PARTS INVOLVED—Blood.

SEX OR AGE MOST AFFECTED—Both sexes; all ages.

SIGNS & SYMPTOMS
- Minor form may produce no symptoms.
- Fatigue.
- Paleness.
- Breathlessness.
- Irregular heartbeat, especially with exertion.
- Bloody or dark urine.
- Jaundice (yellow skin and eyes).
- Deformed bones.
- Enlarged spleen.

CAUSES—The inherited genes affect hemoglobin production. Hemoglobin in healthy people has two pairs of protein chains (alpha and beta); with thalassemia, one of the protein chains is reduced and causes an imbalance between the two chains in the hemoglobin produced.

RISK INCREASES WITH
- Family history of thalassemia.
- Genetic factors, including absence of the gene necessary to manufacture hemoglobin-A.

HOW TO PREVENT
- Cannot be prevented at present. If you have a family history of thalassemia, obtain genetic counseling before having children.
- Prenatal screening is available.

 WHAT TO EXPECT

DIAGNOSTIC MEASURES
- Your health care provider will do a physical exam and ask questions about your symptoms.
- Medical tests will include blood studies and possibly other tests to check for complications.

APPROPRIATE HEALTH CARE
- Patients with thalassemia trait normally require no treatment. Genetic counseling is usually recommended.
- The main form of treatment for severe thalassemia is blood transfusions along with iron chelation (therapy to remove excess iron in the blood).
- Bone marrow transplant (stem cell transplant) may be options for some.
- Surgery to remove the spleen may be recommended.

POSSIBLE COMPLICATIONS
- Infections, worsening of anemia, jaundice, leg ulcers, cholelithiasis (gallstones), pathologic fractures, impaired growth rate, delayed or absent puberty, cardiac disease, and iron overload.
- Transfusion or chelation complications.
- It can cause death by early adulthood or middle age, depending on severity.

PROBABLE OUTCOME—Varies. This condition is currently considered incurable. However, symptoms can be relieved or controlled. Some forms are consistent with a normal or nearly normal lifespan. Research continues for new treatments.

 HOW TO TREAT

GENERAL MEASURES—To learn more: Cooley's Anemia Foundation, 330 Seventh Ave, #200, New York, NY; 10001; (800)522-7222; website www.thalassemia.org.

MEDICATION
- Your health care provider may prescribe:
  - Antibiotics for infections.
  - Vitamin supplements.
  - Deferoxamine by injection for iron chelation.
  - Drugs to prevent blood transfusion reactions.

ACTIVITY—Activity levels are usually not limited unless there are heart problems. You will be advised of any limits.

DIET
- Try to avoid foods rich in iron.
- Drinking coffee or tea may help reduce the iron in the body.

 CALL YOUR DOCTOR IF

- You or a family member has symptoms of thalassemia.
- After diagnosis, any symptoms cause concern.

THORACIC-OUTLET SYNDROME
(Cervical-Rib Syndrome)

GENERAL INFORMATION

DEFINITION—Thoracic outlet syndrome (TOS) is a general term used to describe symptoms that occur due to pressure on nerves and blood vessels in the neck area. The thoracic outlet is a space between the rib cage and the collar-bone.

BODY PARTS INVOLVED—Nerves and blood vessels that supply the neck, shoulders, arms and hands.

SEX OR AGE MOST AFFECTED—Adults between ages 35 and 55, usually women.

SIGNS & SYMPTOMS
• Numbness, tingling, or prickling feelings in the neck, shoulders, arms, or hands.
• There may be no pain or mild to more severe pain.
• Weakness and tiredness in the arms and hands.
• Poor blood flow that causes coldness, swelling, and blueness in the hands and fingers (rare).
• Sense of touch may be lost.

CAUSES—Nerves and blood vessels that supply the shoulder, arms, and hands begin in the neck. They then pass as a bundle near the cervical ribs and collarbone. Pressure on this nerve and blood vessel bundle creates symptoms. There are multiple problems that can lead to the pressure.

RISK INCREASES WITH
• An extra rib in the body. It may have fiber-like bands attached to it.
• Overextending arm or shoulder or repeated overhead arm movements. This may be due to work activities or exercise.
• Carrying heavy loads.
• Fracture of clavicle (collarbone) or first rib.
• Drooping shoulders or head due to poor posture.
• Tumor or blood clots.
• Obesity.
• Pregnancy.
• Other health or emotional disorders may make a person more at risk for TOS.

HOW TO PREVENT—No specific preventive measures. Try to avoid repetitive arm and shoulder activities and overhead arm tasks. Exercise daily to maintain good physical fitness.

WHAT TO EXPECT

DIAGNOSTIC MEASURES
• Your own observation of symptoms.
• Your health care provider will do a physical exam and ask questions about your symptoms and activities.

• You may be asked to make certain movements with the head, arm, and shoulders to help find the cause of the symptoms. Other medical tests may be done to rule out problems that could cause similar symptoms.

APPROPRIATE HEALTH CARE
• Treatment may involve physical therapy, stretching and strengthening exercises, drugs, ultrasound therapy, electrical stimulation, manipulation, or surgery. Your health care provider will discuss an individual plan for you depending on your diagnosis and symptoms.
• Certain forms of TOS may need surgery to relieve pressure.
• Surgery may be an option when other treatments are not helpful.

POSSIBLE COMPLICATIONS
• TOS can recur.
• If surgery is performed, it may have complications.
• Chronic pain syndrome, disability, and depression may occur in some patients.
• Some loss of function in arm and shoulders.

PROBABLE OUTCOME—With treatment, symptoms can be relieved in most patients.

HOW TO TREAT

GENERAL MEASURES
• Use heat to help relieve pain (e.g., heating pad, warm shower, or warm, moist compresses).
• Try to avoid stress if possible.

MEDICATION
• You may use nonprescription drugs, such as acetaminophen, ibuprofen, or aspirin (not for children) to relieve pain. Drugs cannot correct the underlying condition.
• Other drugs or injections for specific symptoms may be prescribed.

ACTIVITY
• Physical therapy and exercise will be prescribed to promote shoulder muscle function and improve any posture faults. These are usually recommended for 2 to 3 months.
• Avoid activities that worsen pain symptoms.

DIET—No special diet. If weight is a problem, a weight-loss diet is recommended.

CALL YOUR DOCTOR IF

• You or a family member has symptoms of thoracic outlet syndrome.
• Symptoms don't improve with treatment.

THROMBOCYTOPENIA

GENERAL INFORMATION

DEFINITION—Thrombocytopenia is a decrease in the number of platelet cells in the blood. Platelets (thrombocytes) play a vital role in the control of bleeding at the site of an injury. With thrombocytopenia, there is a tendency to bleed, mainly from the smaller blood vessels. This causes abnormal bleeding into the skin and other body places. Platelets are normally produced in the bone marrow and are removed or destroyed by the spleen when not needed.

BODY PARTS INVOLVED—Blood, which affects all body parts.

SEX OR AGE MOST AFFECTED—Both sexes; all ages.

SIGNS & SYMPTOMS
- Petechiae. These are small, round, nonraised, purple-red spots on the skin (especially the legs).
- Bruising easily.
- Bleeding in the mouth and nosebleeds.
- Heavy or prolonged menstrual periods.
- Blood in the urine or stool.

CAUSES—Low platelets occur if the bone marrow doesn't make enough platelets or the body destroys the platelets or the spleen holds on to too many platelets.

RISK INCREASES WITH
- Cancer.
- Aplastic anemia.
- Exposure to toxic chemicals.
- Drugs such as diuretics, aspirin, ibuprofen, quinine, sulfa antibiotics, some antiseizures, rifampin, heparin, anticancer drugs, and others.
- Excess alcohol use.
- Viral infection (including HIV).
- Certain inherited conditions.
- Autoimmune disorders (e.g., idiopathic thrombocytopenic purpura, lupus, or rheumatoid arthritis).
- Widespread bacterial infection.
- Surgery.
- Vitamin B-12 or folate deficiency.
- Pregnancy.
- Enlarged spleen (it can be caused by a number of disorders).
- Rare conditions that cause blood clots (e.g., thrombotic thrombocytopenic purpura or disseminated intravascular coagulation).

HOW TO PREVENT—No specific prevention. Avoid risk factors where possible (e.g., excess alcohol use).

WHAT TO EXPECT

DIAGNOSTIC MEASURES
- Your own observation of symptoms.
- Your health care provider will usually do a physical exam and ask questions about your symptoms and activities.
- Medical tests may include blood studies and other tests to check for an underlying disorder.

APPROPRIATE HEALTH CARE
- Treatment will be provided for any specific disorder that is diagnosed.
- Watchful waiting is an option. This means monitoring the symptoms for a time before deciding on treatment.
- Stop using any drug that could be the cause. An alternative drug may be prescribed.
- Surgery to remove the spleen (splenectomy) may be recommended for persistent cases.
- Pregnant women with mild thrombocytopenia usually require no treatment.
- Platelet transfusions may be prescribed. This may be for patients with serious bleeding, those planning major surgery, and those with chronic thrombocytopenia.

POSSIBLE COMPLICATIONS—Severe blood loss can be life-threatening.

PROBABLE OUTCOME—It will depend on the underlying condition. If the cause can be identified and removed, the outlook is generally good. In other cases, the long-term management can be helped with treatment.

HOW TO TREAT

GENERAL MEASURES
- Wear or carry medical ID that shows your medical problem and any drugs you take.
- For patients with thrombocytopenia, avoid injury, and get medical care if injury occurs.
- To learn more: National Heart, Lung, & Blood Institute, PO Box 30105, Bethesda, MD 20824; website:www.nhlbi.nih.gov.

MEDICATION—A number of drugs are used for treatment. Your health care provider will discuss the options, risks, and benefits before prescribing.

ACTIVITY
- If platelet counts are very low, bed rest and reduced activity to avoid injury may be needed.
- Avoid contact sports or activities that put you at risk for bruising or bleeding, Ask your health care provider for advice before starting a new physical activity.

DIET—No special diet. Avoid alcohol or ask your health care provider about its use.

CALL YOUR DOCTOR IF

- You or a family member has symptoms of thrombocytopenia.
- Symptoms worsen during treatment. Severe blood loss is an emergency situation.
- New or unexplained symptoms develop.

THROMBOPHILIA
(Hypercoagulable States; Blood Clotting Disorders)

 GENERAL INFORMATION

DEFINITION—People with thrombophilia have an increased risk for blood clots developing in the arteries (blood vessels that carry blood away from the heart) and the veins (blood vessels that carry blood to the heart). A clot inside a blood vessel is called a thrombus or an embolus.

BODY PARTS INVOLVED—Blood.

SEX OR AGE MOST AFFECTED—Both sexes; all ages.

SIGNS & SYMPTOMS
- People with thrombophilia have no specific symptoms unless a blood clot develops.
- Pain and swelling in a leg occurs if you have a blood clot in a large vein in a leg. This is called deep vein thrombosis (DVT).
- A blood clot may travel to the heart and on into a lung, causing a pulmonary embolus (PE). Possible symptoms are chest pain, pain on deep breathing, shortness of breath or, rarely, collapse.
- Symptoms can occur if a clot forms in other parts of the body.

CAUSES
- Thrombophilia is an inherited or acquired condition (or both). The inherited form means a person is born with the tendency to form blood clots. Acquired conditions are often a result of surgery, trauma, drugs, or a medical condition.
- More common inherited forms include:
  - Factor V Leiden (the most common).
  - Prothrombin 20210 mutation.
  - Elevated levels of homocysteine.
  - Protein C deficiency.
  - Protein S deficiency.
  - Antithrombin deficiency.
  - Elevated levels of fibrinogen or dysfunctional fibrinogen (dysfibrinogenemia).
  - Elevated factor VIII levels.

RISK INCREASES WITH
- Family history for inherited forms.
- Acquired forms: antiphospholipid syndrome, surgery, cancer, being immobile (e.g., bed rest), heart failure, obesity, oral contraceptives, hormone use after menopause, certain drugs, use of a catheter in a vein, pregnancy, and other conditions.

HOW TO PREVENT
- You can't prevent inherited forms. Your health care provider may advise preventive measures, in certain situations that temporarily put you at high risk of having a blood clot.
- The benefits of testing people for thrombophilia who have not had a blood clot is still being researched.

 WHAT TO EXPECT

DIAGNOSTIC MEASURES
- Your health care provider may test for thrombophilia under certain circumstances (e.g., repeated blood clots or clots occur at a younger age, pregnancy, or you are a blood relative of someone with certain types of high-risk thrombophilia).
- Medical tests include thrombophilia screen (basic clotting tests). If the results of this suggest that thrombophilia is possible, then another blood sample will be taken for more detailed tests.

APPROPRIATE HEALTH CARE
- Treatment with drugs may be advised if:
  - You have had a blood clot and need to prevent another one.
  - You have not had a blood clot, but have a high risk of getting one.
  - You have a temporary situation that puts you at high risk of a blood clot. This may be done if you are pregnant, within 6 weeks after childbirth, or are immobile for a long period.

POSSIBLE COMPLICATIONS
- A pulmonary embolus, stroke, heart attack, or a blood clot in the brain or abdomen can all be life-threatening conditions.
- Adverse effects of drug therapy.

PROBABLE OUTCOME—Many forms of thrombophilia are mild, so that most people with thrombophilia have no problems from their condition. Treatment can successfully prevent complications in many cases.

 HOW TO TREAT

GENERAL MEASURES
- Wear or carry medical ID that shows your medical problem and any drugs you take.
- If you are having any medical treatment or surgery, tell your health care provider about the thrombophilia.

MEDICATION—Anticoagulant drugs or low-dose aspirin may be prescribed.

ACTIVITY—Usually no limits.

DIET
- Eat a healthy diet, low in fat.
- Maintain a healthy weight (overweight or obesity increases the risk of blood clots in legs).

 CALL YOUR DOCTOR IF

You or a family member has concerns about thrombophilia.

THROMBOPHLEBITIS, SUPERFICIAL
(Phlebitis)

 GENERAL INFORMATION

DEFINITION—Superficial thrombophlebitis is an inflammation (redness and swelling) in a superficial vein due to a blood clot. Superficial means the vein is near the surface of the skin. It occurs most often in the veins in the legs, and sometimes in the arms or groin.

BODY PARTS INVOLVED—Veins.

SEX OR AGE MOST AFFECTED
- Both sexes, but more common in females.
- All ages, but most common in adults.

SIGNS & SYMPTOMS
- Tenderness, redness, and pain in the affected area. The symptoms usually come on slowly.
- Vein may feel like a tender, hard cord under the skin.
- Fever (sometimes).
- In some cases, there are no symptoms.

CAUSES—Any problem that involves the vein, blood, or blood flow can lead to a blood clot. Over time, as the blood flow slows down, blood cells may clump together and form a clot.

RISK INCREASES WITH
- Varicose veins.
- Illness or surgery with a lot of time spent in bed.
- Personal history or family history of blood-clotting disorder.
- Catheter use (tube inserted into vein).
- Long car rides or airplane trips where you are sitting for long periods.
- Elderly.
- Use of birth control pills.
- Overweight or obesity.
- Injuries, burns, or infections.
- Pregnancy.
- Chronic illnesses, heart problems, and some cancers.
- Intravenous (IV) drug abusers.

HOW TO PREVENT
- Avoid risk factors where possible.
- On long trips, walk when you can, move legs often, and consider support stockings to prevent swollen legs.

 WHAT TO EXPECT

DIAGNOSTIC MEASURES
- Your health care provider will examine the affected area of the leg and ask questions about your symptoms.
- Medical tests may be done to make sure there are no other medical problems. These include blood tests and ultrasound (using sound waves to check the blood flow).

APPROPRIATE HEALTH CARE
- Treatment usually involves rest and elevation of the affected leg or arm and drugs (depending on the cause).
- If varicose veins are a problem, they may need treatment.

POSSIBLE COMPLICATIONS—The main concern is about blood clots forming in deep veins (deep vein thrombosis). They can have serious complications such as pulmonary embolism (clot in the lung).

PROBABLE OUTCOME—Usually curable in several days to 3 weeks.

 HOW TO TREAT

GENERAL MEASURES
- Apply heat with warm compresses. Wet a towel in hot water, wring it out, and place it on the affected area.
- Wearing support stockings may help. Some types can be purchased at a drugstore. Your health care provider may prescribe prescription-type support stockings.

MEDICATION
- Your health care provider may prescribe:
  - Nonsteroidal anti-inflammatory drugs, such as aspirin (not for children) or ibuprofen, to decrease swelling, redness, and pain.
  - Anticoagulants (drugs to prevent blood clots) may be prescribed.
  - Antibiotics may be prescribed if there is an infection.

ACTIVITY
- You may be advised to rest with the affected leg or arm elevated as much as possible for 1 or 2 days. Move the feet, ankles, and legs often.
- When the symptoms begin to get better, resume normal activity slowly. Rest often. Don't sit or stand for prolonged periods, and don't cross your legs.

DIET—No special diet. If overweight, a weight loss diet is often recommended.

 CALL YOUR DOCTOR IF

- You or a family member has symptoms of superficial thrombophlebitis.
- The following occur during treatment: fever of 102°F (38.9°C) or higher, pain gets worse, coughing up blood, shortness of breath, chest pain, or swelling of leg or foot.

THROMBOSIS, DEEP VEIN

GENERAL INFORMATION

DEFINITION—A deep vein thrombosis (DVT) is a blood clot (thrombus) that forms inside a deep vein. It may block the blood flow partially or completely.

BODY PARTS INVOLVED—It most often occurs in the lower legs (calves) or thighs. Less often it occurs in the pelvis or abdomen.

SEX OR AGE MOST AFFECTED—Both sexes (slightly more common in men) and usually occurs in persons over age 40.

SIGNS & SYMPTOMS
- Sometimes no symptoms occur.
- Swelling, tenderness, or pain in the leg, especially the calf muscle.
- Warmth or redness of the leg.
- Soreness or pain when walking. The soreness does not disappear with rest.
- Pain when raising the leg and flexing the foot.

CAUSES—Pooling of blood in the vein, which triggers blood-clotting mechanisms. The pooling may occur after prolonged bed rest, following surgery, or from long-lasting illness, such as heart attack, stroke, or bone fracture.

RISK INCREASES WITH
- Persons over 40.
- Obesity or smoking.
- Estrogen use in birth control pills or for replacement after menopause. More of a risk with smokers.
- Surgery and surgery recovery.
- Long (e.g., over 4 hours) auto or airplane trip.
- During pregnancy and right after childbirth.
- Cancer, heart failure, stroke, and polycythemia.
- Bed rest for an extended time.
- Fractures.
- Intravenous (IV) drug abuse.
- Blood disorders that increase blood clot risk.

HOW TO PREVENT
- Avoid prolonged bed rest if possible. Move legs as often as possible after surgery or during a long illness.
- On long auto or airplane trips, exercise your legs at least once every hour. Elevate legs when possible. Drink fluids. Avoid alcohol.
- Stop smoking, especially if you take estrogen.
- Wear special compression stockings.

WHAT TO EXPECT

DIAGNOSTIC MEASURES
- Your health care provider will do a physical exam of the affected area. Questions will be asked about your symptoms and activities.
- Medical tests such as ultrasound may be done to confirm the diagnosis.

APPROPRIATE HEALTH CARE
- Small clots located in the calf may not need treatment right away. These clots often clear up on their own.
- In many cases, hospital care is required for injections of blood thinning drugs and to watch for complications.
- A surgical procedure may be done to insert a filtering device ("umbrella") into the vena cava (main vein to the lungs). It will trap clots before they reach the lungs.
- Surgery or other procedure may be done to remove a large clot.
- Special compression stockings may be prescribed. They help prevent pain, swelling, and complications.

POSSIBLE COMPLICATIONS
- Pulmonary embolism (blood clot travels to the lung).
- Embolism to another part of the body.
- Post-thrombotic syndrome due to vein damage. Blood pools in lower leg, causing swelling and pain in leg.
- Excessive bleeding from blood thinning drugs.

PROBABLE OUTCOME—Usually curable with treatment. It may depend on an underlying condition.

HOW TO TREAT

GENERAL MEASURES—Follow medical advice.

MEDICATION
- Usually, an intravenous (IV) anticoagulant (blood thinner) drug is prescribed. This stops a clot from growing and prevents new clots. Blood tests will be ongoing to check the anticoagulant level. Oral anticoagulants may be prescribed for 6 months or longer.
- Thrombolytic drugs, which dissolve the clots, may be prescribed in more severe cases.

ACTIVITY
- Rest at home as advised by your health care provider. While resting, make it a habit to move leg muscles, bend ankles, and wiggle toes.
- Elevate the feet higher than the hips when sitting or when in bed. Place a cushion under the feet or raise the foot of the bed higher.

DIET—No special diet.

CALL YOUR DOCTOR IF

- You or a family member has symptoms of deep vein thrombosis.
- The following occur with treatment: any unexpected bleeding, chest pain, coughing up blood, shortness of breath, continued or increased swelling, and pain.

THROMBOSIS & EMBOLUS, ARTERIAL

 GENERAL INFORMATION

DEFINITION—Thrombosis occurs when a blood clot (thrombus) forms in an artery. An embolism is a blood clot (embolus) that travels from the site where it formed to another location in the body. A clot can become stuck in an artery and reduce blood flow (called ischemia) or block blood flow completely (called infarct). This blockage starves tissues of blood and oxygen and can result in damage or tissue death (necrosis). Clots may be substances other than blood (e.g., tissue, fat globule, or air bubble).

BODY PARTS INVOLVED—A clot often occurs in the legs. It may occur in the brain and cause a stroke, or in the heart and cause a heart attack. Less often it occurs in the kidneys, intestines, or eyes.

SEX OR AGE MOST AFFECTED—Adults of both sexes.

SIGNS & SYMPTOMS
- Symptoms depend on where the clot lodges.
- Legs—pain in the calf with exercise; weakness, numbness, burning and tingling sensations; or weak or absent pulse beyond the blocked blood flow. Symptoms ease up with rest.
- Body organs—pain in the part of the body that is involved and decreased organ function.

CAUSES—Clots may form with any condition that damages the smooth lining of the heart or a blood vessel. As the clot grows, small or large portions break away and are carried by the bloodstream to other areas of the body.

RISK INCREASES WITH
- Atherosclerosis (hardening of the arteries).
- Injury to a blood vessel from an accident or from surgery.
- Heart valve disease.
- Heart attack or family history of heart attack or stroke.
- Atrial fibrillation.
- Adults over 60.
- Smoking.
- High blood pressure.
- Diabetes.
- Thrombophilia (blood clotting disorders).

HOW TO PREVENT
- No specific preventive measures.
- Seek medical care for treatable risk factors.
- Anticoagulant (blood thinner) drugs may be prescribed for people at risk for blood clots.
- Exercise regularly to help keep blood vessels healthy.

 WHAT TO EXPECT

DIAGNOSTIC MEASURES
- Your own observation of symptoms.
- Your health care provider will do a physical exam and ask about your activities and symptoms.
- Medical tests may include x-rays of the blood vessels (after injection of a special substance), ultrasound, echocardiogram, or MRI.

APPROPRIATE HEALTH CARE
- Early treatment is needed and usually requires drugs or surgery or other procedure.
- The goals of treatment are to relieve symptoms and to improve the interrupted blood flow to the affected area. Any underlying condition that caused the clot will be treated to prevent further problems.
- Surgery or other procedures may be done:

POSSIBLE COMPLICATIONS—When blood flow is blocked in an artery, it can be life threatening.

PROBABLE OUTCOME—Depends on the location of the clot, size of the affected blood vessel, and size of the clot. Prompt diagnosis and treatment improve outcome.

 HOW TO TREAT

GENERAL MEASURES—Follow medical advice.

MEDICATION
- Drugs to break up the clot may be given through a catheter (tube) directly into the artery involved.
- Anticoagulants or antiplatelets to reduce the risk of clots forming may be prescribed.
- Drugs to widen blood vessels may be prescribed.
- Pain relievers will be prescribed as needed.

ACTIVITY—Complete rest is needed until blood flow is re-established by treatment.

DIET—No special diet.

📞 **CALL YOUR DOCTOR IF**

- You or a family member has symptoms of arterial thrombosis or embolus. This is an emergency! Get medical help immediately.
- Symptoms return after surgery.
- New, unexplained symptoms develop. Drugs used in treatment may produce side effects.

THRUSH
(Oral Candidiasis)

 GENERAL INFORMATION

DEFINITION—Thrush is a fungal infection of the mouth. It is common in newborns and infants. In adults, it is usually a result of an underlying condition.

BODY PARTS INVOLVED—Mouth; gums; tongue; soft palate; cheeks; lips.

SEX OR AGE MOST AFFECTED—Newborns and infants, but may also affect older children and adults.

SIGNS & SYMPTOMS
- Patches (plaques) appear in the mouth.
- Patches are white to creamy-yellow, and slightly raised. They are similar to milk curds, but they don't wipe off.
- Usually no pain, but may have mild discomfort.
- If patches are rubbed off, they can leave small, painful ulcers (sores).
- The mouth is dry.
- Infant may have trouble feeding.

CAUSES—A fungus called *Candida albicans*. It is usually present in small numbers in the mouth. Certain factors may cause it to multiply out of control.

RISK INCREASES WITH
- Treatment with antibiotics. This may upset the natural balance of germs in the mouth and allow thrush to develop.
- Birth. Newborns may acquire the infection during passage through the birth canal, especially if the mother has a vaginal yeast infection.
- Aging.
- People with poor nutrition.
- HIV infection.
- Diabetes.
- Dentures.
- Weak immune system due to illness or drugs.
- Chronic steroid drug use (oral or inhaled).
- Smoking.
- Having conditions that cause dry mouth.

HOW TO PREVENT
- Good oral hygiene, especially if you have dentures.
- Avoid antibiotics, unless prescribed for you.
- People at risk for thrush may be prescribed a preventive drug.
- For dry mouth problems, increase water intake and use nonprescription dry mouth products (e.g., sugar-free gum, mouthwash, or artificial saliva).

 WHAT TO EXPECT

DIAGNOSTIC MEASURES
- Your own observation of symptoms.
- Your health care provider will do a physical exam of the mouth and ask questions about your symptoms and recent use of antibiotics or other drugs.
- Medical tests may include a scraping of the patch for viewing under a microscope.

APPROPRIATE HEALTH CARE
- Infants often need no treatment.
- In others, treatment is aimed at improving the underlying condition and helping the symptoms of thrush.

POSSIBLE COMPLICATIONS—Complications are rare. They are more likely to occur in those with underlying conditions.

PROBABLE OUTCOME—Usually clears up within 2 weeks. Thrush has a tendency to recur.

 HOW TO TREAT

GENERAL MEASURES
- If an infant has the infection, sterilize any objects that may be placed in the baby's mouth.
- Older children and adults:
  - Brush teeth with a soft toothbrush.
  - Rinse the mouth with warm salt water a few times a day. Use one-half teaspoon of salt in one cup of warm water. This may ease the pain.

MEDICATION
- Nystatin oral suspension may be prescribed. Follow instructions that are provided with the product. Mothers who are nursing an infant with thrush should use the prescribed drug on her nipples. This prevents the infection from being spread back to the infant.
- Other antifungal drugs are effective and may be prescribed for adults.

ACTIVITY—No limits.

DIET—No changes in infants. Older children and adults should maintain a good fluid intake with milk, liquid gelatin, ice cream, custard, water, tea, or other beverages and foods that are easy to swallow. Use a straw for drinking if the patches are painful.

 CALL YOUR DOCTOR IF

- You or a family member has symptoms of thrush.
- Dehydration (sunken eyes, poor elasticity of the skin, and lethargy) occurs in a child.
- Fever develops.

THUMB-SUCKING

GENERAL INFORMATION

DEFINITION—Thumb sucking is the placing of the finger or thumb on the roof of the mouth behind the teeth and sucking with lips and teeth closed. Thumb sucking is common in infants and young children and is a behavior, not a disorder.

BODY PARTS INVOLVED—Mouth, teeth, tongue, pharynx, finger, or thumb.

SEX OR AGE MOST AFFECTED—Children of both sexes up to age 12, but most common in young children.

SIGNS & SYMPTOMS—Sucking of the thumb. It is most likely to occur before going to sleep, while watching TV, or when hungry, ill, or tired.

CAUSES—Thumb sucking is one of the first acts that an infant can do that brings pleasure. The need to suck is present in all babies. They will suck on almost anything that they can bring into contact with their mouths.

RISK INCREASES WITH—None known.

HOW TO PREVENT
• Thumb sucking is normal and does not need to be prevented. The behavior is calming and soothing to a baby.
• Provide pacifiers early in infancy if you desire. They cause no health problems. Once your child no longer needs a pacifier for their sucking need, you can start to wean them from pacifier use.

WHAT TO EXPECT

DIAGNOSTIC MEASURES—None needed.

APPROPRIATE HEALTH CARE—No treatment or action is usually necessary. Talk to your child's health care provider if you have any questions or concerns about thumb sucking.

POSSIBLE COMPLICATIONS—Thumb sucking that continues past age 6. It could cause problems with your child's mouth or teeth. Also, the child may get teased by others about the baby-like behavior. Parents should work with the child to change the habit for the sake of appearance and dental health.

PROBABLE OUTCOME—Some babies stop thumb sucking by age one. In most cases, the habit is given up by the time a child is 3 or 4 years old.

HOW TO TREAT

GENERAL MEASURES
• For a child over age 6 or 7 who sucks the thumb or fingers, follow the advice of your child's health care provider, or try those listed here:
  - Give the child extra attention.
  - Watch the child's behavior to see if conflicts or anxiety seems to provoke sucking. Help the child explore other ways to cope with stress.
  - If the child decides to try to stop sucking, help the child set goals. Give rewards for any progress toward the goal. Reward is not a bribe, but something earned through effort.
  - Methods such as scolding, shaming, and nagging are usually of no avail. Other methods do not always work either. These include mittens, bad-tasting substances on the thumb, elbow splints, and others.
  - Consult your child's dentist for help as well. The dentist may fit a training device in the child's mouth to prevent the thumb from touching the roof of the mouth.

MEDICATION—Drugs are not needed.

ACTIVITY—No limits.

DIET—No special diet.

CALL YOUR DOCTOR IF OR DENTIST IF

Your child wishes to stop thumb sucking and self-help methods are not working.

THYROID CANCER

GENERAL INFORMATION

DEFINITION—Thyroid cancer is a cancer that starts in the thyroid gland. The thyroid gland produces hormones that help regulate different body functions. Thyroid cancer is rare compared with other types of cancer. Thyroid cancers are often diagnosed after nodules are found by the patient or during a routine exam.

BODY PARTS INVOLVED—Thyroid gland.

SEX OR AGE MOST AFFECTED—Both sexes (women more than men) and ages over 40.

SIGNS & SYMPTOMS
- May have no symptoms.
- Lump in the neck.
- Neck or throat pain (may extend to the ears).
- Hoarseness or change in voice.
- Trouble swallowing.
- Breathing problems.
- Persistent and unexplained cough.

CAUSES—Exact cause of most thyroid cancers is unknown. Genetic factors may play a role.

RISK INCREASES WITH
- History of exposure of the thyroid to high levels of radiation (but not routine x-ray exposure).
- Family history of thyroid cancer.
- Age over 40 and women more than men.
- Certain inherited genetic syndromes.

HOW TO PREVENT
- No specific preventive measures.
- Be aware of risks (such as previous radiation therapy to the neck or family history). This can allow earlier diagnosis and treatment.
- Some people with a family history may choose to have the thyroid removed to prevent cancer. Your health care provider and a genetic counselor can discuss your risks and your treatment options.

WHAT TO EXPECT

DIAGNOSTIC MEASURES
- Your own observation of any symptoms.
- Your health care provider will perform a physical exam. This may reveal a lump in the thyroid, or swollen lymph nodes in the neck.
- Medical tests are done, first to diagnose the cancer, and then to find out if it has spread to other body organs (staging). Tests may include blood studies, laryngoscopy, iodine scan, biopsy, ultrasound, and thyroid function tests.

APPROPRIATE HEALTH CARE
- Treatment will depend on the type of thyroid cancer. It may include surgery, radioactive iodine treatment, thyroid hormone therapy, radiation, and chemotherapy.

- Treatment plans often use two or more of the above options, but surgery is the main treatment for all thyroid cancers. Surgery may be a thyroidectomy (removal of the thyroid) or removal of only part of the thyroid (thyroid lobectomy). Lymph nodes may need to be removed also.
- Radioactive iodine treatment may be done with or without the surgery.
- External radiation may be used, especially if cancer has spread.
- If the cancer does not respond to surgery or radiation and has spread to other parts of the body, chemotherapy may be used.

POSSIBLE COMPLICATIONS
- Surgery complications may occur.
- Rarely, spread of the cancer to the lungs, bones, or other parts of the body.
- Thyroid cancer may recur after treatment (even if thyroid has been removed). It can happen years later.

PROBABLE OUTCOME—The outcome is generally excellent. Surgery cures most thyroid cancers. In some cases, the cancer can't be cured, but patients can live a long time and still lead a productive life.

HOW TO TREAT

GENERAL MEASURES
- Joining a support group helps many patients.
- See your health care provider on a regular basis for follow up testing to check if the thyroid cancer has returned.
- To learn more: American Thyroid Association, 6066 Leesburg Pike, Suite 650, Falls Church, VA 22041; (800) 849-7643; website: www.thyroid.org.

MEDICATION
- Chemotherapy (anticancer drugs) may be prescribed.
- Lifetime replacement of thyroid hormone will be prescribed.

ACTIVITY—No limits except as advised by your health care provider following treatment. Stay as physically active as possible.

DIET—Eat a healthy diet. After surgery, a soft food diet may help if you have difficulty in swallowing.

CALL YOUR DOCTOR IF

- You or a family member has symptoms of thyroid cancer.
- Any symptoms develop during or after treatment that cause concern.

THYROID NODULE

GENERAL INFORMATION

DEFINITION—A thyroid nodule is a growth (lump) in the thyroid gland located in the front of the neck. The thyroid gland produces hormones that help regulate different body functions. Most often, the nodules are benign (noncancerous). About 5% are malignant (cancerous). Benign nodules are common.

BODY PARTS INVOLVED—Thyroid gland.

SEX OR AGE MOST AFFECTED—Both sexes (women more than men) and all age groups.

SIGNS & SYMPTOMS
* Most nodules have no symptoms. They are sometimes found during routine physical exams.
* Swelling or lump in the throat.
* Pain and tenderness in the thyroid gland.
* Difficulty swallowing if a large nodule is pressing on the windpipe or esophagus.
* Hyperthyroidism (overactive thyroid) symptoms may occur if the nodule produces too much thyroid hormone. Symptoms can include weight loss, sleep problems, and being irritable.
* Hoarseness (rare).

CAUSES—For unknown reasons, the tissue in the thyroid develops into the nodules. There are several different types of nodules that develop. They may be cystic (fluid filled) or solid. There may be one nodule or many. Thyroid nodules can cause a goiter (an enlarged thyroid).

RISK INCREASES WITH
* Aging.
* Females.
* Radiation therapy during childhood, even in small doses, to the head, neck, or upper chest.
* Exposure to radiation.
* Family history of thyroid nodules.
* Certain thyroid conditions (e.g., thyroiditis).

HOW TO PREVENT—No specific preventive measures.

WHAT TO EXPECT

DIAGNOSTIC MEASURES
* Your own observation of any symptoms.
* Your health care provider will do a physical exam and ask about your symptoms and history of radiation exposure.
* Medical tests are usually done to rule out cancer.

APPROPRIATE HEALTH CARE
* Treatment will depend on the type of nodules.
* Watchful waiting is an option if the nodule is benign. This means monitoring the thyroid with testing for a time before deciding if treatment is needed.
* Drug treatment may be prescribed to help shrink benign nodules.
* Surgery (thyroidectomy) is usually performed for malignant nodules. It is usually done also for larger benign nodules or nodules where the diagnosis is unclear if they are or are not cancerous. Thyroid hormone replacement therapy will be required for life after the thyroid is removed.

POSSIBLE COMPLICATIONS
* Side effects of treatment can lead to hypothyroidism or hyperthyroidism.
* Rarely, spread of a malignant tumor to other places in the body.
* Injury to the vocal cords during surgery.
* Permanent hoarseness or loss of voice following surgery.

PROBABLE OUTCOME
* Benign nodules may require no treatment. Others can be treated successfully.
* Most cancerous thyroid nodules are curable.

HOW TO TREAT

GENERAL MEASURES—To learn more: American Thyroid Association, 6066 Leesburg Pike, Suite 650, Falls Church, VA 22041; (800) 849-7643; website: www.thyroid.org.

MEDICATION
* Radioactive iodine or drugs to suppress (stop) the thyroid from producing hormones may be prescribed.
* Injections may be recommended for benign nodules to shrink them. It may require one or more injections over a few months.
* Antithyroid drugs or replacement thyroid hormone may be prescribed.

ACTIVITY—No limits, unless surgery is performed.

DIET—No special diet.

CALL YOUR DOCTOR IF

* You or a family member has symptoms of thyroid nodules or thyroid enlargement.
* New, unexplained symptoms develop. Drugs used in treatment may produce side effects.

THYROIDITIS

 ## GENERAL INFORMATION

DEFINITION
- Thyroiditis is a group of inflammatory thyroid disorders. The thyroid gland is a hormone-producing organ at the base of the neck, next to the trachea (windpipe). Types include:
  - Chronic lymphocytic thyroiditis (Hashimoto's thyroiditis or autoimmune thyroiditis) is the most common type.
  - Subacute granulomatous thyroiditis (DeQuervain's thyroiditis). It is less common.
  - Subacute lymphocytic thyroiditis (silent thyroiditis or postpartum thyroiditis). It occurs more often in women who have recently delivered a baby.
  - Acute suppurative thyroiditis (rarer type).

BODY PARTS INVOLVED—Thyroid gland.

SEX OR AGE MOST AFFECTED—Middle-aged persons of both sexes between ages 30 and 50, but more common in women.

SIGNS & SYMPTOMS
- No symptoms may occur or they may be mild.
- Enlarged thyroid gland (goiter).
- May have trouble swallowing.
- Pain or tenderness in the thyroid (sometimes).
- Fever (sometimes).
- Underactive thyroid (hypothyroidism). It may cause fatigue, weight gain, constipation, depression, and trouble concentrating.
- Overactive thyroid (hyperthyroidism). It is less common, and may cause weight loss, anxiety, heart palpitations, and sleep problems.

CAUSES—Thyroiditis can be brought on by a number of different factors. In the most common type, it is an immune system problem, but why this occurs is unknown. Other factors include viral or bacterial infections.

RISK INCREASES WITH
- Disorder of the body's immune system.
- Pregnancy.
- Family history of thyroid disease.
- Previous thyroid disorders.
- Various viruses, such as mumps or influenza.
- Bacterial infection of the thyroid gland (rare).

HOW TO PREVENT—No specific preventive measures.

 ## WHAT TO EXPECT

DIAGNOSTIC MEASURES
- Your own observation of symptoms.
- Your health care provider will usually do a physical exam and ask about your symptoms.
- Medical tests include blood studies to check your thyroid function. Other tests may be done to confirm the diagnosis.

APPROPRIATE HEALTH CARE
- Treatment, if needed, is with drugs, and will depend on the type of thyroiditis.
- If symptoms are not severe, treatment may involve watchful waiting. This means monitoring thyroid function for a few months before deciding on treatment.

POSSIBLE COMPLICATIONS—Permanent loss of thyroid function. This requires lifelong thyroid hormone replacement.

PROBABLE OUTCOME—Will depend on the type. The chronic type can be treated successfully with thyroid hormone therapy. It may take several weeks of therapy for symptoms to improve. Other types of thyroiditis may clear up on their own in 4 to 6 months.

 ## HOW TO TREAT

GENERAL MEASURES
- With any type of thyroiditis, it is important to follow up with your health care provider for periodic exams.
- To learn more: American Thyroid Association, 6066 Leesburg Pike, Suite 650, Falls Church, VA 22041; (800) 849-7643; website: www.thyroid.org.

MEDICATION
- Antithyroid drugs or thyroid replacement hormones, depending on the activity of your thyroid hormones.
- Beta-adrenergic blockers to suppress symptoms of an overactive thyroid may be prescribed.
- Antibiotics to fight infection, if needed.
- Cortisone drugs to decrease inflammation may rarely be prescribed.
- You may use aspirin (not for children) or ibuprofen to control mild pain.

ACTIVITY—No limits.

DIET—No special diet.

 ## CALL YOUR DOCTOR IF

- You or a family member has symptoms of thyroiditis.
- New, unexplained symptoms develop.

TINEA CRURIS
(Jock Itch)

GENERAL INFORMATION

DEFINITION—Tinea cruris (jock itch) is a fungal infection of the skin in the groin.

BODY PARTS INVOLVED—Groin and nearby skin.

SEX OR AGE MOST AFFECTED—Both sexes (more likely to occur in men than in women) and in adults more than children.

SIGNS & SYMPTOMS
- Scaling red patches (often ring-shaped) on the skin of the groin, thighs, and buttocks.
- Patches have well-defined edges.
- Sometimes small, pus-filled blisters appear.
- Itching of involved areas.
- Pain (if the skin also becomes infected with bacteria).

CAUSES—Infection by fungi called dermatophytes. These germs tend to grow in the darkness, warmth, and moisture of the body's groin area.

RISK INCREASES WITH
- Hot, humid weather.
- Excessive sweating.
- Tight clothing.
- Obesity, which fosters sweating.
- Friction of skin against skin from constant movement.
- Contact with infected surfaces, such as towels or benches.
- Weak immune system due to illness or drugs.
- Diabetes.
- Other fungal infection such as athlete's foot (tinea pedis).
- Crowded conditions (e.g., athletic teams, members of armed forces).

HOW TO PREVENT
- Dry completely after bathing. Use clean towel.
- Don't sit around in a wet bathing suit.
- Wear loose fitting, cotton underwear.
- Wear clean, dry athletic supporters and underwear for each workout.
- Use nonprescription tolnaftate after bathing if you have had tinea cruris before. This powder can help prevent a recurrence.

WHAT TO EXPECT

DIAGNOSTIC MEASURES
- Your own observation of symptoms.
- Your health care provider will do a physical exam of the affected area.
- Medical tests may include a microscopic exam of scraped-off scales.

APPROPRIATE HEALTH CARE—Treatment usually involves drugs applied to the skin and sometimes taken by mouth. Use them for the length of time prescribed, even if the rash goes away.

POSSIBLE COMPLICATIONS
- Recurrences are common.
- Bacterial infection in the affected area.

PROBABLE OUTCOME—Symptoms can be controlled in 2 to 4 weeks with treatment.

HOW TO TREAT

GENERAL MEASURES
- For home care, follow the steps listed in Preventive Measures.
- If you also have an athlete's foot infection, treat both areas with equal care. Put on socks before putting on underwear.

MEDICATION
- You may use nonprescription, topical antifungal drugs for treatment and prevention.
- Other topical or oral (taken by mouth) antifungal drugs may be prescribed.

ACTIVITY—No limits.

DIET—No special diet. If overweight is a problem, a weight loss diet may be recommended.

CALL YOUR DOCTOR IF

- You or a family member has symptoms of tinea cruris.
- Skin symptoms worsen despite treatment.
- Infection recurs after treatment.

TINEA VERSICOLOR

 GENERAL INFORMATION

DEFINITION—Tinea versicolor is an infection caused by a yeast type of skin fungus. It changes the color of skin that it affects.

BODY PARTS INVOLVED—Skin of the chest, back, shoulders, upper arms, trunk or groin. This rarely affects the face.

SEX OR AGE MOST AFFECTED—Both sexes and is more common in teens and young adults.

SIGNS & SYMPTOMS
- Small, scaly spots (or patches) on the skin. They may appear white to pink or tan to dark. They show up differently on light skin as compared to darker skin.
- Affected skin may itch (more likely if the person gets hot).
- Spots begin small and spread. They may join together to form larger patches.
- In hot climates, a person may have the spots all year round. In other climates, they may fade during the cooler months.

CAUSES—A fungus called *Malassezia* (previously named *Pityrosporum orbiculare*). It is present on normal skin, but it can't be seen and it normally causes no problems. Why it grows more active and causes symptoms for some people is unknown. It is not contagious and is not due to poor hygiene.

RISK INCREASES WITH
- Teens and young adults.
- Exposure to heat and high humidity.
- Excess sweating.
- Skin that is more oily.
- Weak immune system due to illness or drugs.

HOW TO PREVENT—No specific preventive measures. Once you have had the infection, retreatment can help stop a recurrence.

 WHAT TO EXPECT

DIAGNOSTIC MEASURES
- Your own observation of symptoms.
- Your health care provider can usually diagnose the disorder by an exam of the affected skin.
- Medical tests may include a microscopic exam of scales scraped from the skin to confirm the diagnosis.

APPROPRIATE HEALTH CARE
- Numerous topical products are effective in clearing tinea versicolor.
- Your health care provider will usually suggest a method to help prevent a recurrence. Several options are available. One method is to repeat treatment every week for 3 to 4 weeks and then once a month for 3 to 4 months.

POSSIBLE COMPLICATIONS
- Recurrence is common. The episodes of recurrence decline with age.
- The cosmetic appearance of the skin may cause some emotional distress, especially in young teens.

PROBABLE OUTCOME—Treatment can clear up the infection. Following treatment, the patches may remain for 6 weeks or longer.

 HOW TO TREAT

GENERAL MEASURES—Self-care involves application of tropical antifungal product.

MEDICATION
- Nonprescription, antifungal, topical products such as shampoos, creams, or lotions may be recommended. They are applied to the affected areas. Use product as directed on label.
- In some cases, antifungal drugs taken by mouth may be prescribed.

ACTIVITY—No limits. Try to avoid activities that cause excess sweating. If heavy sweating occurs, shower as soon as possible.

DIET—No special diet.

 CALL YOUR DOCTOR IF

- You or a family member has symptoms of tinea versicolor.
- Infection doesn't improve despite treatment.

TINNITUS

GENERAL INFORMATION

DEFINITION—Tinnitus is a persistent sound heard in one or both ears when there is no environmental noise. Tinnitus can be a common symptom of nearly all ear disorders, as well as other medical problems.

BODY PARTS INVOLVED—Ears.

SEX OR AGE MOST AFFECTED—Both sexes; all ages.

SIGNS & SYMPTOMS—A noise that may be a ringing, buzzing, humming, roaring, whistling, or hissing sound that is heard in one or both ears. The sound may be continuous, off and on, pulsing, or in time with the heartbeat.

CAUSES—There has probably been some sort of damage to the hearing system, but why this might cause tinnitus is unclear. Tinnitus does not cause deafness, nor does deafness cause tinnitus. They can both occur together in some patients.

RISK INCREASES WITH
- Older age.
- Hearing loss.
- Earache or ear infection.
- Labyrinthitis.
- Ménière's disease.
- Otitis media or externa.
- Otosclerosis.
- Ototoxicity.
- Earwax blockage.
- Aneurysm or tumor in the head (rare).
- Foreign body in the ear.
- Certain drugs (antibiotics, aspirin, antidepressants, diuretics, and others).
- High or low blood pressure.
- Head trauma.
- Anemia.
- Hypothyroidism or hyperthyroidism.
- Allergies.
- Exposure to excessively loud noise, either once or over a period of time.

HOW TO PREVENT—No specific prevention known.

WHAT TO EXPECT

DIAGNOSTIC MEASURES
- Your own observation of symptoms.
- Your health care provider may do a physical exam and an ear exam. Questions will be asked about your symptoms.
- Medical tests may be done to check for an underlying disorder.

APPROPRIATE HEALTH CARE
- If tinnitus is ongoing, the treatment is basically finding methods that help you to cope with the constant noise. Try one method for a time to see if it helps. Sometimes, a combination of different methods will work.
- Dental treatment may be recommended.
- Electrical stimulation with cochlear implant may help tinnitus, but it is usually used only for severe deafness.
- Tinnitus retraining therapy (TRT) may help. It combines counseling with sound therapy.

POSSIBLE COMPLICATIONS—There are usually no medical complications. Emotional problems may develop due to feelings of distress for those who find the noise very difficult to live with.

PROBABLE OUTCOME—Treatment of an underlying disorder may help. Often there is no cure, and learning to cope is the best therapy. Some people tolerate the condition much better than others. Research is ongoing to find the cause and effective treatment.

HOW TO TREAT

GENERAL MEASURES
- Try to ignore the sound by directing your attention to other things and activities. Counseling or biofeedback training may help you learn to do this technique.
- Play music in the background during the day and while falling asleep.
- Learn techniques to control stress in your life. This helps some people with tinnitus.
- Quit smoking. Find a way to stop that works.
- A hearing aid for deafness may help mask tinnitus.
- Wear a tinnitus suppressor or masker. This is a device that fits in the ear like a hearing aid, and presents a more pleasant sound.
- To learn more: American Tinnitus Association, PO Box 5, Portland, OR 97207; (800) 634-8978; website: www.ata.org.

MEDICATION—There are no drugs for tinnitus. Drugs normally prescribed for other conditions may help tinnitus in some people.

ACTIVITY—No limits.

DIET—It may help to eat a low-salt diet. Avoid or limit caffeine (e.g., coffee or chocolate) and alcohol.

CALL YOUR DOCTOR IF

- You or a family member has symptoms of tinnitus.
- Feelings of distress about tinnitus worsen.

TOENAIL, INGROWN

GENERAL INFORMATION

DEFINITION—An ingrown toenail is a common problem in which one or both edges of a nail grows into the flesh of a toe. It usually occurs in the great (big) toe. This can lead to infection and inflammation.

BODY PARTS INVOLVED—Toes.

SEX OR AGE MOST AFFECTED—Both sexes; most common in adolescents and adults.

SIGNS & SYMPTOMS—Pain, tenderness, redness, swelling, and heat in the toe where the sharp nail-edge pierces the nearby fold of tissue. Once tissue around the nail becomes red and sore, infection often develops.

CAUSES—The nail grows sideways or is compressed and pokes into or pinches off the skin. This can cause a break in the skin leading to inflammation (a foreign body reaction) and sometimes, an infection.

RISK INCREASES WITH
- The nail is more curved than normal.
- The toenail is clipped back too far, allowing tissue to grow up over it.
- Shoes fit poorly, forcing the toe of the shoe against the nail and surrounding tissue.
- Injury to the nail, or infection of the nail.
- Sports activities that require sudden stops ("toe jamming").
- Poor blood circulation to feet (such as with diabetes).

HOW TO PREVENT
- Wear roomy, well-fitting shoes and socks.
- Carefully cut toenails straight across, and not too short.
- People with diabetes or blood vessel disease have poor healing abilities. Be very careful in trimming your toenails. Foot injury is a risk with these disorders because of changes in blood flow to the feet.
- If you often handle heavy objects in your work, consider wearing work shoes with steel toe boxes.
- Keep feet clean and dry.

WHAT TO EXPECT

DIAGNOSTIC MEASURES
- Your own observation of symptoms.
- See your health care provider if home care does not help. Diagnosis is confirmed by an exam of the affected toe.

APPROPRIATE HEALTH CARE
- If there is an infection, drugs usually relieve symptoms within 1 week.
- If an ingrown toenail occurs often, then surgery is often the best treatment. The type of surgery will depend on how severe the problem is. It may involve just removing overgrown skin tissue, removing a portion of the toenail, or complete removal of the toenail.

POSSIBLE COMPLICATIONS—An ingrown toenail may become very painful, red, and swollen with pus if treatment for infection is delayed. Sometimes a bloody growth called proud flesh builds up on the side of the nail.

PROBABLE OUTCOME—Curable with treatment.

HOW TO TREAT

GENERAL MEASURES
- The following home treatment may help mild cases:
  - Soak toe for 20 minutes twice a day in a gallon of warm water (may add 2 tablespoons of Epsom salts).
  - Lift the nail corners gently, and wedge a very small piece of cotton under the ingrown nail edges. This will lift the nail slightly so it can grow past the skin tissue it is digging into. Replace the cotton daily. Do not cut a "V" in the middle of the nail. This is not helpful.
  - There are certain products you can buy that may soften the nail and the skin around it, which can help relieve the pain. Follow the directions carefully. These products should not be used if you have diabetes or a blood vessel problem.

MEDICATION
- Antibiotic ointment may be prescribed for infection.
- You may use ibuprofen or acetaminophen for pain.
- A tetanus shot or booster may be recommended.

ACTIVITY
- Resume your normal activities as soon as symptoms improve. You may need to wear sandals or a shoe with the toe cut out until the toe heals.
- If you have surgery, your health care provider will instruct you about aftercare, such as keeping the foot propped up as much as possible.

DIET—No special diet.

CALL YOUR DOCTOR IF

- You have symptoms of an ingrown toenail that persist despite self-treatment.
- The following occur during treatment or after surgery:
  - Signs of infection (pain, redness, heat, swelling, or tenderness) in the toe.
  - Red streaks going up the foot or ankle.

TONGUE INFLAMMATION
(Glossitis)

GENERAL INFORMATION

DEFINITION—Tongue inflammation is an acute or chronic condition due to a variety of causes. It is sometimes contagious, but not cancerous.

BODY PARTS INVOLVED—Tongue and adjacent parts of the mouth.

SEX OR AGE MOST AFFECTED—Both sexes; all ages.

SIGNS & SYMPTOMS
- Bright red, swollen tongue.
- Tongue looks and feels smooth.
- Tongue may be sore and tender.
- Hairy-looking tongue, sometimes with a black surface.
- A tongue with a red tip and edges.

CAUSES—The inflammation can be due to many different causes.

RISK INCREASES WITH
- Bacterial or viral (including herpes) infections.
- Burns.
- Injury from jagged teeth, ill-fitting dentures, tongue or lip piercing, mouth-breathing, or repeated biting during seizures.
- Hot foods or spices.
- Poor dental health.
- Allergy to toothpaste, mouthwash (especially mouthwash containing peroxide), candy, dye, or material used in dental work.
- Adverse reaction to drugs.
- Poor nutrition, especially vitamin deficiencies.
- Smoking.
- Chemical or environmental exposure to irritating or corrosive chemicals.
- Alcoholism.
- Diabetes or other illnesses.
- Topical or inhaled steroids.
- Prolonged antibiotic use leading to yeast infections.
- Dry mouth such as from Sjögren's syndrome.

HOW TO PREVENT
- Practice good oral hygiene. Obtain regular dental check-ups.
- Don't smoke. Avoid irritants (e.g., hot and spicy foods and alcohol).
- Prevent tongue injury by wearing protective headgear for contact sports or cycling.

WHAT TO EXPECT

DIAGNOSTIC MEASURES
- Your own observation of symptoms.
- Your health care provider will do an exam of the mouth and tongue.
- Medical tests may be done to check for cause.

APPROPRIATE HEALTH CARE
- Treatment will be directed at the underlying cause along with self-help measures.
- If tongue symptoms are caused by teeth or denture problems, consult your dentist. The problem won't heal until the cause is eliminated.

POSSIBLE COMPLICATIONS
- Tongue inflammation can become chronic if not adequately treated.
- Tongue may become swollen and block the airway.

PROBABLE OUTCOME—Usually curable in 2 weeks with treatment.

HOW TO TREAT

GENERAL MEASURES
- Notice if there is an connection between eating specific foods and tongue symptoms. Irritating foods may include chocolate, citrus, acidic foods (vinegar, pickles), salted nuts, or potato chips.
- Rinse mouth 3 or more times a day with a salt solution (mix one-half teaspoon of salt in one cup of warm water).

MEDICATION
- For minor pain, you may use nonprescription drugs, such as anesthetic mouthwashes or acetaminophen.
- For infection and pain, antibiotics or antifungals or topical anesthetics may be prescribed.

ACTIVITY—No limits.

DIET
- No special diet, except to avoid foods that may cause the symptoms.
- Drink as many fluids and eat as well-balanced a diet as possible while healing.
- To reduce pain, sip liquids through straws. Foods or fluids that cause the least pain are milk, liquid gelatin, yogurt, ice cream, and custard.

CALL YOUR DOCTOR IF

- You or a family member has symptoms of tongue inflammation.
- Symptoms don't improve in 3 days despite treatment.
- Pain gets worse and isn't relieved by treatment.
- Tongue swells and interferes with swallowing.

TONSILLITIS

GENERAL INFORMATION

DEFINITION—Tonsillitis is an inflammation of the tonsils due to an infection. The tonsils are lymphoid tissue located on each side of the back of the throat. They are small at birth, enlarge during childhood, and become smaller during the teen years. Tonsils usually help prevent infections in the nose, mouth, and throat from spreading to other places in the body. However, they themselves can become infected. Tonsillitis can be spread from person to person.

BODY PARTS INVOLVED—Tonsils; throat.

SEX OR AGE MOST AFFECTED—Both sexes and all ages, but most common in children between ages 5 and 10.

SIGNS & SYMPTOMS
- Sore throat and pain when you swallow.
- Tonsils are redder than normal.
- Throat may have white or yellow patches.
- Swollen glands on either side of the jaw.
- Fever.
- Headache.
- Ear pain.
- Bad breath.
- A very young child may not want to eat.

CAUSES—Most cases are caused by a viral infection. A bacterial infection (often Streptococcus, or "strep" as it is called) may also be a cause. Viral or bacterial germs are spread both by droplets you breathe in (e.g., from a person's cough or sneeze) or through germs on a surface or object that you handle and then touch your nose, mouth, or eyes.

RISK INCREASES WITH
- Young children.
- Daycare centers (both children and teachers).
- Living, working, or being in crowded places.
- Having a chronic illness, such as diabetes.

HOW TO PREVENT—There are no specific preventive measures. Wash hands often to prevent spreading germs. Avoid contact with persons who have strep infections or other infections. Don't share glasses, cups, silverware, or toothbrushes.

WHAT TO EXPECT

DIAGNOSTIC MEASURES
- Your own observation of symptoms.
- Your health care provider will examine your head, neck, and throat.
- Medical tests may include a rapid strep test and a throat culture (to find which germ is the cause). Family members may also need a strep test. A person may carry the strep germ, but not have any symptoms.

APPROPRIATE HEALTH CARE
- Treatment usually involves self-care and drug therapy if needed.
- If tonsillitis is severe and occurs often, your health care provider may suggest surgery (tonsillectomy) to remove the tonsils.

POSSIBLE COMPLICATIONS
- Abscess (an infected sore on the tonsils).
- Chronic tonsillitis. It can cause ear infection and enlarged tonsils. This may lead to breathing problems and snoring.
- Rheumatic fever may occur if the cause is strep and it is not treated, or if treatment is stopped too soon.

PROBABLE OUTCOME—Most cases heal well with no problems. Symptoms generally begin to improve in a few days.

HOW TO TREAT

GENERAL MEASURES
- To relieve the sore throat, gargle frequently with warm or cold double-strength tea or warm salt water (mix one-half teaspoon of salt in one cup of water).
- Suck on throat lozenges or hard candy such as lemon drops, to increase moisture in the mouth.

MEDICATION
- If the cause is a bacterial infection, an antibiotic (e.g., penicillin) is usually prescribed. It is typically taken for 10 days. Antibiotics will not cure a viral infection.
- To relieve pain, you may use acetaminophen or ibuprofen. Don't give aspirin to children under age 18.

ACTIVITY
- Stay away from others until fever, pain, and other symptoms disappear.
- Bed rest if there is fever. Then return to your regular routine.

DIET—Drink plenty of fluids. While the throat is very sore, use liquids for food. This includes milkshakes, soups, and high-protein fluids (diet or instant-breakfast type drinks).

CALL YOUR DOCTOR IF

- You or a family member has symptoms of tonsillitis. If there is any trouble with breathing, call right away.
- Symptoms worsen, or other symptoms occur during treatment.

TOOTH ABSCESS
(Periapical Abscess; Periodontal Abscess)

GENERAL INFORMATION

DEFINITION—A tooth abscess is a pus-filled sac around a tooth root, which is imbedded in bone of the upper or lower jaw.

BODY PARTS INVOLVED—Teeth, gums; jawbone.

SEX OR AGE MOST AFFECTED—Both sexes; all ages.

SIGNS & SYMPTOMS
- Persistent toothache or throbbing, extreme pain upon biting or chewing.
- Swelling and tenderness in the neck glands and on the side of the face.
- Earache.
- Fever.
- General ill feeling.
- Foul taste and bad breath (if the abscess opens spontaneously).

CAUSES—The pulp (nerves and blood vessels that fill the central cavity of a tooth) is invaded by bacteria, usually as a result of dental caries (tooth decay) that destroy a tooth's enamel and dentin, or when a tooth is injured. Abscess also occur from periodontal disease (bacteria invades pockets between the teeth and gums).

RISK INCREASES WITH
- Tooth decay due to plaque.
- Early childhood caries (baby bottle tooth decay).
- Gingivitis.
- Infection following an injury or surgery.
- Weak immune system due to illness or drugs.

HOW TO PREVENT
- Prevent decay with brushing and flossing:
  - Use a soft-bristle toothbrush to remove plaque from the teeth's front and back surfaces, especially at the gum line.
  - Learn to use dental floss correctly. Ask your dentist or hygienist to demonstrate the technique.
- Use fluoride mouthwash, toothpaste, tablets or liquid supplement if recommended by dentist.
- Don't let an infant fall asleep with a bottle of milk, juice, or formula in the mouth.
- Reduce sugar consumption. Tooth decay increases as sugar consumption increases.

WHAT TO EXPECT

DIAGNOSTIC MEASURES
- Your own observation of symptoms.
- Your dental care provider (dentist) will do an exam of the mouth.
- Medical tests may include x-rays of the mouth and a culture of a sample of the pus.

APPROPRIATE HEALTH CARE
- Treatment may include drug therapy, self-care, and/or surgery.
- Surgery may involve a procedure to drain the pus from the affected area. Root canal surgery may be needed to preserve the tooth. The tooth may be extracted if it can't be saved.

POSSIBLE COMPLICATIONS
- If untreated, the abscess can erode a small channel to the gum surface where it forms a gumboil (swelling). If the gumboil bursts, it lets foul-tasting pus into the mouth. The abscess can also erode into the jawbone and produce an infection in the bone itself (osteomyelitis).
- Loss of the tooth.
- Spread of infection through the bloodstream to other body parts.

PROBABLE OUTCOME—With treatment and follow up care, the outlook is good.

HOW TO TREAT

GENERAL MEASURES
- Rinse your mouth with warm salt water (mix one-half teaspoon of salt in one cup of water). Repeat each hour or as often as feels good.
- Don't chew on the affected side of your mouth for at least 2 days.
- Follow medical instructions for home care after any dental surgery.

MEDICATION
- For minor pain, you may use nonprescription drugs such as ibuprofen or acetaminophen.
- Antibiotics for infection or stronger pain relievers may be prescribed.

ACTIVITY—Normally no limits. Activities level may depend on your symptoms.

DIET—A liquid or soft diet may be necessary for 1 or 2 days until pain subsides.

CALL YOUR DENTIST IF

- You or a family member has symptoms of a tooth abscess.
- The following occurs during treatment: fever of 101°F (38.3°C) or higher or pain becomes severe.
- New, unexplained symptoms develop.

TOOTH DECAY
(Cavities)

GENERAL INFORMATION

DEFINITION—Tooth decay is the destruction of enamel (outer surface), allowing injury to the dentin (layer below the enamel). This leads to involvement of the pulp (the layer below the dentin), which contains nerves and blood vessels. Tooth decay (also called caries) and the common cold are the most common human disorders.

BODY PARTS INVOLVED—Teeth.

SEX OR AGE MOST AFFECTED—Both sexes; all ages.

SIGNS & SYMPTOMS
* Tooth sensitivity to heat and cold.
* Tooth discomfort after eating sugar.
* Darkening on or between the teeth (cavity) when the decay has progressed enough to be seen. The most common tooth-cavity sites are the gum line, biting surfaces and surfaces between adjacent teeth.
* Unpleasant taste in the mouth and bad breath because of stagnant food and bacteria trapped in the cavity.
* Persistent tooth pain (in the final stages of decay when the pulp becomes inflamed).

CAUSES—Cavities are caused by acid destruction of tooth material. Acid is produced by bacteria in the mouth. The bacteria feed on food debris—usually sugar—and produce the acid that dissolves tooth material. The combination of sugars from food debris, bacteria and chemicals in the saliva form a substance called plaque. Plaque becomes a localized site of acid production, which forms continuously at the neck of each tooth. This plaque must be thoroughly cleaned away at the gum line daily or it can cause tooth decay.

RISK INCREASES WITH
* Certain foods or drinks that tend to cling to the teeth; frequent snacking or sipping of drinks.
* Poor dental hygiene.
* Eating disorders, heartburn, or certain cancer treatments.
* Dry mouth (can be due to illness or use of certain drugs).
* Teeth that are crowded or rotated.

HOW TO PREVENT
* Brush and floss teeth regularly.
* See your dentist on a regular basis for dental check ups and professional cleaning.
* Ask your dentist about using fluoride mouthwash, liquid, tablets or having fluoride treatments once or twice a year.
* Sealants may help prevent enamel erosion.
* Avoid sugary drinks or sucking on sugary candy.

WHAT TO EXPECT

DIAGNOSTIC MEASURES
* Your own observation of symptoms.
* Your dental care provider (dentist) will do an exam of the teeth. The decayed area feels soft when the dentist probes it with a sharp instrument.
* X-rays of the teeth are usually done.

APPROPRIATE HEALTH CARE
* Treatment may include:
  - Removing all decay in the tooth and replacing it with a restorative material (filling). The filling prevents further decay.
  - A crown may be placed on the tooth if decay is more extensive.
  - A root canal may be done if the nerve in a tooth dies from decay or injury.
  - Fluoride treatment.
  - Tooth extraction if tooth can't be restored.

POSSIBLE COMPLICATIONS
* Abscess around a decayed tooth.
* Pain (may affect activities of daily life).
* Loss of a tooth.
* Infection.

PROBABLE OUTCOME—Usually curable with dental treatment.

HOW TO TREAT

GENERAL MEASURES—No specific instructions.

MEDICATION
* For minor pain, you may use nonprescription drugs such as ibuprofen or acetaminophen.
* Your dentist may prescribe stronger pain relievers or fluoride supplements.

ACTIVITY—No limits.

DIET—Eat a healthy diet. Limit snacking.

CALL YOUR DENTIST IF

* You or a family member has symptoms of tooth decay.
* New or recurring symptoms develop after treatment.

TOOTH GRINDING
(Bruxism)

 GENERAL INFORMATION

DEFINITION—Tooth grinding is the habit of grinding or clenching the teeth. Bruxism is the medical term for the problem. Tooth grinding is often done while asleep, but grinding or tapping teeth during the day is also common. Continual tooth grinding may erode gums and supporting bones in the mouth.

BODY PARTS INVOLVED—Teeth; gums; temporomandibular joints.

SEX OR AGE MOST AFFECTED—Both sexes; all ages.

SIGNS & SYMPTOMS
- Pain in the jaw muscles. Ear aches may occur.
- Clenching of the jaw, or clicking noises in the jaw.
- Annoying tooth grinding noises at night. These may be loud enough to awaken others.
- Teeth may become loose and more sensitive to cold and heat.
- Damage to teeth, supporting gums, and bone (a dentist will notice the changes in a dental exam).
- Headaches.
- Daytime sleepiness.

CAUSES—The cause is unclear. There may be several physical and psychosocial (psychologic and social) factors involved. The causes for daytime (wake) tooth grinding and sleep tooth grinding may be different.

RISK INCREASES WITH
- Alcohol, caffeine, or smoking before bedtime.
- Depression, stress, and/or anxiety.
- Teeth that are not aligned properly.
- Sleep apnea or snoring.
- Some antidepressant or antipsychotic drugs may increase the risk.
- Tooth grinding occurs in children. They may grind their teeth when they have a cold, ear ache, allergies, or other problems. The children usually outgrow the habit, and it typically causes no damage to the teeth.

HOW TO PREVENT—Avoid stressful situations if possible.

 WHAT TO EXPECT

DIAGNOSTIC MEASURES
- Your own or bed partner's observation of symptoms.
- See your dentist if self-help measures aren't working. Your dentist will examine your teeth and the jaw areas of your face.

APPROPRIATE HEALTH CARE
- Several treatment options may be discussed.
- No treatment may be needed if grinding is not causing oral health or well-being problems.
- Dental work can help certain problems (e.g., abnormal bite or crooked or missing teeth).
- A night guard or orthotic device may be prescribed. This is a custom-made plastic device worn at night to stop upper and lower teeth from coming together.
- Biofeedback training (relaxation exercises) or counseling to learn ways to cope more effectively with stress may be needed.
- Physical therapy, hypnosis therapy, or discontinuing drugs that are a risk factor may help some patients.

POSSIBLE COMPLICATIONS
- Teeth, bones, and gums may erode or crack from the grinding pressure.
- Problems with the temporomandibular joint. This is the hinge-like area where your upper jaw connects to the lower jaw.
- Continued problems with disrupted sleep.

PROBABLE OUTCOME—Treatment can help relieve the symptoms and limit any further damage to the teeth or other complications.

 HOW TO TREAT

GENERAL MEASURES
- Self-treatment options may sometimes help.
  - Reduce intake of alcohol and caffeine.
  - Try taking a warm bath before bedtime.
  - Use a warm washcloth to apply heat to the jaw area.
  - Decrease the stress in your life, where possible.
  - Have your bed partner wake you at night when you grind your teeth. Then get up and do some simple activity for about 10 minutes before you go back to sleep.
- Avoid chewing gum. It can increase the clenching and grinding of the jaw muscles.

MEDICATION
- Your health care provider or dentist may prescribe drugs for a short period for certain problems. These include muscle relaxants or mild sleeping aids.
- Botulinum toxin (Botox) injections may be recommended in some cases to temporarily stop the grinding.

ACTIVITY—No limits.

DIET—No special diet.

 CALL YOUR DENTIST IF

- You or a family member grinds teeth at night.
- Call your health care provider if symptoms are due to emotional problems.

TORTICOLLIS
(Wryneck; Cervical Dystonia)

 GENERAL INFORMATION

DEFINITION—Torticollis is a problem of the neck muscles that causes a twisted head movement. Torticollis is a type of movement disorder (dystonia).

BODY PARTS INVOLVED—Brain and central nervous system; muscular system.

SEX OR AGE MOST AFFECTED—Adults ages 30 to 60 (women more than men). Congenital torticollis is a type that affects newborns.

SIGNS & SYMPTOMS
• Symptoms may begin slowly and progress over time or develop suddenly.
• Head turns (or tilts) toward one shoulder while the chin turns toward the opposite shoulder. The head may be pulled forward or backward.
• The head may not move from the abnormal position (tonic), may have jerky head movements (clonic), or may have both types.
• Neck muscles are tense and tender.
• There may be pain in the neck, back, or shoulder.
• In a newborn, a lump may be felt in the neck muscle.

CAUSES
• The nerves and muscles involved are affected by various causes. Sometimes, no cause is found. This is called idiopathic spasmodic torticollis. Genetic factors may play a role.
• In the congenital type, the exact cause is unknown.

RISK INCREASES WITH
• Family history of torticollis.
• Cervical spine problems (injury, fractures, scar tissue, tumor, infections, ligament problems, and others).
• Inflammatory problems (such as myositis and others).
• Certain prescribed drugs.
• Some drugs of abuse.
• Infection in tissues around neck muscles.
• Congenital type risks include position of the baby in the womb, a difficult delivery, or certain birth defects.

HOW TO PREVENT—No specific measures.

 WHAT TO EXPECT

DIAGNOSTIC MEASURES
• Your own observation of symptoms.
• Your health care provider will do a physical exam of the affected area and ask questions about your symptoms and activities.
• Medical tests may include x-rays, MRI, CT, and studies of muscle movements.

APPROPRIATE HEALTH CARE
• Congenital torticollis is initially treated with physical therapy, including daily passive therapy for at least a year. If therapy is not successful, then surgery to lengthen neck muscles is performed.
• For other forms of torticollis, drug therapy may help, along with physical therapy, and other therapies. Mild cases may not need treatment.
• If a drug is causing the problem, it should be stopped.
• A neck brace or collar may be recommended.
• Electrical stimulation may be recommended.
• Rarely, a surgical procedure to denervate (cut the nerves) in the neck muscles may be recommended.

POSSIBLE COMPLICATIONS
• Condition becomes chronic; depression; disability.
• Social phobia.

PROBABLE OUTCOME
• The symptoms often improve with one or more types of treatment. Complete remission may occur. Other patients may have neck problems for months or years.
• Congenital torticollis can usually be corrected with muscle-stretching exercises or surgery.

 HOW TO TREAT

GENERAL MEASURES
• Relieve pain from neck spasms with heat or massage. Take hot showers or use warm, moist compresses, deep-heating ointments, or heating pad.
• "Sensory tricks" may help. Place a hand on the chin, side of face, or back of neck to reduce muscle spasms.
• Stress may worsen symptoms. Learn stress-reduction techniques, including biofeedback.
• To learn more: National Spasmodic Torticollis Association, 9920 Talbot Ave., Suite 233, Fountain Valley, CA 92708; (800) 487-8385; website: www.torticollis.org.

MEDICATION
• Muscle relaxants, anti-inflammatories, or other drugs may be prescribed. They may be taken by mouth or injected by a health care provider.
• Injections of botulinum toxin into the neck muscles may be prescribed.

ACTIVITY—Physical therapy is often prescribed.

DIET—No special diet.

📞 **CALL YOUR DOCTOR IF**

• You or a family member has symptoms of torticollis.
• Symptoms don't improve with treatment.

TOXIC SHOCK SYNDROME

 GENERAL INFORMATION

DEFINITION—Toxic shock syndrome is a rare form of blood poisoning caused by poisons (toxins) released by bacteria. Menstrual toxic shock involves the female reproductive and respiratory systems.

BODY PARTS INVOLVED—Almost all organ systems in the body.

SEX OR AGE MOST AFFECTED—It has been associated with tampon use in menstruating women. Nonmenstrual toxic shock can affect all ages (including children) and both sexes.

SIGNS & SYMPTOMS
- Sudden, high fever in a healthy person.
- Chills.
- Vomiting and watery diarrhea.
- Rash that resembles sunburn.
- Low blood pressure.
- Excessive thirst.
- Rapid pulse.
- Feeling of impending doom.
- Mental changes, such as confusion.
- Extreme fatigue and weakness.
- Headache.
- Sore throat.

CAUSES—Bacteria, usually staphylococcal (staph) or streptococcal (strep) that most commonly grow on the skin and mucous membranes. The bacteria produce toxins that enter the bloodstream, causing an immune reaction in some people.

RISK INCREASES WITH
- Current or recent staph or strep infection.
- Tampon use (more so if left in for a long time or superabsorbent).
- Contraceptives such as a diaphragm or sponge.
- Childbirth.
- Surgery (especially nasal surgery).
- Foreign body, wound packing, or other packing such as stopping nosebleeds.
- Wound infection, bone infection, or burns.

HOW TO PREVENT
- There are no specific preventive measures.
- Avoid tampons or use low-absorbent type. Change tampons frequently, and alternate them at night with sanitary pads.
- Follow how-to-use instructions provided with contraceptive diaphragms and sponges.
- Wash hands carefully before inserting or removing tampons, diaphragms, sponges, or wound packings.
- Keep skin wounds clean. Get medical care for infected wounds.
- Pregnant women or new mothers should seek medical care for any possible staph or strep infection.

 WHAT TO EXPECT

DIAGNOSTIC MEASURES
- Your own observation of symptoms.
- Your health care provider will do a physical exam.
- Medical tests may include blood and urine studies and other tests to check for complications.

APPROPRIATE HEALTH CARE
- Immediate hospital care is required to give intravenous (IV) fluids, antibiotics, and electrolytes to correct fluid and electrolyte loss and dehydration.
- Treatment is provided for kidney or heart problems and mechanical breathing support, if needed.
- Tampons, diaphragms, or other foreign bodies are removed at once.

POSSIBLE COMPLICATIONS
- Severe shock.
- Kidney failure.
- Congestive heart failure.
- Respiratory distress.
- Loss of hair and nails.
- Recurrence of toxic shock syndrome.
- Death in severe cases.

PROBABLE OUTCOME—Many patients recover with early diagnosis and prompt hospital treatment, but some cases are fatal. Skin of the palms and soles often peels during recovery.

 HOW TO TREAT

GENERAL MEASURES—Follow medical advice.

MEDICATION
- Antibiotics, usually given through a vein (IV), for infection.
- Drugs for low blood pressure may be prescribed.
- Intravenous fluids and electrolytes as needed.

ACTIVITY—Resume your normal activities as advised by your health care provider.

DIET—No special diet after recovery.

 CALL YOUR DOCTOR IF

- You or a family member has symptoms of toxic shock syndrome. Call immediately! Shock develops rapidly.
- New, unexplained symptoms develop. Drugs used in treatment may produce side effects.
- Symptoms recur after recovery.

TOXOPLASMOSIS

 ## GENERAL INFORMATION

DEFINITION—Toxoplasmosis is an infection in humans and animals caused by a tiny parasite, *Toxoplasma gondii*. It can live up to a year in water or moist soil. The parasite can infect most types of animals, especially cats. Humans get the Infection in different ways.

BODY PARTS INVOLVED—Nerves, heart, gastrointestinal, skin.

SEX OR AGE MOST AFFECTED—Both sexes: all ages.

SIGNS & SYMPTOMS
- No symptoms usually (80% to 90% of patients). If they do occur, they can begin 1 to 2 weeks after exposure.
- Fever, sore throat, muscle aches, or fatigue.
- Swollen lymph glands (often in head and neck).
- Rash (sometimes).
- Inflammation (redness and soreness) of the retina (retinitis).

CAUSES
- People can get a toxoplasmosis infection by eating foods or drinking water that contain the germs. Infection can occur if you touch something, such as infected cat litter, with your hands then touch your mouth or eyes.
- Pregnant women who get the infection can transmit it to their offspring.
- Rarely, blood transfusion, organ transplantation, or lab accident.

RISK INCREASES WITH
- Eating raw or partially-cooked meat (e.g., pork, lamb, beef, or venison). Eating raw fruits or vegetables grown in infected soil. Handling raw meats, and then touching the mouth.
- Infected cats (who usually have no symptoms). They pass germs in their stools (feces) into litter boxes, the soil in gardens, or in a child's sand box. The germs get on a person's hands when they change litter or garden. The hands then accidentally touch the mouth or eyes. Children who eat the sand or soil can become infected.
- Weak immune system due to illness or drugs.

HOW TO PREVENT
- Cook meat thoroughly. Carefully wash any surface that raw meat has touched, including your hands. Wash raw fruits and vegetables before eating them.
- Persons with weak immune systems and pregnant women should avoid contact with cat feces and litter. Wear gloves when gardening or changing cat litter.
- Change cat litter boxes daily. Feed indoor cats only canned, dry, or cooked meat (no raw meat).
- Protect children's play areas, including sand boxes, from cat and dog feces.

 ## WHAT TO EXPECT

DIAGNOSTIC MEASURES
- Your health care provider may do a physical exam and ask questions about your symptoms and activities.
- A blood test is needed to confirm the diagnosis.

APPROPRIATE HEALTH CARE
- Treatment is usually not needed for a healthy person with no symptoms or if their symptoms are mild.
- For an infected pregnant female, your obstetric provider will discuss the treatment available, the risks involved, and the expected outcomes.
- For a person with a weakened immune system, treatment is usually with drugs.
- HIV infected persons should discuss testing for toxoplasmosis with their health care provider.
- Infected newborns (with or without symptoms) are usually treated with drugs to help prevent complications that may occur as they get older.
- If drugs are prescribed, your health care provider will do frequent blood tests to monitor for side effects.

POSSIBLE COMPLICATIONS
- Complications are rare. Inflammation may occur in the eyes (retinitis), the brain (encephalitis), or heart (myocarditis). People with weak immune systems are more likely to have complications.
- Pregnant women may have a miscarriage or stillbirth.
- Serious health problems or death may result for newborns who get infection from the mother.

PROBABLE OUTCOME—The majority of infected persons have no symptoms. Those with mild symptoms recover on their own.

 ## HOW TO TREAT

GENERAL MEASURES—None specific.

MEDICATION
- Pyrimethamine and sulfadiazine are the drugs most often prescribed to treat toxoplasmosis. These or other drugs may be prescribed for a pregnant woman.
- Corticosteroids, if necessary, for inflammation.

ACTIVITY—Usually no limits.

DIET—No special diet.

 ## CALL YOUR DOCTOR IF

- You or your a family member has symptoms of toxoplasmosis.
- Symptoms worsen.

TRANSIENT ISCHEMIC ATTACK

 GENERAL INFORMATION

DEFINITION—A transient ischemic attack (TIA) is a temporary loss of blood supply (ischemia) to a part of the brain causing a brief decrease in brain function. A TIA is sometimes called a "mini stroke" or a warning stroke. They are a high risk factor for a future stroke. (However, most strokes are not preceded by a TIA.)

BODY PARTS INVOLVED—Blood vessels to the brain and the part of the brain supplied by the affected blood vessels.

SEX OR AGE MOST AFFECTED—Adults over age 40 and men more than women.

SIGNS & SYMPTOMS
- Most attacks last less than an hour and some may last only for minutes. Symptoms are similar to those of a stroke. After the attack, normal function returns.
- Loss of muscle function on one side of the body.
- Sudden onset of headache or dizziness.
- Tingling in the arms and legs.
- Numbness.
- Vision disturbance or temporary blindness in one eye.
- Confusion.
- Faintness without loss of consciousness.
- Slurred speech or inability to speak.

CAUSES—A temporary loss of blood supply (and oxygen) to a part of the brain. It can be due to a blood clot, partially blocked blood vessel, or other less common causes. There is no permanent damage to the brain (as with a stroke).

RISK INCREASES WITH
- Aging; males; and African Americans.
- Personal or family history of high blood pressure, atherosclerosis, stroke, or blood clotting disorders.
- Diabetes, heart disease, carotid artery disease, peripheral artery disease, or migraine.
- High cholesterol levels or high homocysteine levels.
- Obesity.
- Smoking or excess alcohol use.
- Sedentary lifestyle (being physically inactive).

HOW TO PREVENT
- Reduce your risks where possible.
- Get medical care for treatable risk factors. Exercise daily. Maintain a healthy weight. Eat a healthy diet.
- Don't smoke. Avoid excess alcohol use.
- Have your blood pressure checked regularly. If it is high, get medical advice for treatment to reduce it.
- Preventive drug therapy may be prescribed.

 WHAT TO EXPECT

DIAGNOSTIC MEASURES
- If symptoms occur, call 911 for emergency care. Do not ignore symptoms even if they are short-lived. Stroke and TIA symptoms are alike.
- Emergency care will include a physical exam and questions about your symptoms and activities. Medical tests may include studies to check heart, brain, and blood vessel function.

APPROPRIATE HEALTH CARE
- Hospital care may be needed for a short time.
- Treatment may include drugs, taking control of risk factors (diabetes, high blood pressure, heart disease, and others), and lifestyle changes. A treatment plan will be based on your individual case.
- Surgery (endarterectomy) may be needed to remove plaques (fatty deposits) from carotid arteries in the neck. Heart valve replacement surgery may be needed.

POSSIBLE COMPLICATIONS—Stroke. After a TIA, more than one-third of the persons will have a stroke (about half will occur within a year).

PROBABLE OUTCOME
- There are normally no lasting effects (such as weakness on one side) from a TIA. Treatment of TIAs can help reduce your risk for stroke.
- TIAs can recur. Symptoms of each attack may be similar or different from others.

 HOW TO TREAT

GENERAL MEASURES
- Stop smoking and limit alcohol use.
- To learn more: American Stroke Association, 7272 Greenville Ave., Dallas, TX 75231; (888) 478-7653; website: www.strokeassociation.org.

MEDICATION
- To prevent future TIAs or strokes, you may be prescribed anticoagulants, antiplatelets, aspirin, statin drugs, antihypertensives, or other drugs.
- Drugs for other disorders may be prescribed.

ACTIVITY—Routine exercise is helpful. Follow your heath care provider's advice. Try to get 30 to 60 minutes of exercise (e.g., walking) each day for most days of the week.

DIET
- Eat a healthy diet. It should be low in salt and fat and high in fiber and fresh fruits and vegetables.
- A weight-loss diet may be recommended.

☎ CALL YOUR DOCTOR IF

- You or a family member has symptoms of a TIA. Seek emergency help.
- Symptoms recur or new symptoms develop.

TRANSIENT SYNOVITIS OF THE HIP
(Toxic Synovitis)

GENERAL INFORMATION

DEFINITION—Transient synovitis of the hip is inflammation (swelling and pain) of the tissues around the hip joint. It usually affects one hip, not both, and is a common cause of sudden hip pain in young children. Transient is used to describe a condition that lasts a short time. Synovitis describes an inflamed joint in the body.

BODY PARTS INVOLVED—Hip and legs.

SEX OR AGE MOST AFFECTED—It occurs more often in children ages 3 to 10, and most are boys. It can occur in infants and adults.

SIGNS & SYMPTOMS
- Mild or more severe pain in the hip. It may start quickly or come on slowly.
- Some children may have pain in the inner thigh or knee area.
- Difficulty walking or standing.
- Walking with a limp.
- Hip is tender to the touch.
- Mild fever less than 101°F (38.3°C) may occur.

CAUSES—The exact cause is unknown. It sometimes occurs after a viral upper respiratory tract infection. An allergic reaction, a minor injury, or growth abnormality may be involved.

RISK INCREASES WITH—Boys ages 3 to 10.

HOW TO PREVENT—None known.

WHAT TO EXPECT

DIAGNOSTIC MEASURES
- Your own or child's observation of symptoms.
- Your child's health care provider will do a physical exam with careful attention to the painful hip area.
- Medical tests may include blood studies, x-rays, and other tests. These are done to confirm the diagnosis and make sure that there is not another problem involved.

APPROPRIATE HEALTH CARE
- The main treatment is rest at home.
- Rarely, traction (at home or in the hospital) may be recommended.

POSSIBLE COMPLICATIONS—Complications are rare, but may involve other problems with hip or thigh bones.

PROBABLE OUTCOME
- The pain may start to improve within 24 to 48 hours, and is usually gone completely within 2 weeks. Some children may have minor pain for several weeks.
- A few children may get the disorder again. If it does recur, it is usually within 6 months.

HOW TO TREAT

GENERAL MEASURES
- Use heat and massage to help ease the symptoms.
- Check your child's temperature daily to see if high fever develops.

MEDICATION—Naproxen or ibuprofen may be prescribed for treating pain and inflammation.

ACTIVITY—Limit activities until the pain symptoms are gone. Bed rest may be recommended.

DIET—No special diet.

CALL YOUR DOCTOR IF

- Your child has symptoms of transient synovitis of the hip.
- After diagnosis, your child develops a high fever, other symptoms get worse, or symptoms don't improve within 10 days.

TRENCH MOUTH
(Necrotizing Ulcerative Gingivitis; Vincent's Disease)

 GENERAL INFORMATION

DEFINITION—Trench mouth is an infection and inflammation of the gums. It is rare and not contagious or cancerous.

BODY PARTS INVOLVED—Gums. If untreated, trench mouth can spread to: lymph glands in the neck; tonsils; vocal cords; bronchial tubes; rectum; or vagina.

SEX OR AGE MOST AFFECTED—It affects both sexes and all ages, but is most common in young adults (20 to 40 years).

SIGNS & SYMPTOMS
- Painful gums.
- Gums that bleed when pressed.
- Excess saliva.
- Bad breath.
- Ulcers (sores) covered with gray membrane on the gums.
- Swallowing with difficulty.
- Speaking difficulty.

CAUSES—Overgrowth of the normal bacteria found in the mouth, causing an infection of the gums. Why this occurs is unknown.

RISK INCREASES WITH
- Poor nutrition.
- Weak immune system due to illness or drugs.
- Smoking or chewing tobacco.
- Stress.
- Poor oral hygiene. Tartar, plaque, or food debris between teeth.
- Infection in mouth, teeth, or throat.

HOW TO PREVENT
- Maintain good oral hygiene.
  - Brush teeth twice a day or after each meal. Use a soft bristle toothbrush or a power toothbrush. A fluoride toothpaste is often recommended.
  - Floss teeth at least once a day with waxed or unwaxed dental floss or use an interdental cleaner. An oral irrigator may be used in addition to flossing.
  - A tongue scraper can be used to clean the tongue.
  - Use an antiseptic mouthwash if desired.
- Get regular professional dental cleanings.
- Eat a well-balanced diet.
- Don't smoke.

 WHAT TO EXPECT

DIAGNOSTIC MEASURES
- Your own observation of symptoms.
- Your dental care provider or health care provider will do an exam of the gums.
- Dental x-rays or facial x-rays may be done.

APPROPRIATE HEALTH CARE—Treatment involves curing the infection and relieving symptoms. Treatment may include drug therapy, oral hygiene care, and professional dental cleaning.

POSSIBLE COMPLICATIONS—Infection may spread to other areas of the face (cheeks, lips, and jawbone) and cause tissue damage, periodontal disease, and loss of teeth.

PROBABLE OUTCOME—Usually curable in two weeks with treatment. Frequent dental check-ups, up to once a month, are recommended after treatment.

 HOW TO TREAT

GENERAL MEASURES
- Rinse your mouth with warm salt water a few times a day. Use one-half teaspoon of salt in one cup of water.
- Follow steps listed in Preventive Measures on how to brush and floss your teeth.
- Don't smoke. Find a way to quit.
- Find ways to reduce stress in your life.

MEDICATION
- Antibiotics may be prescribed for infection.
- You may use nonprescription drugs, such as acetaminophen, for minor pain.
- A topical pain reliever to apply to the gums may be prescribed.

ACTIVITY—Usually, no limits.

DIET
- A liquid or soft diet may be necessary for two or three days because of gum tenderness. When pain subsides, eat a normal, healthy diet. Avoid spicy or hot (temperature) food.
- Drink plenty of fluids each day.

 CALL YOUR DOCTOR IF

- You or a family member has symptoms of trench mouth.
- One or more of the following occur during treatment—fever, swelling of neck or face, swallowing difficulty, or inability to eat.

TRICHINOSIS

GENERAL INFORMATION

DEFINITION—Trichinosis is a parasitic roundworm infection. It is very uncommon in the United States.

BODY PARTS INVOLVED—The infection affects different places in the body (e.g., gastrointestinal tract, lymphatic system and bloodstream, and large muscles of the body).

SEX OR AGE MOST AFFECTED—Both sexes; all ages.

SIGNS & SYMPTOMS
- People may be infected and never have symptoms.
- Early stages (usually begin in 7 to 10 days):
  - Appetite loss, nausea, and vomiting.
  - Diarrhea and stomach cramps.
- Later stages:
  - Puffy eyelids and face.
  - Muscle pain.
  - Headache.
  - Itching, burning skin.
  - Sweating.
  - High fever (102°F to 104°F or 38.9°C to 40°C).
- Late stages:
  - Symptoms decrease, but some muscle tissues remain permanently infected with microscopic cysts. In rare cases, these cause heart and central nervous system disorders.

CAUSES—Infection with a parasite, *Trichinella spiralis*. It is transmitted to humans when they eat infected animals. Human cases can result from eating undercooked pork or wild animal meat. Thorough cooking kills the parasite and makes infected meat safe to eat. The parasites pass from animal to animal in contaminated food (usually raw garbage).

RISK INCREASES WITH
- Eating improperly cooked or raw pork.
- Weak immune system due to illness or drugs.

HOW TO PREVENT—Don't eat raw or undercooked pork meats (including ready-to-eat pork sausage). Cook all meats thoroughly.

WHAT TO EXPECT

DIAGNOSTIC MEASURES
- Your own observation of symptoms.
- Your health care provider will usually do a physical exam and ask about your symptoms and diet.
- Medical tests including blood studies, and a muscle biopsy may be done to confirm the diagnosis. With a biopsy, a small amount of muscle tissue is removed for viewing under a microscope.

APPROPRIATE HEALTH CARE
- Treatment usually includes antiworm drugs, drugs for pain and fever, and rest at home.
- Hospital care is usually needed for more severe cases. Breathing support and intravenous (IV) fluids may be needed.

POSSIBLE COMPLICATIONS
- Heart and lung complications.
- Central nervous system problems.
- Kidney damage.
- Vision or hearing disorders.
- Some deaths have been reported.

PROBABLE OUTCOME—Usually curable in 5–6 weeks in most persons with rest and treatment and, in severe cases, hospital care.

HOW TO TREAT

GENERAL MEASURES—Follow medical advice for care at home.

MEDICATION
- Anthelmintic (antiworm) drugs to kill the parasites are usually prescribed.
- Corticosteroids may be given to patients with severe symptoms or with central nervous system involvement.
- You may take nonprescription drugs, such as acetaminophen, to reduce fever and discomfort.

ACTIVITY—Rest in bed until symptoms improve. While confined to bed, move legs often to reduce the likelihood of deep vein blood clots. Resume normal activities gradually.

DIET—No special diet. Drink plenty of fluids.

CALL YOUR DOCTOR IF

- You or a family member has symptoms of trichinosis.
- New, unexplained symptoms develop. Drugs used in treatment may produce side effects, especially nausea, vomiting, skin rash, or fever.

TRICHOMONIASIS

GENERAL INFORMATION

DEFINITION—Trichomoniasis is a parasitic infection that affects both sexes, but usually causes symptoms only in women. Trichomoniasis (sometimes called "trich") is a sexually transmitted disease (STD).

BODY PARTS INVOLVED—Reproductive system.

SEX OR AGE MOST AFFECTED—Both sexes, but is more common in women; usually affects sexually active adolescents and adults.

SIGNS & SYMPTOMS
- Women:
  - Discomfort varies from woman to woman and from time to time in the same woman.
  - Foul-smelling, frothy vaginal discharge that is most apparent several days after a menstrual period.
  - Vaginal itching and pain.
  - Pain with intercourse.
  - Redness of the vaginal lips (labia) and vulva.
  - Painful and frequent urination.
- Men:
  - Infected men usually have no symptoms.
  - Rarely may have painful urination and a pale white discharge from the penis.

CAUSES—Infection from a tiny parasite, *Trichomonas vaginalis*. The infection is spread from person to person during sexual intercourse. Symptoms may start 4 to 28 days after being exposed. The parasite may also live in the body for years without producing symptoms. Since it thrives in both men and women, both sexual partners must receive treatment.

RISK INCREASES WITH
- Having multiple sexual partners.
- Having sex with someone who has, or had, multiple sexual partners.
- Engaging in unsafe sex.

HOW TO PREVENT
- Use latex (rubber) condoms during sexual intercourse.
- Limit your sexual partners or practice abstinence. The more sex partners you have, the greater your risk for any sexual transmitted disease.

WHAT TO EXPECT

DIAGNOSTIC MEASURES
- Your own observation of symptoms.
- Your health care provider will do a physical exam and a pelvic exam in women.
- Medical tests may include Pap smear and studies of vaginal discharge and urine. Tests to check for other STDs are often done.

APPROPRIATE HEALTH CARE—Treatment is with drug therapy. Your sexual partner(s) must be treated at the same time. This will prevent you from getting reinfected.

POSSIBLE COMPLICATIONS—If the infection is untreated, it can lead to other problems. Women may be more at risk for HIV infection (if exposed). If pregnant, it may cause early delivery and low birth weight baby. In men, prostate, bladder, or urethra problems may occur.

PROBABLE OUTCOME—Can be cured with treatment.

HOW TO TREAT

GENERAL MEASURES
- Don't douche unless prescribed for you.
- Wear cotton underpants or pantyhose with a cotton crotch.
- Take showers instead of tub baths.
- Don't sit around in wet clothing, especially in a wet bathing suit.
- To learn more: Centers for Disease Control & Prevention (CDC); (800) 232-4636; website: www.cdc.gov/std.

MEDICATION
- Metronidazole (Flagyl) or tinidazole (Tindamax) are usually prescribed for you and your sexual partner. They may be given as a single dose. Don't drink alcohol when you take the drug. If combined, they interact and cause a reaction with nausea, vomiting, sweating, weakness, and other symptoms.
- Topical drugs may be prescribed.

ACTIVITY—Avoid sexual activity until you and your sexual partner complete treatment and have no symptoms.

DIET—No special diet.

CALL YOUR DOCTOR IF

- You or a family member has symptoms of trichomoniasis.
- Symptoms get worse despite treatment.
- Unusual vaginal bleeding or swelling occurs.

TRIGEMINAL NEURALGIA
(Tic Douloureux)

GENERAL INFORMATION

DEFINITION—Trigeminal neuralgia is a condition involving the 5th cranial (trigeminal) nerve that causes episodes of severe facial pain.

BODY PARTS INVOLVED—The nerve and its branches supply sensation to the face, scalp, teeth, mouth, and nose.

SEX OR AGE MOST AFFECTED—The condition is more common in adults over age 40. Women are affected more than men.

SIGNS & SYMPTOMS
- Attacks of severe facial pain, described as "jabbing" or "searing" or like an electrical shock. These attacks (or bouts) of pain usually last for seconds, or sometimes for 1 to 2 minutes. A dull ache may be felt between bouts, or there may be little or no discomfort.
- Facial spasm (or tic) often occurs at the same time as pain.
- Only one side of the face is usually affected, but it may occur at different times on both sides.
- Pain is often triggered by touching or stroking the face, brushing teeth, shaving, exposure to wind, or chewing.
- Attacks may occur several times a day. They may disappear for weeks or months.
- A less common form, called atypical trigeminal neuralgia, may cause less-intense symptoms.

CAUSES—In most cases, the cause is believed to be blood vessels pressing on the trigeminal nerve. Pressure on the nerve may be caused by a tumor or multiple sclerosis. In some cases, the cause is unknown.

RISK INCREASES WITH—Increased age and females.

HOW TO PREVENT—No specific preventive measures.

WHAT TO EXPECT

DIAGNOSTIC MEASURES
- Your own observation of symptoms.
- Your health care provider will do a physical exam of the affected facial area and ask about your symptoms and activities. This is usually enough for diagnosis.
- Medical tests may be done to check for other problems.

APPROPRIATE HEALTH CARE
- Most patients obtain pain relief with drugs. However, as time goes by, the drugs may become ineffective in some patients and the pain then "breaks through."
- Alternate type of treatments have been used by some, but they are not always effective. These include acupuncture, herbal remedies, biofeedback, electrical stimulation, hypnosis, myotherapy (muscle release), and others.
- Surgery may be effective when drugs don't help. The different procedures available will be explained to you.

POSSIBLE COMPLICATIONS—Interference with daily life activities due to the frequent, severe pain episodes.

PROBABLE OUTCOME—Symptom relief is usually possible with treatment. Sometimes surgery may be required. A patient may experience pain-free intervals (lasting from months to years), and then the pain returns exactly as before.

HOW TO TREAT

GENERAL MEASURES
- Keep a daily "pain" log about your symptoms, drug therapy, and possible triggers.
- Learn to control stress. It may trigger or worsen pain.
- To learn more: Facial Pain Association, 925 NW 56th Terr., Suite C, Gainesville, GA 32605; (800) 923-3608; website: www.fpa-support.org.

MEDICATION
- Anticonvulsant (antiseizure) drugs are often prescribed to help relieve the pain.
- Other drugs including antidepressants, muscle relaxants, or antispasmodics may be helpful in some cases. Ordinary pain relievers are not helpful for this disorder.
- Alcohol injections that provide temporary pain relief may be recommended.
- Nonprescription products applied to the skin may help some patients. These include capsaicin (Zostrix) or lidocaine. Ask your health care provider before using.

ACTIVITY—No limits. Avoid blasts of hot or cold air.

DIET—No special diet.

CALL YOUR DOCTOR IF

- You or a family member has symptoms of trigeminal neuralgia.
- New, unexplained symptoms develop. Drugs used in treatment may produce side effects.

TUBERCULOSIS

GENERAL INFORMATION

DEFINITION—Tuberculosis (TB) is a contagious, bacterial infection that mainly involves the lungs. TB is occurring less often in the United States, but it is a major health problem in many parts of the world.

BODY PARTS INVOLVED—Lungs primarily, but may spread to other organs. Childhood TB is usually confined to the middle of the lungs. TB in adults usually affects the top of the lungs.

SEX OR AGE MOST AFFECTED—Both sexes; all ages.

SIGNS & SYMPTOMS
- Early stages:
  - No symptoms (often).
  - Flu-like symptoms.
- Middle and later stages:
  - Cough (lasts 3 weeks or more).
  - Low fever and/or chills.
  - Weight loss.
  - Chronic fatigue.
  - Heavy sweating, especially at night.
  - Cough with sputum that over time becomes bloody, yellow, thick, or gray.
  - Chest pain and/or shortness of breath.
  - Reddish or cloudy urine (sometimes).

CAUSES—Infection by a bacteria, most often *Mycobacterium tuberculosis*. Germs are transmitted in the air from one person to another. Many persons are infected with TB that is inactive and there are no symptoms (called latent TB infection or LTBI). About 1 in 10 of these people will eventually develop active TB.

RISK INCREASES WITH
- Adults over 60.
- Exposure to a TB-infected person.
- HIV infection.
- Weak immune system due to illness or drugs.
- Crowded or unclean living conditions.
- Alcoholism or IV drug abuse.
- Cancer, other lung disorders, or diabetes.
- Coming from countries where TB is common.

HOW TO PREVENT
- Treatment for several months with isoniazid (INH) if a tuberculin skin test is positive.
- Latent TB may be treated to prevent active TB.
- A vaccine called BCG is used in countries where TB is common and less often used in U.S.

WHAT TO EXPECT

DIAGNOSTIC MEASURES
- Your health care provider will do a physical exam and ask about your symptoms.
- Medical tests may include TB skin test, blood studies, sputum study, and chest x-ray.

APPROPRIATE HEALTH CARE
- Treatment is with drugs. It is important to take the drugs as prescribed to be sure the infection is cured.
  - If people stop the drugs once they feel better, but the infection is still active, they can spread the infection to others.
  - Also, this allows the TB bacteria to become resistant to the drugs and they may no longer kill the bacteria.
- Multidrug-resistant TB (MDR-TB) is resistance to at least two TB drugs. Stronger TB drugs have to be used which have serious side effects. MDR-TB is more difficult to cure, and it can be fatal. Extensively drug resistant TB (XDR TB) is a more rare form.
- It is sometimes necessary to isolate (separate from other persons) or have hospital care for a TB patient.

POSSIBLE COMPLICATIONS
- Lung abscess, chronic obstructive pulmonary disease, bronchiectasis, or respiratory failure.
- Spread of infection to brain, bone, spine, and kidneys.
- Without treatment, TB can be fatal.

PROBABLE OUTCOME—Usually curable with treatment.

HOW TO TREAT

GENERAL MEASURES
- If you are infectious, use tissue to cover mouth when coughing, sleep in a separate bed, keep away from others, and don't go to work or school.
- Have regular follow-up visits with your health care provider to see if treatment is working.
- To learn more: CDC (Centers for Disease Control & Prevention); (800) 232-4636; website: www.cdc.gov/tb.

MEDICATION—Antitubercular drugs, usually for 6 to 12 months will be prescribed. Several types are given at the same time to avoid bacterial resistance to the drugs. Patients are probably not infectious after 10 days to 2 weeks of treatment. Drug-resistant TB may need treatment for up to two years.

ACTIVITY
- Get extra rest until symptoms improve. You may need to restrict activities for 6 months.
- You will be advised about restrictions on commercial air travel while infectious.

DIET—No special diet.

CALL YOUR DOCTOR IF

- You or a family member has symptoms of TB.
- Symptoms persist or worsen despite treatment or new symptoms develop.
- You have been exposed to TB-infected person.

TYPHOID FEVER

GENERAL INFORMATION

DEFINITION—Typhoid fever is a bacterial infection of the gastrointestinal tract and bloodstream. In the United States, people affected have usually been traveling internationally.

BODY PARTS INVOLVED—Gastrointestinal tract; skin; central nervous system.

SEX OR AGE MOST AFFECTED—Both sexes; all ages. Infants and persons over 60 usually have the severest cases.

SIGNS & SYMPTOMS
- Fever, headache, fatigue.
- Constipation and dry cough. Diarrhea is less common.
- Bloated abdomen with some discomfort and loss of appetite.
- Confusion and feeling listless.
- Rash (rose spots) on the front of the body.
- May have eye symptoms, (e.g., vision changes).
- Later symptoms may include foul smelling diarrhea, weight loss, weakness, slow pulse, rapid breathing, delirium, and others.

CAUSES—Infection with *Salmonella typhi*, a type of bacteria. The infection is spread by persons who are ill with the infection, or carriers who have been ill and recovered, but still carry the germs. You can become ill if you eat food or drink beverages prepared by one of these persons. Also, the germs may get into sewage and contaminate water that is used for drinking or washing foods. Shellfish from contaminated water or canned meat prepared improperly can cause outbreaks of the infection. Symptoms may appear 10 to 20 days after exposure.

RISK INCREASES WITH
- Travel to countries where typhoid is present.
- Weak immune system due to illness or drugs.

HOW TO PREVENT
- For travel to countries where typhoid is present, consider typhoid vaccine (injection or oral form). It is not 100% protective, so take precautions with food and water. During travel, avoid tap water, salad and raw vegetables, unpeeled fruits, and dairy products. Follow the advice: "boil it, cook it, peel it, or forget it."
- Wash your hands after using the bathroom and before handling food.

WHAT TO EXPECT

DIAGNOSTIC MEASURES
- Your own observation of symptoms.
- Your health care provider will do a physical exam and ask about your symptoms and recent travel.
- Medical tests may include blood, urine, and stool studies.

APPROPRIATE HEALTH CARE
- Hospital care is needed for severe cases; others can be cared for at home. Follow any special instructions provided for preventing infection from being spread to other persons.
- People in certain types of jobs, such as food handlers, health care, or childcare workers, will need to be tested for the germs before they can resume their usual work. They need three negative tests.
- Surgery may be needed in severe cases if complications occur, such as bleeding or an abscess.

POSSIBLE COMPLICATIONS
- Perforation of the intestines.
- Gastrointestinal hemorrhage or abscess.
- Pneumonia.
- Bone infection.
- Congestive heart failure.
- Without treatment, it can be fatal.

PROBABLE OUTCOME—Usually curable in 2 to 3 weeks with treatment. Relapse may occur in 10–20% of patients. Treatment is repeated.

HOW TO TREAT

GENERAL MEASURES
- Use a heating pad or warm compress to relieve abdominal cramps.
- Wash hands carefully and often.
- To learn more: CDC (Centers for Disease Control & Prevention); (800) 232-4636; website: www.cdc.gov.

MEDICATION
- Antibiotics will be prescribed. They may be given by injection or taken by mouth.
- For severe cases, steroids will be prescribed in addition to antibiotics.
- Eye symptoms may require eyedrops or ointments.

ACTIVITY—Bed rest is needed until all symptoms have been gone at least 3 days. The legs should be moved often in bed to prevent deep vein blood clots from forming.

DIET—Diet will be determined by the symptoms.

CALL YOUR DOCTOR IF

- You or a family member has symptoms of typhoid fever.
- New symptoms develop or other symptoms become worse, despite treatment.

ULCER, PEPTIC
(Duodenal Ulcer; Gastric Ulcer)

GENERAL INFORMATION

DEFINITION—A peptic ulcer is an open sore in the lining of the gastrointestinal tract. Ulcers that form in the upper part of the small intestine are duodenal ulcers. They are the most common type. Ulcers that form in the stomach are called gastric ulcers and are less common. Rarely, a third type can occur in the esophagus.

BODY PARTS INVOLVED—Gastrointestinal tract.

SEX OR AGE MOST AFFECTED—Both sexes; all ages, but most common in adults.

SIGNS & SYMPTOMS
* Pain in the upper abdomen or, sometimes, the lower chest. It may be a burning, boring, or gnawing feeling that lasts 30 minutes to 3 hours. It may be worse before or after eating. It often awakens a person during the night. The pain may come and go. Weeks of off-and-on pain may alternate with short, pain-free periods.
* Pain is briefly relieved with use of antacids.
* Appetite loss and weight loss. With duodenal, it may be weight gain, as person eats more to ease discomfort.
* Vomiting (may contain bright red blood or digested blood [looks like coffee grounds]).
* Blood in the stool.

CAUSES
* Damage to the lining of the gastrointestinal tract. This is most often due to either an infection with *Helicobacter pylori* bacteria or the use of aspirin or other nonsteroidal anti-inflammatory drugs (NSAIDs). *Helicobacter pylori* bacteria is present in many healthy people. Why it leads to ulcers in some people is unknown.
* Ulcers are not caused by stress, or anxiety, or eating spicy foods (they may aggravate ulcers).

RISK INCREASES WITH
* Use of nonsteroidal anti-inflammatory drugs (e.g., aspirin).
* *Helicobacter pylori* infection.
* Family history of ulcers.
* Smoking and/or excess alcohol use (possibly).

HOW TO PREVENT—None specific. Avoid those risk factors that you can control.

WHAT TO EXPECT

DIAGNOSTIC MEASURES
* Your own observation of symptoms.
* Your health care provider will do a physical exam and ask about your symptoms and activities.
* Medical tests may include blood and stool tests, endoscopy, and test for *Helicobacter pylori*.

APPROPRIATE HEALTH CARE
* Treatment is with drugs and, sometimes, lifestyle changes.
* Discontinue the use of NSAIDs. If unable to do so, other drugs may be prescribed to prevent side effects.
* Hospital care may be needed for bleeding ulcer, severe perforation, or obstruction.
* Surgery for some patients for complications or if drug treatment is not effective.

POSSIBLE COMPLICATIONS
* Perforation. This is an erosion of the ulcer through the stomach or intestinal wall. It can cause infection or bleeding into the abdomen. Surgery may be required.
* Internal bleeding (which can cause anemia).
* Duodenal ulcers are almost always benign; gastric ulcers may rarely become malignant.
* Intestinal obstruction.

PROBABLE OUTCOME—With treatment, gastric ulcers heal in about 8 weeks and duodenal ulcers in about 4 weeks. Ulcers can recur.

HOW TO TREAT

GENERAL MEASURES
* Quit smoking. Find a way to stop that works.
* If you drink alcohol heavily, stop or cut down.
* If stress is a problem, learn ways to cope.
* To learn more: National Digestive Diseases Information Clearinghouse, 2 Information Way, Bethesda, MD 20892; (800) 891-5389; website: www.digestive.niddk.nih.gov.

MEDICATION
* Your health care provider may prescribe:
  - Antibiotics to treat the *Helicobacter pylori* infection.
  - Antacids to help neutralize stomach acid.
  - Proton pump inhibitors or H-2 blockers to reduce stomach acid. Long-term therapy may be required for some patients.
  - Drugs to coat and protect the lining of the stomach and the small intestine.

ACTIVITY—No limits.

DIET—Eat several small, healthy meals at regular times each day.

CALL YOUR DOCTOR IF

* You or a family member has symptoms of an ulcer.
* Vomiting occurs that is bloody or looks like coffee grounds, or stool is bloody, black, or tarry-looking.
* You feel weak, tired, have pale skin, or back pain.

URETHRITIS

GENERAL INFORMATION

DEFINITION—Urethritis is an inflammation of the urethra. The urethra is the tube that carries urine out of the bladder when you urinate. In women, it is about an inch long. In men, it is the full length of the penis.

BODY PARTS INVOLVED—Urethra; bladder (sometimes).

SEX OR AGE MOST AFFECTED—It can affect all ages and both sexes. In women, it often occurs along with a bladder infection or inflammation (cystitis).

SIGNS & SYMPTOMS
- Painful or burning urination. The pain can be severe.
- Discharge that may be cloudy, yellow-green mucus, or may be watery and white.
- Genital itching, tenderness, or swelling.
- Frequent urge to urinate, even when there is not much urine in the bladder.
- May have blood in urine or semen.
- Men may have no symptoms.

CAUSES
- An infection that is spread by a sexually transmitted disease (STD). The most common cause is a gonorrhea infection. When other infections (e.g., chlamydia or ureaplasma) are the cause, it is called nongonococcal urethritis (NGU).
- Trauma (injury) can be a cause. It may be due to a foreign body insertion or use of a medical instrument.
- Irritation or sensitivity to chemicals used in spermicides or contraceptive creams, foams, or jellies.

RISK INCREASES WITH
- Bacterial infection that spreads and enters the urethra from the skin around the genitals and anal area.
- Contact with an infected sexual partner.
- Multiple sexual partners.
- High-risk sexual behavior.
- Current or previous sexually transmitted disease.
- Use of a urinary catheter (tube used to remove urine).

HOW TO PREVENT—Practicing safe sexual behaviors will help with prevention. This includes abstinence or having only one sexual partner and using rubber (latex) condoms to help protect against infections.

WHAT TO EXPECT

DIAGNOSTIC MEASURES
- Your own observation of symptoms.
- Your health care provider will usually do an exam of the genital area.

- Medical t[...]
culture of u[...]
other STD[...]

APPROP[...]
- Treatme[...]
infection. [...]
60 days [...]
- If traum[...]
avoiding [...]
- Avoid [...]
can cause ure[...]

POSSIBLE COMPLICATIONS
- In women, urinary tract infections, pelvic inflammatory disease (PID), urethral stricture, or infertility may occur. There is also a risk of complications in pregnancy and in a newborn.
- In men, urinary tract infections, urethral stricture, or prostatitis (prostate infection) may occur.

PROBABLE OUTCOME—Proper treatment usually brings complete recovery. Symptoms should improve in about 3 days. Complications are rare.

HOW TO TREAT

GENERAL MEASURES
- To relieve pain, take sitz baths. Sit in a tub of warm water for 15 minutes at least twice a day.
- See your health care provider for follow up testing after treatment to be sure cure is complete.
- Keep the area around the genitals clean. Use unscented, plain soap.

MEDICATION—Antibiotics for infection will usually be prescribed. A single dose is often all that is needed. In some cases, the infection is persistent and drug therapy may be needed for 14 to 28 days.

ACTIVITY—Avoid sexual intercourse until you and your sexual partner are free of symptoms. Otherwise, no limits.

DIET
- Drink plenty of fluids every day.
- Drinking cranberry juice helps acidify urine. Some drugs are more effective with acid urine.

CALL YOUR DOCTOR IF

- You or a family member has symptoms of urethritis.
- Symptoms worsen or new symptoms occur after treatment.

EDING, DYSFUNCTIONAL
(al Abnormal Uterine Bleeding)

AL INFORMATION

Dysfunctional uterine bleeding
eding that is abnormal, irregular,
rt of a normal menstrual period. There
nor, infection, or pregnancy involved.

PARTS INVOLVED—Uterus; vagina.

EX OR AGE MOST AFFECTED—Women
ages 40 to 50 and under age 20.

SIGNS & SYMPTOMS
* Bleeding between periods. Blood flow may be light or heavy, prolonged, or random, and may contain clots.
* Periods last for more than 7 days and/or occur less than 21 days apart and may have extra heavy bleeding.

CAUSES
—The normal menstrual cycle depends on a balance of estrogen and progesterone. Bleeding problems occur if they get out of balance. There is too much estrogen or not enough progesterone. This happens most often due to anovulation (failure of the ovaries to produce or release eggs). Anovulation is more likely to occur in women who are close to menopause and young girls whose menstrual cycles have just started.

RISK INCREASES WITH
* Women ages 40 to 50 and under age 20.
* Polycystic ovary syndrome.
* Obesity.
* Smoking.
* Endocrine disorders.

HOW TO PREVENT—No preventive measures.

WHAT TO EXPECT

DIAGNOSTIC MEASURES
* Your own observation of symptoms.
* Your health care provider will usually do a physical exam and a pelvic exam. Questions will be asked about your symptoms and activities. Dysfunctional uterine bleeding is diagnosed after other causes of abnormal uterine bleeding have been ruled out. These include diseases, drugs, pregnancy, eating disorders, gynecological infections, polyps or other growths, or tumors.
* One or more medical tests are needed to help confirm the diagnosis.

APPROPRIATE HEALTH CARE
* Goals of treatment are to return periods to a normal cycle or stop the bleeding altogether. Treatment will depend on a woman's age, other medical conditions, and the severity of the bleeding.

* If bleeding is severe, a hospital stay may be needed to bring it under control.
* Treatment will be given for anemia if it exists.
* If symptoms are not severe, treatment may involve watchful waiting. This means monitoring the bleeding for a few months before treating it.
* Hormone therapy is usually the first treatment step, particularly in younger women. An intrauterine device (IUD) may be an option.
* If hormones do not help the bleeding, surgery may be needed. Your health care provider will discuss options, benefits, and risks. Together, you'll choose the treatment that will work best for you:
  - Dilation and curettage (D & C) may be the recommended procedure.
  - Other surgery options include endometrial ablation (destruction or removal of the uterine lining), or hysterectomy. These procedures mean a woman can no longer become pregnant. They may be used for women who are close to menopause.

POSSIBLE COMPLICATIONS
* Anemia due to excessive bleeding.
* Increased risk for endometrial cancer.
* Infertility from lack of ovulation.

PROBABLE OUTCOME—Outcome will depend on the woman's medical condition, age, the severity of the problem, and treatment.

HOW TO TREAT

GENERAL MEASURES
—To learn more: National Women's Health Information Center (800) 994-9662;
website: www.womenshealth.gov.

MEDICATION
* Hormone therapy may be prescribed. This includes birth control pills, hormone-replacement therapy, or progesterone.
* Iron supplements may be prescribed for anemia.

ACTIVITY—No limits.

DIET—With anemia, an iron-rich diet may be recommended.

CALL YOUR DOCTOR IF

* You or a family member has abnormal uterine bleeding.
* The following occur during treatment:
  - Bleeding becomes heavy (filling a pad or tampon more often than once an hour).
  - Signs of infection develop, such as fever, a general ill feeling, headache, dizziness, or muscle aches.

UTERINE FIBROIDS
(Myomas; Leiomyomas)

 GENERAL INFORMATION

DEFINITION
• Uterine fibroids (also called myomas or leiomyomas) are tumors that grow in and around the muscular wall of the uterus. There may be one or many fibroids. Fibroids are benign (not cancerous). Fibroid size can be very tiny to the size of a cantaloupe or larger. They are common in women of childbearing age. Major types of fibroids include:
- Subserous (grow outwards from uterine wall).
- Intramural (grow inside the wall of uterus).
- Submucous (grow inward from uterine wall).
- Pedunculated myomas (are attached to the uterine wall by stalks).

BODY PARTS INVOLVED—Uterus.

SEX OR AGE MOST AFFECTED—20-40% of women over 35.

SIGNS & SYMPTOMS
• Often, no symptoms occur. The fibroids may be diagnosed during a pelvic exam.
• Menstruation may be more frequent and may have heavy bleeding or passing of clots.
• Frequent urination; constipation may occur.
• Pressure or pain in abdomen or lower back.
• Pain during intercourse.

CAUSES—Exact cause is unknown. May involve estrogen and progesterone hormones.

RISK INCREASES WITH
• Increasing age until after menopause.
• African American women more than white women.
• Family history of fibroids.
• Obesity.
• Not having given birth, early age for starting menstruation, high blood pressure, or high fat diet may be risks.

HOW TO PREVENT—Cannot be prevented.

 WHAT TO EXPECT

DIAGNOSTIC MEASURES
• Your health care provider will do a physical exam and a pelvic exam.
• Medical tests may include pregnancy test, Pap smear, ultrasound, laparoscopy, hysteroscopy, hysterosalpingogram, or biopsy.

APPROPRIATE HEALTH CARE
• Treatment will vary depending on symptoms and diagnostic tests, location and size of the fibroids, general health, and desire for future pregnancies.
• Treatment is usually not needed if there are no symptoms or symptoms are mild. Regular follow up medical exams will be done.

• Hormone therapy, to suppress natural estrogen, is often the first step or before surgery.
• Surgery may be recommended. Several different surgical procedures are possible. Be sure you understand all aspects of your choices, and the risks and benefits involved. Hysterectomy is surgery to remove the uterus. A myomectomy removes the fibroids.
• Uterine fibroid embolization (UFE), also called uterine artery embolization (UAE), is a nonsurgical procedure. It treats fibroids by cutting off their blood flow.
• Radiofrequency ablation (RFA) or myoma coagulation (called myolysis) uses electric current to treat fibroids.
• Cryomyolysis uses a probe to freeze fibroid.
• Blood transfusion may be done for severe anemia.

POSSIBLE COMPLICATIONS
• Heavy bleeding and anemia (weakness, fatigue, and paleness).
• Complications may occur in a pregnancy.
• Fibroids may return after surgical treatment.
• Fibroids may rarely affect fertility.
• Very rarely, a cancerous type fibroid occurs (leiomyosarcoma).
• Severe symptoms affect daily life activities.

PROBABLE OUTCOME
• Treatment may not be needed. In other cases, drugs help relieve symptoms. Fibroids can be removed with surgery.
• Fibroid size may decrease after menopause.

 HOW TO TREAT

GENERAL MEASURES—Be sure you understand all of your treatment options.

MEDICATION
• Your health care provider may prescribe:
- A gonadotropin-releasing hormone to induce an abrupt, artificial menopause that stops the bleeding and reduces size of the fibroid.
- Nonsteroidal anti-inflammatories for pain.
- Birth control pills or progestins for menstrual bleeding.
- Progestin-releasing intrauterine device (IUD) for heavy bleeding and pain.
- Iron supplements for anemia.

ACTIVITY—No limits usually.

DIET—No special diet.

 CALL YOUR DOCTOR IF

• You or a family member has symptoms of uterine fibroids.
• Symptoms worsen or recur after treatment.

UTERINE MALIGNANCY
(Endometrial Carcinoma)

 GENERAL INFORMATION

DEFINITION—Uterine malignancy is cancer of the uterus. Endometrial cancer is the most common type. It develops in the lining (endometrium) of the uterus. Sarcoma is a less common type of uterine cancer. It involves the muscles and/or other supporting tissues of the uterus.

BODY PARTS INVOLVED—Uterus.

SEX OR AGE MOST AFFECTED—It usually affects postmenopausal women over age 50.

SIGNS & SYMPTOMS
• Bleeding or spotting. This usually happens after menstrual periods have stopped for 12 months or more. A watery or blood-streaked vaginal discharge may occur before bleeding or spotting.
• Bleeding or pain with, or after, sexual intercourse.
• Bleeding between normal periods (premenopause).
• Pain or mass in the pelvic area and weight loss.

CAUSES—Exact cause is unknown. Increased estrogen levels are thought to play a role.

RISK INCREASES WITH
• Postmenopausal women.
• Diabetes, obesity, or high blood pressure.
• Women who have never given birth to a child.
• High estrogen levels from natural or other sources.
• Use of estrogen without also using progesterone.
• Personal or family history of endometrial, breast, ovarian, or colon cancer.
• Endometrial hyperplasia.
• Use of the drug tamoxifen.
• History of uterine polyps, menstrual cycles without ovulation, or other signs of hormone imbalance.
• Early menstruation and late menopause (after age 52).
• Polycystic ovarian syndrome.
• High fat diet; lack of exercise.
• Previous pelvic radiation therapy.

HOW TO PREVENT
• There are no specific measures. Reduce risk factors where possible.
• Pelvic exams every 6 to 12 months may aid in early detection and treatment. Other screening tests may be done for women with high risk factors.
• Seek medical care for any vaginal bleeding or spotting after menopause.
• Control diabetes and high blood pressure.
• Maintain ideal body weight.
• Exercise on a regular basis.

 WHAT TO EXPECT

DIAGNOSTIC MEASURES
• Your own observation of symptoms, especially abnormal bleeding.
• Your health care provider will do a physical exam and a pelvic exam.
• Medical tests are done, first to diagnose the cancer, and then to find out if it has spread to other body organs (staging). Tests will be explained to you. They may include blood tests, Pap smear, liver function tests, chest x-ray, CT scan, mammogram, barium enema, MRI, vaginal ultrasound, endometrial biopsy, and/or dilatation and curettage (D & C).

APPROPRIATE HEALTH CARE
• Treatment will depend on the extent of the disease, your health and your preferences. It may involve one or more of the following: surgery, radiation, chemotherapy (anticancer drugs) or possibly hormone therapy.
• Surgery treatment may include removing the uterus and, usually, the ovaries and fallopian tubes.
• Other disorders, such as diabetes, high blood pressure, or anemia, will also be treated.
• Counseling may help you cope with having cancer.

POSSIBLE COMPLICATIONS
• Cancer treatments can cause side effects.
• Cancer recurs (most recur in first two years).
• Spread of cancer to other parts of the body.

PROBABLE OUTCOME—With early diagnosis and treatment, 90% of patients survive at least 5 years. Older patients and delayed diagnosis have poorer outcomes.

 HOW TO TREAT

GENERAL MEASURES—To learn more: American Cancer Society; (800) ACS-2345; website: www.cancer.org or National Cancer Institute; (800) 4-CANCER; website: www.cancer.gov.

MEDICATION—Chemotherapy or hormone therapy may be prescribed.

ACTIVITY—You will be advised about limits.

DIET—Eat a healthy diet, even if you lose your appetite from radiation or drug therapy.

☎ **CALL YOUR DOCTOR IF**

• You or a family member has symptoms of uterine malignancy.
• Any new or recurring symptoms develop.

UTERINE PROLAPSE

GENERAL INFORMATION

DEFINITION
• Uterine prolapse means the uterus has fallen or dropped from its normal position in the pelvis. This causes it to bulge into or beyond the vagina. Other types of genital prolapse may also occur:
- Cystocele (part of bladder bulges into vagina).
- Enterocele (small bowel bulges into vagina).
- Rectocele (rectum bulges into the vagina).

BODY PARTS INVOLVED—Uterus; ligaments that suspend the uterus; vagina.

SEX OR AGE MOST AFFECTED—Women over age 40.

SIGNS & SYMPTOMS
• A lump in front or back of the vagina, or a lump that extends outside of the vagina.
• Vague discomfort or pressure in the pelvic region.
• Backache that gets worse with lifting.
• Frequent and painful urination.
• Stress incontinence (urine leakage when laughing, sneezing, or coughing) may occur.
• Problem in moving bowels.
• Pain with sexual intercourse.

CAUSES—Prolapse occurs when muscles and ligaments of the pelvic floor become weak and overstretched. Genetics may play a role.

RISK INCREASES WITH
• Being overweight.
• Having one or more vaginal births.
• Obstetrical trauma and lacerations sustained during labor and delivery.
• Normal aging and decreased estrogen.
• Strain on the supportive muscles due to chronic coughing (from smoking or lung disorder) or chronic constipation.
• Previous pelvic surgery.
• Work or other activities requiring heavy lifting.
• Tumors or large fibroids.

HOW TO PREVENT
• May not prevent, but you can reduce the risk.
• Maintain a healthy body weight.
• Practice pelvic floor exercises during pregnancy and after childbirth.
• Exercise on a regular basis.
• Don't smoke.
• Avoid constipation.

WHAT TO EXPECT

DIAGNOSTIC MEASURES
• Your own observation of symptoms.
• Your health care provider can usually diagnose the prolapse with a pelvic exam. Medical tests may be done to check for other pelvic disorders or complications.

APPROPRIATE HEALTH
• Treatment options depend [on] the prolapse. Other facto[rs] patient's age, if pregnan[cy] other pelvic disorders.
• Patients with mild symptoms [can be] treated without surgery. This may include a[n] exercise program (e.g., Kegel), hormone therapy, or use of a pessary.
• A pessary is a small device inserted into the vagina to help maintain the uterus in a normal position. They come in different shapes, and are individually fitted.
• Surgery may be needed for severe prolapse. Several methods are available and it can be performed to save the uterus if desired. Your options will be discussed.

POSSIBLE COMPLICATIONS
• Vaginal ulcer (sore area).
• Surgery complications.
• Prolapse recurs after surgery.
• Problems with bladder, bowel, or sexual functions.

PROBABLE OUTCOME—Mild prolapse usually responds to conservative treatment. A more severe prolapse can be helped with surgery.

HOW TO TREAT

GENERAL MEASURES
• Avoid wearing tight girdles or clothing that increases intra-abdominal pressure.
• Get treatment for any chronic coughing problem.
• Quit smoking. Find a plan that works for you.
• Kegel exercises. Learn to recognize, control, and develop the pelvic muscles. They are the ones you use to interrupt urination in mid-stream.
• To learn more: National Women's Health Information Center (800) 994-9662; website: www.womenshealth.gov.

MEDICATION
• Estrogen (creams, pills, patch, or ring) may be prescribed.
• Stool softeners may be prescribed for constipation.

ACTIVITY
• Avoid heavy lifting.
• After any surgery, follow medical advice.

DIET
• Begin a weight-loss plan if overweight.
• Eat high-fiber diet to prevent constipation.

CALL YOUR DOCTOR IF

• You or a family member has symptoms of uterine prolapse.
• Symptoms don't improve, despite treatment.

GENERAL INFORMATION

DEFINITION—Vaginal or vulvar cancer is the growth of malignant cells in the vagina or on the vulva. These cancers are rare. The vagina is the opening to the birth canal. The vulva is the area surrounding the vagina and extending to the thighs including the clitoris and vaginal lips.

BODY PARTS INVOLVED—Vagina; vulva.

SEX OR AGE MOST AFFECTED—It occurs mostly in women over age 50. One type (rhabdomyosarcoma) occurs in children.

SIGNS & SYMPTOMS
- There are usually no symptoms in early stage.
- Vulvar itching.
- Abnormal vaginal bleeding.
- Discomfort, pain, or bleeding with intercourse.
- Small or large, firm, painless sores on the vulva that may bleed easily.
- Changes in skin color.

CAUSES—The exact cause is unknown. Certain risk factors have been identified.

RISK INCREASES WITH
- Women over age 60.
- Being born between 1938 and 1971 to a mother who took DES to control spotting or bleeding in pregnancy. DES is diethylstilbestrol, a drug prescribed up to 1971.
- Family history of cancer of reproductive organs.
- Human papillomavirus (HPV) (it causes genital warts).
- HIV infection.
- Smoking.
- Precancerous conditions.
- Other cancer.

HOW TO PREVENT
- No specific preventive measures. Avoid risk factors where possible. Have a yearly pelvic exam and Pap smear to detect possible problems early.
- Become familiar with the appearance of your genitals. Use a mirror and examine once a month. Darker spots around the labia are generally not vaginal or vulvar cancer. They may be a sign of melanoma, a skin cancer. See your health care provider for any dark skin change.
- HPV vaccine (approved for ages 9-26). It protects against most, but not all, HPV types that cause genital warts or cervical or vaginal cancer. It is most effective when given before first sexual contact.

WHAT TO EXPECT

DIAGNOSTIC MEASURES
- Your own observation of symptoms.
- Your health care provider will do a physical exam and a pelvic exam and ask questions about your symptoms.
- Medical tests help to diagnose cancer and to check if it has spread to other parts of the body (called staging).

APPROPRIATE HEALTH CARE
- Treatment options include surgery, radiation, laser therapy, and chemotherapy. It depends on the location and stage of the cancer, and the age and physical health of the patient. Precancer conditions may be treated.
- Surgery involves leaving normal skin while removing the cancer. Different options are used depending on the cancer stage. All or part of the vagina and vulva may be removed. Lymph node removal may be needed if cancer has spread.
- Laser therapy may be used for treatment of some vulvar cancer.
- Radiation treatment may be done. External radiation shrinks the primary tumor. Internal radiation (implants) affects cancer that has spread to nearby tissues.

POSSIBLE COMPLICATIONS
- Cancer treatments can cause side effects.
- Cancer recurs.
- Spread of cancer to other parts of the body.

PROBABLE OUTCOME—Early diagnosis and treatment offer a good chance for complete recovery.

HOW TO TREAT

GENERAL MEASURES—To learn more: American Cancer Society, (800) ACS-2345; website: www.cancer.org or National Cancer Institute, (800) 4-CANCER; website: www.nci.nih.gov.

MEDICATION
- Anticancer (chemotherapy) drugs may be given by pill, through a vein, or applied topically.
- Pain relievers (if needed) may be prescribed.
- Use stool softener (if needed) to prevent constipation.

ACTIVITY
- After surgery, resume your normal activities gradually, allowing 6 weeks for full recovery.
- Sexual relations may be resumed when healing is complete or as advised by your health care provider.

DIET—No special diet.

CALL YOUR DOCTOR IF

- You or a family member has symptoms of cancer of the vagina or vulva.
- After treatment, any symptoms cause concern.

VAGINISMUS

GENERAL INFORMATION

DEFINITION
- Vaginismus involves spasms (clenching up) of the pelvic muscles before sexual intercourse. Types are:
  - Primary vaginismus—a woman has never been able to have sexual intercourse.
  - Secondary vaginismus—a woman has had intercourse previously, but is no longer able to because of the spasms.

BODY PARTS INVOLVED—Pelvic muscles.

SEX OR AGE MOST AFFECTED—Females after puberty.

SIGNS & SYMPTOMS
- Muscle spasms around the vagina and rectum. They may be quite painful.
- The vagina closes so tightly that the penis cannot penetrate for sexual intercourse. It also prevents inserting any object into the vagina, such as a tampon, diaphragm, or speculum (used for pelvic exam).

CAUSES—It may be caused by physical or mental (emotional) factors, or a combination of the two.

RISK INCREASES WITH
- An unconscious desire to prevent penile penetration. This may be due to fear of pain, anxiety, hostility, anger, or a distaste for sex.
- Being brought up to think that sex is a sin or dirty.
- Previous sexual trauma (incest, rape, sexual abuse).
- The first sexual experience for a woman.
- A sexual partner who is not sensitive; insufficient or unskillful foreplay.
- Emotional stress.
- Infections, allergic reactions, or a rigid, intact hymen.
- Surgical or postdelivery scarring.
- Endometriosis (a gynecological condition).

HOW TO PREVENT—Pelvic exam by a health care provider and counseling prior to beginning of sexual activity may help.

WHAT TO EXPECT

DIAGNOSTIC MEASURES
- Your own observation of symptoms.
- Your health care provider will do a physical exam and a pelvic exam if possible. Sedation may be needed for a complete exam.
- A sexual history is important. This will include early childhood experiences, family attitudes toward sex, previous and current sexual responses.
- Contraceptive practices, reproductive goals, feelings about your sexual partner, and specifics about the pain you experience will be discussed.

APPROPRIATE HEALTH CARE
- Treatment will be given for any medical problems. This is often followed by therapy to help with emotional problems, and to reduce the muscle spasms.
- One therapy involves dilating (widening) the vaginal opening gently and gradually. This is done with rubber or glass dilators. Treatments may be started at the medical office and then continued at home.
- Prior to dilation therapy or attempted intercourse, sit in a tub of warm water for 10 to 15 minutes. Baths often relax muscles and relieve discomfort.
- Kegel exercises to control the pelvic muscles may be helpful. You will be instructed on how to do them.
- Counseling is helpful for many patients and their partners. It can help resolve any conflicts and concerns in your life, and to improve communication with your partner.

POSSIBLE COMPLICATIONS—Emotional problems caused by guilt, anxiety, loss of self-esteem, and feeling inadequate. Relationship problems with your sexual partner.

PROBABLE OUTCOME—Medical treatment and counseling can help. Treating the underlying cause may clear up the condition.

HOW TO TREAT

GENERAL MEASURES—You and your partner may try other sexual activities. This can include massage, oral sex, or masturbation.

MEDICATION
- Anti-anxiety drugs or muscle relaxants may be prescribed for a short period of time.
- Before attempting intercourse, you and your partner should use a vaginal lubricant.

ACTIVITY—No limits.

DIET—No special diet.

CALL YOUR DOCTOR IF

- You or a family member has symptoms of vaginismus.
- Symptoms don't improve after 3 weeks, despite treatment. Symptoms recur after treatment.

VAGINITIS
(Vulvovaginitis; Vaginitis, Atrophic)

GENERAL INFORMATION

DEFINITION
• Vaginitis is an inflammation (pain, redness, and swelling) of the vagina. Types include:
- Infectious—this is the most common type and is usually caused by a bacterial infection. It may also be due to a yeast or parasitic infection.
- Noninfectious—may be caused by vaginal dryness (atrophic), allergic reaction, or chemical irritation.

BODY PARTS INVOLVED—Vagina; urethra; bladder; skin around the genitals.

SEX OR AGE MOST AFFECTED—Female adolescents and adults. It most often occurs during the reproductive years.

SIGNS & SYMPTOMS
• The vagina normally has a thin, whitish or clear discharge. It change if an infection occurs:
- Texture (thick, thin, or curd-like).
- Color (white, gray, or yellowish).
- Odor (fishy smell).
- Amount (heavy or light).
• Itching, burning, irritation, redness, swelling, and possibly pain in the vagina or vulva (external genitals).
• Vaginal dryness (due to atrophy).
• Pain with sexual intercourse.
• Pain and burning when urinating.
• Symptoms may vary with the menstrual cycle.

CAUSES
• Infectious vaginitis causes include: bacterial vaginosis (most common cause), vulvovaginal candidiasis (a yeast infection), or trichomoniasis (a parasitic infection).
• Noninfectious causes include: a decrease of natural estrogen (at menopause), an irritant (such as clothes that rub), or an allergic reaction (such as a spermicide).

RISK INCREASES WITH
• Use of antibiotic drugs.
• Spermicide or use of intrauterine device (IUD).
• Weak immune system due to illness or drugs.
• Sexual activity.
• Poor or excessive hygiene; douching.
• Changing hormone levels (e.g., pregnancy, breastfeeding, menopause, or birth control pills).

HOW TO PREVENT
• Wear underwear and pantyhose with a cotton crotch. Avoid wearing tight jeans, pants, or panty hose.
• Keep genital area clean and dry. Don't douche.
• Don't sit around in a wet bathing suit.
• Avoid perfumed or deodorant soap, detergents, fabric softeners, bubble baths, powder, and vaginal sprays.
• Always wipe away from the vagina—front to back—after bowel movements.
• Use a latex condom for sexual intercourse unless you and your partner are monogamous (having one mate).

WHAT TO EXPECT

DIAGNOSTIC MEASURES
• Your health care provider will usually do a physical exam, a pelvic exam, and ask questions about your symptoms.
• Tests may be done of the vaginal discharge.

APPROPRIATE HEALTH CARE
• Treatment will depend on the cause of the vaginitis. Drugs are usually prescribed for infections and sometimes for vaginal dryness or irritation. Your sexual partner needs treatment if trichomoniasis is the cause.
• If the vaginitis is due to an irritant or allergic reaction, stop using the offending product.

POSSIBLE COMPLICATIONS
• Vaginitis may recur after treatment.
• Without treatment, infections can lead to more serious medical problems, be a risk factor for sexually transmitted disease, or cause pregnancy complications.

PROBABLE OUTCOME—With proper treatment, full recovery is expected.

HOW TO TREAT

GENERAL MEASURES—Don't assume you have a yeast infection and use antifungal drugs to self-treat without a diagnosis. Those drugs won't help other types of infection. In addition, a vaginal infection should not be self-treated with herbal remedies, douches, or deodorant sprays.

MEDICATION
• For infection, an antibiotic, antifungal, or antiparasitic drug may be prescribed. Take the entire drug course prescribed, even if symptoms improve in a few days.
• For vaginal dryness, estrogen creams or oral tablets may be recommended.
• For vaginal irritation, steroid or hormone creams may be prescribed.

ACTIVITY—It is best to avoid sexual intercourse until treatment is complete.

DIET—No special diet.

CALL YOUR DOCTOR IF

• You or a family member has symptoms of vaginitis.
• Symptoms recur following treatment.

VAGINOSIS, BACTERIAL

GENERAL INFORMATION

DEFINITION—Vaginosis is an infection of the vagina. Bacterial vaginosis (BV) means that bacteria are the cause of the infection. It is not thought to be a sexually transmitted disease (STD), but sexual activity has been linked to this infection. It may cause vaginitis that has symptoms of soreness, itching, and irritation.

BODY PARTS INVOLVED—Vagina and skin.

SEX OR AGE MOST AFFECTED—Females of all ages (most often in the childbearing years).

SIGNS & SYMPTOMS
- About 50% of women have no symptoms.
- Vaginal discharge that may have an unpleasant odor (referred to as a "fishy" smell). The color and amount of discharge varies from woman to woman.

CAUSES—Normally, there are a number of harmless bacteria in the vagina. They may help protect against other infections such as yeast infection. These harmless bacteria sometimes get out of balance and undesirable bacteria are able to grow. Why this occurs is unknown. Undesirable bacteria types are *Gardnerella vaginalis*, *Mycoplasma hominis*, and *Mobiluncus species*.

RISK INCREASES WITH
- Intrauterine contraceptive device (IUD).
- Smokers.
- New sexual partner, or increase in number of sexual partners in the month before diagnosis.
- Women who have sex with women.
- Douching.

HOW TO PREVENT
- There are no specific preventive measures. The following general measures may help to prevent bacterial vaginosis or other vaginal disorders.
- Use condoms with new sexual partners to help protect against infections, possibly bacterial vaginosis.
- Keep genital area clean and dry. Use plain unscented soap. Avoid vaginal douching, hygiene sprays, and deodorant tampons. Be sure sexual partner is clean.
- Take showers rather than tub baths. If you take a bath, don't add oils or bubble bath to the water.
- Wear cotton underwear or pantyhose with a cotton crotch.
- Don't sit around in wet clothes, such as a bathing suit.
- After going to the bathroom, wipe from front to back (vagina to anus).
- Change tampons or sanitary pads frequently.

WHAT TO EXPECT

DIAGNOSTIC MEASURES
- Your health care provider will do a physical exam including a pelvic exam. Because some women have no symptoms of the infection, it may be diagnosed on a routine exam.
- Medical tests may include studies of the vaginal discharge and a Pap smear.

APPROPRIATE HEALTH CARE
- Treatment is usually recommended for women who have symptoms and women who will be having surgical procedures.
- For pregnant women with the infection, your obstetric provider will discuss the diagnosis, risks, and treatment recommendations when needed.

POSSIBLE COMPLICATIONS
- Infection may recur, but it can be retreated.
- Risk of other types of vaginal infection (such as HIV).
- Increased risk of infection with any uterine surgery.
- May cause problems with pregnancy and delivery.

PROBABLE OUTCOME—Mild cases may get better without treatment. Treatment can relieve symptoms in other cases, but recurrence is common.

HOW TO TREAT

GENERAL MEASURES
- If you smoke, find a way to stop.
- Testing and treating male sexual partners is usually not needed.
- Douches or deodorant sprays that mask vaginal odor should not be used to treat BV. They may eliminate the odor, but they will not cure the condition.

MEDICATION—Metronidazole (Flagyl) or clindamycin (Cleocin) are often prescribed for treatment of bacterial vaginosis. They are available in an oral and topical form.

ACTIVITY—No limits.

DIET—No special diet.

CALL YOUR DOCTOR IF

- You or a family member has a vaginal discharge.
- Symptoms persist longer than 1 week or worsen, despite treatment.
- Unusual vaginal bleeding or swelling develops.

VALVULAR HEART DISEASE

 ## GENERAL INFORMATION

DEFINITION—Valvular heart disease occurs when one or more of the heart valves do not function properly. The heart has four valves—mitral, tricuspid, aortic, and pulmonic. Normally the valves open and close to keep blood flowing in one direction through the heart. Narrowed valves (stenosis) can obstruct blood flow. Widened or scarred valves allow blood to leak backward (insufficiency or regurgitation).

BODY PARTS INVOLVED—Heart valves.

SEX OR AGE MOST AFFECTED—Both sexes; all ages.

SIGNS & SYMPTOMS
- No symptoms (sometimes).
- Fatigue and weakness.
- Dizziness or fainting.
- Chest pain.
- Shortness of breath (may wake you out of a sleep).
- Lung congestion.
- Heart rhythm problems.

CAUSES—Heart valve disease can be congenital (present at birth) or acquired during one's lifetime (due to a variety of conditions).

RISK INCREASES WITH
- Aging.
- Family history of heart valve disease.
- Rheumatic fever (a complication of strep throat).
- High blood pressure.
- Congenital (being born with) heart defects.
- Endocarditis (heart inflammation).
- Heart disease risk factors such as smoking, diabetes, high cholesterol, overweight, lack of exercise, and family history of early heart disease.
- Heart attack or heart failure.
- Other less common risk factors.

HOW TO PREVENT—No known preventive measures. Obtain medical care for any disorders that can lead to heart valve problems.

 ## WHAT TO EXPECT

DIAGNOSTIC MEASURES
- Your health care provider will do a physical exam.
- Medical tests may include blood studies, x-rays (of the heart, lungs, and blood flow), electrocardiogram (measures the heart's electrical activity), echocardiogram (uses sound waves to examine the heart), and others.

APPROPRIATE HEALTH CARE
- Treatment will depend on the type of heart valve disease and its severity. Treatment may involve drug therapy, lifestyle changes, and surgery or other medical procedures. Your health care provider will discuss a treatment plan based on your individual situation.
- Drugs will not cure heart valve disease, but can help relieve symptoms and prevent or delay complications.
- Lifestyle changes may involve physical activity, diet changes, smoking cessation, and limits on alcohol use.
- Surgery to repair or replace a valve may be needed for some patients. Others may have a procedure (called balloon valvuloplasty) to increase blood flow in a valve.

POSSIBLE COMPLICATIONS
- Heart valve infection.
- If untreated, advanced valve disease can cause congestive heart failure, blood clots, stroke, or sudden cardiac death.

PROBABLE OUTCOME—The condition is usually lifelong. Some people will need no treatment. In others, conservative treatments can help control the valve problem for many years. For some patients, surgery or other medical procedure can often treat the valve problem successfully.

 ## HOW TO TREAT

GENERAL MEASURES
- Carry or wear medical ID that shows you have heart valve disease. Also, advise any health care provider who treats you in the future.
- See your health care provider on a regular basis even if you feel completely well.
- Don't smoke. Find a way to quit.
- To learn more: American Heart Association, 7272 Greenville Ave., Dallas, TX 75231; (800) 242-8721; website: www.americanheart.org.

MEDICATION
- Drugs may be prescribed to lower blood pressure, treat heart failure, prevent irregular heartbeats (arrhythmias), lower cholesterol, or thin the blood (anticoagulants).
- Antibiotic drugs may be prescribed.

ACTIVITY—A regular exercise plan is usually recommended. You will be advised about any specific limits on physical activity.

DIET—You may be advised to eat a low-fat or low-salt diet, or begin a weight-loss diet.

 ## CALL YOUR DOCTOR IF

- You or a family member has symptoms of valvular heart disease.
- Symptoms worsen or new symptoms develop.

VARICOCELE

GENERAL INFORMATION

DEFINITION—A varicocele is a tangled network of blood vessels, or varicose veins, in the testicles. Varicocele occurs more often in the left testicle than the right, and, less often, in both. It can take up to 20 years to grow large enough to be noticeable. This is a common condition, occurring in about 15% of men.

BODY PARTS INVOLVED—Testicles.

SEX OR AGE MOST AFFECTED—Males (often in their 20s or 30s).

SIGNS & SYMPTOMS
- In most cases, there are no symptoms. It may be diagnosed during a routine physical exam.
- Ache in the testicle or it may cause pain.
- Feeling of heaviness or dragging in the scrotum (the pouch of skin that contains the testicles).
- Small testicle.
- Enlarged veins can be felt (like feeling a "bag of worms"), and the testicle can look lumpy.

CAUSES
- Normally, blood in the testicles travels through a series of small veins into a large vein that goes up through the abdomen. A series of one-way valves in the veins prevents the reverse flow of blood back to the testicles. Sometimes, these one-way valves become damaged or defective. This causes the blood to flow backward. This reverse flow of blood stretches and enlarges the tiny veins around the testicle to cause a varicocele.
- Because of the varicocele, the blood does not cool as it does in a normal vein. The increased temperature of the blood raises the temperature of the testicles. This is believed to contribute to infertility, as heat can damage or destroy sperm. The raised temperature may also block production of new, healthy sperm.

RISK INCREASES WITH—Men in their 20s or 30s.

HOW TO PREVENT—No known preventive measures.

WHAT TO EXPECT

DIAGNOSTIC MEASURES
- Your health care provider will do an exam of the genital area. Varicoceles may be seen with the naked eye or by palpating (feeling) the area while a patient is standing up.
- Small varicoceles may be diagnosed with ultrasound or other medical tests.

APPROPRIATE HEALTH CARE
- No treatment may be needed if there are no symptoms or the symptoms are mild and infertility is not an issue. Wear an athletic supporter or a pair of snug-fitting underwear to provide the scrotum with support.
- Surgery or other treatment may be recommended if the varicocele causes pain, atrophy, or infertility.
- Most varicoceles can be corrected through a surgical procedure called varicocelectomy (tying off the affected spermatic veins). It is usually performed under general or local anesthesia as an outpatient.
- Laparoscopy may be an option. It involves the insertion of a thin, lighted tube (called a laparoscope) through a small incision (cut) in the abdomen to locate and tie off the varicocele.
- A nonsurgical alternative called varicocele embolization may be recommended. A small catheter (tube) is inserted into the groin. Substances that will block the flow of blood are inserted through the catheter. The affected veins are sealed off, causing the blood flow to return to its normal path.

POSSIBLE COMPLICATIONS
- Low sperm count.
- Male infertility.
- Varicocele may recur after treatment.
- Some patients develop a condition called hydrocele. This is a fluid-filled cyst that forms around the testicle. Minor surgery is used to correct the problem.

PROBABLE OUTCOME
- Successful treatment can reduce the swelling and discomfort of varicoceles that cause symptoms.
- Treatment may help with infertility. It takes about 90 days for a sufficient quantity of new sperm to be produced to permit fertilization. Semen study is usually done at 3 and 6 months after treatment.

HOW TO TREAT

GENERAL MEASURES—None specific.

MEDICATION—Drugs are normally not needed.

ACTIVITY—No limits.

DIET—No special diet.

CALL YOUR DOCTOR IF

- You or a family member has symptoms of a varicocele.
- Symptoms recur after treatment.

VARICOSE VEINS

GENERAL INFORMATION

DEFINITION—Varicose veins are veins, usually in the legs and ankles, which become permanently enlarged and often twisted. Varicose veins typically involve the superficial veins (those close to the skin).

BODY PARTS INVOLVED—Veins in the legs, including superficial veins, deep veins and veins that connect superficial and deep veins. Veins in the vaginal lips during pregnancy and those around the anus (hemorrhoids) also may become varicose.

SEX OR AGE MOST AFFECTED—Adults of both sexes, but women more than men.

SIGNS & SYMPTOMS
- Enlarged, bulging, ropelike, bluish veins that are visible under the skin. They appear most often in the back of the calf or on the inside of the leg from the ankle to the groin.
- Vague discomfort and aching, or pain in the legs, especially after standing.
- Fatigue.

CAUSES—The veins of the legs contain one-way valves every few inches to help blood return against gravity to the heart. Varicose veins can develop when valves leak and the blood pressure in the veins prevents blood from draining properly. Blood pools in the veins causing them to stretch, bulge, and be visible.

RISK INCREASES WITH
- Increasing age and females.
- Family history of varicose veins.
- Prolonged sitting or standing (as with certain types of work).
- Pregnancy.
- History of blood clots.
- Overweight, high blood pressure, straining (as with constipation), prior leg surgery or injury, and being less active physically may add to risk.
- Congenital (being born with) abnormal veins.

HOW TO PREVENT
- None specific. Risks may be reduced.
- Exercise regularly (e.g., walking, swimming, or bicycling) to keep circulation healthy.
- Don't sit or stand for long periods.
- Maintain a healthy weight.
- May wear compression hose if at high risk.
- Elevate your legs when possible.

WHAT TO EXPECT

DIAGNOSTIC MEASURES
- Your own observation of symptoms.
- Your health care provider will do a physical exam of the affected veins and ask about your symptoms.
- Medical tests may include an ultrasound.

APPROPRIATE HEALTH CARE
- Simple self-care methods may be recommended.
- Surgery and other treatment methods may be done for pain, recurrent phlebitis (inflamed veins), skin changes, or for cosmetic reasons.
- Veins can be sealed off by using sclerotherapy (injections), laser, intense-pulsed light therapy, or radiofrequency ablation. Veins can also be removed with surgery. Your health care provider will discuss your options, the risks, and benefits of each one with you.
- Spider veins (idiopathic telangiectases) are small superficial veins. They may be treated with a laser or with injections.

POSSIBLE COMPLICATIONS
- Ulcers (deep sores) in the legs or ankles.
- Phlebitis (inflammation) in a vein or thrombophlebitis (small blood clot in a vein).
- Large varicose veins may bleed easily if bumped or scratched.
- Complications may occur with treatment.
- Varicose veins may return after treatment.

PROBABLE OUTCOME—Self-care steps may help symptoms. Medical treatment has a high success rate.

HOW TO TREAT

GENERAL MEASURES
- Take frequent rest periods with legs elevated.
- Use lightweight, elastic compression hosiery. Put them on before getting out of bed.
- Avoid tight clothes around waist, legs, or groin.
- Avoid long periods of sitting or standing. Take breaks and walk around.
- Wear comfortable shoes and avoid high heels.
- Cross legs at ankles and not at the knees.

MEDICATION—A chemical may be injected (sclerotherapy) into small varicose veins to make them collapse and disappear over time. Other veins will take over blood flow.

ACTIVITY
- Exercise regularly.
- After treatment, you will be advised about temporary limits on activity. Compression hose will usually need to be worn for a period of time.

DIET—Consider a weight-loss diet, if overweight.

CALL YOUR DOCTOR IF

- You or a family member has varicose veins.
- After diagnosis, the veins cause problems.

VITAMIN DEFICIENCIES

GENERAL INFORMATION

DEFINITION—Vitamin deficiencies develop when there is insufficient intake or absorption of a vitamin. This deficiency is rare in the U.S. and is usually due to failure of the intestine to absorb enough of the vitamin.

BODY PARTS INVOLVED—Total body tissues.

SEX OR AGE MOST AFFECTED—Both sexes; all ages.

SIGNS & SYMPTOMS
- Vitamin A—night blindness, dry eyes, rough skin, loss of appetite, diarrhea, anemia.
- Vitamin B1—loss of sensation in the legs, weakness, congestive heart failure, lack of urinary control, psychosis, abdominal pain.
- Vitamin B2—cracked lips, pallor, sore tongue.
- Vitamin B3 (Niacin)—fatigue and weakness, poor appetite, sore mouth and tongue, indigestion, nausea, vomiting, diarrhea.
- Vitamin B6—dermatitis, sore mouth and tongue, abdominal pain, vomiting, diarrhea.
- Vitamin B12—weakness, sore tongue, nausea, bleeding gums, numbness in hands and feet, jaundice, headache, poor memory, depression.
- Vitamin C—tender legs, bleeding and bruising under the skin, anemia, bleeding gums, loss of teeth, rough skin, increased susceptibility to infection, weakness and fatigue.
- Vitamin D—restlessness, poor sleep habits, profuse sweating, bowed legs in infants, delayed walking in infants, bone pain, muscle weakness.
- Vitamin E—muscle weakness, swelling of the ankles, abdomen and face in infants, anemia in premature infants.
- Vitamin K—unusual bleeding or bruising.

CAUSES
- Inadequate diet.
- Impaired absorption from disease or drug use.

RISK INCREASES WITH
- Fad diets.
- Use of certain medications.
- Alcohol or drug (including laxative) abuse.
- Malabsorption; disease; pregnancy.
- Poverty; very young or very old.
- Intestinal parasites; gastrointestinal surgery.

HOW TO PREVENT
- Proper diet.
- Supplemental vitamins if needed.

WHAT TO EXPECT

DIAGNOSTIC MEASURES
- Your own observation of symptoms.
- Your health care provider will do a physical exam.
- Medical tests may include blood and urine studies, x-rays of bones, and others.

APPROPRIATE HEALTH CARE
- Treatment will involve correction of the underlying cause.
- Hospital care may be required for severe malnutrition or alcoholism.

POSSIBLE COMPLICATIONS
- Vision problems; infections, death, if untreated (vitamin A deficiency).
- Brain, nerve damage; heart disease (vitamin B deficiency).
- Bone dislocations, osteopenia, osteoporosis, fractures (vitamin C and D deficiency). Difficult or impossible vaginal childbirth in women with flattened pelvic bones. Cesarean section is usually required (vitamin D deficiency).
- Chronic anemia (vitamin E deficiency).
- Severe or fatal hemorrhage (vitamin K deficiency).

PROBABLE OUTCOME—Usually curable with vitamin supplementation.

HOW TO TREAT

GENERAL MEASURES—No specific instructions.

MEDICATION—You may be prescribed vitamin supplements depending on the type of deficiency. Don't take more than the prescribed amount.

ACTIVITY
- Exercise daily if able. Avoid excess bed rest.
- Don't drive at night if you have vision problem.
- Handle children carefully to avoid bone or joint injury until deficiency is corrected.

DIET—Eat a well balanced diet that includes foods rich in vitamins. Take prenatal vitamins if you are pregnant. Provide your infant with vitamin supplements or vitamin fortified formula.

CALL YOUR DOCTOR IF

- You or a family member has symptoms of vitamin deficiency.
- Symptoms don't improv treatment.
- Unexplained bleeding
- Pain or suspected fracti injury, even a minor injury

Illr

...IFORMATION

...oss of skin pigment
...patches. This
...s of any race or
...who get the disorder
are in good general health.

BODY PARTS INVOLVED—It affects skin on the hands, face and lips, arms, armpits, legs, and sometimes, the genitals.

SEX OR AGE MOST AFFECTED—Both sexes. It is more common in late childhood (9 to 12 years) to mid-adulthood.

SIGNS & SYMPTOMS
* White patches on the skin.
* They are flat and can't be felt with the fingers. Skin texture does not change.
* They don't hurt or itch.
* They spread to form very large, irregularly shaped areas without pigment.
* The amount of skin affected differs in each person. Some may have small areas, while others may gradually lose pigment over their entire body.
* Hair color may turn gray prematurely.

CAUSES—Exact cause is unknown. An autoimmune problem is likely involved. The immune system by mistake attacks the body itself. With vitiligo, it attacks the pigment-producing cells (melanocytes), and they become weak or die, resulting in a lack of pigment production. Some people develop vitiligo at the site of skin trauma (e.g., abrasion or surgery site). Genetic factors may play a role.

RISK INCREASES WITH
* Family history of vitiligo.
* Autoimmune disorders (e.g., thyroid disease).

HOW TO PREVENT—Cannot be prevented at present.

WHAT TO EXPECT

DIAGNOSTIC MEASURES
* Your own observation of symptoms.
* Your health care provider will do a physical exam of the affected areas of the skin.
* Medical tests may be done to check for disorders such as a thyroid problem.

APPROPRIATE HEALTH CARE
* Treatment is sometimes not needed. The disorder is benign and often more of a cosmetic concern.
* If treatment is desired, your health care provider will discuss several options. Treatment can be done to repigment the affected skin or depigment the non-affected skin.
* Treatment measures may include drugs, phototherapy (use of light), PUVA (light therapy combined with drugs), lasers, or surgery.
* Counseling may be helpful for patients if the disorder is causing emotional problems.

POSSIBLE COMPLICATIONS
* Disorder may never disappear completely, causing permanent white skin areas.
* Emotional problems may occur.
* Eye problems.
* Increased risk for autoimmune disorders.

PROBABLE OUTCOME—It is impossible to predict how much improvement will occur with treatment. Some skin areas may improve, but other new areas may develop. Younger individuals (under 30) and those who obtain treatment early usually respond best. Allow 1 year to evaluate results.

HOW TO TREAT

GENERAL MEASURES
* Some patients with limited disease may choose to use a makeup product. Cover the affected skin with opaque makeup, self-tanning products, or dyes to help make it less noticeable. Use hair dye if hair affected.
* To learn more: National Vitiligo Foundation, PO Box 23226, Cincinnati, OH 45223; (513) 541-3903 (not toll free); website: www.nvfi.org.

MEDICATION
* Drugs to apply to the skin for repigmenting (e.g., corticosteroids, immunomodulators, or repigmenting agents) may be prescribed.
* Drugs to apply to the skin for depigmenting (e.g., monobenzylether of hydroquinone) may be prescribed.
* Oral drugs (e.g., corticosteroids) may be prescribed.
* Use a sunscreen with SPF of 30 or higher.

ACTIVITY—No limits.

DIET—No special diet.

CALL YOUR DOCTOR IF

* You or a family member has symptoms of vitiligo.
* Skin appearance does not improve with treatment.

...isorders

VOCAL CORD NODULES
(Singer's Nodes)

 GENERAL INFORMATION

DEFINITION—Vocal cord nodules are benign (noncancerous) overgrowths of tissue on the vocal cords.

BODY PARTS INVOLVED—Larynx (voicebox).

SEX OR AGE MOST AFFECTED—The condition can be common in children and occurs in women more than men.

SIGNS & SYMPTOMS
- Persistent hoarseness without pain.
- Breathy or scratchy voice.
- Singers may notice they have a voice alteration.

CAUSES—The vocal cords are located in the voice box (larynx) in the middle of the throat. They are made up of two fibrous bands that vibrate to produce sound. The bands are covered with skin-like tissue. This tissue becomes thickened when the vocal cords are used a lot. A part of the thickened tissue can grow and produce nodules. They appear as red, swollen bumps and may be the size of a pinhead up to a small pea. When nodules occur, the vocal cords cannot close completely. This causes the voice to sound hoarse.

RISK INCREASES WITH
- Continued overuse of the voice by singing, shouting, yelling, lecturing, or other forms of talking too loudly or too much.
- Excessive coughing or throat clearing.
- Using the voice incorrectly.
- People who use the voice a lot such as singers, teachers, ministers, auctioneers, cheerleaders, aerobic instructors, and others.
- Smoking or exposure to smoke.
- Chronic infection caused by allergies or irritants.
- Reflux (stomach acid backs up into throat).

HOW TO PREVENT
- Take voice or speech lessons to learn proper techniques for speaking or singing.
- Don't smoke. Avoid being around smokers.
- Drink plenty of fluids.
- Try not to use the voice too long or too loudly.
- Rest your voice for a while when it appears to have been overused.

 WHAT TO EXPECT

DIAGNOSTIC MEASURES
- Your own observation of symptoms.
- Your health care provider will do a physical exam of the throat and vocal cords and ask questions about your symptoms and how you use your voice.
- A laryngoscope (a small, narrow tube with a light) is often used to view the throat and vocal cords. It may be inserted through the nose or the mouth.

APPROPRIATE HEALTH CARE
- Any underlying disorder, such as reflux, will be treated as needed.
- Treatment usually involves voice therapy (voice behavior).
  - This may include voice rest (using your voice less, controlling the loudness, and not talking much for a few days).
  - It can include behavior training on healthy use of the voice and proper voice techniques.
  - Therapy may take 1 to 2 sessions a week for 5 to 6 weeks.
- Surgery (rarely) to remove nodules may be needed if voice therapy is not effective. Surgery is usually not done in children under age 12.

POSSIBLE COMPLICATIONS
- Without treatment, permanent hoarseness or voice change may occur.
- Nodules may regrow after treatment if voice continues to be overused.

PROBABLE OUTCOME—Almost always curable with voice therapy treatment or surgery.

 HOW TO TREAT

GENERAL MEASURES
- Don't smoke; avoid smoky environments.
- Don't whisper (it can irritate the vocal cords). Write notes to communicate.

MEDICATION—Drugs are usually not needed for this disorder.

ACTIVITY—No limits except those for voice usage.

DIET—No special diet.

 CALL YOUR DOCTOR IF

- You or a family member is hoarse for more than 2 weeks.
- Symptoms recur after treatment.

VULVOVAGINAL CANDIDIASIS
(Vaginal Yeast Infection)

 GENERAL INFORMATION

DEFINITION—Vulvovaginal candidiasis is an infection of the vagina and vulva (external genitals). It is a common disorder.

BODY PARTS INVOLVED—Vagina; cervix; vulva (vaginal lips); skin around the genitals.

SEX OR AGE MOST AFFECTED—It can affect women of all ages but occurs most often in the childbearing years. Men may have candidiasis infection with no symptoms.

SIGNS & SYMPTOMS
- The symptoms vary among women and from time to time, in the same woman.
- White, "curdy" vaginal discharge (resembles lumps of cottage cheese). Odor may be unpleasant, but not foul.
- Swollen, red, tender, itching vaginal lips (labia) and surrounding skin.
- Burning during urination.
- Change in vaginal color from pale pink to red.
- Pain during sexual intercourse (dyspareunia).

CAUSES—Most often, the cause is a yeast-like fungus called *Candida albicans*. Healthy women can have this yeast in their vagina (and the mouth and intestines). If the normal conditions of the vagina change, the yeast can overgrow and cause infection. Rarely, *Candida* may be passed from person to person, by sexual intercourse.

RISK INCREASES WITH
- Pregnancy.
- Diabetes.
- Certain drugs (e.g., antibiotics, corticosteroids, and birth control pills).
- Weak immune system from drugs or disease.

HOW TO PREVENT
- There are no specific preventive measures. The following steps may reduce the risks.
- Use condoms with new sexual partners to help protect against some infections.
- Keep the genital area clean and dry. Use plain unscented soap. Be sure sexual partner is clean. Avoid vaginal douching.
- Take showers rather than tub baths. If you take a bath, don't add oils or bubble bath to the water.
- Wear cotton underwear or pantyhose with a cotton crotch. Avoid tight fitting clothing (such as jeans).
- Don't sit around in wet clothes, such as bathing suits.
- After going to the bathroom, wipe from front to back (vagina to anus).
- Change tampons or sanitary pads frequently.
- Take antibiotics only when prescribed for you.

 WHAT TO EXPECT

DIAGNOSTIC MEASURES
- Your own observation of symptoms.
- Your health care provider will usually do a physical exam and a pelvic exam and ask questions about your symptoms.
- Medical test of vaginal discharge may be done.

APPROPRIATE HEALTH CARE—Treatment is with topical or oral drugs. Sexual partners do not need to be treated.

POSSIBLE COMPLICATIONS
- Vaginitis (soreness, itching, and irritation).
- Some women may develop recurrent vulvovaginal candidiasis (RVVC). This is when four or more episodes of vulvovaginal candidiasis have occurred in one year.

PROBABLE OUTCOME—Symptoms will normally clear up with treatment.

 HOW TO TREAT

GENERAL MEASURES
- If urinating causes burning, urinate through a tubular device, such as a toilet paper roll or plastic cup with the bottom cut out, or pour a cup of warm water over the genital area while you urinate.
- To learn more: Women's Health Information Center; (800) 994-9662; website: www.womenshealth.gov.

MEDICATION
- Antifungal drugs, either in vaginal creams or suppositories or in oral form, may be recommended. Some nonprescription examples are miconazole nitrate (Monistat-7) and clotrimazole (Gyne-Lotrimin, Mycelex-7, and FemCare). Follow the instructions on the product. If you have tried one of these drugs and it has not worked for you, your health care provider may prescribe a prescription-only drug.
- Recurrent vulvovaginal candidiasis treatment usually involves two weeks of intensive antifungal drugs, then up to six months of a lower "maintenance" dose.

ACTIVITY—Delay sexual relations until symptoms clear up.

DIET—No special diet.

 CALL YOUR DOCTOR IF

- You or a family member has symptoms of vulvovaginal candidiasis.
- Symptoms get worse or recur after treatment.

VULVOVAGINITIS BEFORE PUBERTY

GENERAL INFORMATION

DEFINITION—Vulvovaginitis before puberty is an inflammation (redness and soreness) of the vagina or vulva before a young girl reaches puberty. Mild cases are common. Before puberty, the skin around the vaginal area can be very sensitive, and it can easily become red and inflamed.

BODY PARTS INVOLVED—Vagina; cervix; vulva (vaginal lips); skin around the genitals.

SEX OR AGE MOST AFFECTED—Female infants and children.

SIGNS & SYMPTOMS
- Redness, pain, and itching in the genital area.
- Vaginal discharge (may have an odor).
- Pain with urination.
- Bleeding from the affected area (sometimes).

CAUSES
- Infections caused by bacteria, parasites (including pinworms), yeast-like fungi, or virus.
- Allergies to synthetic fabrics, soap, or other items in contact with the genitals.
- Scratches, abrasions, or genital injury from foreign body in the vagina (this could be some toilet paper).
- Genital injury from sexual abuse.
- Irritation from bubble bath or oils put in bath water.

RISK INCREASES WITH
- Poor hygiene such as infrequent bathing, not wiping, or wiping incorrectly after urinating or bowel movement.
- Diabetes.
- Trauma or injury to the vaginal area.
- Overweight.
- Wearing tight leotards, jeans, underwear, or bathing suits, or using bubble bath.

HOW TO PREVENT
- Teach the child to wipe from the vagina toward the anus after bowel movements.
- Don't let the child sit around in wet clothing, especially a wet bathing suit. Avoid tight clothing.
- Have the child bathe or shower frequently. No soap is needed in the genital area.
- Don't use scented or antibacterial soap or any bubble bath, or dyed or perfumed toilet tissue.
- Provide the child with cotton underpants or underpants with a cotton crotch. Change underpants daily.
- Teach your child to resist and report any attempted sexual contact by anyone.
- Don't wash your child's hair in the bath. Shampoo the hair over a sink instead. If you do it in the bath, wash it at the end of the bath. Be sure to rinse off any shampoo that may have gotten on the genital area.
- Use a bland ointment for skin protection.

WHAT TO EXPECT

DIAGNOSTIC MEASURES
- Your own observation of symptoms.
- Your child's health care provider will usually do a physical exam, including a gentle exam of the genital area.
- Medical tests may include blood studies and a culture of any vaginal discharge.

APPROPRIATE HEALTH CARE
- Treatment will depend on the cause.
- It may involve removing any foreign object in the vagina.
- Stop the use of any product that may cause irritation or allergy, such as soap or bubble bath.
- Your child's health care provider will discuss any possibility of child abuse with you.

POSSIBLE COMPLICATIONS—Symptoms may persist or other skin infections may develop. Rarely, an infection may worsen.

PROBABLE OUTCOME—Symptoms often clear up by using preventive measures. In cases of infection, drugs will relieve symptoms.

HOW TO TREAT

GENERAL MEASURES
- Follow steps in Preventive Measures.
- Prevent urine from stinging the inflamed skin. The child may urinate while in the shower. Urinate through a toilet paper roll or plastic cup with the bottom cut out. Pour a cup of warm water over the genital area while urinating.
- Taking sitz baths (warm water baths) in clear water 2 to 4 times a day may help symptoms.

MEDICATION
- Nonprescription topical ointments, or 0.5% or 1% hydrocortisone cream, 3 to 4 times a day may be recommended to relieve burning and itching.
- Drugs for infection (including antibiotics, antifungal, or antiparasitic drugs) may be prescribed.

ACTIVITY—No limits.

DIET—No special diet.

☎ CALL YOUR DOCTOR IF

- Your child has symptoms of vulvovaginitis.
- You suspect a child has been sexually abused.
- Symptoms don't improve in 7 to 10 days or symptoms worsen, despite treatment.

WARTS
(Verruca Vulgaris)

GENERAL INFORMATION

DEFINITION—Warts (called common warts) are noncancerous skin growths caused by a virus. They are mildly contagious from person to person and from one area to another on the same person. They can appear anywhere on the skin (e.g., fingers, hands, arms, and knees). Verruca vulgaris is the medical term for warts. Note—genital warts are a separate topic.

BODY PARTS INVOLVED—Skin.

SEX OR AGE MOST AFFECTED—Both sexes; most common in children and young adults between ages 1 and 30, but occur at any age.

SIGNS & SYMPTOMS
- A small, raised bump on the skin.
- Warts begin very small and grow larger.
- Warts have a rough surface and clearly defined borders. They are usually the same color as the skin, but sometimes darker.
- Warts often appear in clusters around a "mother wart."
- If you cut into the wart surface, it contains small black dots or bleeding points.
- Warts are painless and typically don't itch.
- Plantar warts appear on the soles of the feet.

CAUSES—Infection of the outer skin layer (epidermis) by the human papillomavirus (HPV) family. The virus causes some cells to grow more rapidly than normal. Warts are very common.

RISK INCREASES WITH
- Children and young adults.
- Skin that is injured, cracked, or moist.
- Chronic exposure to water (e.g., dishwashing).
- Jobs that involve handling meat and fish.
- Weak immune system due to drugs or illness.

HOW TO PREVENT
- None specific. Reduce risks where possible.
- To keep from spreading warts, don't scratch them. Warts spread readily to small cuts and scratches. Don't bite fingernails (can spread warts to fingertips).
- Wear thong sandals in public showers. Don't share towels.

WHAT TO EXPECT

DIAGNOSTIC MEASURES
- Your own observation of symptoms.
- Health care provider skin exam if needed.

APPROPRIATE HEALTH CARE
- There are a variety of nonprescription products and home (or folk) remedies for warts. Family members or friends may recommend trying different treatments.

- Your health care provider has other options for treatment. These can be done during an office visit. Some treatments may be somewhat painful, so be sure to discuss the risks and benefits. Options:
  - Cryotherapy (freezing) with liquid nitrogen. Freezing causes a blister to form that heals in about a week. More than one treatment may be needed for complete wart removal.
  - Electrosurgery (using heat). This treatment is often done in one office visit. An electric needle is used to cut away the wart or destroy it.
  - Surgery with a knife (scalpel) or laser.
  - Injection of a drug into the wart.

POSSIBLE COMPLICATIONS
- Spread to other places in the body.
- Scars where warts were removed.
- Recurrence of warts after treatment.

PROBABLE OUTCOME—There is no one specific treatment for warts that works for everybody. Most warts eventually go away on their own. Some are cured with nonprescription drugs. Some may require medical care that could include surgery. There are also many "home remedies" that may work for some people. Nonsurgical treatment for warts may take some time, so be patient.

HOW TO TREAT

GENERAL MEASURES—Follow instructions from your health care provider for home care after any medical treatment.

MEDICATION
- There are nonprescription drugs for treatment of warts. Most are applied to skin daily for several weeks. Also available is a freezing aerosol product. Follow the instructions provided with any product that you buy.
- Your health care provider may prescribe stronger drugs or injections for removing warts.

ACTIVITY—No limits. Cover warts if activity involves skin-to-skin contact.

DIET—No special diet.

CALL YOUR DOCTOR IF

- You or your child has warts that cause concern or warts appear on the face or genital area.
- Self-treatment for warts has not worked.
- After treatment, the treated skin becomes hot, red, and painful.
- Warts don't disappear completely after treatment.
- Other warts appear after treatment.

WARTS, GENITAL
(Condylomata Acuminata; Ve

GENERAL INFORMATION

DEFINITION—Genital warts are growths on the genitals caused by a virus. Genital warts often have no symptoms and many people (especially females) do not know they are infected. 30% to 50% of sexually active people in the United States have genital warts.

BODY PARTS INVOLVED—Urethra; genitals; rectum.

SEX OR AGE MOST AFFECTED—Both sexes of sexually active young people and adults. Women are affected more often than men.

SIGNS & SYMPTOMS
● Warts appear on moist surfaces of the genital area. They are thin, flexible, solid raised areas of the skin, growing in stalks or clusters. They are taller than they are wide. They may be tiny or grow in larger masses.
● In women, they may be on the inside and outside of the vagina, on the cervix, or around the anus.
● Men may have warts on the tip or shaft of the penis or around the anus.
● They don't hurt or itch.
● Women may have a vaginal discharge.

CAUSES
● Genital warts are caused by certain types of the human papillomavirus (HPV). More than 80 types of HPV have been identified and most are harmless. About 30 types are spread through sexual contact.
● Genital warts spread very easily from one person to another. They are spread through oral, genital, or anal sex with an infected person. Genital warts can be transmitted even when there are no visible warts or other symptoms. They have an incubation period of 1 to 6 months. Genital warts are considered a sexually transmitted disease (STD).

RISK INCREASES WITH
● Having other STD.
● Having sex with multiple sexual partners or having sex with a partner who has had many sexual partners.
● Early age for first sexual intercourse.

HOW TO PREVENT
● Abstinence (no sexual activity) or having sex with one partner known to be disease-free.
● Use rubber (latex) condoms during sexual intercourse. They reduce risks, but don't fully prevent HPV.
● HPV vaccine for females and males. It protects against HPV strains that cause 90% of genital warts. It is most effective when given before first sexual contact.

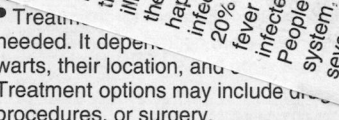

WEST NILE VIRUS

GENERAL INFOR

DEFINITION—West Nile virus
that can cause a mild or, les
illness in humans. Outbrea
the summer and continu
happen year round. M
infected will not hav
20% will have a mi
fever that lasts a
infected perso
People with
system, or
severe ill

BODY

SE

● Treatm
needed. It depe
warts, their location, and
Treatment options may include d
procedures, or surgery.
● Warts may be treated with drugs applied to the skin.
● Warts may be frozen (cryotherapy), burned (electrocautery), or removed with laser therapy.
● Large warts that have not responded to other treatment may need surgical removal.
● Pregnant women with genital warts will be examined by their obstetric providers. The possible problems for mother and for the baby and options for treatment will be discussed.

POSSIBLE COMPLICATIONS
● Treatment complications (rare).
● Genital warts do not cause cancer. But, some types of HPV that cause genital warts can also cause, or be a risk factor for, genital cancers.

PROBABLE OUTCOME—Warts often clear up on their own. Treatment can remove the warts, but the HPV infection remains in the body. Recurrence of warts after treatment is common.

HOW TO TREAT

GENERAL MEASURES—Don't pick, squeeze, or scratch the warts. You can spread them to other places in your body.

MEDICATION—There are several types of drugs that can be used on the warts. Some are applied at a medical office and others can be used at home. Your health care provider will discuss the options. Follow instructions carefully.

ACTIVITY—No limits unless advised.

DIET—No special diet.

CALL YOUR DOCTOR IF

● You or a family member has symptoms of genital warts.
● Warts recur after treatment.

...is an infection
...s often, a serious
...ks usually occur in
...e into the fall, but can
...st people (80%) who are
...any symptoms. About
...d infection called West Nile
...ew days. A few (1 in 150
...s) will develop a severe illness.
...hronic disease, weak immune
...he elderly are more likely to have
...ess.

PARTS INVOLVED—Whole body.

OR AGE MOST AFFECTED—Both sexes;
ages.

SIGNS & SYMPTOMS
- Mild symptoms may include:
  - Fever, chills, headache, or eye pain.
  - Body aches and feeling tired.
  - Nausea and vomiting and loss of appetite.
  - Swollen lymph glands.
  - Skin rash on the chest, stomach, and back.
- Severe symptoms can include high fever, headache, neck stiffness, stupor, disorientation, coma, tremors, convulsions, muscle weakness, vision loss, numbness, and paralysis.

CAUSES—Bite of an infected mosquito. Mosquitoes are carriers that become infected when they feed on infected birds. Infected mosquitoes can then spread the infection to humans and other animals when they bite. In rare cases, it has spread through blood transfusions, organ transplants, breastfeeding, during pregnancy from mother to baby, and lab work. It is not spread through casual contact such as touching or kissing a person with the virus. People may develop symptoms between 3 and 14 days after being bitten by an infected mosquito.

RISK INCREASES WITH
- People who spend a lot of time outdoors.
- Presence of mosquitoes in or around the home.
- Time of year (usually early spring to late fall).

HOW TO PREVENT
- When outdoors, use mosquito repellent containing DEET on the skin. Wear protective, light-colored clothing. Spray clothing with DEET or permethrin products.
- Put screens on windows and doors. Drain standing water from buckets, flower pots, and other items.
- Don't handle dead birds. Call local health department.
- Mosquito control programs in communities can help.

 WHAT TO EXPECT

DIAGNOSTIC MEASURES
- See your health care provider if you have any concern about the symptoms. A physical exam may be done and questions asked about your symptoms and activities.
- A blood test may be done if needed to confirm diagnosis.

APPROPRIATE HEALTH CARE
- Most people will not seek or need medical care. Mild symptoms are similar to other virus infections that people usually treat themselves.
- No treatment is available to cure the infection. Drugs may help relieve symptoms such as fever or headache.
- Severe symptoms require hospital care. Treatment can include fluids given through a vein (IV), breathing support (sometimes with a machine), and steps to prevent more complications.

POSSIBLE COMPLICATIONS
- Encephalitis (inflammation of the brain).
- Meningitis (inflammation of the brain's lining).
- Meningoencephalitis (having both of the above).
- Permanent brain damage, muscle weakness, or death (rare).

PROBABLE OUTCOME—Mild symptoms clear up without treatment. In severe cases, most patients recover with hospital care.

 HOW TO TREAT

GENERAL MEASURES
- Follow instructions from your health care provider for home care after any medical treatment.
- To learn more: Centers for Disease Control and Prevention; (800) 232-4636; website: www.cdc.gov, or call your local health department.

MEDICATION—Use nonprescription drugs for mild symptoms such as fever, pain, or headache. Antibiotics do not help virus infections.

ACTIVITY—No limits (with mild symptoms).

DIET—No special diet.

 CALL YOUR DOCTOR IF

- You or a family member has symptoms of West Nile virus infection that cause concern.
- If symptoms are severe, get emergency care.
- After recovery, new symptoms develop (e.g., mental changes, weakness, breathing problems, chest pain, or yellow skin or eyes).

WHIPLASH
(Cervical Sprain or Strain)

 GENERAL INFORMATION

DEFINITION—Whiplash (cervical sprain or strain) is a common neck injury. It is caused by a sudden movement of the head backward and then forward (or vice versa). Whiplash is often the result of a rear-end car accident. Symptoms may develop right away, within 2 to 3 days, or have a delayed onset of weeks. Symptoms vary from person to person.

BODY PARTS INVOLVED—Muscles, tendons, ligaments, discs, and nerves in the neck.

SEX OR AGE MOST AFFECTED—Both sexes (women more than men); all ages.

SIGNS & SYMPTOMS
- Pain in the back and/or front of the neck.
- Neck stiffness or difficulty in moving neck.
- Pain may occur in lower back, shoulder, or arm.
- Headache.
- Vision changes.
- Hearing noises in the ear (tinnitus).
- Dizziness.
- Arm weakness, tingling, numbness, or heaviness.
- Trouble sleeping due to pain.
- Problems with memory or concentration.

CAUSES—The sudden head movement forces the neck to move beyond its normal range of motion. As this occurs, it causes trauma (over-stretching and tearing) to the muscles, tendons, and ligaments in the neck. A herniated disc and nerve compression can also occur.

RISK INCREASES WITH
- Motor vehicle accident (can be at a slow or high speed).
- Contact sports.
- Amusement park rides (e.g., roller coaster).
- Being punched or being hit by a falling object.
- Females.
- Child abuse (e.g., shaken baby syndrome).

HOW TO PREVENT
- Use seatbelts and the padded headrests in your car. Drive carefully and defensively. Don't drink and drive.
- Wear proper head gear for contact sports.
- Appropriate methods to prevent child abuse.

 WHAT TO EXPECT

DIAGNOSTIC MEASURES
- Your own observation of symptoms.
- Your health care provider will do a physical exam and ask questions about your symptoms and the cause of your injury.
- X-rays or other tests may be done to rule out injury to the spine.

APPROPRIATE HEALTH CARE
- There are different treatment options that can relieve symptoms and often lead to full recovery. A treatment plan is based on severity of symptoms and your individual needs.
- Treatments can include drugs, ice or heat therapy, physical therapy, and neck exercises.
- In some cases, radiofrequency therapy (uses radio waves and heat), transcutaneous electric nerve stimulation (TENS), or traction may be options. Very rarely, disc surgery is needed.
- Other treatments help some people (e.g., massage, chiropractor care, or acupuncture).
- Counseling can be helpful if problems such as depression, stress, or anxiety develop. Insurance or legal factors may add to stress.

POSSIBLE COMPLICATIONS
- Symptoms may continue up to 2 years or more.
- Symptoms may affect person's quality of life.
- Depression or other emotional problems.
- Chronic pain syndrome may develop.

PROBABLE OUTCOME—Different treatments work for different people. Many patients heal fully or have symptom relief in a week to 3 months.

 HOW TO TREAT

GENERAL MEASURES
- You may try applying ice packs (over a towel) to injured area for 10 to 20 minutes each hour for first 24 hours. After 24 hours, use heat if desired. Take warm showers twice a day or apply warm soaks to the neck several times a day for 10 to 15 minutes.
- Use of a soft foam cervical (neck) collar may or may not help symptoms. Get medical advice.

MEDICATION
- Oral or injected pain relievers, muscle relaxants, or drugs for specific symptoms may be prescribed.
- You may use ibuprofen, naproxen, or acetaminophen for minor pain.

ACTIVITY
- Exercises (e.g., stretching) for the neck and range-of-motion exercises are often prescribed. A physical therapist can provide help and instructions.
- Maintaining normal life activities and remaining active will help most patients in recovering.

DIET—No special diet.

 CALL YOUR DOCTOR IF

- You or a family member has symptoms of whiplash. If severe, get emergency help!
- Symptoms don't improve with treatment.
- Any new symptoms develop.

WHOOPING COUGH
(Pertussis)

GENERAL INFORMATION

DEFINITION—Whooping cough is a serious and highly contagious infection of the nose, throat, and lungs. Pertussis is the medical name. Use of a vaccine has greatly reduced the occurrence of the disease.

BODY PARTS INVOLVED—Bronchial tubes; larynx; lungs.

SEX OR AGE MOST AFFECTED—Both sexes; all ages, but most common in children.

SIGNS & SYMPTOMS
- Early stages:
  - Runny nose.
  - Dry cough that leads to cough with thick sputum.
  - Slight fever.
- Late stages:
  - Severe, ongoing coughing bouts that last up to 1 minute. The face turns red or blue from lack of oxygen while coughing. At the end of each coughing effort, the person gasps for breath with a "whooping" sound.
  - Vomiting (especially with severe coughing).
  - Little or no fever.

CAUSES—*Bordetella pertussis* bacteria. Germs are spread by contact with an infected person, breathing in germs in the air, or touching an object with germs on it. The time from being exposed to the germs to having symptoms is about 7 to 10 days, and not more than 21 days.

RISK INCREASES WITH
- Children who have not been immunized or have not completed the whole series of vaccine shots.
- The vaccine protection fades as children get older. Teens and adults can easily get the infection if exposed.
- A person who does not know they have the infection may spread the germs. This can happen during the first 21 days of their cough.
- Close contact with an infected person.

HOW TO PREVENT
- Pertussis vaccine starting in infancy.
- Consult your health care provider about booster vaccine for teens and adults.
- Keep infants away from persons who are ill.

WHAT TO EXPECT

DIAGNOSTIC MEASURES
- Your own observation of symptoms.
- Your health care provider will do a physical exam. The diagnosis can be made based on the symptoms and knowing about contact with an infected person.
- Medical tests include blood and mucus tests.

APPROPRIATE HEALTH CARE
- Treatment depends on how severe the symptoms are.
- Severely ill infants will need hospital care.
- Children can usually be treated at home. They should get extra rest, drink plenty of fluids, take any prescribed drugs, and be watched for any complications.

POSSIBLE COMPLICATIONS
- Children under age one are at high risk for complications. They are less likely in older children and adults.
- Complications include severe ear infection, nose-bleeds, dehydration, pneumonia, convulsions, and in rare cases, brain damage and death.

PROBABLE OUTCOME—Usually curable in about 6 weeks with treatment (may range from 3 weeks to 3 months). The usual course of illness is: 2 weeks with the cough; 2 weeks with bouts of the "whooping" cough; and 2 weeks for recovery. Some persistent coughs may continue for months.

HOW TO TREAT

GENERAL MEASURES—Keep an ill person at home and away from others when possible.

MEDICATION
- An antibiotic is usually prescribed. If started early in the infection, it helps improve symptoms. It also reduces the risk of spreading germs.
- Close contacts of an infected person are usually prescribed antibiotics to help prevent the infection (even if they have had the vaccine).

ACTIVITY
- Keep the child in bed or resting until the fever disappears. Normal activity should be resumed slowly, according to strength.
- Return to daycare, school, or work is permitted after taking antibiotics for five days. Without antibiotics, it will be 3 to 4 weeks after the start of symptoms.

DIET
- Drink extra fluids, such as fruit juice, tea, carbonated drinks, and clear soups.
- No special diet. Small, frequent meals may decrease vomiting.

CALL YOUR DOCTOR IF

- You or a family member has symptoms of whooping cough or has been exposed to anyone with it.
- You are concerned about any symptoms.
- Vomiting persists more than 1 or 2 days.
- You are concerned about any symptoms.

WILMS' TUMOR
(Nephroblastoma)

GENERAL INFORMATION

DEFINITION—Wilms' tumor is a malignant, mixed tumor (one that contains several cell types) of the kidneys. Only one kidney is affected in 90% of cases. The kidneys are a pair of organs that are shaped like kidney beans. They are located on either side of the backbone. Kidneys filter and clean the blood in the body and make urine.

BODY PARTS INVOLVED—Kidneys.

SEX OR AGE MOST AFFECTED—It usually affects children of both sexes under age 7 (most often ages 2 to 5). Very rarely, it may not appear until teen years or adulthood.

SIGNS & SYMPTOMS
- Enlarged abdomen. A large, firm, smooth tumor can usually be felt within the abdominal wall.
- Blood in the urine (urine may appear cloudy).
- Abdominal pain (sometimes).
- Nausea or repeated vomiting.
- Fever.
- Weight loss and loss of appetite.
- Constipation.
- High blood pressure (this may have no symptoms).

CAUSES—Exact cause is unknown. It often occurs along with other congenital (being born with) abnormalities. These include urinary tract problems, absence of iris in the eyes (aniridia), and enlargement of one side of the body.

RISK INCREASES WITH
- Congenital abnormalities.
- African Americans are more often affected.
- Girls are more often affected than boys.
- Family history of Wilms' tumor.

HOW TO PREVENT—Cannot be prevented.

WHAT TO EXPECT

DIAGNOSTIC MEASURES
- Your own observation of symptoms.
- Your child's health care provider will do a physical exam.
- Different medical tests are done to verify the diagnosis and to determine if the cancer has spread to other places in the body (called staging).

APPROPRIATE HEALTH CARE
- The treatment plan will be determined by the stage of the cancer, the type of cancer cells, the size of the tumor, and your child's age and health status. Your child's health care provider will discuss all aspects of treatment with you.

- Surgery is usually needed for treatment. It may involve removal of the tumor and the whole affected kidney or less often, a portion of the kidney. Body tissue around the kidney and lymph nodes may need to be removed.
- Chemotherapy (anticancer drugs) may be done before and/or after surgery. Radiation may be done for certain stages of the tumor.

POSSIBLE COMPLICATIONS
- Cancer may recur.
- Tumor may slowly spread to lungs, bones, liver, or brain, if untreated.
- Adverse reactions, including hair loss, from radiation treatment and chemotherapy.
- Surgery procedures may have complications.
- Kidney function problems.
- Chemotherapy and radiation treatment are risk factors for developing other types of cancer.

PROBABLE OUTCOME—With appropriate treatment, the outlook is good. In most cases, Wilms' tumor is curable with surgery, radiation treatment, and chemotherapy (anticancer) drugs. Long-term follow-up care is needed to watch for any late effects of treatment.

HOW TO TREAT

GENERAL MEASURES—To learn more: American Cancer Society; (800) ACS-2345; website: www.cancer.org or National Cancer Institute; (800) 4-CANCER; website: www.cancer.gov.

MEDICATION—Your child's health care provider may prescribe anticancer drugs, antinausea drugs, pain relievers, antibiotics (if infection occurs), and stool softeners to prevent constipation following surgery.

ACTIVITY—An active lifestyle is possible with one kidney. Sports activities that carry a risk of kidney injury (e.g., hockey or boxing) should be avoided.

DIET—No special diet.

CALL YOUR DOCTOR IF

- Your child has symptoms of Wilms' tumor.
- The following occur during treatment:
  - Vomiting, abdominal pain, or constipation.
  - Shortness of breath.
  - Swelling in feet or ankles.
- New, unexplained symptoms develop. Drugs used in treatment may cause side effects.

WILSON DISEASE

GENERAL INFORMATION

DEFINITION—Wilson disease is an inherited disorder in which excessive amounts of copper accumulate in the body. Although the accumulation of copper begins at birth, symptoms of the disorder appear later in life, between the ages of 6 and 40. The liver of a person who has Wilson disease does not release copper into bile as it should. Bile is a liquid produced by the liver that helps with digestion. As the intestines absorb copper from food, the copper builds up in the liver and injures liver tissue. Eventually, the damage causes the liver to release the copper into the bloodstream, which carries the copper throughout the body. The copper buildup leads to damage in the kidneys, brain, and eyes.

BODY PARTS INVOLVED—The liver, blood, central nervous system, urinary system and/or musculoskeletal system.

SEX OR AGE MOST AFFECTED—Both sexes, all ages.

SIGNS & SYMPTOMS
- Jaundice (yellowing of the eyes and skin).
- Vomiting blood.
- Speech and language problems.
- Tremors in the arms and hands.
- Rigid muscles.
- Difficulty in walking and swallowing.
- Menstrual problems, infertility, or miscarriage.
- Abnormal eye movements.
- Mental, behavior and/or personality changes.
- Many signs may be detected by a doctor. The Kayser-Fleischer ring—a rusty brown ring around the cornea of the eye that can be seen only through an eye exam. Others signs include swelling of the liver and spleen; fluid buildup in the lining of the abdomen; anemia; low platelet and white blood cell count in the blood; high levels of amino acids, protein, uric acid, and carbohydrates in urine; and softening of bones.

CAUSES—Both parents must carry the gene that each passes to the affected child. A person with one abnormal gene is a carrier.

RISK INCREASES WITH—Family history of Wilson disease (but most patients have no family history).

HOW TO PREVENT—There are no known preventive measures. Genetic testing may be helpful in diagnosing a patient's relatives.

WHAT TO EXPECT

DIAGNOSTIC MEASURES
- Your own observation of symptoms.
- Your health care provider will do a physical exam. It is usually diagnosed through tests that measure the amount of copper in the blood, urine, and liver. An eye exam would detect the Kayser-Fleischer ring.
- Other tests may include x-ray, MRI, CT, liver biopsy, and genetic testing.

APPROPRIATE HEALTH CARE
- Treatment generally consists of anti-copper agents to remove excess copper from the body and to prevent it from building up again.
- Other symptoms will be treated as needed.
- In rare cases in which there is severe liver disease, a liver transplant may be needed.

POSSIBLE COMPLICATIONS
- The primary consequence for approximately 40% of patients is liver disease. The onset of liver disease is usually at age 8-16 years.
- Damage to the nervous system and disabling symptoms.
- Without proper treatment, Wilson disease is generally fatal, usually by the age of 30.

PROBABLE OUTCOME—Lifelong treatment is required. If treatment is begun early enough, symptomatic recovery is usually complete, and a life of normal length and quality can be expected.

HOW TO TREAT

GENERAL MEASURES
- Follow medical advice for home care after diagnosis.
- To learn more: Wilson's Disease Association, 5572 N Diversey Blvd, Milwaukee, WI; 53217; (866) 961-0533;
website: www.wilsonsdisease.org.

MEDICATION
- Drug therapy may include trientine, D-penicillamine, or tetrathiomolydate. Zinc for maintenance therapy stops the intestines from absorbing copper and promotes copper excretion.
- Other drugs as needed for complications.
- Patients may also need to take vitamin B6.

ACTIVITY
- Activities may be limited until symptoms improve. Return to normal activities gradually.
- Exercise or physical therapy may help improve some muscular symptoms.

DIET—A low copper diet may be prescribed. You will be advised about what foods to avoid or limit (e.g., shellfish or liver).

CALL YOUR DOCTOR IF

- You or a family member has symptoms of Wilson disease.
- Symptoms worsen despite treatment.
- Drugs used in treatment cause unexpected side effects.

ZINC DEFICIENCY

GENERAL INFORMATION

DEFINITION—Zinc deficiency is an inadequate amount of zinc in the body's cells. This affects the function of the testicles, liver, and muscles, and affects the structure of bones, teeth, hair, and skin. Zinc is a vital part of many enzymes that aid chemical reactions needed for normal body function. This includes immune function and skin healing. Mild zinc deficiency may be common, but it is difficult to diagnose and the symptoms can be subtle. Severe zinc deficiency is less common, but has known symptoms.

BODY PARTS INVOLVED—All body cells.

SEX OR AGE MOST AFFECTED—Both sexes; all ages.

SIGNS & SYMPTOMS
- Poor appetite and diarrhea.
- Children have poor growth and delayed sexual development.
- Sensations of unpleasant tastes and odors, or decreased senses of taste and smell.
- Decreased sex drive.
- Rough skin.
- Eye problems (e.g., poor night vision).
- Sparse hair growth.
- Deformed nails.
- Poor wound healing.
- Increase in number of infections.
- Mental or emotional changes.
- Pregnancy problems, such as spontaneous abortion or failure to gain adequate weight.

CAUSES—Zinc deficiency is caused by an increased need, increased loss, decreased absorption, or diet problems.

RISK INCREASES WITH
- A need for an increase in zinc requirements:
  - Pregnancy.
  - Rapid growth in children.
  - Burns or major trauma.
- Increased loss of zinc:
  - Diabetes, cirrhosis, renal disease, sickle cell anemia.
  - Malabsorption disorders.
  - Diuretic drug use.
- Decreased absorption:
  - Certain inherited disorders.
  - Parasite infection.
  - Diet high in phytates (plant fiber).
  - Certain drugs (e.g., tetracyclines and quinolones).
  - Bariatric (weight-loss) surgery.
- Insufficient amount of zinc in diet:
  - Being a vegetarian.
  - Breastfeeding.
  - Being fed through a vein (parenteral feeding).
  - Alcoholism.
  - Elderly persons living in institutions.

HOW TO PREVENT
- Eat a normal, healthy diet.
- Use zinc supplements if needed.

WHAT TO EXPECT

DIAGNOSTIC MEASURES
- Your own observation of symptoms.
- Your health care provider may do a physical exam and ask questions about your symptoms and diet. A diagnosis is usually based on the person's signs and symptoms, medical history, and risk factors.
- Medical studies may be done on blood or urine to determine zinc levels. However, these studies do not completely measure zinc status because of the way zinc is stored in the body. Other medical tests may be done to determine any underlying disorder.

APPROPRIATE HEALTH CARE—Treatment usually consists of treating the underlying cause, zinc supplements, and diet changes if needed.

POSSIBLE COMPLICATIONS—Complications are similar to Signs & Symptoms. Death can occur in severe zinc deficiency.

PROBABLE OUTCOME—In many cases, zinc supplementation is sufficient to resolve the deficiency. In some cases, the outcome depends on the underlying cause.

HOW TO TREAT

GENERAL MEASURES—Follow medical instructions. Compliance with your medical treatment plan is essential for the best outcome.

MEDICATION—Oral or injected zinc supplements will be prescribed.

ACTIVITY—No limits.

DIET
- Eat foods high in zinc such as red meat or pork, seafood, milk, eggs, grains, beans, or nuts. A dietitian can be of help with meal planning.
- Avoid excessive intake of foods with high phytate content (e.g., raw cereals).

CALL YOUR DOCTOR IF

- You or a family member has zinc deficiency symptoms.
- Symptoms worsen or don't improve with treatment.

Surgeries

ABDOMINAL AORTIC ANEURYSM REPAIR

 GENERAL INFORMATION

DEFINITION—An aneurysm is a weakened, dilated (widened) segment of an artery. The surgery replaces a segment of the dilated aorta in the abdomen with graft material to strengthen the wall.

BODY PARTS INVOLVED—Abdominal cavity, aorta, and sometimes the iliac arteries.

REASONS FOR SURGERY—To prevent a rupture of the abdominal aortic aneurysm which usually results in massive hemorrhage and death.

SURGICAL RISK INCREASES WITH
- Age.
- Diabetes.
- Poor kidney function.
- High blood pressure.
- Poor nutrition.
- Chronic lung disease.

 WHAT TO EXPECT

WHO OPERATES—General surgeon, vascular surgeon, cardiothoracic surgeon.

WHERE PERFORMED—Hospital.

DIAGNOSTIC TESTS
- Before surgery: Blood tests, chest x-ray, CT scan, EKG (see Glossary for these two terms).
- After surgery: Blood tests.

ANESTHESIA—General anesthesia.

DESCRIPTION OF OPERATION
- The abdomen is opened through a long vertical midline incision from the ribcage to the pubis.
- The bowels are mobilized and pulled off to the side to expose the aneurysm.
- Control of blood flow in the aorta is obtained above and below the aneurysm with clamps.
- The aneurysm is opened and inspected. A graft is sewn to the upper end just below the arteries to the kidneys and to the lower end just above the split going to the legs. Sometimes the graft must be sewn to the individual leg arteries if the aneurysm extends too close to or beyond the split. The walls of the original aorta are sewn over the graft.
- The wound is closed once all bleeding is controlled.
- Infrequently the aneurysm is resected and removed.
- Another option for repair may be placement of an endovascular graft inside the intact aneurysm. This can be done with a nonsurgical technique.

POSSIBLE COMPLICATIONS
- Bleeding from the graft site.
- Kidney failure.
- Poor circulation to the intestines which can lead to gangrene.
- Poor circulation to the lower extremities.
- Incisional hernia.

AVERAGE HOSPITAL STAY—Usually 5-10 days with the first day or two in the intensive care unit.

PROBABLE OUTCOME—Expect full recovery in 8-12 weeks with no recurrence of the aneurysm. Older patients may take many months (or years) to regain strength.

 POSTOPERATIVE CARE

GENERAL MEASURES
- Hard ridges will form along the incisions. As they heal, the ridges will gradually recede.
- Shower as usual. You may wash the incisions gently with mild soap. After showering, replace any dressings with a new dry dressing.
- Wear compression stockings when up for the first few weeks after surgery.

MEDICATION
- Your doctor may prescribe pain relievers. Use only as much as you need to be comfortable.
- You may use nonprescription pain relievers such as acetaminophen for minor pain. Ask your doctor if it is okay to take ibuprofen or aspirin.

ACTIVITY
- Start ambulating (walking) as soon as you are home. Take frequent naps as needed during the day when tired. Avoid strenuous activity for 6 to 8 weeks.
- You may swim once all sutures are out.
- Resume sexual relations when comfortable and when advised by your surgeon.

DIET—No special diet.

 CALL YOUR DOCTOR IF

- Pain, swelling, redness, drainage, or bleeding increases in the surgical area.
- You develop symptoms of infection including headache, muscle aches, dizziness, fever, or a general ill feeling.
- You develop nausea and vomiting.
- You have prolonged constipation.
- Legs are cold, numb, or painful.
- New unexplained symptoms develop.

ABDOMINAL AORTIC ANEURYSM REPAIR

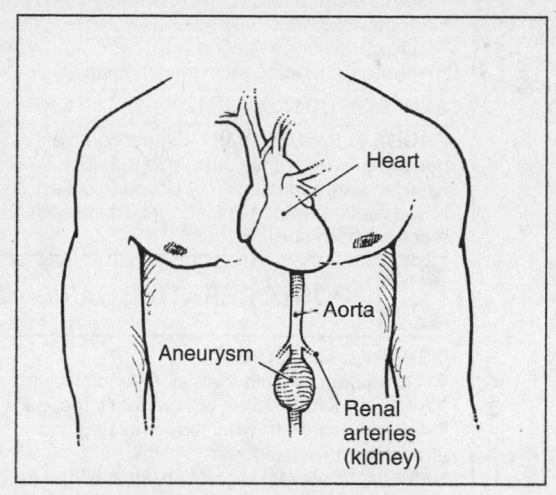

Most aortic aneurysms occur between the renal arteries and the bifurcation (split) which goes to the legs.

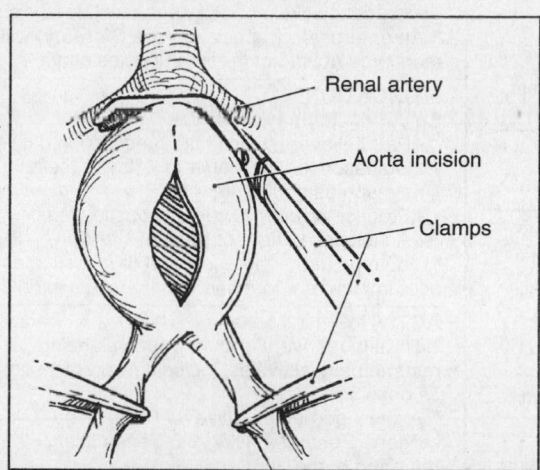

The aorta is clamped above and below the aneurysm and opened.

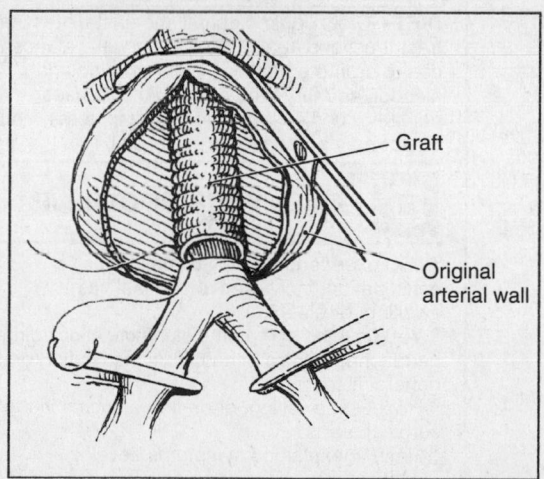

The graft is sewn inside the aorta and the wall of the aneurysm is closed over the graft.

ABDOMINOPERINEAL RESECTION

GENERAL INFORMATION

DEFINITION—Removal of cancerous cells in the rectum and anus through an incision in the lower abdomen and the perineum. Because the anus and rectum are removed, the intestines cannot be reconnected. A colostomy (see Colostomy in Surgery section) is performed at the same time so that digestive function is not disrupted.

BODY PARTS INVOLVED—Rectum, anus, sigmoid colon, perineum, abdomen.

REASONS FOR SURGERY—Cancer of the rectum or anus.

SURGICAL RISK INCREASES WITH
- Adults over 60.
- Diabetes.
- Obesity; smoking.
- Poor nutrition.
- Recent illness.
- Alcoholism or other chronic illness.
- Use of some prescription and nonprescription drugs. Inform your doctor of any drugs, medications, or vitamin and herb supplements you are using or have used in the last month.

WHAT TO EXPECT

WHO OPERATES—Proctologist, general surgeon, or colon and rectal surgeon.

WHERE PERFORMED—Hospital.

DIAGNOSTIC TESTS
- Before surgery: Colonoscopy, sigmoidoscopy, barium enema, ultrasound, CT scan (see Glossary for these terms), blood and urine studies.
- After surgery: Laboratory examination of removed tissue, blood studies.

ANESTHESIA—General anesthesia by injection and inhalation with an airway tube placed in the windpipe.

DESCRIPTION OF OPERATION
- An incision is made in the abdomen. The abdominal muscles are divided and the peritoneal cavity is entered. The sigmoid colon is located, isolated and divided. The colon above the sigmoid is brought to the skin surface for a colostomy.
- The distal bowel portion is closed and placed deep in the pelvis.
- Incisions are made in the perineum.
- The rectum, anus and end of the bowel (intestine) are isolated and cut free of connective tissue.
- Tubes are left in to allow drainage.
- The skin edges of both incisions are closed with sutures or clips, which usually can be removed in 7 to 10 days after surgery.
- The colostomy bag is fitted and placed in position.

POSSIBLE COMPLICATIONS
- Excessive bleeding.
- Hernia around colostomy or surgery incision.
- Impotence.
- Surgical-wound infection.
- Adhesions leading to intestinal obstruction.

AVERAGE HOSPITAL STAY—7 to 10 days.

PROBABLE OUTCOME—Expect complete healing of surgical wounds. You will need to wear an external colostomy pouch to collect bowel movements. Allow about 3 months for recovery from surgery.

POSTOPERATIVE CARE

GENERAL MEASURES
- A hard ridge should form along each incision. As they heal, the ridges will gradually recede.
- Ask your surgeon when you may begin to shower or bathe as usual.
- Move and elevate legs often while in bed to decrease the likelihood of deep-vein blood clots.
- An enterostomy specialist (see Glossary) will teach you how to care for your colostomy.

MEDICATION
- Your doctor may prescribe:
  - Pain relievers. Don't take prescription pain medication longer than 4 to 7 days. Use only as much as you need.
  - Stool softeners to prevent constipation.
  - Antibiotics to fight or prevent infection.
- You may use nonprescription drugs, such as acetaminophen, for minor pain. Avoid aspirin.

ACTIVITY
- To help recovery and aid your well-being, resume daily activities, including work, as soon as possible.
- Avoid vigorous exercise for 6 weeks after surgery. Resume driving 2-3 weeks after returning home.

DIET—Clear liquid diet until the gastrointestinal tract functions again. Then eat a well-balanced diet to promote healing. Avoid caffeine and alcohol, and any food or spice that causes painful or unpleasant digestive symptoms. Your doctor may prescribe a special diet.

CALL YOUR DOCTOR IF

- You experience nausea, vomiting, constipation, increased abdominal pain, swelling, or bleeding.
- You develop symptoms of infection including headache, muscle aches, dizziness, fever, or a general ill feeling.
- Redness, swelling, or drainage occurs in the surgical areas.
- New, unexplained symptoms develop.

ABDOMINOPERINEAL RESECTION

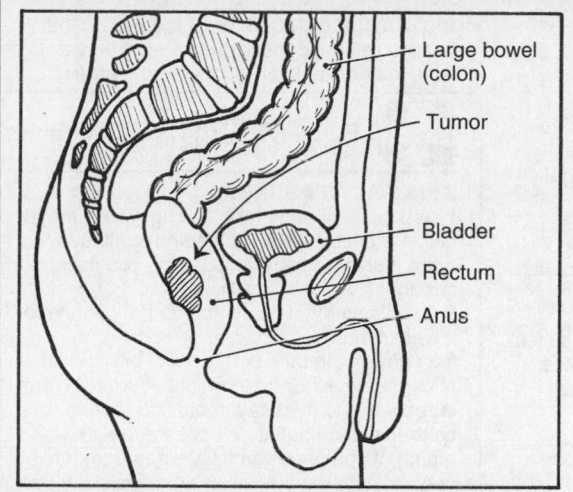

Large bowel (colon)

Tumor

Bladder

Rectum

Anus

An illustration of the appearance and anatomical relationships of the large bowel with representation of a rectal tumor.

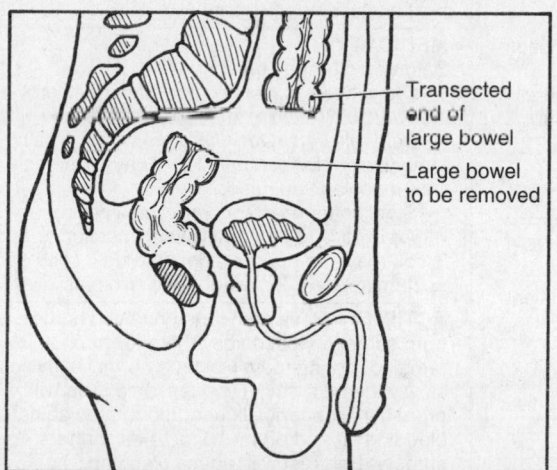

Transected end of large bowel

Large bowel to be removed

The large bowel is transected above the tumor. The distal segment is closed prior to removal.

Colostomy

Drainage tube

• Tumor removed, along with rectum, large bowel and anus.
• Drainage tube left in place to be removed after healing.
• The proximal transected end of large bowel is brought out through the abdominal wall and skin to form a colostomy.

ABORTION
(Suction Curettage)

GENERAL INFORMATION

DEFINITION—Removal of a fetus and accompanying tissue from the uterus. It can be used to terminate a pregnancy, or to remove a fetus that has died in utero, and is usually performed in pregnancies of 12 weeks duration or less.

BODY PARTS INVOLVED—Uterus, placenta, vagina (route for surgery).

REASONS FOR SURGERY
- Missed or incomplete miscarriage.
- Elective termination of pregnancy. The patient should receive competent counseling before making this decision.

SURGICAL RISK INCREASES WITH
- Obesity.
- Smoking.
- Poor nutrition.
- Recent or chronic illness.
- Use of some prescription and nonprescription drugs. Inform your doctor of any drugs, medications, or vitamin and herb supplements you are using or have used in the last month.

WHAT TO EXPECT

WHO OPERATES—General surgeon or obstetrician-gynecologist.

WHERE PERFORMED—Hospital or outpatient surgical facility.

DIAGNOSTIC TESTS
- Before surgery: Pregnancy test, psychological counseling and testing, blood and urine studies.
- After surgery: Laboratory examination of removed tissue.

ANESTHESIA—Local anesthesia by injection, sometimes accompanied by sedation.

DESCRIPTION OF OPERATION
- The opening of the cervix is dilated by the use of instruments or laminaria (see Glossary).
- A small plastic tube is passed through the vagina and cervix into the uterus. The tube is connected to a suction apparatus.
- Gentle suction through the tube removes the uterine contents. You may feel cramps in the lower abdomen, nausea, sweating and faintness.
- The tube is removed, and the lining of the uterus is scraped with a curette to be sure all the placental tissue is removed.

POSSIBLE COMPLICATIONS
- Excessive bleeding.
- Perforation or infection of the uterus.
- Potential psychological problems.

AVERAGE HOSPITAL STAY—None.

PROBABLE OUTCOME—Expect complete healing without complications. Allow several days to one week for recovery from surgery.

POSTOPERATIVE CARE

GENERAL MEASURES
- Use sanitary pads for bleeding, which may last for several days. If bleeding continues for more than 14 days after surgery, you may use tampons.
- Avoid sexual relations and do not douche for 2 weeks after surgery.
- If you wish to take birth-control pills, begin taking them either on the night you return from surgery or the next day, a backup form of contraception should be used for the first month. If you prefer an IUD, diaphragm, or cervical cap, the fitting can be made during your next doctor's appointment.

MEDICATION
- Your doctor may prescribe:
  - Drugs such as methylergonovine (Methergine) or oxytocin (Pitocin) to help uterus contract.
  - Pain relievers. Don't take prescription pain medication longer than 4 to 7 days. Use only as much as you need.
  - Stool softeners to prevent constipation.
  - Antibiotics to fight or prevent infection.
- You may use nonprescription drugs, such as acetaminophen, for minor pain. Avoid aspirin.

ACTIVITY—Have someone drive you home from surgery. Rest quietly there for the remainder of the day. Resume normal activities slowly the next day, if you feel able. You will probably experience light or moderate vaginal bleeding on and off for 10 to 14 days after surgery. Bed rest will reduce bleeding.

DIET—No special diet.

CALL YOUR DOCTOR IF

- You develop symptoms of infection including headache, muscle aches, dizziness, fever, or a general ill feeling.
- A foul smelling vaginal discharge develops after several days.
- You experience nausea, vomiting, constipation, or abdominal swelling.
- New, unexplained symptoms develop.

ABORTION
(Suction Curettage)

Uterus
Fetus
Bladder
Vagina
Suction tube
Leg

- A side view of an adult female showing a small fetus within the uterus (womb).
- Suction tube in place. One end of the tube is attached to the suction machine and the other end is passed through the vagina and cervix into the uterus.

Gentle suction through the tube removes the fetus and placenta.

Suction tube removed. Uterus is now empty. Pregnancy terminated.

ABSCESS DRAINAGE SUPERFICIAL

GENERAL INFORMATION

DEFINITION—To open and drain an abscess.

BODY PARTS INVOLVED—Abscesses may occur anywhere in the body. The most common areas include: female breast during lactation, armpit, anal area, groin, vaginal lips, face, area around the tonsils, scrotum, back, and arms, legs, hands and feet.

REASONS FOR SURGERY—Treatment of infections. If an abscess breaks open and drains spontaneously, surgery is often still required to assure complete drainage.

SURGICAL RISK INCREASES WITH
- Obesity.
- Smoking.
- Poor nutrition.
- Diabetes.
- Recent or chronic illness.
- Use of some prescription and nonprescription drugs. Inform your doctor of any drugs, medications, or vitamin and herb supplements you are using or have used in the last month.

WHAT TO EXPECT

WHO OPERATES—Family doctor or general surgeon.

WHERE PERFORMED—Doctor's office, outpatient surgical facility, hospital, or emergency room.

DIAGNOSTIC TESTS
- Before surgery: Blood and urine studies (sometimes).
- After surgery: Laboratory examination of removed pus (sometimes).

ANESTHESIA
- Local anesthesia by injection.
- General anesthesia by injection and inhalation.

DESCRIPTION OF OPERATION
- An incision is made over the abscess.
- The incision is spread apart, and a sterile-gloved finger or instrument is inserted inside the abscess to break up small pockets. The pus is drained and the cavity is irrigated.
- Gauze is packed into the space left by the abscess. Sometimes a soft rubber drain may be left in the incision, either method allows the cavity to heal from the bottom outward. The drain is usually removed 24 to 48 hours after surgery.
- The skin is left open to prevent recurrence of the abscess.
- A gauze dressing is applied over the wound.

POSSIBLE COMPLICATIONS
- Excessive bleeding.
- Surgical-wound infection.
- Recurrence of the abscess.

AVERAGE HOSPITAL STAY—0 to 1 day.

PROBABLE OUTCOME—Expect complete healing without complications. Allow about 2 weeks for recovery from surgery. Further surgery may be indicated.

POSTOPERATIVE CARE

GENERAL MEASURES
- Bathe or shower as usual. You may wash the wound gently with mild, unscented soap after the gauze or drain is removed.
- Change the gauze dressing at least daily after bathing, or more frequently if saturated with drainage.

MEDICATION
- Your doctor may prescribe:
  - Pain relievers. Don't take prescription pain medication longer than 4 to 7 days. Use only as much as you need.
  - Antibiotics to fight infection.
- You may use nonprescription drugs, such as acetaminophen, for minor pain. Avoid aspirin.

ACTIVITY
- Avoid vigorous exercise for 1 week after surgery.
- Resume driving 1 to 2 days after returning home.

DIET—Eat a well-balanced diet to promote healing.

CALL YOUR DOCTOR IF

- You experience nausea or vomiting.
- Pain, swelling, redness, drainage, or bleeding increases in the surgical area.
- You develop symptoms of infection including headache, muscle aches, dizziness, fever, or a general ill feeling.
- New, unexplained symptoms develop.

ABSCESS DRAINAGE SUPERFICIAL

A side view of an adolescent male face showing an abscess.

Abscess

Abscess is incised, the incision spread apart, and a gloved finger or instrument is inserted into abscess cavity to break up small pockets.

Gauze inserted into space left by the abscess. This provides a drain that allows the abscess cavity to heal from the bottom outward.

ADHESIONS, SEPARATION OF

 GENERAL INFORMATION

DEFINITION—Separation of adhesions (fibrous bands of tissue) that cause parts of the abdomen and pelvis to cling together abnormally. Adhesions can result from: previous abdominal surgery, congenital defects, pelvic inflammatory disease, endometriosis, ruptured ectopic pregnancy, radiation treatment, or any ruptured organ that has caused infection and scarring.

BODY PARTS INVOLVED—Abdominal or pelvic organs.

REASONS FOR SURGERY—Relief of a partial or complete intestinal obstruction caused by adhesions.

SURGICAL RISK INCREASES WITH
- Adults over 60, obesity, smoking.
- Excess alcohol consumption.
- Poor nutrition.
- Multiple previous surgeries.
- Diabetes.
- Recent or chronic illness.
- Use of some prescription and nonprescription drugs. Inform your doctor of any drugs, medications, or vitamin and herb supplements you are using or have used in the last month.

 WHAT TO EXPECT

WHO OPERATES—General surgeon.

WHERE PERFORMED—Hospital.

DIAGNOSTIC TESTS
- Before surgery: Blood and urine studies, abdominal x-rays; sometimes a barium enema or small bowel series (see Glossary).
- After surgery: Blood studies.

ANESTHESIA—General anesthesia by injection and inhalation with an airway tube placed in the windpipe.

DESCRIPTION OF OPERATION
- An incision is made in the abdomen over the obstruction.
- The obstruction is isolated and the adhesions are divided carefully.
- The bowel is examined for strangulation (lost blood supply). Any strangulated portion is removed, and the normal ends are joined.
- The abdominal contents are then inspected for undetected disease. Other surgeries may be performed at this time.
- The abdominal contents are replaced. Muscle layers are closed with sutures, and skin is closed with sutures or clips, which can usually be removed in 1 week.

POSSIBLE COMPLICATIONS
- Excessive bleeding, blood clots.
- Surgical-wound infection.
- Incisional hernia.
- Inadvertent bowel injury.
- Recurrence of obstruction (25% chance).

AVERAGE HOSPITAL STAY—5 to 7 days.

PROBABLE OUTCOME—Expect complete healing without complications. Allow about 6 weeks for recovery from surgery.

 POSTOPERATIVE CARE

GENERAL MEASURES
- A hard ridge should form along the incision. As it heals, the ridge will gradually recede.
- Shower as usual. You may wash the incision gently with mild, unscented soap beginning 24 to 48 hours after surgery. Avoid bathing until your sutures are removed.
- Move and elevate legs often while resting in bed to decrease the likelihood of deep-vein blood clots.

MEDICATION
- You may use nonprescription drugs, such as acetaminophen, for minor pain. Avoid aspirin.
- Your doctor may prescribe:
  - Pain relievers. Don't take prescription pain medication longer than 4 to 7 days. Use only as much as you need.
  - Stool softeners to prevent constipation.
  - Antibiotics to fight or prevent infection.

ACTIVITY
- To help recovery and aid your well-being, resume daily activities, including work, as soon as you are able. Avoid heavy lifting and heavy exercise until your doctor advises that it is okay to resume these activities.
- Resume driving 3 weeks after returning home.
- Resume sexual relations when your doctor determines that healing is complete.

DIET—Clear liquid diet until the gastrointestinal tract begins to function again. Then eat a well-balanced diet to promote healing.

 CALL YOUR DOCTOR IF

- Pain, swelling, redness, bleeding, or drainage increases in the surgical area.
- You develop symptoms of infection including headache, muscle aches, dizziness, fever, or a general ill feeling.
- You experience nausea, vomiting, constipation or abdominal swelling.
- New, unexplained symptoms develop.

ADHESIONS, SEPARATION OF

An illustration of the surgical incision to enter the abdomen.

Incision site

The adhesion causes the small bowel to be obstructed. Here a surgical instrument cuts the adhesions free.

Adhesions

The bowel is manually inspected for other disease.

Small bowel

ADRENAL GLAND REMOVAL
(Adrenalectomy)

 GENERAL INFORMATION

DEFINITION—Removal of one or both of the adrenal glands.

BODY PARTS INVOLVED—Adrenal glands.

REASONS FOR SURGERY
- Cushing's syndrome.
- Pheochromocytoma (a tumor).
- Other adrenal gland tumors.

SURGICAL RISK INCREASES WITH
- Adults over 60.
- Obesity.
- Smoking.
- Stress.
- Poor nutrition.
- Diabetes.
- Recent illness.
- Alcoholism or other chronic illness.
- Use of some prescription and nonprescription drugs. Inform your doctor of any drugs, medications, or vitamin and herb supplements you are using or have used in the last month.

 WHAT TO EXPECT

WHO OPERATES—General surgeon.

WHERE PERFORMED—Hospital.

DIAGNOSTIC TESTS
- Before surgery: Blood and urine studies, x-rays of kidneys, CT scan (see Glossary) of adrenal area.
- After surgery: Blood studies, laboratory examination of removed tissue.

ANESTHESIA—General anesthesia by injection and inhalation with an airway tube placed in the windpipe.

DESCRIPTION OF OPERATION
- The adrenal glands can frequently be removed using Laparoscopy (see in Surgery section), rather than open surgery.
- When open surgery is required, the incision may be in the abdomen or the flank (on the back, near the kidneys).
- The adrenal glands are located, isolated, cut free and removed.
- The skin incisions are closed with sutures or clips, which usually can be removed about 1 week after surgery.

POSSIBLE COMPLICATIONS
- Excessive bleeding.
- Surgical-wound infection.
- Adrenal-hormone shortage.
- Fluid retention.
- Increased risk of life-threatening infections.

AVERAGE HOSPITAL STAY—5 to 7 days for open surgery, 1 to 2 days for laparoscopic surgery.

PROBABLE OUTCOME—Expect complete healing without complications. Allow about 6 weeks for recovery from surgery.

 POSTOPERATIVE CARE

GENERAL MEASURES
- Hard ridges should form along the incisions. As they heal, the ridges will gradually recede.
- Shower as usual beginning 24-48 hours after surgery. Avoid baths until sutures are removed. You may wash the incisions gently with mild, unscented soap.
- Weigh daily. Report a weight gain of 2 or more pounds in any 24-hour period to your doctor.
- Move and elevate legs often while resting in bed to decrease the likelihood of deep-vein blood clots.

MEDICATION
- Your doctor may prescribe:
  - Pain relievers. Don't take prescription pain medication longer than 4 to 7 days. Use only as much as you need.
  - Stool softeners to prevent constipation.
  - Antibiotics to fight or prevent infection.
  - Steroids to replace those formerly manufactured by the adrenal glands.
- You may use nonprescription drugs, such as acetaminophen, for minor pain. Avoid aspirin.

ACTIVITY
- To help recovery and aid your well-being, resume daily activities, including work, as soon as you are able.
- Avoid vigorous exercise for 6 weeks after surgery.
- Resume driving when your doctor advises that it is okay to do so.
- Resume sexual relations when your doctor determines that healing is complete.

DIET—A low-salt diet may be prescribed.

 CALL YOUR DOCTOR IF

- Pain, swelling, redness, drainage, or bleeding increases in the surgical area.
- You develop symptoms of infection including headache, muscle aches, dizziness, fever, or a general ill feeling. If any of these do develop, even after recovery, call your doctor.
- Nausea, vomiting, dizziness, fatigue, weakness, fluid retention, or weight gain occurs.
- New unexplained symptoms develop.

ADRENAL GLAND REMOVAL
(Adrenalectomy)

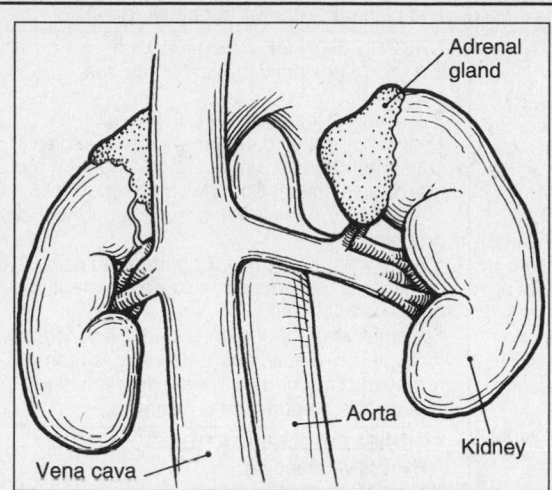

An illustration of the adrenal glands.

Adrenal gland

Aorta

Kidney

Vena cava

The adrenal gland is freed from the kidney on the left side of the patient.

Adrenal gland removed.

AMNIOCENTESIS

 GENERAL INFORMATION

DEFINITION—Removal of fluid from the amniotic sac during pregnancy.

BODY PARTS INVOLVED—Uterus, amniotic sac.

REASONS FOR SURGERY
- Laboratory examination of amniotic fluid helps diagnose abnormalities of the unborn child. Although genetic testing may be done as early as the 11th week of pregnancy, the best time is usually between the 14th and 20th weeks of pregnancy. There is ample fluid, time to treat certain problems before the baby is born, and enough time exists to terminate the pregnancy if necessary. Amniocentesis may also be done in the third trimester to assess fetal development. Amniocentesis is often done for one or more of the following reasons:
- Mother is over 35 years old.
- Either parent has a chromosome abnormality.
- Mother previously had a child with a chromosome abnormality (e.g., Down syndrome).
- Patient had abnormal results from a blood screening test, such as maternal serum alpha-fetoprotein (MSAFP or AFP) test.
- Mother produces antibodies, most commonly to the fetal blood cells, that can cause the unborn child to be very anemic. The amniotic fluid is tested for a chemical (bilirubin) that serves as a marker for fetal anemia.
- To evaluate pregnancy for infection.
- To remove excess amniotic fluid, most often in twins when one baby has too much amniotic fluid and the other has too little.
- Mother carries a sex-linked abnormality, and the unborn child's sex must be determined.
- To evaluate fetal lung maturity.
- Unborn child's maturity or other conditions must be determined late in pregnancy.

SURGICAL RISK INCREASES WITH
- Obesity.
- Previous abdominal surgery.
- Previous infection in pelvic organs.

 WHAT TO EXPECT

WHO OPERATES—Obstetrician-gynecologist or family doctor.

WHERE PERFORMED—Outpatient surgical facility or hospital.

DIAGNOSTIC TESTS
- Before surgery: Blood and urine studies.
- During surgery: Ultrasonography (see Glossary).
- After surgery: Laboratory examination of the amniotic fluid.

ANESTHESIA—Local anesthesia by injection. To ensure the unborn child's safety, sedatives and pain relievers will not be used.

DESCRIPTION OF OPERATION
- A local anesthetic is injected into the abdomen.
- A hollow needle is inserted through the abdominal wall into the uterus. The needle will cause temporary pain, but should not hurt more than any injection. Some women report mild cramping, or a feeling of pressure, during the procedure.
- Amniocentesis is usually performed using continuous ultrasound to allow a constant view of the needle's path.
- A small amount of amniotic fluid is suctioned through the needle, and the needle is then removed. Your body will make more fluid to replace the amount that is removed.

POSSIBLE COMPLICATIONS
- Excessive bleeding.
- Surgical-wound infection.
- Unwanted abortion triggered by procedure in 1 out of 150 to 200 cases.
- Injury to the fetus (rare).

AVERAGE HOSPITAL STAY—None.

PROBABLE OUTCOME—More than 95% of amniocentesis tests indicate no abnormalities. Some couples at high risk want the procedure done to reduce their anxiety during pregnancy. However, normal amniocentesis results cannot guarantee a child without defects. At present, there are no tests for all abnormalities.

 POSTOPERATIVE CARE

GENERAL MEASURES—Bathe or shower as usual. You may wash the injection site gently with mild, unscented soap.

MEDICATION—Medicine is usually not necessary.

ACTIVITY—No restrictions after 2 or 3 hours following the procedure.

DIET—No special diet.

 CALL YOUR DOCTOR IF

- You experience nausea or vomiting.
- You develop pain or cramping in the lower abdomen or shoulder.
- You experience vaginal bleeding or a loss of fluid from the vagina.
- You develop symptoms of infection including headache, muscle aches, dizziness, fever, or a general ill feeling.

AMNIOCENTESIS

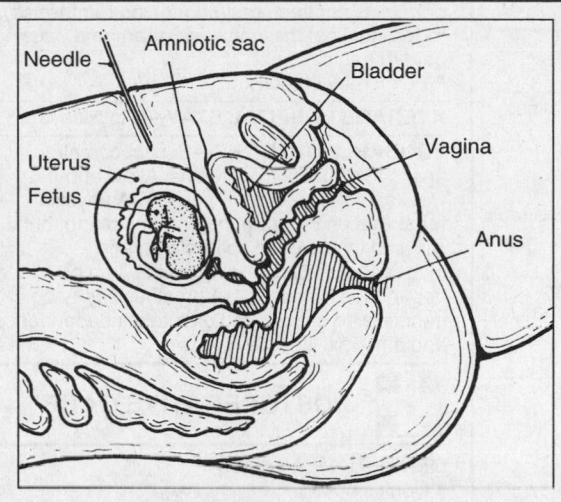

- An illustration of the structures near any amniocentesis procedure.
- Hollow needle inserted through the skin and abdominal wall.

Hollow needle penetrates the cavity of the uterus.

Amniotic fluid suctioned through the needle and collected for study.

AMPUTATION

GENERAL INFORMATION

DEFINITION—Removal of a limb or appendage.

BODY PARTS INVOLVED—Arms, legs, hands, feet, fingers, or toes.

REASONS FOR SURGERY
* Tumor or pain (severe and chronic).
* Injury to blood vessels that cannot be repaired or reconstructed.
* Hardening or obstructions of the arteries.
* Impaired blood circulation due to diabetes.
* Buerger's disease, Raynaud's phenomena.
* Severe infection with gangrene.
* Severe frostbite.

SURGICAL RISK INCREASES WITH
* Adults over 60.
* Smoking, obesity, stress, poor nutrition.
* Excess alcohol consumption.
* Coronary artery disease.
* Diabetes.
* Disease that increases coagulability of blood.
* Use of some prescription and nonprescription drugs. Inform your doctor of any drugs, medications, or vitamin and herb supplements you are using or have used in the last month.

WHAT TO EXPECT

WHO OPERATES—General surgeon, vascular surgeon, or orthopedic surgeon.

WHERE PERFORMED—Hospital.

DIAGNOSTIC TESTS
* Before surgery: Blood and urine studies, x-ray of part to be amputated, arterial doppler studies or arteriography (see Glossary for both).
* After surgery: Blood studies.

ANESTHESIA—General anesthesia by injection and inhalation with an airway tube placed in the windpipe or spinal anesthesia.

DESCRIPTION OF OPERATION
* An incision is made around the part to be amputated.
* Tissue, muscles, blood vessels, nerves and bone are severed.
* The bone is filed smooth, and the bone end is covered with connective tissue. Frequently tubes are left in the wound to allow drainage.
* Muscles are closed with large sutures. The skin is closed with fine sutures, which are left in place for 2 to 4 weeks after surgery.
* A snug bandage is often wrapped around the affected area of the body, and may be left in place for several days following surgery.
* In some cases, an immediate, temporary prosthesis (artificial limb) is fitted.

POSSIBLE COMPLICATIONS
* Excessive bleeding, surgical-wound infection, or muscle contractures (shortening of muscles).
* Feelings that the limb is still there and causing pain ("phantom limb").
* Pulmonary embolism.

AVERAGE HOSPITAL STAY—2 to 7 days.

PROBABLE OUTCOME—Expect complete healing without complications. Allow about 6 weeks for recovery from surgery. A physical rehabilitation program may be frustrating, but it will lead to improved self-esteem and independence. Depending on the limb or appendage amputated, a prosthesis may be beneficial in helping you maintain independence and a normal lifestyle.

POSTOPERATIVE CARE

GENERAL MEASURES
* Don't smoke.
* Keep stump slightly elevated to reduce swelling.
* Shower as usual. You may wash the surgical wound gently with mild, unscented soap.

MEDICATION
* Your doctor may prescribe:
  - Pain relievers. Don't take prescription pain medication longer than 4 to 7 days. Use only as much as you need.
  - Stool softeners to prevent constipation.
  - Antibiotics to fight or prevent infection.
* You may use nonprescription drugs, such as acetaminophen, for minor pain. Avoid aspirin.

ACTIVITY
* To help recovery and aid your well-being, resume daily activities, including work, as soon as you are able.
* Ask your doctor when you may resume driving or engaging in vigorous exercise.

DIET—Eat a well-balanced diet to promote healing.

CALL YOUR DOCTOR IF

* Pain, swelling, redness, drainage, or bleeding increases in the surgical area.
* You develop symptoms of infection including headache, muscle aches, dizziness, fever, or a general ill feeling.
* You experience nausea, vomiting, or constipation.
* New, unexplained symptoms develop.

AMPUTATION

An illustration of an above-the-knee amputation.

Upper leg

Femur

Kneecap

Incision

Knee joint

Tibia

Skin, connective tissue, muscles, blood vessels, nerves, and bone are severed.

Femur

- Bone end filed smooth and covered with connective tissue.
- Muscles closed with large sutures, skin closed with fine sutures.
- Drains remain in place.

ANAL FISSURE TREATMENT

 ## GENERAL INFORMATION

DEFINITION—A crack or tear in the membrane that lines the anus, by relieving the spasm in the anal sphincter muscle which causes the tear.

BODY PARTS INVOLVED—Anus and lining membrane, anal muscles (sphincter).

REASONS FOR SURGERY—Relief of pain.

SURGICAL RISK INCREASES WITH
- Obesity, smoking.
- Recent or chronic illness.
- Diabetes.
- Use of some prescription and nonprescription drugs. Inform your doctor of any drugs, medications, or vitamin and herb supplements you are using or have used in the last month.

 ## WHAT TO EXPECT

WHO OPERATES—General surgeon or proctologist.

WHERE PERFORMED—Hospital or outpatient surgical facility.

DIAGNOSTIC TESTS—Before surgery: Blood and urine studies, anoscopy, sigmoidoscopy (see Glossary for both).

ANESTHESIA
- Local anesthesia by injection.
- Spinal anesthesia by injection.
- General anesthesia by injection and inhalation with an airway tube placed in the windpipe.

DESCRIPTION OF OPERATION
- Sometimes dilatation (see Glossary) of the sphincter muscles is sufficient to treat the problem.
- In other cases, one of the outer sphincter muscles is cut to prevent recurrence.
- Rarely, the fissure is cut from the surrounding tissue and removed.
- Bleeding vessels are tied or closed with electrocauterization.
- The surgical area may be left open to hasten healing. Bandages are applied.

POSSIBLE COMPLICATIONS
- Excessive bleeding or pain.
- Surgical-wound infection.
- Inability to control bowel movements until healing is complete.
- Incontinence.

AVERAGE HOSPITAL STAY—0 to 1 day.

PROBABLE OUTCOME—Expect complete healing without complications. Allow about 3 weeks for recovery from surgery.

 ## POSTOPERATIVE CARE

GENERAL MEASURES
- Sit in a tub of warm water for 15 to 20 minutes several times a day to relieve discomfort.
- Use soft moistened tissue to clean the anal area after bowel movements.

MEDICATION
- Your doctor may prescribe:
  - Pain relievers. Don't take prescription pain medication longer than 4 to 7 days. Use only as much as you need.
  - Stool softeners to prevent constipation.
- You may use nonprescription drugs, such as acetaminophen, for minor pain. Avoid aspirin.

ACTIVITY
- To help recovery and aid your well-being, stay off your feet and in bed for several days following surgery.
- Avoid vigorous exercise for 4 weeks after surgery.
- Resume driving 1 week after returning home.

DIET—Eat a well-balanced diet to promote healing. Increase fiber and fluid intake to prevent constipation.

 ## CALL YOUR DOCTOR IF

- Pain, swelling, redness, drainage, or bleeding increases in the surgical area.
- You experience nausea, vomiting, or constipation.
- You develop symptoms of infection including headache, muscle aches, dizziness, fever, or a general ill feeling.
- New, unexplained symptoms develop

ANAL FISSURE TREATMENT

An illustration of an anal fissure. This view places the patient lying on back with legs extended.

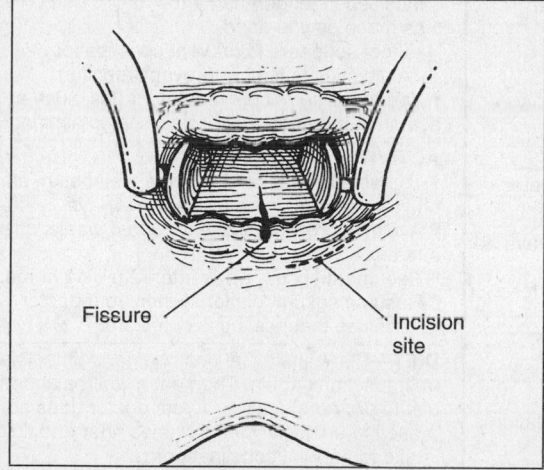

Sphincter muscle is expanded with special instrument. The incision site is indicated above the sphincter muscle.

Fissure cut free from surrounding tissue and removed. Sphincter muscle has been cut.

ANAL FISTULA REPAIR

GENERAL INFORMATION

DEFINITION—Opening or removal of an anal fistula, an abnormal tract extending from inside the rectum to the skin outside of the anus.

BODY PARTS INVOLVED—Rectum, skin and underlying tissue around the rectum and anus.

REASONS FOR SURGERY
• Repeated abscesses in the anal and rectal areas.
• Chronic drainage from a fistula.

SURGICAL RISK INCREASES WITH
• Diabetes.
• Poor nutrition.
• Recent or chronic illness.
• Obesity.
• Smoking.
• Use of some prescription and nonprescription drugs. Inform your doctor of any drugs, medications, or vitamin and herb supplements you are using or have used in the last month.

WHAT TO EXPECT

WHO OPERATES—General surgeon or proctologist.

WHERE PERFORMED—Outpatient surgical facility or hospital.

DIAGNOSTIC TESTS—Before surgery: x-rays of lower gastrointestinal tract, colonoscopy, anoscopy or sigmoidoscopy (see Glossary for all 3).

ANESTHESIA
• Local anesthesia by injection.
• Spinal anesthesia by injection.
• General anesthesia by injection and inhalation with an airway tube placed in the windpipe.

DESCRIPTION OF OPERATION
• Abscesses are drained, if necessary.
• The fistula is located with a delicate probe, and the skin and tissue over the fistula is opened.
• The surgical wound is left open to heal from inside out.
• Occasionally, the internal opening of the fistula may be located very high inside the rectum. In this case, it may be necessary to perform the operation in two stages a few weeks apart.

POSSIBLE COMPLICATIONS
• Excessive bleeding.
• Surgical-wound infection.
• Slow healing or recurrence.
• Incontinence.

AVERAGE HOSPITAL STAY—0 to 3 days.

PROBABLE OUTCOME—Expect complete healing without complications in 4 to 5 weeks for small fistulas, and up to 16 weeks for fistulas that are deeper.

POSTOPERATIVE CARE

GENERAL MEASURES
• Take warm sitz baths (see Glossary) several times a day to relieve discomfort.
• Move and elevate legs often while confined to bed to decrease the likelihood of deep-vein blood clots.
• Change bandages or sanitary pads 4 to 5 times a day or as directed by your doctor.
• Clean the rectal area with soap and water after bowel movements.

MEDICATION
• Your doctor may prescribe:
 - Pain relievers. Don't take prescription pain medication longer than 4 to 7 days. Use only as much as you need.
 - Stool softeners to prevent constipation.
 - Antibiotics to fight or prevent infection.
• You may use nonprescription drugs, such as acetaminophen, for minor pain. Avoid aspirin.

ACTIVITY
• To help recovery and aid your well-being, stay off your feet and in bed for several days.
• Avoid vigorous exercise for 3 to 4 weeks after surgery.
• Resume driving 1 week after returning home.
• Resume sexual relations when your doctor determines that healing is complete.

DIET—Clear liquid diet until the gastrointestinal tract functions again. Then eat a well-balanced diet to promote healing, if your doctor does not prescribe a special diet. Increase fiber and fluid intake to prevent constipation.

CALL YOUR DOCTOR IF

• Pain, swelling, redness, drainage, or bleeding increases in the surgical area.
• You develop symptoms of infection including headache, muscle aches, dizziness, fever, or a general ill feeling.
• You experience nausea, vomiting, or constipation.
• New, unexplained symptoms develop.

ANAL FISTULA REPAIR

Anus

Fistula

An illustration of an anal fistula. The opening of the tract that appears on the skin may occur in various places in the area surrounding the anus.

Anus retracted to expose the fistula tract. A probe is inserted to locate the inner opening of the fistula.

Fistula is opened and the surgical wound is then left open to allow healing from inside out.

Rectal mucosa (lining)

Internal opening

Anal verge

External opening

ANEURYSM REPAIR, VENTRICULAR

GENERAL INFORMATION

DEFINITION—A surgical procedure to remove an aneurysm (a swelling or ballooning of the heart wall) due to weakening that is caused by disease or muscle damage from a heart attack.

BODY PARTS INVOLVED—Usually the left ventricle of the heart.

REASONS FOR SURGERY
- Prevent rupture and uncontrolled bleeding.
- Increase the efficiency of the remaining heart muscle.
- Reduce risk of blood clots.

SURGICAL RISK INCREASES WITH
- Obesity, smoking.
- Recent or chronic illness such as heart attack, high blood pressure, thyroid disease, diabetes, or kidney disease.
- Chronic obstructive pulmonary disease (COPD).
- Chronic congestive heart failure (advanced).
- Use of some prescription and nonprescription drugs. Inform your doctor of any drugs, medications, or vitamin and herb supplements you are using or have used in the last month.

WHAT TO EXPECT

WHO OPERATES—Cardiovascular surgeon.

WHERE PERFORMED—Hospital.

DIAGNOSTIC TESTS
- Before surgery: Blood studies, chest x-ray, cardiac catheterization, ECG, sonogram, arteriogram (see Glossary for all).
- After surgery: ECG, chest x-ray, blood tests.

ANESTHESIA—General anesthesia by injection and inhalation with an airway tube placed in the windpipe. The heart is placed on heart-lung bypass.

DESCRIPTION OF OPERATION
- The patient is connected to the heart-lung equipment to allow the heart to be stopped temporarily so surgery can be performed on the diseased tissue.
- The heart is made to stop by cooling and weak electrical shock.
- The aneurysm is removed along with a border of normal heart tissue.
- The edges of the heart are sewn together. A graft may be sewn into place between the two cut edges.
- The heart is warmed, then the heartbeat is restored by a weak electrical shock.
- Note: Coronary artery bypass surgery is frequently performed at the same time.

POSSIBLE COMPLICATIONS
- Surgical wound infection.
- Excessive bleeding.
- Blood clot to leg or kidney and other areas.
- Stroke.
- Kidney failure.
- Continued heartbeat irregularities.

AVERAGE HOSPITAL STAY—7 to 10 days.

PROBABLE OUTCOME—Improved effectiveness of heart function and reduced likelihood of heartbeat irregularities. Allow 6 weeks for recovery from surgery.

POSTOPERATIVE CARE

GENERAL MEASURES
- No smoking.
- A hard ridge should form along the incision. As it heals, the ridge will gradually recede.
- Shower as usual after discharge. You may wash the incision gently with mild, unscented soap.
- Move and elevate legs frequently while resting in bed to decrease the likelihood of deep-vein blood clots.

MEDICATION
- Your doctor may prescribe:
  - Pain relievers. Don't take prescription pain medication longer than 4 to 7 days. Use only as much as you need.
  - Stool softeners to prevent constipation.
  - Antibiotics to fight or prevent infection.
  - Heart medications to prevent rhythm disturbances and strengthen heart muscle contractions.
  - Medications to reduce blood pressure.
- You may use nonprescription drugs, such as acetaminophen, for minor pain. Avoid aspirin.

ACTIVITY
- To help recovery and aid your well-being, resume daily activities as soon as possible.
- Resume driving 1 month after returning home.
- Resume sexual relations when your doctor determines that healing is complete.
- Ask your doctor for advice about an exercise rehabilitation program.

DIET—As directed by your doctor.

CALL YOUR DOCTOR IF
- Pain, swelling, redness, drainage, or bleeding increases in the surgical area.
- You develop symptoms of infection including headache, muscle aches, dizziness, fever, or a general ill feeling.
- You experience a cough, irregular heartbeat, constipation, or leg pain.
- New, unexplained symptoms develop.

ANEURYSM REPAIR, VENTRICULAR

An illustration of the heart as seen after the chest wall has been opened showing the ballooning out of the left ventricle representing the aneurysm as well as the proposed incision site.

Aneurysm

Incision site

The aneurysm is incised and any blood clot inside is removed. The weakened scarred area is excised and the remaining heart muscle closed in layers.

The appearance of the heart after the aneurysm has been excised and the remaining heart muscle closed with the sutures.

ANGIOPLASTY, CORONARY
(Percutaneous Transluminal Coronary Angioplasty)

GENERAL INFORMATION

DEFINITION—A nonsurgical shaping or alteration of blood vessels. In this procedure, a catheter with an inflatable balloon is inserted into a blocked or partially blocked coronary artery.

BODY PARTS INVOLVED—Coronary arteries (the blood vessels that supply nourishment to the heart muscle).

REASONS FOR SURGERY—To open a block or partial block of a coronary artery.

SURGICAL RISK INCREASES WITH
- Obesity, smoking.
- Excess alcohol consumption.
- Angina (for more than 1 year).
- Calcification of blood vessels.
- Use of some prescription and nonprescription drugs. Inform your doctor of any drugs, medications, or vitamin and herb supplements you are using or have used in the last month.

WHAT TO EXPECT

WHO OPERATES—Cardiologist.

WHERE PERFORMED—Hospital.

DIAGNOSTIC TESTS
- Before surgery: EKG (see Glossary), chest x-ray, blood tests, heart catheterization with x-ray and fluoroscopic examinations (see Glossary).
- During surgery: X-rays after injection of dye through the catheter into various parts of the heart.
- After surgery: EKG, chest x-ray, blood tests.

ANESTHESIA—Local, with sedation.

DESCRIPTION OF OPERATION
- The cardiac balloon catheter is inserted into an artery in the arm or leg. Fluoroscopy (see Glossary) provides guidance for the catheter to pass through the artery to the heart.
- Blood-pressure readings are taken, and the heart's ability to pump blood is tested.
- The catheter is guided into the coronary-artery system. Fluoroscopy allows identification of any disease in the coronary arteries.
- The catheter is passed through the occlusion, the balloon is inflated, and the occlusion is compressed, allowing blood to flow through once again.
- Stents may be placed to keep the artery open.
- When all examinations have been completed, the catheter balloon is withdrawn. The insertion site is compressed until bleeding stops.

POSSIBLE COMPLICATIONS
- Break or rupture in the dilated artery lining.
- Dislodged plaque that blocks the artery further downstream.
- Coronary spasm.
- Reaction to the dye used in x-ray studies.
- Complete coronary artery blockage. This requires immediate open-heart surgery to remove blockage and prevent a heart attack.
- Irregular heartbeat (arrhythmia).

AVERAGE HOSPITAL STAY—0 to 1 day.

PROBABLE OUTCOME—Opening of blockage in occluded coronary artery.

POSTOPERATIVE CARE

GENERAL MEASURES
- No smoking.
- A hard ridge usually forms beneath the puncture site in the groin. As it heals, the ridge will gradually recede.
- Discoloration under the skin where the catheter was inserted should disappear in 2 weeks.
- Shower as usual. You may wash the insertion site gently with mild, unscented soap.
- Between showers, keep the wound dry with a bandage for the first 2 or 3 days after the procedure. If a bandage gets wet, change it promptly.
- If the wound bleeds during the first 24 hours after surgery, press a clean tissue or cloth to it for 10 to 15 minutes continuously.

MEDICATION
- Your doctor may prescribe pain relievers.
- You may use nonprescription drugs, such as acetaminophen, for minor pain. Avoid aspirin.

ACTIVITY
- To help recovery and aid your well-being, resume daily activities, including work, as soon as possible. This procedure requires much less time for recovery than coronary bypass surgery.
- Avoid vigorous exercise for 2 weeks after surgery.
- Resume driving 2 days after returning home.

DIET—As directed by your doctor.

CALL YOUR DOCTOR IF

- You experience sudden or severe chest pain.
- You develop shortness of breath.
- Pain, swelling, redness, drainage, or bleeding increases in the surgical area.
- You develop symptoms of infection including headache, muscle aches, dizziness, fever, or a general ill feeling.
- New, unexplained symptoms develop.

ANGIOPLASTY, CORONARY
(Percutaneous Transluminal Coronary Angioplasty)

Balloon catheter

Blockage

An illustration of the cardiac balloon catheter about to enter the right coronary artery.

Fluoroscopy allows identification of any disease in the coronary arteries and the catheter is passed through the occlusion.

Then the balloon is inflated, the plaque is broken, and the occlusion is dilated allowing blood to flow freely once again. After all examinations have been completed, the catheter balloon is withdrawn.

ANTERIOR CRUCIATE LIGAMENT RECONSTRUCTION

 GENERAL INFORMATION

DEFINITION—Surgery to reconstruct a torn anterior cruciate ligament (ACL) using a graft to replace the damaged ligament. The ACL is one of four major knee ligaments and helps stabilize the knee. It runs from the thigh bone (femur) to the shin bone (tibia).

BODY PARTS INVOLVED—ACL and possibly other knee ligaments or other parts of the knee.

REASONS FOR SURGERY
- To restore near normal stability, function, range of motion, and strength to the knee.
- Prevent degeneration or injury to other parts of the knee.

SURGICAL RISK INCREASES WITH
- Age.
- Obesity.
- Smoking.
- Knee joint disease.
- History of thrombophlebitis.
- Chronic lung disease.

 WHAT TO EXPECT

WHO OPERATES—Orthopedic surgeon.

WHERE PERFORMED—Hospital or outpatient surgical facility.

DIAGNOSTIC TESTS
- Before surgery: Blood tests; knee x-ray and MRI (see Glossary).
- After surgery: Usually none.

ANESTHESIA—General or spinal anesthesia.

DESCRIPTION OF OPERATION
- One type of arthroscopic surgery is described. Other variations or open surgery are also used.
- A tendon in your knee or hamstring is taken for the graft to reconstruct the torn ligament. This is called autograft. The graft may also be taken from a deceased donor (called allograft).
- One or two small incisions are made on the top of the knee. An arthroscope (see Glossary) and tiny tools are inserted into the knee joint.
- The torn ACL is removed. Other damage to the knee is trimmed or repaired. In order to reconstruct the tendon, holes are drilled through bone structures in the thigh and shin. The new graft will be placed through these holes.
- The graft is secured with screws or staples, or other hardware. The surgeon will check the tension of the graft and verify the knee has full range of motion.
- The incisions are then closed with stitches or tape. Dressings, and sometimes a brace, are applied to the knee.

POSSIBLE COMPLICATIONS
- Surgical complications are rare, but can include infection, bleeding, blood clots, reaction to anesthesia, or failure of ligament to heal.
- After the surgery, a few patients may experience knee instability, stiffness, pain, or numbness. Loss of range of motion may occur.

AVERAGE HOSPITAL STAY—Usually done as an outpatient procedure, but some patients may require a 1 or 2 day hospital stay.

PROBABLE OUTCOME—ACL reconstruction is usually quite successful. Most patients who follow rehabilitation guidelines will have a stable knee that is as near normal as possible. Recovery typically takes 4 to 6 months, but may take longer in some cases.

 POSTOPERATIVE CARE

GENERAL MEASURES
- For the first few days after surgery, use RICE method (rest, ice, elevation, compression [with ace bandage]) for the knee. Don't place a pillow behind the knee—put it under the calf for support.
- Change or remove the dressing as instructed.
- You can shower 48 hours after surgery (but follow your doctor's instructions if different). Don't take tub baths until advised.

MEDICATION
- You may be prescribed pain relievers, antibiotics, or anti-inflammatory drugs.
- You may use nonprescription pain reliever such as acetaminophen for minor pain. Ask your doctor about taking ibuprofen or aspirin.

ACTIVITY
- There are a number of options for ACL rehabilitation after surgery. Each individual is different. Follow your doctor's instructions.
- Use crutches for walking as advised.
- A knee brace or CPM (a motion machine) may be recommended.
- You will work with a physical therapist to help regain knee function, strength, and range of motion. This may take several months.
- You will be advised when to return to work or resume sports or other physical activities.

DIET—No special diet.

 CALL YOUR DOCTOR IF

- Pain, swelling, redness, drainage, or bleeding increases in the surgical area.
- You develop signs of infection, including headache, muscle aches, dizziness, fever, or a general ill feeling.
- New unexplained symptoms develop.

ANTERIOR CRUCIATE LIGAMENT RECONSTRUCTION

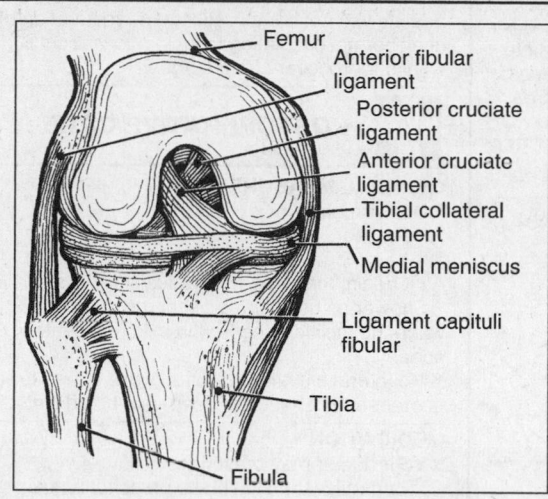

Femur
Anterior fibular ligament
Posterior cruciate ligament
Anterior cruciate ligament
Tibial collateral ligament
Medial meniscus
Ligament capituli fibular
Tibia
Fibula

An illustration of normal knee anatomy.

Incision sites

Torn anterior cruciate ligament

Torn ACL.

Autograft ligament

The new graft replaces the torn ACL.

AORTOILIAC BYPASS GRAFT

 GENERAL INFORMATION

DEFINITION—Placement of an artificial graft to bypass a blood clot or narrowing in the arteries that supply blood to the abdomen, genital area, and legs.

BODY PARTS INVOLVED—Aorta, iliac arteries.

REASONS FOR SURGERY—Restoration of normal blood circulation in the legs.

SURGICAL RISK INCREASES WITH
- Alcoholism, obesity, smoking.
- Diabetes, coronary artery disease, or atherosclerosis.
- Use of some prescription and nonprescription drugs. Inform your doctor of any drugs, medications, or vitamin and herb supplements you are using or have used in the last month.

 WHAT TO EXPECT

WHO OPERATES—General surgeon or vascular surgeon.

WHERE PERFORMED—Hospital.

DIAGNOSTIC TESTS
- Before surgery: Blood and urine studies, ultrasound, arteriograms (see Glossary for both).
- After surgery: Blood studies.

ANESTHESIA—General anesthesia by injection and inhalation with an airway tube placed in the windpipe.

DESCRIPTION OF OPERATION
- An incision is made in the abdomen.
- The abdominal muscles are separated to expose the abdominal organs, which are inspected for undetected disease. (Other surgeries may be performed at this time.)
- The aorta and iliac arteries are located and clamped to isolate the obstruction.
- An artificial graft is selected and fitted in place. One end attaches to the aorta and the other two ends to the iliac arteries.
- The graft is sewn in place and the clamps are released. Blood can now circulate freely.
- The muscles of the abdomen are closed in layers. The skin is closed with sutures or clips, which usually can be removed about 1 week after surgery.

POSSIBLE COMPLICATIONS
- Excessive bleeding.
- Surgical-wound infection, graft infection.
- Incisional hernia.
- Inadvertent injury to the ureter.
- Impotence.
- Occlusion of arteries beyond the grafted vessels.

AVERAGE HOSPITAL STAY—5 to 7 days.

PROBABLE OUTCOME—Expect complete healing without complications and restoration of near-normal circulation to legs. Allow about 6 weeks for recovery from surgery.

 POSTOPERATIVE CARE

GENERAL MEASURES
- Don't smoke.
- Keep feet clean and dry.
- A hard ridge should form along the incision. As it heals, the ridge will gradually recede.
- Shower as usual after discharge. You may wash the incision gently with mild, unscented soap.
- Move and elevate legs often while in bed to decrease the chance of deep-vein blood clots.

MEDICATION
- Your doctor may prescribe:
  - Pain relievers. Don't take prescription pain medication longer than 4 to 7 days. Use only as much as you need.
  - Stool softeners to prevent constipation.
  - Antibiotics to fight or prevent infection.
- You may use nonprescription drugs, such as acetaminophen, for minor pain. Avoid aspirin.

ACTIVITY
- To help recovery and aid your well-being, resume daily activities, including work, as soon as you are able.
- Avoid vigorous exercise for 6 weeks after surgery. Your doctor will prescribe an exercise program.
- Resume driving 5 weeks after returning home.
- Resume sexual relations when your doctor has determined that healing is complete.

DIET—Clear liquid diet until the gastrointestinal tract begins to function again. Then eat a well-balanced diet to promote healing. Your doctor may recommend a diet low in fat and sodium (see Appendix for both diets).

 CALL YOUR DOCTOR IF

- Pain, swelling, redness, drainage, or bleeding increases in the surgical area.
- You develop symptoms of infection including headache, muscle aches, dizziness, fever, or a general ill feeling.
- You experience nausea, vomiting, constipation, or abdominal swelling.
- Your legs or feet become cold, discolored, numb or painful.
- New, unexplained symptoms develop.

AORTOILIAC BYPASS GRAFT

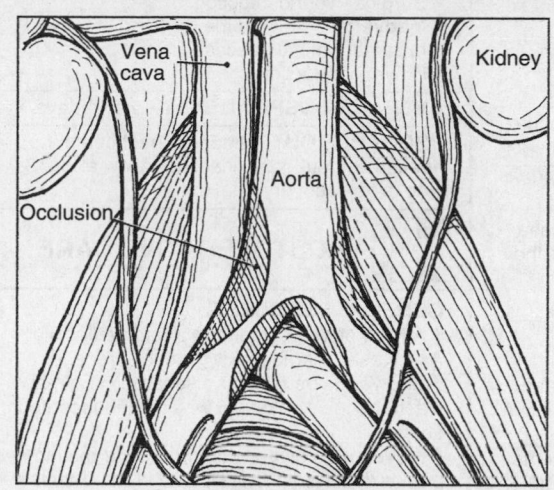

An illustration of the aorta, iliac arteries, and the occlusions to be bypassed.

The aorta and iliac arteries are clamped to isolate the obstruction.

● Polyester graft fitted in place. The upper end fits the aorta and the two lower ends fit the iliac arteries.
● After the graft is in place, the clamps are released. Blood can now again circulate freely.

APPENDECTOMY

GENERAL INFORMATION

DEFINITION—Removal of the appendix, an outgrowth of tissue from the cecum, the first part of the large intestine.

BODY PARTS INVOLVED—Appendix, cecum, peritoneum.

REASONS FOR SURGERY—Treatment of an infected appendix. Signs and symptoms of infection can include: abdominal pain, nausea or vomiting, loss of appetite, tenderness in the right lower abdomen, low-grade fever, or elevated white blood-cell count.

SURGICAL RISK INCREASES WITH
- Alcoholism, obesity, smoking.
- Chronic heart, lung, liver, or kidney disease.
- Use of some prescription and nonprescription drugs. Inform your doctor of any drugs, medications, or vitamin and herb supplements you are using or have used in the last month.

WHAT TO EXPECT

WHO OPERATES—General surgeon.

WHERE PERFORMED—Hospital.

DIAGNOSTIC TESTS
- Before surgery: Blood and urine studies, x-ray of abdomen, ultrasound and CT scan (see Glossary).
- After surgery: Blood studies and examination of removed tissue.

ANESTHESIA
- General anesthesia by injection and inhalation with an airway tube placed in the windpipe.
- Spinal anesthesia by injection.

DESCRIPTION OF OPERATION
- An incision is made in the lower abdomen.
- The abdominal muscles and organs are separated and the appendix is isolated, cut free and removed.
- The area around the appendix is inspected for undetected diseases. Other surgeries may be performed at this time.
- Any fluid or pus from the infected appendix is suctioned away.
- Sometimes, a drain is placed in the area left by the removed appendix. The drain is usually removed 2 to 3 days following surgery.
- The abdominal cavity is closed, and the skin is closed with sutures, which usually can be removed 1 week after surgery.
- Alternatively, surgery may be performed using a laparoscope (see Glossary). In this case, several small incisions would be made in the abdomen to facilitate viewing and removal of the appendix.

POSSIBLE COMPLICATIONS
- Excessive bleeding.
- Surgical-wound infection.
- Inadvertent injury to the ureter.
- Intra-abdominal abscess.
- Bowel obstruction.

AVERAGE HOSPITAL STAY—2 to 4 days.

PROBABLE OUTCOME—Expect complete healing without complications. Allow about 3 weeks for recovery from surgery.

POSTOPERATIVE CARE

GENERAL MEASURES
- A hard ridge should form along the incision. As it heals, the ridge will gradually recede.
- Shower as usual after discharge. You may wash the incision gently with mild, unscented soap.
- Move and elevate legs often while resting in bed to decrease the likelihood of deep-vein blood clots.

MEDICATION
- Your doctor may prescribe:
  - Pain relievers. Don't take prescription pain medication longer than 4 to 7 days. Use only as much as you need.
  - Stool softeners to prevent constipation.
  - Antibiotics to fight or prevent infection.
- You may use nonprescription drugs, such as acetaminophen, for minor pain. Avoid aspirin.

ACTIVITY
- To help recovery and aid your well-being, resume daily activities, including work, as soon as you are able.
- Avoid vigorous exercise for 6 weeks after surgery.
- Resume driving 2 weeks after returning home.

DIET—Clear liquid diet until the gastrointestinal tract begins to function again. Then eat a well-balanced diet to promote healing.

CALL YOUR DOCTOR IF

- Pain, swelling, redness, drainage, or bleeding increases in the surgical area.
- You develop symptoms of infection including headache, muscle aches, dizziness, fever, or a general ill feeling.
- You experience nausea, vomiting, constipation or abdominal swelling.
- New, unexplained symptoms develop.

APPENDECTOMY

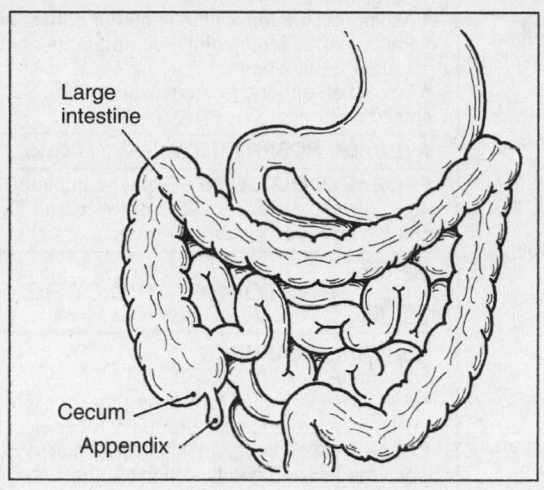

An illustration of the vermiform appendix attached to the cecum (the first part of the large intestine).

Large intestine

Cecum

Appendix

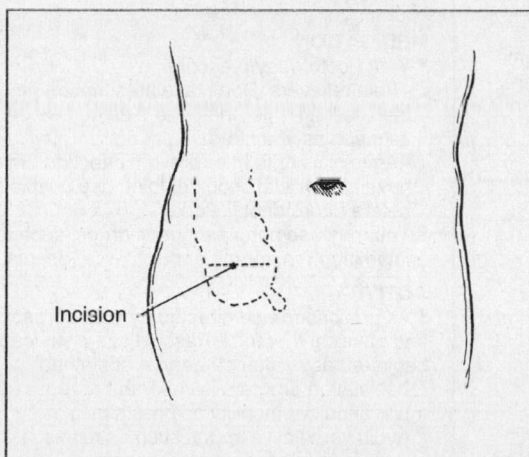

The incision is usually made at a point approximately 2/3 the distance between the navel and the point of the hip.

Incision

Appendix isolated, cut free and removed. The stump is then cauterized and sterilized to prevent infection.

ARTHROPLASTY, SHOULDER

GENERAL INFORMATION

DEFINITION—Surgical replacement and repair of an injured or diseased shoulder to restore function of the movable joint.

BODY PARTS INVOLVED—Shoulder joint, muscles, ligaments, bones, cartilage and bursa forming the shoulder joint.

REASONS FOR SURGERY—Diseased or injured shoulder causing chronic pain or disability impairing the quality of life. Disorders treated include rheumatoid arthritis, osteoarthritis, rotator cuff arthropathy, avascular necrosis, congenital defects, old trauma, and failed shoulder prosthesis.

SURGICAL RISK INCREASES WITH
- Obesity, smoking.
- Excess alcohol consumption.
- Recent or chronic illness.
- Diabetes.
- Use of some prescription and nonprescription drugs. Inform your doctor of any drugs, medications, or vitamin and herb supplements you are using or have used in the last month.

WHAT TO EXPECT

WHO OPERATES—Orthopedic surgeon.

WHERE PERFORMED—Hospital.

DIAGNOSTIC TESTS
- Before surgery: X-rays of joint, CT scan, or MRI (see Glossary for both), joint aspiration (to check for active infection), blood and urine studies.
- During surgery: X-rays.
- After surgery: X-rays, blood tests, and examination of tissue removed.

ANESTHESIA—General anesthesia by injection and inhalation with an airway tube placed in the windpipe.

DESCRIPTION OF OPERATION
- An incision is made into the affected shoulder.
- The surgeon will do any repair work necessary, there may be a need to remove tissue fragments, reattach tendons to bones and muscles, stitch or staple torn tissue.
- A total shoulder replacement may be necessary for severe shoulder disability. One type is designed to maintain and reproduce the normal anatomy of the shoulder joint. Another type may be used if there is rotator cuff damage that cannot be repaired.
- The incision is closed with stitches and bandaged. The shoulder is immobilized in a sling, splint, or cast that is left on for 2 to 3 weeks.

POSSIBLE COMPLICATIONS
- Excessive bleeding, blood clots.
- Surgical-wound infection.
- Accidental fracture of the shoulder bones.
- Failure or loosening of the components of the shoulder replacement.
- Formation of bone in areas where there should be none.

AVERAGE HOSPITAL STAY—2 to 4 days.

PROBABLE OUTCOME—Expect complete healing without complications. Allow about 6 months for recovery from surgery.

POSTOPERATIVE CARE

GENERAL MEASURES
- No smoking.
- A hard ridge should form along the incision. As it heals, the ridge will gradually recede.
- Shower as usual after discharge. You may wash the incision gently with mild, unscented soap.

MEDICATION
- Your doctor may prescribe:
  - Pain relievers. Don't take prescription pain medication longer than 4 to 7 days. Use only as much as you need.
  - Antibiotics to fight or prevent infection. If you have an artificial shoulder joint, use antibiotics before future dental work.
- You may use nonprescription drugs, such as acetaminophen, for minor pain. Avoid aspirin.

ACTIVITY
- As prescribed and directed by your surgeon and physical therapist. Passive exercises can begin 3-6 days after surgery. A sustained rehabilitation program is important to regain as much shoulder mobility as possible.
- Avoid very active sports such as tennis, skiing, swimming, or contact sports.
- Resume driving when your doctor determines that healing is complete.

DIET—Eat a well-balanced diet to promote healing.

CALL YOUR DOCTOR IF

- Pain, swelling, redness, drainage, or bleeding increases in the surgical area.
- You develop symptoms of infection including headache, muscle aches, dizziness, fever, or a general ill feeling.
- New, unexplained symptoms develop.

ARTHROPLASTY, SHOULDER

Shoulder is prepared for incision.

Incision site

Diseased head

Humerus
(arm)

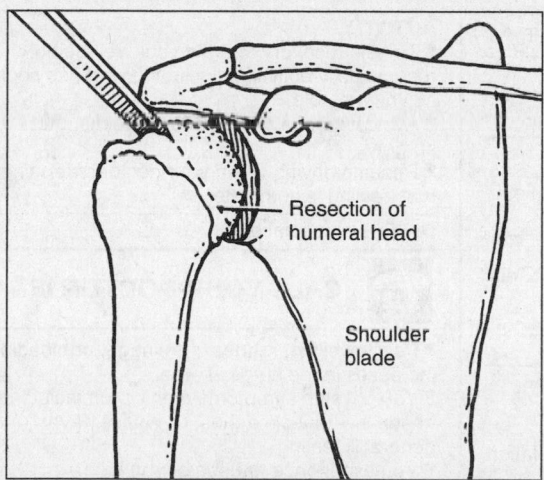

After the humeral head has been
surgically exposed, the diseased
surface is removed.

Resection of
humeral head

Shoulder
blade

A prosthetic device is inserted into
the humeral base. Cement is used to
adhere device to the bone. Shoulder
is closed and immobilized for a period
of time (not illustrated).

Prosthetic shoulder
replacement

Humeral head
base

ARTHROSCOPY

GENERAL INFORMATION

DEFINITION—Visual examination of a joint with an arthroscope, a fiber-optic instrument with a lighted tip (with or without repair of damaged tissue).

BODY PARTS INVOLVED—Joint, usually in the knee, but often performed in the shoulder.

REASONS FOR SURGERY
- Diagnosis of disease or injury inside a joint.
- Removal of bone or cartilage or repair of tendons or ligaments.

SURGICAL RISK INCREASES WITH
- Adults over 60.
- Obesity, smoking.
- Poor nutrition.
- Recent or chronic illness.
- Diabetes.
- Use of some prescription and nonprescription drugs. Inform your doctor of any drugs, medications, or vitamin and herb supplements you are using or have used in the last month.

WHAT TO EXPECT

WHO OPERATES—Orthopedist.

WHERE PERFORMED—Hospital or outpatient surgical facility.

DIAGNOSTIC TESTS
- Before surgery: Blood and urine studies, x-ray of joint.
- After surgery: Blood studies, x-ray, examination of removed fluid or tissue.

ANESTHESIA
- Local anesthesia by injection.
- Spinal anesthesia by injection.
- General anesthesia by injection and inhalation with an airway tube placed in the windpipe.

DESCRIPTION OF OPERATION
- A small incision is made at the side of the joint to be examined (several openings may be made for a complete examination). The arthroscope is inserted into the joint. Diagnostic and/or surgical procedures are then performed, depending on the problem.
- The arthroscope is removed. The skin is closed with sutures or clips, which usually can be removed about 7 to 10 days after surgery.

POSSIBLE COMPLICATIONS
- Bleeding into joint.
- Surgical-wound infection.
- Slow healing.

AVERAGE HOSPITAL STAY—0 to 1 day.

PROBABLE OUTCOME—Expect complete healing without complications. Allow about 6 weeks to 3 months for recovery from surgery.

POSTOPERATIVE CARE

GENERAL MEASURES
- Shower as usual. You may wash the incision gently with mild, unscented soap.
- Move and elevate legs often while resting in bed to decrease the likelihood of deep-vein blood clots.
- Following a knee arthroscopy, use crutches or a cane to walk until your doctor determines that healing is complete.
- Physical therapy may hasten healing and restore strength. Ask your doctor.

MEDICATION
- Your doctor may prescribe:
  - Pain relievers. Don't take prescription pain medication longer than 4 to 7 days. Use only as much as you need.
  - Antibiotics to fight or prevent infection.
- You may use nonprescription drugs, such as acetaminophen, for minor pain. Avoid aspirin.

ACTIVITY
- To help recovery and aid your well-being, resume daily activities, including work, as soon as you are able.
- Avoid vigorous exercise for 6 weeks after surgery.
- Resume driving when your doctor determines that healing is complete.

DIET—No special diet.

CALL YOUR DOCTOR IF

- Pain, swelling, redness, drainage, or bleeding increases in the surgical area.
- You develop symptoms of infection including headache, muscle aches, dizziness, fever, or a general ill feeling.
- You experience nausea or vomiting.
- New, unexplained symptoms develop.

ARTHROSCOPY

An illustration of the knee joint area frequently examined by arthroscopy.

Femur

Patella

Knee joint

Incision

Fibula

Tibia

Arthroscope

- After an incision is made at the side of the joint to be examined, the arthroscope is inserted into the joint.
- The operator inspects the joint and performs whatever surgical procedures are indicated.

After the arthroscope is removed, the small incisions in the skin are closed.

BAKER'S CYST REMOVAL

 GENERAL INFORMATION

DEFINITION—Removal of Baker's cyst, a benign cystic tumor on the back of the knee joint. The cyst consists of accumulated fluid that protrudes between two groups of muscles behind the knee. Baker's cyst may result from injury or from diseases, such as arthritis, gout, or inflammation of the membrane lining the knee joint.

BODY PARTS INVOLVED—Space behind the knee joint on either or both sides of the knee.

REASONS FOR SURGERY—If the cyst has resulted from disease, it may disappear after successful treatment of the underlying disease. Often, local steroid injections are successful in treating a Baker's cyst. Otherwise, the cyst is removed when it becomes painful or unsightly. In children, the cyst is usually left to heal by itself, and is not removed unless it presses on nerves or blood vessels.

SURGICAL RISK INCREASES WITH
- Obesity; smoking.
- Poor nutrition.
- Recent or chronic illness.
- Diabetes.
- Use of some prescription and nonprescription drugs. Inform your doctor of any drugs, medications, or vitamin and herb supplements you are using or have used in the last month.

 WHAT TO EXPECT

WHO OPERATES—General surgeon or orthopedist.

WHERE PERFORMED—Outpatient surgical facility or hospital.

DIAGNOSTIC TESTS
- Before surgery: Blood and urine studies; x-rays of both knees; ultrasound; venography; arthrograms (see Glossary for all).
- After surgery: Blood studies; examination of tissue removed.

ANESTHESIA
- Local anesthesia by injection.
- Spinal anesthesia by injection.
- General anesthesia by injection and inhalation with an airway tube placed in the windpipe.

DESCRIPTION OF OPERATION
- An incision is made over the cyst.
- The cyst is located, cut free from surrounding tissue and removed.
- A synthetic patch is sometimes sutured in place to cover the defect left from removal of the cyst.
- The skin is closed with fine sutures, which usually can be removed about 2 weeks after surgery.

POSSIBLE COMPLICATIONS
- Excessive bleeding.
- Surgical-wound infection.
- Slow healing and continued pain.
- Damage to nerves or arteries behind knee.
- Recurrence (rare).

AVERAGE HOSPITAL STAY—0 to 1 day.

PROBABLE OUTCOME—Expect complete healing without complications. Allow about 4 weeks for recovery from surgery.

 POSTOPERATIVE CARE

GENERAL MEASURES
- A hard ridge should form along the incision. As it heals, the ridge will gradually recede.
- Shower as usual after discharge. You may wash the incision gently with mild, unscented soap.
- Keep legs elevated as much as possible for the first several days following surgery.

MEDICATION
- Your doctor may prescribe:
  - Pain relievers. Don't take prescription pain medication longer than 4 to 7 days. Use only as much as you need.
  - Antibiotics to fight or prevent infection.
- You may use nonprescription drugs, such as acetaminophen, for minor pain. Avoid aspirin.

ACTIVITY
- To help recovery and aid your well-being, resume daily activities, including work, as soon as you are able.
- Use crutches or a cane to walk (as directed by your doctor).
- Avoid vigorous exercise for 6 weeks after surgery.
- Resume driving 2 weeks after returning home if you have adequate range-of-motion in knee.

DIET—Eat a well-balanced diet to promote healing.

 CALL YOUR DOCTOR IF

- Pain, swelling, redness, drainage, or bleeding increases in the surgical area.
- You develop symptoms of infection including headache, muscle aches, dizziness, fever, or a general ill feeling.
- You experience nausea or vomiting.
- New, unexplained symptoms develop.

BAKER'S CYST REMOVAL

Baker's cyst

Popliteal space

An illustration of a Baker's cyst located in the popliteal space behind the knee joint.

Cyst origin

Muscles pulled apart to expose the area where the cyst begins.

Graft

Synthetic patch sutured in place to cover the defect left after surgical removal of the cyst.

BARIATRIC SURGERY
(Gastric Bypass)

 GENERAL INFORMATION

DEFINITION—A surgical procedure to limit food intake and absorption with the ultimate goal of losing weight.

BODY PARTS INVOLVED—Abdominal cavity, stomach, small intestines.

REASONS FOR SURGERY—To treat obesity.

SURGICAL RISK INCREASES WITH
* Age.
* Diabetes.
* Poor kidney function.
* High blood pressure.
* Chronic lung disease.
* Degree of obesity.

 WHAT TO EXPECT

WHO OPERATES—General surgeon.

WHERE PERFORMED—Hospital.

DIAGNOSTIC TESTS
* Before surgery: Blood tests, chest x-ray, EKG (see Glossary).
* After surgery: Blood tests.

ANESTHESIA—General anesthesia.

DESCRIPTION OF OPERATION
* There are two main types of surgery done for weight loss—restrictive operations to limit the stomach size and bypass operations to limit the absorption of food. Sometimes a combination of the two is done.
* The most common restrictive operations involve a small upper abdominal incision. A "band-like" device is placed around the upper stomach to limit the flow of food through the stomach and into the intestines. This is usually adjustable to permit more food or less food if needed. Another method of restriction is performed using staples across the stomach with a small opening for food to pass through. These procedures can often be done using laparoscopy rather than an incision.
* The bypass procedure is often combined with making the stomach pouch smaller. The small intestine is then brought up to this shortened stomach so that only the last couple of feet of intestine is exposed to the food passing through, severely limiting absorption of potential calories.

POSSIBLE COMPLICATIONS
* Bleeding.
* Kidney failure.
* Failure of bowel connections to heal with leakage of intestinal contents.
* Blood clots.
* Incisional hernia.
* Respiratory failure.

AVERAGE HOSPITAL STAY—Usually 3-10 days (depending on the procedure done).

PROBABLE OUTCOME—Expect full recovery in 6-8 weeks with continued weight loss over 1-2 years.

 POSTOPERATIVE CARE

GENERAL MEASURES
* Hard ridges will form along the incisions. As they heal, the ridges will gradually recede.
* Use heat on the incision to help relieve incisional pain.
* Shower as usual. You may wash the incisions gently with mild soap. After showering, replace any dressings with a new dry dressing.
* Wear compression stockings when up for the first few weeks after surgery.
* Discuss diet with your surgeon.

MEDICATION
* Your doctor may prescribe pain relievers. Use only as much as you need to be comfortable.
* You may use nonprescription pain relievers such as acetaminophen for minor pain. Ask your doctor if it is okay to take ibuprofen or aspirin.

ACTIVITY
* Start ambulating (walking) as soon as you are home. Take frequent naps as needed during the day when tired. Avoid strenuous activity for 6 to 8 weeks.
* You may swim once all sutures are out.
* Resume sexual relations when comfortable and when advised by your surgeon.

DIET—Consult your surgeon.

 CALL YOUR DOCTOR IF

* Pain, swelling, redness, drainage, or bleeding increases in the surgical area.
* You develop symptoms of infection including headache, muscle aches, dizziness, fever, or a general ill feeling.
* You develop nausea and vomiting.
* Prolonged constipation occurs.
* New, unexplained symptoms develop.

BARIATRIC SURGERY
(Gastric Bypass)

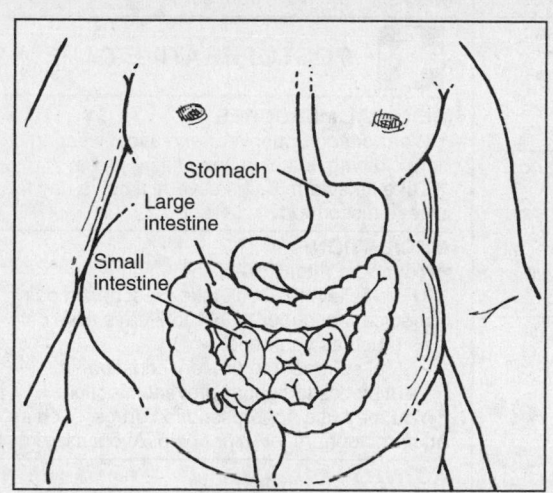

An illustration of the stomach and surrounding structures.

Stomach

Large intestine

Small intestine

One method of restricting food passage is a mechanical banding of the upper stomach. The port is used to adjust the constriction of the band.

Gastric band

Adjustable port

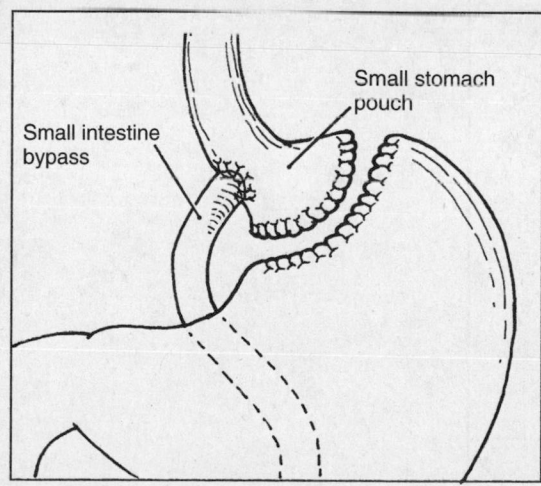

Another method is to reduce the size of the stomach pouch and reattach it to a shortened segment of the small intestine.

Small stomach pouch

Small intestine bypass

BARTHOLIN'S GLAND ABSCESS DRAINAGE

GENERAL INFORMATION

DEFINITION—Removal of a blockage of the Bartholin's glands caused by a cyst or an abscess (on accumulation of mucus or infection). These two small glands are located in the base of the vaginal lips.

BODY PARTS INVOLVED—Bartholin's glands, lips of vagina.

REASONS FOR SURGERY—Appropriate treatment of an abscess or cyst which will result in near immediate relief of symptoms and will reduce the risk of subsequent infection.

SURGICAL RISK INCREASES WITH
- Obesity.
- Smoking.
- Poor nutrition.
- Recent illness.
- Alcoholism or chronic illness.
- Diabetes.
- Use of some prescription and nonprescription drugs. Inform your doctor of any drugs, medications, or vitamin and herb supplements you are using or have used in the last month.

WHAT TO EXPECT

WHO OPERATES—Obstetrician-gynecologist, family doctor, or general surgeon.

WHERE PERFORMED—Doctor's office, outpatient surgical facility, or hospital.

DIAGNOSTIC TESTS
- Before surgery: Blood and urine studies, laboratory examination of vaginal discharge.
- After surgery: Laboratory examination of pus or secretions from opened glands.

ANESTHESIA
- Local anesthesia by injection.
- Regional anesthesia by injection.
- General anesthesia, usually by inhalation.

DESCRIPTION OF OPERATION
- A small incision is made in the labia over the area of the abscess. A catheter is placed through the incision, and is allowed to drain into the vagina. The catheter is left in place for approximately 2 weeks.
- The alternate method is marsupialization. In this procedure, the edges of the glands are opened and the linings are folded back and sewn open. This forms a small pouch that drains easily. Sutures that will be absorbed by the body are used to form the pouch.

POSSIBLE COMPLICATIONS
- Excessive bleeding.
- Surgical-wound infection.

AVERAGE HOSPITAL STAY—0 to 1 day.

PROBABLE OUTCOME—Expect complete healing without complications. Allow about 2 weeks for recovery from surgery.

POSTOPERATIVE CARE

GENERAL MEASURES
- Wear cotton underwear and avoid wearing tight clothing, such as snug-fitting jeans.
- Take lukewarm baths several times a day to relieve discomfort.

MEDICATION
- Your doctor may prescribe:
  - Pain relievers. Don't take prescription pain medication longer than 4 to 7 days. Use only as much as you need.
  - Stool softeners to prevent constipation.
  - Antibiotics to fight or prevent infection.
- You may use nonprescription drugs, such as acetaminophen, for minor pain. Avoid aspirin.

ACTIVITY
- To help recovery and aid your well-being, resume daily activities, including work, as soon as you are able.
- Avoid vigorous exercise for 4 weeks after surgery.
- Resume driving 4 days after returning home.
- Resume sexual relations when your doctor determines that healing is complete.

DIET—No special diet.

CALL YOUR DOCTOR IF

- Pain, swelling, redness, drainage, or bleeding increases in the surgical area.
- You develop symptoms of infection including headache, muscle aches, dizziness, fever, or a general ill feeling.
- New, unexplained symptoms develop.

BARTHOLIN'S GLAND, ABSCESS DRAINAGE

An illustration showing the normal appearance of the Bartholin's glands, which are two small glands located at the base of the vaginal lips.

Bartholin's glands

The appearance of a Bartholin's gland which is blocked because of a cyst or abscess.

Blocked gland

A small incision has been placed in the labia over the area of the abscess. A catheter has been placed in the incision to facilitate continued drainage.

Drainage tube

BLADDER (URINARY) REMOVAL
(Cystectomy)

GENERAL INFORMATION

DEFINITION—Removal of the urinary bladder and adjacent tissues and organs, and diversion of the urinary stream. This involves an artificial opening, which is called an ostomy or stoma.

BODY PARTS INVOLVED
• Males: Bladder, prostate, urethra, ureters, seminal vesicles, small intestine.
• Females: Urinary bladder, urethra, ureters, cervix, vagina, small intestine.

REASONS FOR SURGERY—Cancer of the bladder.

SURGICAL RISK INCREASES WITH
• Poor nutrition.
• Obesity.
• Repeated surgeries on the bladder.
• Diabetes.
• Use of some prescription and nonprescription drugs. Inform your doctor of any drugs, medications, or vitamin and herb supplements you are using or have used in the last month.

WHAT TO EXPECT

WHO OPERATES—Urologist.

WHERE PERFORMED—Hospital.

DIAGNOSTIC TESTS
• Before surgery: Blood and urine studies, x-ray of kidneys and chest, ultrasound, CT scan, cystoscopy (see Glossary for all).
• During surgery: Cystoscopy (see Glossary).

ANESTHESIA—General anesthesia by injection and inhalation with an airway tube placed in the windpipe.

DESCRIPTION OF OPERATION
• An incision is made in the abdomen. The muscles are separated and the abdominal cavity is entered.
• The blood supply and the ureters are cut and tied.
• The bladder and adjacent tissues and organs are cut free and removed.
• The ureters are diverted through an intestinal pouch (called an ileal conduit) to an opening made in the skin (the stoma).
• The muscles are replaced and sewn together with sutures. The skin is closed with sutures or clips, which usually can be removed about 1 week after surgery.

POSSIBLE COMPLICATIONS
• Excessive bleeding, blood clots.
• Incisional hernia or infection.
• Impotence in males.
• Recurring urinary tract infections.
• Obstruction of the ureter, leakage of urine.

AVERAGE HOSPITAL STAY—7 to 10 days.

PROBABLE OUTCOME—Expect complete healing of surgical wounds. You will need to wear an external pouch to collect urine. The stoma will heal and shrink to its permanent size in 2 to 4 months after surgery. Allow about 6 to 8 weeks for recovery from surgery.

POSTOPERATIVE CARE

GENERAL MEASURES
• A hard ridge should form along the incision. As it heals, the ridge will gradually recede.
• Shower as usual aer discharge. You may wash the incision gently with mild, unscented soap.
• Move and elevate legs often while resting in bed to decrease the likelihood of deep-vein blood clots.
• An enterostomy specialist (see Glossary) will help you and your family learn to cope with new urination habits.
• Dry the area around the stoma by patting, not rubbing.

MEDICATION
• Your doctor may prescribe:
  - Pain relievers. Don't take prescription pain medication longer than 4 to 7 days. Use only as much as you need.
  - Stool softeners to prevent constipation.
  - Antibiotics to fight or prevent infection.
• You may use nonprescription drugs, such as acetaminophen, for minor pain. Avoid aspirin.

ACTIVITY
• To help recovery and aid your well-being, resume daily activities, including work, as soon as possible.
• Avoid vigorous exercise for 6 weeks after surgery. Avoid heavy lifting indefinitely.
• Resume driving 3 weeks after returning home.

DIET—Clear liquid diet until the gastrointestinal tract functions again. Then eat a well-balanced diet to promote healing.

CALL YOUR DOCTOR IF

• Pain, swelling, redness, drainage, or bleeding increases in the surgical area.
• You develop symptoms of infection including headache, muscle aches, dizziness, fever, or a general ill feeling.
• You experience nausea, vomiting, constipation, or abdominal swelling.
• You wish to discuss treatment for impotence.
• New, unexplained symptoms develop.

BLADDER (URINARY) REMOVAL
(Cystectomy)

An illustration of the bladder and other parts of the urinary tract.

- The bladder and adjacent tissues and organs are cut free and removed.
- The ureters are divided and an intestinal pouch is created by isolating a small/short segment of small bowel (ileum).

After the bladder has been removed, the ureters are connected to an ileal conduit to drain the kidneys.

BONE GRAFT

GENERAL INFORMATION

DEFINITION—Filling space between fragments of a broken bone.

BODY PARTS INVOLVED—Bone.

REASONS FOR SURGERY
* Joining of two or more parts of a bone that have broken and not grown back together.
* Fusion of the spine after injury or surgery.

SURGICAL RISK INCREASES WITH
* Adults over 60.
* Obesity.
* Smoking.
* Poor nutrition.
* Diabetes.
* Rheumatoid arthritis.
* Recent or chronic illness.
* Use of some prescription and nonprescription drugs. Inform your doctor of any drugs, medications, or vitamin and herb supplements you are using or have used in the last month.

WHAT TO EXPECT

WHO OPERATES—Orthopedist.

WHERE PERFORMED—Hospital.

DIAGNOSTIC TESTS
* Before surgery: X-rays of area to be grafted, blood and urine studies.
* After surgery: Blood studies, x-rays of grafted area.

ANESTHESIA—General anesthesia by injection and inhalation with an airway tube placed in the windpipe.

DESCRIPTION OF OPERATION
* If bone for the graft is to be an autograft (taken from the patient), it is usually removed from the top of the hip bone, the spine, or the ribs. Otherwise, bone is obtained from a bone bank (see Glossary).
* An incision is made over the affected bone. The bone is located and isolated.
* The bone to be grafted is shaped to fit the affected area. The bone is held in place with wire or screws.
* The skin is closed with sutures or clips, which usually can be removed about 1 week after surgery.
* A splint or plaster cast keeps the affected part rigid and promotes healing (sometimes).

POSSIBLE COMPLICATIONS
* Excessive bleeding.
* Surgical-wound infection.
* Rejection of transplanted bone.
* Continued non-healing.

AVERAGE HOSPITAL STAY—7 to 10 days.

PROBABLE OUTCOME—Expect complete healing without complications. Allow about 6 months for recovery from surgery.

POSTOPERATIVE CARE

GENERAL MEASURES—Move and elevate legs often while resting in bed to decrease the likelihood of deep-vein blood clots.

MEDICATION
* Your doctor may prescribe:
  - Pain relievers. Don't take prescription pain medication longer than 4 to 7 days. Use only as much as you need.
  - Stool softeners to prevent constipation.
  - Antibiotics to fight or prevent infection.
* You may use nonprescription drugs, such as acetaminophen, for minor pain. Avoid aspirin.

ACTIVITY
* To help recovery and aid your well-being, resume daily activities, including work, as soon as your doctor advises that you are able.
* Avoid vigorous exercise for 3 months after surgery.
* Resume driving when able.

DIET—No special diet.

CALL YOUR DOCTOR IF

* Pain, swelling, redness, drainage, or bleeding increases in the surgical area.
* You develop symptoms of infection including headache, muscle aches, dizziness, fever, or a general ill feeling.
* New, unexplained symptoms develop.

BONE GRAFT

Ileum

Graft site

An illustration of a frequent bone graft site. In this case, located on the crest of the ileum (hip bone).
(These illustrations are used as examples. The principles and techniques are similar for bone grafts in other locations.)

Graft

After muscles and covering tissues are separated, the segment of bone is removed from its normal site.

Graft

The bone graft is transplanted into another part of the body (in this example, the spine) where it will provide stabilization.

BONE MARROW ASPIRATION & BIOPSY

 ## GENERAL INFORMATION

DEFINITION—Drawing tissue and cells from the marrow of one of the large bones in order to study the number and types of cells present.

BODY PARTS INVOLVED—Usually pelvis bone, sometimes sternum or leg bone.

REASONS FOR SURGERY—To determine if there are abnormal cells, such as tumor cells, or to see if there are adequate numbers of the cells which make up the various blood components. The two most common indications are to look for cancer cells like leukemias or to try to determine a cause for anemia..

SURGICAL RISK INCREASES WITH—Blood clotting disorders.

 ## WHAT TO EXPECT

WHO OPERATES—Hematologist-oncologist or internist.

WHERE PERFORMED—Hospital or outpatient facility or physician's office.

DIAGNOSTIC TESTS
* Before procedure: None other than those to work up underlying disease process.
* After procedure: Laboratory study of removed tissue and cells.

ANESTHESIA—Local anesthesia, local with sedation, or general anesthesia.

DESCRIPTION OF OPERATION
* The biopsy/aspiration is usually performed in the posterior portion of the pelvis bone.
* A local anesthetic is injected over the site and a large bore needle is pushed down against the outer cortex of the bone. The needle is then pushed through the outer bone and enters the marrow space. A syringe is used to aspirate tissue and cells from the marrow and the needle is withdrawn.
* There is frequently sharp pain elicited by the aspiration of cells. No sutures are required.

POSSIBLE COMPLICATIONS
* Bleeding from the puncture site.
* Injury to structures adjacent to the bone.
* Infection of the puncture site.

AVERAGE HOSPITAL STAY—None.

PROBABLE OUTCOME—Expect full recovery in 1-2 days.

 ## POSTOPERATIVE CARE

GENERAL MEASURES
* Slight swelling may occur under the puncture site.
* Use ice on the puncture site for 12-24 hours to minimize bleeding and swelling if advised by your physician.
* Shower as usual. You may wash the puncture site gently with mild soap. After showering, replace any dressings with a new dry dressing for the first few days.

MEDICATION
* Your doctor may prescribe pain relievers. Use only as much as you need to be comfortable.
* You may use nonprescription pain relievers such as acetaminophen for minor pain. Ask your doctor if it is okay to take ibuprofen or aspirin.

ACTIVITY—Start ambulating (walking) as soon as you are home.

DIET—No special diet.

 ## CALL YOUR DOCTOR IF

* Pain, swelling, redness, drainage, or bleeding increases in the surgical area.
* You develop symptoms of infection including headache, muscle aches, dizziness, fever, or a general ill feeling.
* New unexplained symptoms develop.

BONE MARROW ASPIRATION & BIOPSY

A site is chosen on the posterior and lateral portion of the pelvis bone.

Aspiration site

Pelvis

A needle is inserted through the skin and pushed through the outer layer of the bone.

Needle aspiration

Pelvis

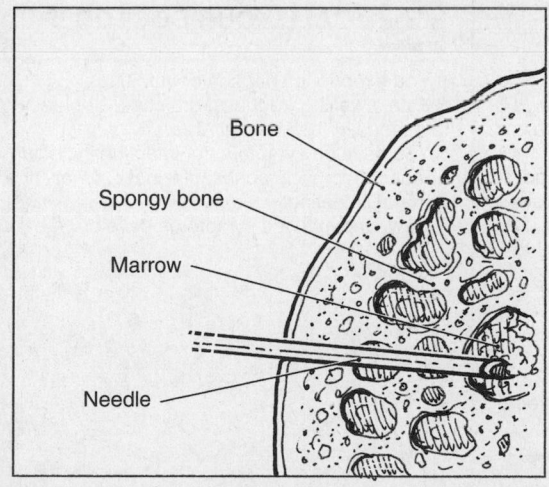

Cells and fluid are aspirated from the soft marrow of the pelvic bone.

Bone

Spongy bone

Marrow

Needle

BREAST ABSCESS DRAINAGE

GENERAL INFORMATION

DEFINITION—To open and drain an abscess in the female breast.

BODY PARTS INVOLVED—Lactating breast, nipple, lactiferous ducts.

REASONS FOR SURGERY—Relief of pain and prevention of the spread of infection.

SURGICAL RISK INCREASES WITH
• Obesity.
• Smoking.
• Poor nutrition.
• Recent or chronic illness.
• Diabetes.
• Use of some prescription and nonprescription drugs. Inform your doctor of any drugs, medications, or vitamin and herb supplements you are using or have used in the last month.

WHAT TO EXPECT

WHO OPERATES—General surgeon or obstetrician-gynecologist.

WHERE PERFORMED—Hospital, emergency room, doctor's office or outpatient surgical facility.

DIAGNOSTIC TESTS
• Before surgery: Blood and urine studies, ultrasound, mammogram, aspiration (see Glossary for all).
• After surgery: Laboratory examination of removed pus.

ANESTHESIA
• Local anesthesia by injection.
• General anesthesia by injection and inhalation with an airway tube placed in the windpipe.

DESCRIPTION OF OPERATION
• An incision is made in the breast over the abscess. The incision is deepened and pus is removed.
• An instrument is forced into the abscess. Pockets of pus are broken up by the surgeon's finger. The opening is enlarged and the area is irrigated with a salt solution.
• Gauze packing is inserted to allow drainage. A small, plastic tube may be placed in the incision to collect additional pus and allow drainage. The drain or gauze packing is usually removed 3 to 5 days following surgery.

POSSIBLE COMPLICATIONS
• Excessive bleeding.
• Surgical-wound infection.
• Slow healing.
• Breast engorgement, if breast is not emptied regularly of milk. Leakage of milk through incision.
• Recurrence of abscess.

AVERAGE HOSPITAL STAY—0 to 2 days.

PROBABLE OUTCOME—Expect complete recovery without complications. Nursing can usually be resumed on the affected side in about 2 weeks. Allow about 3 weeks for complete recovery from surgery.

POSTOPERATIVE CARE

GENERAL MEASURES
• A hard ridge should form along the incision. As it heals, the ridge will gradually recede.
• Shower as usual. After removal of the drain, You may wash the incision gently with mild, unscented soap.
• Change dressings daily after a shower.
• Wearing a loose bra at bedtime may make you more comfortable.
• If you continue nursing, use a breast pump on the abscessed side to prevent engorgement. Continue to nurse from the unaffected breast. The infant is unlikely to become infected.

MEDICATION
• Your doctor may prescribe:
  - Pain relievers. Don't take prescription pain medication longer than 4 to 7 days. Use only as much as you need.
  - Antibiotics to fight infection.
• You may use nonprescription drugs, such as acetaminophen, for minor pain. Avoid aspirin.

ACTIVITY
• To help recovery and aid your well-being, resume daily activities, including work, as soon as you are able.
• Avoid vigorous exercise for 3 weeks after surgery.
• Resume driving 2 days after returning home.

DIET—Eat a well-balanced diet to promote healing. Drink at least 8 glasses of water daily.

CALL YOUR DOCTOR IF

• You experience nausea or vomiting.
• Pain, swelling, redness, drainage, or bleeding increases in the surgical area.
• You develop symptoms of infection including headache, muscle aches, dizziness, fever, or a general ill feeling.
• New, unexplained symptoms develop.

BREAST ABSCESS DRAINAGE

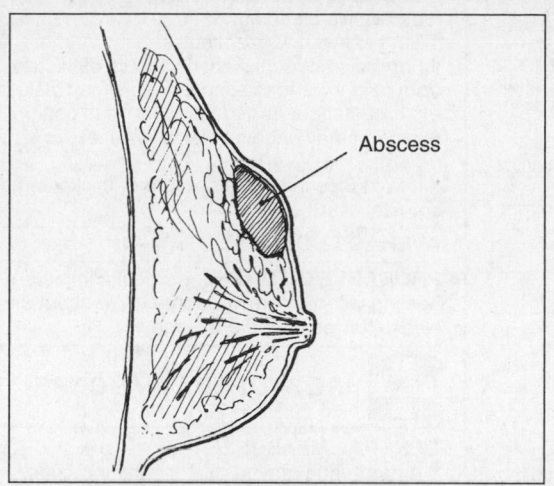

A side illustration of a breast abscess that has become red, warm and fluctuant.

Abscess

The incision is made into the abscess cavity, a pocket is created, the incision is deepened and pus is removed. An instrument having been forced into the abscess, pockets of pus are now broken up by the surgeon's finger. The opening is enlarged and the area is irrigated with a salt solution. Gauze packing is inserted for drainage.

A small, plastic drain may be placed in the incision to collect additional pus and allow drainage. The drain or gauze packing remains in place for several days and is then removed.

Drain tube

BREAST AUGMENTATION
(Augmentation Mammoplasty)

GENERAL INFORMATION

DEFINITION—Implantation of artificial material inside the female breasts to enlarge them or give them a different shape.

BODY PARTS INVOLVED—Female breasts, underlying muscles.

REASONS FOR SURGERY
- Enlargement of the breasts in patients who have less breast tissue than they desire.
- Correction of asymmetry of the breasts.

SURGICAL RISK INCREASES WITH
- Smoking.
- Obesity.
- Excess alcohol consumption.
- Recent or chronic illness.
- Diabetes.
- Use of some prescription and nonprescription drugs. Inform your doctor of any drugs, medications, or vitamin and herb supplements you are using or have used in the last month.

WHAT TO EXPECT

WHO OPERATES—Plastic and reconstructive surgeon.

WHERE PERFORMED—Hospital, doctor's office, or outpatient surgical facility.

DIAGNOSTIC TESTS
- Before surgery: Blood studies, mammogram (see Glossary).
- After surgery: Usually none.

ANESTHESIA
- General anesthesia by injection and inhalation.
- Local anesthesia with sedation.

DESCRIPTION OF OPERATION
- Incisions may be made under the breast, through the nipple or in the armpit.
- The breast tissue is brought forward by raising muscles from below the breast or the muscles next to the chest wall.
- A pocket is created, and the implant (a mammary prosthesis filled with saline) is inserted. The procedures are usually repeated on the other breast.
- The skin is closed with sutures or clips, which usually can be removed about 1 week after surgery. A light bandage is applied.
- Occasionally, a drain may be left in place for several days to promote healing.
- A bra or elastic bandage is fitted to give support and to reduce possible bleeding.

POSSIBLE COMPLICATIONS
- Excessive bleeding.
- Surgical-wound infection.
- Formation of a thickened capsule of tissue from scar around the implant. This may make the breast more firm to the touch than usual.
- Implant may become dislodged, leak, or rupture.
- Keloid (see in Illness section) or thickening of surgical scars.

AVERAGE HOSPITAL STAY—0 to 1 day.

PROBABLE OUTCOME—Expect complete healing without complications. Allow about 2 weeks for recovery from surgery.

POSTOPERATIVE CARE

GENERAL MEASURES
- A hard ridge may form along the incisions. The ridges will heal and gradually recede without treatment.
- Bathe or shower as usual. You may wash the incisions gently with mild, unscented soap.
- Use ice packs to reduce swelling and to relieve incisional pain.
- You should wear a support bra both during the day and while you sleep, until your doctor determines that healing is complete.

MEDICATION
- Your doctor may prescribe:
  - Pain relievers. Don't take prescription pain medication longer than 4 to 7 days. Use only as much as you need.
  - Antibiotics to fight or prevent infection.
- You may use nonprescription drugs, such as acetaminophen, for minor pain. Avoid aspirin.

ACTIVITY
- Resume daily activities and work as soon as possible.
- Avoid vigorous exercise for 6 weeks after surgery.
- Resume driving 1 week after returning home.

DIET—No special diet.

CALL YOUR DOCTOR IF

- Pain, swelling, redness, drainage, or bleeding increases in the surgical area.
- You develop symptoms of infection including headache, muscle aches, dizziness, fever, or a general ill feeling.
- You experience nausea or vomiting.
- New, unexplained symptoms develop.

BREAST AUGMENTATION
(Augmentation Mammoplasty)

Incisions for the implant may be made under the breast, through the nipple or in the armpit. In this example, it is under the breast line in the chest wall skin.

Incision site

After the pocket is created, a prosthesis is inserted. The procedure is usually repeated on the other breast.

Breast

Prosthesis

Skin is closed with sutures that absorb or that can be removed about 1 week after surgery. A light bandage is usually all that is necessary for a dressing following surgery.

Prosthesis

BREAST BIOPSY BY EXCISION

GENERAL INFORMATION

DEFINITION—Removal of suspected abnormal tissue from the breast.

BODY PARTS INVOLVED—Female breast, male breast (rare).

REASONS FOR SURGERY—Clinical or mammographic signs or symptoms that may indicate breast cancer.

SURGICAL RISK INCREASES WITH
- Obesity.
- Smoking.
- Poor nutrition.
- Recent or chronic illness.
- Diabetes.
- Use of some prescription and nonprescription drugs. Inform your doctor of any drugs, medications, or vitamin and herb supplements you are using or have used in the last month.

WHAT TO EXPECT

WHO OPERATES—General surgeon.

WHERE PERFORMED—Hospital or outpatient surgical facility.

DIAGNOSTIC TESTS
- Before surgery: Blood and urine studies, mammogram, ultrasound (see Glossary for both).
- After surgery: Laboratory examination of removed tissue.

ANESTHESIA
- Local anesthesia often with sedation.
- General anesthesia by injection and inhalation with an airway tube placed in the windpipe.

DESCRIPTION OF OPERATION
- A special wire (the size of a thin guitar string) with a hooked tip may be inserted into the breast to localize the abnormality.
- An incision is made over the tissue to be removed. It is often possible to make a very cosmetic incision by cutting at the edge of the areola.
- The suspect tissue is cut free of the surrounding breast tissue and removed.
- Bleeding is controlled with ties or electrocautery.
- The skin is closed with sutures, which usually can be removed about 1 week after surgery.
- The removed tissue is sent to the pathology laboratory for microscopic examination.

POSSIBLE COMPLICATIONS
- Excessive bleeding.
- Surgical-wound infection.
- Unsightly scar on breast (rare).
- In cases of a large biopsy, or if the tissue removed is close to the skin, there may be some changes to the contour of the breast.

AVERAGE HOSPITAL STAY—Usually none.

PROBABLE OUTCOME—Expect complete healing without complications. Allow about 2 weeks for recovery from surgery.

POSTOPERATIVE CARE

GENERAL MEASURES
- A hard ridge may form along or beneath the incision. As it heals, the ridge will gradually recede.
- Shower as usual. You may wash the incision gently with mild, unscented soap.
- Wear a supportive bra. Apply bandages to the surgical wound and change them as directed by your doctor.
- Wearing a loose bra at bedtime may make you more comfortable.

MEDICATION
- Your doctor may prescribe pain relievers. Don't take prescription pain medication longer than 4 to 7 days. Use only as much as you need.
- You may use nonprescription drugs, such as acetaminophen, for minor pain. Avoid aspirin.

ACTIVITY
- To help recovery and aid your well-being, resume daily activities, including work, as soon as possible.
- Avoid vigorous exercise for 2 weeks after surgery.
- Resume driving the day after surgery.

DIET—No special diet.

CALL YOUR DOCTOR IF

- Pain, swelling, redness, drainage, or bleeding increases in the surgical area.
- You develop symptoms of infection including headache, muscle aches, dizziness, fever, or a general ill feeling.
- New, unexplained symptoms develop.

BREAST BIOPSY BY EXCISION

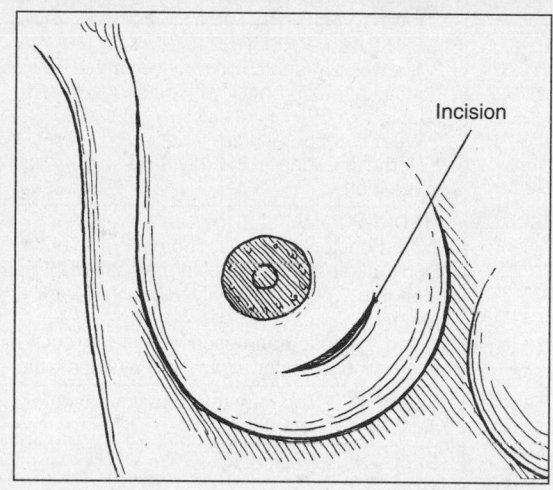

An illustration of a typical incision over the site of suspected abnormal breast tissue.

Incision

The suspect tissue is cut free of the surrounding breast tissue and removed.

Suspect tissue

Appearance of the breast after closure of the skin, following tissue removal.

BREAST BIOPSY BY NEEDLE ASPIRATION

 ## GENERAL INFORMATION

DEFINITION—Removal of fluid or tissue from the breasts.

BODY PARTS INVOLVED—Breast.

REASONS FOR SURGERY—Diagnosis of a thickening or lump. Needle biopsy is often the best first step for diagnosis of a lump in the breast.

SURGICAL RISK INCREASES WITH—Bleeding disorders.

 ## WHAT TO EXPECT

WHO OPERATES—Family doctor, general surgeon, or pathologist.

WHERE PERFORMED—Hospital, doctor's office or outpatient surgical facility.

DIAGNOSTIC TESTS
* Before surgery: Medical history and physical examination, ultrasound, mammogram (see Glossary for both).
* After surgery: Laboratory examination of removed fluid or tissue.

ANESTHESIA—Local anesthesia by injection (sometimes). Often, no anesthetic is necessary.

DESCRIPTION OF OPERATION
* A small, hollow needle is inserted into the thickening or lump.
* If the thickening or lump is a cyst, fluid usually can be removed and the cyst will shrink or disappear. This is often considered both therapeutic and diagnostic.
* In some cases, the removed fluid is sent to the laboratory to be examined for abnormal cells.
* If a solid tumor is detected, the tissue is recovered by passing the needle through the suspicious tissue several times, while using a syringe to aspirate as large a sample of cells as possible. The tissue is sent to the laboratory for microscopic examination.
* The needle is withdrawn and pressure is exerted on the site of the biopsy, a bandage is then applied.

POSSIBLE COMPLICATIONS
* Infection in surgical area (rare).
* Collection of blood (hematoma) under the skin where needle was inserted.

AVERAGE HOSPITAL STAY—Outpatient.

PROBABLE OUTCOME—Expect complete healing without complications. No recovery time is required.

 ## POSTOPERATIVE CARE

GENERAL MEASURES
* Shower as usual. You may wash the area of needle insertion gently with mild, unscented soap.
* Wear a supportive bra if desired.
* Remove bandage the day after surgery and leave it off.

MEDICATION
* Your doctor may prescribe pain relievers. Don't take prescription pain medication longer than 4 to 7 days. Use only as much as you need.
* You may use nonprescription drugs, such as acetaminophen, for minor pain. Avoid aspirin.

ACTIVITY—You may return to your usual activities immediately.

DIET—No special diet.

 ## CALL YOUR DOCTOR IF

* Pain, swelling, redness, drainage, or bleeding increases in the surgical area.
* You develop symptoms of infection including headache, muscle aches, dizziness, fever, or a general ill feeling.
* New, unexplained symptoms develop.

BREAST BIOPSY BY NEEDLE ASPIRATION

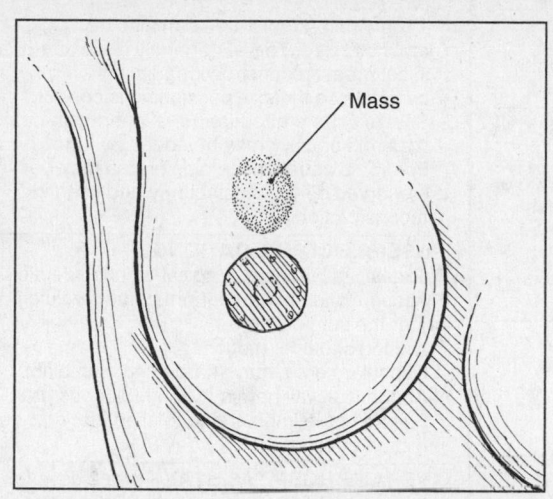

An illustration of a typical mass within the breast.

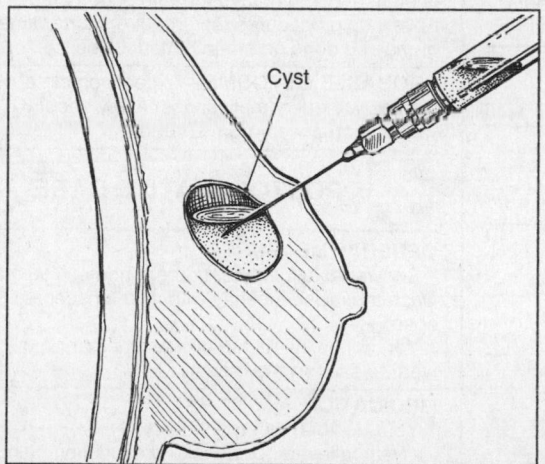

A small, hollow needle is inserted into the thickening or lump. Fluid is aspirated if the lump is a cyst.

If a solid tumor is detected, tissue is aspirated through the needle and a laboratory examination is done to determine whether the tissue is benign or malignant.

BREAST RECONSTRUCTION

GENERAL INFORMATION

DEFINITION—Rebuilding the female breast after mastectomy by using an implant or other body tissue.

BODY PARTS INVOLVED—Breasts, chest wall muscles, abdominal wall or back.

REASONS FOR SURGERY—Reconstruction of the breast following a mastectomy for breast cancer is usually done for psychological and cosmetic reasons. It also helps to reestablish symmetry. In most states, health insurance is required to cover reconstruction.

SURGICAL RISK INCREASES WITH
- Obesity, smoking.
- Excess alcohol consumption.
- Recent or chronic illness or diabetes.
- Previous radiation to the breast.
- Use of some prescription and nonprescription drugs. Inform your doctor of any drugs, medications, or vitamin and herb supplements you are using or have used in the last month.

WHAT TO EXPECT

WHO OPERATES—Plastic surgeon, general surgeon or oncology surgeon (sometimes).

WHERE PERFORMED—Hospital.

DIAGNOSTIC TESTS
- Before surgery: As required for the mastectomy procedure.
- After surgery: As required for follow up of cancer therapy or monitoring.

ANESTHESIA—General anesthesia by injection and inhalation, with an airway tube placed in the windpipe.

DESCRIPTION OF OPERATION
- Several options are available and additional methods are undergoing development. You and your surgeon should have a clear understanding of what is to be done during surgery, but the surgeon will need some leeway in case unexpected problems occur.
- Expander/implant reconstruction is the most common. It consists of placement of an expander (empty or partially filled plastic shell) under the muscle either at the time of mastectomy or after the mastectomy surgery has healed. The expander is slowly inflated with saline over 2 to 3 months and eventually replaced by a permanent implant filled with saline. The opposite breast may need a reduction or "lift" to achieve symmetry.
- Autologous graft is a more complex reconstruction which can achieve a superior cosmetic result without the need for any "foreign" implant. Tissue is moved to the chest wall from the lower abdomen or back to

reconstruct the breast. This can also be done at the time of the mastectomy or as a delayed procedure.
- The nipple-areola area can also be reconstructed. This is generally done after the initial breast reconstruction healing is complete so that the positioning is correct. Skin may be grafted from the inner thigh near the groin or color may be added by tattooing. For some patients, the nipple area may be preserved during mastectomy and used in reconstruction.

POSSIBLE COMPLICATIONS
- Excessive bleeding, surgical-wound infection.
- Accumulation of blood (hematoma) or fluid under the surgical area.
- Limited shoulder motion.
- Capsular contracture (hardening of implant).
- Abdominal wall hernia (with autologous graft).
- Failure of the implant due to slippage, rupture, infection or scarring.

AVERAGE HOSPITAL STAY—1 to 2 days for implant and 4 to 6 days for autologous graft. Follow up procedures may require shorter times or may be done on an outpatient basis.

PROBABLE OUTCOME—Expect complete healing without complications. Allow about 6 weeks for recovery from surgery.

POSTOPERATIVE CARE

GENERAL MEASURES
- Shower as usual after you are home. You may wash the incision gently with mild, unscented soap.
- You will be instructed on the type of bra to wear to support the breast.

MEDICATION
- Your doctor may prescribe:
  - Pain relievers. Don't take prescription pain medication longer than 4 to 7 days. Use only as much as you need.
  - Antibiotics to fight or prevent infection.
- You may use nonprescription drugs, such as acetaminophen, for minor pain. Avoid aspirin.

ACTIVITY
- Return to work and normal activity as soon as possible.
- Your doctor may recommend special exercises to aid in recovery of arm mobility.

DIET—No special diet.

CALL YOUR DOCTOR IF

- Pain, swelling, redness, drainage, or bleeding increases in the surgical area.
- You develop symptoms of infection including headache, muscle aches, dizziness, fever, or a general ill feeling.

BREAST RECONSTRUCTION

Illustration shows the appearance of right breast after mastectomy.

A pocket is prepared for an implant.

Muscles

Side view of the breast showing the implant in position.

Skin

Fat

Implant

BREAST REDUCTION
(Reduction Mammoplasty)

GENERAL INFORMATION

DEFINITION—Removal of excess tissue and overlying skin from the female breasts. Usually this surgery also includes reconstruction of breast shape.

BODY PARTS INVOLVED—Breasts.

REASONS FOR SURGERY
- Reduction of overly large breasts to improve appearance and/or emotional well-being.
- Relief of back and neck pain from weight of overly large breasts.
- Reconstruction of a breast to match a surgical change made in the other breast.

SURGICAL RISK INCREASES WITH
- Obesity.
- Smoking.
- Excess alcohol consumption.
- Diabetes.
- Poor nutrition.
- Use of some prescription and nonprescription drugs. Inform your doctor of any drugs, medications, or vitamin and herb supplements you are using or have used in the last month.

WHAT TO EXPECT

WHO OPERATES—Plastic and reconstructive surgeon.

WHERE PERFORMED—Hospital.

DIAGNOSTIC TESTS
- Before surgery: Blood and urine studies, mammogram (see Glossary).
- After surgery: Blood studies.

ANESTHESIA—General anesthesia by injection and inhalation with an airway tube placed in the windpipe.

DESCRIPTION OF OPERATION
- The breast is marked where the skin will be removed and where the nipple will be after tissue is removed.
- The skin between the new nipple location and the natural nipple location is incised and removed. The nipple stays attached to underlying tissue.
- Another incision is made below the nipple. Excess tissue is removed through this incision.
- The removed tissue is sent to a pathology laboratory to be examined and analyzed for any early signs of breast cancer.
- Drains are sometimes left in place to prevent fluid or blood from accumulating under the sutures.
- The skin is closed with fine sutures, which usually can be removed about 10 to 14 days after surgery.

POSSIBLE COMPLICATIONS
- Excessive bleeding, blood clots.
- Surgical-wound infection.
- Discoloration of healing skin edges.
- Abnormal scarring (called keloids) may necessitate a second surgery for scar revision.
- Development of small, tumor-like cysts (seromas) or collections of blood and serum in the breast tissue as it heals.

AVERAGE HOSPITAL STAY—4 to 5 days.

PROBABLE OUTCOME—Expect complete healing without complications. The breasts may take 3 to 12 weeks to assume their final shape. Allow about 4 weeks for recovery from surgery. Some women experience a change in nipple sensation following surgery.

POSTOPERATIVE CARE

GENERAL MEASURES
- A small ridge may form along the incisions. As they heal, the ridges will gradually recede.
- Shower as usual. You may wash the incision gently with mild, unscented soap.
- Move and elevate your legs often while resting in bed to decrease the likelihood of deep-vein clots.
- Women over age 30 should have a mammogram both before and 6 months following surgery. The postoperative mammogram will serve as a baseline for future mammograms.

MEDICATION
- Your doctor may prescribe:
  - Pain relievers. Don't take prescription pain medication longer than 4 to 7 days. Use only as much as you need.
  - Antibiotics to fight or prevent infection.
- You may use nonprescription drugs, such as acetaminophen, for minor pain. Avoid aspirin.

ACTIVITY
- To help recovery and aid your well-being, resume daily activities, including work, as soon as you are able.
- Avoid vigorous exercise for 6 weeks after surgery.
- Resume driving 1 month after returning home.

DIET—No special diet.

CALL YOUR DOCTOR IF

- Pain, swelling, redness, drainage, or bleeding increases in the surgical area.
- You develop symptoms of infection including headache, muscle aches, dizziness, fever, or a general ill feeling.
- New, unexplained symptoms develop.

BREAST REDUCTION
(Reduction Mammoplasty)

New nipple location

Excess to be removed

An illustration showing markings on the breast where skin will be removed and the nipple will be placed after the reduction procedure.

Skin between the new nipple location and the natural nipple location is incised and removed. The nipple stays attached to the underlying tissue.

Another incision is made below the nipple. Excess tissue is removed, drains are left in place to prevent collection of fluid, and skin is closed with fine sutures. Sutures are usually removed about 10 to 14 days after surgery.

BRONCHOSCOPY

 ## GENERAL INFORMATION

DEFINITION—Visual examination of the lining of the bronchial tubes and removal of tissue and secretions. The procedure is performed with a flexible bronchoscope, an optical instrument with a lighted tip.

BODY PARTS INVOLVED—Windpipe (trachea), larynx, bronchial tree.

REASONS FOR SURGERY
- Suspected cancer in the bronchial tubes.
- Foreign matter that has been inhaled accidentally.
- Bleeding in the bronchial tubes.
- X-ray studies (bronchograms) to diagnose diseases of the lung, such as bronchiectasis or emphysema.

SURGICAL RISK INCREASES WITH
- Obesity.
- Smoking.
- Recent or chronic illness, especially chronic lung disease.
- Diabetes.
- Alcoholism.
- Use of some prescription and nonprescription drugs. Inform your doctor of any drugs, medications, or vitamin and herb supplements you are using or have used in the last month.

 ## WHAT TO EXPECT

WHO OPERATES—Thoracic surgeon, general surgeon, pulmonary specialist, or otolaryngologist (ear, nose and throat doctor).

WHERE PERFORMED—Hospital or outpatient surgical facility.

DIAGNOSTIC TESTS
- Before surgery: Blood and urine studies, x-ray of chest, CT scan (see Glossary).
- During surgery: Bronchogram (see Glossary).
- After surgery: Laboratory examination of removed tissue and secretions, x-rays to check for complications.

ANESTHESIA
- Local anesthesia with sedation.
- General anesthesia by injection and inhalation with an airway tube placed in the windpipe.

DESCRIPTION OF OPERATION
- The bronchoscope is inserted through the nose or mouth, past the back of the tongue, into the main bronchial tube and its branches. Supplemental oxygen is supplied during the procedure.
- Foreign matter is removed, if necessary. Tissue is gathered and secretions are collected.
- The bronchoscope is removed.

POSSIBLE COMPLICATIONS
- Excessive bleeding.
- Infection in lung or bronchial tubes.
- Injury to wall of a bronchus.
- Aspiration of mucus into the lower bronchial tissues.
- Heart rhythm disturbances.

AVERAGE HOSPITAL STAY—Usually outpatient, but depends on underlying disease.

PROBABLE OUTCOME—Tissue and secretions obtained successfully without complications in almost all cases. Allow about 24 hours for recovery from the procedure.

 ## POSTOPERATIVE CARE

GENERAL MEASURES
- Don't smoke.
- Use of a vaporizer will help increase moisture in the air you breathe for the first 3 to 4 nights after the procedure.

MEDICATION
- Your doctor may prescribe:
  - Pain relievers. Don't take prescription pain medication longer than 4 to 7 days. Use only as much as you need.
  - Antibiotics to fight or prevent infection.
- You may use nonprescription drugs, such as acetaminophen, for minor pain. Avoid aspirin.

ACTIVITY
- To help recovery and aid your well-being, resume daily activities, including work, as soon as you are able.
- Avoid vigorous exercise for 7 days after the procedure.
- Resume driving 24 hours after returning home.

DIET—No special diet (unless one is required by an underlying disorder).

 ## CALL YOUR DOCTOR IF

- You experience excessive bleeding.
- You experience shortness of breath, increasing cough, or chest pain.
- You develop symptoms of infection including headache, muscle aches, dizziness, fever, or a general ill feeling.
- New, unexplained symptoms develop.

BRONCHOSCOPY

An illustration of the bronchoscope inserted into the mouth past the tongue and into the main bronchial tube and its branches.

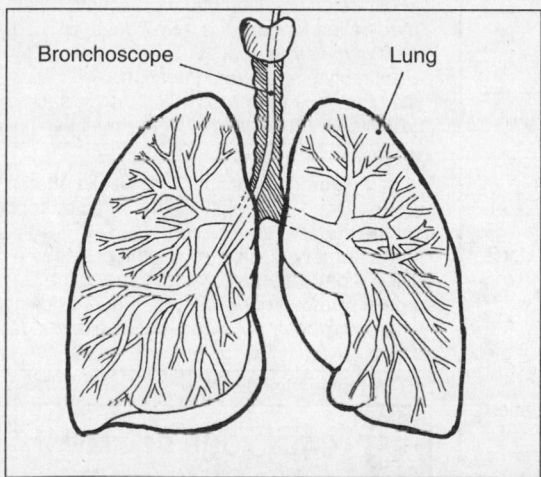

- The flexible bronchoscope can be passed into either of the main stem bronchial branches.
- Foreign matter is removed by suction. If necessary, tissue is gathered and secretions are collected to be studied microscopically.

Fluid being suctioned from the bronchoscope while still in place.

BUNION REMOVAL

GENERAL INFORMATION

DEFINITION—Removal of a bunion, a bony and fibrous outgrowth at the base of the big toe.

BODY PARTS INVOLVED—Foot, joint between the metatarsal bone and big toe, fluid sac that surrounds the joint.

REASONS FOR SURGERY
- Relief of pain.
- Correction of deformity.

SURGICAL RISK INCREASES WITH
- Poor nutrition.
- Recent illness.
- Alcoholism or chronic illness.
- Diabetes.
- Vascular disease.
- Use of some prescription and nonprescription drugs. Inform your doctor of any drugs, medications, or vitamin and herb supplements you are using or have used in the last month.

WHAT TO EXPECT

WHO OPERATES—General surgeon, orthopedist or podiatrist.

WHERE PERFORMED—Doctor's office, outpatient surgical facility or hospital.

DIAGNOSTIC TESTS
- Before surgery: X-rays of foot, blood and urine studies.
- After surgery: X-rays of foot.

ANESTHESIA
- Local anesthesia by injection.
- Spinal anesthesia by injection.
- General anesthesia by injection and inhalation with an airway tube placed in the windpipe.

DESCRIPTION OF OPERATION
- An incision is made over the bunion.
- The capsule of the joint connecting the metatarsal bone and the big toe is opened.
- A section from the metatarsal bone is cut or filed away and removed. Another small bone (the sesamoid bone) attached to a tendon is removed also.
- Tendons attached to the base of the metatarsal and toe bones are cut. This allows the bones to straighten when healed.
- A pin (metal rod) may be placed in the great toe.
- The skin is closed with sutures, which usually can be removed about 10 days after surgery.

POSSIBLE COMPLICATIONS
- Excessive bleeding.
- Surgical-wound infection.
- Slow healing.

AVERAGE HOSPITAL STAY—0 to 1 day.

PROBABLE OUTCOME—Expect complete healing without complications. Allow about 6 weeks for recovery from surgery.

POSTOPERATIVE CARE

GENERAL MEASURES
- A hard ridge should form along the incision. As it heals, the ridge will gradually recede.
- Shower as usual. You may wash the incision gently with mild, unscented soap.
- Between showers, keep the wound dry and covered with a bandage for the first 2 or 3 days after surgery. If a bandage gets wet, change it promptly.
- Apply nonprescription antibiotic ointment to the wound before applying bandages.
- If the wound bleeds, press a clean tissue or cloth to it.

MEDICATION
- Your doctor may prescribe:
  - Pain relievers. Don't take prescription pain medication longer than 4 to 7 days. Use only as much as you need.
  - Antibiotics to prevent infection.
- You may use nonprescription drugs, such as acetaminophen, for minor pain. Avoid aspirin.

ACTIVITY
- Avoid vigorous exercise for 6 weeks after surgery. Don't put weight on the affected foot until the surgical area heals.
- If the surgery was on your left foot, resume driving 4 days after returning home. If the surgery was on your right foot, resume driving when your doctor advises that it is okay to do so.

DIET—No special diet.

CALL YOUR DOCTOR IF

- Pain, swelling, redness, drainage, or bleeding increases in the surgical area.
- You develop symptoms of infection including headache, muscle aches, dizziness, fever, or a general ill feeling.
- New, unexplained symptoms develop.

BUNION REMOVAL

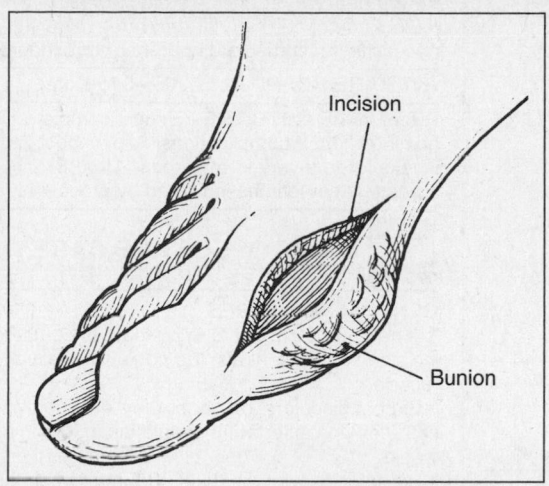

An illustration of a typical bunion. An incision is made over the bunion.

Overgrown section from the metatarsal bone is cut or filed away and removed.

Tendons attached to the base of the metatarsal bone and toe bones are cut to allow bones to straighten when healed.

CARDIAC CATHETERIZATION & ANGIOGRAM

GENERAL INFORMATION

DEFINITION—Diagnostic procedures to examine functions of the heart.

BODY PARTS INVOLVED—Heart muscle, heart valves, coronary arteries, large artery in arm or leg.

REASONS FOR SURGERY
- Evaluation of chest pain.
- Diagnosis of a congenital heart defect and valvular-heart disease.
- Measurement of the heart muscle's ability to pump blood.
- Identification of narrowing or obstruction in the coronary arteries.

SURGICAL RISK INCREASES WITH
- Stress, obesity, smoking.
- Recent or chronic illness.
- Alcoholism.

WHAT TO EXPECT

WHO OPERATES—Cardiologist.

WHERE PERFORMED—Hospital.

DIAGNOSTIC TESTS
- Before surgery: Blood and urine studies, ECG (see Glossary), chest x-ray.
- During surgery: Intracardiac pressures, cardiac output, cinematography, fluoroscopy, ECG (see Glossary for all).
- After surgery: ECG, blood studies.

ANESTHESIA—Local anesthesia by injection, usually accompanied by sedation.

DESCRIPTION OF OPERATION
- The cardiac catheter is inserted into an artery in the patient's arm or leg. Fluoroscopy provides guidance for the catheter to pass through the artery to the heart.
- Blood-pressure readings are taken, and the heart's ability to pump blood is tested.
- The catheter is guided into the coronary-artery system. Dye is injected through the catheter and into the coronary arteries. Multiple images will be taken to allow identification of any disease in the coronary arteries.
- When all examinations have been completed, the catheter is withdrawn, and the artery into which it was inserted is compressed until bleeding stops. If an arm artery was used, it may need to be repaired. A tight bandage is placed over the entry site for the catheter, and you will be expected to keep that area of your body flat for approximately 6 hours.

POSSIBLE COMPLICATIONS
- Excessive bleeding, blood clot in an artery.
- Reaction to dye (allergy).
- Surgical-wound infection.

- Development of hematomas (collections of blood) where skin was pierced to enter artery.
- Heartbeat disturbance, cardiac arrest (rare).
- Blockage of coronary artery (rare) necessitating immediate open-heart procedure.

AVERAGE HOSPITAL STAY—0 to 1 day.

PROBABLE OUTCOME—Expect complete healing without complications. Allow about 2 weeks for recovery from surgery. Urgent surgery is sometimes indicated by procedure.

POSTOPERATIVE CARE

GENERAL MEASURES
- A hard ridge should form beneath the catheter incision site. As it heals, the ridge will gradually recede.
- Expect discoloration under the skin where the catheter was inserted. It should disappear in 2 weeks.
- Bathe or shower as usual. You may wash the incision gently with mild, unscented soap.
- Between showers, keep the wound dry and covered with a bandage for the first 2 or 3 days after surgery. If a bandage gets wet, change it promptly. Apply nonprescription antibiotic ointment to the wound before applying new bandages.
- If the wound bleeds during the first 24 hours after surgery, press a clean tissue or cloth to it for 10 to 15 minutes continuously.

MEDICATION
- Your doctor may prescribe pain relievers. Don't take prescription pain medication longer than 4 to 7 days. Use only as much as you need.
- You may use nonprescription drugs, such as acetaminophen, for minor pain. Avoid aspirin.

ACTIVITY
- Avoid vigorous exercise for 2 weeks after surgery.
- Resume driving 2 days after returning home.

DIET—No special diet.

CALL YOUR DOCTOR IF

- You experience sudden or severe chest pain.
- Pain, swelling, redness, drainage, or bleeding increases in the surgical area.
- You develop symptoms of infection including headache, muscle aches, dizziness, fever, or a general ill feeling.
- You develop decreased sensation or pain in the limb where artery was entered.

CARDIAC CATHETERIZATION & ANGIOGRAM

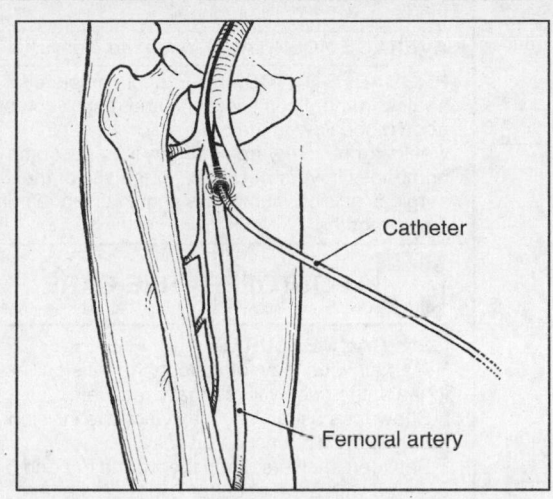

An illustration of a typical location for catheter insertion in the large artery of the leg. The catheter may also be placed in a large vessel in the arm.

- When the catheter is in place, accurate blood pressure measurements may be made continuously.

Catheter

Femoral artery

The catheter is guided into the coronary artery system. Pressure readings are made in various chambers of the heart and great blood vessels for later interpretation.

Catheter

Heart

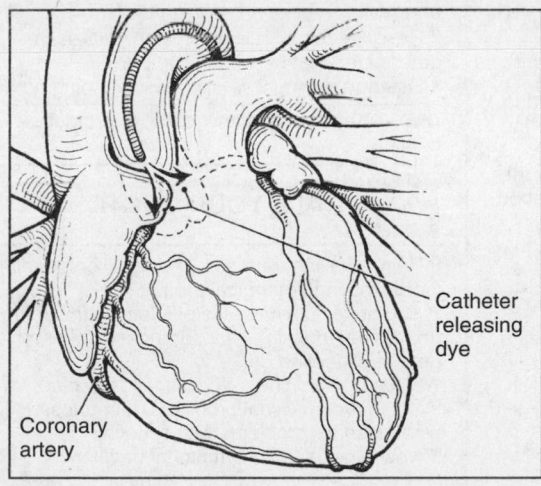

Dye is injected through the catheter to fill the coronary arteries to accurately locate any narrowing or obstructions in the coronary artery system.

- When all examinations have been completed, the catheter is withdrawn and the artery it was inserted into is compressed until bleeding stops.

Catheter releasing dye

Coronary artery

CAROTID ARTERY ENDARTERECTOMY

GENERAL INFORMATION

DEFINITION—Removal of obstruction in carotid (neck) artery usually due to hardening of arteries (arteriosclerosis).

BODY PARTS INVOLVED—Carotid arteries.

REASONS FOR SURGERY—Prevention of stroke and transient ischemic attacks (see Glossary).

SURGICAL RISK INCREASES WITH
- Adults over 80.
- Obesity, smoking.
- Poor nutrition.
- Excess alcohol consumption.
- Recent or chronic illness.
- Atherosclerosis, coronary artery disease.
- Diabetes.
- Use of some prescription and nonprescription drugs. Inform your doctor of any drugs, medications, or vitamin and herb supplements you are using or have used in the last month.

WHAT TO EXPECT

WHO OPERATES—General surgeon, neurosurgeon, cardiovascular surgeon, or peripheral vascular surgeon.

WHERE PERFORMED—Hospital.

DIAGNOSTIC TESTS
- Before surgery: Blood and urine studies, chest x-ray, ECG, arteriograms, CT scan of head (see Glossary for all).
- After surgery: Blood studies.

ANESTHESIA
- Local anesthetic by injection and sedation.
- General anesthesia by injection and inhalation with an airway tube placed in the windpipe.

DESCRIPTION OF OPERATION
- An incision is made in the neck over the obstruction.
- The obstructed area is isolated. A tube is often placed in the carotid artery and is used to circulate blood around the obstruction while the blockage is being cleared.
- A small incision is made in the artery over the obstruction which is scraped away. The opened area is sometimes patched with a graft fashioned from a vein from another part of the body or a cloth-like material.
- The temporary bypass tube is removed as the artery is closed.
- The skin is closed with sutures or clips, which usually can be removed in 2 weeks.
- A drain is frequently left in for 24 hours.

POSSIBLE COMPLICATIONS
- Excessive bleeding, hematoma (blood clot).
- Surgical-wound infection.

- Stroke, heart problems, pneumonia.
- Inadvertent injury to a branch of the nerves to the face, vocal cord or tongue.

AVERAGE HOSPITAL STAY—2 to 3 days.

PROBABLE OUTCOME—Expect complete healing without complications and restoration of good blood flow to the brain. Allow about 2 weeks for recovery from surgery. Expect some numbness in your neck area at the site of the surgical incision, numbness should disappear in 3 to 4 months.

POSTOPERATIVE CARE

GENERAL MEASURES
- A small ridge may form along the incision. As it heals, the ridge will gradually recede.
- Shower as usual. You may wash the incision gently with mild, unscented soap.
- Between showers, keep the wound dry and covered with a bandage for 2 to 3 days after surgery. If bandage gets wet, change it promptly.
- Move and elevate legs often while in bed to decrease the likelihood of deep-vein blood clots.

MEDICATION
- Your doctor may prescribe:
  - Pain relievers. Don't take prescription pain relievers for longer than 4 to 7 days. Use only as much as you need.
  - Stool softeners to prevent constipation.
  - Antibiotics to fight or prevent infection.
  - Anticoagulants to prevent blood clots.
- You may use nonprescription drugs, such as acetaminophen, for minor pain. Avoid aspirin.

ACTIVITY
- To help recovery and aid your well-being, resume daily activities, including work, as soon as you are able.
- Avoid vigorous exercise for 6 weeks after surgery.
- Resume sexual relations when your doctor determines that healing is complete.
- Resume driving 3 weeks after returning home.

DIET—Eat a well-balanced diet to promote healing.

CALL YOUR DOCTOR IF

- Pain, swelling, redness, drainage, or bleeding increases in the surgical area.
- You develop symptoms of infection including headache, muscle aches, dizziness, fever, or a general ill feeling.
- Nausea, vomiting, or constipation occurs.
- You develop visual problems, numbness, weakness, or problems with speech.
- New, unexplained symptoms develop.

CAROTID ARTERY ENDARTERECTOMY

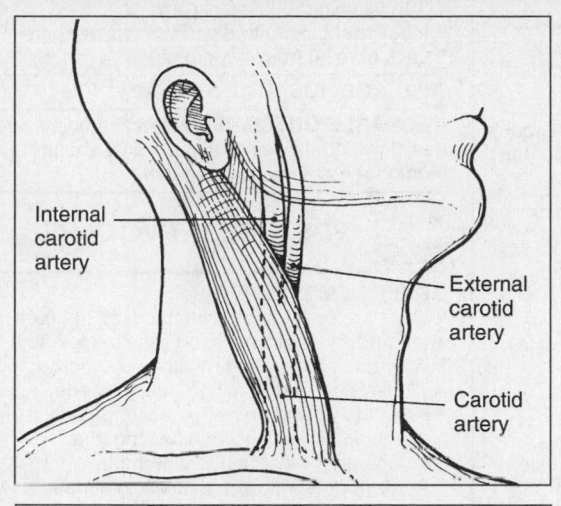

Illustration shows the anatomical locations of the carotid artery, external carotid artery and internal carotid artery.

Internal carotid artery

External carotid artery

Carotid artery

The arterial debris causing the obstruction (which was located by previous special studies) is removed.

Obstruction

A patch is grafted in place to close the artery that has been cleared of obstruction.

Graft patch

CARPAL TUNNEL SYNDROME REPAIR

 ## GENERAL INFORMATION

DEFINITION—Cutting the transverse carpal ligament, the fibrous tissue extending across the wrist.

BODY PARTS INVOLVED—Transverse carpal ligament, median nerve and surrounding fibrous tissue, wrist joint.

REASONS FOR SURGERY—Relief of pain or numbness caused by compression of the median nerve.

SURGICAL RISK INCREASES WITH
- Obesity.
- Smoking.
- Poor nutrition.
- Recent or chronic illness.
- Alcoholism.
- Diabetes.
- Use of some prescription and nonprescription drugs. Inform your doctor of any drugs, medications, or vitamin and herb supplements you are using or have used in the last month.

 ## WHAT TO EXPECT

WHO OPERATES—Hand surgeon, general surgeon, orthopedist neurosurgeon, or plastic and reconstructive surgeon.

WHERE PERFORMED—Hospital or outpatient surgical facility.

DIAGNOSTIC TESTS
- Before surgery: Blood and urine studies, x-ray of wrist, nerve-conduction tests (see Glossary).
- After surgery: Blood studies.

ANESTHESIA
- Local anesthesia by injection.
- Regional anesthesia by injection.
- General anesthesia by injection and inhalation with an airway tube placed in the windpipe.

DESCRIPTION OF OPERATION
- A tourniquet is applied above the wrist to prevent bleeding in the surgical area.
- An incision is made in the underside of the wrist.
- The transverse carpal ligament is located and cut, releasing the compressed median nerve.
- The skin is closed with fine sutures, which usually can be removed about 10 days after surgery. Absorbable stitches are not removed.
- A bandage is applied, and a splint is used to hold the wrist in position. In some instances, the stitched wound may be left uncovered.
- For some patients, the surgery may be done using an arthroscope (see Glossary) inserted through small incisions to minimize scarring and pain, and to speed recovery.

POSSIBLE COMPLICATIONS
- Excessive bleeding.
- Surgical-wound infection.
- Inadvertent injury to blood vessels or nerves.
- Lack of relief from symptoms.

AVERAGE HOSPITAL STAY—0 to 1 day.

PROBABLE OUTCOME—Expect complete healing without complications. Allow about 1 month for recovery from surgery.

 ## POSTOPERATIVE CARE

GENERAL MEASURES
- If the wound bleeds during the first 24 hours after surgery, press a clean tissue or cloth to it.
- A hard ridge should form along the incision. As it heals, the ridge will gradually recede.
- Keep the wound dry with a bandage until it has healed. Protect it when bathing. If a bandage gets wet, change it promptly.
- Apply nonprescription antibiotic ointment to the wound before applying new bandages.
- Keep the hand elevated for the first 1 to 2 days following surgery. Place one or two pillows under the hand and arm when you are sitting or sleeping.
- If your fingers are not wrapped in the dressing, try to keep them moving to reduce stiffness.

MEDICATION
- Your doctor may prescribe:
  - Pain relievers. Don't take prescription pain medication longer than 4 to 7 days. Use only as much as you need.
  - Antibiotics to fight or prevent infection.
- You may use nonprescription drugs, such as acetaminophen, for minor pain. Avoid aspirin.

ACTIVITY
- To help recovery and aid your well-being, resume daily activities, including work, as soon as you are able.
- Resume driving when your doctor determines that healing is complete.

DIET—No special diet.

 ## CALL YOUR DOCTOR IF

- Pain, swelling, redness, drainage, or bleeding increases in the surgical area.
- You develop symptoms of infection including headache, muscle aches, dizziness, fever, or a general ill feeling.
- New, unexplained symptoms develop.

CARPAL TUNNEL SYNDROME REPAIR

An illustration of the incision site at the wrist area where compression of the median nerve occurs.

Incision

After the skin is incised, the transverse carpal ligament is exposed.

Transverse carpal ligament

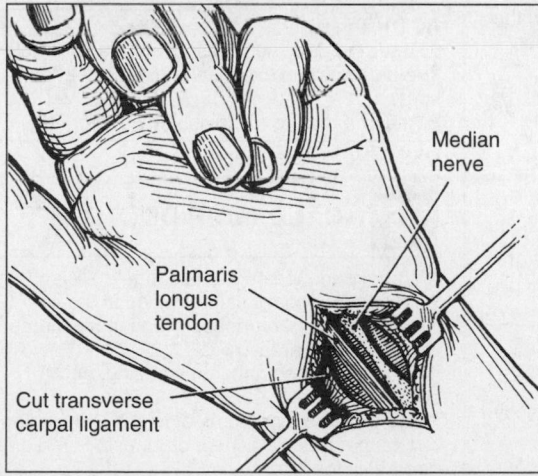

Carpal ligament is located and cut, releasing the compressed median nerve. This usually cures symptoms.

Median nerve

Palmaris longus tendon

Cut transverse carpal ligament

CATARACT EXTRACTION

 GENERAL INFORMATION

DEFINITION—Removal of cataracts, an opacity or clouding of the lens of the eye. This procedure is almost always performed in conjunction with an intraocular (within the eye) lens implant. Several surgical techniques are available, the doctor will choose the one that is most appropriate to your age and eye condition.

BODY PARTS INVOLVED—Eye, cornea, lens, eyelid membrane lining.

REASONS FOR SURGERY—Restoration of normal or near-normal vision.

SURGICAL RISK INCREASES WITH
- Obesity, smoking.
- Newborns and infants.
- Recent or chronic illness.
- Diabetes.
- Use of some prescription and nonprescription drugs. Inform your doctor of any drugs, medications, or vitamin and herb supplements you are using or have used in the last month.

 WHAT TO EXPECT

WHO OPERATES—Ophthalmologist.

WHERE PERFORMED—Hospital or outpatient facility.

DIAGNOSTIC TESTS
- Before surgery: Blood and urine studies, eye examinations, ultrasound (see Glossary).
- After surgery: Eye examinations.

ANESTHESIA—Local anesthesia by injection. One injection prevents eyelid blinking and another one immobilizes the eyeball.

DESCRIPTION OF OPERATION
- A special instrument is used to hold the eyelids apart.
- A small incision is made in the cornea and the diseased lens is removed through the incision. Often, the lens is first fragmented with ultrasound and the debris is simply suctioned away.
- An artificial lens, known as an intraocular lens, is usually inserted in the eye to replace the discarded lens.
- Few or no stitches (sutures) are required to close the wound.
- Pilocarpine or atropine eye-drop solutions are placed in the eye to keep the pupil open. Bandages are applied.

POSSIBLE COMPLICATIONS
- Surgical-wound infection.
- Postoperative inflammation.
- Lens capsule thickens causing hazy or cloudy vision.
- Dislocation of intraocular lens implant.
- Astigmatism.
- Retinal detachment.
- Increased pressure within the eyeball (glaucoma).

AVERAGE HOSPITAL STAY—0 to 1 day.

PROBABLE OUTCOME—Expect complete healing and improved vision without complications. Allow about 3-4 days for recovery from surgery. Vision may remain blurred for awhile, but will gradually clear over a 4 to 10 week period.

 POSTOPERATIVE CARE

GENERAL MEASURES
- Have someone drive you home following surgery.
- Sleep with your head elevated on two pillows.
- When changing the bandage, you should gently clean the eye using a warm, wet washcloth. Do not press or rub the eye. The new bandage can then be positioned and taped in place.
- Move and elevate legs often while resting in bed to decrease the likelihood of deep-vein blood clots.
- Avoid bending, straining, or lying flat. These cause pressure inside the eye.

MEDICATION
- Your doctor may prescribe:
  - Pain relievers. Don't take prescription pain medication longer than 4 to 7 days. Use only as much as you need.
  - Stool softeners to prevent constipation.
  - Antibiotic eye drops or ointment to fight or prevent eye infection. Keep eye drops cold, but not frozen, in the refrigerator.
  - Anti-inflammatory drops or ointment.
  - Eye drops to keep pupil dilated.
- You may use nonprescription drugs, such as acetaminophen, for minor pain. Avoid aspirin.

ACTIVITY
- Return to daily activities as soon as possible.
- Avoid vigorous exercise for 6 weeks after surgery.
- Resume driving as advised by doctor.

DIET—No special diet.

 CALL YOUR DOCTOR IF

- You experience sudden change in vision.
- You have a sharp pain or blood in the eye.
- Pain, swelling, redness, or drainage increases in the surgical area.
- You experience nausea, vomiting, or constipation.
- You develop symptoms of infection including headache, muscle aches, dizziness, fever, or a general ill feeling.

CATARACT EXTRACTION

Surgical incision site below the iris.

Incision
site

The diseased lens is removed and an intraocular lens is inserted.

Intraocular
lens

Artificial lens is in place. Incision is closed with fine sutures. Sometimes, no sutures are required.

CERVIX, BIOPSY OF

GENERAL INFORMATION

DEFINITION—Removal of tissue from the cervix (the lower third of the uterus).

BODY PARTS INVOLVED—Cervix, vagina (as route for surgery).

REASONS FOR SURGERY
• Investigation of diseases of the cervix. Laboratory examination of the removed tissue aids in diagnosis.
• Usually follows a visual examination or a Pap smear (see Glossary) of the cervix that revealed a possible abnormality (dysplasia).
• May be done for exploratory purposes for conditions such as infertility.
• Sometimes done as a follow-up in women who have previously been treated for early cervical cancer or dysplasia (atypical cells) of the cervix.

SURGICAL RISK INCREASES WITH
• Bleeding disorders.
• Use of drugs such as anticoagulants or aspirin.

WHAT TO EXPECT

WHO OPERATES—Obstetrician-gynecologist, family doctor, or general surgeon.

WHERE PERFORMED—Doctor's office or outpatient surgical facility.

DIAGNOSTIC TESTS
• Before surgery: Pap smear (see Glossary), pelvic exam, blood and urine tests.
• During surgery: Your doctor may stain the cervix before removing any sample tissue. Areas that do not hold the stain are the most important ones to examine. The staining is harmless and painless.
• After surgery: Laboratory examination of removed tissue.

ANESTHESIA—Local anesthesia by injection.

DESCRIPTION OF OPERATION
• A speculum is inserted into the vagina to hold it open and to bring the cervix into view.
• Your physician may perform a colposcopic biopsy, in which a slender, optical instrument with a lighted tip is used to pinpoint the areas of the cervix to be biopsied.
• Another instrument is used to gather the tissue. The instrument used will vary, depending on the type of biopsy being performed. In a punch biopsy, the clinician will use a small instrument resembling a paper punch to punch out a small sample of cervical tissue. Several punches may be necessary. Another common form of biopsy uses a curette (a thin, metal instrument with a spoon-shaped tip) to scrape tissue from the cervix. Still another technique

that may be used is called LEEP (loop excision electrosurgical procedure). In this procedure, a thin, hand-held wire loop, activated by an electrosurgical generator, is used to make a very precise and uniform cut across the cervix.
• The instruments are removed and the tissue is then sent to a laboratory for microscopic analysis.
• Usually, the procedure is concluded by applying silver nitrate, or a similar agent, to the biopsy sites to prevent bleeding by chemically cauterizing the wounds.

POSSIBLE COMPLICATIONS—Excessive bleeding or infection.

AVERAGE HOSPITAL STAY—Usually none.

PROBABLE OUTCOME—Tissue obtained successfully without complications in virtually all cases. There may be some spotting of blood for several days, followed by a vaginal discharge, as the biopsy sites heal. Allow several days for recovery from the procedure.

POSTOPERATIVE CARE

GENERAL MEASURES
• Wear cotton panties or pantyhose with a cotton crotch. Avoid panties made from nylon, polyester, silk or other nonventilating materials.
• Use a sanitary pad to protect your clothing. Avoid tampons, as they may lead to infection.
• Shower as usual. Use nonperfumed soap.
• Don't douche unless it is recommended by your doctor.

MEDICATION
• Your doctor may prescribe vaginal creams to relieve discomfort.
• You may use nonprescription drugs, such as acetaminophen, for minor pain or cramps. If the cramps are severe, your doctor may prescribe additional medication to relieve the pain.

ACTIVITY
• Resume driving 24 hours after the procedure.
• Resume sexual relations 1 to 2 weeks after surgery, unless otherwise specified by your doctor.

DIET—No special diet.

CALL YOUR DOCTOR IF

• You develop symptoms of infection including headache, muscle aches, dizziness, fever, or a general ill feeling.
• Vaginal discharge increases or begins to have an unpleasant odor.
• You experience discomfort that simple pain medication does not relieve quickly.
• Unusual vaginal swelling or bleeding develops.

CERVIX, BIOPSY OF

Side view of the vagina, cervix and uterus. This illustration shows a speculum inserted into the vagina to stretch it open and expose the cervix (the lower third of the uterus). A colposcope is used to pinpoint the areas to be biopsied.

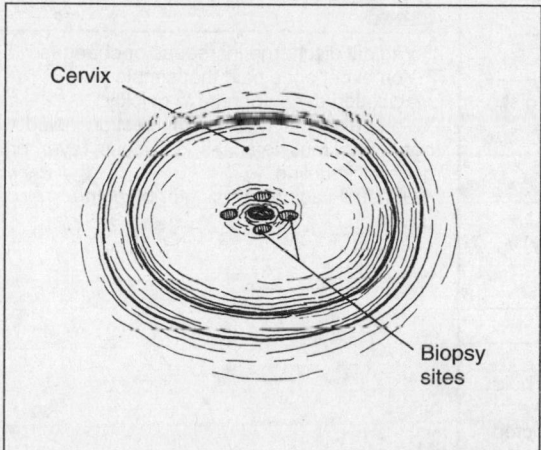

A closer view of the cervix shows the different sites where biopsies are taken. Biopsy sites are usually chosen on the basis of the appearance of the cervix.

A curette is inserted and is used to remove small amounts of tissue in the suspected areas of the cervix.

CERVIX, CRYOSURGERY OF

 GENERAL INFORMATION

DEFINITION—Destruction of abnormal (infected or damaged) cells in the cervix, the lower third of the uterus. An instrument called a cryosurgery probe is used to freeze abnormal cells with liquid nitrogen.

BODY PARTS INVOLVED—Cervix, vagina (as route for surgery).

REASONS FOR SURGERY
● Primary treatment of mild to moderate cervical dysplasia (abnormal cell growth).
● Sometimes used to treat severe cervical dysplasia.
● Treatment of benign (noncancerous) growths on the cervix (such as polyps) or genital warts.
● Treatment of cervicitis (inflammation of the cervix).

SURGICAL RISK INCREASES WITH—None expected.

 WHAT TO EXPECT

WHO OPERATES—Obstetrician-gynecologist, family doctor or general surgeon.

WHERE PERFORMED—Doctor's office or outpatient surgical facility.

DIAGNOSTIC TESTS
● Before surgery: Pap smear (see Glossary), vaginal exam.
● After surgery: Pap smear in 2 to 3 months.

ANESTHESIA—Usually none.

DESCRIPTION OF OPERATION
● A speculum is inserted into the vagina to hold it open and to bring the cervix into view.
● The cryosurgery probe is held on the affected areas long enough to freeze and destroy abnormal cells.
● The instruments are removed. Discomfort during surgery may vary from one person to the next but should not cause much distress.

POSSIBLE COMPLICATIONS
● Surgical wound infection (rare).
● Cervical stenosis (narrowing).
● Failure of the procedure to destroy all of the cervical dysplasia, particularly with severe dysplasia.

AVERAGE HOSPITAL STAY—Usually none.

PROBABLE OUTCOME—Expect complete healing without complications. You may experience mild uterine cramping and facial flushing. Vaginal discharge is common. The discharge may be profuse, foul-smelling, and last for 7 to 10 days or longer. Allow about 3 weeks for recovery from surgery.

 POSTOPERATIVE CARE

GENERAL MEASURES
● Wear cotton panties or pantyhose with a cotton crotch. Avoid panties made from nylon, polyester, silk or other nonventilating materials.
● Use a sanitary pad to protect your clothing. Avoid tampons, as they may lead to infection.
● Shower as usual. Use nonperfumed soap.
● Don't douche unless it is recommended by your doctor.

MEDICATION—You may use nonprescription drugs, such as acetaminophen, to relieve minor pain. Avoid aspirin.

ACTIVITY—No restrictions. Resume sexual relations when your doctor determines healing is complete.

DIET—No special diet.

 CALL YOUR DOCTOR IF

● Vaginal discharge increases or changes.
● You experience pain that simple pain medication does not relieve quickly.
● You develop symptoms of infection including headache, muscle aches, dizziness, fever, or a general ill feeling.
● Unusual vaginal swelling or bleeding develops.

CERVIX, CRYOSURGERY OF

- This view illustrates a female patient with extended legs in stirrups on an examining table to allow examination of the genital area.
- The speculum is inserted into the vagina to stretch it open and expose the cervix.

Cervix

Speculum

- A side view of the pelvic structures.
- The cryosurgery probe, which has been brought to temperatures well below zero, is held on the affected areas long enough to freeze and destroy the abnormal cervical cells.

Cryosurgical probe

Probe removed after suspicious cells have been destroyed.

Probe

Abnormal cells

CERVIX, ELECTROCAUTERIZATION OF

GENERAL INFORMATION

DEFINITION—Destruction of abnormal (infected or damaged) cells in the cervix, in the lower third of the uterus. An instrument called an electrocautery uses electric current to destroy the abnormal tissue.

BODY PARTS INVOLVED—Cervix, vagina (as route for surgery).

REASONS FOR SURGERY
- Presence of abnormal cells in the cervix.
- Inflammation or infection of the cervix.

SURGICAL RISK INCREASES WITH
- Diabetes.
- Use of some prescription and nonprescription drugs. Inform your doctor of any drugs, medications, or vitamin and herb supplements you are using or have used in the last month.

WHAT TO EXPECT

WHO OPERATES—Obstetrician-gynecologist, general surgeon or family doctor.

WHERE PERFORMED—Doctor's office or outpatient surgical facility.

DIAGNOSTIC TESTS
- Before surgery: Pap smear (see Glossary), vaginal-discharge study.
- After surgery: Vaginal-discharge study, Pap smear in about 2 months.

ANESTHESIA—Usually none.

DESCRIPTION OF OPERATION
- A speculum is inserted into the vagina to hold it open and to bring the cervix into view.
- The electrocautery probe is inserted into the cervix. The flow of electric current is applied through the probe to destroy abnormal cells. You may experience some mild cramping.
- The instruments are removed. Discomfort after surgery will vary from one person to another, but any pain or cramping should be minor.

POSSIBLE COMPLICATIONS
- Surgical-wound infection.
- Inadvertent damage to normal vaginal tissue.
- Cervical stenosis (narrowing).

AVERAGE HOSPITAL STAY—None.

PROBABLE OUTCOME—Healing requires up to 2 months. During this time, you will have a frequent, watery vaginal discharge. Allow about 6 weeks for recovery from surgery.

POSTOPERATIVE CARE

GENERAL MEASURES
- Wear cotton panties or pantyhose with a cotton crotch. Avoid panties made from nylon, polyester, silk or other nonventilating materials.
- Wear a sanitary pad to protect clothing. Avoid tampons, as they may lead to infection.
- Bathe or shower as usual. Use mild, unscented soap.
- Do not douche unless prescribed by your doctor.
- Following this procedure, you should have a Pap smear (see Glossary) twice a year for 2 years, and then annually thereafter.

MEDICATION
- Your doctor may prescribe:
  - Pain relievers. Don't take prescription pain medication longer than 4 to 7 days. Use only as much as you need.
  - Vaginal creams or medicated douches.
  - Antibiotics to fight or prevent infection.
- You may use nonprescription drugs, such as acetaminophen, for minor pain. Avoid aspirin.

ACTIVITY
- To help recovery and aid your well-being, resume daily activities, including work, as soon as you are able.
- Delay sexual relations until your doctor determines that healing is complete.

DIET—No special diet.

CALL YOUR DOCTOR IF

- Vaginal discharge increases or begins to have an unpleasant odor.
- You experience pain that simple pain medication does not relieve quickly.
- Unusual vaginal swelling or bleeding develops.
- You develop symptoms of infection including headache, muscle aches, dizziness, fever, or a general ill feeling.
- New, unexplained symptoms develop.

CERVIX, ELECTROCAUTERIZATION OF

Cervix

Speculum

- This view illustrates a female patient with extended legs in stirrups on an examining table to allow examination of the genital area.
- The speculum is inserted into the vagina to stretch it open and expose the cervix.

Electrocautery probe

- A side view of the pelvic structures showing the speculum in the vagina.
- The electrocautery probe is inserted through the speculum to reach the uterine opening in the cervical area.

Probe

A view showing the electrocautery probe touching abnormal cervical cells. A flow of electric current is applied through the electrocautery probe to destroy the cells.

CESAREAN SECTION

GENERAL INFORMATION

DEFINITION—Delivery of a baby through an incision in the mother's lower abdominal and uterine walls.

BODY PARTS INVOLVED—Uterus, abdominal wall, placenta, placental membranes, fetus.

REASONS FOR SURGERY
- Danger to the mother or baby from one or more of many causes, including:
  - Baby's head too large to pass through the birth canal.
  - Breech presentation (see Glossary).
  - Insufficient contractions of the uterus.
  - Abnormal attachment of placenta.
  - Severe preeclampsia (see in Illness section).
  - Fetal distress.
  - Failure of normal labor in a patient who had a previous cesarean section.
  - Acute herpes genitalis infection.

SURGICAL RISK INCREASES WITH
- Obesity, smoking, poor nutrition.
- Excess alcohol consumption.
- Placenta previa with excessive blood loss.
- Preeclampsia or eclampsia of pregnancy (see in Illness section).
- Prior cesarean section.
- Chronic heart or lung disease.
- Use of some prescription and nonprescription drugs. Inform your doctor of any drugs, medications, or vitamin and herb supplements you are using or have used in the last month.

WHAT TO EXPECT

WHO OPERATES—Obstetrician-gynecologist.

WHERE PERFORMED—Hospital.

DIAGNOSTIC TESTS
- Before surgery: Blood and urine studies, sonogram (see Glossary).
- After surgery: Blood and urine studies.

ANESTHESIA
- Local anesthesia by injection.
- Spinal anesthesia by injection.
- General anesthesia by injection and inhalation with an airway tube placed in the windpipe (sometimes).

DESCRIPTION OF OPERATION
- An incision is made in the abdomen.
- Another incision is made in the uterus.
- Baby and placenta are removed.
- The uterus is closed and the abdominal contents are replaced. Connective tissue, muscles and skin are closed. The skin is closed with sutures or clips, which usually can be removed 2 to 7 days after surgery.

POSSIBLE COMPLICATIONS
- Excessive bleeding or surgical-wound infection.
- Postoperative anemia.
- Endomyometritis (inflammation of the muscular substance of the uterus).
- Endometritis (inflammation of the lining of the uterus).

AVERAGE HOSPITAL STAY—3 to 5 days.

PROBABLE OUTCOME—No complications expected. Allow 4 to 6 weeks for recovery from surgery.

POSTOPERATIVE CARE

GENERAL MEASURES
- A hard ridge should form along the incision. As it heals, the ridge will gradually recede.
- Shower as usual. You may wash the incision gently with mild, unscented soap. You may resume tub baths 2 to 3 weeks after surgery.
- Don't douche unless it is recommended by your doctor.
- Move and elevate your legs often while resting in bed to improve circulation and decrease the likelihood of deep-vein clots.

MEDICATION
- Your doctor may prescribe:
  - Pain relievers. Use only as much as you need.
  - Vaginal cream, if vaginal discharge develops an unpleasant odor.
  - Antibiotics to fight or prevent infection.
- You may use nonprescription drugs, such as acetaminophen, for minor pain. Avoid aspirin.

ACTIVITY
- To help recovery and aid your well-being, resume daily activities, including work, as soon as you are able.
- Resume driving 2 to 4 weeks after surgery.
- Avoid sexual intercourse for 4 to 6 weeks.

DIET—No special diet.

CALL YOUR DOCTOR IF

- Bleeding soaks more than 1 pad or tampon each hour.
- Pain, swelling, redness, drainage, or bleeding increases in the surgical area.
- Vaginal discharge or the urge to urinate frequently persists beyond 1 month after surgery.
- You develop symptoms of infection including headache, muscle aches, dizziness, fever, or a general ill feeling.
- New, unexplained symptoms develop.

CESAREAN SECTION

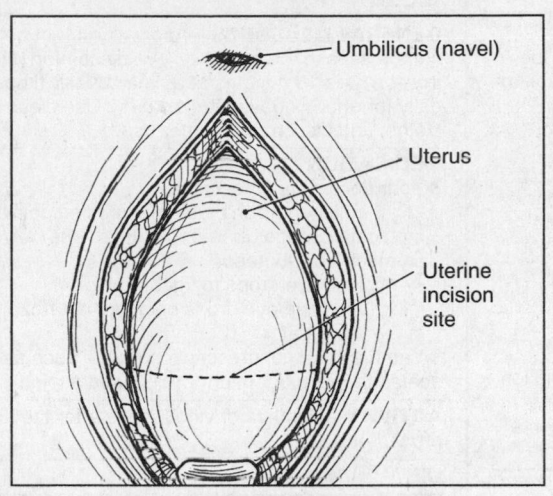

Umbilicus (navel)

Uterus

Uterine
incision
site

- An illustration, looking from above, of a patient lying flat on an operating table.
- A vertical (as illustrated) or transverse incision is made exposing the uterus. A transverse incision is made in the uterus.

Uterus

The baby and the placenta are removed.

The uterus is closed, followed by closure of connective tissue, muscles and skin of the abdominal wall.

Uterine
closure

CHALAZION REMOVAL

GENERAL INFORMATION

DEFINITION—Removal of a chalazion, a nontender inflammation in the cartilage of the eyelid. Chalazions are caused by a blockage in the meibomian glands (see Glossary).

BODY PARTS INVOLVED—Eyelids (upper or lower), meibomian glands.

REASONS FOR SURGERY—A chalazion is not cancerous or infectious. It is removed to improve appearance or to relieve pressure on an eyeball. Surgery is performed only after simpler treatment has failed.

SURGICAL RISK INCREASES WITH
- Diabetes.
- Use of some prescription and nonprescription drugs. Inform your doctor of any drugs, medications, or vitamin and herb supplements you are using or have used in the last month.

WHAT TO EXPECT

WHO OPERATES—Ophthalmologist.

WHERE PERFORMED—Doctor's office or outpatient surgical facility.

DIAGNOSTIC TESTS—Complete eye examination before surgery.

ANESTHESIA—Local anesthesia by injection.

DESCRIPTION OF OPERATION
- The eyelid is turned inside out and held to expose its underside.
- The chalazion is identified.
- An incision is made on the surface of the chalazion.
- The chalazion is cut free and removed.
- The eye is bandaged.

POSSIBLE COMPLICATIONS
- Excessive bleeding.
- Surgical-wound infection.

AVERAGE HOSPITAL STAY—None.

PROBABLE OUTCOME—Expect complete healing without complications. Allow about 1 week for recovery from surgery. Chalazions may recur.

POSTOPERATIVE CARE

GENERAL MEASURES—Apply warm (not hot) compresses to the eye to relieve discomfort. Do this for 10 to 15 minutes at a time several times daily for about 2 days after surgery. Use clean cloths, and discard them after use.

MEDICATION
- Your doctor may prescribe:
  - Pain relievers. Don't take prescription pain medication longer than 4 to 7 days. Use only as much as you need.
  - Antibiotic eye drops to fight or prevent infection. Keep eye drops cold, but not frozen, in the refrigerator.
- You may use nonprescription drugs, such as acetaminophen, for minor pain. Avoid aspirin.

ACTIVITY—Resume driving 2 days after the procedure.

DIET—No special diet.

CALL YOUR DOCTOR IF

- Pain, swelling, redness, drainage, or bleeding increase in the surgical area.
- You develop symptoms of infection including headache, muscle aches, dizziness, fever, or a general ill feeling.
- Your vision changes.
- New, unexplained symptoms develop.

CHALAZION REMOVAL

Appearance of the chalazion seen through the eyelid skin.

Chalazion

The eyelid is turned inside out and held to expose its underside. The chalazion is identified on the inverted lid.

An incision made on the membranous lining of the eyelid allows the chalazion to be cut free and removed.

CIRCUMCISION

 ## GENERAL INFORMATION

DEFINITION—Removal of the foreskin of the penis. This section describes circumcision performed at times other than at birth or several days after birth.

BODY PARTS INVOLVED—Penis, foreskin of the penis.

REASONS FOR SURGERY
- Correction of inability to retract the foreskin completely (phimosis).
- Treatment of infection of the penis (balanitis).
- Urinary tract infection (sometimes).

SURGICAL RISK INCREASES WITH
- Poor nutrition.
- Recent or chronic illness.
- Alcoholism.
- Use of some prescription and nonprescription drugs. Inform your doctor of any drugs, medications, or vitamin and herb supplements you are using or have used in the last month.

 ## WHAT TO EXPECT

WHO OPERATES—Family doctor, general surgeon, or urologist.

WHERE PERFORMED—Hospital or outpatient surgical facility.

DIAGNOSTIC TESTS
- Before surgery: Blood and urine studies.
- After surgery: Blood studies.

ANESTHESIA
- Local anesthesia by injection.
- General anesthesia (sometimes) by injection and inhalation with an airway tube placed in the windpipe.

DESCRIPTION OF OPERATION
- The foreskin is carefully retracted from the tip of the penis.
- A clamp is placed under the foreskin.
- The clamped foreskin is slit in two places on the top and bottom of the penis.
- The foreskin between the two slits is cut free and removed.
- The mucous membrane of the foreskin is folded back on itself and sewn to the remaining skin of the penis, usually with sutures that will be absorbed by the body.
- Petroleum jelly and a bandage are applied.

POSSIBLE COMPLICATIONS
- Excessive bleeding.
- Surgical-wound infection.

AVERAGE HOSPITAL STAY—0 to 1 day.

PROBABLE OUTCOME—Expect complete healing without complications. Allow about 3 weeks for recovery from surgery.

 ## POSTOPERATIVE CARE

GENERAL MEASURES
- If the wound bleeds during the first 24 hours after surgery, press a clean tissue or cloth to it for 10 minutes.
- Use ice packs to relieve pain in the surgical area for the first 24 hours after surgery.
- Wear underwear that will keep you the most comfortable (jockey or boxers).
- Shower as usual. You may wash the surgical wound gently with mild, unscented soap.
- Change the bandage as recommended by your doctor. Between showers, keep the wound dry for the first 2 or 3 days after surgery. If a bandage gets wet, change it promptly.
- Apply nonprescription antibiotic ointment to the wound before applying new bandages.
- Avoid conditions that may cause you to become sexually aroused. Until healed, a penile erection can be painful and can put unnecessary strain on the stitches.

MEDICATION
- Your doctor may prescribe:
  - Pain relievers. Don't take prescription pain medication longer than 4 to 7 days. Use only as much as you need.
  - Antibiotics to fight or prevent infection.
  - Medications to relax you and decrease the likelihood of developing an erection during recovery.
- You may use nonprescription drugs, such as acetaminophen, for minor pain. Avoid aspirin.

ACTIVITY
- To help recovery and aid your well-being, resume daily activities, including work, as soon as you are able.
- Avoid vigorous exercise for 4 weeks after surgery.
- Resume driving 5 days after returning home.
- Resume sexual relations when your doctor determines that healing is complete.

DIET—No special diet.

 ## CALL YOUR DOCTOR IF

- Pain, swelling, redness, drainage, or bleeding increases in the surgical area.
- You develop symptoms of infection including headache, muscle aches, dizziness, fever, or a general ill feeling.
- You have difficulty urinating.
- New, unexplained symptoms develop.

CIRCUMCISION

An illustration of the foreskin being carefully retracted and stretched from the tip of the penis with clamps.

The foreskin between slits is cut free and removed.

Mucus membrane of foreskin is folded back on itself and sewn to the remaining skin of the penis. Healing is rapid and sutures drop out without painful removal.

CLEFT LIP REPAIR

GENERAL INFORMATION

DEFINITION—Repair of a hereditary deformity of the upper lip called a "cleft lip," in which lip, nose and palate structures do not fuse correctly prior to birth. Frequently, this defect extends to the roof of the mouth (palate) and can hamper development of normal speech. Surgery is usually performed when the patient is about 3 months old. If a cleft palate exists, it is usually repaired in a separate surgery when the patient is 12 to 18 months old.

BODY PARTS INVOLVED—Upper lip, muscles surrounding the mouth, membrane lining the mouth, roof of the mouth (palate).

REASONS FOR SURGERY
- Prevention of nursing and feeding problems that can retard normal growth.
- Rearrangement of the distorted tissues to make the lip and palate function normally and appear as normal as possible.

SURGICAL RISK INCREASES WITH
- Other congenital abnormalities.
- Poor nutrition. This often results from inability to nurse properly because of the deformity.
- Use of some prescription and nonprescription drugs. Inform your doctor of any drugs, medications, or vitamin and herb supplements you have given your child in the last month.

WHAT TO EXPECT

WHO OPERATES—Plastic and reconstructive surgeon.

WHERE PERFORMED—Hospital.

DIAGNOSTIC TESTS
- Before surgery: Blood and urine studies.
- After surgery: Blood studies.

ANESTHESIA
- Local anesthesia by injection.
- General anesthesia by a combination of injection and inhalation with an airway tube placed in the windpipe.

DESCRIPTION OF OPERATION
- The areas are marked where the lip, mouth and palate should be.
- The skin to be relocated is cut free from its underlying tissue. Bleeding is controlled with clamps, medication (epinephrine) or cautery.
- The skin flaps are adjusted to their desired position.
- The muscles and skin edges are reconstructed with fine sutures, which usually can be removed about 7 to 10 days after surgery.

POSSIBLE COMPLICATIONS
- Excessive bleeding.
- Surgical-wound infection.

AVERAGE HOSPITAL STAY—5 to 7 days.

PROBABLE OUTCOME—Expect complete healing without complications. Allow about 4 weeks for recovery from surgery.

POSTOPERATIVE CARE

GENERAL MEASURES
- A hard ridge should form along the incision. As it heals, the ridge will gradually recede.
- Bathe the child as usual. You may wash the incision gently with mild, unscented soap.
- Your child may have difficulty with his or her speech and should be under the close supervision of a speech and language pathologist.
- Babies with cleft lip and cleft palate often have middle ear problems. Therefore, your child should be seen by an otolaryngologist (ear, nose and throat specialist).
- Cleft lip can sometimes be associated with other problems or defects. Therefore, it is important that you and your baby be seen by a genetic specialist (geneticist) to determine the cause of the cleft lip.

MEDICATION
- Your doctor may prescribe:
  - Pain relievers. Don't give your child prescription pain medication longer than 4 to 7 days. Use only as much as your child needs.
  - Antibiotics to fight or prevent infection.
- You may give your child nonprescription drugs, such as acetaminophen, for minor pain. Avoid aspirin.

ACTIVITY—No restrictions.

DIET—No special diet.

CALL YOUR DOCTOR IF

- Pain, swelling, redness, drainage, or bleeding increases in the surgical area.
- Your child develops symptoms of infection including headache, muscle aches, dizziness, fever, or a general ill feeling.
- Your child develops vomiting, constipation, or abdominal swelling.
- New, unexplained symptoms develop.

CLEFT LIP REPAIR

An illustration of mouth and lip skin between the lip and the nose showing the cleft lip deformity.

Cleft lip

Skin to be relocated is cut free from its underlying tissue.

Skin flaps are adjusted to their desired new position and skin edges approximated and sewn.

COCHLEAR IMPLANT

 GENERAL INFORMATION

DEFINITION—Installation of a microelectronic (tiny electrodes) system designed to improve hearing in some persons with hearing impairments. A cochlear implant consists of 3 parts: a microphone, a microcomputer, and a cochlear electrode.

BODY PARTS INVOLVED—Cochlea (an organ in the inner ear that transforms sound vibrations into nerve impulses for transmission to the brain), skin behind the ear.

REASONS FOR SURGERY—Treatment for profound hearing loss. The sensitive structures within the cochlea may have been damaged by trauma, toxic effect of drugs, or infection. The auditory nerve carrying sound signals to the brain is intact, but it receives no stimulus. The implant provides signals which can be taken up by the auditory nerve. It improves, but cannot restore, normal hearing.

SURGICAL RISK INCREASES WITH
- Recent or chronic illness, diabetes.
- Use of some prescription and nonprescription drugs. Inform your doctor of any drugs, medications, or vitamin and herb supplements you are using or have used in the last month.

 WHAT TO EXPECT

WHO OPERATES—Ear, nose and throat specialist (otolaryngologist).

WHERE PERFORMED—Hospital.

DIAGNOSTIC TESTS
- Before surgery: Auditory testing.
- After surgery: Auditory testing.

ANESTHESIA—General anesthesia by injection and inhalation, with an airway tube placed in the windpipe.

DESCRIPTION OF OPERATION
- An incision is made behind and slightly above the ear. A burr-type instrument is used to drill a circular hole in the bone for preparation for implanting the internal coil.
- The mastoid bone in the ear is opened to gain access for the electrodes that will be led from the internal coil into the inner ear.
- The internal coil is then positioned in the prepared site and secured with stitches.
- The electrodes are then inserted deep in the inner ear.
- Once the surgical wound is healed, an external unit consisting of a stimulator with built-in microphone is provided for wearing behind the ear. It may be attached to eyeglasses or a headband or special magnets between the internal and external components.

- A microcomputer is connected to the microphone by a wire, and is worn in a pouch attached to the belt. The microcomputer turns sound into an electrical code which is sent by radio wave to the cochlear electrodes.

POSSIBLE COMPLICATIONS
- Vertigo (feeling as if the room is spinning).
- Surgical-wound infection, bleeding.
- Facial nerve damage during surgery.
- Technical failure of the implant.

AVERAGE HOSPITAL STAY—2 to 3 days.

PROBABLE OUTCOME—Expect complete healing without complications. Stitches will be removed a few days after surgery. One or more follow up visits to your doctor will be needed to program the implant. The hearing capability with the implant will vary from person to person and cannot be reliably predicted.

 POSTOPERATIVE CARE

GENERAL MEASURES
- A hard ridge should form along the incision. As it heals, the ridge will gradually recede.
- Bathe or shower as usual. You may wash the incision gently with mild, unscented soap. Use an ear plug or shower cap to avoid getting water inside the ear.

MEDICATION
- Your doctor may prescribe:
  - Pain relievers. Don't take prescription pain medication longer than 4 to 7 days. Use only as much as you need.
  - Antibiotics to fight or prevent infection. Use antibiotics before any future dental work.
- You may use nonprescription drugs, such as acetaminophen, for minor pain. Avoid aspirin.

ACTIVITY
- Avoid sudden head movements as they can cause dizziness.
- Avoid bending over for the first few days following surgery.
- Try not to blow your nose or sneeze for the first two weeks.
- Resume work, driving and other normal activities in 2 to 3 weeks.

DIET—While in the hospital, you may progress from a liquid diet to a soft diet to a regular diet.

 CALL YOUR DOCTOR IF

- Pain, swelling, redness, drainage, or bleeding increases in the surgical area.
- You develop symptoms of infection including headache, muscle aches, dizziness, fever, or a general ill feeling.
- New, unexplained symptoms develop.

COCHLEAR IMPLANT

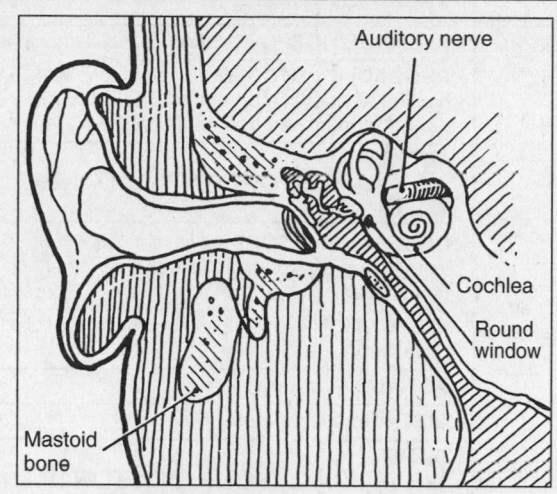

Illustration demonstrating anatomy of the ear where the implant is inserted.

Cochlear implant devices are surgically positioned. Wiring from internal transmitter runs through the middle ear and round window into the cochlea.

After surgery, the external stimulator is positioned. The illustration shows a wire to the power source.

COLONOSCOPY

GENERAL INFORMATION

DEFINITION—Visual examination of the inside of the rectum and the colon (large intestine) with a fiber-optic scope, in order to identify abnormalities and remove tissue for laboratory examination.

BODY PARTS INVOLVED—Anus, rectum, colon.

REASONS FOR SURGERY—Examination of the rectum and lower intestinal tract for disorders that may include: fissures, fistulas, narrowed sections of the intestine, unexplained blood in stools, benign or cancerous tumors, or precancerous polyps.

SURGICAL RISK INCREASES WITH
- Adults over 60.
- Obesity.
- Smoking.
- Poor nutrition.
- Recent or chronic illness.
- Use of some prescription and nonprescription drugs. Inform your doctor of any drugs, medications, or vitamin and herb supplements you are using or have used in the last month.

WHAT TO EXPECT

WHO OPERATES—General surgeon, family doctor, proctologist, or gastroenterologist.

WHERE PERFORMED—Hospital, outpatient surgical facility, or well-equipped doctor's office.

DIAGNOSTIC TESTS
- Before surgery: Blood and urine studies, stool examinations, x-rays of lower gastrointestinal tract.
- After surgery: Laboratory examination of removed tissue and other material.

ANESTHESIA—Intravenous sedation.

DESCRIPTION OF OPERATION
- The examination is best accomplished after thorough cleansing of large bowel with laxatives and enemas. Your physician will instruct you on how to cleanse your bowel.
- The colonoscope is lubricated, inserted into the rectum and passed into the colon.
- The colonoscope will be inserted through the full length of the large intestine.
- Affected areas are located, examined or treated. Polyps or tumors are removed for laboratory examination, and other biopsies of the colon wall may also be performed.
- Other necessary minor surgical procedures may be performed. The colonoscope is removed.

POSSIBLE COMPLICATIONS
- Excessive bleeding.
- Perforation of the colon.

AVERAGE HOSPITAL STAY—Usually none.

PROBABLE OUTCOME—Expect complete healing without complications. Allow about 4 days for recovery from surgery.

POSTOPERATIVE CARE

GENERAL MEASURES—No special instructions except those listed under other headings.

MEDICATION—Medicine is usually not necessary.

ACTIVITY—No restrictions.

DIET—No special diet.

CALL YOUR DOCTOR IF

- You experience abdominal pain or bloating which increases after the procedure.
- You have rectal bleeding which is excessive or lasts more than 24 hours.
- You experience pain or swelling in your rectum or have blood in your stools.
- You develop symptoms of infection including headache, muscle aches, dizziness, fever, or a general ill feeling.
- You experience nausea or vomiting.

COLONOSCOPY

Colonoscope

An illustration of a draped patient and the colonoscope inserted into the anal opening and rectum.

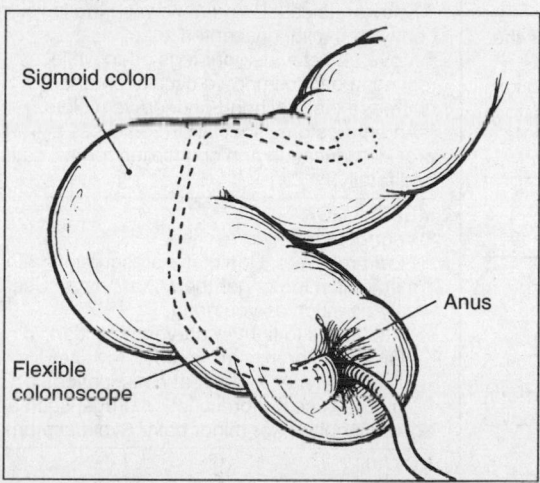

Sigmoid colon

Anus

Flexible colonoscope

The colonoscope is advanced through the rectum into the sigmoid colon.

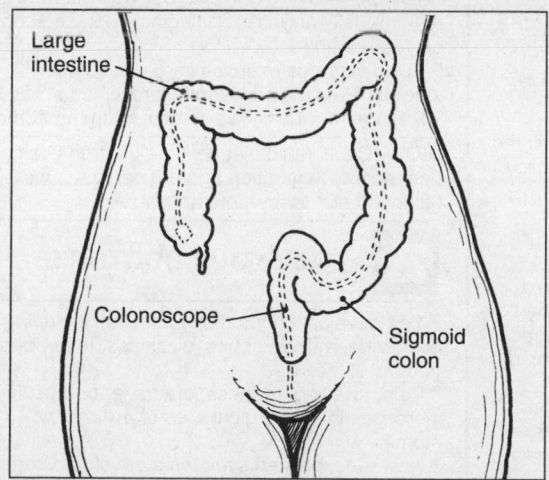

Large intestine

Colonoscope

Sigmoid colon

The colonoscope is inserted to the full length of the large intestine. This procedure locates possible affected areas to be examined or treated. Suspicious areas may be biopsied for microscopic examination.

COLOSTOMY

GENERAL INFORMATION

DEFINITION—Creation of an artificial opening between a part of the colon (large intestine) and the surface of the body. All feces will leave the body through this opening, which is called an ostomy or stoma.

BODY PARTS INVOLVED—Large intestine.

REASONS FOR SURGERY
- Injury or infection which has caused perforation and peritonitis (see Glossary).
- Intestinal blockage, usually caused by cancer or scarring from a chronic infection.
- Colon or rectal surgery which weakens an area of the bowel and necessitates a temporary bypass of the colon until the bowel has healed.
- Anal or rectal cancer.
- Radiation therapy to colon or rectum.

SURGICAL RISK INCREASES WITH
- Obesity, poor nutrition.
- Excess alcohol consumption, smoking.
- Recent illness, diabetes, chronic illness of the heart, lungs, liver or gastrointestinal tract.
- Use of some prescription and nonprescription drugs. Inform your doctor of any drugs, medications, or vitamin and herb supplements you are using or have used in the last month.

WHAT TO EXPECT

WHO OPERATES—General surgeon, colon-rectal surgeon.

WHERE PERFORMED—Hospital.

DIAGNOSTIC TESTS
- Before surgery: Blood and urine studies, chest and gastrointestinal x-rays, ECG, colonoscopy, or sigmoidoscopy (see Glossary for all).
- After surgery: Blood studies.

ANESTHESIA—General anesthesia by injection and inhalation with an airway tube placed in the windpipe.

DESCRIPTION OF OPERATION
- An incision is made in the abdomen. The abdominal muscles are separated to expose the abdominal organs, which are inspected for any undetected disease.
- The colon section that is to be opened is isolated and clamped on both sides, then cut between the clamps. The end of the colon closer to the stomach is brought out of the abdomen and clamped outside the skin. The end farther from the stomach is usually closed, but may be brought out as a separate opening (mucous fistula).
- The abdominal contents are replaced, and muscles are closed around the stoma. Skin is closed with sutures or clips, which usually can be removed in about 1 week.

POSSIBLE COMPLICATIONS
- Excessive bleeding, blood clots.
- Surgical-wound infection, incisional hernia.
- Skin irritation around the stoma.
- Hernia around the stoma (stomal hernia).
- Diarrhea.

AVERAGE HOSPITAL STAY—5 to 7 days.

PROBABLE OUTCOME—Expect complete healing without complications. You can look forward to a relatively normal life, except that bowel movements will now pass through the stoma instead of the rectum. You will need to wear an external colostomy pouch to collect bowel movements. Allow about 6 weeks for recovery from surgery.

POSTOPERATIVE CARE

GENERAL MEASURES
- A hard ridge should form along the incision. As it heals, the ridge will gradually recede.
- Shower as usual. You may wash the incision gently with mild, unscented soap.
- Move and elevate your legs often while resting in bed to improve circulation and decrease the likelihood of deep-vein clots.
- An enterostomy specialist (see Glossary) will provide education and counseling for the patient and family.

MEDICATION
- Your doctor may prescribe:
  - Pain relievers. Don't take prescription pain medication for longer than 4 to 7 days. Use only as much as you need.
  - Antibiotics to fight or prevent infection.
  - Ointment for skin around ostomy site.
  - Stool softener to prevent constipation.
- You may use nonprescription drugs, such as acetaminophen, for minor pain. Avoid aspirin.

ACTIVITY
- To help recovery and aid your well-being, resume daily activities, including work, as soon as you are able.
- Avoid vigorous exercise for 6 weeks after surgery. Resume sexual relations when able.
- Resume driving 3 weeks after returning home.

DIET—Clear liquid diet until the gastrointestinal tract begins to function again. Then eat a well-balanced diet to promote healing.

CALL YOUR DOCTOR IF

- You develop symptoms of infection including headache, muscle aches, dizziness, fever, or a general ill feeling.
- Pain, swelling, redness, drainage, or bleeding increases in the surgical area or around the stoma.
- New, unexplained symptoms develop. Drugs in treatment may produce side effects.

COLOSTOMY

An illustration of the incision site in the abdominal wall. The "x's" mark common areas for colon transection.

Incision

Colon

The abdominal muscle is separated to expose the abdominal organs. The colon section to be opened is isolated, clamped on both sides, then cut between the clamps.

Colon

Skin

Muscle

Colostomy

Closed colon

• The proximal end of the colon (closer to the stomach) is brought out of the abdomen and clamped outside the skin. The distal end (farther from the stomach) is usually closed, but may also be brought out to the skin.
• After the operation, bowel movements will emerge through the open end of the colostomy, which has been sewn to the skin through an opening in the abdominal wall.

COLOVAGINAL FISTULA REPAIR

 GENERAL INFORMATION

DEFINITION—Repair of a fistula (an abnormal tract) between the colon and vagina that usually results from diverticulitis, cervical cancer, inflammatory bowel disease, radiation therapy, or surgical procedures.

BODY PARTS INVOLVED—Sigmoid colon, vagina, and rectum.

REASONS FOR SURGERY
- Prevention of fecal matter from contaminating the vagina or urinary tract.
- Discomfort and embarrassment caused by feces and gas passing through the vagina.

SURGICAL RISK INCREASES WITH
- Obesity, smoking.
- Poor nutrition, alcoholism.
- Recent or chronic illness.
- Diabetes.
- Use of some prescription and nonprescription drugs. Inform your doctor of any drugs, medications, or vitamin and herb supplements you are using or have used in the last month.

 WHAT TO EXPECT

WHO OPERATES—Obstetrician-gynecologist, proctologist, colon-rectal surgeon or general surgeon.

WHERE PERFORMED—Hospital.

DIAGNOSTIC TESTS
- Before surgery: Blood and urine studies, x-ray of lower gastrointestinal tract and kidneys.
- After surgery: Blood studies.

ANESTHESIA—General anesthesia by injection and inhalation with an airway tube placed in the windpipe.

DESCRIPTION OF OPERATION
- The abdomen is explored and the involved area of the colon is isolated. The colon is separated from the vaginal opening.
- The segment of colon involved is resected (removed) and the colon is sewn back together.
- Sometimes, a temporary colostomy (see in Surgery section) is necessary for proper healing. This is closed at a later time.
- The skin and muscles are closed with sutures. The skin sutures are removed in about a week.

POSSIBLE COMPLICATIONS
- Excessive bleeding.
- Surgical-wound infection.
- Failure to heal completely.

AVERAGE HOSPITAL STAY—5 to 7 days.

PROBABLE OUTCOME—Expect complete healing without complications. Allow about 6 weeks for recovery from surgery.

 POSTOPERATIVE CARE

GENERAL MEASURES
- A hard ridge should form along the incision. As it heals, the ridge will gradually recede.
- Shower as usual. Avoid baths until the incision has completely healed. You may wash the incision gently with mild, unscented soap.
- Avoid constipation and straining during bowel movements.

MEDICATION
- Your doctor may prescribe:
  - Pain relievers. Don't take prescription pain medication longer than 4 to 7 days. Use only as much as you need.
  - Stool softeners to prevent constipation.
  - Antibiotics to fight or prevent infection.
- You may use nonprescription drugs, such as acetaminophen, for minor pain. Avoid aspirin.

ACTIVITY
- To help recovery and aid your well-being, resume daily activities, including work, as soon as you are able.
- Avoid vigorous exercise for 6 weeks after surgery. Resume sexual relations when your doctor determines that healing is complete.
- Resume driving 3 weeks after returning home.

DIET—Nothing by mouth until the gastrointestinal tract functions again. Then, gradually progress to a well-balanced diet to promote healing. Increase dietary fiber and fluid intake to help prevent constipation.

 CALL YOUR DOCTOR IF

- Pain, swelling, redness, drainage, or bleeding increases in the surgical area.
- You develop signs of infection including headache, muscle aches, dizziness, fever, or a general ill feeling.
- You experience nausea, vomiting, constipation, or diarrhea.
- New, unexplained symptoms develop.

COLOVAGINAL FISTULA REPAIR

An illustration of the side view of the normal female urogenital tract.
The uterus is absent from a previous hysterectomy.

A view of a fistula (an abnormal tract) which has formed between the sigmoid colon and the vagina.

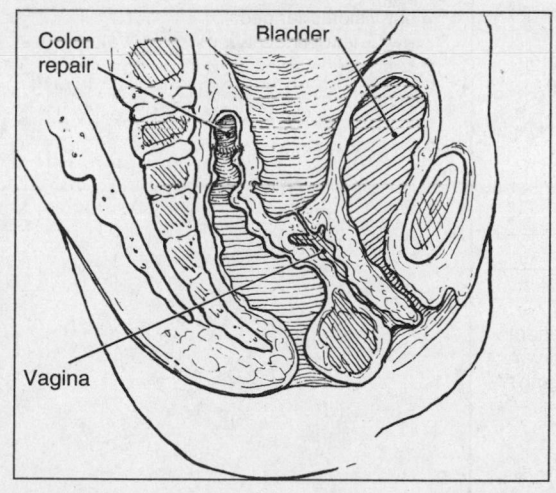

The involved area of the colon is isolated and separated from the vagina. The segment of the colon involved is removed and the colon is then sewn back together.

CORNEA TRANSPLANT
(Keratoplasty)

 GENERAL INFORMATION

DEFINITION—Removing a diseased or injured cornea and replacing it with a healthy cornea from a donor.

BODY PARTS INVOLVED—Cornea (the front part of the eyeball).

REASONS FOR SURGERY—Restoration of vision or prevention of blindness.

SURGICAL RISK INCREASES WITH
- Obesity.
- Smoking.
- Poor nutrition.
- Recent or chronic illness.
- Alcoholism.
- Diabetes.
- Use of some prescription and nonprescription drugs. Inform your doctor of any drugs, medications, or vitamin and herb supplements you are using or have used in the last month.

 WHAT TO EXPECT

WHO OPERATES—Ophthalmologist.

WHERE PERFORMED—Hospital.

DIAGNOSTIC TESTS
- Before surgery: Blood and urine studies, eye examination.
- After surgery: Eye examination.

ANESTHESIA
- Local anesthesia by injection.
- General anesthesia by injection and inhalation with an airway tube placed in the windpipe.

DESCRIPTION OF OPERATION
- The diseased or injured cornea is cut free with scissors and removed.
- The donor cornea (usually from an eye bank) is grafted into the area with tiny sutures.
- The sutures holding the transplanted cornea are removed when healing has taken place, usually about 3 to 4 weeks after surgery.

POSSIBLE COMPLICATIONS
- Surgical-wound infection.
- Rejection of transplant (rare).
- Secondary glaucoma.

AVERAGE HOSPITAL STAY—2 days.

PROBABLE OUTCOME—Expect complete healing without complications. Allow 3 to 4 weeks for recovery from surgery. Some patients can see better within a day or two of surgery, others may not gain optimum vision for months or even a year or more.

 POSTOPERATIVE CARE

GENERAL MEASURES—Avoid getting water in the eye.

MEDICATION
- Your doctor may prescribe:
  - Pain relievers. Don't take prescription pain medication longer than 4 to 7 days. Use only as much as you need.
  - Stool softeners to prevent constipation.
  - Eyedrops containing a topical steroid to help prevent rejection and an antibiotic to prevent or treat infection.
- You may use nonprescription drugs, such as acetaminophen, for minor pain. Avoid aspirin.

ACTIVITY
- To help recovery and aid your well-being, resume daily activities, including work, as soon as you are able.
- Avoid vigorous exercise. Don't bend over or lift heavy objects until transplant is healed completely.
- Resume driving when your doctor determines that healing is complete.
- You will probably wear an eye shield at night for 2 to 3 months.

DIET—No special diet. Increase dietary fiber and fluid intake to help prevent constipation.

 CALL YOUR DOCTOR IF

- Pain, swelling, redness, drainage, or bleeding increases in the surgical area.
- You develop symptoms of infection including headache, muscle aches, dizziness, fever, or a general ill feeling.
- You experience nausea, vomiting, or constipation.
- Your vision changes.
- New, unexplained symptoms develop.

CORNEA TRANSPLANT
(Keratoplasty)

An illustration of the incision site and cornea, which covers the pupil of the eye.

Incision site

Diseased or injured cornea is cut free with scissors and removed.

Cornea

The donor cornea is fastened into the area with sutures. Sutures can be removed when healing has taken place, usually about 3 to 4 weeks after surgery.

Donor cornea

CORONARY ARTERY BYPASS GRAFT
(Heart Bypass)

GENERAL INFORMATION

DEFINITION—Using a section of the patient's leg vein or an artery in the chest wall to bypass a partial or complete blockage in the coronary artery system.

BODY PARTS INVOLVED—Heart, coronary arteries, chest wall, large veins of legs.

REASONS FOR SURGERY
- Angina pectoris.
- Restoration of blood to the heart muscle after a heart attack.
- Prevention of a possible heart attack, if coronary arteries have narrowed.

SURGICAL RISK INCREASES WITH
- Obesity, smoking.
- Recent or chronic illness, diabetes.
- Chronic obstructive pulmonary disease (COPD), heart failure.
- Use of some prescription and nonprescription drugs. Inform your doctor of any drugs, medications, or vitamin and herb supplements you are using or have used in the last month.

WHAT TO EXPECT

WHO OPERATES—Cardiovascular surgeon.

WHERE PERFORMED—Hospital.

DIAGNOSTIC TESTS
- Before surgery: Blood studies, chest x-ray, cardiac catheterization, ECG, sonogram (see Glossary for all).
- During surgery: ECG, angiograms (see Glossary).
- After surgery: ECG, chest x-ray, sonogram.

ANESTHESIA—General anesthesia by injection and inhalation with an airway tube placed in the windpipe.

DESCRIPTION OF OPERATION
- A section of the patient's large leg vein, or a section of the mammary artery (located in the chest), is removed and set aside to be used as the bypass vein graft.
- An incision is made through the breastbone, and the chest is spread open to expose the heart.
- The heart is stopped with a chemical solution that temporarily paralyzes the heart muscle fibers and the heart's temperature is reduced. Circulation and breathing are then performed by a heart-lung machine.
- The bypass vein graft is sutured in place to allow blood flow to resume beyond the blocked area.
- After reheating the heart, it is given a mild electric shock that causes heartbeat to resume.

- The heart-lung machine is then stopped and disconnected.
- The breastbone edges are rejoined with metal suture material, and muscles, tissue and skin are closed with lighter sutures.

POSSIBLE COMPLICATIONS
- Heart rhythm abnormalities.
- Excessive bleeding, blood clots.
- Occlusion (blockage) of grafted vessels.
- Infection, kidney failure.
- New area of injury to the heart muscle, stroke.

AVERAGE HOSPITAL STAY—6-10 days.

PROBABLE OUTCOME—Angina pectoris is cured in almost all cases, and the probability of future heart attacks is reduced. Allow 6 weeks for recovery from surgery.

POSTOPERATIVE CARE

GENERAL MEASURES
- A hard ridge should form along the incision. As it heals, the ridge will gradually recede.
- Shower as usual after discharge. You may wash the incision gently with mild soap.
- Move and elevate legs frequently while resting in bed to decrease the likelihood of deep-vein blood clots.

MEDICATION—Your doctor may prescribe:
- Pain relievers. Don't take prescription pain medication for longer than 4 to 7 days. Use only as much as you need.
- Antiarrhythmics to prevent heartbeat irregularities.
- Digitalis to strengthen the heart muscle.
- Anticoagulants to decrease the likelihood of blood clots.

ACTIVITY
- To help recovery and aid your well-being, resume daily activities, including driving or work, as soon as your doctor determines that you are able.
- Resume sexual relations when your doctor determines that healing is complete.
- Ask your doctor for advice about an exercise rehabilitation program.

DIET—Low-salt, low-fat, high-fiber (see Appendix for diets).

CALL YOUR DOCTOR IF

- Pain, swelling, redness, drainage, or bleeding increases in the surgical area.
- You develop symptoms of infection including headache, muscle aches, dizziness, fever, or a general ill feeling.
- You develop a cough, heartbeat irregularities, leg pain or constipation, or any other new symptoms.

CORONARY ARTERY BYPASS GRAFT
(Heart Bypass)

Left coronary artery

Right coronary artery

Heart

An illustration of the heart showing the coronary artery circulation.

Blockage

The blocked area in this illustration is the left anterior descending coronary artery, a common site for such blockage to occur.

Bypass graft

Blockage

A bypass vein or artery grafted in place allows blood flow to resume beyond the blocked area and thus restore more normal circulation to some of the damaged heart muscle.

CRANIOTOMY

GENERAL INFORMATION

DEFINITION—Cutting through the skull (cranium) to expose and treat disorders in the brain or associated tissues.

BODY PARTS INVOLVED—Scalp, skull, brain and membrane coverings.

REASONS FOR SURGERY
- Removal of blood clots, aneurysms, or tumors.
- Repair of tears in the brain's membrane coverings.
- Drainage of a brain abscess.

SURGICAL RISK INCREASES WITH
- Smoking, excess alcohol consumption.
- Chronic illness.
- Recent illness, especially upper respiratory infection.
- Diabetes.
- Use of some prescription and nonprescription drugs. Inform your doctor of any drugs, medications, or vitamin and herb supplements you are using or have used in the last month.

WHAT TO EXPECT

WHO OPERATES—Neurosurgeon.

WHERE PERFORMED—Hospital.

DIAGNOSTIC TESTS
- Before surgery: Blood and urine studies, x-ray of skull, MRI, angiogram, EEG, ECG, CT scan (see Glossary for all).
- After surgery: EEG, x-rays of skull, blood studies, CT scan, angiogram (sometimes).

ANESTHESIA—General anesthesia by injection and inhalation with an airway tube placed in the windpipe.

DESCRIPTION OF OPERATION
- A portion of the head area is shaved. An incision is made in the scalp over the area of suspected disorder.
- A flap of bone is cut away from the skull and set aside.
- The disorder is located and treated as necessary.
- The bone flap is replaced.
- The scalp is closed with sutures or clips, which usually can be removed about 1 week after surgery.

POSSIBLE COMPLICATIONS
- Stroke, seizure.
- Excessive bleeding, blood clots.
- Surgical-wound infection.
- Brain damage.
- Swelling of the brain caused by the trauma of surgery.

AVERAGE HOSPITAL STAY—10 to 14 days.

PROBABLE OUTCOME—Expect complete healing of surgical wounds. Allow about 8 weeks for recovery from surgery.

POSTOPERATIVE CARE

GENERAL MEASURES
- A hard ridge should form along the incision. As it heals, the ridge will gradually recede.
- Shower as usual after discharge. You may wash the incision gently with mild, unscented soap.
- After bathing or showering, replace any wet dressings with clean, dry ones.
- Move and elevate legs often while resting in bed to decrease the likelihood of deep-vein blood clots.

MEDICATION
- Your doctor may prescribe:
  - Pain relievers. Don't take prescription pain medication longer than 4 to 7 days. Use only as much as you need.
  - Stool softeners to prevent constipation.
  - Antibiotics to fight or prevent infection.
- You may use nonprescription drugs, such as acetaminophen, for minor pain. Avoid aspirin.

ACTIVITY
- To help recovery and aid your well-being, resume daily activities, including work, as soon as you are able.
- Avoid vigorous exercise for 6 weeks after surgery.
- Resume driving about 3 weeks (or as advised) after returning home (can depend on underlying disorder).
- Resume sexual relations when your doctor determines that healing is complete.

DIET—Clear liquid diet until the gastrointestinal tract functions again. Then eat a well-balanced diet to promote healing.

CALL YOUR DOCTOR IF

- Pain, swelling, redness, drainage, or bleeding increases in the surgical area.
- You experience nausea, vomiting, or constipation.
- You develop symptoms of infection including headache, muscle aches, dizziness, fever, or a general ill feeling.
- You develop speech difficulties, weakness or paralysis of the face, arms, or legs.
- New, unexplained symptoms develop.

CRANIOTOMY

Incision

An illustration of a shaved head and a typical incision site on the scalp.

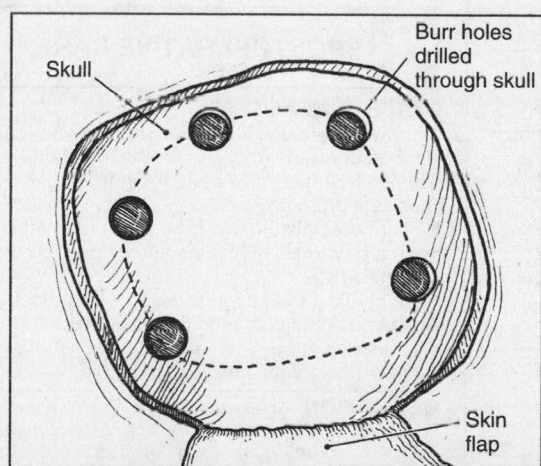

Skull

Burr holes drilled through skull

Skin flap

Skin over the scalp is incised, exposing the skull bone, and a flap is formed.

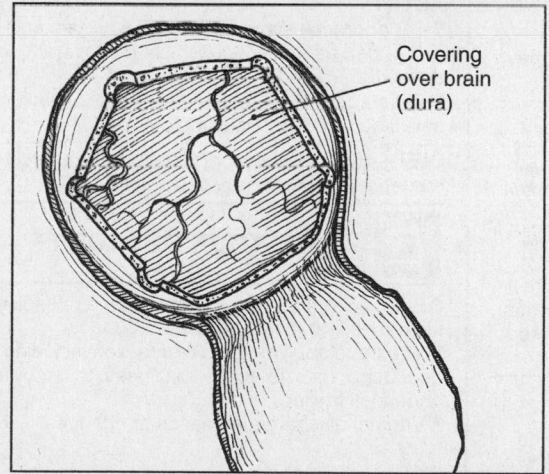

Covering over brain (dura)

Skin and bone flap are retracted to expose the brain covering where the suspected area of pathology is located.

CRYOSURGERY

GENERAL INFORMATION

DEFINITION—Thermal destruction of abnormal or diseased tissue by freezing, usually with liquid nitrogen.

BODY PARTS INVOLVED—Skin, anus, cervix.

REASONS FOR SURGERY
- Removal of skin lesions such as actinic keratoses (precancerous conditions caused by the sun) and warts.
- Treatment of cervicitis (inflammation of the cervix).
- Treatment of mild to moderate cervical dysplasia (abnormal cell growth).
- Sometimes used to treat severe cervical dysplasia.
- Treatment of benign (noncancerous) growths on the cervix (such as polyps) or genital warts.
- Moderate hemorrhoids.
- Anal fissures.

SURGICAL RISK INCREASES WITH—None expected.

WHAT TO EXPECT

WHO OPERATES—Dermatologist or family doctor (to treat skin lesions), obstetrician-gynecologist (to treat cervicitis or other cervical abnormalities), or general surgeon (for hemorrhoids or fissures).

WHERE PERFORMED—Hospital, outpatient surgical facility, doctor's office, or emergency room.

DIAGNOSTIC TESTS
- Before surgery: Blood and urine studies (occasionally).
- After surgery: None expected.

ANESTHESIA—Usually none. For skin lesions, the area to be treated is sometimes anesthetized with an injection of local anesthetic. A general or spinal anesthesia may be used for anorectal lesions.

DESCRIPTION OF OPERATION
- For small skin lesions, liquid nitrogen is applied to a cotton-tipped applicator. The applicator is held to the skin lesions until they are frozen and destroyed.
- For surgery on the cervix or anus, a special probe instrument is used. Liquid nitrogen circulates in the tip of this instrument causing it to become almost as cold as the liquid nitrogen itself. The instrument tip is held on the affected areas until the abnormal tissue is frozen.

POSSIBLE COMPLICATIONS
- Surgical-wound infection (rare).
- Failure of the procedure to destroy all of the abnormal tissue.

- For anorectal surgery: constipation, urinary retention, recurrence of hemorrhoids.
- When cryosurgery is performed on the cervix, cervical stenosis (narrowing) can occur.

AVERAGE HOSPITAL STAY—Usually none.

PROBABLE OUTCOME
- For skin lesions: Initial swelling and redness become a blister in 2 or 3 days. The blister will rupture by itself about 2 weeks after surgery. It will leave a scab, but little or no scar after complete healing.
- For surgery of the cervix: Expect complete healing without complications. There may be mild uterine cramping and facial flushing. Vaginal discharge is common, discharge may be profuse, foul-smelling, and last for 7 to 10 days. Allow about 3 weeks for recovery from surgery.
- For anorectal surgery (hemorrhoids or fissure): There may be moderate discharge for 2 to 3 weeks, and considerable swelling for 1 week.

POSTOPERATIVE CARE

GENERAL MEASURES
- Shower as usual. If appropriate, keep any skin wounds dry with bandages for the first 2 or 3 days after surgery. If a bandage gets wet, change it promptly.
- For anorectal surgery: Take warm sitz baths twice a day to aid in healing and help to relieve discomfort.
- For cervical therapy, discuss with your doctor when you should be seen for a follow-up examination to be sure healing is complete and that treatment was effective.

MEDICATION—You may use nonprescription drugs, such as acetaminophen, to relieve minor pain.

ACTIVITY
- For anorectal surgery: Stay off your feet and rest in bed as much as possible for several days.
- For surgery of the cervix: Avoid any sexual activity until healing is complete.

DIET—High-fiber diet or Metamucil for anorectal surgery. Otherwise, no special diet.

CALL YOUR DOCTOR IF

- Pain, swelling, redness, drainage, or bleeding increases in the surgical area.
- You develop symptoms of infection including headache, muscle aches, dizziness, fever, or a general ill feeling.
- Vaginal discharge increases or changes.

CRYOSURGERY

An illustration of a skin lesion on the neck to be treated with cryosurgery (very low temperature).

Lesion

A cotton-tipped applicator that has been dipped in liquid nitrogen is held against the lesion to destroy abnormal cells.

Cotton-tipped applicator

Large treated areas should be covered with bandages until healing is complete.

CULDOCENTESIS

GENERAL INFORMATION

DEFINITION—Piercing the "cul-de-sac," the space deep in the vagina behind and under the cervix, in order to obtain a fluid sample for laboratory examination.

BODY PARTS INVOLVED—Vagina, lowest part of pelvis behind the uterus and cervix.

REASONS FOR SURGERY—Investigation of possible ailments in the abdomen and pelvis, including: bleeding inside the lower pelvic cavity, ruptured ectopic pregnancy, ruptured ovarian cyst, ovarian cancer, or pelvic inflammatory disease. Laboratory examination of the removed fluid aids in diagnosis.

SURGICAL RISK INCREASES WITH
- Recent or chronic illness.
- Diabetes.
- Use of some prescription and nonprescription drugs. Inform your doctor of any drugs, medications, or vitamin and herb supplements you are using or have used in the last month.

WHAT TO EXPECT

WHO OPERATES—Obstetrician-gynecologist, general surgeon, or family doctor.

WHERE PERFORMED—Doctor's office, outpatient surgical facility, or hospital.

DIAGNOSTIC TESTS
- Before surgery: Pap smear, vaginal and abdominal exam, x-rays of lower abdomen.
- After surgery: Laboratory examination of removed fluid.

ANESTHESIA—Local anesthesia by injection.

DESCRIPTION OF OPERATION
- A speculum is inserted into the vagina to hold it open.
- The rear lip of the cervix is raised.
- A local anesthetic is applied to the farthest back portion of the vagina (cul-de-sac).
- The posterior wall of the vagina is penetrated with a needle and syringe.
- Fluid, if present, is aspirated. No sutures are necessary.

POSSIBLE COMPLICATIONS
- Perforation of bladder or bowel (rare).
- Excessive bleeding.
- Surgical-wound infection.

AVERAGE HOSPITAL STAY—Usually none.

PROBABLE OUTCOME
- A fluid sample is obtained successfully without complications in virtually all cases. If fluid or blood confirms other findings that suggest a serious disease or condition, you may need further surgery.
- If no fluid is obtained and there are no complications, but you still have your original symptoms, expect further observation or tests to diagnose your conditions.
- Allow about 1 week for recovery from the procedure.

POSTOPERATIVE CARE

GENERAL MEASURES
- Resume your usual activities as soon as possible, if symptoms that caused the need for surgery disappear. If symptoms recur, see your doctor.
- Continue to use your usual birth-control methods. Your periods should not be disturbed.
- Use sanitary pads for your next menstrual period. Avoid tampons temporarily; they may lead to infection.

MEDICATION
- Your doctor may prescribe medicines according to diagnosis.
- You may use nonprescription drugs, such as acetaminophen, to relieve minor pain. Avoid aspirin.

ACTIVITY—Resume normal activities gradually. Resume sexual relations when able. This will depend on various underlying causes. Ask your doctor.

DIET—No special diet.

CALL YOUR DOCTOR IF

- You experience vaginal bleeding that is heavier than expected.
- Symptoms recur or worsen.
- You develop symptoms of infection including headache, muscle aches, dizziness, fever, or a general ill feeling.

CULDOCENTESIS

- This view illustrates a female patient with extended legs in stirrups on an examining table to allow examination of the genital area.
- The speculum is inserted into the vagina to stretch it open and expose the cervix.

Cervix

Speculum

Forceps grasp the rear lip of the cervix to expose the cul-de-sac (the farthest back portion of the vagina).

Uterus

Rectum

Cul-de-sac

The cul-de-sac is penetrated with needle and syringe. Fluid, if present, is aspirated.

CYSTOSCOPY

GENERAL INFORMATION

DEFINITION—Visual examination of the lower urinary tract and collection of a urine sample from the bladder. The examination is performed with a cystoscope, a thin fiber-optic instrument with a lighted tip.

BODY PARTS INVOLVED—Urethra, bladder, openings into the bladder.

REASONS FOR SURGERY
- Blood in the urine (hematuria).
- Inability to control urination (incontinence).
- Recurrent urinary tract infections.
- Congenital abnormalities of the urinary tract.
- Tumors of the bladder.
- Bladder or kidney stones.
- Tightening of the urethra or the ureters.

SURGICAL RISK INCREASES WITH
- Obesity.
- Smoking.
- Recent or chronic illness.
- Diabetes.
- Use of some prescription and nonprescription drugs. Inform your doctor of any drugs, medications, or vitamin and herb supplements you are using or have used in the last month.

WHAT TO EXPECT

WHO OPERATES—Urologist.

WHERE PERFORMED—Hospital, doctor's office, or outpatient surgical facility.

DIAGNOSTIC TESTS
- Before surgery: Blood and urine tests, x-rays of kidneys, ureters (see Glossary) and bladder, CT scan (see Glossary).
- During surgery: Retrograde pyelograms (see Glossary).
- After surgery: Blood studies.

ANESTHESIA
- Spinal anesthesia (sometimes) by injection or injected general anesthesia.
- Local anesthesia with or without sedation.

DESCRIPTION OF OPERATION
- The patient urinates before surgery so that urine remaining in the bladder can be measured.
- The cystoscope is lubricated and inserted through the urethra into the bladder. A urine sample is collected.
- Fluid is pumped through the cystoscope to inflate the bladder, which allows visual examination of the entire bladder wall.
- Bladder or kidney stones are removed, if necessary. Tissue samples are gathered and, if necessary, lesions are treated.

- Catheters are passed through the cystoscope and guided to the openings into the ureters. A harmless dye is injected through the catheters into the ureters to perform x-ray studies.
- The cystoscope is removed.

POSSIBLE COMPLICATIONS
- Excessive bleeding.
- Damage to the urethra.
- Perforation of bladder.
- Urinary tract infection.
- Injury to the penis.

AVERAGE HOSPITAL STAY—0 to 3 days.

PROBABLE OUTCOME—Examination completed and urine sample collected successfully in virtually all cases. If the procedure is confined to inspection and manual manipulation, recovery is usually rapid and should take only 2 to 4 days.

POSTOPERATIVE CARE

GENERAL MEASURES
- Warm baths for 10 to 15 minutes several times a day may help to relieve discomfort.
- You may notice a small amount of blood in your urine following the exam; this should last no more than 24 hours.
- Drink eight 8 ounce glasses of water a day.

MEDICATION
- Your doctor may prescribe:
  - Pain relievers. Don't take prescription pain medication longer than 4 to 7 days. Use only as much as you need.
  - Antibiotics to fight or prevent infection.
- You may use nonprescription drugs, such as acetaminophen, for minor pain.

ACTIVITY
- Avoid vigorous exercise for 2 weeks after surgery.
- Resume sexual relations when your doctor determines that healing is complete.
- Resume driving 2 days after returning home.

DIET—No special diet.

CALL YOUR DOCTOR IF

- Pain, swelling, redness, drainage, or bleeding increases in the surgical area.
- You develop symptoms of infection including headache, muscle aches, dizziness, fever, or a general ill feeling.
- You experience nausea or vomiting.
- You have painful or difficult urination.
- New, unexplained symptoms develop.

CYSTOSCOPY

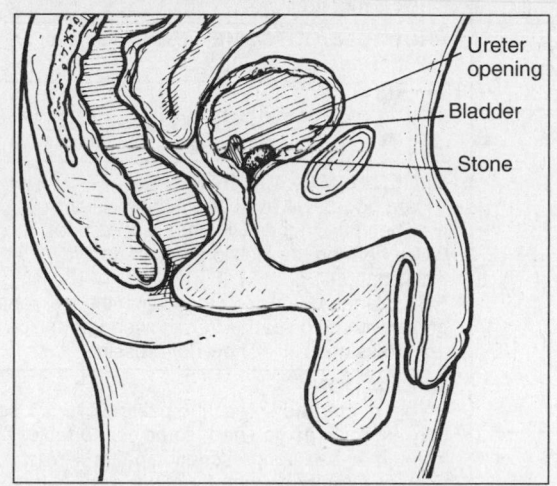

A cross-section of the male pelvis showing the urethra, bladder and openings into the bladder. A typical stone inside the bladder is illustrated.

Ureter opening

Bladder

Stone

A lubricated cystoscope is inserted through the urethra into the bladder to allow removal of the stone. If needed, a catheter can be passed through the cystoscope.

Bladder

Cystoscope

A catheter passed through the cystoscope toward the opening of the ureter. The catheter can be passed through the ureteral opening to remove other stones higher in the urinary tract.

Bladder wall

Ureter opening

Cystoscope

Catheter

DEFIBRILLATOR IMPLANTATION

GENERAL INFORMATION

DEFINITION—Permanent placement of device to automatically "shock" the heart in the event of a dangerous arrhythmia or cardiac arrest.

BODY PARTS INVOLVED—Heart, subclavian vein.

REASONS FOR SURGERY—To prevent fatal arrhythmia or cardiac arrest.

SURGICAL RISK INCREASES WITH
- Age.
- Diabetes.
- Poor kidney function.
- High blood pressure.
- Poor nutrition.
- Chronic lung disease.
- Obesity.

WHAT TO EXPECT

WHO OPERATES—Cardiologist, cardiothoracic surgeon.

WHERE PERFORMED—Hospital or outpatient facility.

DIAGNOSTIC TESTS
- Before surgery: Blood tests, chest x-ray, EKG (see Glossary).
- After surgery: EKG, chest x-ray.

ANESTHESIA—General anesthesia or local anesthesia with sedation.

DESCRIPTION OF OPERATION
- The defibrillator is implanted in a manner similar to a pacemaker. The subclavian vein is accessed just under the clavicle. A wire is threaded into the vein and a catheter placed over the wire. The pacing wires are passed through the catheter and wedged into the ventricle of the heart. The wires are then connected to the defibrillator.
- A pocket is created between the skin and chest wall muscle (subcutaneous space) near the insertion site and the defibrillator is placed in the pocket.
- The pocket is closed with sutures and the defibrillator is tested to make sure it is functioning properly.

POSSIBLE COMPLICATIONS
- Bleeding around the insertion site or pocket.
- Infection.
- Migration (movement) or dislodging of wires (leads).
- Pneumothorax (air in chest cavity outside the lung).
- Hemothorax (bleeding into chest cavity).
- Blockage of subclavian vein.

AVERAGE HOSPITAL STAY—Usually outpatient, but may need short hospital stay for medical monitoring.

PROBABLE OUTCOME—Expect full recovery in 2 to 3 weeks.

POSTOPERATIVE CARE

GENERAL MEASURES
- Hard ridges will form along the incisions. As they heal, the ridges will gradually recede.
- Use heat on the incision to help relieve incisional pain.
- Shower as usual. You may wash the incisions gently with mild soap. After showering, replace any dressings with a new dry dressing.

MEDICATION
- Your doctor may prescribe pain relievers. Use only as much as you need to be comfortable.
- You may use nonprescription pain relievers such as acetaminophen for minor pain. Ask your doctor if it is okay to take ibuprofen or aspirin.
- Heart medications to control the rate or rhythm of the heart may be prescribed.

ACTIVITY
- Start ambulating (walking) as soon as you are home.
- You may swim once all sutures are out.

DIET—No special diet.

CALL YOUR DOCTOR IF

- Pain, swelling, redness, drainage, or bleeding increases in the surgical area.
- You develop symptoms of infection including headache, muscle aches, dizziness, fever, or a general ill feeling.
- You develop chest pain or shortness of breath.
- Arm becomes cold, numb, painful, or swollen.
- New unexplained symptoms develop.

DEFIBRILLATOR IMPLANTATION

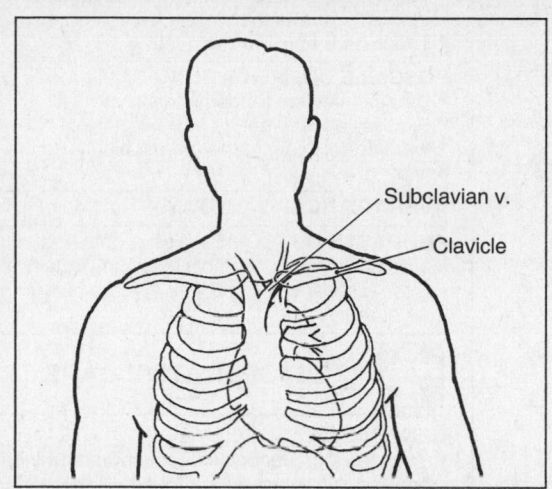

The subclavian vein can be accessed on either side right behind the clavicle.

Once the vein is punctured, a catheter sheath is placed to allow insertion of the pacing wires into the heart muscle.

A subcutaneous pocket is created below the clavicle. The defibrillator is attached to the pacing wires and placed in the pocket.

DILATATION & CURETTAGE OF THE UTERUS (D & C)

 GENERAL INFORMATION

DEFINITION—Opening the cervix and scraping the lining (endometrium) and contents of the uterus. The D & C is often both a diagnostic and a therapeutic procedure.

BODY PARTS INVOLVED—Uterus, cervix, vagina (as route for surgery).

REASONS FOR SURGERY
- Diagnosis of abnormal bleeding or possible cancer inside the uterus.
- Incomplete spontaneous miscarriage.
- Treatment of minor diseases of the uterus.
- Prevent or stop hemorrhage or subsequent infection following miscarriage.
- Removal of membranes and placenta after childbirth in cases where they fail to deliver spontaneously (retained placenta).
- Elective abortion during early pregnancy.

SURGICAL RISK INCREASES WITH
- Obesity, smoking, alcoholism.
- Cervical infection or ongoing uterine infection.
- Recent or chronic illness, diabetes.
- Use of some prescription and nonprescription drugs. Inform your doctor of any drugs, medications, or vitamin and herb supplements you are using or have used in the last month.

 WHAT TO EXPECT

WHO OPERATES—Obstetrician-gynecologist, general surgeon or family doctor.

WHERE PERFORMED—Outpatient surgical facility or hospital.

DIAGNOSTIC TESTS
- Before surgery: Pap smear (see Glossary), pregnancy test, blood and hormonal studies.
- After surgery: Blood studies, Pap smear in 2 months.

ANESTHESIA—Local anesthesia by injection, or general anesthesia by injection and inhalation with an airway tube placed in the windpipe.

DESCRIPTION OF OPERATION
- The vagina is cleansed with an antiseptic.
- The cervix is carefully opened (dilated), either by inserting a series of tapered metal rods, each with a progressively larger diameter, into the cervical opening at the time of the procedure, or in advance by the use of laminaria (freeze-dried seaweed), which are placed in the cervix 8 to 12 hours prior to surgery. The laminaria will swell and gradually open the cervix to 1 to 2 centimeters.
- A curette is inserted into the uterus. The curette can be a suction device or a looped knife.

- The curette is used to scrape or suction the endometrium from the uterine wall.
- The instruments are removed.

POSSIBLE COMPLICATIONS
- Uterine infection (endometritis).
- Excessive bleeding.
- Inadvertent injury to the uterus, bladder or bowel.

AVERAGE HOSPITAL STAY—0 to 1 day.

PROBABLE OUTCOME—Tissue obtained successfully without complications in virtually all cases. Allow about 4 to 6 weeks for recovery from surgery.

 POSTOPERATIVE CARE

GENERAL MEASURES
- You may experience mild to moderate uterine cramping or backache for 2 to 3 days following surgery.
- Don't douche unless your physician recommends it.
- Expect slight vaginal bleeding during recovery from surgery. Use a sanitary pad to protect clothing. Avoid tampons temporarily, as they may lead to infection.
- Your first menstrual period following the procedure may be earlier or later than normal.

MEDICATION
- Your doctor may prescribe:
  - Hormones, if necessary to correct an imbalance.
  - Pain relievers. Don't take prescription pain medication longer than 4 to 7 days. Use only as much as you need.
  - Antibiotics to fight or prevent infection.
- You may use nonprescription drugs, such as acetaminophen, for minor pain. Avoid aspirin.

ACTIVITY
- Resume driving in 1 to 2 days.
- To help recovery and aid your well-being, resume daily activities, including work, as soon as you are able.
- Avoid sexual relations until spotting ceases.

DIET—No special diet.

 CALL YOUR DOCTOR IF

- Vaginal discharge increases or smells unpleasant.
- You experience pain that simple pain medication does not relieve quickly.
- Unusual vaginal swelling or bleeding develops.
- You develop symptoms of infection including headache, muscle aches, dizziness, fever, or a general ill feeling.
- New, unexplained symptoms develop.

DILATATION & CURETTAGE OF THE UTERUS (D & C)

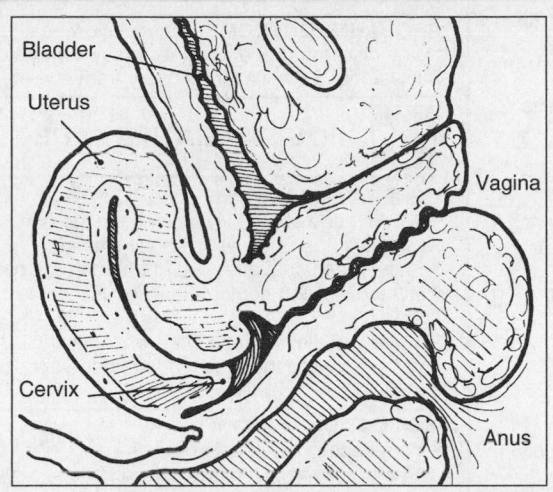

Bladder

Uterus

Vagina

Cervix

Anus

A side view of the female genital area.

Dilator

Forceps grasp the anterior portion of the cervix and a dilator is inserted into uterus.

Curette

After the cervix has been dilated, a curette is passed into the cavity of the uterus. The curette is used to scrape or suction away the uterine lining for laboratory analysis or therapeutic reasons.

DISC REMOVAL, HERNIATED
(Laminectomy)

GENERAL INFORMATION

DEFINITION—Removal of part or all of an intervertebral disc that has protruded from its normal position.

BODY PARTS INVOLVED—Spine, intervertebral disc.

REASONS FOR SURGERY—Relief of painful symptoms caused by pressure on nerves or spinal cord.

SURGICAL RISK INCREASES WITH
- Adults over 60.
- Obesity, poor nutrition, smoking.
- Chronic illness, especially back pain or alcoholism.
- Diabetes.
- Use of some prescription and nonprescription drugs. Inform your doctor of any drugs, medications, or vitamin and herb supplements you are using or have used in the last month.

WHAT TO EXPECT

WHO OPERATES—Neurosurgeon, orthopedist.

WHERE PERFORMED—Hospital.

DIAGNOSTIC TESTS
- Before surgery: Blood and urine tests, x-rays of back and lungs, CT scan and/or MRI, ECG (see Glossary for all).
- After surgery: Blood studies, back x-rays.

ANESTHESIA—General anesthesia by injection and inhalation with an airway tube placed in the windpipe.

DESCRIPTION OF OPERATION
- An incision is made over the protruded disc.
- The arches of the spine are cut away and removed to allow visualization of the disc.
- The protruding disc is scooped out.
- Sometimes, the vertebral bone around the affected area is joined together with normal bone taken from your hip area and inserted into the space from which the disc was removed. This procedure is called fusion.
- The skin is closed with sutures or clips, which usually can be removed about 1 week after surgery.

POSSIBLE COMPLICATIONS
- Excessive bleeding, blood clots.
- Surgical-wound infection.
- Injury to nerve roots, which can lead to paralysis.
- Incomplete disc removal.
- Unrelieved or worsened pain.
- Impaired bladder function (rare).

AVERAGE HOSPITAL STAY—2 to 6 days.

PROBABLE OUTCOME—Expect slow healing. Some discomfort and weakness may continue. Allow about 5 weeks for recovery from surgery.

POSTOPERATIVE CARE

GENERAL MEASURES
- A hard ridge should form along the incision. As it heals, the ridge will gradually recede.
- Shower as usual after you are home. You may wash the incision gently with mild, unscented soap.
- Move and elevate legs often while resting in bed to decrease the likelihood of deep-vein blood clots.

MEDICATION
- Your doctor may prescribe:
  - Pain relievers. Don't take prescription pain medication longer than 4 to 7 days. Use only as much as you need.
  - Stool softeners to prevent constipation.
  - Antibiotics to fight or prevent infection.
- You may use nonprescription drugs, such as acetaminophen, for minor pain. Avoid aspirin.

ACTIVITY
- To help recovery and aid your well-being, resume daily activities, including work, as soon as you are able.
- Avoid vigorous exercise or lifting for 6 weeks after surgery. Then begin back exercises (physical therapy) under medical supervision.
- Resume driving 6 weeks after returning home.
- Resume sexual relations when able.

DIET—Clear liquid diet until the gastrointestinal tract begins to function again. Then eat a well-balanced diet to promote healing.

CALL YOUR DOCTOR IF

- Pain, swelling, redness, drainage, or bleeding increases in the surgical area.
- You develop symptoms of infection including headache, muscle aches, dizziness, fever, or a general ill feeling.
- You experience nausea, vomiting, constipation, or abdominal swelling.
- You have weakness, numbness, or pain in the back, buttocks, or legs.
- You experience loss of bladder or bowel control.
- New, unexplained symptoms develop.

DISC REMOVAL, HERNIATED
(Laminectomy)

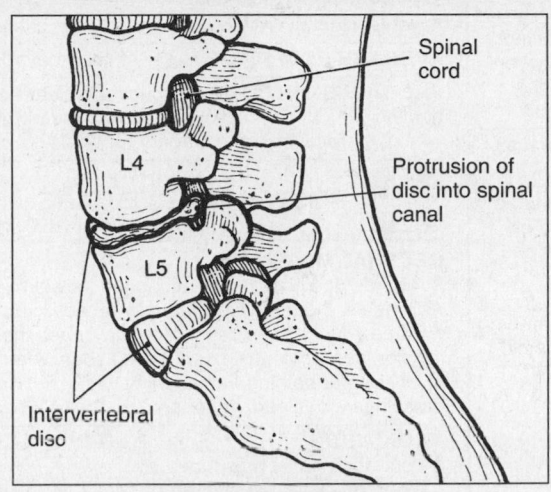

Spinal cord

Protrusion of disc into spinal canal

L4

L5

Intervertebral disc

An illustration of the bony spine, the spinal cord and the protruding intervertebral disc. This example shows the disc separating the 4th and 5th vertebral bodies.

Spinal cord

Protruding disc

After the skin has been incised, the arches of the bone are located, cut away and partially or totally removed allowing the protruding disc to be scooped out.

Disc removed

Appearance after the disc has been removed.

DUCTUS ARTERIOSUS CLOSURE

GENERAL INFORMATION

DEFINITION—Closure of an abnormal opening in the ductus arteriosus, a blood vessel between the heart's aorta and the pulmonary artery that usually closes in the first few days of life.

BODY PARTS INVOLVED—Ductus arteriosus, pulmonary artery, aorta.

REASONS FOR SURGERY—For unknown reasons, closure does not always happen. The surgery is performed so that normal growth and development may occur. If the abnormal opening is large, surgery is performed during the first few days after birth. Otherwise, surgery may be delayed until the child is 1 to 2 years old.

SURGICAL RISK INCREASES WITH
- Preterm infants.
- Obesity.
- Recent or chronic illness.
- Use of some prescription and nonprescription drugs. Inform your doctor of any drugs, medications, or vitamin and herb supplements your child is using or has used in the last month.

WHAT TO EXPECT

WHO OPERATES
- Cardiovascular surgeon.
- Pediatric surgeon.

WHERE PERFORMED—Hospital.

DIAGNOSTIC TESTS
- Before surgery: Blood and urine studies, x-ray of chest, echocardiogram, cardiac catheterization (sometimes), ECG (see Glossary for all).
- During surgery: ECG monitor (see Glossary).
- After surgery: Blood studies.

ANESTHESIA—General anesthesia by injection and inhalation with an airway tube placed in the windpipe.

DESCRIPTION OF OPERATION
- An incision is made in the chest. The muscles are divided and the chest is spread open.
- The lung is deflated to expose the ductus arteriosus.
- The ductus arteriosus is tied tightly or clamped in two places, cut between the clamps and tied. The ends are sewn shut to prevent bleeding from the pulmonary artery or the aorta.
- Tubes are left in place to drain fluid. A catheter is left in place to remove air from the chest so that the lung can reinflate itself within 24 to 48 hours.
- The muscles are sewn together in layers with strong sutures.
- The skin is closed with sutures or clips, which usually can be removed about 1 week after surgery.

POSSIBLE COMPLICATIONS
- Excessive bleeding.
- Surgical-wound infection.
- Nerve injury.

AVERAGE HOSPITAL STAY—About 4 days.

PROBABLE OUTCOME—Expect complete healing without complications. Allow about 4 weeks for recovery from surgery.

POSTOPERATIVE CARE

GENERAL MEASURES
- A hard ridge should form along the incision. As it heals, the ridge will gradually recede.
- Bathe your child as usual. You may wash the incision gently with mild, unscented soap. After showering or bathing, replace any wet dressings with clean, dry ones.

MEDICATION
- Your doctor may prescribe:
  - Pain relievers. Don't give your child prescription pain medication longer than 4 to 7 days. Use only as much as your child needs.
  - Antibiotics to fight or prevent infection.
- You may give your child nonprescription drugs, such as acetaminophen, for minor pain. Avoid aspirin.

ACTIVITY
- Avoid vigorous exercise for 6 weeks after surgery.
- Don't let your child ride in a car for 2 weeks after returning from the hospital.

DIET—Clear liquid diet until the gastrointestinal tract functions again. Then provide a well-balanced diet to promote healing.

CALL YOUR DOCTOR IF

- You observe excessive bleeding.
- You observe symptoms of infection including headache, muscle aches, dizziness, fever, or a general ill feeling.
- Your child experiences nausea, vomiting, constipation, or abdominal swelling.
- New, unexplained symptoms develop.

DUCTUS ARTERIOSUS CLOSURE

An illustration of the surgical site to expose the heart and great blood vessels. The patient is usually placed on the side with arm extended over the head.

Rib cage

Incision site

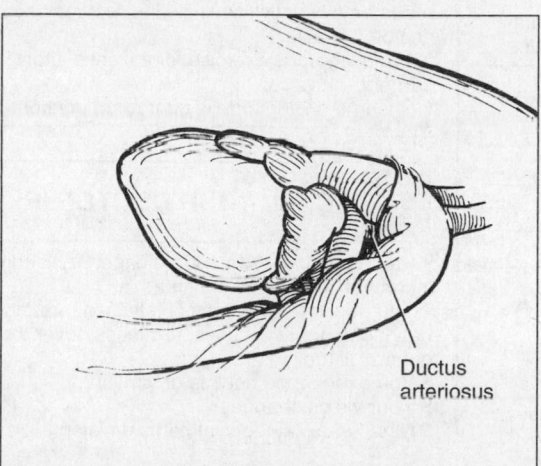

Shown is the ductus arteriosus, which is a blood vessel between the aorta and the pulmonary artery that usually closes at birth.

Ductus arteriosus

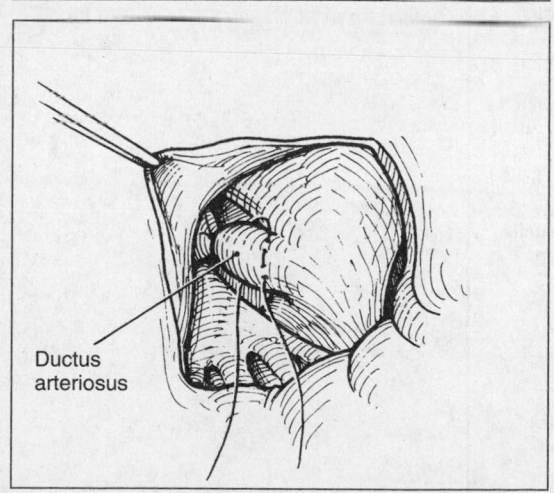

Ductus arteriosus is tied and endo sewn to prevent bleeding from the pulmonary artery or the aorta.

Ductus arteriosus

ECTROPION REPAIR

 ## GENERAL INFORMATION

DEFINITION—Repair of an ectropion (see Illness section) by removal of excess cartilage in the edge of the eyelid.

BODY PARTS INVOLVED—Lower eyelid.

REASONS FOR SURGERY
- Improved appearance.
- Relief of redness, irritation and discomfort.
- Reduced likelihood of infection in the membrane surrounding the eye.

SURGICAL RISK INCREASES WITH
- Smoking.
- Stress.
- Poor nutrition.
- Recent or chronic illness.
- Alcoholism.
- Diabetes.
- Use of some prescription and nonprescription drugs. Inform your doctor of any drugs, medications, or vitamin and herb supplements you are using or have used in the last month.

 ## WHAT TO EXPECT

WHO OPERATES—Ophthalmologist.

WHERE PERFORMED—Hospital, ophthalmologist's office, or outpatient surgical facility.

DIAGNOSTIC TESTS
- Before surgery: Blood and urine studies, eye examination.
- After surgery: Eye examination, laboratory examination of removed tissue.

ANESTHESIA—Local anesthesia by injection.

DESCRIPTION OF OPERATION
- An incision is made in the eyelid.
- The cartilage is cut close to the outer eyelid edge. A small wedge of cartilage is cut free and removed. The cartilage is sewn back together with fine sutures.
- Another wedge of cartilage is cut free and removed from the side of the eyelid close to the nose.
- The remaining cartilage is sewn together with fine sutures.
- The skin is closed with sutures, which usually can be removed about 10 days after surgery.

POSSIBLE COMPLICATIONS
- Surgical-wound infection.
- Recurrence.

AVERAGE HOSPITAL STAY—0 to 2 days.

PROBABLE OUTCOME—Expect complete healing without complications. Allow about 2 weeks for recovery from surgery.

 ## POSTOPERATIVE CARE

GENERAL MEASURES
- Bathe or shower as usual, but keep the eye area dry for 4 to 5 days after surgery.
- Sleep for several nights on 2 pillows to decrease swelling. An eye shield to be worn at night may be prescribed.

MEDICATION
- Your doctor may prescribe:
  - Pain relievers. Don't take prescription pain medication longer than 4 to 7 days. Use only as much as you need.
  - Antibiotic eye drops to fight or prevent infection. Keep drops cold, but not frozen, in the refrigerator.
- You may use nonprescription drugs, such as acetaminophen, for minor pain. Avoid aspirin.

ACTIVITY
- To help recovery and aid your well-being, resume daily activities, including work, as soon as you are able.
- Avoid vigorous exercise for 2 weeks after surgery.
- Resume driving 2 days after returning home.

DIET—No special diet.

 ## CALL YOUR DOCTOR IF

- Pain, swelling, redness, drainage, or bleeding increases in the surgical area.
- You develop symptoms of infection including headache, muscle aches, dizziness, fever, or a general ill feeling.
- You experience nausea or vomiting.
- Your vision changes.
- New, unexplained symptoms develop.

ECTROPION REPAIR

An illustration of the eye, eyelid and typical incision site for ectropion repair.

Incision site

Cartilage is cut close to the outer eyelid edge. A small wedge of cartilage is cut free and removed.

The cartilage is sewn back together and skin closed with small sutures, which are usually removed about 10 days after surgery.

ELECTROCAUTERIZATION
(Electrocoagulation; Electrosurgery; Fulguration)

 GENERAL INFORMATION

DEFINITION—Removal of abnormal or diseased tissue, or control of bleeding in small blood vessels, with controlled electric current.

BODY PARTS INVOLVED—Skin, blood vessels in surgical area.

REASONS FOR SURGERY
- Removal of lesions on the skin.
- Control of bleeding from small blood vessels during other surgeries.
- Stop bleeding from lesions in the lining of the stomach, small intestine, or colon during endoscopy.
- Remove lesions in bladder.

SURGICAL RISK INCREASES WITH—None expected.

 WHAT TO EXPECT

WHO OPERATES—Family doctor, urologist, dermatologist, plastic and reconstructive surgeon, gastroenterologist, or general surgeon.

WHERE PERFORMED—Hospital, outpatient surgical facility, or doctor's office.

DIAGNOSTIC TESTS—Usually none.

ANESTHESIA—Local anesthesia by injection.

DESCRIPTION OF OPERATION
- The procedure described here is used for dermatological lesions.
  - Usually, a lesion is numbed with local anesthesia, and removed with a curette (see Glossary) or excised.
  - Electrocauterization with an electric instrument destroys abnormal tissue that the curette does not remove.

POSSIBLE COMPLICATIONS
- Surgical-wound infection.
- Damage to underlying structure.
- Perforation (in bladder and bowel procedures).

AVERAGE HOSPITAL STAY—Usually none.

PROBABLE OUTCOME—Expect complete healing without complications. The scab will drop off spontaneously and the scar should be small. Allow 2 to 3 weeks for healing and recovery from surgery.

 POSTOPERATIVE CARE

GENERAL MEASURES
- If the wound bleeds during the first 24 hours after surgery, press a clean tissue or cloth to it for 10 minutes.
- When appropriate, cover the surgical wound with a small bandage to protect it.
- Shower as usual. Avoid baths until the wound has completely healed. Between showers, keep the wound dry with a bandage for the first 2 or 3 days after surgery. If a bandage gets wet, change it promptly.
- Apply nonprescription antibiotic ointment to the wound before applying new bandages.

MEDICATION—You may use nonprescription drugs, such as acetaminophen, for minor pain. Avoid aspirin.

ACTIVITY
- Avoid vigorous exercise for about 1 week after surgery, depending on other surgeries performed. Ask your doctor.
- Resume driving when able.

DIET—No special diet.

 CALL YOUR DOCTOR IF

- Pain, swelling, redness, drainage, or bleeding increases in the surgical area.
- You develop abdominal pain or swelling after endoscopy.
- You develop symptoms of infection including headache, muscle aches, dizziness, fever, or a general ill feeling.
- New, unexplained symptoms develop.

ELECTROCAUTERIZATION
(Electrocoagulation; Electrosurgery; Fulguration)

Skin lesion

- After local anesthesia, the skin lesion is cleansed thoroughly.
- The location of the skin lesion in this illustration is on the hand and used as an example. The principles and techniques are similar for electrocauterization of skin lesions in other locations.

Electrocautery

The electrocautery destroys the cells of the skin lesion and prevents excessive bleeding.

Curette

A curette removes the destroyed tissue. After tissue removal, the electrocautery is once again used to destroy cells at the base of the site where the lesion was removed.

ENDOMETRIAL BIOPSY

GENERAL INFORMATION

DEFINITION—A diagnostic procedure that involves removal of tissue from the endometrium, the inner lining of the uterus.

BODY PARTS INVOLVED—Inner lining of the uterus, vagina (as route for surgery).

REASONS FOR SURGERY—Investigation of bleeding between menstrual periods or postmenopausal bleeding. Also used to investigate infertility. Laboratory examination of the removed tissue aids in diagnosis. If appropriate, the surgery is performed during the last few days of the patient's menstrual cycle. This is the best time to identify possible hormonal problems and, for patients undergoing fertility evaluation, to determine if ovulation is occurring.

SURGICAL RISK INCREASES WITH—None expected.

WHAT TO EXPECT

WHO OPERATES—Obstetrician-gynecologist, general surgeon, or family doctor.

WHERE PERFORMED—Doctor's office, outpatient surgical facility, or hospital.

DIAGNOSTIC TESTS
* Before surgery: Pap smear, pregnancy test.
* After surgery: Laboratory examination of removed tissue.

ANESTHESIA—Usually none. Your doctor may prescribe a mild tranquilizer before surgery to calm you.

DESCRIPTION OF OPERATION
* A speculum is inserted into the vagina to hold it open and to bring the cervix into view. In some cases, it is necessary to use a tenaculum, a hooklike instrument that holds and helps stabilize the cervix.
* A small, straw-shaped instrument (or other biopsy instrument) is inserted through the cervix into the uterus. It is gently scraped against the inner lining of the uterus to gather tissue.
* An alternate method involves obtaining the tissue sample with a suction instrument, this procedure is sometimes referred to as vacuum aspiration.
* The instruments are removed. The surgery may cause slight pain, but it should be minor and temporary.

POSSIBLE COMPLICATIONS
* Excessive bleeding.
* Infection of the uterine lining (endometritis).
* Inadvertent injury to the uterus (rare).

AVERAGE HOSPITAL STAY—Usually none.

PROBABLE OUTCOME—Tissue obtained successfully without complications in virtually all cases. Laboratory testing can confirm whether ovulation has occurred, and may identify other causes of infertility, such as infection. Laboratory examination will generally determine if there are any abnormal cells found in the uterine lining. Allow about 1 week for recovery from surgery. During this time, you should expect vaginal discharge.

POSTOPERATIVE CARE

GENERAL MEASURES
* Bathe or shower as usual.
* Wear sanitary pads for the rest of this menstrual period. Avoid tampons temporarily, as they may lead to infection. Your menstrual flow may be heavier than usual.
* Wear cotton panties or pantyhose with a cotton crotch. Avoid panties made from nylon, polyester, silk, or other nonventilating materials.
* Don't douche unless it is prescribed for you.

MEDICATION
* Your doctor may prescribe:
  - Hormones, if a hormone imbalance exists.
  - Antibiotics to fight or prevent infection.
* You may use nonprescription drugs, such as acetaminophen, for minor pain. Avoid aspirin.

ACTIVITY
* Resume daily activities and work as soon as possible.
* You may resume sexual relations once all bleeding has stopped and medical clearance is given.

DIET—No special diet.

CALL YOUR DOCTOR IF

* Vaginal discharge increases or begins to have an unpleasant odor.
* You experience pain that simple medication does not relieve quickly.
* Vaginal swelling or bleeding develops.
* You experience abdominal or lower back pain.
* You develop symptoms of infection including headache, muscle aches, dizziness, fever, or a general ill feeling.
* New, unexplained symptoms develop.

ENDOMETRIAL BIOPSY

- This view illustrates a female patient with extended legs in stirrups on an examining table to allow examination of the genital area.
- The speculum is inserted into the vagina to stretch it open and expose the cervix.

Shown are the uterus, the endometrium (inner lining of the uterus), the operating curette and the forceps holding the upper lip of the cervix to allow introduction of the curette.

The curette removes a sample of the endometrium. The removed tissue is submitted to the laboratory for study.

ENDOVASCULAR SURGERY

GENERAL INFORMATION

DEFINITION—Repair of a narrowed (stenosed) or dilated (aneurysmal) artery using a special graft placed inside the artery. It is usually performed using a percutaneous (needle puncture) technique.

BODY PARTS INVOLVED—Various arteries in the body.

REASONS FOR SURGERY—To prevent rupture of an abdominal aortic aneurysm which usually results in massive hemorrhage and death, or to obtain better blood flow in a narrowed artery.

SURGICAL RISK INCREASES WITH
* Age.
* Diabetes.
* Poor kidney function.
* High blood pressure.
* Poor nutrition.
* Chronic lung disease.

WHAT TO EXPECT

WHO OPERATES—General surgeon, vascular surgeon, radiologist, cardiologist, or neurosurgeon.

WHERE PERFORMED—Hospital.

DIAGNOSTIC TESTS
* Before surgery: Blood tests, chest x-ray, CT scan, and EKG (see Glossary).
* After surgery: Blood tests.

ANESTHESIA—General anesthesia, local anesthesia with sedation.

DESCRIPTION OF OPERATION
* The following is a description of an endo-vascular repair of an abdominal aortic aneurysm.
* The femoral artery is punctured in the groin and a large cannula (tube) is placed.
* The blood is thinned with anticoagulants.
* The endovascular graft is inserted through the cannula in the groin and positioned across the dilated aneurysmal portion of the abdominal aorta.
* A balloon inside the graft is inflated to seat the graft.
* The catheters and cannula are removed. The hole in the femoral artery may need to be repaired.

POSSIBLE COMPLICATIONS
* Bleeding from the groin site.
* Kidney failure.
* Poor circulation to the intestines which can lead to gangrene.
* Poor circulation to the lower extremities.
* Incisional hernia.
* Rupture or bleeding from the aorta.

AVERAGE HOSPITAL STAY—Usually 1 to 2 days.

PROBABLE OUTCOME—Expect full recovery in 2 to 3 weeks with no recurrence of the aneurysm.

POSTOPERATIVE CARE

GENERAL MEASURES
* A hard ridge may form in the groin over the puncture site. As it heals, the ridge will gradually recede.
* Shower as usual. You may wash the incisions gently with mild soap. After showering, replace any dressings with a new dry dressing.

MEDICATION
* Your doctor may prescribe pain relievers. Use only as much as you need to be comfortable.
* You may use nonprescription pain relievers such as acetaminophen for minor pain. Ask your doctor if it is okay to take ibuprofen or aspirin.

ACTIVITY
* Start ambulating (walking) as soon as you are home. Avoid strenuous activity for 2-3 weeks.
* You may swim once all sutures are out.
* Resume sexual relations when comfortable and when advised by your surgeon.

DIET—No special diet.

CALL YOUR DOCTOR IF
* Pain, swelling, redness, drainage, or bleeding increases in the surgical area.
* You develop symptoms of infection including headache, muscle aches, dizziness, fever, or a general ill feeling.
* You develop nausea and vomiting or abdominal pain.
* Prolonged constipation occurs.
* Legs are cold, numb, or painful.
* New unexplained symptoms develop.

ENDOVASCULAR SURGERY

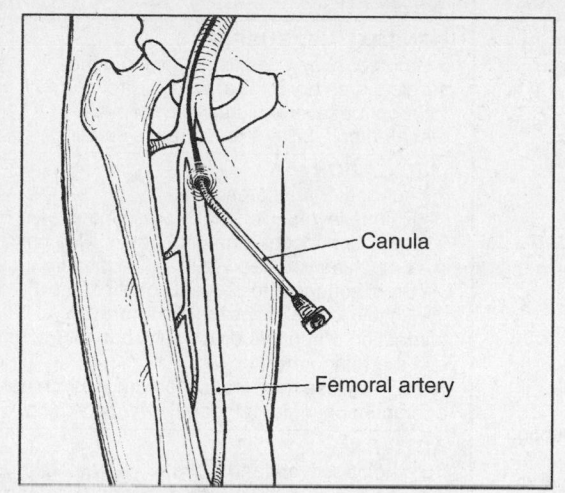

The femoral artery is accessed in the groin. A sheath or canula is placed to pass the graft.

Canula

Femoral artery

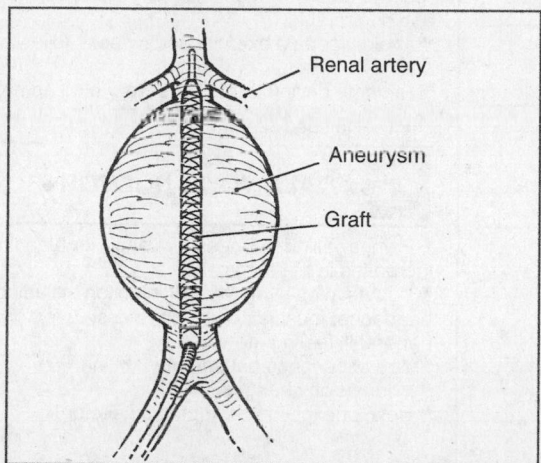

X-ray is used to position the graft in the exact location before the balloon is inflated.

Renal artery

Aneurysm

Graft

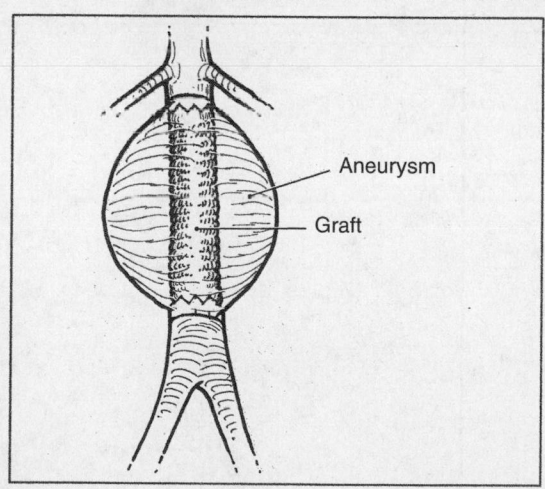

The graft is pressed into place inside the aorta when the balloon is inflated. The balloon is then deflated and removed allowing blood to flow through the graft.

Aneurysm

Graft

ENTROPION REPAIR

 ## GENERAL INFORMATION

DEFINITION—Shortening of excess tissue in the edge of the eyelid by removal of excess cartilage.

BODY PARTS INVOLVED—Skin and cartilage of the upper eyelid.

REASONS FOR SURGERY
- Improved appearance.
- Relief of redness, irritation and discomfort.

SURGICAL RISK INCREASES WITH
- Stress.
- Smoking.
- Poor nutrition.
- Recent or chronic illness.
- Alcoholism.
- Diabetes.
- Use of some prescription and nonprescription drugs. Inform your doctor of any drugs, medications, or vitamin and herb supplements you are using or have used in the last month.

 ## WHAT TO EXPECT

WHO OPERATES—Ophthalmologist.

WHERE PERFORMED—Hospital, ophthalmologist's office or outpatient surgical facility.

DIAGNOSTIC TESTS
- Before surgery: Blood and urine studies, eye examination.
- After surgery: Laboratory examination of removed tissue.

ANESTHESIA—Local anesthesia by injection.

DESCRIPTION OF OPERATION
- An incision is made in the eyelid.
- The cartilage is partially cut about midway between the two sides of the eyelid.
- A small amount of the cartilage is cut free of connective tissue and removed.
- The remaining cartilage is closed with silk sutures. The skin is closed over the cartilage with fine sutures that usually can be removed about 10 days after surgery.

POSSIBLE COMPLICATIONS—Surgical-wound infection.

AVERAGE HOSPITAL STAY—1 to 2 days.

PROBABLE OUTCOME—Expect complete healing without complications. Allow about 2 weeks for recovery from surgery.

 ## POSTOPERATIVE CARE

GENERAL MEASURES
- Bathe or shower as usual but keep the surgical area dry for 4 or 5 days after surgery.
- Sleep for several nights with the head elevated on 2 pillows to decrease swelling.

MEDICATION
- Your doctor may prescribe:
  - Pain relievers. Don't take prescription pain medication longer than 4 to 7 days. Use only as much as you need.
  - Stool softeners to prevent constipation.
  - Antibiotic eye drops to fight or prevent infection. Keep eye drops cold, but not frozen, in the refrigerator.
- You may use nonprescription drugs, such as acetaminophen, for minor pain. Avoid aspirin.

ACTIVITY
- To help recovery and aid your well-being, resume daily activities, including work, as soon as you are able.
- Avoid vigorous exercise for 2 weeks following surgery.
- Resume driving 2 days after returning home.

DIET—No special diet.

 ## CALL YOUR DOCTOR IF

- Pain, swelling, redness, drainage, or bleeding increases in the surgical area.
- You develop symptoms of infection including headache, muscle aches, dizziness, fever, or a general ill feeling.
- You experience nausea or vomiting.
- Your vision changes.
- New, unexplained symptoms develop.

ENTROPION REPAIR

An illustration of excess tissue in the edge of the eyelid.

Entropion

Incision site made in the skin overlying the eyelid.

Incision site

- The cartilage in the upper eyelid is cut about midway between the two sides of the eyelid and removed.
- Bleeding is controlled and skin is closed with small sutures, which can be removed in about 10 days following surgery.

EPISIOTOMY
(Perineotomy)

 GENERAL INFORMATION

DEFINITION—Surgical incision at the exterior of the vaginal opening to create enlargement.

BODY PARTS INVOLVED—Vagina, perineum.

REASONS FOR SURGERY—Usually performed during childbirth, just before the widest diameter of the baby's head passes through the outlet of the birth canal. This allows easier passage of the baby's head to reduce the potential of damage to the mother's vagina, bladder and rectum. Also helps expedite delivery in the case of forceps or vacuum use, or when there is maternal exhaustion or fetal distress, such as in a case of shoulder dystocia (when the shoulders of the baby get stuck after the head has already delivered).

SURGICAL RISK INCREASES WITH
- Obesity.
- Diabetes.

 WHAT TO EXPECT

WHO OPERATES—Obstetrician-gynecologist, family doctor, or midwife.

WHERE PERFORMED—Hospital or outpatient surgical facility.

DIAGNOSTIC TESTS
- Before surgery: Blood and urine studies.
- After surgery: Blood studies.

ANESTHESIA—Local anesthesia by injection.

DESCRIPTION OF OPERATION
- An incision is made in the perineum (the small area between the vaginal opening and the anus), just before the widest part of the baby's head is to be delivered. The size of the incision depends on how large an opening is required for the baby's head to pass through safely.
- The baby and placenta are delivered.
- The surgical area is repaired with sutures that will be absorbed by the body.

POSSIBLE COMPLICATIONS
- Excessive bleeding.
- Surgical-wound infection (rare).
- Inadvertent injury to sphincter or rectum (rare).

AVERAGE HOSPITAL STAY—2 days.

PROBABLE OUTCOME—Expect complete healing without complications. Allow about 6 weeks for recovery from childbirth.

 POSTOPERATIVE CARE

GENERAL MEASURES
- Shower as usual. You may wash the incision gently with mild, unscented soap.
- Cleanse the surgical area with warm (not hot) water after urination or bowel movements.
- Use ice packs made of gauze soaked in ice-cold witch hazel to relieve discomfort during the first 24 hours after delivery.

MEDICATION
- Your doctor may prescribe:
  - Stool softeners to prevent constipation.
  - Antibiotics to fight infection.
- You may use nonprescription drugs, such as acetaminophen, for minor pain. Avoid aspirin.

ACTIVITY
- Follow your doctor's advice on resuming, or beginning, a postpartum exercise program.
- Resume driving 10 days after returning home.
- Resume sexual relations when your doctor determines that healing is complete (usually about 3 to 6 weeks).

DIET—Eating a high-fiber diet will help prevent constipation, which is common after childbirth. Increase your fluid intake as you increase your fiber intake.

 CALL YOUR DOCTOR IF

- Pain, swelling, redness, drainage, or bleeding increases in the surgical area.
- You develop symptoms of infection including headache, muscle aches, dizziness, fever, or a general ill feeling.
- You experience nausea, vomiting, constipation, or abdominal swelling.
- New, unexplained symptoms develop.

EPISIOTOMY
(Perineotomy)

Incision site

Baby's head

Anus

- This view illustrates a female patient with extended legs in stirrups on an examining table to allow examination of the genital area.
- The female genital area with a baby's head crowning at the entrance to the vagina and the incision site for the episiotomy.

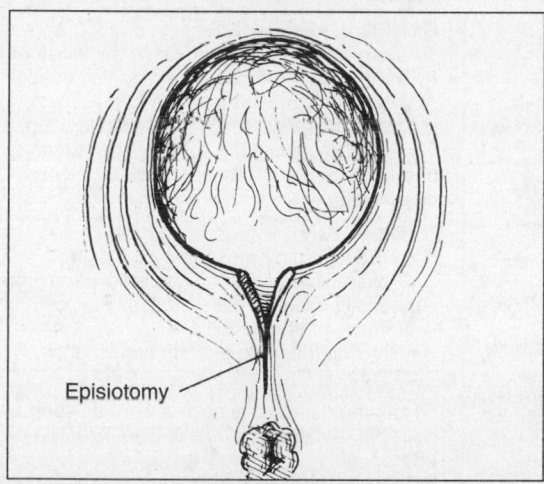

Episiotomy

Incision is made in the perineum just before the widest part of the baby's head is delivered.

After the baby and placenta have been delivered, the episiotomy site is repaired with absorbable sutures.

ESOPHAGECTOMY

GENERAL INFORMATION

DEFINITION—Removal of part of the esophagus, the tubular passage from the back of the throat to the stomach.

BODY PARTS INVOLVED—Esophagus, stomach, colon (sometimes).

REASONS FOR SURGERY
- Cancer of the esophagus (see Esophagus Cancer in Illness section).
- Burns and scarring of the esophagus.
- Opening a closure of the esophagus in a newborn (usually an inherited defect).

SURGICAL RISK INCREASES WITH
- Adults over 60, newborns and infants.
- Obesity, smoking, poor nutrition.
- Excess alcohol consumption.
- Chronic or recent illness, especially lung disease, pneumonia, or diabetes.
- Use of some prescription and nonprescription drugs. Inform your doctor of any drugs, medications, or vitamin and herb supplements you are using or have used in the last month.

WHAT TO EXPECT

WHO OPERATES—General surgeon or thoracic surgeon.

WHERE PERFORMED—Hospital.

DIAGNOSTIC TESTS
- Before surgery: Blood and urine tests, x-rays of chest and upper gastrointestinal tract, esophagogram, esophagoscopy, bronchoscopy (see Glossary for all).
- After surgery: Blood and urine studies, x-rays of chest and upper gastrointestinal tract.

ANESTHESIA—General anesthesia by injection and inhalation with an airway tube placed in the windpipe.

DESCRIPTION OF OPERATION
- Incisions are made in the abdomen and chest to expose the esophagus.
- The esophagus is isolated and examined.
- Abnormal tissues are removed. If the surgery is performed to treat cancer, nearby lymph glands are also removed.
- The bottom end of the remaining part of the esophagus is joined with the stomach. Sometimes the colon is used to bridge the gap.
- The chest and abdomen are closed in layers. The skin is closed with sutures or clips, which can usually be removed about 1 week later.
- During the operation, a thin, plastic tube (called a jejunostomy tube) may be placed in your intestine and brought to the outside. It will be used to provide you with nourishment until you are able to take food by mouth.

- The operation can sometimes be done through an abdominal incision and a small incision at the base of the neck.

POSSIBLE COMPLICATIONS
- Excessive bleeding; blood clots.
- Surgical-wound infection; incisional hernia.
- Leakage of digestive material from new junction of esophagus and intestinal tract.
- Scarring at operation site prevents normal passage of food and fluids.
- Pneumonia.

AVERAGE HOSPITAL STAY—7 to 14 days.

PROBABLE OUTCOME—If the surgery was performed to treat cancer, the 5-year survival is about 50%. If the surgery was performed for other reasons, expect complete healing without complications. Allow 8 to 12 weeks for recovery from surgery.

POSTOPERATIVE CARE

GENERAL MEASURES
- A hard ridge should form along the incisions. As they heal, the ridges will gradually recede.
- Shower as usual after you are home. You may wash the incision gently with mild soap.
- Move and elevate legs often while resting in bed to decrease the likelihood of deep-vein blood clots.

MEDICATION
- Your doctor may prescribe:
  - Pain relievers. Don't take prescription pain medication longer than 4 to 7 days. Use only as much as you need.
  - Stool softeners to prevent constipation.

ACTIVITY
- Resume daily activities and work as soon as possible. Avoid vigorous exercise for 12 weeks after surgery.
- Resume driving 3 weeks after returning home.
- Resume sexual relations when able.

DIET—Nothing by mouth for the first 6 to 7 days to allow healing of the connection between the esophagus and the stomach. Then, start with liquids and gradually progress to a well-balanced diet to promote healing. Avoid coffee, tea, cocoa, cola drinks, alcoholic beverages, and any food or spice that cause indigestion.

CALL YOUR DOCTOR IF

- Pain, swelling, redness, drainage, or bleeding increases in the surgical area.
- You develop symptoms of infection including headache, muscle aches, dizziness, fever, or a general ill feeling.
- You experience excessive weakness or black, tarry stools.

ESOPHAGECTOMY

An illustration of the sites where incisions are made in order to expose the esophagus and the stomach.

Incision sites

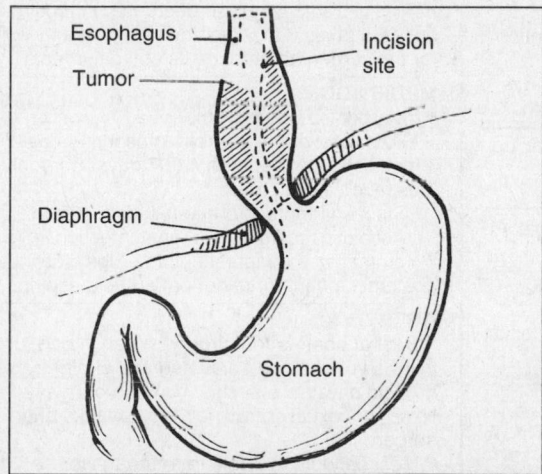

Esophagus

Incision site

Tumor

Diaphragm

Stomach

A portion of the esophagus is removed on both sides of the tumor or other defect.

The bottom end of the remaining part of the esophagus is joined with the stomach. Sometimes the colon is used to replace the missing portion of the esophagus.

FACE LIFT & BLEPHAROPLASTY

GENERAL INFORMATION

DEFINITION
- Face lift (rhytidectomy): Removal of excess skin, fat and tissue from the face in order to tighten sagging skin and eliminate wrinkles, jowls, or a double chin.
- Blepharoplasty: Removal of excess fat and skin from around the eyelids to reduce puffiness, bags under the eyes, and wrinkles.

BODY PARTS INVOLVED—Skin and underlying tissue of the face and eyelids.

REASONS FOR SURGERY
- Improved appearance of the face.
- Improved appearance and function of the eyelids.

SURGICAL RISK INCREASES WITH
- Obesity; smoking; poor nutrition.
- Recent or chronic illness.
- Diabetes.
- Alcoholism.
- Use of some prescription and nonprescription drugs. Inform your doctor of any drugs, medications, or vitamin and herb supplements you are using or have used in the last month.

WHAT TO EXPECT

WHO OPERATES—Plastic and reconstructive surgeon.

WHERE PERFORMED—Doctor's office, outpatient surgical facility, or hospital.

DIAGNOSTIC TESTS
- Before surgery: Blood and urine studies.
- After surgery: Blood studies.

ANESTHESIA
- Local anesthesia by injection.
- General anesthesia by injection and inhalation with an airway tube placed in the windpipe.

DESCRIPTION OF OPERATION
- A number of different face lift procedures are available. Your doctor will explain the options.
- Usually a face lift involves incisions that are made where scarring will be less visible.
- Care is taken to clamp and tie tiny bleeding vessels during the procedure to prevent collection of scar tissue under the skin.
- Flaps of skin are cut away around the eyes and face. The skin is separated from underlying tissues. The muscles are tightened and excess fat and tissue are removed.
- The skin is closed with fine sutures, which usually can be removed about 1 week after surgery. Drains may be placed in the incision and left for a day.
- Compression dressings are applied to reduce swelling and bleeding.

POSSIBLE COMPLICATIONS
- Excessive bleeding; blood clots.
- Surgical-wound infection.
- Collection of blood (hematoma) under areas where skin has been removed.
- Scarring or facial muscles are asymmetrical.
- Facial nerve damage.

AVERAGE HOSPITAL STAY—0 to 3 days.

PROBABLE OUTCOME—Expect complete healing and improved appearance without complications. Allow about 6 weeks or more for recovery from surgery.

POSTOPERATIVE CARE

GENERAL MEASURES
- Dressings or wraps will be applied.
- Shower as usual the day after or as directed.
- Apply nonprescription antibiotic ointment if prescribed.
- Bruising and swelling are to be expected, and may take 2 to 3 weeks to decrease. In most cases, it takes 3 to 6 months following a face lift for the surgery to produce its optimal effects.

MEDICATION
- Your doctor may prescribe:
  - Pain relievers. Don't take prescription pain medication longer than 4 to 7 days. Use only as much as you need.
  - Stool softeners to prevent constipation.
  - Antibiotics to fight or prevent infection.
- You may use nonprescription drugs, such as acetaminophen, for minor pain. Avoid aspirin.

ACTIVITY
- Rest at home after surgery. When in bed, use pillows to keep head elevated and straight.
- Avoid physical exercise, bending or heavy lifting, or sexual activity for 1 to 2 weeks after surgery.
- Most patients are able to return to work in 7 to 10 days.
- Resume driving 3 to 7 days after surgery or as directed.

DIET—Liquid to soft diet for the first few days after surgery. Then, no special diet.

CALL YOUR DOCTOR IF

- Pain, swelling, redness, drainage, or bleeding increases in the surgical area.
- You develop symptoms of infection including headache, muscle aches, dizziness, fever, or a general ill feeling.
- You experience nausea or vomiting.
- New, unexplained symptoms develop.

FACE LIFT & BLEPHAROPLASTY

Incision site

Flaps of skin cut away around the eyes and face. Excess tissue is removed from underlying areas and excess skin is trimmed away.

Skin is closed with fine sutures.

Incision sites

An illustration of excessive tissue surrounding the eye and the incision sites generally used.

FIBROID TUMOR REMOVAL
(Myomectomy)

GENERAL INFORMATION

DEFINITION—Removal of fibroid tumors (leiomyoma, myoma) from the uterus through an incision in the lower abdomen.

BODY PARTS INVOLVED—Uterus.

REASONS FOR SURGERY
- Pelvic pain or back pain.
- Pressure on the bladder.
- Abnormal uterine bleeding; anemia.
- Difficulty in becoming pregnant.
- Discomfort with sexual intercourse.

SURGICAL RISK INCREASES WITH
- Obesity.
- Smoking.
- Poor nutrition, especially inadequate iron intake that has led to anemia.
- Recent or chronic illness.
- Diabetes.
- Use of some prescription and nonprescription drugs. Inform your doctor of any drugs, medications, or vitamin and herb supplements you are using or have used in the last month.

WHAT TO EXPECT

WHO OPERATES—General surgeon or obstetrician-gynecologist.

WHERE PERFORMED—Hospital.

DIAGNOSTIC TESTS
- Before surgery: Blood studies; dilatation and curettage of the uterus (D & C); laparoscopy; x-ray of abdomen; barium-enema x-rays; intravenous pyelogram (see Glossary for all).
- After surgery: Blood studies.

ANESTHESIA—General anesthesia by injection and inhalation with an airway tube placed in the windpipe.

DESCRIPTION OF OPERATION
- One or more incisions are made in the lower abdomen.
- The muscles are separated and connective tissues are cut free to expose the uterus.
- Fibroid tumors are located and each tumor is removed separately, and each excision is repaired.
- The internal structures are closed in layers.
- The skin is closed with sutures or skin clips, which can be removed about 4 to 7 days later.

POSSIBLE COMPLICATIONS
- Excessive bleeding.
- Surgical-wound infection.
- Recurrence of the tumor.
- Perforation of the uterus or bowel during surgery.
- Bowel obstruction.

AVERAGE HOSPITAL STAY—2 to 3 days.

PROBABLE OUTCOME—The uterus is left intact, and you will still have menstrual periods. Your next period may be heavier than usual but should occur at about the expected time. Allow about 6 weeks for recovery from surgery.

POSTOPERATIVE CARE

GENERAL MEASURES
- A hard ridge should form along the incision. As it heals, the ridge will gradually recede.
- Shower as usual once at home. You may wash the incision gently with a mild soap.
- Wear sanitary pads to absorb blood.

MEDICATION
- Your doctor may prescribe:
  - Pain relievers. Don't take prescription pain medication longer than 4 to 7 days. Use only as much as you need.
  - Vaginal creams or medicated douches, if vaginal discharge develops an unpleasant odor.
  - Antibiotics to fight or prevent infection.
- You may use nonprescription drugs, such as acetaminophen, for minor pain. Avoid aspirin.

ACTIVITY
- To help recovery and aid your well-being, resume daily activities, including work, as soon as you are able.
- Resume driving about 2 weeks after surgery.
- Resume sexual relations when your doctor determines that healing is complete.

DIET—Clear liquid diet until the gastrointestinal tract functions again. Then eat a well-balanced diet to promote healing.

CALL YOUR DOCTOR IF

- You experience vaginal bleeding that soaks more than 1 pad per hour.
- You develop symptoms of infection including headache, muscle aches, dizziness, fever, or a general ill feeling.
- You have abdominal swelling or severe abdominal pain.
- The urge to urinate frequently persists longer than 1 month.
- Excessive vaginal discharge persists beyond 1 month after surgery.
- Symptoms recur after surgery.
- New, unexplained symptoms develop.

FIBROID TUMOR REMOVAL
(Myomectomy)

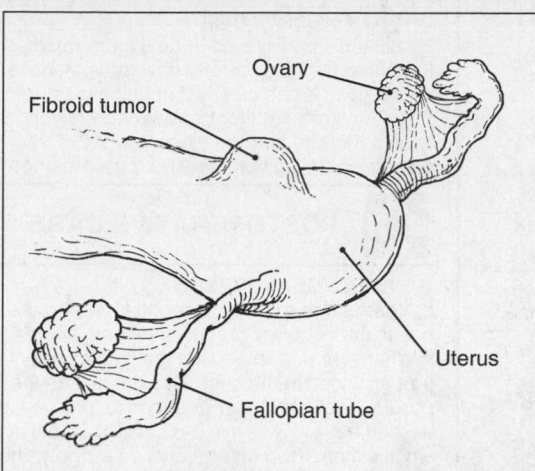

Fibroid tumor

Ovary

Uterus

Fallopian tube

In this example, the fibroid tumor is on the front surface of the uterus.

After the skin has been incised and muscles retracted, the uterus and fibroid tumor are visible through the incision site.

Fibroid removed

The fibroid tumor is removed and the surgical site is repaired with absorbable sutures.

FRACTURE REPAIR
(Fracture Reduction)

GENERAL INFORMATION

DEFINITION—Realigning ends of a fractured (broken) bone. Open reduction is when an incision is made to fix the bone fragments. Closed reduction is when the bones are realigned by traction and fixed externally by a cast or splint.

BODY PARTS INVOLVED—Any bone in the body.

REASONS FOR SURGERY—Restoration of normal position and function of a broken bone.

SURGICAL RISK INCREASES WITH
- Adults over 60.
- Obesity; smoking; poor nutrition; alcoholism.
- Recent or chronic illness.
- Diabetes.
- Use of some prescription and nonprescription drugs. Inform your doctor of any drugs, medications, or vitamin and herb supplements you are using or have used in the last month.

WHAT TO EXPECT

WHO OPERATES—Orthopedist, general surgeon, or family doctor.

WHERE PERFORMED—Hospital, outpatient facility, doctor's office, or emergency room.

DIAGNOSTIC TESTS
- Before surgery: Blood and urine studies; x-ray of affected area.
- During surgery: X-rays.
- After surgery: X-rays through cast or splint to determine if rejoined pieces remain in good position for healing.

ANESTHESIA
- Local anesthesia by injection.
- General anesthesia by injection and inhalation with an airway tube placed in the windpipe.

DESCRIPTION OF OPERATION
- In an open reduction, one or more incisions may be made in the skin over the fracture.
- The bone fragments are aligned as close as possible to their normal position.
- Sometimes, metal pins, screws or plates are used to re-join the areas of the fracture.
- Once the broken ends of bone are set, the affected part is kept rigid with a cast or splint.

POSSIBLE COMPLICATIONS
- Excessive bleeding.
- Improper alignment of joined bone ends.
- Failure of bones to heal (non-union).
- Pressure on nearby nerves, nerve damage.
- Infection.

AVERAGE HOSPITAL STAY—0 to 6 days.

PROBABLE OUTCOME
- Children's bones tend to heal more rapidly. Fractured bones of elderly patients may never heal properly, particularly if nutrition is poor.
- The time required for healing depends on the type of fracture and the extent of tissue damage. Healing time may be quite prolonged.

POSTOPERATIVE CARE

GENERAL MEASURES
- A hard ridge will form along the incision. As it heals, the ridge will gradually recede.
- Whenever possible, raise the limb or body part enclosed in the cast. This decreases the possibility of swelling. For example, prop a leg cast on a pillow when in bed, and on a footstool when sitting. Prop an arm cast on a pillow on your chest.
- Follow medical instructions for care of the cast or splint.

MEDICATION
- Your doctor may prescribe:
  - Pain relievers. Don't take prescription pain medication longer than 4 to 7 days. Use only as much as you need.
  - Antibiotics to fight or prevent infection.
- You may use nonprescription drugs, such as acetaminophen, for minor pain. Avoid aspirin.

ACTIVITY
- Special exercises, physical therapy, or rehabilitation therapy may be needed. Follow all medical instructions to assure complete healing.
- Crutches, a walker, or other mechanical aids may be used during recovery.
- Resume driving when your doctor determines that it is safe to do so.
- To help recovery and aid your well-being, resume daily activities, including work, as soon as you are able.

DIET—Eat a well-balanced diet to promote healing. Increase fiber and fluid intake if constipation occurs due to decreased activity.

CALL YOUR DOCTOR IF

- You experience severe, persistent pain under the cast.
- You observe color change, coldness, or numbness in tissues beyond the cast.
- Tissue swelling is greater than before the cast was applied.
- You develop symptoms of infection including headache, muscle aches, dizziness, fever, or a general ill feeling.
- New, unexplained symptoms develop.

FRACTURE REPAIR
(Fracture Reduction)

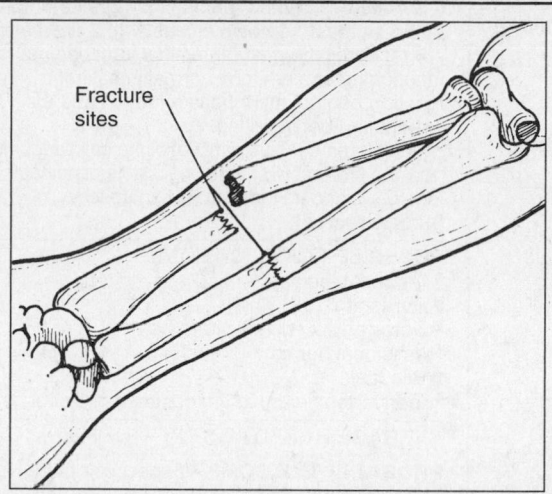

An illustration of fractures of the forearm bones.

Fracture sites

When possible, the fractured bone ends are aligned by manipulation from the outside. If this cannot be done, the bone fragments can be aligned by surgical procedures to produce the same result.

Bones aligned

After the broken ends of bone are aligned, the affected part is held in place with a plaster cast or splint.

Cast

GALLBLADDER REMOVAL
(Cholecystectomy, Open)

 GENERAL INFORMATION

DEFINITION—Removal of the gallbladder though an incision in the abdomen.

BODY PARTS INVOLVED—Gallbladder, bile ducts.

REASONS FOR SURGERY
- Gallstones.
- Suspected gallbladder tumors.
- Chronic gallbladder infection.
- Sudden, severe infection of the gallbladder that does not respond rapidly to treatment.

SURGICAL RISK INCREASES WITH
- Obesity, smoking.
- Recent or chronic illness.
- Alcoholism, cirrhosis of the liver, diabetes, heart disease, or chronic obstructive pulmonary disease (COPD).
- Use of some prescription and nonprescription drugs. Inform your doctor of any drugs, medications, or vitamin and herb supplements you are using or have used in the last month.

 WHAT TO EXPECT

WHO OPERATES—General surgeon.

WHERE PERFORMED—Hospital.

DIAGNOSTIC TESTS
- Before surgery: Blood studies, x-rays of the gallbladder, ultrasound, ECG, radionuclide excretion scan (see Glossary for all).
- During surgery: Cholangiogram (see Glossary).
- After surgery: Blood studies.

ANESTHESIA—General anesthesia by injection and inhalation with an airway tube placed in the windpipe.

DESCRIPTION OF OPERATION
- An incision is made under the right rib cage or down the center of the abdomen. Abdominal muscles are separated to expose abdominal organs, which are inspected for undetected disease. Other surgeries may be performed at this time.
- The gallbladder is cut free and removed from under the liver.
- A cholangiogram is done to determine if gallstones are lodged in the bile ducts. If necessary, the gallstones are removed.
- The incision is closed with sutures, skin clips or staples, which usually can be removed about 1 week after surgery. Occasionally, a drainage tube is left in place to drain bile around the liver. If stones are removed from the bile duct, a second tube (T-tube) is placed to drain this duct and allow x-rays to be taken later of the bile duct.

- Sometimes, a tube running through the nose to the stomach remains at least 1 to 2 days after surgery until the gastrointestinal tract begins functioning again. Once normal intestinal function begins, the tube is removed and the patient can begin eating.
- Note: Laparoscopic removal of the gallbladder is now the preferable surgery in suitable candidates (see Gallbladder Removal By Laparoscopy in Surgery section).

POSSIBLE COMPLICATIONS
- Internal bleeding.
- Peritonitis.
- Surgical-wound infection.
- Incisional hernia.
- Bile leak.
- Inadvertent injury to the common bile duct.

AVERAGE HOSPITAL STAY—3 to 5 days.

PROBABLE OUTCOME—Expect complete healing without complications. The surgery relieves symptoms in 90% of patients. Allow about 6 weeks for recovery from surgery.

 POSTOPERATIVE CARE

GENERAL MEASURES
- A hard ridge should form along the incision. As it heals, the ridge will gradually recede.
- Shower as usual after you are home. You may wash the incision gently with mild, unscented soap.

MEDICATION
- Your doctor may prescribe pain relievers. Don't take prescription pain medication longer than 4 to 7 days. Use only as much as you need.
- You may use nonprescription drugs, such as acetaminophen, to relieve minor pain. Avoid aspirin.

ACTIVITY
- Take short walks as soon as possible.
- Resume driving 3 weeks after returning home.
- Resume sexual relations when able.

DIET—Your doctor will prescribe a diet.

 CALL YOUR DOCTOR IF

- Pain, swelling, redness, drainage, or bleeding increases in the surgical area.
- You develop symptoms of infection including headache, muscle aches, dizziness, fever, or a general ill feeling.
- You experience constipation, abdominal swelling, or unrelieved hiccups.
- You develop signs of jaundice (yellow skin or eyes).
- New, unexplained symptoms develop.

GALLBLADDER REMOVAL
(Cholecystectomy, Open)

An illustration of the liver and gallbladder located just under the right rib cage. The liver must be retracted upward in order to expose the gallbladder.

Gallbladder is cut free and removed. Catheter is inserted into bile duct to inject contrast dye for a cholangiography.

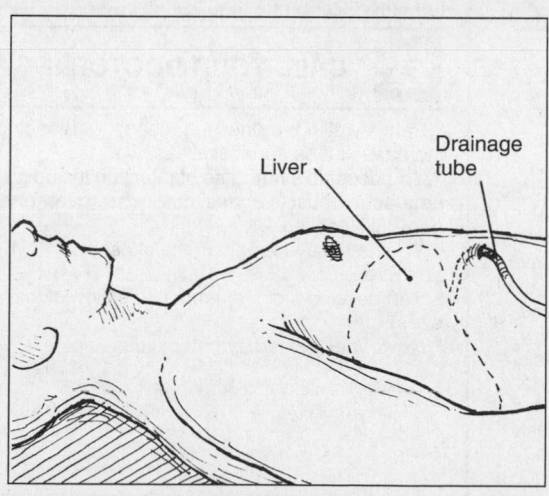

Occasionally, a drainage tube is left in place to drain bile around the liver.

GALLBLADDER REMOVAL BY LAPAROSCOPY
(Cholecystectomy, Laparoscopic)

 GENERAL INFORMATION

DEFINITION—Removal of the gallbladder with a laparoscope (a lighted scope attached to a video camera).

BODY PARTS INVOLVED—Gallbladder, bile ducts, liver.

REASONS FOR SURGERY
• Treatment of gallstones.
• Acute inflammation of the gallbladder.
• Benign and malignant tumors of the gallbladder.
• Chronic gallbladder infection.

SURGICAL RISK INCREASES WITH
• Obesity, smoking.
• Excess alcohol consumption.
• Recent or chronic illness.
• Cirrhosis of the liver.
• Diabetes.
• Use of some prescription and nonprescription drugs. Inform your doctor of any drugs, medications, or vitamin and herb supplements you are using or have used in the last month.

 WHAT TO EXPECT

WHO OPERATES—General surgeon.

WHERE PERFORMED—Hospital, outpatient surgical facility.

DIAGNOSTIC TESTS
• Before surgery: Blood studies, x-rays, ECG, ultrasound, radionuclide excretion scan (see Glossary for all).
• After surgery: Blood tests.

ANESTHESIA—General anesthesia by injection and inhalation with an airway tube placed in the windpipe.

DESCRIPTION OF OPERATION
• Four small incisions are made in the abdomen. A small needle is inserted into one incision to inflate the abdomen with carbon dioxide so the surgeon can see clearly.
• The laparoscope is inserted into one incision near the naval and the surgeon looks at a video monitor to see inside the abdomen. Surgical instruments are inserted into the other incisions.
• The gallbladder and the ducts running from it are located and separated. The gallbladder duct is clipped and the gallbladder is cut away and removed through one of the small incisions.
• The laparoscope and surgical instruments are removed and the carbon dioxide is allowed to escape from the abdomen.
• Small sutures under the skin and an adhesive bandage are used to close the wounds.

POSSIBLE COMPLICATIONS
• Surgical wound infection.
• Inadvertent injury to the common bile duct or to the small intestine.
• Bile leak.
• Excessive bleeding, blood clots.
• Unexpected findings such as adhesions, severe infection, or inflammation may make it necessary to stop the laparoscopy procedure and use an open surgical procedure (see Gallbladder Removal in Surgery section).

AVERAGE HOSPITAL STAY—0 to 2 days.

PROBABLE OUTCOME—Expect complete healing without complications. Allow 1 to 2 weeks for recovery from surgery.

 POSTOPERATIVE CARE

GENERAL MEASURES—Shower as usual. You may wash the incision gently with mild, unscented soap. After the shower, replace any wet dressings with clean, dry ones.

MEDICATION
• Your doctor may prescribe pain relievers. Don't take prescription pain medication longer than 4 to 7 days. Use only as much as you need.
• You may use nonprescription drugs, such as acetaminophen, for minor pain. Avoid aspirin.

ACTIVITY
• Resume work and normal activity as soon as possible.
• Avoid vigorous activity for 6 weeks after surgery.

DIET—The use of a general anesthetic and abdominal surgery may require a liquid or soft diet for a few days. Your doctor will advise you if this is necessary. Generally, you should avoid fatty foods for a month following surgery.

 CALL YOUR DOCTOR IF

• Pain, swelling, redness, drainage, or bleeding increases in the surgical areas.
• You develop symptoms of infection including headache, muscle aches, dizziness, fever, or a general ill feeling.
• You have severe pain in the chest or abdomen.
• You develop signs of jaundice (yellow skin or eyes).
• New, unexplained symptoms develop.

GALLBLADDER REMOVAL BY LAPAROSCOPY
(Cholecystectomy, Laparoscopic)

Carbon dioxide is used to inflate the abdomen to separate the organs.

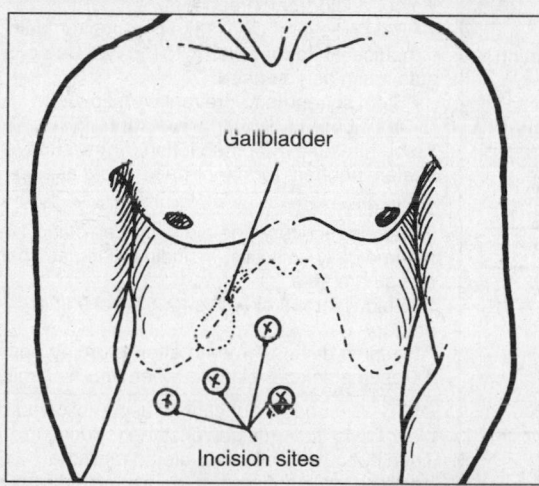

Small incisions are made in the abdomen to allow insertion of the laparoscope and surgical instruments.

The gallbladder is held in position while the cystic duct is separated and clipped. The gallbladder is cut away and removed.

GASTROENTEROSTOMY FOR PYLORIC OBSTRUCTION

GENERAL INFORMATION

DEFINITION—Creation of an artificial passage between the stomach and the small intestine to bypass obstructions caused by ulcer scar tissue.

BODY PARTS INVOLVED—Stomach, duodenum, jejunum (usually).

REASONS FOR SURGERY—Restoration of normal function of the gastrointestinal tract.

SURGICAL RISK INCREASES WITH
- Adults over 60.
- Newborns and infants.
- Stress.
- Obesity.
- Smoking.
- Excess alcohol consumption.
- Poor nutrition.
- Recent or chronic illness.
- Diabetes.
- Use of some prescription and nonprescription drugs. Inform your doctor of any drugs, medications, or vitamin and herb supplements you are using or have used in the last month.

WHAT TO EXPECT

WHO OPERATES—General surgeon.

WHERE PERFORMED—Hospital.

DIAGNOSTIC TESTS
- Before surgery: Blood and urine studies, gastroscopy, x-rays of upper gastrointestinal tract, serum electrolytes (see Glossary).
- After surgery: Blood and urine studies.

ANESTHESIA—General anesthesia by injection and inhalation with an airway tube placed in the windpipe.

DESCRIPTION OF OPERATION
- An incision is made in the upper abdomen.
- The abdominal muscles are separated to expose the abdominal organs, which are inspected for any undetected disease. Other surgeries may be performed at this time.
- The stomach and jejunum are isolated. A small opening is made in each, and they are joined with sutures at the openings.
- The abdominal muscles are closed with sutures. The skin is closed with sutures or clips, which usually can be removed in about 1 week.

POSSIBLE COMPLICATIONS
- Excessive bleeding, surgical-wound infection.
- Spillage of stomach contents into abdomen.
- Slow digestion and emptying of the stomach.
- Incisional hernia.

AVERAGE HOSPITAL STAY—7 to 10 days.

PROBABLE OUTCOME—Expect complete healing without complications. Allow about 6 weeks for recovery from surgery.

POSTOPERATIVE CARE

GENERAL MEASURES
- A hard ridge should form along the incision. As it heals, the ridge will gradually recede.
- Shower as usual. Avoid baths until the incision has completely healed. You may wash the incision gently with mild, unscented soap. After showering, replace any wet dressings with clean, dry ones.
- Move and elevate legs often while resting in bed to decrease the likelihood of deep-vein blood clots.

MEDICATION
- Your doctor may prescribe:
  - Pain relievers. Don't take prescription pain medication longer than 4 to 7 days. Use only as much as you need.
  - Stool softeners to prevent constipation.
  - Antibiotics to fight or prevent infection.
- You may use nonprescription drugs, such as acetaminophen, for minor pain. Avoid aspirin.

ACTIVITY
- To help recovery and aid your well-being, resume daily activities, including work, as soon as you are able.
- Avoid vigorous exercise for 6 weeks after surgery.
- Resume driving 1 month after returning home.
- Resume sexual relations when you feel able.

DIET—Nasogastric suction is used, followed by clear liquid diet until bowel starts to function. Then eat a well-balanced diet to promote healing. Avoid coffee, tea, cocoa, cola drinks, alcoholic beverages, and any food or spice that causes indigestion.

CALL YOUR DOCTOR IF

- Pain, swelling, redness, drainage, or bleeding increases in the surgical area.
- You develop symptoms of infection including headache, muscle aches, dizziness, fever, or a general ill feeling.
- You experience nausea, vomiting, constipation, abdominal swelling, or black, tarry stools.
- New, unexplained symptoms develop.

GASTROENTEROSTOMY FOR PYLORIC OBSTRUCTION

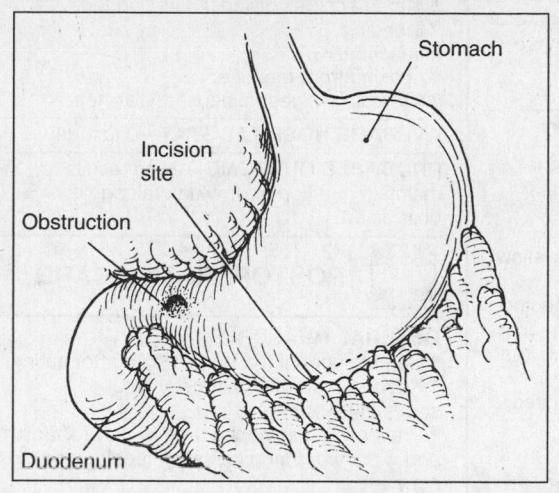

An illustration of a typical obstruction site in the lower end of the stomach, just before the duodenum (beginning of the first part of the intestine).

After the stomach and a small loop of small intestine are isolated, an opening is made in each.

The cut end of the stomach is then joined with the surgically opened part of the jejunum, once again establishing a clear channel for the passage of food and fluids.

GASTROSTOMY

GENERAL INFORMATION

DEFINITION—Making a surgical opening into the stomach for placement of a feeding or drainage tube.

BODY PARTS INVOLVED—Stomach, skin, structures of the abdominal wall.

REASONS FOR SURGERY
- Prevention of pneumonia in patients with swallowing disorders.
- Provide nutrition to those who cannot swallow.
- Blockage of esophagus.
- To provide access to the stomach for feeding or drainage of stomach contents. It is frequently used in patients who cannot eat or will not eat adequate amounts of food, or to drain the stomach when prolonged drainage is required.

SURGICAL RISK INCREASES WITH
- Obesity, poor nutrition.
- Recent or chronic illness, especially chronic lung disease.
- Diabetes.
- Excess alcohol consumption.
- Use of some prescription and nonprescription drugs. Inform your doctor of any drugs, medications, or vitamin and herb supplements you are using or have used in the last month.

WHAT TO EXPECT

WHO OPERATES—General surgeon or gastroenterologist.

WHERE PERFORMED—Hospital or outpatient surgical facility.

DIAGNOSTIC TESTS—Before surgery: Blood and urine studies, x-rays of gastrointestinal tract, endoscopy (see Glossary).

ANESTHESIA
- Local anesthesia by injection.
- General anesthesia by injection and inhalation with an airway tube placed in the windpipe.

DESCRIPTION OF OPERATION
- An incision is made in the abdominal wall.
- The stomach is isolated and an opening is made into it.
- The tube (usually polyvinyl chloride or rubber) is secured by sutures to hold it in place. The tube is held within the stomach by a balloon that is filled with water.
- The other end of the tube is pulled to the outside through a separate puncture site.
- The abdominal incision is closed and the tube is stitched to the skin.
- The procedure may also be accomplished with gastroscopy (see Gastrostomy, Percutaneous Endoscopic in Surgery section).

POSSIBLE COMPLICATIONS
- Skin irritation around the gastrostomy tube.
- Tube becomes dislodged or clogged.
- Bleeding.
- Infection.
- Leaking from the tube.
- Cramping, bloating, nausea, diarrhea.

AVERAGE HOSPITAL STAY—0 to 1 day.

PROBABLE OUTCOME—Good results to maintain nutrition or provide drainage if obstructed.

POSTOPERATIVE CARE

GENERAL MEASURES
- Remain upright for 1/2 to 1 hour after eating.
- Keep skin around gastrostomy tube scrupulously clean.
- Prevent dislodging the tube by careful taping and vigilance during dressing, feeding and activities.
- If used for drainage, make sure gastrostomy tube doesn't become obstructed (use water irrigations).
- Shower as usual after you are home. You may wash the incision gently with mild, unscented soap. After showering, replace any wet dressings with clean, dry ones.
- Move and elevate legs often while resting in bed to decrease the likelihood of deep-vein blood clots.

MEDICATION
- Your doctor may prescribe:
  - Pain relievers.
  - Don't take prescription pain medication longer than 4 to 7 days. Use only as much as you need.
- You may use nonprescription drugs, such as acetaminophen, for minor pain. Avoid aspirin.

ACTIVITY—Resume normal activity as soon as possible to promote healing.

DIET
- Your doctor will prescribe a diet.
- Vitamin and mineral supplements (sometimes).

CALL YOUR DOCTOR IF

- Pain, swelling, redness, drainage, or bleeding increases in the surgical area.
- You develop symptoms of infection including headache, muscle aches, dizziness, fever, or a general ill feeling.
- You experience constipation, abdominal swelling, nausea, or vomiting.
- The skin around the tube becomes raw or irritated.
- The tube falls out.
- New, unexplained symptoms develop.

GASTROSTOMY

An illustration of the abdomen with proposed incision site for gastrostomy.

Stomach

Incision site

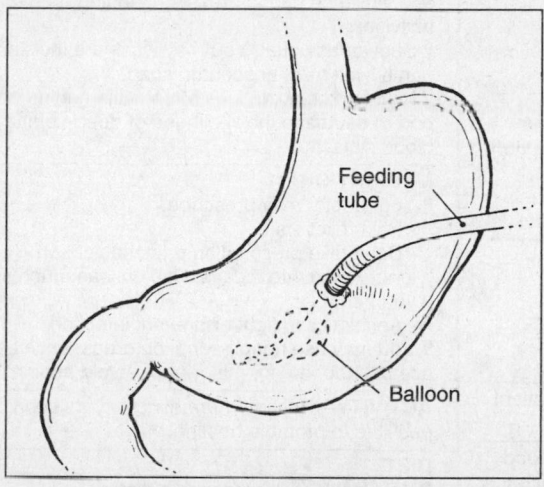

After the stomach has been located, a small opening is made into it and the stomach tube is pushed into the cavity of the stomach. The tube is secured by a balloon within the stomach.

Feeding tube

Balloon

The other end of the tube is pulled to the outside through a separate small incision.

GASTROSTOMY, PERCUTANEOUS ENDOSCOPIC (P.E.G. Procedure)

 GENERAL INFORMATION

DEFINITION—Technique for placing a feeding tube without having to perform an open laparotomy (operation on the abdomen). This procedure is less costly and time consuming than a surgical gastrostomy (see in Surgery section).

BODY PARTS INVOLVED—Stomach, skin, structures of the abdominal wall.

REASONS FOR SURGERY
- To provide nutrition for those who cannot swallow.
- To provide nutrition to those who cannot or will not eat adequate amounts of food.
- Blockage of esophagus.
- Prevention of pneumonia in patients with swallowing disorders.

SURGICAL RISK INCREASES WITH
- Stress, obesity, poor nutrition.
- Recent or chronic illness, especially chronic lung disease.
- Diabetes.
- Excess alcohol consumption.
- Use of some prescription and nonprescription drugs. Inform your doctor of any drugs, medications, or vitamin and herb supplements you are using or have used in the last month.

 WHAT TO EXPECT

WHO OPERATES—General surgeon or gastroenterologist.

WHERE PERFORMED—Hospital or outpatient surgical facility.

DIAGNOSTIC TESTS—Before surgery: Blood and urine studies, x-rays of gastrointestinal tract.

ANESTHESIA—Local anesthesia (usually lidocaine injection).

DESCRIPTION OF OPERATION
- The endoscopist anesthetizes the throat with lidocaine or other local anesthesia.
- The endoscopist passes the endoscope to the appropriate point in the stomach.
- A small incision is made in the skin and an intravenous cannula is pushed through the skin into the stomach.
- A string is passed into the stomach through the cannula, the string is grasped inside the stomach and is brought back out through the mouth.
- The gastrostomy tube is tied to the string, then pulled back into the stomach and out through the abdominal wall.
- The gastrostomy tube is then fixed to the abdominal wall.

POSSIBLE COMPLICATIONS
- Abscess formation, wound infection.
- Inadvertent tube dislodgement.
- Catheter malfunction.
- Clogging of tube.
- Drainage around tube.

AVERAGE HOSPITAL STAY—0 to 1 day for procedure. Total time varies according to underlying disorder.

PROBABLE OUTCOME—Satisfactory alternate method of feeding.

 POSTOPERATIVE CARE

GENERAL MEASURES
- Remain upright for 1/2 to 1 hour after eating.
- Keep skin around gastrostomy tube scrupulously clean.
- Prevent dislodging the tube by careful taping and vigilance during dressing, feeding and activities.
- Shower as usual. You may wash the incision gently with mild, unscented soap.
- Move and elevate legs often while resting in to bed to decrease the likelihood of deep-vein blood clots.

MEDICATION
- Your doctor may prescribe:
  - Pain relievers.
  - Don't take prescription pain medication longer than 4 to 7 days. Use only as much as you need.
  - Antibiotics to fight or prevent infection.
- You may use nonprescription drugs, such as acetaminophen, for minor pain. Avoid aspirin.

ACTIVITY—Resume normal activity as soon as possible to promote healing.

DIET
- Your doctor will prescribe a diet.
- Vitamin and mineral supplements may be recommended.

 CALL YOUR DOCTOR IF

- Pain, swelling, redness, drainage, or bleeding increases in the surgical area.
- You develop symptoms of infection including headache, muscle aches, dizziness, fever, or a general ill feeling.
- You experience constipation, abdominal swelling, nausea, or vomiting.
- The tube falls out.
- New, unexplained symptoms develop.

GASTROSTOMY, PERCUTANEOUS ENDOSCOPIC (P.E.G. Procedure)

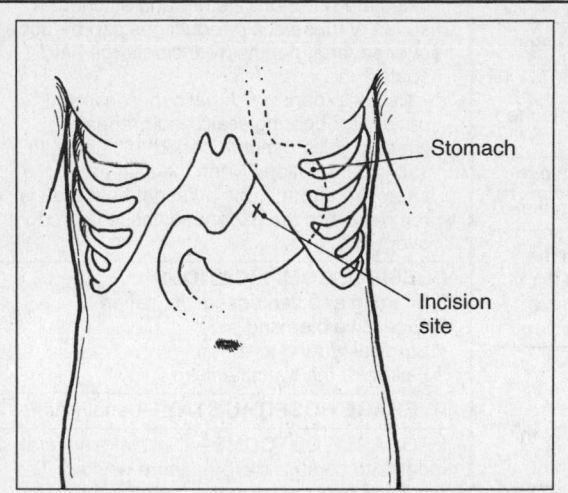

An illustration of the incision site in the abdomen over the position in the stomach chosen for the gastrostomy.

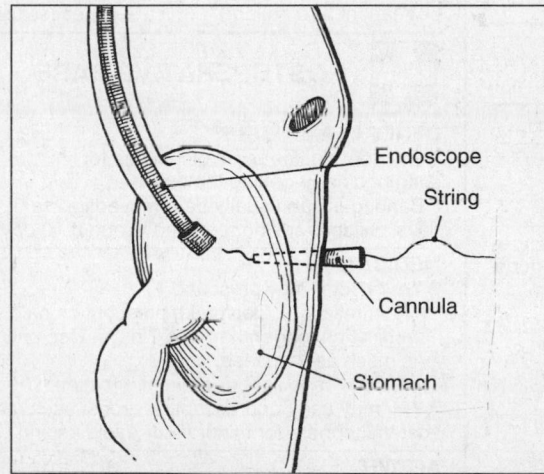

Shown are the endoscope at the upper end of the stomach and a tube inside the endoscope. The doctor makes a small incision into the skin and pushes an intravenous cannula through the skin into the stomach.

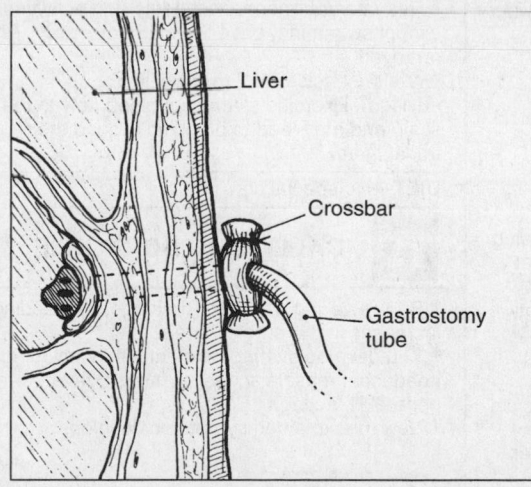

Final appearance with the feeding tube in place. The external end of the feeding tube is clamped to provide access for feeding in the future (not illustrated).

HAIR TRANSPLANT

GENERAL INFORMATION

DEFINITION—Relocating scalp hair and hair follicles from an area of thick hair growth to balding or thinning areas. More than one treatment session may be needed to create the best results.

BODY PARTS INVOLVED—Hair and scalp.

REASONS FOR SURGERY—Male or female pattern baldness (see in Illness section), an inherited trait. The hair loss is typically on the front or top of the scalp. Person will need thick hair on the back or sides of the scalp to have enough hair follicles to move.

SURGICAL RISK INCREASES WITH
- Certain skin conditions.
- Some chronic illnesses.
- Poor quality hair on the back and sides of the head.
- Hair transplants that are performed before hair loss has come to a standstill.

WHAT TO EXPECT

WHO OPERATES—Hair transplant surgeon.

WHERE PERFORMED—Doctor's office, outpatient surgical facility, or special hair-transplant clinic.

DIAGNOSTIC TESTS
- Before surgery: Laboratory tests may be done to check for any underlying medical problem.
- After surgery: None required.

ANESTHESIA—Local anesthetic injected into both the donor and recipient sites. Sedation may be used for comfort and relaxation.

DESCRIPTION OF OPERATION
- Several procedures are available. You and your doctor will decide the most appropriate one depending on the degree and location of your baldness:
  - Punch grafts (plugs): A round graft is punched out of a donor site and fitted into a hole in the bald area. Each punch contains about 15 hairs plus skin and fatty tissue.
  - Mini-plugs: About half the size of punch grafts and used to fill in spaces between larger grafts.
  - Micro-plugs: Made by splitting one large plug into 4 to fill in spaces. Adds a more irregular natural look to hairline.
  - Strip grafts: Similar to punch grafts except the graft is long and thin. May be used to finish hairline once plugs have filled in bald spot.
  - Flaps: A flap of hair on the back or side is cut out and swiveled onto the bald spot. The cut edges of the donor site are brought together and stitched closed.
  - Scalp reduction: An area of bald skin (2 inches by six inches) is cut out and the two sides are brought together and stitched. A series of these scalp reductions can be done over several months, reducing large bald spots.
  - Tissue expansion: A balloon is inserted under hair-bearing scalp and gradually (weekly, for a 2 month period) inflated with saltwater solution. When the skin has stretched enough, the adjacent bald area is removed and the expanded tissue is brought over to cover it.

POSSIBLE COMPLICATIONS
- Scarring and decreased circulation.
- Excessive bleeding.
- Surgical-wound infection.
- Failure of the transplant.

AVERAGE HOSPITAL STAY—Usually none.

PROBABLE OUTCOME—It will take several months to be sure the procedure worked. The results of hair replacement surgery are permanent and no long-term care is necessary.

POSTOPERATIVE CARE

GENERAL MEASURES
- Ask your doctor about guidelines for shampooing or getting the hair wet.
- Bandages can usually be removed in 2 to 5 days. Stitches will be removed in about 10 days.

MEDICATION
- Your doctor may prescribe:
  - Pain relievers. Don't take prescription pain medication longer than 4 to 7 days. Use only as much as you need.
  - Antibiotics to fight or prevent infection.
- You may use nonprescription drugs, such as acetaminophen, for minor pain. Avoid aspirin.

ACTIVITY
- Resume your normal schedule and activities, except swimming, once the bandages are removed.
- Avoid exercise for 2 to 3 weeks (or as advised). Exercise stimulates blood flow to the scalp and may lead to bleeding around the transplants.

DIET—No special diet.

CALL YOUR DOCTOR IF

- Pain, swelling, redness, drainage, or bleeding increases in the surgical area.
- You develop symptoms of infection including headache, muscle aches, dizziness, fever, or a general ill feeling.
- New, unexplained symptoms develop.

HAIR TRANSPLANT

The surgical area before a plug transplant.

Donor site

Transplant site

A round plug is removed from a donor site and prepared for insertion into the transplant site.

Hair plug in place

Hair plug is in place.

HAMMERTOE CORRECTION

GENERAL INFORMATION

DEFINITION—Removal of tendons and joining of middle joints in the toes to correct hammertoe, a deformity in which the toes bend downward. This causes the tops of the toes to become calloused from rubbing against the inside of shoes. Hammertoe probably results from wearing shoes that do not fit properly, especially high-heeled shoes that place pressure on the front part of the foot and compress the smaller toes together tightly.

BODY PARTS INVOLVED—All toes except the big toes, tendons, blood vessels and nerves connected to these toes, and overlying skin.

REASONS FOR SURGERY
- Relief of painful calluses.
- Prevention of permanent deformity.

SURGICAL RISK INCREASES WITH
- Obesity.
- Smoking.
- Excess alcohol consumption.
- Diabetes.
- Use of some prescription and nonprescription drugs. Inform your doctor of any drugs, medications, or vitamin and herb supplements you are using or have used in the last month.

WHAT TO EXPECT

WHO OPERATES—General surgeon (sometimes), podiatrist, or orthopedic surgeon.

WHERE PERFORMED—Hospital or outpatient surgical facility.

DIAGNOSTIC TESTS
- Before surgery: Blood and urine studies, x-ray of feet.
- After surgery: Blood studies.

ANESTHESIA
- Local anesthesia by injection.
- Regional anesthesia by injection.

DESCRIPTION OF OPERATION
- After local anesthesia is injected, a tourniquet is applied above the ankle to keep the surgical area from bleeding.
- An incision is made through the skin.
- The tendons that attach to the toes are located, cut free of connective tissue to foot bones, and realigned so that they no longer bend downward.
- The middle joints of the affected toes are often fused together permanently with fine pins and wire sutures.
- The skin is closed with fine sutures, which usually can be removed about 7 to 10 days after surgery.
- A dressing is placed over the toes to help maintain their new position.

POSSIBLE COMPLICATIONS
- Excessive bleeding.
- Surgical-wound infection.
- Bones may return to previous position.
- Excessive swelling which can last for several months.

AVERAGE HOSPITAL STAY—None.

PROBABLE OUTCOME—Expect complete healing and relief of symptoms without complications. Allow about 4 weeks for recovery from surgery.

POSTOPERATIVE CARE

GENERAL MEASURES
- A hard ridge should form along the incision. As it heals, the ridge will gradually recede.
- Shower as usual. You may wash the incision gently with mild, unscented soap. After a shower, replace any wet dressings with clean, dry ones.
- Wear shoes that fit well and do not cramp the toes or put undue stress on the front of the foot.
- While healing, wear flat shoes and cotton socks.
- Your doctor may prescribe a special shoe to be worn while healing.
- Your doctor may prescribe crutches or a cane to be used until healing is complete.

MEDICATION
- Your doctor may prescribe pain relievers. Don't take prescription pain medication longer than 4 to 7 days. Use only as much as you need.
- You may use nonprescription drugs, such as acetaminophen, for minor pain. Avoid aspirin.

ACTIVITY
- Avoid vigorous exercise for 6 weeks after surgery.
- Resume driving 1 week after returning home.

DIET—No special diet.

CALL YOUR DOCTOR IF

- Pain, swelling, redness, drainage, or bleeding increases in the surgical area.
- You develop symptoms of infection including headache, muscle aches, dizziness, fever, or a general ill feeling.
- You experience nausea or vomiting.
- New, unexplained symptoms develop.

HAMMERTOE CORRECTION

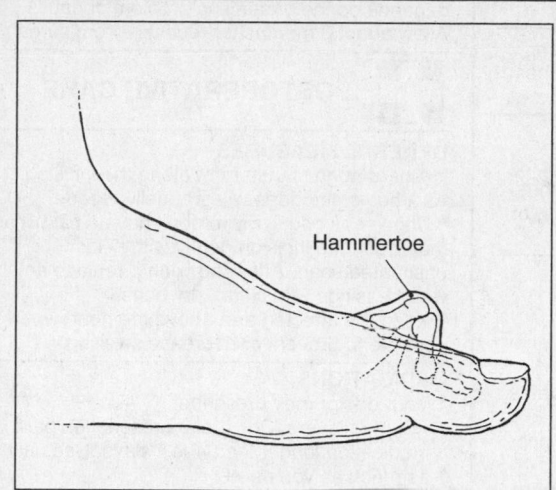

An illustration of a typical hammer toe (a deformity in which the toes bend downward).

Hammertoe

After local anesthesia is injected, tendons are located and divided so toes no longer bend downward.

Tendon

Bone

The portion of bone is removed and toes can return to normal shape.

Bone

HAND SURGERY

GENERAL INFORMATION

DEFINITION—Any operation performed to restore or preserve the normal function of the hand.

BODY PARTS INVOLVED—Hand.

REASONS FOR SURGERY—Preservation or restoration of normal function of the hand that has been lost or impaired by disease, injury, or malformation.

SURGICAL RISK INCREASES WITH
- Obesity.
- Smoking.
- Poor nutrition.
- Excess alcohol consumption.
- Recent or chronic illness, especially diabetes, peripheral vascular disease and arthritis.
- Use of some prescription and nonprescription drugs. Inform your doctor of any drugs, medications, or vitamin and herb supplements you are using or have used in the last month.

WHAT TO EXPECT

WHO OPERATES—General surgeon, hand surgeon, plastic surgeon, or orthopedic surgeon.

WHERE PERFORMED—Doctor's office, outpatient surgical facility, hospital, or emergency room.

DIAGNOSTIC TESTS
- Before surgery: Blood and urine studies, x-ray of hands.
- After surgery: Blood studies.

ANESTHESIA
- Local anesthesia (sometimes) by injection.
- Regional anesthesia by injection.
- General anesthesia by injection and inhalation with an airway tube placed in the windpipe.

DESCRIPTION OF OPERATION
- The arm of the affected hand is elevated and wrapped with a blood-pressure cuff inflated to higher than normal blood pressure. This prevents the surgical area from bleeding.
- The procedures depend on the injury or disease in the hand.
- The wound is covered with gauze and padded dressings.

POSSIBLE COMPLICATIONS
- Excessive bleeding.
- Surgical-wound infection.
- Nerve damage.
- Scarring of tendons which limits motion.

AVERAGE HOSPITAL STAY—0 to 2 days.

PROBABLE OUTCOME—Expect complete healing of surgical wound. Success of surgery depends on the underlying problem or cause. Allow about 3 months for recovery from surgery.

POSTOPERATIVE CARE

GENERAL MEASURES
- A hard ridge should form along the incision. As it heals, the ridge will gradually recede.
- Shower as usual, if you don't have a cast. You may wash the incision gently with mild, unscented soap. After showering, replace any wet dressings with clean, dry ones.
- Keep the affected arm above the heart when possible to prevent or decrease swelling.

MEDICATION
- Your doctor may prescribe:
  - Pain relievers. Don't take prescription pain medication longer than 4 to 7 days. Use only as much as you need.
  - Antibiotics to fight or prevent infection.
- You may use nonprescription drugs, such as acetaminophen, for minor pain. Avoid aspirin.

ACTIVITY
- To help recovery and aid your well-being, resume daily activities, including work, as soon as you are able.
- Your doctor will prescribe a physical therapy rehabilitation program.
- Avoid vigorous exercise for 3 weeks after surgery.
- Resume driving when the hand has healed.

DIET—Eat a well-balanced diet to promote healing.

CALL YOUR DOCTOR IF

- You develop pain or a throbbing sensation in the affected hand.
- Swelling, redness, drainage, or bleeding increases in the surgical area.
- You develop symptoms of infection including headache, muscle aches, dizziness, fever, or a general ill feeling.
- You experience nausea or vomiting.
- New, unexplained symptoms develop.

HAND SURGERY

- A typical hand injury with a deep laceration.
- Hand injuries may include severed nerves or blood vessels, severed or injured tendons or connective tissue, or amputated fingers.

Severed tendon

The ragged injury is made into a clean surgical incision and muscles and connective tissue retracted for exposure. A severed tendon can be seen and repaired.

Skin is carefully closed after repair to the injured hand tissue. The hand and forearm are usually kept rigid with a plaster cast or splint.

HEART TRANSPLANTATION

 GENERAL INFORMATION

DEFINITION—Replacement of a diseased heart with a healthy heart.

BODY PARTS INVOLVED—Diseased or abnormal heart and a healthy heart from donor.

REASONS FOR SURGERY
- Heart failure from coronary artery disease.
- Heart failure from cardiomyopathy.
- Valvular heart disease with congestive heart failure.
- Heart failure from severe congenital heart disease.

SURGICAL RISK INCREASES WITH
- Adults over 60, obesity, poor nutrition.
- Recent or chronic illness, diabetes.
- Alcoholism, smoking.
- Use of some prescription and nonprescription drugs. Inform your doctor of any drugs, medications, or vitamin and herb supplements you are using or have used in the last month.

 WHAT TO EXPECT

WHO OPERATES—Cardiovascular surgeon.

WHERE PERFORMED—Hospital.

DIAGNOSTIC TESTS
- Before surgery: Blood and urine studies, chest x-ray, studies of the immune system, ECG, cardiac catheterization, ultrasound (see Glossary for all).
- During surgery: Cardiac monitoring.
- After surgery: Blood studies, ECG.

ANESTHESIA—General anesthesia by injection and inhalation with an airway tube placed in the windpipe.

DESCRIPTION OF OPERATION
- A healthy heart is obtained from a donor who has died from an accident or a disease other than heart disease, HIV, or hepatitis (see Glossary for both).
- An incision is made in the recipient's chest to expose the heart.
- A heart-lung machine sustains life while the diseased heart is cut free and removed, and until the donor heart has been transplanted.
- The donor heart is sewn into place. The aorta, pulmonary artery, superior vena cava and inferior vena cava are connected to the new heart.
- The skin is closed with sutures or clips, which are removed about 1 week after surgery.

POSSIBLE COMPLICATIONS
- Excessive bleeding, surgical-wound infection.
- Life-threatening general infections.
- Rejection of the transplanted heart.
- Cancer which develops as an adverse effect of immunosuppressant drugs.

AVERAGE HOSPITAL STAY—10 to 21 days.

PROBABLE OUTCOME—A successful transplantation prolongs life and improves the quality of life for patients who might otherwise have died. Allow about 6 weeks for recovery from surgery. Rejection of the transplant remains a life-long risk. Life expectancy varies depending on each individual patient.

 POSTOPERATIVE CARE

GENERAL MEASURES
- A hard ridge should form along the incision. As it heals, the ridge will gradually recede.
- Shower as usual. Avoid baths until the incision has completely healed. You may wash the incision gently with mild, unscented soap. After showering, replace any wet dressings with clean, dry ones.
- Move and elevate legs often while resting in bed to decrease the chance of deep-vein blood clots.

MEDICATION
- Your doctor may prescribe:
  - Pain relievers. Don't take prescription pain medication longer than 4 to 7 days. Use only as much as you need.
  - Stool softeners to prevent constipation.
  - Antibiotics to fight or prevent infection.
  - Immunosuppressant drugs to decrease the likelihood of rejection.
- You may use nonprescription drugs, such as acetaminophen, for minor pain. Avoid aspirin.

ACTIVITY
- To help recovery and aid your well-being, resume daily activities, including work, as soon as you are able.
- Avoid vigorous exercise for 6 weeks after surgery. Resume exercise after consulting your doctor.
- Resume sexual relations when your doctor determines that healing is complete.

DIET—Your doctor may prescribe a diet.

 CALL YOUR DOCTOR IF

- Pain, swelling, redness, drainage, or bleeding increases in the surgical area.
- You develop symptoms of infection including headache, muscle aches, dizziness, fever, or a general ill feeling.
- You experience nausea, vomiting, constipation, abdominal swelling, heartbeat irregularities, or extreme fatigue.
- New, unexplained symptoms develop.

HEART TRANSPLANTATION

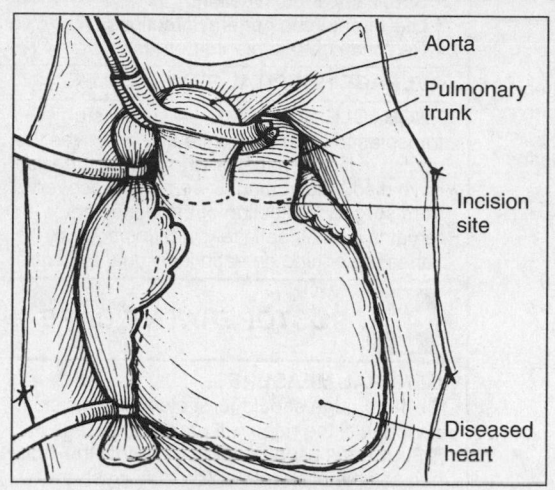

Aorta

Pulmonary trunk

Incision site

Diseased heart

- An illustration of a diseased heart. The major blood vessels into and away from the heart are clamped and incision sites for the heart transplant indicated.
- A heart-lung machine sustains life while the diseased heart is cut free and removed, and until the donor heart has been transplanted.

Vena cava

Aorta

Pulmonary trunk

After major vessels have been severed, the diseased heart is now ready to be removed from the chest and discarded.

- The donor heart is sewn in place. The aorta, pulmonary arteries, superior vena cava and inferior vena cava are connected to the new heart.
- The donor heart, which had been kept motionless by cooling, is now stimulated to resume beating with warming and a weak electrical current.

HEART-LUNG TRANSPLANTATION

GENERAL INFORMATION

DEFINITION—Replacement of poorly functioning lungs and a damaged or healthy heart with donor organs. If the recipient's heart is normal, it may be extracted and donated to another patient in need of a heart transplantation only (see Heart Transplantation in Surgery section).

BODY PARTS INVOLVED—Lungs, heart, trachea and blood vessels.

REASONS FOR SURGERY—Chronic lung disorders such as pulmonary hypertension, emphysema, cystic fibrosis and other lung conditions causing pulmonary fibrosis.

SURGICAL RISK INCREASES WITH
- Adults over 60, obesity, poor nutrition.
- Recent or chronic illness.
- Alcoholism, smoking.
- Diabetes.
- Use of some prescription and nonprescription drugs. Inform your doctor of any drugs, medications, or vitamin and herb supplements you are using or have used in the last month.

WHAT TO EXPECT

WHO OPERATES—Cardiovascular surgeon or thoracic surgeon.

WHERE PERFORMED—Hospital.

DIAGNOSTIC TESTS
- Before surgery: Blood and urine studies, studies of the immune system, ECG, cardiac catheterization, echocardiography, ultrasound, biopsy, pulmonary angiography, lung function studies (see Glossary for all).
- During surgery: Cardiac monitoring (see Glossary).
- After surgery: Repeat of some tests for monitoring of the new organs.

ANESTHESIA—General anesthesia by injection and inhalation, with an airway tube placed in the windpipe.

DESCRIPTION OF OPERATION
- An incision is made in the recipient's chest to expose the heart and lungs.
- A heart-lung machine sustains life while the diseased organs are cut free and removed, and until the donor organs have been transplanted.
- The donor organs are sewn into place. The new lungs are connected to the trachea.
- The skin is closed with sutures or clips, which usually can be removed about 1 week after surgery.

POSSIBLE COMPLICATIONS
- Excessive bleeding, blood clots.
- Surgical-wound infection.
- Life-threatening general infections.
- Rejection of transplanted organs.

AVERAGE HOSPITAL STAY—3 weeks.

PROBABLE OUTCOME—A successful transplantation prolongs life and improves the quality of life for patients who might otherwise have died. Allow about 6 weeks for recovery from surgery. Rejection of the transplant remains a risk indefinitely. Life expectancy varies depending on each individual patient.

POSTOPERATIVE CARE

GENERAL MEASURES
- A hard ridge should form along the incision. As it heals, the ridge will gradually recede.
- Shower as usual. Avoid baths until the incision has completely healed. You may wash the incision gently with mild, unscented soap. After showering, replace any wet dressings with clean, dry ones.
- Move and elevate legs often while resting in bed to decrease the chance of deep-vein blood clots.

MEDICATION
- Your doctor may prescribe:
  - Pain relievers. Don't take prescription pain medication longer than 4 to 7 days. Use only as much as you need.
  - Stool softeners to prevent constipation.
  - Antibiotics to fight or prevent infection.
  - Immunosuppressant drugs to decrease the likelihood of rejection.
- You may use nonprescription drugs, such as acetaminophen, for minor pain. Avoid aspirin.

ACTIVITY
- Rehabilitation will begin after surgery.
- Resume normal activity as soon as possible.
- Avoid vigorous exercise for 6 weeks after surgery.
- Resume sexual relations when your doctor determines that healing is complete.

DIET—Your doctor will prescribe a diet.

CALL YOUR DOCTOR IF

- Pain, swelling, redness, drainage, or bleeding increases in the surgical area.
- You develop symptoms of infection including headache, muscle aches, dizziness, fever, or a general ill feeling.
- You develop shortness of breath or bloody sputum.
- You have fluid retention.
- New, unexplained symptoms develop.

HEART-LUNG TRANSPLANTATION

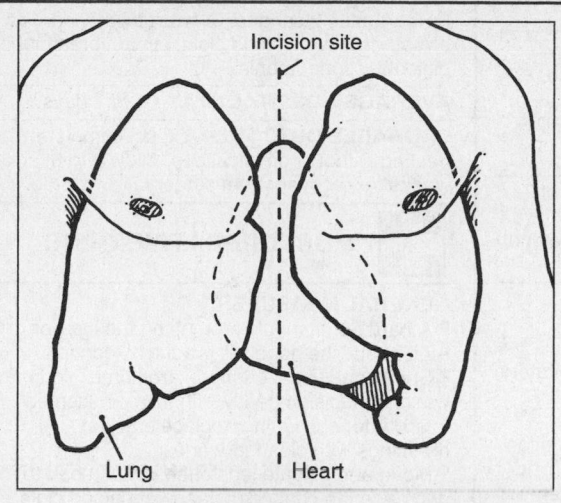

Illustration demonstrating surgical anatomy. Mid-line incision is made and recipient's heart and lungs are exposed.

Incision site

Lung   Heart

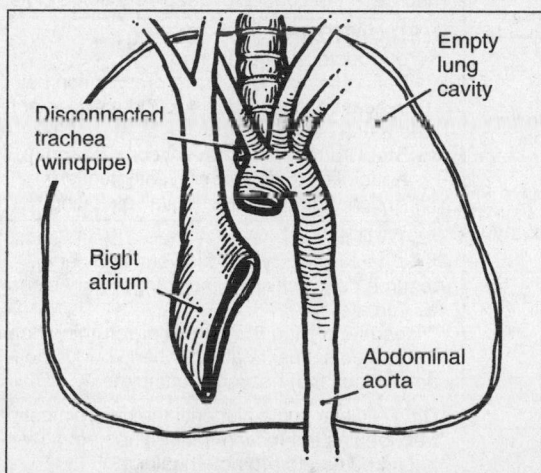

Recipient's heart and lungs are removed, leaving an empty cavity where new organs will be attached.

Empty lung cavity

Disconnected trachea (windpipe)

Right atrium

Abdominal aorta

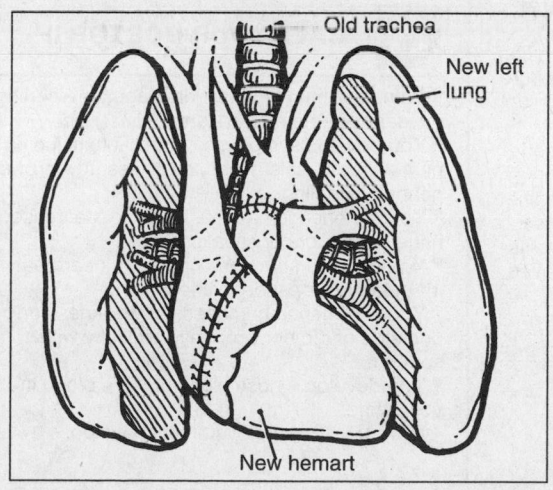

Donor's heart and lungs are sewn into position. The surgical site is examined for any leaks prior to closing of the chest.

Old trachea

New left lung

New hemart

HEART VALVE REPLACEMENT

GENERAL INFORMATION

DEFINITION—Replacement of one or more diseased heart valves with porcine (derived from swine) or artificial valves.

BODY PARTS INVOLVED—Valves that separate major sections of the heart.

REASONS FOR SURGERY—Prevention of complications resulting from valvular heart disease, especially congestive heart failure and bacterial endocarditis.

SURGICAL RISK INCREASES WITH
- Adults over 60.
- Obesity, smoking, poor nutrition.
- Recent illness such as acute upper respiratory infection.
- Alcoholism or chronic illness.
- Use of some prescription and nonprescription drugs. Inform your doctor of any drugs, medications, or vitamin and herb supplements you are using or have used in the last month.

WHAT TO EXPECT

WHO OPERATES—Cardiovascular surgeon.

WHERE PERFORMED—Hospital.

DIAGNOSTIC TESTS
- Before surgery: Blood and urine studies, x-ray of chest, ECG, cardiac catheterization (see Glossary for both).
- During surgery: ECG monitor.
- After surgery: Blood studies, ECG.

ANESTHESIA—General anesthesia by injection and inhalation with an airway tube placed in the windpipe.

DESCRIPTION OF OPERATION
- An incision is made in the chest, and the breastbone is divided. The chest is opened to expose the heart.
- A heart-lung machine circulates enough blood to sustain life throughout the surgical procedure.
- The diseased heart valves are located through delicate incisions made in the heart.
- Diseased valves are removed and replaced with artificial or porcine valves.
- The incisions in the heart are closed with fine sutures, and the chest cavity is reconstructed with wire sutures. The skin is closed with lighter sutures or clips, which usually can be removed about 1 week after surgery.
- Drains may be left in place for several days following the surgery.

POSSIBLE COMPLICATIONS
- Excessive bleeding, blood clots.
- Surgical-wound infection.
- Failure of the heart to resume normal heartbeat (rare).
- Clotting or infection of valve.
- Kidney damage or kidney failure.
- Heart attack, congestive heart failure, cardiac arrest, deep-vein blood clots, stroke, breathing difficulties, pneumonia.

AVERAGE HOSPITAL STAY—5 to 7 days.

PROBABLE OUTCOME—Expect complete healing without complications. Allow 4 to 6 weeks for recovery from surgery.

POSTOPERATIVE CARE

GENERAL MEASURES
- A hard ridge should form along the incision. As it heals, the ridge will gradually recede.
- Shower as usual after you are home. You may wash the incision gently with mild, unscented soap. After showering, replace any wet dressings with clean, dry ones.
- Move and elevate legs often while in bed to decrease the chance of deep-vein blood clots.

MEDICATION
- Your doctor may prescribe:
  - Pain relievers. Don't take prescription pain medication longer than 4 to 7 days. Use only as much as you need.
  - Stool softeners to prevent constipation.
  - Antibiotics to fight or prevent infection.
  - Anticoagulant to prevent valve clotting.

ACTIVITY
- To help recovery and aid your well-being, resume daily activities, including work, as soon as you are able.
- Resume driving 5 weeks after returning home.
- Resume sexual relations when your doctor determines that healing is complete.

DIET—Clear liquid diet until the gastrointestinal tract begins to function again. Then eat a well-balanced diet to promote healing.

CALL YOUR DOCTOR IF

- Pain, swelling, redness, drainage, or bleeding increases in the surgical area.
- You develop symptoms of infection including headache, muscle aches, dizziness, fever, or a general ill feeling.
- You experience nausea, vomiting, decreased urine output, or constipation.
- You develop shortness of breath, heartbeat irregularities, or sudden chest pain.
- You experience numbness or weakness on one side of the body, or have difficulty with speech.
- You develop a nose bleed or have blood in your urine.
- New, unexplained symptoms develop.

HEART VALVE REPLACEMENT

Incision site

- An illustration of the incision site over the breast bone, which will be spread to allow exposure of the heart.
- A heart-lung machine circulates enough blood to sustain life throughout the surgical procedure.

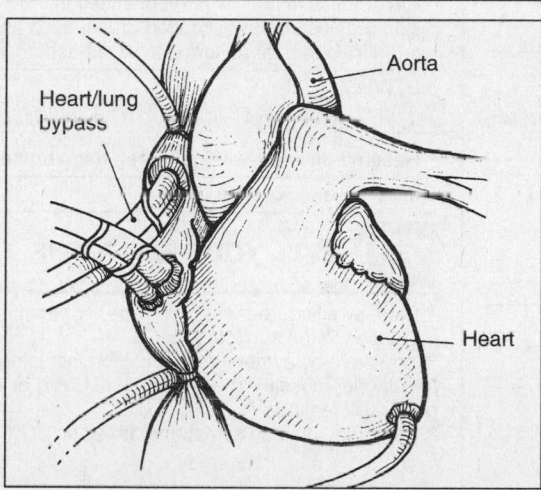

Aorta

Heart/lung bypass

Heart

The diseased heart valves are located through delicate incisions made in the heart.

Valve replacement

- Diseased valves are removed and replaced with artificial or porcine valves.
- The incisions made in the heart are closed with fine sutures. The chest cavity is reconstructed with wire sutures in the chest muscle and breast bone.

HEEL SPUR REMOVAL

 ## GENERAL INFORMATION

DEFINITION—Removal of a heel spur, a sharp outgrowth on the bone of the heel.

BODY PARTS INVOLVED—Bottom of the heel bone.

REASONS FOR SURGERY—Relief of pain.

SURGICAL RISK INCREASES WITH
- Obesity.
- Smoking.
- Poor nutrition.
- Excess alcohol consumption.
- Recent or chronic illness.
- Diabetes.
- Use of some prescription and nonprescription drugs. Inform your doctor of any drugs, medications, or vitamin and herb supplements you are using or have used in the last month.

 ## WHAT TO EXPECT

WHO OPERATES—General surgeon, orthopedist, or podiatrist.

WHERE PERFORMED—Outpatient surgical facility or doctor's office.

DIAGNOSTIC TESTS
- Before surgery: Blood and urine studies, x-rays of both feet.
- After surgery: Blood studies, laboratory examination of removed tissue.

ANESTHESIA
- Local anesthesia by injection.
- Spinal anesthesia by injection (sometimes).

DESCRIPTION OF OPERATION
- Different surgical options are available for treatment. One option is described here.
- An incision is made over the spur.
- The spur is cut free and removed with special instruments.
- The skin is closed with sutures, which usually can be removed about 10 to 14 days after surgery.

POSSIBLE COMPLICATIONS
- Excessive bleeding.
- Surgical-wound infection.
- Numbness.
- Recurrence of the heel problem.
- Scar tissue from the incision becomes tender or painful.

AVERAGE HOSPITAL STAY—Usually none.

PROBABLE OUTCOME—Expect complete healing without complications. Allow about 6 months for complete recovery from surgery.

 ## POSTOPERATIVE CARE

GENERAL MEASURES
- If the wound bleeds during the first 24 hours after surgery, press a clean tissue or cloth to it for 10 minutes.
- A hard ridge should form along the incision. As it heals, the ridge will gradually recede.
- Shower as usual. You may wash the incision gently with mild, unscented soap.
- Use crutches or a cane to walk until your doctor determines that healing is complete.
- Between baths, keep wound dry with a bandage for the first 2 or 3 days after surgery. If a bandage gets wet, change it promptly.

MEDICATION
- Your doctor may prescribe:
  - Pain relievers. Don't take prescription pain medication longer than 4 to 7 days. Use only as much as you need.
  - Antibiotics to fight or prevent infection.
- You may use nonprescription drugs, such as acetaminophen, for minor pain. Avoid aspirin.

ACTIVITY
- Avoid vigorous exercise for 3 months after surgery.
- Resume driving 1 week after returning home.

DIET—No special diet.

 ## CALL YOUR DOCTOR IF

- Pain, swelling, redness, drainage, or bleeding increases in the surgical area.
- You develop symptoms of infection including headache, muscle aches, dizziness, fever, or a general ill feeling.
- New, unexplained symptoms develop.

HEEL SPUR REMOVAL

An illustration of a typical bone spur on the heel bone.

Heel bone

Bone spur

A typical incision site to enable removal of the bone spur, which is cut free and removed with special instruments.

Incision site

Skin is closed with sutures, which can usually be removed about 10 to 14 days after surgery.

HEMORRHOID BANDING

GENERAL INFORMATION

DEFINITION—Destruction of hemorrhoids (varicose veins that occur inside or outside the anus) by a technique that uses a rubber band over the stalk of the hemorrhoid to cut off blood flow.

BODY PARTS INVOLVED—Anus, rectum, dilated veins in anus and rectum (hemorrhoids).

REASONS FOR SURGERY—Pain, excessive bleeding, itching, or prolapse of dilated veins in the rectum and anus.

SURGICAL RISK INCREASES WITH
- Obesity.
- Smoking.
- Poor nutrition.
- Adults over 60.
- Excess alcohol consumption.
- Recent or chronic illness.
- Diabetes.
- Inflammatory bowel disease.
- Use of some prescription and nonprescription drugs. Inform your doctor of any drugs, medications, or vitamin and herb supplements you are using or have used in the last month.

WHAT TO EXPECT

WHO OPERATES—Proctologist, colon-rectal surgeon, or general surgeon.

WHERE PERFORMED—Doctor's office, hospital, or outpatient surgical facility.

DIAGNOSTIC TESTS
- Before surgery: Blood and urine studies, anoscopy, sigmoidoscopy (see Glossary for both).
- After surgery: Blood studies.

ANESTHESIA
- Local anesthesia by injection.
- Spinal anesthesia by injection.
- General anesthesia by injection and inhalation with an airway tube placed in the windpipe.

DESCRIPTION OF OPERATION
- The doctor inserts several fingers to dilate the anal muscles. Sometimes anal muscles must be dilated vigorously to expose the hemorrhoids.
- The hemorrhoid is visualized and grasped with a special instrument.
- A small rubber band is slipped over the stalk of the hemorrhoid to bind it and cut off blood flow.

POSSIBLE COMPLICATIONS
- Excessive bleeding.
- Surgical-wound infection.
- Severe pain, especially with bowel movements.
- Urinary retention.

AVERAGE HOSPITAL STAY—0 to 1 day.

PROBABLE OUTCOME—Curable in most patients, no matter what age. Allow about 2 weeks for recovery from surgery.

POSTOPERATIVE CARE

GENERAL MEASURES
- Take warm sitz baths about every 4 hours and following bowel movements to relieve pain and help keep the rectal area clean. Sit in warm water for 10 to 20 minutes as often as it feels good.
- Avoid heavy lifting. If not possible, learn proper body mechanics to reduce strain contributing to recurrence.
- Don't strain with bowel movements or urination.
- Wipe gently after bowel movements with soft, moist, white toilet paper or absorbent, moist cotton.
- Expect drainage from the rectum for 2 to 3 weeks.

MEDICATION
- Your doctor may prescribe:
  - Pain relievers. Don't take prescription pain medication for longer than 4 to 7 days. Use only as much as you need.
  - Stool softeners or laxatives to prevent constipation.
  - Analgesic ointment to relieve pain.
  - Vitamins to encourage healing.
- You may use nonprescription drugs, such as acetaminophen, for minor pain. Avoid aspirin.

ACTIVITY
- Resume driving 1 week after returning home.
- Avoid sitting for long periods of time.
- Resume sexual relations as soon as you wish.

DIET
- No special diet. Increase dietary fiber and fluid intake to prevent constipation. Straining during bowel movements can cause hemorrhoids to recur.
- Vitamin and mineral supplements (sometimes).

CALL YOUR DOCTOR IF

- Pain, swelling, redness, drainage, or bleeding increase in the surgical area.
- You develop symptoms of infection including headache, muscle aches, dizziness, fever, or a general ill feeling.
- You become constipated.
- New, unexplained symptoms develop.

HEMORRHOID BANDING

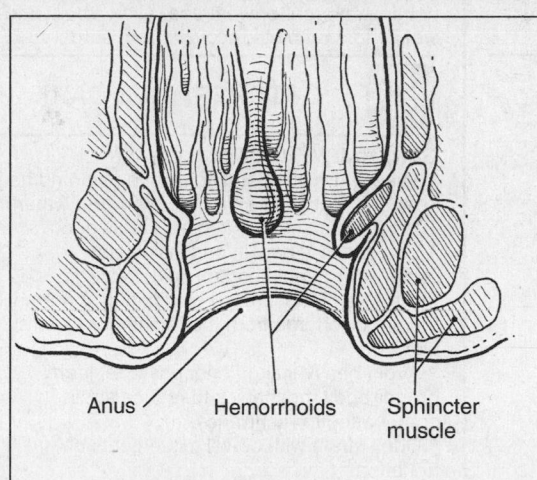

Anus | Hemorrhoids | Sphincter muscle

An illustration of a cross-sectional view of the region of the body containing the anus, the sphincter muscle of the anus and a view of an internal hemorrhoids just inside the anus.

Rubber band

A hemorrhoid is found and grasped with a special instrument.

Rubber band

A small rubber band is slipped over the stalk of the hemorrhoid to bind it and cut off the blood flow.

HEMORRHOID REMOVAL
(Hemorrhoidectomy)

 GENERAL INFORMATION

DEFINITION—Removal of hemorrhoids (varicose veins that occur inside or on the outside of the anus).

BODY PARTS INVOLVED—Dilated veins around the anus or just inside the rectum.

REASONS FOR SURGERY
- Relief of excessive itching, pain, or bleeding.
- Relief of a painful thrombosed hemorrhoid (hemorrhoid containing a blood clot).

SURGICAL RISK INCREASES WITH
- Adults over 60.
- Obesity.
- Smoking.
- Poor nutrition.
- Excess alcohol consumption.
- Chronic illness.
- Inflammatory bowel disease.
- Bleeding problems.

 WHAT TO EXPECT

WHO OPERATES—Proctologist, colon-rectal surgeon, or general surgeon.

WHERE PERFORMED—Outpatient surgical facility or hospital.

DIAGNOSTIC TESTS
- Before surgery: Blood and urine studies, anoscopy: sigmoidoscopy (see Glossary for both).
- After surgery: Blood studies.

ANESTHESIA
- Local anesthesia by injection.
- Spinal anesthesia by injection.
- General anesthesia by injection and inhalation with an airway tube placed in the windpipe.

DESCRIPTION OF OPERATION
- The dilated veins from around the anus and inside the rectum are cut free and removed, with care taken not to damage the sphincter muscle. Sometimes anal muscles must be dilated vigorously to expose the hemorrhoids.
- The surgical area may be sewn closed or left open, and medicated gauze is used to cover it.

POSSIBLE COMPLICATIONS
- Excessive bleeding.
- Surgical-wound infection.
- Urinary retention (common).
- Stricture of anus.
- Severe pain, especially with bowel movements.
- Constipation.

AVERAGE HOSPITAL STAY—2 to 3 days.

PROBABLE OUTCOME—Curable in most patients, no matter what age. Allow about 6 to 8 weeks for complete recovery from surgery.

 POSTOPERATIVE CARE

GENERAL MEASURES
- Take warm sitz baths to relieve pain and help keep the rectal area clean. Sit in warm water for 10 to 20 minutes as often as it feels good.
- Use sanitary napkin/pad inside your underwear to help control fluid drainage, discharge of mucus and bleeding. It is normal to have a discharge from the rectum for several weeks.
- Avoid heavy lifting. If not possible, learn proper body mechanics to reduce strain contributing to recurrence.
- Don't strain with bowel movements or urination.
- Wipe anal area gently after bowel movements with soft, white toilet paper.

MEDICATION
- Your doctor may prescribe:
  - Pain relievers. Don't take prescription pain medication for longer than 4 to 7 days. Use only as much as you need.
  - Stool softeners or laxatives to prevent constipation.
  - Analgesic ointment to relieve pain.
  - Vitamins to encourage healing.
- You may use nonprescription drugs, such as acetaminophen, for minor pain. Avoid aspirin.

ACTIVITY
- Rest at home as needed and take it easy for 7 to 10 days before you return to full schedule.
- Resume driving 1 week after returning home.
- Avoid sitting for long periods of time.
- Resume sexual relations as soon as you wish.

DIET—No special diet. Increase dietary fiber and fluid intake to prevent constipation. Straining during bowel movements can cause hemorrhoids to recur.

 CALL YOUR DOCTOR IF

- Pain, swelling, redness, drainage, or bleeding increase in the surgical area.
- You develop symptoms of infection including headache, muscle aches, dizziness, fever, or a general ill feeling.
- You become constipated.
- You begin urinating frequently in small amounts or are unable to urinate.
- New, unexplained symptoms develop.

HEMORRHOID REMOVAL
(Hemorrhoidectomy)

Internal hemorrhoid extending through the anus

Anus

An illustration of a typical internal hemorrhoid arising from inside the anus and extending through the anal opening.

Dilated veins around the anus and inside the rectum are cut free and removed, with care taken not to damage the sphincter muscles.

The surgical area is sewn closed or left open and medicated gauze is used to cover.

HERNIA REPAIR, FEMORAL
(Femoral Herniorrhaphy)

 GENERAL INFORMATION

DEFINITION—Closing or repairing a femoral hernia, an internal defect or weakness in the muscles of the abdominal wall. Sometimes, some fatty tissue or an intestine protrudes through the hernia defect, causing a noticeable bulge. If the intestine or other tissue becomes trapped in the hernia defect, it is called an incarcerated hernia. If the blood supply to the trapped intestine or tissue is blocked, it is called a strangulated hernia.

BODY PARTS INVOLVED—Groin (muscles and ligaments inside the lower abdomen next to the genitals), abdominal muscles, the opening allowing the femoral artery to pass from the abdomen to the leg.

REASONS FOR SURGERY
- Incarcerated hernia. This is an emergency!
- Strangulated hernia. This is an emergency!
- Uncomplicated hernia. Most surgeons recommend operating on a femoral hernia, even if no symptoms are present, in order to prevent the serious complications of incarceration or strangulation.

SURGICAL RISK INCREASES WITH
- Adults over 60, obesity, smoking.
- Excess alcohol consumption.
- Recent or chronic illness, especially chronic lung disease or diabetes.
- Use of some prescription and nonprescription drugs. Inform your doctor of any drugs, medications, or vitamin and herb supplements you are using or have used in the last month.

 WHAT TO EXPECT

WHO OPERATES—General surgeon; urologist.

WHERE PERFORMED—Hospital or outpatient surgical facility.

DIAGNOSTIC TESTS
- Before surgery: Blood and urine studies, chest x-ray; ECG (see Glossary).
- After surgery: Blood studies.

ANESTHESIA
- Spinal anesthesia by injection.
- Local anesthesia by injection.
- General anesthesia by injection and inhalation with an airway tube placed in the windpipe.

DESCRIPTION OF OPERATION
- An incision is made in the groin area. The muscles and tissue are separated and the hernia sac is opened.
- The contents of the hernia sac are replaced in the abdominal cavity. The neck of the sac is sutured and a "plug" of plastic webbing is used to close the defect.
- The groin wall is sewn shut. The skin is closed with sutures or clips, which can usually be removed about 1 week after surgery.

POSSIBLE COMPLICATIONS
- Recurrence of hernia.
- Damage to the testicle's blood or nerve supply, if the patient is male.
- Compression of the femoral vein.
- Injury to nerve to groin and thigh area.
- Urinary retention.

AVERAGE HOSPITAL STAY—0 to 4 days.

PROBABLE OUTCOME—Expect complete healing without complications. Male virility should not be affected. Allow about 6 weeks for recovery from surgery.

 POSTOPERATIVE CARE

GENERAL MEASURES
- A hard ridge should form along the incision. As it heals, the ridge will gradually recede.
- Avoid heavy lifting.
- Don't strain with urination or bowel movements.

MEDICATION
- Your doctor may prescribe:
  - Pain relievers. Don't take prescription pain medication longer than 4 to 7 days. Use only as much as you need.
  - Antibiotics to fight or prevent infection.
- You may use nonprescription drugs, such as acetaminophen, for minor pain. Avoid aspirin.

ACTIVITY
- Avoid vigorous exercise and don't lift anything heavier than 5 pounds for 6 weeks after surgery.
- Resume driving 3 to 4 weeks after surgery.
- Resume sexual relations when able.

DIET—Clear liquid diet until the gastrointestinal tract functions again. Then eat a well-balanced diet to promote healing. Increase dietary fiber and fluid intake to prevent constipation and straining during bowel movements.

 CALL YOUR DOCTOR IF

- Pain, swelling, redness, drainage, or bleeding increases in the surgical area.
- You develop symptoms of infection including headache, muscle aches, dizziness, fever, or a general ill feeling.
- A bulge appears in the groin, the thigh, scrotum, vaginal lips, or surgical area.
- You become constipated.
- New, unexplained symptoms develop.

HERNIA REPAIR, FEMORAL
(Femoral Herniorrhaphy)

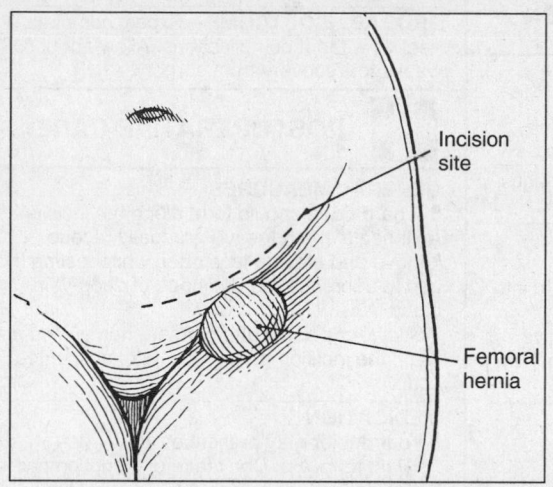

An illustration of a typical femoral hernia located in the groin.

Incision site

Femoral hernia

- Skin has been incised and the muscles retracted disclosing the hernia sac.
- Contents of the hernia sac are replaced in the abdominal cavity.
- Muscles and fascia are used to cover the defect that allowed the hernia to protrude.
- Sometimes a plug of mesh or patch of mesh is used to bolster the defect.

Hernia sac

Muscle layers are sewn together followed by skin closure with sutures or clips, which can usually be removed about 1 week after surgery.

HERNIA REPAIR, HIATAL
(Hiatal Herniorrhaphy)

 GENERAL INFORMATION

DEFINITION—Repair of a hiatal hernia, an abnormal weakness or opening in the diaphragm, where the esophagus enters the abdomen.

BODY PARTS INVOLVED—Lower esophagus, diaphragm, upper part of stomach.

REASONS FOR SURGERY
- Relief of painful symptoms.
- Prevent the stomach from shifting upward into the chest cavity.
- Prevent the stomach from spilling digestive acid into the esophagus, causing infection, pain and scarring.

SURGICAL RISK INCREASES WITH
- Adults over 60, newborns and infants.
- Obesity or poor nutrition.
- Smoking, alcoholism.
- Recent or chronic illness, especially diabetes or chronic lung disease.
- Use of some prescription and nonprescription drugs. Inform your doctor of any drugs, medications, or vitamin and herb supplements you are using or have used in the last month.

 WHAT TO EXPECT

WHO OPERATES—General surgeon.

WHERE PERFORMED—Hospital.

DIAGNOSTIC TESTS
- Before surgery: Blood and urine studies, x-rays of chest and upper gastrointestinal tract, ECG, endoscopy (see Glossary for both).
- After surgery: Blood studies.

ANESTHESIA—General anesthesia by injection and inhalation with an airway tube placed in the windpipe.

DESCRIPTION OF OPERATION
- An incision is made in the abdomen or the chest.
- The hernia in the diaphragm is located and, in some cases, closed with sutures.
- The top of the stomach is wrapped around the lower part of the esophagus and sutured in place.
- The skin is closed with sutures or clips, which usually can be removed about 1 week after surgery.
- Laparoscopic repair is now available for some patients (see Laparoscopy in Surgery section).

POSSIBLE COMPLICATIONS
- Excessive bleeding or surgical-wound infection.
- Incisional hernia.
- Injury to esophagus or stomach.

AVERAGE HOSPITAL STAY—5 to 7 days.

PROBABLE OUTCOME—Expect complete healing without complications. Allow about 6 weeks for recovery from surgery.

 POSTOPERATIVE CARE

GENERAL MEASURES
- A hard ridge should form along the incision. As it heals, the ridge will gradually recede.
- Move and elevate legs often while resting in bed to decrease the likelihood of deep-vein blood clots.
- Shower as usual after you are home. You may wash the incision gently with mild, unscented soap.

MEDICATION
- Your doctor may prescribe:
  - Pain relievers. Don't take prescription pain medication longer than 4 to 7 days. Use only as much as you need.
  - Stool softeners to prevent constipation.
  - Antibiotics to fight or prevent infection.
- You may use nonprescription drugs, such as acetaminophen, for minor pain. Avoid aspirin.

ACTIVITY
- To help recovery and aid your well-being, resume daily activities, including work, as soon as you are able.
- Avoid heavy lifting for 6 weeks after surgery. Learn proper body mechanics to avoid strain contributing to recurrence and to prevent incisional hernia.
- Avoid vigorous exercise for 6 weeks after surgery. Resume driving 4 weeks after returning home.

DIET—Clear liquid diet until the gastrointestinal tract begins to function again. Then eat a well-balanced diet to promote healing. Avoid coffee, tea, cocoa, cola drinks, alcoholic beverages, and any food or spice that aggravates symptoms.

 CALL YOUR DOCTOR IF

- Pain, swelling, redness, drainage, or bleeding increase in the surgical area.
- You develop symptoms of infection including headache, muscle aches, dizziness, fever, or a general ill feeling.
- You experience nausea, vomiting, constipation, black tarry stools, difficulty in swallowing, or abdominal swelling.
- New, unexplained symptoms develop.

HERNIA REPAIR, HIATAL
(Hiatal Herniorrhaphy)

An illustration of a typical incision site to allow exposure of the lower end of the esophagus, the upper end of the stomach, and the diaphragm (a large muscle that separates the chest from the abdominal cavity).

Incision site

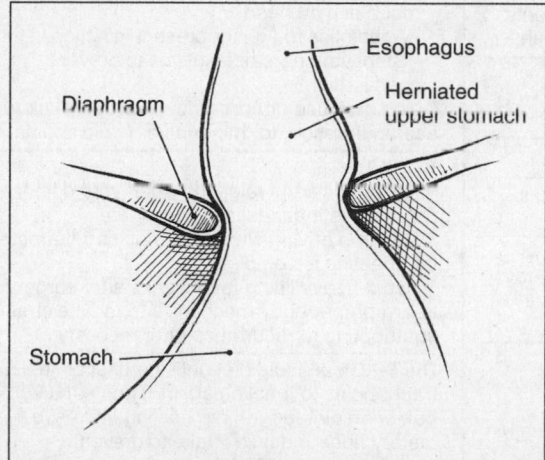

Esophagus

Herniated upper stomach

Diaphragm

Stomach

The herniated upper stomach through the widened opening in the diaphragm.

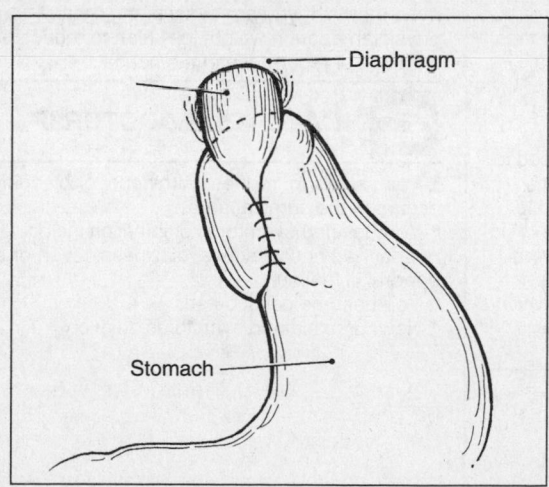

Diaphragm

Stomach

The top of the stomach is wrapped around the lower part of the esophagus and sutured in place.

HERNIA REPAIR, INCISIONAL
(Incisional Herniorrhaphy)

 GENERAL INFORMATION

DEFINITION—Repair of a defect in the abdominal wall created by a previous surgical incision. It is called an incisional hernia or ventral hernia.

BODY PARTS INVOLVED—Abdomen and intestines where previous surgery has been performed.

REASONS FOR SURGERY
• Possible strangulation of bowel.
• Painful lump in the abdomen.

SURGICAL RISK INCREASES WITH
• Obesity, poor nutrition.
• Excess alcohol consumption, smoking.
• Recent or chronic illness, especially chronic lung disease or diabetes.
• Use of some prescription and nonprescription drugs. Inform your doctor of any drugs, medications, or vitamin and herb supplements you are using or have used in the last month.

 WHAT TO EXPECT

WHO OPERATES—General surgeon.

WHERE PERFORMED—Outpatient surgical facility or hospital.

DIAGNOSTIC TESTS
• Before surgery: Blood and urine studies, x-rays of the abdomen and chest, ECG (see Glossary).
• After surgery: Blood studies.

ANESTHESIA
• Local anesthesia by injection.
• Spinal anesthesia by injection.
• General anesthesia by injection and inhalation with an airway tube placed in the windpipe.

DESCRIPTION OF OPERATION
• An incision is made in the abdomen over the defect. The area is examined for protruding intestine.
• The intestine is replaced in the abdominal cavity. Usually, plastic mesh is used to strengthen the repair. The mesh can be used to cover the defect in the abdominal wall or the muscles can be closed and the mesh used to reinforce them.
• A drain is sometimes left in place for several days.
• The skin is closed with sutures or clips, which usually can be removed about 1 week after surgery.

POSSIBLE COMPLICATIONS
• Surgical-wound infection.
• Inadvertent injury to intestinal tract.
• Bowel obstruction.
• Recurrent hernia.

AVERAGE HOSPITAL STAY—0 to 4 days.

PROBABLE OUTCOME—Curable in most patients, no matter what age. Allow 2 to 4 weeks for recovery from surgery.

 POSTOPERATIVE CARE

GENERAL MEASURES
• A hard ridge should form along the incision. As it heals, the ridge will gradually recede.
• Shower as usual. You may wash the incision gently with mild, unscented soap. After showering, change any wet dressings and replace them with clean, dry ones.
• Don't strain with bowel movements or urination.

MEDICATION
• Your doctor may prescribe:
  - Pain relievers. Don't take prescription pain medicine longer than 4 to 7 days. Use only as much as you need.
  - Antibiotics to fight or prevent infection.
  - Stool softeners or laxatives to prevent constipation.
• You may use nonprescription drugs, such as acetaminophen, for minor pain. Avoid aspirin.

ACTIVITY
• Resume sexual relations when your doctor determines that healing is complete.
• Resume driving when your doctor determines that healing is complete.
• Avoid heavy lifting for 6 weeks after surgery. Learn proper body mechanics to reduce strain contributing to recurrence after recovery.

DIET—Clear liquid diet until the gastrointestinal tract begins to function again. Then eat a well-balanced diet to promote healing. Increase dietary fiber and fluid intake to prevent constipation and straining during bowel movements. If you are overweight, consult your physician about a weight loss plan to reduce the chances of recurrence of the hernia.

 CALL YOUR DOCTOR IF

• Pain, swelling, redness, drainage, or bleeding occurs in the surgical area.
• You develop symptoms of infection including headache, muscle aches, dizziness, fever, or a general ill feeling.
• You become constipated.
• New, unexplained symptoms develop.

HERNIA REPAIR, INCISIONA
(Incisional Herniorrhaphy)

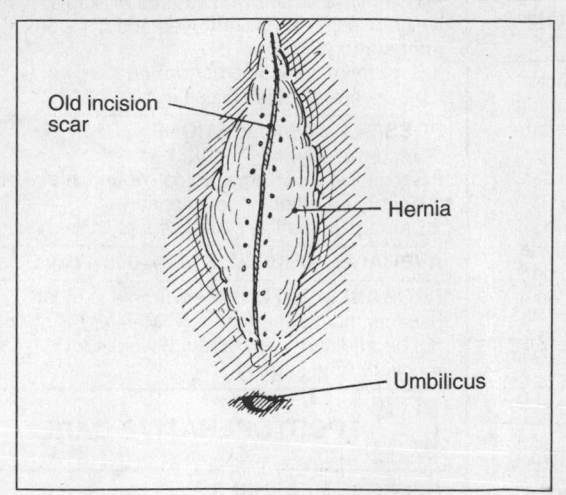

An illustration of an incisional hernia in the abdominal wall protruding through an old incision scar.

Old incision scar

Hernia

Umbilicus

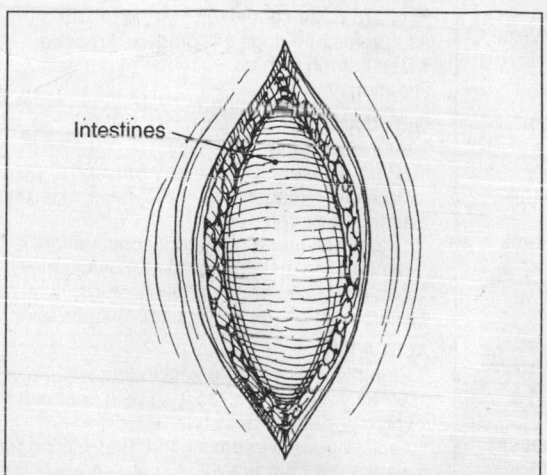

Abdominal muscles retracted to reveal intestines pushing through the abdominal muscles.

Intestines

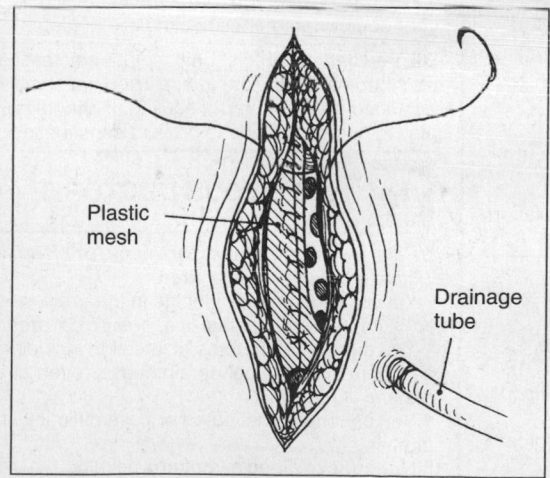

The intestine is replaced in the abdominal cavity. Usually a plastic mesh is used to strengthen the repair.

Plastic mesh

Drainage tube

HERNIA REPAIR, INGUINAL
(Inguinal Herniorrhaphy)

 GENERAL INFORMATION

DEFINITION—Closing or repairing a defect (opening) in the muscle layer of the abdominal wall in the inguinal (groin) area. A sac (of fatty tissue or an intestine) protrudes through the hernia defect, causing a noticeable bulge. If intestine or other abdominal contents are caught in the hernia and cannot be pushed back, it is called an incarcerated hernia. If the opening is so tight that it has cut off the blood supply to the incarcerated tissue, it is called a strangulated hernia.

BODY PARTS INVOLVED—Groin muscles and ligaments inside the lower abdomen next to the genitals, abdominal muscles.

REASONS FOR SURGERY
- Incarcerated hernia: This is an emergency!
- Strangulated hernia: This is an emergency!
- The hernia is getting larger or it is painful.
- To prevent future complications of the hernia.

SURGICAL RISK INCREASES WITH
- Adults over 60, newborns and infants.
- Excess alcohol consumption, smoking.
- Chronic lung disease, prostatism, constipation, or family history of hernias.
- Use of some prescription and nonprescription drugs. Inform your doctor of any drugs, medications, or vitamin and herb supplements you are using or have used in the last month.

 WHAT TO EXPECT

WHO OPERATES—General surgeon or urologist.

WHERE PERFORMED—Hospital or outpatient surgical facility.

DIAGNOSTIC TESTS
- Before surgery: Blood and urine studies, possible x-rays of abdomen and chest, ECG (see Glossary).
- After surgery: Blood studies.

ANESTHESIA
- Spinal anesthesia by injection.
- Local anesthesia by injection.
- General anesthesia by injection and inhalation with an airway tube placed in the windpipe.

DESCRIPTION OF OPERATION
- There are options for performing this surgery. Described here is an open hernia repair:
- An incision is made in the abdomen. The abdominal muscles are separated.
- The hernia is located and any sac is reduced (pushed back into place) or removed.
- A plastic mesh is generally used to reinforce and cover the defect in the muscles.

- The skin is closed with sutures or staples, which usually can be removed about 1 week after surgery.
- Surgery may also be performed laparoscopically (see Glossary).

POSSIBLE COMPLICATIONS
- Recurrent hernia.
- Excessive bleeding, surgical-wound infection.
- Urinary retention or constipation.
- Damage to testicle's blood supply or nerves.

AVERAGE HOSPITAL STAY—0 to 4 days.

PROBABLE OUTCOME—Curable in most patients, no matter what age. Male virility should not be affected. Allow about 6 weeks for recovery from surgery.

 POSTOPERATIVE CARE

GENERAL MEASURES
- A hard ridge should form along the incision. As it heals, the ridge will gradually recede.
- Don't strain with bowel movements or urination.

MEDICATION
- Your doctor may prescribe:
  - Pain relievers. Don't take prescription pain medication longer than 4 to 7 days. Use only as much as you need.
  - Stool softeners to prevent constipation.
  - Antibiotics to fight or prevent infection.
- You may use nonprescription drugs, such as acetaminophen, for minor pain. Avoid aspirin.

ACTIVITY
- Resume daily activities, including work, as soon as you are able (as long as it does not involve strenuous activity).
- Avoid vigorous exercise and heavy lifting for 6 weeks after surgery.
- Resume driving and sexual relations when your doctor determines healing is complete.

DIET—Clear liquid diet until the gastrointestinal tract begins to function again. Then eat a well-balanced diet to promote healing. It should be high in fiber and fluids to prevent constipation.

 CALL YOUR DOCTOR IF

- Pain, swelling, redness, drainage, or bleeding increases in the surgical area.
- You develop pain or a bulge in the groin, scrotum, testicle, vaginal lips, or surgical area.
- You develop symptoms of infection including headache, muscle aches, dizziness, fever, or a general ill feeling.
- You become constipated or have difficulty in urinating.
- New, unexplained symptoms develop.

HERNIA REPAIR, INGUINAL
(Inguinal Herniorrhaphy)

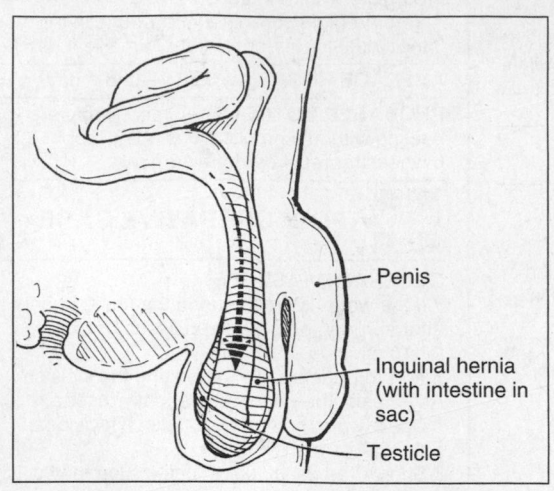

- A side view of the male pelvic region.
- A typical inguinal hernia in which a loop of intestine has dropped down into the scrotum.

Penis

Inguinal hernia (with intestine in sac)

Testicle

The hernia is located and the herniated material is pushed back into the abdomen. The sac is closed.

Herniated material

Spermatic cord

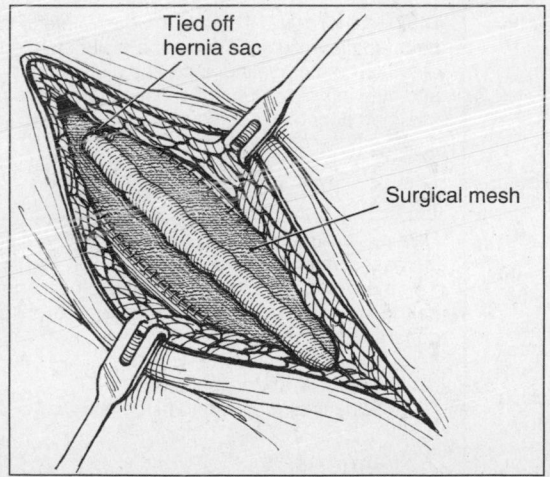

Mesh or other patch material is used to cover any defect and the outer muscles are closed over the top.

Tied off hernia sac

Surgical mesh

GENERAL INFORMATION

FINITION—Closure of an umbilical hernia, a ~akening in the muscles around the umbilicus avel) that allows abdominal contents to otrude prominently.

BODY PARTS INVOLVED—Abdominal muscular wall around the navel.

REASONS FOR SURGERY
- Improved appearance.
- Relief of pain.
- Prevention of incarceration or strangulation of the intestines (see Hernia Repair, Inguinal in Surgery section).

SURGICAL RISK INCREASES WITH
- Newborns and infants.
- Obesity, poor nutrition.
- Smoking, alcoholism.
- Recent or chronic illness.
- Diabetes.
- Use of some prescription and nonprescription drugs. Inform your doctor of any drugs, medications, or vitamin and herb supplements you are using or have used in the last month.

WHAT TO EXPECT

WHO OPERATES—General surgeon or pediatric surgeon.

WHERE PERFORMED—Hospital or outpatient surgical facility.

DIAGNOSTIC TESTS
- Before surgery: Blood and urine studies, possible abdominal and chest x-rays, ECG (see Glossary).
- After surgery: Blood studies.

ANESTHESIA
- Local anesthesia by injection.
- Spinal anesthesia by injection.
- General anesthesia by injection and inhalation with an airway tube placed in the windpipe.

DESCRIPTION OF OPERATION
- An incision is made slightly above or below the navel.
- Sometimes, an incision is made in the peritoneum to open the peritoneal cavity. The contents of the hernia sac are located and replaced in the abdominal cavity. The peritoneum is closed.
- The large abdominal muscle is pulled over the defect. The membrane covering the muscle is overlapped and tied to close the defect Plastic mesh (or other patch material) may be used to reinforce the muscles.
- The skin is closed with sutures or clips, which usually can be removed about 10 days after surgery. Drains may be placed temporarily around the incision to drain off excess fluid.

POSSIBLE COMPLICATIONS
- Excessive bleeding.
- Surgical-wound infection.
- Seroma (fluid collects at the wound site).
- Incisional hernia or recurrent umbilical hernia.

AVERAGE HOSPITAL STAY—0 to 1 day.

PROBABLE OUTCOME—Expect complete healing without complications. Allow about 3 to 6 weeks for recovery from surgery.

POSTOPERATIVE CARE

GENERAL MEASURES
- If the wound bleeds during the first 24 hours after surgery, press a clean tissue or cloth to it for 10 minutes.
- A hard ridge should form along the incision. As it heals, the ridge will gradually recede.
- Use a warm compress to relieve incisional pain.
- Shower as usual. Avoid baths. You may wash the incision gently with mild, unscented soap. Between showers, keep the wound dry with a bandage for the first 2 or 3 days after surgery. If a bandage gets wet, change it promptly.

MEDICATION
- Your doctor may prescribe:
  - Pain relievers. Don't use prescription pain medication longer than 4 to 7 days. Use only as much as you need.
  - Stool softeners to prevent constipation.
  - Antibiotics to fight or prevent infection.
- You may use nonprescription drugs, such as acetaminophen, for minor pain. Avoid aspirin.

ACTIVITY
- You can usually return to work in 2 to 4 weeks. Avoid vigorous exercise and heavy lifting for 6 weeks after surgery.
- Resume driving about 10 after surgery.
- Resume sexual relations in about 1 to 2 weeks, or as advised by your doctor.

DIET—Clear liquid diet until the gastrointestinal tract functions again. Then eat a well-balanced diet to promote healing. Increase dietary fiber and fluid intake to prevent constipation and straining during bowel movements.

CALL YOUR DOCTOR IF

- Pain, swelling, redness, drainage, or bleeding increases in the surgical area.
- You develop symptoms of infection including headache, muscle aches, dizziness, fever, or a general ill feeling.
- You experience nausea, vomiting, constipation, or abdominal swelling.
- New, unexplained symptoms develop.

HERNIA REPAIR, UMBILICAL

An illustration of a typical umbilical (navel) hernia and the incision site for the hernia repair.

Umbilical hernia

Umbilicus

Incision site

- The incision is sometimes extended through the peritoneum to open the cavity.
- Contents of the hernia sac are located and replaced in the abdominal cavity.

Peritoneal sac

Defect in muscle

The peritoneum is closed. The large abdominal muscles will be pulled over the defect, when possible, and covered with mesh. Finally the skin is closed over the mesh.

HIP NAILING FOR HIP FRACTURE

GENERAL INFORMATION

DEFINITION—A surgical procedure to reattach the broken fragments of the fractured femur near the hip.

BODY PARTS INVOLVED—The head and neck of the femur and the acetabulum (the socket of the pelvis that receives the femur to form the hip joint).

REASONS FOR SURGERY
- To make early movement of the hip joint possible after fracture.
- To prevent prolonged bed confinement, which is usually dangerous in the elderly age group when hip fractures become more common.

SURGICAL RISK INCREASES WITH
- Adults over 60, obesity, poor nutrition.
- Smoking.
- Excess alcohol consumption.
- Recent or chronic illness.
- Diabetes.
- Use of some prescription and nonprescription drugs. Inform your doctor of any drugs, medications, or vitamin and herb supplements you are using or have used in the last month.

WHAT TO EXPECT

WHO OPERATES—Orthopedic surgeon or general surgeon (sometimes).

WHERE PERFORMED—Hospital.

DIAGNOSTIC TESTS—Before surgery: Blood and urine studies, x-rays of hip and lung.

ANESTHESIA—General anesthesia by injection and inhalation with an airway tube placed in the windpipe. Spinal anesthesia may be used in some cases.

DESCRIPTION OF OPERATION
- After anesthesia, the area adjacent to the fractured hip is cleaned, shaven and draped.
- An incision is made at a point allowing access to the fractured parts.
- The broken fragments are realigned under direct vision and with x-ray.
- Plates are fitted to hold the nail to be inserted into the fractured fragments.
- The nail is hammered into the broken parts to hold them together and give strength to the injured area of the bone.
- The plate is attached to healthy bone to hold the nail in place.

POSSIBLE COMPLICATIONS
- Surgical-wound infection.
- Excessive bleeding.
- Blood clots breaking loose and traveling to the lungs (pulmonary embolism).
- Refracture at the hip.

AVERAGE HOSPITAL STAY—4 to 7 days, depending on the condition of the patient prior to hip fracture.

PROBABLE OUTCOME—Usually satisfactory recovery with surgery and rehabilitation.

POSTOPERATIVE CARE

GENERAL MEASURES
- Keep incision clean and dry.
- A hard ridge should form along the incision. As it heals, the ridge will gradually recede. Clean the incision daily with plain soap and water.
- Move and elevate legs often while resting in bed to decrease the likelihood of deep-vein blood clots.
- Avoid lifting heavy objects.

MEDICATION
- Your doctor may prescribe:
  - Pain relievers. Don't take prescription pain medication longer than 4 to 7 days. Use only as much as you need.
  - Antibiotics to fight or prevent infection.
  - Stool softeners or laxatives to prevent constipation.
  - Blood thinners to help prevent blood clots.
- You may use nonprescription drugs, such as acetaminophen, for minor pain. Avoid aspirin.

ACTIVITY
- A physical therapy program will be prescribed by your doctor. Usually you will start by using a walker, then crutches, followed by a cane if necessary.
- Avoid vigorous exercise for 12 weeks after surgery or until your doctor determines healing is complete.
- Your doctor will advise you when it is safe to resume driving.
- Resume sexual activity when your doctor determines that healing is complete.

DIET
- As prescribed by your doctor.
- Vitamin and mineral supplements (sometimes).
- Increase dietary fiber and fluid intake to help prevent constipation.

CALL YOUR DOCTOR IF

- Pain, swelling, redness, drainage, or bleeding increases in the surgical area.
- You develop symptoms of infection including headache, muscle aches, dizziness, fever, or a general ill feeling.
- You experience nausea, vomiting, or constipation.
- New, unexplained symptoms develop.

HIP NAILING FOR HIP FRACTURE

An illustration of an incision made over the affected hip showing the head of the femur that is fractured.

Head of femur

Incision site

A closer view of the fractured femur.

Femur

Fracture

The bone fragments are realigned, and a plate, which is attached to healthy bone by a number of screws, is used to hold the nail in place. The nail is hammered into the broken parts of the femur, giving strength to the broken area of the bone.

Nail

Screws

Plate

HIP REPLACEMENT, TOTAL

GENERAL INFORMATION

DEFINITION—Surgical replacement of the hip joint. A metal ball replaces the worn head of the thigh bone and a cup (often plastic) replaces the worn socket.

BODY PARTS INVOLVED—Hip joint; muscles, ligaments, bones and bursa forming the hip joint.

REASONS FOR SURGERY—Diseased or injured hip with pain and stiffness causing an altered gait and impaired quality of life.

SURGICAL RISK INCREASES WITH
- Obesity, smoking.
- Excess alcohol consumption.
- Recent or chronic illness, diabetes.
- Use of some prescription and nonprescription drugs. Inform your doctor of any drugs, medications, or vitamin and herb supplements you are using or have used in the last month.

WHAT TO EXPECT

WHO OPERATES—Orthopedic surgeon.

WHERE PERFORMED—Hospital.

DIAGNOSTIC TESTS
- Before surgery: X-rays of joint, CT scan or MRI (see Glossary for both), joint aspiration (to check for active infection), blood and urine studies.
- During surgery: X-rays.
- After surgery: X-rays, blood tests, and examination of removed tissue.

ANESTHESIA
- General anesthesia by injection and inhalation with an airway tube placed in the windpipe.
- Spinal anesthesia by injection.

DESCRIPTION OF OPERATION
- An incision is made over the affected hip.
- The head and neck of the femur are removed.
- The femoral canal is reamed to accept the metal femoral component (head, neck and stem). The femoral component is cemented in place using a special form of bone cement.
- The acetabulum is shaped to accept a plastic cup. The cup is held in place with metal screws.
- The ball and socket are replaced into normal position.

POSSIBLE COMPLICATIONS
- Excessive bleeding, blood clots.
- Surgical-wound infection.
- Dislocation of hip.
- Pneumonia.
- Loosening of components.

AVERAGE HOSPITAL STAY—5 to 7 days.

PROBABLE OUTCOME—Expect complete healing without complications. Allow about 3 to 6 months for recovery from surgery.

POSTOPERATIVE CARE

GENERAL MEASURES
- Use self-help devices, such as a raised toilet seat, bath bench, and long-handled grippers, to limit hip bending.
- Use handrails and wear low-heel shoes.
- Learn and abide by your safe range of motion.
- Cough and deep breathe as instructed.
- A hard ridge should form along the incision. As it heals, the ridge will gradually recede.
- Shower as usual after discharge. You may wash the incision gently with mild, unscented soap.
- Move and elevate legs often while resting in bed to decrease the likelihood of deep-vein blood clots.
- Use crutches, a walker, or a cane to walk until your doctor determines that healing is complete.
- Physical therapy may hasten healing and restore strength. Ask your doctor.

MEDICATION
- Your doctor may prescribe:
  - Pain relievers. Don't take prescription pain medication longer than 4 to 7 days. Use only as much as you need.
  - Antibiotics to fight or prevent infection. You may be advised to use antibiotics before future dental work.
- You may use nonprescription drugs, such as acetaminophen, for minor pain. Avoid aspirin.

ACTIVITY
- As prescribed and directed by your doctor and physical therapist.
- Avoid very active sports such as tennis, skiing, or contact sports.
- Resume driving when your doctor advises that it is safe to do so.

DIET—Eat a well-balanced diet to promote healing.

CALL YOUR DOCTOR IF

- Pain, swelling, redness, drainage, or bleeding increases in the surgical area.
- You develop symptoms of infection including headache, muscle aches, dizziness, fever, or a general ill feeling.
- New, unexplained symptoms develop.

HIP REPLACEMENT, TOTAL

An illustration of an incision made over the affected hip showing the head of the femur that is diseased or injured.

Iliac crest

Head of femur

Incision

A closer view of a diseased hip joint. After the diseased bone has been removed, the artificial ball and socket are placed into normal position.

Diseased bone

The appearance of the hip after the metal prosthesis has been inserted.

Replacement hip

HYDROCELECTOMY

GENERAL INFORMATION

DEFINITION—Removal of a hydrocele, fluid that has collected in a small sac usually on the testicle or in the membrane covering the testicle. Hydroceles frequently occur in infants, but may also occur in adults.

BODY PARTS INVOLVED—Scrotum, spermatic cord, membrane covering the testicle (tunica vaginalis), blood vessels, and nerves connected to the scrotum.

REASONS FOR SURGERY
* In infants: completion of the repair of a congenital inguinal hernia, which frequently accompanies a congenital hydrocele.
* In adults: removal of an uncomfortable and unsightly scrotal cyst that may conceal a tumor in the testicle.

SURGICAL RISK INCREASES WITH
* Obesity, poor nutrition.
* Smoking, alcoholism.
* Chronic or recent illness.
* Diabetes.
* Use of some prescription and nonprescription drugs. Inform your doctor of any drugs, medications, or vitamin and herb supplements you are using or have used in the last month.

WHAT TO EXPECT

WHO OPERATES—General surgeon or urologist.

WHERE PERFORMED—Hospital or outpatient surgical facility.

DIAGNOSTIC TESTS
* Before surgery: Blood and urine studies, ultrasound (see Glossary).
* After surgery: Usually none.

ANESTHESIA
* General anesthesia by injection and inhalation with an airway tube placed in the windpipe in infants.
* Local anesthesia by injection.
* Spinal anesthesia by injection (sometimes).

DESCRIPTION OF OPERATION
* An incision is made in the scrotum over the testicle.
* The hydrocele is located and cut free from the scrotal contents.
* The hydrocele is incised, and the fluid inside it is drained. The skin edges of the hydrocele are tucked under and sewn together to prevent refilling.
* The scrotal contents are replaced. The skin is closed with fine suture material that will be absorbed by the body.

POSSIBLE COMPLICATIONS
* Excessive bleeding.
* Surgical-wound infection.
* Urinary retention.
* Damaged blood supply to the testicle.
* Twisting of the testicle.
* Recurrent hydrocele.

AVERAGE HOSPITAL STAY—0 to 1 day.

PROBABLE OUTCOME—Expect complete healing without complications. Allow about 2 weeks for recovery from surgery. Post-surgical swelling may last as long as 6 months.

POSTOPERATIVE CARE

GENERAL MEASURES
* A hard ridge should form along the incision. As it heals, the ridge will gradually recede.
* Shower as usual. You may wash the incision gently with mild, unscented soap. After showering, replace any wet dressings with clean, dry ones.
* Children and adults should wear an athletic supporter for 3 to 6 weeks after surgery. Infants should wear double diapers to provide support during healing.

MEDICATION
* Your doctor may prescribe pain relievers. Don't take prescription pain medication longer than 4 to 7 days. Use only as much as you need.
* You may use nonprescription drugs, such as acetaminophen, for minor pain. Avoid aspirin.

ACTIVITY
* Avoid vigorous exercise for 6 weeks after surgery.
* Resume driving 1 week after returning home.
* Resume sexual relations when your doctor determines that healing is complete.

DIET—Clear liquid diet until the gastrointestinal tract begins to function again. Then eat a well-balanced diet to promote healing.

CALL YOUR DOCTOR IF

* Pain, swelling, redness, drainage, or bleeding increases in the surgical area.
* You develop symptoms of infection including headache, muscle aches, dizziness, fever, or a general ill feeling.
* You experience nausea or vomiting.
* New, unexplained symptoms develop.

HYDROCELECTOMY

An illustration of a typical hydrocele distending one portion of the scrotum.

Hydrocele

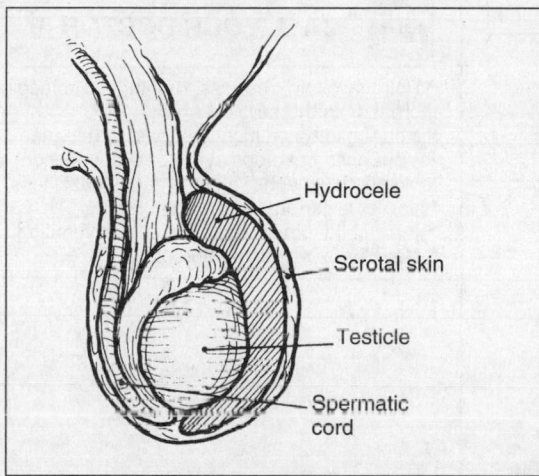

A hydrocele and surrounding tissues including the spermatic cord, testicle and scrotum.

Hydrocele

Scrotal skin

Testicle

Spermatic cord

• After the hydrocele has been incised and the fluid inside drained, the edges of the hydrocele are tucked under and sewn together to prevent refilling.
• The scrotal contents are then replaced and the skin closed with fine absorbable sutures that need not be removed.

HYPOSPADIAS REPAIR & URETHROPLASTY

 ## GENERAL INFORMATION

DEFINITION—Creation of a new urethra to correct hypospadias, a congenital disorder in which the urethra opening is in an abnormal location on the penis. Surgery is usually done in infancy or early childhood.

BODY PARTS INVOLVED—Urethra.

REASONS FOR SURGERY
- Prevention of urinary-tract infections.
- Establishment of sexual function.
- Correction of abnormal urination patterns.

SURGICAL RISK INCREASES WITH
- Obesity.
- Poor nutrition.
- Recent or chronic illness.
- Diabetes.
- Use of some prescription and nonprescription drugs. Inform your doctor of any drugs, medications, or vitamin and herb supplements your child is using or has used in the last month.

 ## WHAT TO EXPECT

WHO OPERATES—Urologist.

WHERE PERFORMED—Hospital.

DIAGNOSTIC TESTS
- Before surgery: Blood and urine studies.
- After surgery: Blood studies, laboratory examination of removed tissue.

ANESTHESIA—General anesthesia by injection and inhalation, with an airway tube placed in the windpipe.

DESCRIPTION OF OPERATION
- An incision is made over the abnormal opening of the urethra.
- An instrument is passed through the urethra and extended along its full length. Abnormal scar tissue is cut free and removed. A new urethra is fashioned from existing tissue and sewn around a catheter, which will remain in place until healing is complete.
- After healing, the catheter is removed.
- The skin is closed with sutures that will be absorbed by the body.

POSSIBLE COMPLICATIONS
- Excessive bleeding.
- Surgical-wound infection.
- Scarring of urethra.

AVERAGE HOSPITAL STAY—2 to 7 days.

PROBABLE OUTCOME—Expect complete healing without complications. Allow about 3 months for recovery from surgery.

 ## POSTOPERATIVE CARE

GENERAL MEASURES
- A ridge should form along the incision. As it heals, the ridge will gradually recede.
- Bathe your child as usual. You may wash the incision gently with mild, unscented soap.

MEDICATION
- Your doctor may prescribe:
  - Pain relievers. Don't take prescription pain medication longer than 4 to 7 days. Use only as much as your child needs.
  - Antibiotics to fight or prevent infection.
- You may give your child nonprescription drugs, such as acetaminophen, for minor pain. Avoid aspirin.

ACTIVITY—Vigorous exercise should be avoided for 6 weeks after surgery.

DIET—No special diet.

 ## CALL YOUR DOCTOR IF

- Pain, swelling, redness, drainage, or bleeding increases in the surgical area.
- Your child has difficulty or pain in urination.
- Your child develops symptoms of infection including headache, muscle aches, dizziness, fever, or a general ill feeling.
- Your child experiences nausea or vomiting.
- New, unexplained symptoms develop.

HYPOSPADIAS REPAIR & URETHROPLASTY

- A typical hypospadias with opening of the urethra under the head of the penis.
- Openings of the urethra may occur in various other places on the penis other than its normal opening.

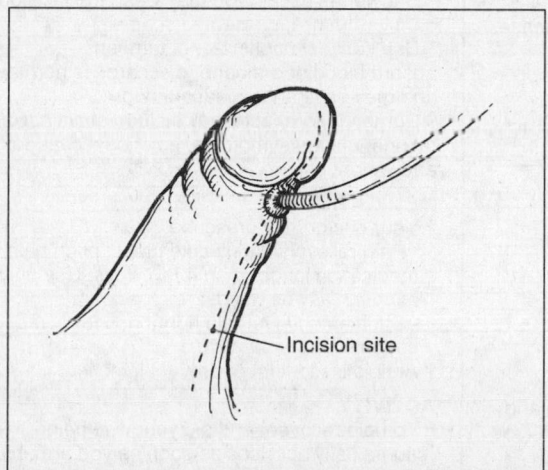

- An instrument is placed through the urethra and is extended along its full length. Abnormal scar tissue is cut free and removed.
- A new urethra is fashioned from existing tissue and sewn around a catheter which will remain in place until healing is complete.

After healing, the catheter is removed.

HYSTERECTOMY (ABDOMINAL) WITH SALPINGO-OOPHORECTOMY

GENERAL INFORMATION

DEFINITION—Removal of the uterus, cervix, fallopian tubes, and ovaries, through an incision in the abdomen.

BODY PARTS INVOLVED—Uterus, cervix, fallopian tubes, ovaries, vagina.

REASONS FOR SURGERY
- Uterus: Cancer or suspected cancer, fibroid tumors, chronic bleeding, prolapsed (dropped) uterus, endometriosis, chronic pelvic infection, severe menstrual pain, or voluntary sterilization.
- Fallopian tubes and ovaries: Cancer or suspected cancer of the ovaries, precancerous or twisted ovarian cysts, ovarian pregnancy, ovarian abscess, damage to the ovaries from severe endometriosis.

SURGICAL RISK INCREASES WITH
- Obesity, smoking.
- Iron-deficiency anemia, heart or lung disease, or diabetes.
- Use of some prescription and nonprescription drugs. Inform your doctor of any drugs, medications, or vitamin and herb supplements you are using or have used in the last month.

WHAT TO EXPECT

WHO OPERATES—General surgeon or obstetrician-gynecologist.

WHERE PERFORMED—Hospital.

DIAGNOSTIC TESTS
- Before surgery: Blood and urine studies, x-rays of abdomen and kidneys, dilatation and curettage of the uterus (D & C), ultrasound (see Glossary for both).
- After surgery: Blood studies.

ANESTHESIA—Spinal anesthesia or general anesthesia by injection and inhalation with an airway tube placed in the windpipe.

DESCRIPTION OF OPERATION
- An incision is made in the abdomen.
- The abdominal organs are examined.
- The uterus is freed from its attachments to the bladder and upper vagina. The uterus is removed along with the fallopian tubes and ovaries.
- The vagina is closed with sutures at its deeper end, the surgical wound is closed.
- The procedure may also be performed by laparoscopy (see in Surgery section).

POSSIBLE COMPLICATIONS
- Excessive bleeding, surgical-wound infection.
- Urinary tract infection.
- Inadvertent injury to the bowel, bladder or ureters.
- Urinary obstruction or bowel obstruction.

AVERAGE HOSPITAL STAY—2 to 5 days.

PROBABLE OUTCOME
- The vagina will be shortened slightly. This should cause no lasting problem. Expect permanent sterility. Allow about 6 weeks for recovery from surgery.
- Removal of the ovaries in premenopausal women will result in menopause (sometimes called surgical menopause).

POSTOPERATIVE CARE

GENERAL MEASURES
- Shower as usual. You may wash the incision gently with mild, unscented soap.
- Use sanitary napkins—not tampons—to absorb blood or drainage (discharge is normal, and may have an unpleasant odor).
- Surgery aftereffects may include constipation, fatigue, urinary symptoms, emotional changes, and weight gain.

MEDICATION
- Your doctor may prescribe:
  - Pain relievers. Don't take prescription pain medication longer than 4 to 7 days. Use only as much as you need.
  - Supplemental female hormones for some patients.
- Antibiotics to fight or prevent infection.

ACTIVITY
- To help recovery and aid your well-being, resume daily activities as soon as you are able.
- Resume driving 2 weeks after returning home.
- Resume sexual relations in 4 to 6 weeks.

DIET—Clear liquid diet until the gastrointestinal tract functions again. Then eat a well-balanced diet to promote healing.

CALL YOUR DOCTOR IF

- Vaginal bleeding soaks more than 1 pad per hour.
- You experience a frequent urge to urinate or have excessive vaginal discharge that persists longer than 1 month.
- Pain or swelling increases in the surgical area.
- You develop symptoms of infection including headache, muscle aches, dizziness, fever, or a general ill feeling.

HYSTERECTOMY (ABDOMINAL) WITH SALPINGO-OOPHORECTOMY

Shown are parts of the female reproductive tract including the uterus, fallopian tubes, ovaries and vagina.

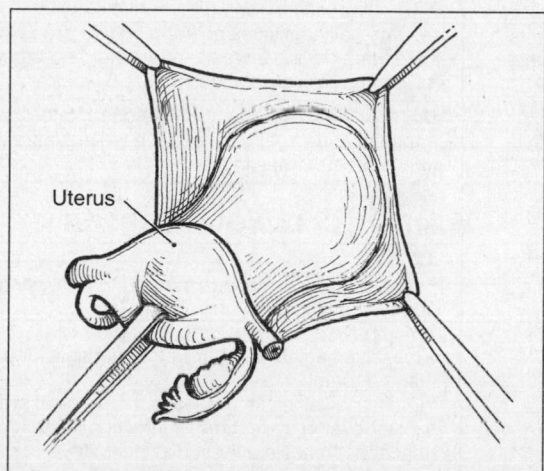

After an incision (either vertical or transverse) has been made in the lower abdomen and the muscles retracted, the uterus, cervix, fallopian tubes and ovaries are cut free and removed.

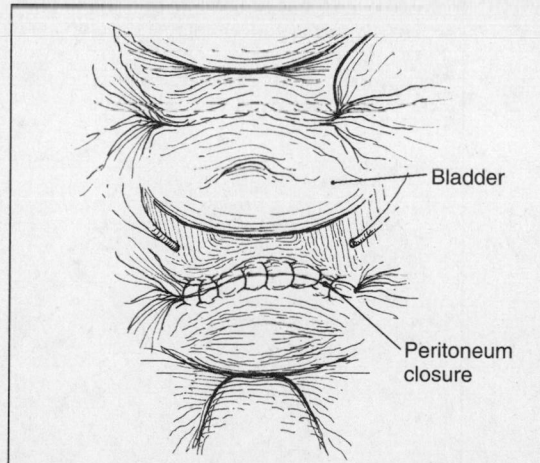

• The peritoneum is closed with sutures.
• The abdominal wall is closed in layers and the skin is closed with sutures that usually can be removed in 10 to 14 days (not illustrated).

HYSTERECTOMY (VAGINAL)

GENERAL INFORMATION

DEFINITION—Removal of the uterus and cervix through an incision in the deepest recesses of the vagina. This surgery is frequently accompanied by reconstructive surgery (colporrhaphy), to repair weakened bladder.

BODY PARTS INVOLVED—Bladder muscles, rectal muscles, uterus, cervix, fallopian tubes, vagina.

REASONS FOR SURGERY—Cancer or suspected cancer, fibroid tumors, chronic bleeding, prolapsed (dropped) uterus, endometriosis, chronic pelvic infection, or severe menstrual pain.

SURGICAL RISK INCREASES WITH
- Obesity, smoking.
- Iron-deficiency anemia, heart or lung disease, or diabetes.
- Use of some prescription and nonprescription drugs. Inform your doctor of any drugs, medications, or vitamin and herb supplements you are using or have used in the last month.

WHAT TO EXPECT

WHO OPERATES—General surgeon or obstetrician-gynecologist.

WHERE PERFORMED—Hospital.

DIAGNOSTIC TESTS
- Before surgery: Blood and urine studies, x-rays of abdomen and kidneys, dilatation and curettage of the uterus (D & C), ultrasound (see Glossary for both).
- After surgery: Blood studies.

ANESTHESIA
- Spinal anesthesia by injection.
- General anesthesia by injection and inhalation with an airway tube placed in the windpipe.

DESCRIPTION OF OPERATION
- The deepest recesses of the vagina are opened. The cervix and uterus are cut free and removed. The rear part of the vagina is closed with sutures.
- A small foley catheter may be in the bladder for several days.
- The procedure may also be performed in conjunction with a laparoscopy (see in Surgery section) to remove the fallopian tubes or ovaries.

POSSIBLE COMPLICATIONS
- Excessive bleeding.
- Surgical-wound infection.
- Inadvertent injury to bladder, rectum or ureters.
- Urinary tract infection.

AVERAGE HOSPITAL STAY—1 to 3 days.

PROBABLE OUTCOME—The vagina will be shortened slightly. This should cause no lasting problem. Expect permanent sterility. Allow about 6 weeks for recovery from surgery.

POSTOPERATIVE CARE

GENERAL MEASURES—Use sanitary napkins—not tampons—to absorb blood or drainage (discharge is normal, and may have an unpleasant odor).

MEDICATION
- Your doctor may prescribe:
  - Pain relievers. Don't take prescription pain medication longer than 4 to 7 days. Use only as much as you need.
  - Supplemental female hormones, unless there are reasons why you should not take them.
- Antibiotics to fight or prevent infection.

ACTIVITY
- To help recovery and aid your well-being, resume daily activities as soon as you are able.
- Resume driving 2 weeks after returning home.
- Resume sexual relations in 4 to 6 weeks.

DIET—Clear liquid diet until the gastrointestinal tract functions again. Then eat a well-balanced diet to promote healing.

CALL YOUR DOCTOR IF

- Vaginal bleeding soaks more than 1 pad per hour.
- You have a frequent urge to urinate or excessive vaginal discharge that persists longer than 1 month.
- Pain or swelling increases in the surgical area.
- You develop symptoms of infection including headache, muscle aches, dizziness, fever, or a general ill feeling.
- You experience abdominal swelling or pain.
- New, unexplained symptoms develop.

HYSTERECTOMY (VAGINAL)

Vaginal wall

Cervix

● This view illustrates a female patient with extended legs in stirrups on an examining table to allow examination of the genital area.
● An illustration of the vagina and cervix showing the first incision made to separate the cervix from the lowest layers of the bladder.

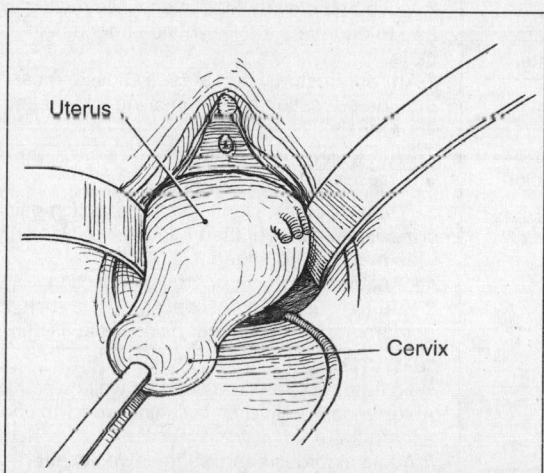

Uterus

Cervix

The deepest recesses of the vagina are opened. The cervix and uterus are cut free and removed. The bladder may also be repaired (not illustrated).

Catheter

A small catheter is left in the bladder to remain there several days until swelling subsides.

ILEOSTOMY

GENERAL INFORMATION

DEFINITION—Creation of an opening in the ileum, the lower part of the small intestine. After surgery, all feces leave the body through this opening, which is called an ostomy or stoma.

BODY PARTS INVOLVED—Ileum, cecum.

REASONS FOR SURGERY
- Ulcerative colitis.
- Multiple colon cancers.
- Colon surgery which weakens an area of the colon and necessitates a temporary bypass of the intestine until the colon has healed.

SURGICAL RISK INCREASES WITH
- Adults over 60, newborns and infants.
- Obesity, smoking, poor nutrition.
- Excess alcohol consumption.
- Recent or chronic illness, especially heart or lung disease or diabetes.
- Use of some prescription and nonprescription drugs. Inform your doctor of any drugs, medications, or vitamin and herb supplements you are using or have used in the last month.

WHAT TO EXPECT

WHO OPERATES—General surgeon or colon-rectal surgeon.

WHERE PERFORMED—Hospital.

DIAGNOSTIC TESTS
- Before surgery: Blood and urine studies, x-rays, ECG, sigmoidoscopy, colonoscopy (see Glossary for all).
- After surgery: Blood and urine studies.

ANESTHESIA—General anesthesia by injection and inhalation with an airway tube placed in the windpipe.

DESCRIPTION OF OPERATION
- An incision is made in the abdomen over the diseased intestinal tract.
- The muscles of the abdominal wall are separated to expose the abdominal organs, which are inspected for undetected disease. Other surgeries may be performed at this time.
- The ileum is clamped on both sides of the area to be opened and cut between the clamps. The part closer to the stomach is brought through another small incision in the abdominal wall to accept the stoma.
- The part of the intestinal tract below the ileum, usually around the diseased part of the intestine, is closed with sutures or is removed with the diseased colon. The abdominal contents are replaced. The muscles and skin are closed with sutures, which usually can be removed about 1 week after surgery.

POSSIBLE COMPLICATIONS
- Excessive bleeding.
- Surgical-wound infection, abscess.
- Incisional or stomal hernia.
- Skin irritation around the stoma.
- Intestinal obstruction.
- Scarring.
- Leakage of the ileal pouch.

AVERAGE HOSPITAL STAY—5 to 7 days.

PROBABLE OUTCOME—Expect complete cure without complications. Allow about 6 weeks for recovery. You will need to wear an external pouch to collect bowel movements.

POSTOPERATIVE CARE

GENERAL MEASURES
- A hard ridge should form along the incision. As it heals, the ridge will gradually recede.
- Shower as usual after discharge. You may wash the incision gently with mild soap.
- Move and elevate legs often while resting in bed to decrease the likelihood of deep-vein clots.
- An "enterostomy nurse" (see Glossary) can provide education and counseling for you and your family.

MEDICATION
- Your doctor may prescribe:
  - Pain relievers. Don't take prescription pain medication longer than 4 to 7 days. Use only as much as you need.
  - Antibiotics to fight or prevent infection.
- You may use nonprescription drugs, such as acetaminophen, for minor pain. Avoid aspirin.

ACTIVITY
- To help recovery and aid your well-being, resume daily activities, including work, as soon as you are able.
- Avoid vigorous exercise for 6 weeks after surgery.
- Resume driving 3 to 4 weeks after surgery.
- Resume sexual relations when able.

DIET—Clear liquid diet until the gastrointestinal tract begins to function again. Then eat a well-balanced diet to promote healing.

CALL YOUR DOCTOR IF

- Pain, swelling, redness, drainage, or bleeding increases in the surgical area.
- You have abdominal swelling or pain.
- You develop symptoms of infection including headache, muscle aches, dizziness, fever, or a general ill feeling.
- Skin around the stoma becomes inflamed and painful.
- New, unexplained symptoms develop.

ILEOSTOMY

The muscles of the abdominal wall are separated to expose the abdominal organs, which are inspected for disease (not illustrated). The ileum is clamped on both sides of the area to be opened and cut between the clamps.

Ileum

Clamps

Abdominal wall

* The part closer to the stomach is brought through another small incision in the abdominal wall to accept the stoma.
* The part of the intestinal tract below the ileum, usually around the diseased part of the intestine, is removed with the diseased colon.

The stoma is shown in a frequently used location extending through the abdominal wall. After surgery, fecal contents will pass into an ileostomy bag.

Stoma

KIDNEY REMOVAL
(Nephrectomy)

 GENERAL INFORMATION

DEFINITION—Removal of a kidney.

BODY PARTS INVOLVED—Kidney, blood vessels connected to kidney, ureter.

REASONS FOR SURGERY
- Cancer or suspected cancer of the kidney.
- Severe kidney trauma.
- Dysfunctional kidney due to infection.

SURGICAL RISK INCREASES WITH
- Adults over 60, newborns and infants.
- Obesity, poor nutrition.
- Smoking, alcoholism.
- Recent or chronic illness.
- Diabetes.
- Renal (kidney failure).
- Use of some prescription and nonprescription drugs. Inform your doctor of any drugs, medications, or vitamin and herb supplements you are using or have used in the last month.

 WHAT TO EXPECT

WHO OPERATES—General surgeon or urologist.

WHERE PERFORMED—Hospital.

DIAGNOSTIC TESTS
- Before surgery: Blood and urine studies, x-rays of kidneys, lower gastrointestinal tract and chest, ECG, ultrasound, cystoscopy, IVP, MRI, CT scan (see Glossary for all).
- After surgery: Blood studies.

ANESTHESIA—General anesthesia by injection and inhalation with an airway tube placed in the windpipe.

DESCRIPTION OF OPERATION
- An incision is made, usually in the left or right flank, but sometimes in the abdomen.
- The vein leading from the kidney is located, isolated and tied.
- The ureter is located, tied and cut away from the kidney.
- The artery that supplies blood to the kidney is tied and transected.
- The kidney is freed of adhesions or adjoining connective tissue and removed; surrounding lymph nodes may also be removed.
- All disconnected blood vessels are tied, and the muscles are closed with sutures. The skin is closed with sutures or clips, which usually can be removed in about 1 week after surgery.
- A urinary catheter (Foley) will be left in place for several days to make it easier to measure the amount of urine you are producing.
- Surgery may also be done by laparoscopy (see in Surgery section).

POSSIBLE COMPLICATIONS
- Excessive bleeding, blood clots.
- Surgical-wound infection.
- Inadvertent injury to the vena cava or other organs near the kidney.

AVERAGE HOSPITAL STAY—3 to 5 days.

PROBABLE OUTCOME—Expect complete healing without complications. Allow about 4 weeks for recovery from surgery.

 POSTOPERATIVE CARE

GENERAL MEASURES
- A hard ridge should form along the incision. As it heals, the ridge will gradually recede.
- Shower as usual. Avoid baths until the incision has healed. You may wash the incision gently with mild, unscented soap.
- Move and elevate legs often while resting in bed to decrease the likelihood of deep-vein blood clots.

MEDICATION
- Your doctor may prescribe:
  - Pain relievers. Don't take prescription pain medication longer than 4 to 7 days. Use only as much as you need.
  - Stool softeners to prevent constipation.
  - Antibiotics to fight or prevent infection.
- You may use nonprescription drugs, such as acetaminophen, for minor pain. Avoid aspirin.

ACTIVITY
- Resuming daily activities, including work, as soon as you are able can help the healing process.
- Avoid vigorous exercise for 6 weeks after surgery.
- Resume driving 5 weeks after returning home.
- Resume sexual relations when your doctor determines that healing is complete.

DIET—Clear liquid diet until the gastrointestinal tract begins to function again. Then eat a well-balanced diet to promote healing.

 CALL YOUR DOCTOR IF

- Pain, swelling, redness, drainage, or bleeding increases in the surgical area.
- You develop symptoms of infection including headache, muscle aches, dizziness, fever, or a general ill feeling.
- You experience nausea, vomiting, abdominal swelling, or constipation.
- New, unexplained symptoms develop.

KIDNEY REMOVAL
(Nephrectomy)

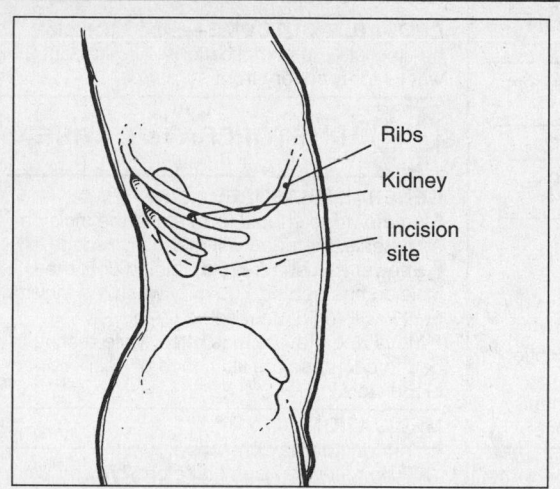

Ribs

Kidney

Incision site

The usual incision for kidney removal in the flank below the last rib.

Kidney

Renal artery

Renal vein

Ureter

Clamps

- The vein leading from the kidney is located, isolated and tied.
- The ureter is located, tied and cut away from the kidney.
- The artery that supplies blood to the kidney is clamped in 2 places and cut between the clamps.
- The kidney is removed.

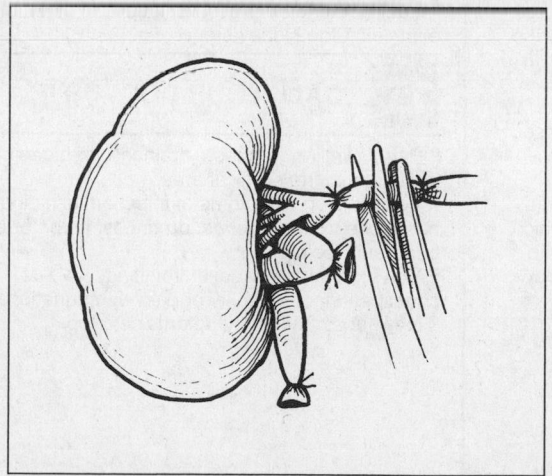

All disconnected blood vessels are tied. The abdominal muscles are closed (not illustrated).

KIDNEY STONE REMOVAL
(Ureterolithotomy)

GENERAL INFORMATION

DEFINITION—Removal of a kidney stone from one of the ureters.

BODY PARTS INVOLVED—Ureter, kidney.

REASONS FOR SURGERY—Restoration of normal urine flow in the ureter.

SURGICAL RISK INCREASES WITH
- Obesity, smoking, alcoholism.
- Poor nutrition.
- Recent or chronic illness.
- Diabetes.
- Use of some prescription and nonprescription drugs. Inform your doctor of any drugs, medications, or vitamin and herb supplements you are using or have used in the last month.

WHAT TO EXPECT

WHO OPERATES—Urologist or general surgeon.

WHERE PERFORMED—Hospital.

DIAGNOSTIC TESTS
- Before surgery: Blood and urine studies, x-rays of chest, ECG, intravenous pyelogram, ultrasound: CT scan (see Glossary for all).
- During surgery: Retrograde pyelogram (see Glossary).
- After surgery: Blood studies, urine tests.

ANESTHESIA—General anesthesia by injection and inhalation with an airway tube placed in the windpipe.

DESCRIPTION OF OPERATION
- An incision is made in the flank. The muscles are separated and the ureter is exposed.
- A small incision is made in the ureter. The kidney stone is pulled free and removed.
- After the ureter is closed, a tube is left in the wound for drainage, and a tube is inserted in the ureter to restore urine flow. This tube is removed after healing.
- Muscle layers are closed. The skin is closed with sutures or clips, which usually can be removed about 1 week after surgery.
- Some kidney stones may also be removed with lithotripsy (see in Surgery section), which involves the use of shockwaves to crush the stone so that it can be passed from the body with your urine.

POSSIBLE COMPLICATIONS
- Excessive bleeding.
- Surgical-wound infection.
- Urine leakage.
- Scarring at operative site causing obstruction or partial obstruction.

AVERAGE HOSPITAL STAY—4 to 5 days.

PROBABLE OUTCOME—Expect complete healing without complications. Allow about 2 weeks for recovery from surgery.

POSTOPERATIVE CARE

GENERAL MEASURES
- A hard ridge should form along the incision. As it heals, the ridge will gradually recede.
- Shower as usual. Avoid bathing until the incision has healed You may wash the incision gently with mild, unscented soap.
- Move and elevate legs often while resting in bed to decrease the likelihood of deep-vein blood clots.

MEDICATION
- Your doctor may prescribe:
  - Pain relievers. Don't take prescription pain medication longer than 4 to 7 days. Use only as much as you need.
  - Stool softeners to prevent constipation.
  - Antibiotics to fight or prevent infection.
- You may use nonprescription drugs, such as acetaminophen, for minor pain. Avoid aspirin.

ACTIVITY
- To help recovery and aid your well-being, resume daily activities, including work, as soon as you are able.
- Avoid vigorous exercise for 6 weeks after surgery.
- Resume driving 2 weeks after returning home.
- Resume sexual relations when your doctor determines that healing is complete.

DIET
- Clear liquid diet until the gastrointestinal tract begins to function. Then eat a well-balanced diet to promote healing.
- Be sure to drink plenty of water every day.
- Your doctor may prescribe a special diet after examining the kidney stone.

CALL YOUR DOCTOR IF

- Pain, swelling, redness, drainage, or bleeding increases in the surgical area.
- You develop symptoms of infection including headache, muscle aches, dizziness, fever, or a general ill feeling.
- You experience nausea, vomiting, constipation, or difficulty or pain with urination.
- New, unexplained symptoms develop.

KIDNEY STONE REMOVAL
(Ureterolithotomy)

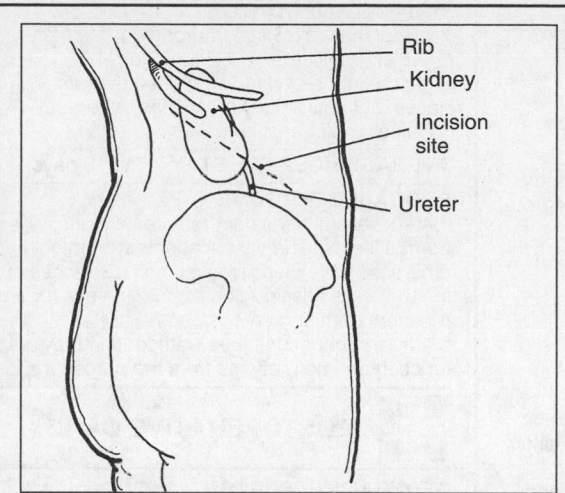

Rib

Kidney

Incision site

Ureter

Incision site on the skin in the flank under the last rib.

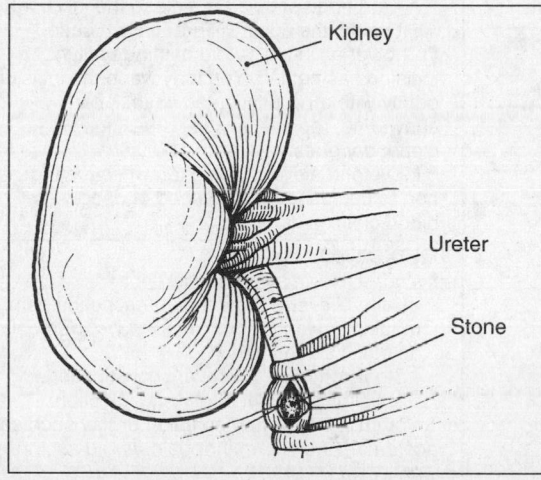

Kidney

Ureter

Stone

After a small incision has been made in the ureter, the kidney stone is pulled free and removed.

Drainage tube

A tube is inserted for drainage. The tissues under the skin are closed with large absorbable sutures. The skin is closed with sutures or clips that usually can be removed about 1 week after surgery.

KIDNEY TRANSPLANTATION

GENERAL INFORMATION

DEFINITION—Replacement of a diseased kidney with a healthy kidney obtained from a healthy donor with compatible immunological characteristics. The donated kidney may come from a living person or deceased donor.

BODY PARTS INVOLVED—Diseased kidney, healthy donor kidney, blood vessels to and from the kidney, ureters.

REASONS FOR SURGERY—Restoration of normal kidney function.

SURGICAL RISK INCREASES WITH
- Adults over 60.
- Obesity, poor nutrition.
- Recent or chronic illness, diabetes.
- Alcoholism, smoking.
- Use of some prescription and nonprescription drugs. Inform your doctor of any drugs, medications, or vitamin and herb supplements you are using or have used in the last month.

WHAT TO EXPECT

WHO OPERATES—General surgeon or urologist.

WHERE PERFORMED—Hospital.

DIAGNOSTIC TESTS
- Before surgery: Blood and urine studies, x-rays of kidneys, ECG, CT scan, ultrasound.
- After surgery: Blood studies.

ANESTHESIA—General anesthesia by injection and inhalation with an airway tube placed in the windpipe.

DESCRIPTION OF OPERATION
- The diseased kidney from the recipient may be removed several weeks in advance. During this time, dialysis (see Glossary) provides artificial kidney function.
- Often, the recipients kidneys are not removed, they are left in place and the donor kidney is placed in the lower right part of the abdomen.
- A kidney is removed from the donor, then chilled and preserved for up to 12 hours.
- An incision is made in the abdomen of the recipient. The abdominal cavity is examined. The new kidney is placed and sewn in position.
- The blood vessels and ureters are connected to the new kidney.
- The peritoneum and abdominal muscles are closed.
- The skin is closed with sutures or clips, which usually can be removed about 1 week after surgery.

POSSIBLE COMPLICATIONS
- Excessive bleeding.
- Surgical-wound infection.
- Ureter leak, blockage of ureter.
- Occasionally, the new kidney does not function right away and continued dialysis is necessary until kidney function is restored.
- Rejection of transplant.

AVERAGE HOSPITAL STAY—7 to 10 days.

PROBABLE OUTCOME
- A successful transplant restores almost normal life expectancy in patients who might otherwise have died. Transplants are successful in 70-80% of cases. Allow about 4 weeks for recovery from surgery.
- A living donor continues with good kidney function and no ill effects from the procedure.

POSTOPERATIVE CARE

GENERAL MEASURES
- A hard ridge should form along the incision. As it heals, the ridge will gradually recede.
- Shower as usual. Avoid bathing until the incision has healed. You may wash the incision gently with mild, unscented soap. After showering, replace any wet dressings with clean, dry ones.
- Move and elevate legs often while resting in bed to decrease the likelihood of deep-vein blood clots.

MEDICATION
- Your doctor may prescribe:
  - Pain relievers. Don't take prescription pain medication longer than 4 to 7 days. Use only as much as you need.
  - Stool softeners to prevent constipation.
  - Antibiotics to fight or prevent infection.
- You may use nonprescription drugs, such as acetaminophen, for minor pain. Avoid aspirin.

ACTIVITY
- To help recovery and aid your well-being, resume daily activities, including work, as soon as you are able.
- Avoid vigorous exercise for 6 weeks after surgery. Resume sexual relations when you feel able.
- Resume driving 2 weeks after returning home.

DIET—Your doctor will prescribe a diet.

CALL YOUR DOCTOR IF

- Pain, swelling, redness, drainage, or bleeding increases in the surgical area.
- You develop symptoms of infection including headache, muscle aches, dizziness, fever, or a general ill feeling.
- You experience nausea or vomiting.
- New, unexplained symptoms develop.

KIDNEY TRANSPLANTATION

Shown are the kidneys and the adjoining body structures involved in the transplantation.

Kidney

Vena cava

Ureter

Aorta

A kidney is removed from the donor, chilled and preserved for up to 12 hours.

Removal of donor kidney

• New kidney is placed and sewn into position. The blood vessels and ureters are connected to the new kidney.
• The abdominal muscles and skin are closed in layers (not illustrated).

New kidney

External iliac artery

External iliac vein

Ureter

KNEE REPLACEMENT, TOTAL

GENERAL INFORMATION

DEFINITION—Surgical replacement of an injured or diseased knee to reestablish a pain-free, movable joint.

BODY PARTS INVOLVED—Knee joint, muscles, ligaments, bones, cartilage and bursa forming the knee joint.

REASONS FOR SURGERY—Diseased or injured knee causing chronic pain or disability impairing the quality of life.

SURGICAL RISK INCREASES WITH
- Obesity, smoking.
- Excess alcohol consumption.
- Recent or chronic illness.
- Diabetes.
- Use of some prescription and nonprescription drugs. Inform your doctor of any drugs, medications, or vitamin and herb supplements you are using or have used in the last month.

WHAT TO EXPECT

WHO OPERATES—Orthopedic surgeon.

WHERE PERFORMED—Hospital.

DIAGNOSTIC TESTS
- Before surgery: X-rays of joint, MRI or CT scan (see Glossary for both), joint aspiration (to check for active infection), blood and urine studies.
- During surgery: X-rays.
- After surgery: X-rays, blood tests, and examination of tissue removed.

ANESTHESIA—General anesthesia by injection and inhalation with an airway tube placed in the windpipe.

DESCRIPTION OF OPERATION
- An incision is made into the affected knee.
- The arthritic or diseased surfaces of the femoral condyles and tibial plateau are removed.
- The above areas are replaced by durable prosthetic components that are fixed firmly in place with a special form of bone cement.
- The new knee joint may be hinged (for unstable knees) or unhinged.

POSSIBLE COMPLICATIONS
- Excessive bleeding, blood clots.
- Surgical-wound infection.
- Pneumonia.
- Limited range-of-motion of the knee.
- Loosening of joint components at a future time.

AVERAGE HOSPITAL STAY—3 to 5 days.

PROBABLE OUTCOME—Expect complete healing without complications. Allow about 6 months for recovery from surgery.

POSTOPERATIVE CARE

GENERAL MEASURES
- No smoking.
- Buy and use self-help devices, such as a raised toilet seat, bath bench and long-handled grippers, to limit knee bending.
- Use handrails and wear low shoes.
- Learn and abide by your safe range of motion.
- Cough and deep breathe as instructed.
- A hard ridge should form along the incision. As it heals, the ridge will gradually recede.
- Shower as usual. You may wash the incision gently with mild, unscented soap.
- Move and elevate legs often while resting in bed to decrease the likelihood of deep-vein blood clots.
- Use crutches or a cane to walk until your doctor determines that healing is complete.
- Physical therapy may hasten healing and restore strength. Ask your doctor.

MEDICATION
- Your doctor may prescribe:
  - Pain relievers. Don't take prescription pain medication longer than 4 to 7 days. Use only as much as you need.
  - Antibiotics to fight or prevent infection. Use antibiotics before future dental work.
- You may use nonprescription drugs, such as acetaminophen, for minor pain. Avoid aspirin.

ACTIVITY
- As prescribed and directed by your surgeon and physical therapist.
- Avoid very active sports such as tennis, skiing, or contact sports.
- Resume driving when your doctor advises that it is safe to do so and range-of-motion has returned sufficiently.

DIET—Eat a well-balanced diet to promote healing.

CALL YOUR DOCTOR IF

- Pain, swelling, redness, drainage, or bleeding increases in the surgical area.
- You develop symptoms of infection including headache, muscle aches, dizziness, fever, or a general ill feeling.
- New, unexplained symptoms develop.

KNEE REPLACEMENT, TOTAL

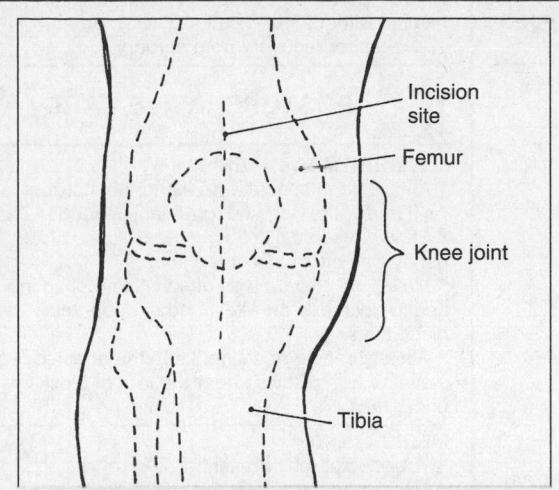

An illustration of the knee joint and a normal site for incision when a replacement procedure is planned.

Incision site

Femur

Knee joint

Tibia

The diseased bone to be removed.

Diseased bone removed

After the diseased surfaces of the femur and tibia have been removed, they are replaced by a durable prosthetic component fixed firmly in place with a special form of bone cement (sometimes).

Knee replacement

KNEECAP REMOVAL
(Patellectomy)

GENERAL INFORMATION

DEFINITION—Removal of the kneecap (patella).

BODY PARTS INVOLVED—Kneecap, knee joint, muscles and ligaments attached to kneecap.

REASONS FOR SURGERY
- Fracture of the kneecap.
- Recurrent dislocations of the kneecap.
- Painful degenerative arthritis in the kneecap.

SURGICAL RISK INCREASES WITH
- Obesity.
- Smoking.
- Poor nutrition.
- Recent or chronic illness.
- Diabetes.
- Use of some prescription and nonprescription drugs. Inform your doctor of any drugs, medications, or vitamin and herb supplements you are using or have used in the last month.

WHAT TO EXPECT

WHO OPERATES—Orthopedist.

WHERE PERFORMED—Hospital or outpatient surgical facility.

DIAGNOSTIC TESTS
- Before surgery: Blood and urine studies, x-rays of both knees.
- After surgery: Blood studies, x-rays of the affected knee.

ANESTHESIA
- Local anesthesia by injection.
- Spinal anesthesia by injection.
- General anesthesia by injection and inhalation with an airway tube placed in the windpipe.

DESCRIPTION OF OPERATION
- An incision is made around the kneecap.
- The muscles and tendons attached to the kneecap are cut, and the kneecap is removed.
- The muscles are sewn back together with strong suture material.
- The skin is closed with sutures or clips, which usually can be removed about 1 week after surgery.

POSSIBLE COMPLICATIONS
- Excessive bleeding.
- Surgical-wound infection.
- Rupture of patellar tendon.
- Blood clots which can break loose and travel to the lung.

AVERAGE HOSPITAL STAY—3 to 6 days.

PROBABLE OUTCOME—Expect complete healing without complications. Allow about 6 to 12 weeks for recovery from surgery.

POSTOPERATIVE CARE

GENERAL MEASURES
- A hard ridge should form along the incision. As it heals, the ridge will gradually recede.
- Shower as usual. You may wash the incision gently with mild, unscented soap.
- Move and elevate legs often while resting in bed to decrease the likelihood of deep-vein blood clots.
- While sleeping or sitting, keep the affected leg elevated with pillows under the foot or blocks under the bed.

MEDICATION
- Your doctor may prescribe:
  - Pain relievers. Don't take prescription pain medication longer than 4 to 7 days. Use only as much as you need.
  - Blood thinners to help reduce the risk of blood clots.
  - Antibiotics to fight or prevent infection.
- You may use nonprescription drugs, such as acetaminophen, for minor pain. Avoid aspirin.

ACTIVITY
- To help recovery and aid your well-being, resume daily activities, including work, as soon as you are able.
- Use crutches or a cane to walk as directed by your doctor. Don't stand for prolonged periods.
- Avoid vigorous exercise for 6 weeks after surgery. A physical therapist can teach you exercises that will restore strength to the knee.
- Resume driving as advised by your doctor. If surgery is on the right leg, it may require a longer recovery period before driving.

DIET—Clear liquid diet until the gastrointestinal tract functions again. Then eat a well-balanced diet to promote healing.

CALL YOUR DOCTOR IF

- Pain, swelling, redness, drainage, or bleeding increases in the surgical area.
- Toes become cold, discolored or numb.
- Excessive pain or swelling develops in calf below operated knee.
- You develop symptoms of infection including headache, muscle aches, dizziness, fever, or a general ill feeling.
- You experience nausea or vomiting.
- New, unexplained symptoms develop.

KNEECAP REMOVAL
(Patellectomy)

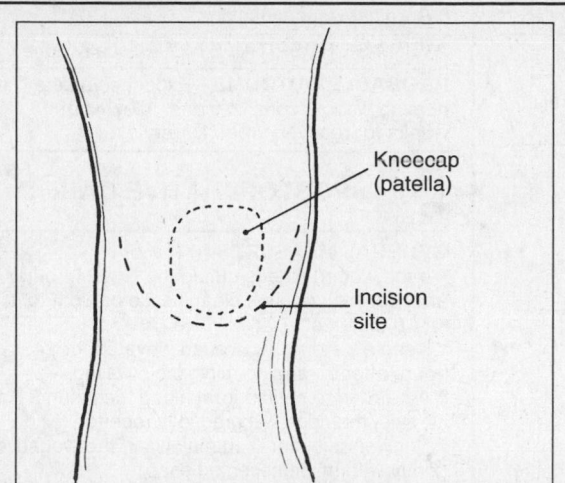

The kneecap and the proposed incision site for kneecap removal.

Kneecap (patella)

Incision site

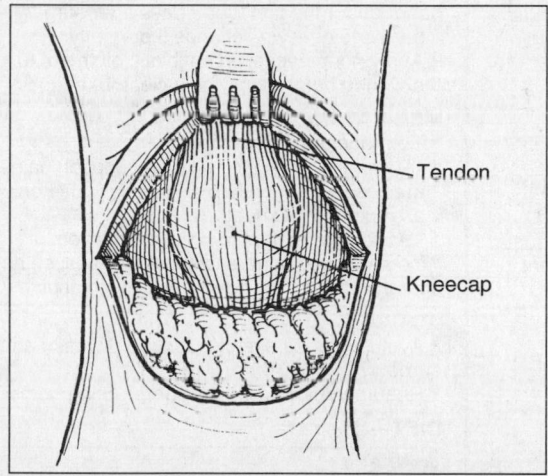

Muscles and tendons attached to the kneecap are cut and the kneecap is removed.

Tendon

Kneecap

The muscles are sewn back together with strong suture material and the skin is closed with sutures or clips that usually can be removed about 1 week after surgery.

LACERATION REPAIR

GENERAL INFORMATION

DEFINITION—Repair of lacerations (open wounds in the skin extending to underlying tissue and sometimes muscle, blood vessels and nerves).

BODY PARTS INVOLVED—Skin, muscle, connective tissue.

REASONS FOR SURGERY
- Prevention of bleeding and infection.
- Examination to identify underlying injuries.
- Closure of the skin to hasten healing.

SURGICAL RISK INCREASES WITH
- Obesity.
- Smoking.
- Poor nutrition.
- Recent or chronic illness.
- Diabetes.
- Use of some prescription and nonprescription drugs. Inform your doctor of any drugs, medications, or vitamin and herb supplements you are using or have used in the last month.

WHAT TO EXPECT

WHO OPERATES—Family doctor, general surgeon, plastic and reconstructive surgeon, orthopedist, emergency room doctor, or hand surgeon.

WHERE PERFORMED—Hospital, outpatient surgical facility, or emergency room.

DIAGNOSTIC TESTS
- Before surgery: Blood and urine studies.
- After surgery: Blood studies.

ANESTHESIA
- Local anesthesia by injection.
- General anesthesia by a combination of injection and inhalation with an airway tube placed in the windpipe.

DESCRIPTION OF OPERATION
- The wound is cleansed and irrigated. The wound is inspected for possible tendon or nerve injury.
- The skin edges are examined. Shredded tissue and debris are removed. Sometimes, a ragged edge is trimmed for better cosmetic results.
- The underlying tissue is closed with sutures that will be absorbed by the body. The skin is closed with small sutures, which usually can be removed about 1 week after surgery.
- A bandage may be used to control bleeding.
- You may need an injection to prevent tetanus. Ask your doctor.

POSSIBLE COMPLICATIONS
- Excessive bleeding.
- Surgical-wound infection.

AVERAGE HOSPITAL STAY—Usually none.

PROBABLE OUTCOME—Expect complete healing without complications. Allow about 3 weeks for recovery from surgery.

POSTOPERATIVE CARE

GENERAL MEASURES
- If the wound bleeds during the first 24 hours after surgery, press a clean tissue or cloth to it for 10 minutes.
- Keep an arm or leg wound elevated for 24 hours after surgery to minimize swelling.
- A hard ridge should form along the wound. As it heals, the ridge will gradually recede.
- Shower as usual. You may wash the wound gently with mild unscented soap.
- Between showers, keep the wound dry with a bandage for the first 2 or 3 days after surgery. If a bandage gets wet, change it promptly.
- Apply nonprescription antibiotic ointment to the wound before applying a clean bandage.

MEDICATION
- Your doctor may prescribe:
  - Pain relievers. Don't take prescription pain medication longer than 4 to 7 days. Use only as much as you need.
  - Antibiotics to fight or prevent infection.
- You may use nonprescription drugs, such as acetaminophen, for minor pain. Avoid aspirin.

ACTIVITY
- Avoid vigorous exercise for 3 to 6 weeks after surgery.
- Resume driving 2 days after returning home.

DIET—No special diet.

CALL YOUR DOCTOR IF

- Pain, swelling, redness, drainage, or bleeding increases in the wound area.
- You develop symptoms of infection including headache, muscle aches, dizziness, fever, or a general ill feeling.
- New, unexplained symptoms develop.

LACERATION REPAIR

Laceration

A typical laceration on the side of the hand and finger.

Shredded tissue and debris are removed. Sometimes a ragged edge of skin is trimmed for better cosmetic results.

The underlying tissue is closed with sutures that will be absorbed by the body. Skin is closed with small sutures that usually can be removed about 1 week after surgery.

LAPAROSCOPY

GENERAL INFORMATION

DEFINITION—Procedure that allows visual examination and some treatments of the pelvic and abdominal organs. The procedure is performed with a laparoscope, a fiber-optic instrument.

BODY PARTS INVOLVED—Abdomen and all its contents.

REASONS FOR SURGERY
- Evaluation and treatment of infertility in women.
- Evaluation of known or suspected endometriosis.
- Complications from pelvic disease.
- Masses or cysts in the pelvis.
- Undiagnosed pelvic or abdominal pain.
- Fibroid tumors of the uterus.
- Hysterectomy, voluntary sterilization.
- Diagnosis and treatment of an ectopic pregnancy (see Glossary).
- Diagnosis and treatment for a variety of abdominal disorders.

SURGICAL RISK INCREASES WITH
- Obesity, smoking, heart or lung disease.
- Advanced pregnancy.
- Previous abdominal surgery for intra-abdominal infections (such as ruptured appendicitis), previous bowel surgery.
- Use of some prescription and nonprescription drugs. Inform your doctor of any drugs, medications, or vitamin and herb supplements you are using or have used in the last month.

WHAT TO EXPECT

WHO OPERATES—General surgeon, obstetrician-gynecologist, or specially trained family doctor.

WHERE PERFORMED—Outpatient surgical facility or hospital.

DIAGNOSTIC TESTS—Before surgery: Blood studies.

ANESTHESIA
- General anesthesia by injection and inhalation with an airway tube placed in the windpipe.
- Local anesthesia.

DESCRIPTION OF OPERATION
- A small incision is made in or below the patient's navel. A needle is inserted to inflate the abdomen with carbon dioxide.
- The operating table is tilted to allow the bowel and carbon dioxide to float up toward the chest. The laparoscope is then inserted through the incision and is used to examine the abdomen visually. Occasionally, other small incisions are made in order to insert other surgical instruments.

- The laparoscope is can also be used to used to perform surgeries, including gallbladder removal, appendectomy, tubal ligation, aspiration and excision of an ovarian cyst, and multiple other gynecological procedures.
- The laparoscope and any other instruments are removed, and the carbon dioxide is allowed to escape from the abdomen.
- Small sutures under the skin and an adhesive bandage are used to close the wound(s).

POSSIBLE COMPLICATIONS—Perforation of the bowel or liver (rare).

AVERAGE HOSPITAL STAY—0 to 2 days.

PROBABLE OUTCOME—Expect full recovery without complications. You may experience slight discomfort for 24 to 48 hours. You may have aches in your shoulders and chest from the carbon dioxide that was used to inflate your abdomen. No treatment is necessary. Allow 1 week for full recovery from surgery.

POSTOPERATIVE CARE

GENERAL MEASURES
- Change the adhesive bandage daily.
- Shower as usual. You may wash the incision gently with mild soap.
- If surgery was for sterilization and you were taking birth-control pills, finish your present package, then you no longer need birth-control.
- Use sanitary pad (not tampons) to stop slight vaginal bleeding which may occur after surgery.

MEDICATION—Your doctor may prescribe pain relievers. Don't take prescription pain medication longer than 4 to 7 days. Use only as much as you need.

ACTIVITY
- To help recovery and aid your well-being, resume daily activities, including work, as soon as you are able.
- Resume driving 24 hours after recovery from surgery.
- Sexual relations may be resumed 2 or 3 days after surgery.

DIET—No special diet. You should avoid carbonated beverages for 48 hours after surgery.

CALL YOUR DOCTOR IF

- You develop symptoms of infection including headache, muscle aches, dizziness, fever, or a general ill feeling.
- You have excessive bleeding or discharge from either the surgical area or the vagina.
- You experience abdominal swelling or pain.
- New, unexplained symptoms develop.

LAPAROSCOPY

A hollow needle is inserted through the abdominal wall to inflate the abdomen with carbon dioxide.

Carbon dioxide

The laparoscope is inserted through a small incision to allow examination of the abdominal contents under direct vision.

Laparoscope

Carbon dioxide

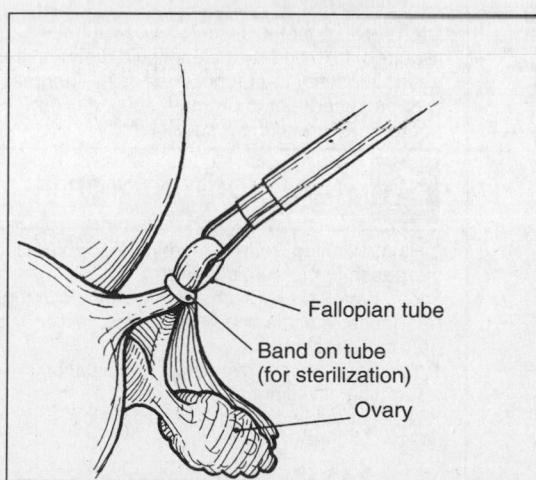

- The laparoscope may be used to provide passage of other instruments for doctors to perform surgical procedures (e.g., a female tubal ligation in this illustration).
- After the laparoscope is removed, carbon dioxide is allowed to escape from the abdomen. The small amount remaining will be readily absorbed by the body.
- Sutures under the skin and adhesive bandages are used to close the wound (not illustrated).

Fallopian tube

Band on tube (for sterilization)

Ovary

LAPAROTOMY

GENERAL INFORMATION

DEFINITION—Exploratory abdominal surgery to identify, diagnose, or treat a variety of conditions.

BODY PARTS INVOLVED—Skin, abdominal muscles, peritoneum, abdominal organs.

REASONS FOR SURGERY
- Diagnostic examination of the abdominal organs.
- Collection of tissue samples for diagnosis.
- Closure of hernias in the abdominal wall.
- Repair or removal of abnormal tissue.
- Removal of diseased organs.
- Correction of unsightly or disfiguring abnormalities.

SURGICAL RISK INCREASES WITH
- Stress, obesity, smoking.
- Excess alcohol consumption.
- Poor nutrition.
- Recent acute respiratory infection.
- Chronic illness.
- Diabetes.
- History of prior abdominal surgery, particularly if it occurred at the site of the current surgery.
- Use of some prescription and nonprescription drugs. Inform your doctor of any drugs, medications, or vitamin and herb supplements you are using or have used in the last month.

WHAT TO EXPECT

WHO OPERATES—General surgeon or obstetrician-gynecologist.

WHERE PERFORMED—Hospital.

DIAGNOSTIC TESTS
- Before surgery: Blood and urine studies, x-rays of kidneys and chest, ECG, ultrasound, MRI, CT scan, laparoscopy (see Glossary for all).
- After surgery: Blood studies.

ANESTHESIA—Spinal or general anesthesia by injection and inhalation with an airway tube placed in the windpipe.

DESCRIPTION OF OPERATION
- An incision is made in the abdomen. The abdominal muscles are separated, and the peritoneum (see Glossary) is opened.
- Blood vessels cut during the surgery are cauterized or clamped and tied. Wound edges are retracted with a special instrument.
- Fluid in the abdominal cavity is often removed for laboratory examination.
- The abdominal organs are examined. Other surgeries may be performed at this time.
- Samples of suspicious tissue are gathered or diseased areas are treated.
- The peritoneum is closed, and the muscles are reconstructed with heavy sutures.

- The skin is closed with sutures or clips, which usually can be removed about 3 to 7 days after surgery.

POSSIBLE COMPLICATIONS
- Excessive bleeding.
- Surgical-wound infection.
- Incisional hernia, excessive scar formation.
- Abscess formation.
- Bowel obstruction, injury to bowel.

AVERAGE HOSPITAL STAY—3 to 5 days.

PROBABLE OUTCOME—Expect complete healing without complications. Allow about 4 weeks for recovery from surgery.

POSTOPERATIVE CARE

GENERAL MEASURES
- A hard ridge should form along the incision. As it heals, the ridge will gradually recede.
- Shower as usual. You may wash the incision gently with mild, unscented soap.
- Move and elevate legs often while resting in bed to decrease the chance of deep-vein blood clots.

MEDICATION
- Your doctor may prescribe:
  - Pain relievers. Don't take prescription pain medication longer than 4 to 7 days. Use only as much as you need.
  - Stool softeners to prevent constipation.
  - Antibiotics to fight or prevent infection.
- You may use nonprescription drugs, such as acetaminophen, for minor pain. Avoid aspirin.

ACTIVITY
- To help recovery and aid your well-being, resume daily activities as soon as you are able.
- Avoid vigorous exercise for 6 weeks after surgery. Resume sexual relations when doctor's exam reveals complete healing.
- Resume driving about 3 weeks after surgery.

DIET—Nasogastric suction is occasionally required, followed by a clear liquid diet until the gastrointestinal tract functions again. Then eat a well-balanced diet to promote healing. Your doctor may prescribe a special diet.

CALL YOUR DOCTOR IF

- Pain, swelling, redness, drainage, or bleeding increases in the surgical area.
- You develop symptoms of infection including headache, muscle aches, dizziness, fever, or a general ill feeling.
- You have nausea, vomiting, constipation, abdominal swelling, or severe pain.
- New, unexplained symptoms develop.

LAPAROTOMY

The incision site frequently used for a laparotomy (any opening made into the abdomen).

Incision sites

- Wound edges are retracted with special instruments.
- Fluid in the abdominal cavity is often removed for laboratory examination.
- The abdominal organs are examined.
- Samples of suspicious tissue are gathered or diseased areas are treated (not illustrated).

Rectus muscle

Intestine

After inspection of all abdominal contents (the intestine is examined here between the surgeon's fingers), the abdominal contents are replaced into normal position. The muscles are closed, and the skin is closed with sutures that can be removed after 3 to 7 days.

LARYNGOSCOPY

GENERAL INFORMATION

DEFINITION—Procedure that allows visual examination and some treatment of the larynx (voice box).

BODY PARTS INVOLVED—Larynx, structure at the top of the windpipe that controls the voice.

REASONS FOR SURGERY
* To remove laryngeal polyps, singer's nodules, and other benign growths.
* To remove enough tissue to biopsy.
* To assess vocal cord mobility.

SURGICAL RISK INCREASES WITH—None expected.

WHAT TO EXPECT

WHO OPERATES—Ear, nose and throat specialist (otolaryngologist).

WHERE PERFORMED—Hospital, outpatient surgical facility, or doctor's office.

DIAGNOSTIC TESTS
* Before surgery: None.
* After surgery: Microscopic examination of removed tissue.

ANESTHESIA—Local anesthesia spray or general anesthesia.

DESCRIPTION OF OPERATION
* A rigid laryngoscope is passed through the mouth and pharynx to extend to the larynx (voice-box).
* The larynx is examined visually by the operator.
* Specimens may be removed by snare for further study (e.g., malignant changes). Minor surgery, such as removing nodules or polyps, may be done at this time.
* The procedure can also be done with a flexible fiberoptic scope.

POSSIBLE COMPLICATIONS
* Excessive bleeding.
* Swelling of tissues in the neck.
* Laryngospasm (closing of larynx).

AVERAGE HOSPITAL STAY—Usually no more than 1 day.

PROBABLE OUTCOME—Complete recovery if growth is benign. If growth is malignant, larynx removal may be necessary (see in Surgery section).

POSTOPERATIVE CARE

GENERAL MEASURES
* Keep your head elevated.
* Don't try to talk. Communicate by writing messages.
* Consult a speech therapist if your doctor recommends.
* No smoking.

MEDICATION
* Your doctor may prescribe pain relievers. Don't take prescription pain medication longer than 4 to 7 days. Use only as much as you need.
* You may use nonprescription drugs, such as acetaminophen, for minor pain. Avoid aspirin.

ACTIVITY
* Return to daily activities and work as soon as possible.
* Avoid strenuous exercise that would cause heavy breathing for several days.

DIET—No special diet.

CALL YOUR DOCTOR IF

* You develop symptoms of infection including headache, muscle aches, dizziness, fever, or a general ill feeling.
* You develop swelling in neck, coughing up of blood, or difficulty in breathing.

LARYNGOSCOPY

An illustration of a patient lying on his back. Instrumentation is in place and a rigid laryngoscope is passed through the mouth and pharynx to examine the larynx.

Vocal cord

Abnormal growth

An illustration of an abnormal growth on the patient's vocal cord.

Biopsy forceps

Tissue specimens are removed with biopsy forceps for further study.

LARYNX REMOVAL
(Laryngectomy)

GENERAL INFORMATION

DEFINITION—Removal of the larynx.

BODY PARTS INVOLVED—Larynx (voice box), organ at the top of the windpipe that controls the voice.

REASONS FOR SURGERY—Cancer of the larynx.

SURGICAL RISK INCREASES WITH
- Adults over 60.
- Obesity, smoking, poor nutrition.
- Recent or chronic illness, alcoholism.
- Diabetes.
- Use of some prescription and nonprescription drugs. Inform your doctor of any drugs, medications, or vitamin and herb supplements you are using or have used in the last month.

WHAT TO EXPECT

WHO OPERATES—Ear, nose and throat specialist (otolaryngologist).

WHERE PERFORMED—Hospital.

DIAGNOSTIC TESTS
- Before surgery: Blood and urine studies, laryngoscopy (see in Surgery section), CT scan, MRI, ECG (see Glossary for all).
- After surgery: Blood studies.

ANESTHESIA—General anesthesia by injection and inhalation with an airway tube placed in the windpipe.

DESCRIPTION OF OPERATION
- An incision is made in the neck. The muscles that attach the larynx to the windpipe are divided.
- The blood vessels and nerves that supply the larynx are located and cut.
- The larynx is cut free and removed with surrounding lymph node tissue (e.g., neck dissection) if indicated.
- A tracheostomy tube (see Glossary) is fitted and positioned.
- The muscles and skin edges are closed around the tube with sutures or clips, which usually can be removed about 1 week after surgery.

POSSIBLE COMPLICATIONS
- Excessive bleeding, surgical-wound infection.
- Inadvertent injury to the esophagus or trachea.
- Difficulty swallowing (usually temporary).

AVERAGE HOSPITAL STAY—5 to 7 days.

PROBABLE OUTCOME—Expect complete healing of the surgical wound. Allow about 4 weeks for recovery from surgery.

POSTOPERATIVE CARE

GENERAL MEASURES
- Keep your head elevated.
- Don't try to talk. Communicate by writing messages. Consult a speech therapist if prescribed by doctor.
- Move and elevate legs often while resting in bed to decrease the likelihood of deep-vein blood clots.
- Treat crusting and secretions around the surgical wound with petroleum jelly, antibiotic ointment, and gauze.
- A hard ridge should form along the incision. As it heals, the ridge will gradually recede.
- Take baths, rather than showers, until your doctor advises that showering may be resumed. When showering, it will be necessary to wear a bib-like cover over the opening to the tracheostomy to prevent water from entering the opening.
- Use a humidifier to add humidity to your home, especially your bedroom.

MEDICATION
- Your doctor may prescribe:
  - Pain relievers. Don't take prescription pain medication longer than 4 to 7 days. Use only as much as you need.
  - Stool softeners to prevent constipation.
  - Antibiotics to fight or prevent infection.
- You may use nonprescription drugs, such as acetaminophen, for minor pain. Avoid aspirin.

ACTIVITY
- To help recovery and aid your well-being, resume daily activities, including work, as soon as you are able.
- Avoid vigorous exercise for 6 weeks after surgery.
- Avoid swimming. Water could enter the stoma and you could drown.
- Resume driving 2 weeks after returning home.
- Rehabilitation may require learning new method for oral communication.

DIET—Tube or intravenous feedings for first 2 days after surgery. Then resume your normal diet gradually.

CALL YOUR DOCTOR IF

- Pain, swelling, redness, drainage, or bleeding increases in the surgical area.
- You develop symptoms of infection including headache, muscle aches, dizziness, fever, or a general ill feeling.
- New, unexplained symptoms develop.

LARYNX REMOVAL
(Laryngectomy)

Structures in the neck. The larynx (voice box) is at the top of the windpipe.

Incision site

Thyroid cartilage

Trachea (windpipe)

● After an incision has been made in the neck, the muscles that attach the larynx to the windpipe are divided.
● The larynx has been cut free and removed

Thyroid cartilage

Trachea

The trachea is sutured to the skin, allowing for a permanent tracheostomy. The muscle and skin edges are closed around the tube with sutures or clips that usually can be removed about 1 week after surgery.

LASER IN-SITU KERATOMILEUSIS (LASIK)

GENERAL INFORMATION

DEFINITION—Removal of a thin layer of tissue from the center of the cornea in order to change the shape of the cornea and improve vision.

BODY PARTS INVOLVED—Cornea.

REASONS FOR SURGERY—To improve vision in patients with nearsightedness, farsightedness, or astigmatism. The goal is to eliminate the need for corrective lenses (glasses or contacts).

SURGICAL RISK INCREASES WITH
* Vascular disease, autoimmune disease.
* Progressive myopia, hyperopia, or amblyopia (lazy eye).
* Women who are pregnant, nursing, or planning on becoming pregnant within 6 months.
* Active or recurrent eye disease, especially glaucoma.
* Diabetes.
* Use of some prescription and nonprescription drugs. Inform your doctor of any drugs, medications, or vitamin and herb supplements you are using or have used in the last month.

WHAT TO EXPECT

WHO OPERATES—Specially trained ophthalmologist.

WHERE PERFORMED—Doctor's office or outpatient surgical facility.

DIAGNOSTIC TESTS—Eye examination to determine degree of correction required.

ANESTHESIA—Topical anesthesia.

DESCRIPTION OF OPERATION
* The surgery involves folding back a thin layer of the outer corneal tissue.
* A thin layer of internal corneal tissue is then removed with the excimer laser. This causes the center of the cornea to flatten (for nearsightedness) or steepen (for farsightedness) or become more rounded (for astigmatism).
* Following removal of the tissue, the flap is replaced. It will usually adhere back in place without the need for sutures.

POSSIBLE COMPLICATIONS
* Infection.
* Difference in power between the two eyes.
* Double vision, hazy vision.
* Increased or decreased sensitivity to light.
* Loss of vision (rare).
* Over or under correction.

AVERAGE HOSPITAL STAY—None.

PROBABLE OUTCOME—Expect complete healing without complications. Usually, corrective lenses will no longer be needed, but sometimes they will still be required with less correction.

POSTOPERATIVE CARE

GENERAL MEASURES
* The entire procedure usually takes no more than 15 minutes.
* An eye patch or shield should be worn at night to protect the eye while sleeping.
* Avoid rubbing the eye.
* Avoid exposing the eye to nonsterile water, such as bath or tap water, to help prevent infection.
* Wear protective eyewear while engaging in sports or other activities (e.g., shop work) where eye injury may occur.
* You may experience temporary side effects such as dry eyes and halos around bright lights at night.
* Recovery is quick. Most patients will see clearly within 1 or 2 days.

MEDICATION
* Your doctor may prescribe:
  - Antibiotics to fight or prevent infection.
  - Anti-inflammatory and moisturizing eye drops.
* You may use nonprescription drugs, such as acetaminophen, for minor pain. Avoid aspirin.

ACTIVITY—Resume driving only after you are sure your vision is adequate (usually within 2 days).

DIET—No special diet.

CALL YOUR DOCTOR IF

* You experience increased pain, redness, or drainage from the eye.
* You have decreased visual acuity or a loss of vision, even temporarily.
* You develop symptoms of infection including headache, muscle aches, dizziness, fever, or a general ill feeling.
* New, unexplained symptoms develop.

LASER IN-SITU KERATOMILEUSIS (LASIK)

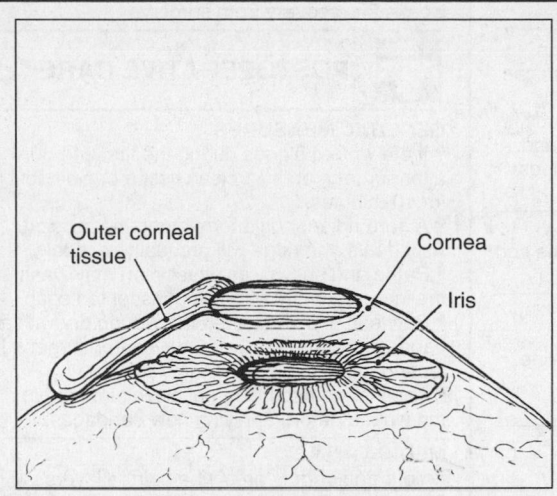

An illustration of the eye, showing a thin layer of outer corneal tissue which has been cut and folded back.

Outer corneal tissue

Cornea

Iris

- A thin layer of internal corneal tissue is then removed with an excimer laser.
- The laser beam can be used to change the shape of the cornea in a number of ways, depending on the type of refractive error which is affecting the patient's vision.

Excimer laser beam

Following removal of the tissue, the flap is replaced. It will usually adhere back in place without the need for sutures.

Corneal flap returned

LIPOMA REMOVAL

GENERAL INFORMATION

DEFINITION—Removal of a lipoma (benign, fatty tumor). Lipomas vary in size. A lipoma can be pea-sized or larger than a grapefruit. Lipomas can be found anywhere on the body, but are most commonly found in the front and back of the chest and abdomen, or in the legs and arms.

BODY PARTS INVOLVED—Skin and underlying tissue, usually on the back, arms and legs.

REASONS FOR SURGERY
- Improved appearance.
- If lipoma is bothersome, e.g., at the belt-line.
- Diagnosis of lipoma is not certain.
- Prevention of cancer (rare).

SURGICAL RISK INCREASES WITH
- Recent or chronic illness.
- Diabetes.
- Use of some prescription and nonprescription drugs. Inform your doctor of any drugs, medications, or vitamin and herb supplements you are using or have used in the last month.

WHAT TO EXPECT

WHO OPERATES—Family doctor, general surgeon, dermatologist, or plastic and reconstructive surgeon.

WHERE PERFORMED—Doctor's office or outpatient surgical facility.

DIAGNOSTIC TESTS
- Before surgery: Blood and urine studies, ultrasound, CT scan (see Glossary for both).
- After surgery: Laboratory examination of removed tissue.

ANESTHESIA
- Local anesthesia by injection.
- General anesthesia by injection and inhalation with an airway tube placed in the windpipe (for larger lipomas).

DESCRIPTION OF OPERATION
- An incision is made over the lipoma.
- The lipoma is cut free from surrounding connective tissue and removed.
- The skin is closed with sutures or clips, which usually can be removed about 1 week after surgery.
- Lipomas can also be removed by liposuction (see in Surgery section).

POSSIBLE COMPLICATIONS
- Excessive bleeding.
- Surgical-wound infection.
- Seroma (fluid collects under the skin).

AVERAGE HOSPITAL STAY—None.

PROBABLE OUTCOME—Expect complete healing without complications. Allow about 3 weeks for recovery from surgery.

POSTOPERATIVE CARE

GENERAL MEASURES
- If the wound bleeds during the first 24 hours after surgery, press a clean tissue or cloth to it for 10 minutes.
- A hard ridge should form along the incision. As it heals, the ridge will gradually recede.
- Bathe and shower as usual. You may wash the incision gently with mild, unscented soap.
- Between showers, keep the wound dry with a bandage for the first 2 or 3 days after surgery. If a bandage gets wet, change it promptly.
- Apply nonprescription antibiotic ointment to the wound before applying new bandages.

MEDICATION
- Your doctor may prescribe pain relievers. Don't take prescription pain medication longer than 4 to 7 days. Use only as much as you need.
- You may use nonprescription drugs, such as acetaminophen, for minor pain. Avoid aspirin.

ACTIVITY—No restrictions.

DIET—No special diet.

CALL YOUR DOCTOR IF

- Pain, swelling, redness, drainage, or bleeding increases in the surgical area.
- You develop symptoms of infection including headache, muscle aches, dizziness, fever, or a general ill feeling.
- New, unexplained symptoms develop.

LIPOMA REMOVAL

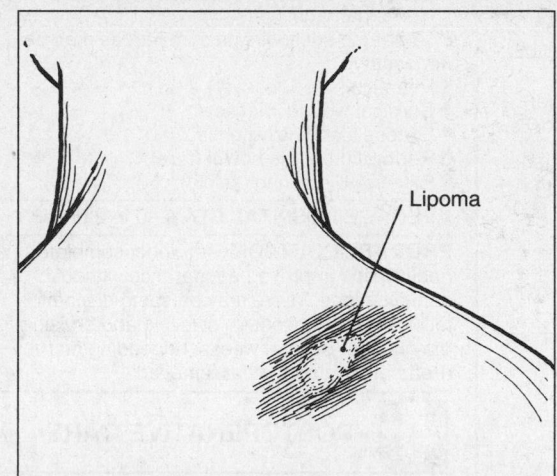

A typical lipoma situated just under the skin. Lipomas may be found in scattered locations over the entire body.

Lipoma

The lipoma is cut free from surrounding connective tissue and removed.

Lipoma

After the lipoma has been excised, the skin is closed with sutures or clips, which usually can be removed about 1 week after surgery (not illustrated).

LIPOSUCTION
(Suction Lipectomy)

GENERAL INFORMATION

DEFINITION—A surgical technique using suction equipment to permanently remove fat deposits, usually from the thighs, hips, buttocks, abdomen or chin.

BODY PARTS INVOLVED—Thighs and hips, buttocks, fat cells of the abdominal wall, chin, or other small areas.

REASONS FOR SURGERY—Cosmetic improvement of fat deposits that are resistant to diet and/or exercise.

SURGICAL RISK INCREASES WITH
- Extreme obesity, smoking.
- Recent or chronic illness.
- Diabetes.
- Excess alcohol consumption.
- History of phlebitis.
- Use of some prescription and nonprescription drugs. Inform your doctor of any drugs, medications, or vitamin and herb supplements you are using or have used in the last month.

WHAT TO EXPECT

WHO OPERATES—Plastic surgeon.

WHERE PERFORMED—Outpatient surgical facility, hospital, or doctor's office.

DIAGNOSTIC TESTS
- Before surgery: Blood and urine studies.
- After surgery: Blood and urine studies.

ANESTHESIA
- Local anesthesia and sedation for small areas.
- General anesthesia by injection and inhalation with an airway tube placed in the windpipe is usually used for larger areas of fat.

DESCRIPTION OF OPERATION
- The plastic surgeon marks areas to be operated on.
- Incisions (about 1/4 inch each) are made in suction areas.
- A suction tube, with one end attached to suction equipment, is repeatedly pushed through the incision into the excess fat and moved back and forth (20 to 30 times at each site) until the desired amount of fat is removed.
- Each incision is stapled or stitched closed, and a pressure dressing is placed over the wounds.
- Drains may be left in place under the skin for several days following surgery.

POSSIBLE COMPLICATIONS
- Nerve damage.
- Repeated suctioning in some areas may be necessary.
- Phlebitis (see Glossary).
- Surgical wound infection.
- Excess bleeding, anemia.
- Perforation of the bowel (rare).
- Excessive scarring (keloid).

AVERAGE HOSPITAL STAY—0 to 2 days.

PROBABLE OUTCOME—Expect complete healing and improved appearance without complications. There may be some discomfort following the procedure, swelling and bruising may last for several weeks, depending on the areas and amount of fat removed.

POSTOPERATIVE CARE

GENERAL MEASURES
- A hard ridge should form along each incision. As they heal, the ridges will gradually recede.
- Don't be concerned about small amounts of straw-colored drainage at the surgical sites.
- Shower as usual. Avoid baths until healing is complete. You may wash the incision gently with mild, unscented soap. After showering, replace any wet dressings with clean, dry ones.
- It may take several weeks or months for tenderness to subside. Allow time for healing and for appearance to improve.

MEDICATION
- Your doctor may prescribe:
  - Pain relievers. Don't take prescription pain medicine longer than 4 to 7 days. Use only as much as you need.
  - Antibiotics to fight or prevent infection.
- You may use nonprescription drugs, such as acetaminophen, for minor pain. Avoid aspirin.

ACTIVITY
- Resume driving 2 weeks after surgery.
- Resume sexual relations when you feel able to.

DIET
- No special diet required.
- Vitamin and mineral supplements (sometimes).

CALL YOUR DOCTOR IF

- Pain, swelling, redness, drainage, or bleeding occurs in the surgical area.
- You develop symptoms of infection including headache, muscle aches, dizziness, fever, or a general ill feeling.
- You become constipated.
- Leg becomes swollen or painful.
- New, unexplained symptoms develop.

LIPOSUCTION
(Suction Lipectomy)

An illustration of fatty deposits under the skin in the buttocks area.

Skin

Fat

Cannula

Very small incisions are made in suction areas and a suction tube with one end attached to suction equipment is pushed through the incision into the excess fat and moved back and forth repeatedly.

Liposuction complete on the patient's right side and progressing to the left side.

LITHOTRIPSY
(Shock Wave Treatment for Kidney Stones)

GENERAL INFORMATION

DEFINITION—A technique to crush kidney stones inside the body without a surgical incision. These stones are too large to pass by normal elimination. Seventy percent of patients pass stones spontaneously, 30% require urological treatment. This technique is one of the available treatments.

BODY PARTS INVOLVED—Kidney, ureter, bladder.

REASONS FOR SURGERY
* Kidney stones that are too large to pass by normal elimination. They are usually lodged in the kidney or upper third of the ureter.
* Relieve blocked urine flow.
* Decrease chance of infection.
* Relieve pain from kidney stone.
* Decrease chance of damage to kidney.

SURGICAL RISK INCREASES WITH
* Poor heart or respiratory function.
* Presence of a cardiac pacemaker.
* Pregnancy.
* Bleeding disorders.
* Use of some prescription and nonprescription drugs. Inform your doctor of any drugs, medications, or vitamin and herb supplements you are using or have used in the last month.

WHAT TO EXPECT

WHO OPERATES—Urologist.

WHERE PERFORMED—A special center for lithotripsy. Usually in an outpatient surgical facility of a regional referral center.

DIAGNOSTIC TESTS
* Before surgery: Cystoscopy (see in Surgery section), x-rays of kidneys, ultrasound, CT scan (see Glossary for both), blood and urine studies.
* During surgery: Ultrasound (see Glossary).
* After surgery: Blood and urine studies, x-rays, ultrasound (see Glossary).

ANESTHESIA—Usually none. Sedation is used in most cases.

DESCRIPTION OF OPERATION
* For one method, the patient rests in a tub of warm water after being sedated.
* Another method avoids the water by using a membrane coupling device applied directly to the skin overlying the kidney.
* The lithotripsy unit sends out high frequency sound waves directed toward the stone. The shock waves pulverize the stones and the small particles then pass spontaneously in your urine over 2-5 days.

POSSIBLE COMPLICATIONS—May require more than 1 treatment.

AVERAGE HOSPITAL STAY—Usually none.

PROBABLE OUTCOME—Mild pain as fragments of stone pass.

POSTOPERATIVE CARE

GENERAL MEASURES
* If you are pregnant, or may be pregnant, advise your doctor. Lithotripsy cannot be performed on pregnant women.
* Soak in tub of warm water once or twice a day to relieve mild back pain.
* Strain urine for 1 to 2 weeks. Place fragments in envelope to return to lithotripsy center or as directed.

MEDICATION
* Your doctor may prescribe antibiotics to fight or prevent infection.
* You may use nonprescription drugs, such as acetaminophen, for minor pain. Avoid aspirin.

ACTIVITY
* Resume normal activity as soon as possible to promote healing.
* Avoid vigorous exercise until your doctor advises that healing is complete.

DIET—Your doctor may recommend a special diet to help prevent recurrence of stones. Increase dietary fiber and fluid intake to prevent constipation.

CALL YOUR DOCTOR IF

* You develop symptoms of infection including headache, muscle aches, dizziness, fever, or a general ill feeling.
* You experience, constipation, abdominal swelling, nausea, or vomiting.
* There is blood or pus in your urine or urination is frequent or painful.
* New, unexplained symptoms develop.

LITHOTRIPSY
(Shock Wave Treatment for Kidney Stones)

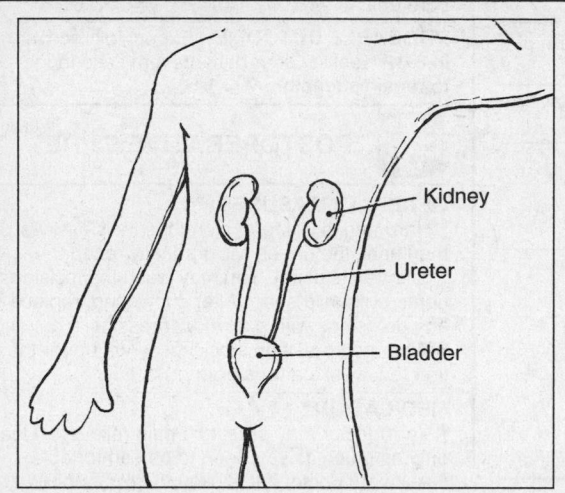

An illustration of the urinary tract.

Kidney

Ureter

Bladder

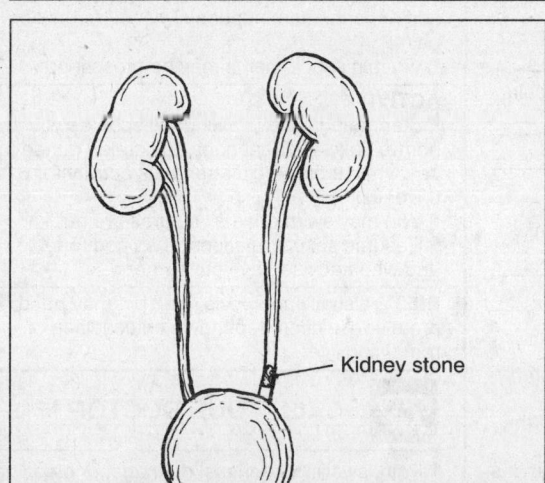

A stone is shown in the ureter leading from the left kidney.

Kidney stone

The lithotripsy unit turns out high frequency sound waves directed toward the stone. The shock waves pulverize the stone into small particles which then pass spontaneously in the patient's urine.

Ureter

Kidney stone breaking up

Sonographic shock waves

LIVER RESECTION

GENERAL INFORMATION

DEFINITION—Surgical removal of a portion of the liver.

BODY PARTS INVOLVED—Abdominal cavity, liver, gallbladder.

REASONS FOR SURGERY—Usually performed to remove an abnormal growth (tumor). May be necessary in trauma to stop excessive bleeding.

SURGICAL RISK INCREASES WITH
- Age.
- Diabetes.
- Poor kidney function.
- High blood pressure.
- Poor nutrition.
- Chronic lung disease.
- Obesity.
- Liver disease such as cirrhosis.

WHAT TO EXPECT

WHO OPERATES—General surgeon, vascular surgeon.

WHERE PERFORMED—Hospital.

DIAGNOSTIC TESTS
- Before surgery: Blood tests, chest x-ray, CT scan, EKG (see Glossary for these 2 terms).
- After surgery: Blood tests.

ANESTHESIA—General anesthesia.

DESCRIPTION OF OPERATION
- The abdomen is opened through a long vertical (up and down) or transverse incision.
- The portion of the liver to be removed is isolated and anatomical planes (sections of the liver) are identified to minimize bleeding.
- Blood vessels and bile ducts are ligated as the liver is separated.
- Up to three-fourths of the liver can usually be removed safely with sufficient liver function from the remaining portion.
- Drains are usually left to minimize collections of bile and blood which typically ooze from the raw edge of the remaining liver for several days or weeks after surgery.

POSSIBLE COMPLICATIONS
- Bleeding from the remaining liver.
- Liver failure and or kidney failure.
- Poor circulation to the remaining liver.
- Prolonged bile leak.
- Incisional hernia.

AVERAGE HOSPITAL STAY—Usually 7-10 days with the first day or two in the intensive care unit.

PROBABLE OUTCOME—Expect full recovery in 8-12 weeks. Older patients may take longer to regain strength.

POSTOPERATIVE CARE

GENERAL MEASURES
- Hard ridges will form along the incisions. As they heal, the ridges will gradually recede.
- Shower as usual. You may wash the incisions gently with mild soap. After showering, replace any dressings with a new dry dressing.
- Wear compression stockings when up for the first few weeks after surgery.

MEDICATION
- Your doctor may prescribe pain relievers. Use only as much as you need to be comfortable.
- Ask your doctor if it is okay to take ibuprofen, aspirin, or acetaminophen (Tylenol) for milder pain.
- Vitamin supplements may be prescribed.

ACTIVITY
- Start ambulating (walking) as soon as you are home. Take frequent naps as needed during the day when tired. Avoid strenuous activity for 6 to 8 weeks.
- You may swim once all sutures are out.
- Resume sexual relations when comfortable and when advised by your surgeon.

DIET—Usually no special diet, but may need protein restriction depending on condition of remaining liver.

CALL YOUR DOCTOR IF

- Pain, swelling, redness, drainage, or bleeding increases in the surgical area.
- You develop symptoms of infection including headache, muscle aches, dizziness, fever, or a general ill feeling.
- You develop nausea and vomiting.
- Prolonged constipation occurs.
- Jaundice (yellow skin or eyes) develops.
- New unexplained symptoms develop.

LIVER RESECTION

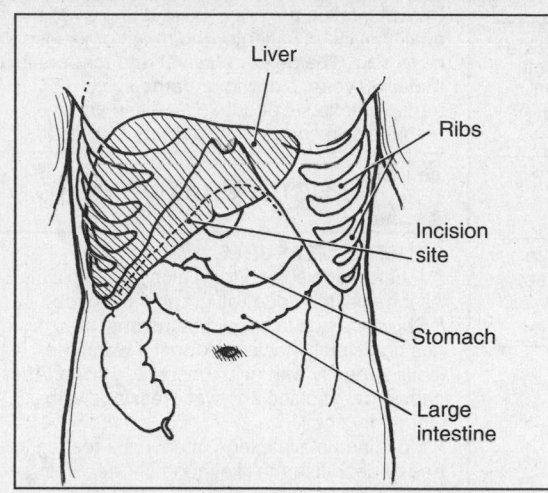

An illustration of the anatomy of the liver and surrounding structures. An incision is usually made below the right rib margin.

Liver

Ribs

Incision site

Stomach

Large intestine

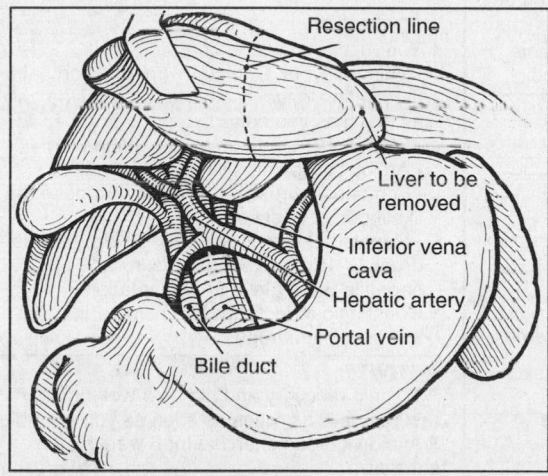

A line of resection is chosen to get adequate margins but maintain circulation in the remaining liver.

Resection line

Liver to be removed

Inferior vena cava

Hepatic artery

Portal vein

Bile duct

The resected liver margin is sutured to control bleeding.

Resected liver

LIVER TRANSPLANTATION

GENERAL INFORMATION

DEFINITION—Replacement of a diseased liver with a healthy liver obtained from a donor with compatible immunological characteristics. In some cases, a segment of the liver of a living, related donor may be used.

BODY PARTS INVOLVED—Diseased or abnormal liver, healthy donor liver, blood vessels, and bile ducts connected to liver.

REASONS FOR SURGERY—End-stage liver failure from liver cancer or other liver disease, such as chronic hepatitis or primary biliary cirrhosis (see Glossary for both).

SURGICAL RISK INCREASES WITH
- Adults over 60, infants.
- Obesity, smoking, poor nutrition.
- Excess alcohol consumption.
- Recent or chronic illness, diabetes.
- Kidney failure.
- Use of some prescription and nonprescription drugs. Inform your doctor of any drugs, medications, or vitamin and herb supplements you are using or have used in the last month.

WHAT TO EXPECT

WHO OPERATES—General surgeon with transplant experience and training.

WHERE PERFORMED—Hospital.

DIAGNOSTIC TESTS
- Before surgery: Immune-system and liver-matching procedures, studies of body systems.
- After surgery: Blood studies.

ANESTHESIA—General anesthesia by injection and inhalation with an airway tube placed in the windpipe.

DESCRIPTION OF OPERATION
- Liver is removed from donor, then chilled and preserved until surgery.
- An incision is made under the recipient's ribs. The abdominal muscles are separated or split, and the peritoneal cavity is opened.
- The liver and its bile ducts are isolated.
- The liver is cut free and removed. The donor liver is positioned and sewn in place. Blood vessels and bile ducts are connected.
- The peritoneum and abdominal muscles are closed. The skin is closed with sutures or clips, which usually can be removed about 1 week after surgery.

POSSIBLE COMPLICATIONS
- Excessive bleeding.
- Surgical-wound infection.
- Rejection of transplant.
- Bile-duct obstruction.
- Recurrence of hepatitis B or C in the new, previously healthy liver.

AVERAGE HOSPITAL STAY—3 weeks.

PROBABLE OUTCOME—A successful transplantation prolongs life and improves the quality of life in patients who might otherwise have died. The 5-year survival rate for people under 60 years old who undergo liver transplantation is about 75%. Allow about 6 months for recovery from surgery.

POSTOPERATIVE CARE

GENERAL MEASURES
- A hard ridge should form along the incision. As it heals, the ridge will gradually recede.
- Shower as usual. Avoid baths until the incision has completely healed. You may wash the incision gently with mild, unscented soap. After showering, replace any wet dressings with clean, dry ones.
- Move and elevate legs often while resting in bed to decrease the likelihood of deep-vein blood clots.

MEDICATION
- Your doctor may prescribe:
  - Pain relievers. Don't take prescription pain medication longer than 4 to 7 days. Use only as much as you need.
  - Stool softeners to prevent constipation.
  - Antibiotics to fight or prevent infection.
  - Immunosuppressant drugs to decrease the likelihood of rejection.
  - Hepatitis B immunoglobulin (HBIg) or other drugs to help prevent the recurrence of hepatitis B after liver transplantation.
- Consult your doctor before using any nonprescription drugs.

ACTIVITY
- To help recovery and aid your well-being, resume daily activities as soon as you are able.
- Avoid vigorous exercise for 6 weeks after surgery.
- Resume driving when your doctor determines that healing is complete.

DIET—Your doctor will prescribe a diet.

CALL YOUR DOCTOR IF

- Pain, swelling, redness, drainage, or bleeding increases in the surgical area.
- You develop symptoms of infection including headache, muscle aches, dizziness, fever, or a general ill feeling.
- You experience nausea, vomiting, constipation, abdominal swelling, or back pain.
- Jaundice occurs (yellow skin or eyes).
- Fluid builds up in abdomen or ankles.
- New, unexplained symptoms develop.

LIVER TRANSPLANTATION

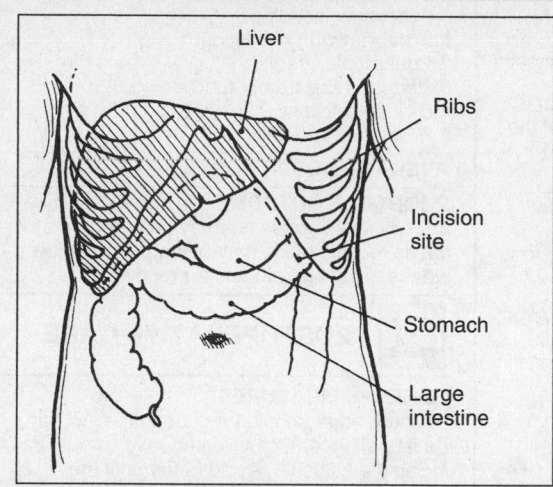

Liver

Ribs

Incision site

Stomach

Large intestine

An illustration of the liver showing its anatomical relationship to other parts of the chest and abdomen.

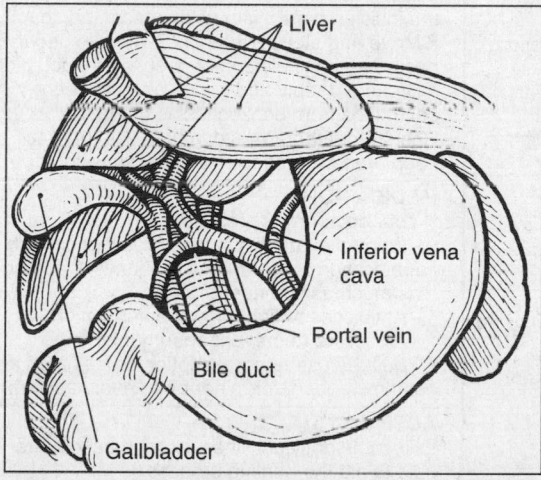

Liver

Inferior vena cava

Portal vein

Bile duct

Gallbladder

The liver and its bile ducts are isolated, cut free and removed.

Transplanted liver

The donor liver is positioned and sewn into place. Blood vessels and bile ducts are connected.

LUNG RESECTION
(Lobectomy; Pneumonectomy)

GENERAL INFORMATION

DEFINITION—Removal of tissue from the lungs. If part of a lung (usually called a lobe) is removed, the surgery is called lobectomy. If the entire lung is removed, the surgery is called pneumonectomy.

BODY PARTS INVOLVED—Lung, bronchial tubes, blood vessels in chest, ribs.

REASONS FOR SURGERY
- Cancer or suspected cancer of the lung.
- Diseased lobes of the lung caused by several chronic conditions, especially bronchiectasis.

SURGICAL RISK INCREASES WITH
- Adults over 60, obesity, poor nutrition.
- Excess alcohol consumption, smoking.
- Recent illness, especially upper-respiratory infection.
- Chronic illness, especially diabetes or lung disease.
- Use of some prescription and nonprescription drugs. Inform your doctor of any drugs, medications, or vitamin and herb supplements you are using or have used in the last month.

WHAT TO EXPECT

WHO OPERATES—Thoracic surgeon.

WHERE PERFORMED—Hospital.

DIAGNOSTIC TESTS
- Before surgery: Blood and urine studies, x-rays of chest and lungs, ECG, CT scan, bronchoscopy (see Glossary for all), pulmonary function studies.
- During surgery: ECG monitor.
- After surgery: Blood studies.

ANESTHESIA—General anesthesia by injection and inhalation with an airway tube placed in the windpipe.

DESCRIPTION OF OPERATION
- An incision is made in the chest. The ribs are spread apart for better exposure to the lungs.
- The blood supply to the diseased area is isolated and tied off.
- The diseased area is located and examined. The growth, the lobe in which it appears or the entire lung is cut free and removed along with lymph nodes in the area (if appropriate).
- A tube is inserted to drain fluid and air from the surgical area.
- The muscles are reconstructed with strong sutures. The skin is closed with sutures or clips, which usually can be removed about 1 week after surgery.

POSSIBLE COMPLICATIONS
- Excessive bleeding.
- Surgical-wound infection.
- Pneumonia.
- Reduced respiratory functioning.
- Bronchial fistula.
- Prolonged air leak.

AVERAGE HOSPITAL STAY—7 to 10 days.

PROBABLE OUTCOME—In some cases, underlying lung disease may be cured. In other cases, quality of life may be improved. Allow 6 weeks to several months for recovery.

POSTOPERATIVE CARE

GENERAL MEASURES
- A hard ridge should form along the incision. As it heals, the ridge will gradually recede.
- Shower as usual. Avoid baths until the incision has completely healed. You may wash the incision gently with mild, unscented soap.
- Move and elevate legs often while in bed to decrease the likelihood of deep-vein blood clots.
- Breathe deeply and cough often to keep secretions from pooling inside the lungs. Respiratory therapists can help you learn to keep bronchial tubes clear. Ask your doctor.

MEDICATION
- Your doctor may prescribe:
  - Pain relievers. Don't take prescription pain medication longer than 4 to 7 days. Use only as much as you need.
  - Antibiotics to fight or prevent infection.
  - A vaccine to prevent pneumonia.
- You may use nonprescription drugs, such as acetaminophen, for minor pain. Avoid aspirin.

ACTIVITY
- Resume daily activities as soon as you are able to aid the healing process.
- Avoid vigorous exercise for 6 weeks after surgery. Resume sexual relations when able.
- Resume driving 5 weeks after returning home.

DIET—Clear liquid diet until the gastrointestinal tract begins to function again. Then eat a well-balanced diet to promote healing.

CALL YOUR DOCTOR IF

- Pain, swelling, redness, drainage, or bleeding increases in the surgical area.
- You develop symptoms of infection including headache, muscle aches, dizziness, fever, or a general ill feeling.
- You experience nausea, vomiting, or shortness of breath, or you develop a "bubbly" feeling under the skin of your chest.
- New, unexplained symptoms develop.

LUNG RESECTION
(Lobectomy; Pneumonectomy)

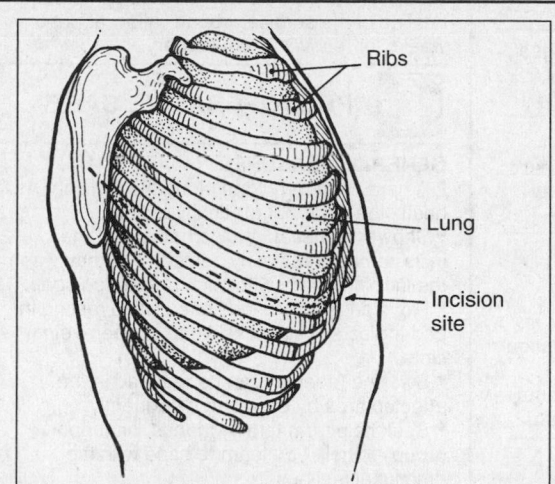

An illustration showing the usual incision site across the chest.

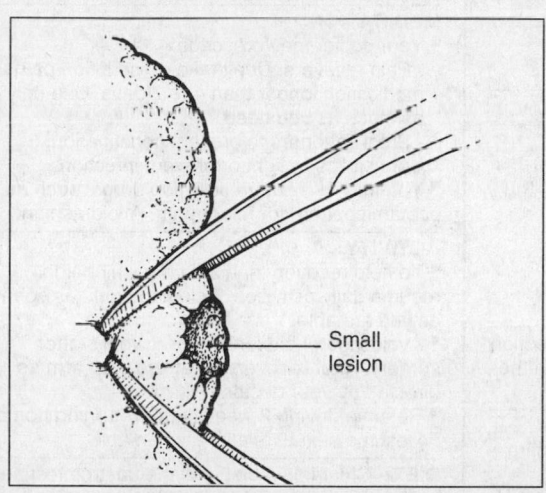

The diseased area on the lung is located and examined. The tumor, the lobe in which it appears, or the entire lung may be cut free and removed.

Muscles of the chest wall are reconstructed with strong sutures. A tube is usually left in place to drain fluid and air from the surgical area and to help the lung reinflate following surgery.

MASTECTOMY, MODIFIED RADICAL

GENERAL INFORMATION

DEFINITION—Complete removal of the breast, including the nipple, and removal of axillary nodes.

BODY PARTS INVOLVED—Breast, lymph glands.

REASONS FOR SURGERY—Cancer of the breast.

SURGICAL RISK INCREASES WITH
- Obesity or poor nutrition.
- Smoking, stress, adults over 60.
- Recent or chronic illness, diabetes.
- Use of some prescription and nonprescription drugs. Inform your doctor of any drugs, medications, or vitamin and herb supplements you are using or have used in the last month.

WHAT TO EXPECT

WHO OPERATES—General surgeon or oncological surgeon.

WHERE PERFORMED—Hospital.

DIAGNOSTIC TESTS
- Before surgery: Blood and urine studies, mammogram, needle biopsy (see Glossary for both).
- During surgery: Laboratory examination of removed tissue by frozen section.
- After surgery: Blood studies, laboratory examination of removed tissue.

ANESTHESIA—General anesthesia by injection and inhalation with an airway tube placed in the windpipe.

DESCRIPTION OF OPERATION
- An incision is made encompassing the entire breast.
- The underlying tissue is cut free and removed in one piece, along with the lymph glands from the armpit. Bleeding is controlled with sutures and electrocauterization. A tube is inserted for drainage, and will be left in place for 1 to 2 weeks.
- The skin is closed with sutures or clips, which usually can be removed about 1 week after surgery.
- See Breast Reconstruction in Surgery section.

POSSIBLE COMPLICATIONS
- Excessive bleeding.
- Surgical-wound infection.
- Depression.
- Accumulation of blood or serum under the skin in the surgical area.
- Limited shoulder motion, nerve damage.
- Lymphedema (see Glossary).
- Skin loss over mastectomy site.

AVERAGE HOSPITAL STAY—0 to 2 days.

PROBABLE OUTCOME—Expect complete healing of the surgical wound. Allow about 6 weeks for recovery from surgery.

POSTOPERATIVE CARE

GENERAL MEASURES
- A hard ridge may form along the incision. As it heals, the ridge will gradually recede.
- Shower as usual. Avoids baths until the incision has completely healed. You may wash the incision gently with mild, unscented soap.
- Move and elevate legs often while resting in bed to decrease the likelihood of deep-vein clots.
- Swelling (edema) can be reduced in the affected area by elevating it frequently.
- Seek help from family, friends, or support groups to help you learn to cope with the emotional feelings.

MEDICATION
- Your doctor may prescribe:
  - Pain relievers. Don't take prescription pain medication longer than 4 to 7 days. Use only as much as you need.
  - Stool softeners to prevent constipation.
  - Antibiotics to fight or prevent infection.
- You may use nonprescription drugs, such as acetaminophen, for minor pain. Avoid aspirin.

ACTIVITY
- To help recovery and aid your well-being, resume daily activities, including work, as soon as you are able.
- Avoid vigorous exercise for 6 weeks after surgery. After recovery, exercise your arm as directed by your doctor.
- Resume driving 2 weeks after returning home.
- Resume sexual relations when able.

DIET—Clear liquid diet until the gastrointestinal tract functions again. Then eat a well-balanced diet to promote healing.

CALL YOUR DOCTOR IF

- Pain, swelling, redness, drainage, or bleeding increases in the surgical area.
- You develop symptoms of infection including headache, muscle aches, dizziness, fever, or a general ill feeling.
- You experience nausea, vomiting, or constipation.
- You develop redness, warmth, swelling, stiffness, or hardness in the affected arm or hand.
- New, unexplained symptoms develop.

MASTECTOMY, MODIFIED RADICAL

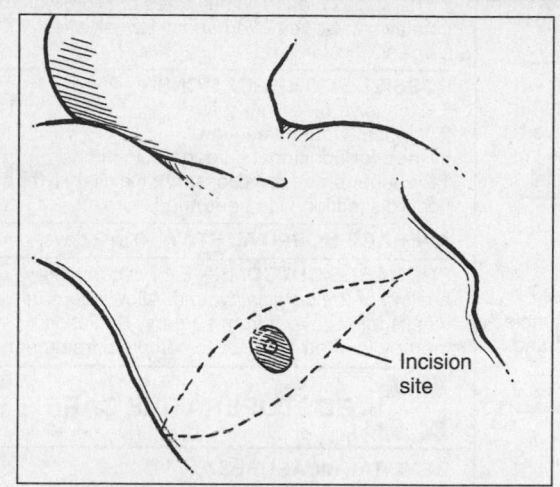

The usual site and elliptical form of the incision to remove the breast and underlying tissue.

Incision site

Underlying breast tissue is cut free and removed in one block with lymph glands from the armpit. The underlying muscle is left in place.

Pectoralis muscle

A tube is inserted for drainage. The tissues under the skin are closed with large, absorbable sutures. The skin is closed with sutures or clips that usually can be removed about 1 week after surgery.

Drainage tube

MASTECTOMY, PARTIAL
(Lumpectomy)

 GENERAL INFORMATION

DEFINITION—Removal of a lump from the female breast that is known or suspected to be cancerous. Lumpectomy is the least invasive procedure for breast cancer surgery, and is the most likely to leave the breast looking normal.

BODY PARTS INVOLVED—Breast.

REASONS FOR SURGERY—Cancer or suspected cancer of the breast. There is frequently more than one option for surgical treatment. Be sure you understand the rationale for any recommended procedure, the risks and benefits involved, as well as any possible alternative treatments.

SURGICAL RISK INCREASES WITH
- Obesity, smoking, stress.
- Poor nutrition.
- Recent or chronic illness.
- Diabetes.
- Use of some prescription and nonprescription drugs. Inform your doctor of any drugs, medications, or vitamin and herb supplements you are using or have used in the last month.

 WHAT TO EXPECT

WHO OPERATES—General surgeon or oncological surgeon.

WHERE PERFORMED—Hospital.

DIAGNOSTIC TESTS
- Before surgery: Blood and urine studies, x-rays of chest, mammograms (see Glossary).
- During surgery: Laboratory examination of the removed lump by a pathologist.
- After surgery: Blood studies, laboratory examination of removed tissue, sometimes bone scans.

ANESTHESIA
- Local anesthesia by injection, accompanied by sedation.
- General anesthesia by injection and inhalation with an airway tube placed in the windpipe.

DESCRIPTION OF OPERATION
- An incision is made over the lump to be removed.
- The lump and a small surrounding area of normal tissue are cut free and removed. Bleeding is controlled with ties and electrocauterization.
- It is frequently necessary to perform axillary node dissection in conjunction with lumpectomy. If lymph node dissection is necessary, a separate incision in the axilla (under the armpit) is made to sample or significantly remove the axillary lymph nodes.

- The skin is closed with sutures or clips, which usually can be removed about 1 week after surgery.

POSSIBLE COMPLICATIONS
- Excessive bleeding.
- Surgical-wound infection.
- Need for additional surgery (sometimes).
- Lymphedema (see Glossary), if axillary lymph node dissection was performed.

AVERAGE HOSPITAL STAY—0 to 2 days.

PROBABLE OUTCOME—Expect complete healing of the surgical wound. Allow about 2 weeks for recovery from surgery. Radiation therapy is often required to complete treatment.

 POSTOPERATIVE CARE

GENERAL MEASURES
- A firm area will appear where the lump was removed. This may remain for several months.
- Shower as usual. Avoid baths until the incision is healed. You may wash the incision gently with mild, unscented soap.

MEDICATION
- Your doctor may prescribe:
  - Pain relievers. Don't take prescription pain medication longer than 4 to 7 days. Use only as much as you need.
  - Stool softeners to prevent constipation.
  - Antibiotics to fight or prevent infection.
- You may use nonprescription drugs, such as acetaminophen, for minor pain. Avoid aspirin.

ACTIVITY
- To help recovery and aid your well-being, resume daily activities, including work, as soon as you are able.
- Avoid vigorous exercise for 2 weeks after surgery.
- Resume driving 1 day after returning home.

DIET—Eat lightly for the remainder of the day. Then eat a well-balanced diet to promote healing.

 CALL YOUR DOCTOR IF

- Pain, swelling, redness, drainage, or bleeding increases in the surgical area.
- You develop symptoms of infection including headache, muscle aches, dizziness, fever, or a general ill feeling.
- You experience nausea or vomiting.
- New, unexplained symptoms develop.

MASTECTOMY, PARTIAL
(Lumpectomy)

A breast lump in a typical location.

Lump

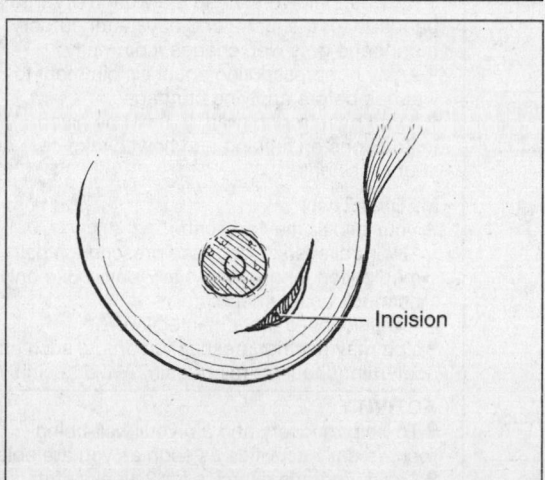

After the skin has been incised, the lump and a small surrounding area of normal tissue are cut free.

Incision

The lump is removed. Afterwards, the remaining breast is carefully palpated for any additional suspicious areas or suspicious lymph nodes.

MELANOMA REMOVAL

GENERAL INFORMATION

DEFINITION—Removal of any lesion on the skin that might be malignant melanoma, the most dangerous form of skin cancer.

BODY PARTS INVOLVED—Skin.

REASONS FOR SURGERY—Treatment of malignant melanoma.

SURGICAL RISK INCREASES WITH
- Obesity, smoking, poor nutrition.
- Recent or chronic illness.
- Diabetes.
- Use of some prescription and nonprescription drugs. Inform your doctor of any drugs, medications, or vitamin and herb supplements you are using or have used in the last month.

WHAT TO EXPECT

WHO OPERATES—General surgeon, dermatologist, or plastic and reconstructive surgeon.

WHERE PERFORMED—Hospital or outpatient surgical facility.

DIAGNOSTIC TESTS
- Before surgery: Blood and urine studies.
- During surgery: Microscopic examination of skin margins to determine how much skin to remove.
- After surgery: Laboratory examination of removed tissue. Possibly, CT scan, MRI, bone scans, PET scan (see Glossary for all).

ANESTHESIA
- Local anesthesia by injection.
- General anesthesia by injection and inhalation with an airway tube placed in the windpipe.

DESCRIPTION OF OPERATION
- Surgery is directed primarily toward cure and secondarily toward preservation of normal appearance.
- The tumor is removed along with a surrounding portion of normal, healthy skin to ensure complete removal of all cancer cells.
- Skin grafts (see in Surgery section) are frequently needed to close large skin defects.
- The skin is closed with fine suture material or clips, which usually can be removed about 10 days after surgery.

POSSIBLE COMPLICATIONS
- Surgical-wound infection.
- Excessive bleeding.
- Residual cancer due to not removing enough diseased skin.

AVERAGE HOSPITAL STAY—0 to 2 days.

PROBABLE OUTCOME—Expect complete healing of the surgical wounds. Examination of removed skin and tissue may reveal that additional treatment will be necessary. Further treatment such as radiation, additional surgery, or anticancer drugs depends on each patient's case. Allow about 2 weeks for recovery from surgery.

POSTOPERATIVE CARE

GENERAL MEASURES
- If the wound bleeds during the first 24 hours after surgery, press a clean tissue or cloth to it for 10 minutes.
- A hard ridge should form along the incisions. As they heal, the ridges will gradually recede.
- If you do not have a skin graft, you may shower as usual. Avoid bathing until the incision has completely healed. You may wash the incision gently with mild, unscented soap.
- Between showers, keep the wound dry with a bandage for the first 2 or 3 days after surgery. If a bandage gets wet, change it promptly.
- Apply nonprescription antibiotic ointment to wounds before applying bandages.
- If you have a skin graft, you will be given instructions on bathing and how to take care of your dressings.

MEDICATION
- Your doctor may prescribe:
  - Pain relievers. Don't take prescription pain medication longer than 4 to 7 days. Use only as much as you need.
  - Antibiotics to prevent infection.
- You may use nonprescription drugs, such as acetaminophen, for minor pain. Avoid aspirin.

ACTIVITY
- To help recovery and aid your well-being, resume daily activities as soon as you are able.
- Avoid vigorous exercise for 2 weeks after surgery.
- Resume driving when your doctor determines you are able. This will vary depending on the size of the melanoma removed and the extent of the surgery.

DIET—No special diet.

CALL YOUR DOCTOR IF

- Pain, swelling, redness, drainage, or bleeding increases in the surgical area.
- You develop symptoms of infection including headache, muscle aches, dizziness, fever, or a general ill feeling.
- New, unexplained symptoms develop.

MELANOMA REMOVAL

Malignant melanoma

- A large lesion on the skin, in this case, on the top of the foot at the base of the toes.
- Melanomas may also appear on other skin locations.

The tumor is removed along with the surrounding portion of normal, healthy skin (usually 2-3 centimeters) to ensure complete removal of all cancerous cells.

- If possible, the skin is closed without grafting, but frequently a skin graft from another site must be used to completely close large lesion sites.
- Sutures used for closure or for skin grafting can usually be removed about 10 days after surgery.

MENISCECTOMY

GENERAL INFORMATION

DEFINITION—Removal of torn cartilage in the knee.

BODY PARTS INVOLVED—Knee and all its parts.

REASONS FOR SURGERY
• Prevention of permanent damage to the knee joint.
• Stop "locking" of knee joint.
• Relieve pain and swelling of knee.

SURGICAL RISK INCREASES WITH
• Obesity.
• Smoking.
• Recent or chronic illness.
• Diabetes.
• Use of some prescription and nonprescription drugs. Inform your doctor of any drugs, medications, or vitamin and herb supplements you are using or have used in the last month.

WHAT TO EXPECT

WHO OPERATES—Orthopedist.

WHERE PERFORMED—Hospital or outpatient surgical facility.

DIAGNOSTIC TESTS
• Before surgery: Blood and urine studies, x-rays of both knees, MRI, arthrogram (see Glossary for both).
• After surgery: X-rays of affected knee, blood studies.

ANESTHESIA
• Spinal anesthesia by injection.
• General anesthesia by injection and inhalation with an airway tube placed in the windpipe.

DESCRIPTION OF OPERATION
• The affected area can be approached by arthroscopy (see Glossary) or by incision into the knee joint. Either approach exposes the injured cartilage.
• If the torn cartilage can be repaired, it will be sutured. Or, if the torn cartilage cannot be repaired, the torn portion will be removed. Any injured ligaments are sewn together.
• The skin is closed with sutures or clips, which usually can be removed about 1 week after surgery.

POSSIBLE COMPLICATIONS
• Excessive bleeding, blood clots.
• Surgical-wound infection.
• Weakened knee joint and subsequent arthritis.

AVERAGE HOSPITAL STAY—0 to 2 days.

PROBABLE OUTCOME—Expect complete recovery without complications. Allow about 6 weeks for recovery from surgery.

POSTOPERATIVE CARE

GENERAL MEASURES
• A hard ridge should form along the incision. As it heals, the ridge will recede gradually.
• Shower as usual. Avoid baths until the incision has completely healed. You may wash the incision gently with mild, unscented soap. After showering, replace any wet dressings with clean, dry ones.
• Use an ice bag on the knee to reduce swelling. The ice bag should be used for 20 minutes, 4 to 5 times a day.
• Move and elevate legs often while resting in bed to decrease the likelihood of deep-vein blood clots.
• When sleeping or sitting, keep the affected leg elevated with pillows under the foot or blocks under the bed to help reduce pain and swelling.

MEDICATION
• Your doctor may prescribe:
  - Pain relievers. Don't take prescription pain medication longer than 4 to 7 days. Use only as much as you need.
  - Antibiotics to fight or prevent infection.
• You may use nonprescription drugs, such as acetaminophen, for minor pain. Avoid aspirin.

ACTIVITY
• To help recovery and aid your well-being, resume daily activities, including work, as soon as you are able.
• Use crutches or a cane to walk as directed by your doctor. Don't stand for prolonged periods.
• Avoid vigorous exercise for 4 weeks after surgery. A physical therapist can teach you exercises that will restore strength to the knee.
• Resume driving after 3 weeks or when your doctor determines that healing is complete.

DIET—Clear liquid diet until the gastrointestinal tract functions again. Then eat a well-balanced diet to promote healing.

CALL YOUR DOCTOR IF

• Pain, swelling, redness, drainage, or bleeding increases in the surgical area.
• Toes become cold, discolored, or numb.
• You develop symptoms of infection including headache, muscle aches, dizziness, fever, or a general ill feeling.
• You experience nausea or vomiting.
• New, unexplained symptoms develop.

MENISCECTOMY

An arthroscope inserted into a knee joint. The illustration shows surgical drapes around the joint.

The surgeon can visualize through the arthroscope any tear in either meniscus.

- The torn meniscus is removed with forceps and extracted through the opening in the skin.
- Skin is closed with sutures or clips that usually can be removed about 1 week after surgery (not illustrated).

MORTON'S NEUROMA REMOVAL

GENERAL INFORMATION

DEFINITION—Removal of Morton's neuroma, a small benign tumor in the nerve that serves the toes. Its cause is unknown and it produces severe pain.

BODY PARTS INVOLVED—A small tumor between the 2nd and 3rd toes or the 3rd and 4th toes. It may occur in either or both feet.

REASONS FOR SURGERY—Relief of pain caused by the neuroma.

SURGICAL RISK INCREASES WITH
- Obesity.
- Smoking.
- Poor nutrition.
- Recent or chronic illness.
- Diabetes.
- Use of some prescription and nonprescription drugs. Inform your doctor of any drugs, medications, or vitamin and herb supplements you are using or have used in the last month.

WHAT TO EXPECT

WHO OPERATES—Orthopedist, podiatrist.

WHERE PERFORMED—Hospital, outpatient surgical facility, doctor's office, or emergency room.

DIAGNOSTIC TESTS
- Before surgery: Blood and urine studies, x-ray of the foot.
- After surgery: Laboratory examination of removed tissue.

ANESTHESIA
- Local anesthesia by injection.
- General anesthesia by injection and inhalation with an airway tube placed in the throat.

DESCRIPTION OF OPERATION
- A tourniquet is wrapped around the leg to decrease bleeding in the surgical area.
- The neuroma is located, cut free from surrounding tissue and removed.
- The skin is closed with sutures, which usually can be removed about 10 to 14 days after surgery. The tourniquet is removed.

POSSIBLE COMPLICATIONS
- Excessive bleeding.
- Surgical-wound infection.
- Numbness in toes due to cut nerve (less bothersome for many patients than the previous pain caused by the neuroma).

AVERAGE HOSPITAL STAY—0 to 1 day.

PROBABLE OUTCOME—Expect complete healing without complications. Allow about 3 weeks for recovery from surgery.

POSTOPERATIVE CARE

GENERAL MEASURES
- If the wound bleeds during the first 24 hours after surgery, press a clean tissue or cloth to it for 10 minutes.
- A hard ridge should form along the incision. As it heals, the ridge will gradually recede.
- Shower as usual. You may wash the incision gently with mild unscented soap.
- Between showers, keep the wound dry with a bandage for the first 2 or 3 days after surgery. If a bandage gets wet, change it promptly. Apply nonprescription antibiotic ointment to the wound before applying new bandages.
- Keep the foot elevated as much as possible during recovery.

MEDICATION
- Your doctor may prescribe:
  - Pain relievers. Don't take prescription pain medication longer than 4 to 7 days. Use only as much as you need.
  - Antibiotics to fight or prevent infection.
- You may use nonprescription drugs, such as acetaminophen, for minor pain. Avoid aspirin.

ACTIVITY
- To help recovery and aid your well-being, resume daily activities, including work, as soon as you are able.
- Avoid vigorous exercise for 6 weeks after surgery.
- Resume driving 1 week after returning home.

DIET—No special diet.

CALL YOUR DOCTOR IF

- Pain, swelling, redness, drainage, or bleeding increases in the surgical area.
- You develop symptoms of infection including headache, muscle aches, dizziness, fever, or a general ill feeling.
- New, unexplained symptoms develop.

MORTON'S NEUROMA REMOVAL

A typical location between the 3rd and 4th toes for a Morton's neuroma (a small benign tumor of nerve tissue).

Neuroma

After a tourniquet has been wrapped around the leg to decrease bleeding in the surgical area, an incision is made through the skin.

Incision site

● The neuroma is located, cut free from the surrounding tissue and removed.
● After removal, skin is closed with sutures that usually can be removed about 10 to 14 days after surgery (not illustrated).
● The tourniquet is removed to allow normal circulation to the leg and foot (not illustrated).

Neuroma

MYRINGOTOMY

GENERAL INFORMATION

DEFINITION—Opening the eardrum (tympanic membrane) to remove fluid in the middle ear. This fluid consists of blood, pus, water, and debris, and usually collects because of infection or allergy. Frequently, a small tube is inserted in the middle ear to maintain drainage.

BODY PARTS INVOLVED—Eardrum, middle ear, external ear canal (route for surgery).

REASONS FOR SURGERY
- Relief of pain caused by pressure.
- Prevent recurrent infections.
- Prevention of temporary or permanent hearing loss.

SURGICAL RISK INCREASES WITH
- Smoking.
- Recent illness, especially upper-respiratory infection.
- Chronic illness, especially diabetes.
- Previous perforation of the eardrum.
- Use of some prescription and nonprescription drugs. Inform your doctor of any drugs, medications, or vitamin and herb supplements you are using or have used in the last month.

WHAT TO EXPECT

WHO OPERATES—Ear, nose and throat specialist (otolaryngologist).

WHERE PERFORMED—Hospital or outpatient surgical facility.

DIAGNOSTIC TESTS
- Before surgery: Blood and urine studies, hearing tests, tympanogram (see Glossary).
- After surgery: Blood studies, hearing tests.

ANESTHESIA
- Local anesthesia by topical application.
- General anesthesia by injection and inhalation with an airway tube placed in the windpipe.

DESCRIPTION OF OPERATION
- An instrument called an ear speculum is placed in the external ear canal, and the operative microscope is positioned.
- An tiny incision is made around the eardrum, with care taken not to injure the small bones in the middle ear.
- The fluid is drained, and a tiny small tube (about the size of a grain of rice) is usually left in place to continue drainage.
- No sutures are placed in the eardrum. It will heal by itself, if infection is minimal or absent.

- The tube will prevent premature closure of the eardrum and allow the middle ear to heal. The tube will usually fall out by itself in 6 to 12 months. Occasionally, it will need to be surgically removed.
- The procedure is often repeated in the other ear.

POSSIBLE COMPLICATIONS
- Excessive bleeding.
- Surgical-wound infection.
- Hearing loss.

AVERAGE HOSPITAL STAY—0 to 1 day.

PROBABLE OUTCOME—Expect complete healing without complications. Hearing should improve noticeably. Allow about 4 weeks for recovery from surgery.

POSTOPERATIVE CARE

GENERAL MEASURES
- Keep the ear dry.
- If future middle ear infections do develop, medicated drops can be placed in the ear canal where they will flow through the tube and into the ear to treat the infection.

MEDICATION
- Your doctor may prescribe:
  - Pain relievers. Don't take prescription pain medication longer than 4 to 7 days. Use only as much as you need.
  - Antibiotics to fight or prevent infection.
- You may use nonprescription drugs, such as acetaminophen, for minor pain. Avoid aspirin.

ACTIVITY
- To help recovery and aid your well-being, resume daily activities, including work, as soon as you are able.
- Your doctor will advise you about limits on certain activities (e.g., swimming).
- Resume driving about 1 week after returning home.

DIET—Liquid diet the first day after surgery, then no special diet.

CALL YOUR DOCTOR IF

- Pain, swelling, redness, drainage, or bleeding increases in the surgical area.
- You develop symptoms of infection including headache, muscle aches, dizziness, fever, or a general ill feeling.
- You experience nausea or vomiting.

MYRINGOTOMY

External ear

Ear canal

Speculum

An illustration of parts of the ear, including cartilage and skin of the external ear. The ear canal, which goes from the outside inward to reach the eardrum, can be seen through a speculum inserted into the ear canal.

Ear drum

Middle ear bone

Pus

A tiny incision is made in a low section of the eardrum allowing fluid to drain.

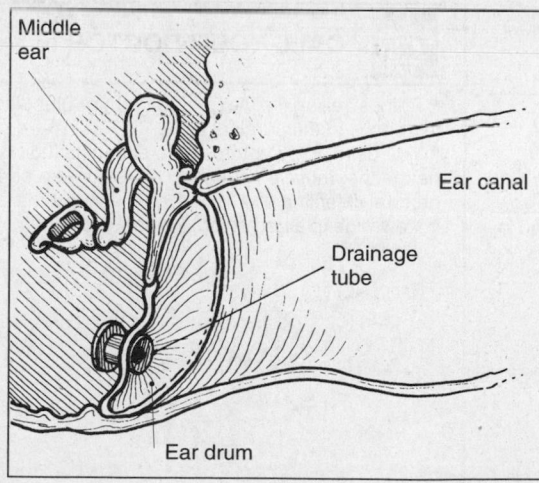

Middle ear

Ear canal

Drainage tube

Ear drum

- A drainage tube is usually left in place to continue drainage.
- No sutures are placed in the eardrum; it will heal by itself if infection is minimal or absent.
- The tubes will prevent premature closure of the eardrum and allow the middle ear to heal. Usually the tubes will come out by themselves 6 to 12 months following surgery.

NAIL REMOVAL

 ## GENERAL INFORMATION

DEFINITION—Removal of part or all of a toenail or fingernail.

BODY PARTS INVOLVED—Toenail, usually in the big toe, any fingernail.

REASONS FOR SURGERY
- Relief of painful symptoms of an ingrown toenail or fingernail, with or without an infection.
- Nails may be removed due to injury (with part of the nail torn away), splinters that cannot be removed without removing the nail, or warts under the nail.
- Nail infection (usually fungus).
- Correction of abnormal nail growth.

SURGICAL RISK INCREASES WITH
- Poor circulation in extremities.
- Diabetes.
- Use of some prescription and nonprescription drugs. Inform your doctor of any drugs, medications, or vitamin and herb supplements you are using or have used in the last month.

 ## WHAT TO EXPECT

WHO OPERATES—General surgeon, family doctor, dermatologist, or podiatrist.

WHERE PERFORMED—Doctor's office or outpatient surgical facility.

DIAGNOSTIC TESTS—None required.

ANESTHESIA—Local anesthesia by injection.

DESCRIPTION OF OPERATION
- A section of skin is cut on the affected side of the toe.
- Part or all of the nail is pulled up along its bed and cut free of its underlying tissue.
- The nail bed along the affected side is scraped.
- A special nonstick bandage is applied tightly to prevent bleeding. Usually, no sutures are needed.

POSSIBLE COMPLICATIONS
- Excessive bleeding.
- Surgical-wound infection.

AVERAGE HOSPITAL STAY—None.

PROBABLE OUTCOME—Expect complete healing without complications. Allow about 3 weeks for recovery from surgery. The nail should eventually grow back.

 ## POSTOPERATIVE CARE

GENERAL MEASURES
- Keep the surgical area dry until after the dressing is changed for the first time at the doctor's office.
- After the dressing is changed for the first time, you may bathe or shower with the dressing on. After bathing, remove the wet dressing and replace it with a clean, dry one.
- After the dressing is changed the first time, soak the affected area in plain or salt water at 101° to 104°F (38.3° to 40°C) for 10 to 20 minutes several times a day to reduce pain and swelling.
- Elevate the affected area as much as possible for the first 24 to 48 hours following surgery, in order to help reduce pain.
- If a toenail is involved, avoid shoes that fit tightly, especially those with narrow toes. Wear white cotton socks.
- To prevent a recurrence of ingrown toenail, when the toenail grows back, cut it straight across instead of rounding off at the corners.

MEDICATION
- Your doctor may prescribe:
  - Pain relievers. Don't take prescription pain medication longer than 4 to 7 days. Use only as much as you need.
  - Antibiotics or antifungal medication to fight or prevent infection.
- You may use nonprescription drugs, such as acetaminophen, for minor pain. Avoid aspirin.

ACTIVITY
- Following toenail removal, avoid vigorous exercise until the nail heals. Don't put any weight on the affected foot for 24 hours, then resume walking gradually.
- No restrictions following fingernail removal.

DIET—No special diet.

 ## CALL YOUR DOCTOR IF

- Pain, swelling, redness, drainage, or bleeding increases in the surgical area.
- You develop symptoms of infection including headache, muscle aches, dizziness, fever, or a general ill feeling.
- New, unexplained symptoms develop.

NAIL REMOVAL

An ingrown toenail in the great toe.

Ingrown nail

- A section of the skin is cut on the affected side of the toe.
- Part or all of the nail is pulled up along its bed and cut free of its underlying tissue.

The toenail is removed and the nailbed along the affected side is scraped to prevent recurrence, if possible. The nailbed hardens slowly. A new nail usually grows to replace the removed one.

NASAL POLYPS REMOVAL
(Nasal Polypectomy)

GENERAL INFORMATION

DEFINITION—Removal of nasal polyps, accumulations of fluid under the membrane lining inside the nose.

BODY PARTS INVOLVED—Nose and its membrane lining.

REASONS FOR SURGERY—Restoration of normal breathing.

SURGICAL RISK INCREASES WITH—Use of some prescription and nonprescription drugs. Inform your doctor of any drugs, medications, or vitamin and herb supplements you are using or have used in the last month.

WHAT TO EXPECT

WHO OPERATES—Ear, nose and throat specialist (otolaryngologist).

WHERE PERFORMED—Doctor's office, hospital, or outpatient surgical facility.

DIAGNOSTIC TESTS—Often, none required. Sometimes, blood and urine studies are done before surgery.

ANESTHESIA
* General anesthesia.
* Local anesthesia by topical application.
* Local anesthesia by injection.

DESCRIPTION OF OPERATION
* The nose is held open with a speculum.
* The polyps are located, clamped and removed with a wire loop.
* Bleeding is controlled with electrocautery.
* An absorbent or non-absorbent packing usually placed in the nose to help reduce bleeding risk. The absorbent packing dissolves on its own. The non-absorbent is usually removed in 1 to 2 days.

POSSIBLE COMPLICATIONS
* Excessive bleeding.
* Surgical-wound infection.

AVERAGE HOSPITAL STAY—0 to 1 day.

PROBABLE OUTCOME—Expect complete healing without complications. Allow about 2 weeks for recovery from surgery.

POSTOPERATIVE CARE

GENERAL MEASURES
* Follow your doctor's instructions about specific follow-up care (such as when it is safe to blow your nose).
* Use saline nasal spray as directed. It is usually started the third day after surgery and is done 3 times a day.

MEDICATION
* Your doctor may prescribe:
  - Pain relievers. Don't take prescription pain medication longer than 4 to 7 days. Use only as much as you need.
  - Antibiotics to fight or prevent infection.
* You may use nonprescription drugs, such as acetaminophen, to relieve pain. Avoid aspirin.

ACTIVITY—Usually, no limits.

DIET—Eat a well-balanced diet to promote healing. Drink plenty of fluids.

CALL YOUR DOCTOR IF

* Pain, swelling, redness, drainage, or bleeding increase in the surgical area.
* You develop symptoms of infection including headache, muscle aches, dizziness, fever, or a general ill feeling.
* You experience nausea or vomiting.
* New, unexplained symptoms develop.

NASAL POLYPS REMOVAL
(Nasal Polypectomy)

A speculum is used to visualize polyps inside the nose.

Speculum

The polyps are visually located by the operator.

Polyps

Wire loop around polyp

- The polyps are clamped and removed with a wire snare.
- Following surgery, the nose is generally packed with petroleum jelly and gauze to prevent bleeding. This pack will be removed at a later time by your doctor.

NECK, RADICAL DISSECTION OF

GENERAL INFORMATION

DEFINITION—Removal of the lymph nodes, a large muscle, and some of the nerves along the side of the neck.

BODY PARTS INVOLVED—Neck muscles, lymph glands, windpipe.

REASONS FOR SURGERY—Cancer in the oral cavity or neck, which will spread to other parts of the body if not removed.

SURGICAL RISK INCREASES WITH
- Adults over 60, obesity, smoking.
- Poor nutrition.
- Recent illness, especially respiratory illness.
- Alcoholism.
- Chronic illness, especially diabetes.
- Use of some prescription and nonprescription drugs. Inform your doctor of any drugs, medications, or vitamin and herb supplements you are using or have used in the last month.

WHAT TO EXPECT

WHO OPERATES—Ear, nose and throat specialist (otolaryngologist), or general surgeon.

WHERE PERFORMED—Hospital.

DIAGNOSTIC TESTS
- Before surgery: Blood and urine studies, x-ray of chest, ECG, CT scan, needle biopsy, open biopsy (see Glossary for all).
- After surgery: Blood studies.

ANESTHESIA—General anesthesia by injection and inhalation with an airway tube placed in the windpipe.

DESCRIPTION OF OPERATION
- An incision shaped like an "H" is made in the neck. Skin flaps are separated from the underlying tissue.
- The lymph glands, muscles, jugular vein, and connective tissue are cut free and removed.
- Sometimes, a tracheostomy (see in Surgery section) is performed. In other cases, part of the jaw and tongue are also removed.
- Tubes are left in the surgical area to drain secretions, the tubes are usually removed 3 to 5 days following surgery.
- The connective tissue is closed, and the skin is closed with sutures or clips, which usually can be removed about 1 week after surgery.

POSSIBLE COMPLICATIONS
- Excessive bleeding.
- Surgical-wound infection.
- Restricted breathing.
- Permanent weakness of lower lip.
- Inadvertent injury to the large blood vessels and nerves in the neck, tip of the lung, thoracic duct, or laryngeal nerve.

AVERAGE HOSPITAL STAY—3 to 5 days.

PROBABLE OUTCOME—Expect complete healing. Removing tissue in the neck may cause some unavoidable disfigurement. However, some cancers can be cured completely with this surgery. Allow about 4 weeks for recovery from surgery. Depending on the muscles removed, you may have decreased movement in the shoulder area on the affected side.

POSTOPERATIVE CARE

GENERAL MEASURES
- A hard ridge should form along the incision. As it heals, the ridge will gradually recede.
- Shower as usual. Avoid baths until the incisions have completely healed. You may wash the incision gently with mild, unscented soap. After showering, replace any wet dressings with clean, dry ones.
- Move and elevate legs often while resting in bed to decrease the likelihood of deep-vein blood clots.

MEDICATION
- Your doctor may prescribe:
  - Pain relievers. Don't take prescription pain medication longer than 4 to 7 days. Use only as much as you need.
  - Stool softeners to prevent constipation.
  - Antibiotics to fight or prevent infection.
- You may use nonprescription drugs, such as acetaminophen, to relieve pain. Avoid aspirin.

ACTIVITY
- To help recovery and aid in your well-being, resume daily activities as soon as you are able.
- Avoid vigorous exercise for 6 weeks after surgery.
- Resume driving 5 weeks after returning home.

DIET—Clear liquid diet until the gastrointestinal tract begins to function again. Then eat a well-balanced diet to promote healing. Increase your fiber and fluid intake to help decrease the likelihood of constipation.

CALL YOUR DOCTOR IF

- Pain, swelling, redness, drainage, or bleeding increases in the surgical area.
- You develop symptoms of infection including headache, muscle aches, dizziness, fever, or a general ill feeling.
- You experience nausea or vomiting, constipation, abdominal swelling, hoarseness, or have difficulty with breathing.
- New, unexplained symptoms develop.

NECK, RADICAL DISSECTION OF

The lymph nodes, muscle and bone in the neck.

Lymph nodes

Sternocleido-mastoid muscle

Clavicle

An illustration of the usual incision sites for radical neck dissection.

Incision sites

- The lymph glands, muscles and connective tissue are cut free and removed.
- Tracheostomy is performed when laryngectomy is done.
- Tubes are left in the surgical area to drain secretions (not illustrated).
- The connective tissues are closed and the skin is closed with sutures or clips, which usually can be removed about 1 week after surgery (not illustrated).

NEPHROSTOMY, PERCUTANEOUS
(Nephrolithotomy, Percutaneous)

 GENERAL INFORMATION

DEFINITION—Creating a puncture wound through the skin and muscles of the back directly into the collecting system of the kidney (where urine is collected before traveling down the ureter to the bladder) and placing a tube for access or drainage.

BODY PARTS INVOLVED—Kidney, ureter.

REASONS FOR SURGERY
• To create an opening into the kidney to maintain temporary or permanent urinary drainage when there is a temporary blockage downstream toward the bladder.
• To provide access to remove or break up stones in the collecting system of the kidney.

SURGICAL RISK INCREASES WITH
• Adults over 60, newborns and infants.
• Obesity, smoking, poor nutrition.
• Recent or chronic illness, especially diabetes or alcoholism.
• Use of some prescription and nonprescription drugs. Inform your doctor of any drugs, medications, or vitamin and herb supplements you are using or have used in the last month.

 WHAT TO EXPECT

WHO OPERATES—General surgeon or urologist.

WHERE PERFORMED—Hospital.

DIAGNOSTIC TESTS
• Before surgery: Blood and urine studies, ultrasound, CT scan, IVP, cystoscopy (see Glossary for all).
• After surgery: Blood and urine studies.

ANESTHESIA—General anesthesia by injection and inhalation with an airway tube placed in the windpipe.

DESCRIPTION OF OPERATION
• A small incision is made, usually in the left or right flank, but sometimes in the abdomen.
• A special needle-like device is passed into the kidney.
• A catheter is passed through the puncture wound into the collecting system of the kidney.
• Stone removal may be accomplished with this procedure, or by pulverization by lithotripsy (see in Surgery section).
• Urine produced by this kidney reaches the outside through the catheter.

POSSIBLE COMPLICATIONS
• Excessive bleeding, blood clots.
• Surgical-wound infection.
• Inadvertent injury to the vena cava or other organs near the kidney.

AVERAGE HOSPITAL STAY—0 to 3 days.

PROBABLE OUTCOME—Expect complete healing without complications. You will need to wear a urine collection bag, either temporarily or permanently, depending on the underlying cause. Allow 4 weeks for recovery from surgery.

 POSTOPERATIVE CARE

GENERAL MEASURES
• Shower as usual. Avoid baths until the incision has completely healed You may wash the incision gently with mild, unscented soap. After showering, replace any wet dressings with clean, dry ones.
• Move and elevate legs often while resting in bed to decrease the likelihood of deep-vein blood clots.
• Your doctor will instruct you in emptying and caring for the catheter tube and collection bag.

MEDICATION
• Your doctor may prescribe:
  - Pain relievers. Don't take prescription pain medication longer than 4 to 7 days. Use only as much as you need.
  - Stool softeners to prevent constipation.
  - Antibiotics to fight or prevent infection.
• You may use nonprescription drugs, such as acetaminophen, to relieve pain. Avoid aspirin.

ACTIVITY
• Return to normal daily activities as soon as possible to promote healing.
• Avoid vigorous exercise for 2 weeks after surgery.
• Resume driving 1 week after returning home.
• Resume sexual relations when your doctor determines that healing is complete.

DIET
• Clear liquid diet until the gastrointestinal tract begins to function again. Then eat a well-balanced diet to promote healing.
• Vitamin and mineral supplements (sometimes).

 CALL YOUR DOCTOR IF

• Pain, swelling, redness, drainage, or bleeding increases in the surgical area.
• You develop symptoms of infection including headache, muscle aches, dizziness, fever, or a general ill feeling.
• You experience constipation, abdominal swelling, nausea, or vomiting.
• The urine in the collection bag becomes red, cloudy, or foul-smelling.
• The catheter tube is dislodged.
• There is very little urine in the collection bag.
• New, unexplained symptoms develop.

NEPHROSTOMY, PERCUTANEOUS
(Nephrolithotomy, Percutaneous)

An illustration of a patient's right flank showing the kidney and surrounding structures.

Ribs

Kidney

Ureter

Bladder

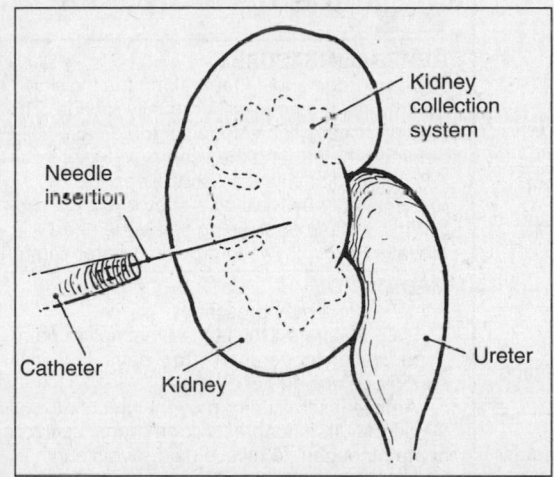

Kidney collection system

Needle insertion

Catheter

Kidney

Ureter

• A special needle-like device is passed into the kidney. A catheter is passed through the puncture wound and into the collecting system of the kidney
• The ureter as shown has become dilated (widened) due to obstruction between the kidney and the bladder.

Urine produced by this kidney reaches the outside through the catheter.

OTOPLASTY
(Ear Plastic Surgery)

GENERAL INFORMATION

DEFINITION—Cosmetic or reconstructive surgery on the outer ear.

BODY PARTS INVOLVED—Ears.

REASONS FOR SURGERY
- Improve appearance of the outer ear (usually to flatten protruding ears).
- To construct or repair a missing or badly damaged ear.

SURGICAL RISK INCREASES WITH
- Previous severe ear injury such as burn or extensive laceration.
- Diabetes.
- Use of some prescription and nonprescription drugs. Inform your doctor of any drugs, medications, or vitamin and herb supplements you are using or have used in the last month.

WHAT TO EXPECT

WHO OPERATES—Plastic surgeon, reconstructive surgeon, or otolaryngologist (ear, nose and throat specialist).

WHERE PERFORMED—Hospital, outpatient facility, well-equipped doctor's office.

DIAGNOSTIC TESTS
- Before surgery: Blood and urine studies.
- After surgery: Usually none necessary.

ANESTHESIA
- Local anesthesia by injection.
- General anesthesia by injection and inhalation with an airway tube placed in the windpipe.

DESCRIPTION OF OPERATION
- To flatten protruding ears (several procedures are available, one is described here):
  - A flap of skin is removed from the back of each ear.
  - The underlying cartilage is remolded and the two edges of the wound stitched together. This brings the ear closer to the head.
  - Bulky dressings are applied to the ear and left on for a few days. They are replaced by a headband that is worn for several weeks.
  - Stitches are removed about a week later.
- For a missing or badly damaged ear:
  - The procedure is extensive and complex and normally involves more than one operation with long intervals of healing inbetween.
  - A piece of rib cartilage is removed and sculptured to resemble a normal ear.
  - The cartilage is transferred to a pocket of skin at the site where the ear will be located. Sometimes a skin graft is necessary.

- Dressings are applied to the ear and left on for 10-14 days until healing is completed and the stitches are removed.
- Hearing in the reconstructed ear may not be normal. When the hearing is normal in the other ear, there is usually no attempt made to improve the hearing in the reconstructed ear.

POSSIBLE COMPLICATIONS
- Sensitivity to cold weather, especially in the first year following surgery.
- Excessive bleeding (rare).
- Excessive scarring (keloid).
- Skin graft failure.
- Surgical wound infection (rare).

AVERAGE HOSPITAL STAY—0 to 1 day.

PROBABLE OUTCOME—Expect complete healing without complications. Allow about 2 weeks for recovery from surgery.

POSTOPERATIVE CARE

GENERAL MEASURES
- A hard ridge should form along the incision. As it heals, the ridge will gradually recede. The resulting scar will be hidden in the crease between the ear and the scalp.
- Bathe and shower as usual. Keep the dressings dry by wearing a shower cap.
- While resting or sleeping, keep the head elevated on 2 pillows to provide greater comfort.

MEDICATION
- Your doctor may prescribe:
  - Pain relievers. Don't take prescription pain medication longer than 4 to 7 days. Use only as much as you need.
  - Antibiotics to fight or prevent infection.
- You may use nonprescription drugs, such as acetaminophen, to relieve pain. Avoid aspirin.

ACTIVITY
- Resume work and everyday activity as soon as possible (usually 5 days for adults, 1 week for children).
- Resume mild exercise 2 to 3 weeks after surgery.
- Avoid vigorous exercise, swimming or contact sports for 6 weeks after surgery.

DIET—No special diet. Eat soft foods if chewing causes discomfort.

CALL YOUR DOCTOR IF

- You experience nausea or vomiting.
- Pain, swelling, redness, drainage, or bleeding increases in the surgical area.
- You develop symptoms of infection including headache, muscle aches, dizziness, fever, or a general ill feeling.
- New, unexplained symptoms develop.

OTOPLASTY
(Ear Plastic Surgery)

Anatomy and incision site on the back of the ear are identified and marked prior to surgery.

Back of ear

Incision site

Skin is opened revealing underlying cartilage, which is remolded to bring ear closer to the head.

Cartilage folded and sewn

Skin is sewn closed and a dressing is applied.

Dressing sewn into position

OVARIAN CYST OR TUMOR REMOVAL

GENERAL INFORMATION

DEFINITION—Removal of cysts or tumors in the ovary.

BODY PARTS INVOLVED—Ovary, pelvis.

REASONS FOR SURGERY
- Tumor or suspected cancer in the ovaries.
- Rupture or twisting of an ovarian cyst.

SURGICAL RISK INCREASES WITH
- Adults over 60, stress, obesity.
- Poor nutrition, alcoholism, smoking.
- Recent or chronic illness, especially diabetes.
- Use of some prescription and nonprescription drugs. Inform your doctor of any drugs, medications, or vitamin and herb supplements you are using or have used in the last month.

WHAT TO EXPECT

WHO OPERATES—Obstetrician-gynecologist or general surgeon.

WHERE PERFORMED—Hospital.

DIAGNOSTIC TESTS
- Before surgery: Blood and urine studies, CT scan of pelvic organs, laparoscopy or culdoscopy, ultrasound, x-rays of chest, lower abdomen and lower intestinal tract, culdocentesis (see Glossary for all).
- During surgery: Laboratory examination of removed tissue by frozen section (see Glossary).
- After surgery: Blood studies.

ANESTHESIA—General anesthesia by injection and inhalation with an airway tube placed in the windpipe.

DESCRIPTION OF OPERATION
- An incision is made in the abdomen. The abdominal muscles are separated and the peritoneum is opened.
- Blood vessels supplying the ovaries are located, clamped and tied.
- The tumor or cyst in the ovary is located, cut free and removed or the cyst may be destroyed by electrocauterization (see Glossary).
- If examination reveals signs of cancer, the ovary is removed.
- The peritoneum is closed, and the abdominal muscles are sewn together with heavy sutures.
- The skin is closed with sutures or clips, which usually can be removed 10 days after surgery.
- This surgery, under many conditions, can be performed laparoscopically (see Glossary). Your doctor can determine which approach is best for your circumstances.

POSSIBLE COMPLICATIONS
- Excessive bleeding.
- Surgical-wound infection.
- Recurrent tumor.
- Excessive scarring (keloid).

AVERAGE HOSPITAL STAY—3 to 5 days. However, if surgery is performed laparoscopically, patients are often not admitted at all or go home the next day.

PROBABLE OUTCOME—Expect complete healing of surgical wound. If cancer is detected, your doctor will prescribe treatment with radiation or anticancer drugs. Allow about 4 weeks for recovery from surgery.

POSTOPERATIVE CARE

GENERAL MEASURES
- A hard ridge should form along the incision. As it heals, the ridge will gradually recede.
- Shower as usual. Avoid baths until the incision is completely healed. You may wash the incision gently with mild, unscented soap. After showering, replace any wet dressings with clean, dry ones.
- Move and elevate legs often while resting in bed to decrease the likelihood of deep-vein blood clots.

MEDICATION
- Your doctor may prescribe:
  - Pain relievers. Don't take prescription pain medication longer than 4 to 7 days. Use only as much as you need.
  - Stool softeners to prevent constipation.
  - Hormone supplements.
  - Antibiotics to fight or prevent infection.
- You may use nonprescription drugs, such as acetaminophen, for minor pain. Avoid aspirin.

ACTIVITY
- To help recovery and aid your well-being, resume daily activities, including work, as soon as you are able.
- Avoid vigorous exercise for 6 weeks after surgery.
- Resume sexual relations when your doctor determines that healing is complete.

DIET—Clear liquid diet until the gastrointestinal tract functions again. Then eat a well-balanced diet to promote healing.

CALL YOUR DOCTOR IF

- Pain, swelling, redness, drainage, or bleeding increases in the surgical area.
- You develop symptoms of infection including headache, muscle aches, dizziness, fever, or a general ill feeling.
- You experience nausea, vomiting, constipation, abdominal swelling, or hot flashes.
- New, unexplained symptoms develop.

OVARIAN CYST OR TUMOR REMOVAL

The organs of the female reproductive tract and the usual abdominal incision for this surgical procedure.

Incision

Fallopian tube

Ovary

Uterus

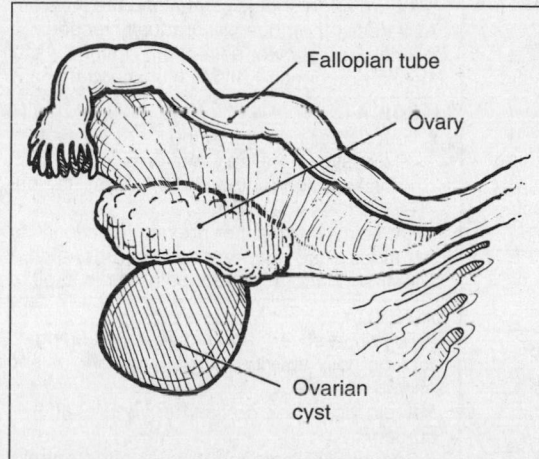

After the incision has been made through the skin and underlying tissue, the tumor or cyst in the ovary is located, cut free and removed.

Fallopian tube

Ovary

Ovarian cyst

- The bed of the ovarian cyst or tumor is sutured closed to prevent bleeding and adhesions.
- The peritoneum is closed. The abdominal muscles are sewn together with heavy sutures and the skin is closed with sutures or clips, which usually can be removed about 10 days after surgery (not illustrated).

PACEMAKER IMPLANTATION

GENERAL INFORMATION

DEFINITION—Placement of a temporary or permanent pacemaker into the chest wall. A pacemaker is an electronic device consisting of an electrode connected to the heart muscle and a regulatory device and power source implanted under the skin. It provides regular, mild electric shocks that stimulate the heart muscle and maintain normal heartbeat.

BODY PARTS INVOLVED—Veins in neck or under collarbone, tissue under the skin below the collarbone, heart.

REASONS FOR SURGERY
● Regulation of heartbeat that has slowed due to heart disease.
● Treatment of heart block.
● Following cardiac surgery to regulate heart rate.

SURGICAL RISK INCREASES WITH
● Adults over 60.
● Obesity.
● Smoking.
● Excess alcohol consumption.
● Recent or chronic illness.
● Diabetes.
● Use of some prescription and nonprescription drugs. Inform your doctor of any drugs, medications, or vitamin and herb supplements you are using or have used in the last month.

WHAT TO EXPECT

WHO OPERATES—Cardiovascular surgeon, cardiologist (sometimes).

WHERE PERFORMED—Outpatient surgical facility or hospital.

DIAGNOSTIC TESTS
● Before surgery: Blood and urine studies, x-ray of chest, ECG (see Glossary).
● During surgery: ECG, fluoroscopy (see Glossary for both).
● After surgery: ECG (see Glossary), x-rays of chest.

ANESTHESIA
● Local anesthesia by injection.
● General anesthesia by injection and inhalation with an airway tube placed in the windpipe.

DESCRIPTION OF OPERATION
● A needle is inserted in a vein under the collarbone. An electrode is passed through the vein into the heart. The implantation site is confirmed.
● The electrode is attached to the power and regulating units. A small incision is made below the collarbone, and the entire device is inserted into the incision and placed under the skin in a pouch created from tissue.

● The skin is closed with suture material, which usually can be removed about 1 week after surgery.

POSSIBLE COMPLICATIONS
● Excessive bleeding.
● Surgical-wound infection.
● Perforation of the heart muscle (rare).
● Pacemaker malfunction.
● Migration of pacing wire.
● Some pacemakers may be affected by radiation from microwave ovens. Ask your doctor.

AVERAGE HOSPITAL STAY—0 to 2 days.

PROBABLE OUTCOME—Expect complete healing without complications. Allow about 2 weeks for recovery from surgery.

POSTOPERATIVE CARE

GENERAL MEASURES
● A hard ridge should form along the incision. As it heals, the ridge will gradually recede.
● Bathe and shower as usual. You may wash the incision gently with mild, unscented soap.

MEDICATION
● Your doctor may prescribe:
  - Pain relievers. Don't take prescription pain medication longer than 4 to 7 days. Use only as much as you need.
  - Antibiotics to fight or prevent infection.
● You may use nonprescription drugs, such as acetaminophen, for minor pain. Avoid aspirin.

ACTIVITY
● To help recovery and aid your well-being, resume daily activities, including work, as soon as you are able.
● Avoid vigorous exercise for 2 weeks after surgery.
● Resume driving about 1 week after returning home.
● Resume sexual relations when able.

DIET—No special diet.

CALL YOUR DOCTOR IF

● Pain, swelling, redness, drainage, or bleeding increases in the surgical area.
● You develop symptoms of infection including headache, muscle aches, dizziness, fever, or a general ill feeling.
● You develop heartbeat irregularities, or your original symptoms return.
● New, unexplained symptoms develop.

PACEMAKER IMPLANTATION

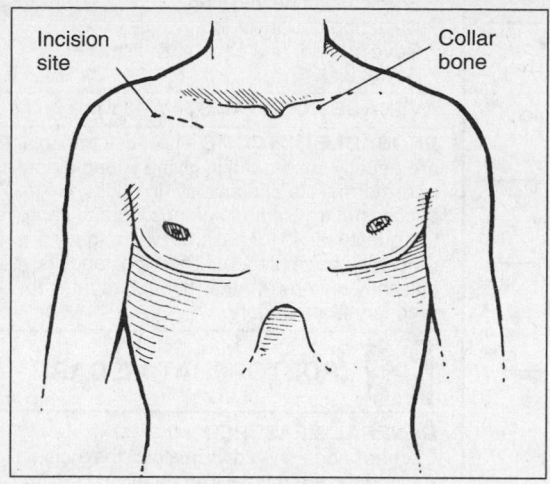

Incision site

Collar bone

An illustration of the chest, collarbone and incision site generally used for pacemaker insertion.

Pacemaker

Electrode

Heart

• An electrode is passed through a vein near the incision site, which ends inside the heart cavity.
• The electrode is attached to the power and regulating units. The entire device is inserted under the skin into a pouch created from tissue under the collarbone.

Pacemaker

The pacemaker in place. The skin has been closed with sutures that usually can be removed about 1 week after surgery.

PANCREAS TRANSPLANTATION

GENERAL INFORMATION

DEFINITION—Replacement of a diseased pancreas with a healthy pancreas obtained from a donor with compatible immunological characteristics. The duodenum is also replaced to allow drainage of pancreatic secretions into the gastrointestinal tract.

BODY PARTS INVOLVED—Diseased or abnormal pancreas and duodenum, healthy donor pancreas and duodenum.

REASONS FOR SURGERY—Prevention of complications of severe diabetes (such as kidney failure and damage to the retinas) or severe chronic pancreatitis.

SURGICAL RISK INCREASES WITH
- Obesity, smoking, stress.
- Poor nutrition.
- Excess alcohol consumption.
- Recent or chronic illness, diabetes.
- Use of some prescription and nonprescription drugs. Inform your doctor of any drugs, medications, or vitamin and herb supplements you are using or have used in the last month.

WHAT TO EXPECT

WHO OPERATES—General surgeon.

WHERE PERFORMED—Hospital.

DIAGNOSTIC TESTS
- Before surgery: Evaluation of all body systems, immune-system and pancreas matching procedures.
- After surgery: Blood studies.

ANESTHESIA—General anesthesia by injection and inhalation with an airway tube placed in the windpipe.

DESCRIPTION OF OPERATION
- The pancreas is removed from the donor, chilled and preserved up to 12 hours until surgery.
- An incision is made under the ribs.
- The abdominal muscles are divided and the peritoneal cavity is entered.
- The pancreas and duodenum are cut free and removed.
- The donor pancreas and duodenum are positioned and connected to blood vessels.
- Sometimes, only the cells of the pancreas that produce insulin (islet cells) are transplanted. In some patients, this is all that is necessary to reestablish normal function.
- The peritoneum and muscles are closed. The skin is closed with sutures or clips, which usually can be removed in 1 week.

POSSIBLE COMPLICATIONS
- Excessive bleeding.
- Surgical-wound infection.
- Rejection of transplant.
- Development of a pancreatic fistula.
- Bowel leak.

AVERAGE HOSPITAL STAY—3 weeks.

PROBABLE OUTCOME—Islet-cell transplants are usually successful in giving young diabetics near-normal life expectancy. In adults, a successful transplant prolongs life and improves the quality of life for patients who might otherwise have died, but life expectancy is currently unknown. Allow about 6 months for recovery from surgery.

POSTOPERATIVE CARE

GENERAL MEASURES
- A hard ridge should form along the incision. As it heals, the ridge will gradually recede.
- Shower as usual. Avoid baths until the incision has completely healed. You may wash the incision gently with mild, unscented soap. After showering, replace any wet dressings with clean, dry ones.
- Move and elevate legs often while resting in bed to decrease the chance of deep-vein blood clots.

MEDICATION
- Your doctor may prescribe:
  - Pain relievers. Don't take prescription pain medication longer than 4 to 7 days. Use only as much as you need.
  - Stool softeners to prevent constipation.
  - Antibiotics to fight or prevent infection.
  - Immunosuppressant drugs to decrease the likelihood of rejection.
- You may use nonprescription drugs, such as acetaminophen, for minor pain. Avoid aspirin.

ACTIVITY
- To help recovery and aid your well-being, resume daily activities as soon as you are able.
- Avoid vigorous exercise for 6 months.

DIET—You doctor will prescribe a diet.

CALL YOUR DOCTOR IF

- Pain, swelling, redness, drainage, or bleeding increases in the surgical area.
- You develop symptoms of infection including headache, muscle aches, dizziness, fever, or a general ill feeling.
- You experience nausea, vomiting, abdominal swelling, or constipation.
- You experience increased frequency of urination or increased thirst.
- New, unexplained symptoms develop.

PANCREAS TRANSPLANTATION

An illustration of the normal location and anatomy of the pancreas.

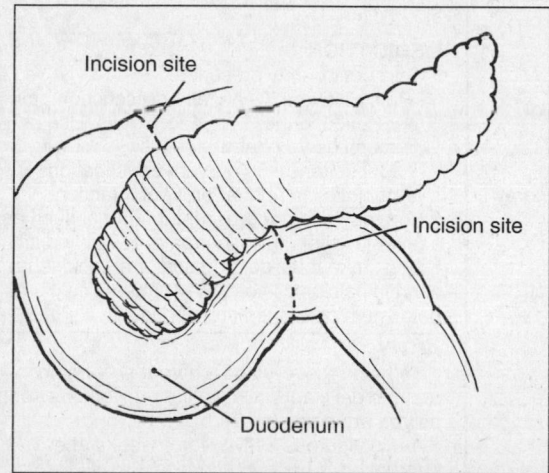

The diseased pancreas and the duodenum are cut free and removed.

- The donor pancreas and duodenum are positioned and connected to the blood vessels.
- Following transplant, muscles and skin are closed with sutures or clips that usually can be removed about 1 week after surgery (not illustrated).

PARATHYROIDECTOMY

GENERAL INFORMATION

DEFINITION—Removal of parathyroid tumors or the parathyroid glands.

BODY PARTS INVOLVED—The two pair (four in total) parathyroid glands (a part of the body's endocrine gland system).

REASONS FOR SURGERY
- Hyperparathyroidism (see Illness section).
- Parathyroid adenoma (a benign tumor).
- Parathyroid cancer (very rare).

SURGICAL RISK INCREASES WITH
- Obesity or smoking.
- Poor nutrition, alcoholism.
- Recent or chronic illness.
- Diabetes.
- Use of some prescription and nonprescription drugs. Inform your doctor of any drugs, medications, or vitamin and herb supplements you are using or have used in the last month.

WHAT TO EXPECT

WHO OPERATES—General surgeon.

WHERE PERFORMED—Hospital.

DIAGNOSTIC TESTS
- Before surgery: Blood and urine studies, x-ray of upper gastrointestinal tract, CT scan, ultrasound, fine needle biopsy, thyroid scan, (see Glossary for all).
- During surgery: Laboratory examination of removed tissue by frozen section (see Glossary).
- After surgery: Blood studies, laboratory examination of removed tissue.

ANESTHESIA—General anesthesia by injection and inhalation with an airway tube placed in the windpipe.

DESCRIPTION OF OPERATION
- An incision is made in the neck just under the Adam's apple. Layers of skin and muscle are lifted up. The parathyroid glands are located.
- If one gland is enlarged (adenoma), it is removed and the rest are left in place.
- If all the glands are equally enlarged, 3 or 3 1/2 of the glands are removed. This leaves enough parathyroid tissue to prevent hypoparathyroidism (low parathyroid hormone production).
- The muscle and skin layers are replaced and the surgical incision is closed.

POSSIBLE COMPLICATIONS
- Excessive bleeding, surgical-wound infection.
- Hypoparathyroidism.
- Inadvertent injury to thyroid gland or vocal-cord nerves.
- Recurrent hyperparathyroidism.
- Repeat surgery if not enough tissue removed.

AVERAGE HOSPITAL STAY—1 to 2 days.

PROBABLE OUTCOME—Expect complete healing without complications. You will probably experience a sore throat and raspy voice following surgery. These are usually temporary symptoms and should diminish as you recover. Allow about 4 weeks for recovery from surgery. Calcium levels may be low temporarily.

POSTOPERATIVE CARE

GENERAL MEASURES
- A hard ridge should form along the incision. As it heals, the ridge will gradually recede.
- Shower as usual. You may wash the incision gently with mild, unscented soap. After showering, replace any wet dressings with clean, dry ones.
- Elevate the head of your bed for the first 2 to 3 nights.
- Move and elevate legs often while resting in bed to decrease the likelihood of deep-vein blood clots.

MEDICATION
- Your doctor may prescribe:
  - Pain relievers. Don't take prescription pain medication longer than 4 to 7 days. Use only as much as you need.
  - Stool softeners to prevent constipation.
  - Antibiotics to fight or prevent infection.
- You may use nonprescription drugs, such as acetaminophen, for minor pain. Avoid aspirin.
- Don't take thiazide diuretics or antacids that contain calcium. These may cause a calcium, potassium or sodium imbalance.

ACTIVITY
- To help recovery and aid your well-being, resume daily activities, including work, as soon as you are able.
- Avoid vigorous activity for 6 weeks after surgery.
- Resume driving 2 weeks after returning home.

DIET—Your doctor will prescribe a diet.

CALL YOUR DOCTOR IF

- Pain, swelling, redness, drainage, or bleeding increases in the surgical area.
- You develop signs of infection including headache, muscle aches, dizziness, fever, or a general ill feeling.
- You experience nausea, vomiting, constipation, or abdominal swelling.
- You have numbness or tingling around the mouth or hands.
- New, unexplained symptoms develop.

PARATHYROIDECTOMY

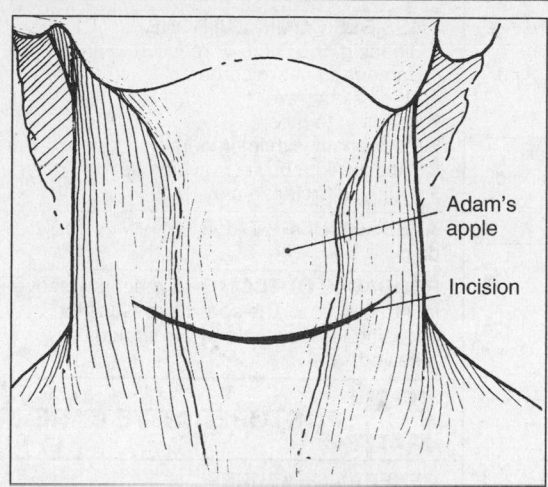

The incision site in the lower part of the neck below the protruding cartilage called the Adam's apple.

Adam's apple

Incision

Parathyroid glands are located. Abnormal ones are removed. If the surgery is being performed because of overactivity of the parathyroid glands, rather than a tumor, all except one of the visualized parathyroid glands are cut free and removed.

Para-
thyroid
gland

Thyroid
gland

- One parathyroid gland removed.
- After the surgery is finished, neck muscles are rejoined, the tissue below the skin is closed with suture material, and the skin is closed.

PELVIC PROLAPSE REPAIR—LAPAROSCOPIC

 GENERAL INFORMATION

DEFINITION—Laparoscopic surgery to restore prolapsed pelvic organs to their natural position and reinforce the pelvic floor muscles in the weakened area to avoid further damage.

BODY PARTS INVOLVED—Pelvic prolapse is a general terms that describes the weakening of the tissues and ligaments that give support to the uterus, vagina, bladder, and rectum.

REASONS FOR SURGERY
- Severity of prolapse.
- Prolapse causes pain.
- Bladder and bowel problems.
- Symptoms affect daily activities, sexual function, or exercise.

SURGICAL RISK INCREASES WITH
- Age.
- Previous pelvic surgery.
- Chronic lung or heart disease.
- Diabetes.
- Obesity.

 WHAT TO EXPECT

WHO OPERATES—Gynecologist, urologist, or urogynecologist.

WHERE PERFORMED—Hospital.

DIAGNOSTIC TESTS
- Before surgery: Blood and urine tests, possibly a proctoscopy or cystogram (see Glossary for both).
- After surgery: None usually.

ANESTHESIA—General anesthesia.

DESCRIPTION OF OPERATION
- Pelvic prolapse laparoscopic surgeries vary. One option is described here.
- An incision is made inside the naval (belly button). A laparoscope (see Glossary) is inserted into the incision. It uses a small camera to view the pelvic structures and magnifies them on video monitors.
- The abdomen is inflated with carbon dioxide gas for better viewing of the organs.
- Three to four small, quarter-inch incisions are made for insertion of additional surgical instruments. (Traditional surgery requires one large incision several inches in length.)
- The vagina and pelvic organs are viewed and suspended internally with permanent sutures. A supportive mesh or fascial graft may be used.
- If needed, a bladder suspension, vaginal hysterectomy, or rectum repair can be done at the same time.
- The instruments are removed, the gas is released, and the incisions are closed with Steri-Strips or stitches.
- A bladder catheter may be placed temporarily to drain the bladder.

POSSIBLE COMPLICATIONS
- Bleeding, Infection, or reaction to anesthesia.
- Damage to nearby organs.
- Blood clots (rare).
- Reaction to mesh.
- Future pain with intercourse.
- Difficulty with bowel movements.
- Rarely, a prolapse may recur.

AVERAGE HOSPITAL STAY—May be 1 to 5 days.

PROBABLE OUTCOME—Expect full recovery in 4 to 6 weeks. The specific reasons for choosing to have the surgery should be resolved.

 POSTOPERATIVE CARE

GENERAL MEASURES
- Shower as usual after 24 hours. The incisions can get wet—pat them dry. Wait a week to take tub baths (or as advised).
- Be sure to keep follow up appointments with your surgeon.

MEDICATION
- Your doctor may prescribe pain relievers. Use only as much as you need to be comfortable.
- You may use nonprescription pain reliever such as acetaminophen for minor pain. Ask your doctor about taking ibuprofen or aspirin.
- To avoid constipation, stool softeners may be recommended.

ACTIVITY
- Start short walks as soon as you are home. Take frequent naps when tired. Avoid prolonged time sitting or lying in bed.
- Return to work after 1 to 3 weeks. The time may depend on the extent of the procedure and person's fitness.
- Resume driving when you feel able or as advised.
- Avoid heavy lifting for 4 to 5 weeks.
- Sexual relations may be resumed in 6 weeks.

DIET—No special diet.

 CALL YOUR DOCTOR IF

- Pain, swelling, redness, drainage, or bleeding increases in the surgical area.
- You develop signs of infection, including headache, muscle aches, dizziness, fever, or a general ill feeling.
- You have difficulty urinating or having a bowel movement.
- New unexplained symptoms develop.

PELVIC PROLAPSE REPAIR—LAPAROSCOPIC

An illustration of the normal position of the pelvic organs. This is a cross section view.

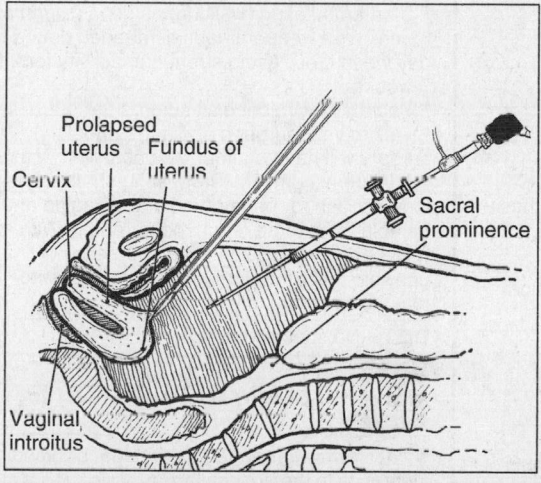

The fundus (dome) of the uterus is grasped and the uterus is pulled back from where it has prolapsed down to the introitus (opening) of the vagina.

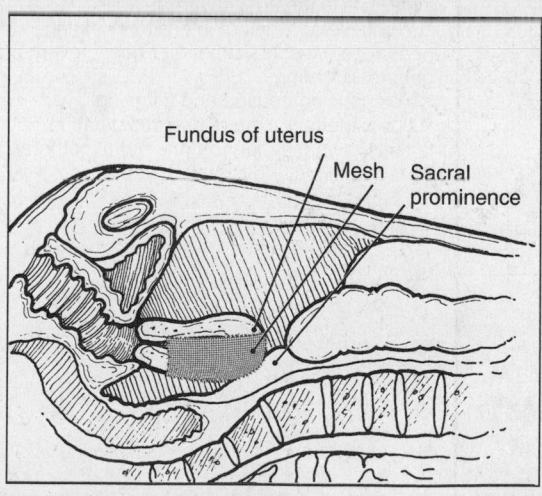

The fundus of the uterus is attached to the sacral prominence to keep it suspended in the pelvis. In this illustration a piece of cloth like material (mesh) has been used to attach the uterus more securely.

PENECTOMY
(Penis Removal)

GENERAL INFORMATION

DEFINITION—Removal of part or all of the shaft and all of the head of the penis with creation of a new outlet for urine.

BODY PARTS INVOLVED—Penis, sometimes perineum.

REASONS FOR SURGERY—Usually done for malignant tumors of the penis. Occasionally done for trauma.

SURGICAL RISK INCREASES WITH
* Age.
* Diabetes.
* Poor kidney function.
* High blood pressure.
* Poor nutrition.
* Chronic lung disease.
* Obesity.

WHAT TO EXPECT

WHO OPERATES—Urologist.

WHERE PERFORMED—Hospital.

DIAGNOSTIC TESTS
* Before surgery: Blood tests, chest x-ray, CT scan, cystoscopy, EKG (see Glossary for these 3 terms).
* After surgery: Blood tests.

ANESTHESIA—General anesthesia or spinal anesthesia.

DESCRIPTION OF OPERATION
* The shaft of the penis is encircled with a tourniquet to minimize bleeding. An incision is made through the skin and the urethra (tube that carries urine from the bladder to the outside) and corpora (blood filled cavities that facilitate erectile function) are identified. These are transected (cut) and vessels are ligated (sewn off).
* If enough shaft is remaining, the urethra is sutured to the skin edges. If insufficient shaft is left, the urethra is brought out through an opening in the perineum. Sphincter function (continence) is usually preserved but erectile function is usually lost.
* A foley catheter (see Glossary) is usually left in the bladder.

POSSIBLE COMPLICATIONS
* Bleeding from the surgery site.
* Urethral stricture (narrowing).
* Infection.

AVERAGE HOSPITAL STAY—Usually 3-5 days.

PROBABLE OUTCOME
* Removal of catheter in 7-14 days.
* Expect full recovery in 6-8 weeks.

POSTOPERATIVE CARE

GENERAL MEASURES
* Hard ridges will form along the incisions. As they heal, the ridges will gradually recede.
* Shower as usual. You may wash the incisions gently with mild soap. After showering, replace any dressings with a new dry dressing.

MEDICATION
* Your doctor may prescribe pain relievers. Use only as much as you need to be comfortable.
* You may use nonprescription pain relievers such as acetaminophen for minor pain. Ask your doctor if it is okay to take ibuprofen or aspirin.

ACTIVITY
* Start ambulating (walking) as soon as you are home. Take frequent naps as needed during the day when tired. Avoid strenuous activity for 2 to 3 weeks.
* You may swim once all sutures are out.
* Talk to your surgeon about the effect the surgery will have on your sexual ability. With a partial penectomy, the remaining shaft may be long enough for penetration of the vagina and be able to become erect upon arousal. With a total penectomy, sexual intercourse is not possible, but other forms of sexual pleasure may be available to you.

DIET—No special diet.

CALL YOUR DOCTOR IF

* Pain, swelling, redness, drainage, or bleeding increases in the surgical area.
* You develop signs of infection including headache, muscle aches, dizziness, fever, or a general ill feeling.
* You develop nausea and vomiting.
* You experience prolonged constipation, difficulty urinating, or no urine out of catheter.
* New unexplained symptoms develop.

PENECTOMY
(Penis Removal)

An illustration of the anatomy with a tumor on the glans.

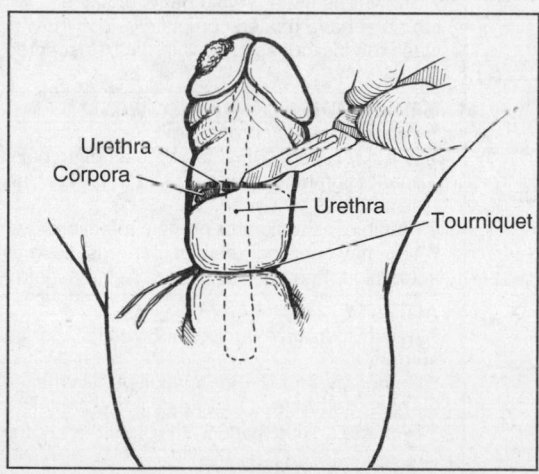

A tourniquet is applied to control bleeding and the incision is made through the shaft of the penis and urethra.

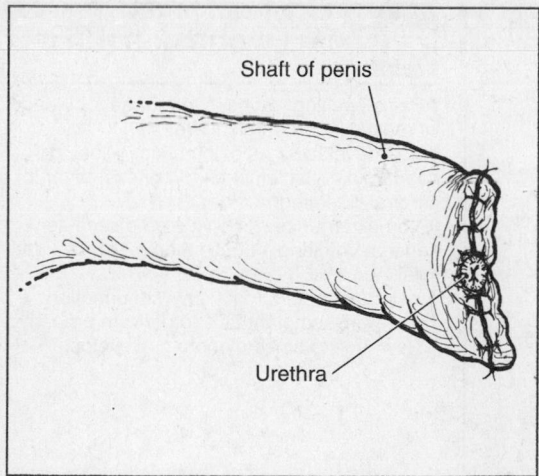

The end of the shaft is closed and the urethra is sutured to the skin edges.

PENILE IMPLANT

GENERAL INFORMATION

DEFINITION—Insertion of semiflexible plastic bars or an inflatable prosthesis in the penis. The former produces a permanent, partial erection. The latter can be inflated at will.

BODY PARTS INVOLVED—Penis.

REASONS FOR SURGERY—Impotence.

SURGICAL RISK INCREASES WITH
- Obesity.
- Smoking.
- Stress.
- Poor nutrition.
- Recent or chronic illness.
- Alcoholism.
- Diabetes.
- Use of some prescription and nonprescription drugs. Inform your doctor of any drugs, medications, or vitamin and herb supplements you are using or have used in the last month.

WHAT TO EXPECT

WHO OPERATES—Urologist.

WHERE PERFORMED—Hospital.

DIAGNOSTIC TESTS
- Before surgery: Blood and urine studies, chest x-ray, ultrasound (see Glossary).
- After surgery: Blood studies.

ANESTHESIA
- Spinal anesthesia by injection.
- General anesthesia by injection and inhalation with an airway tube placed in the windpipe.

DESCRIPTION OF OPERATION
- Plastic implant:
  - An incision is made in the underside of the penis.
  - The tissues on both sides of the urethra are expanded to allow placement of the implants.
  - An implant is placed on each side of the urethra.
  - The skin is closed with sutures that will be absorbed by the body.
- Inflatable prosthesis:
  - Incisions are made in the underside of the penis, the side of the scrotum, and on the abdomen, several inches above the base of the penis.
  - The penile tissue is stretched to allow placement of the prosthesis. The fluid reservoir for the prosthesis is implanted under the skin above the bladder at the base of the pelvis. The prosthesis can be inflated by applying pressure on the reservoir.
  - The skin is closed with sutures that will be absorbed by the body.

POSSIBLE COMPLICATIONS
- Surgical-wound infection.
- Excessive bleeding.
- Urinary retention.
- Rejection of synthetic implants.
- Erosion of skin or urethra.
- Mechanical failure.

AVERAGE HOSPITAL STAY—1 to 2 days.

PROBABLE OUTCOME—Expect complete recovery without complications. Allow about 4 weeks for recovery from surgery. Following recovery, penile sensations and sexual arousal should be near normal.

POSTOPERATIVE CARE

GENERAL MEASURES
- A hard ridge should form along the incision. As it heals, the ridge will gradually recede. After healing, the prosthesis should cause no discomfort.
- Shower as usual. Avoid baths until the incisions have healed completely. You may wash the incisions gently with mild, unscented soap.

MEDICATION
- Your doctor may prescribe:
  - Pain relievers. Don't take prescription pain medication longer than 4 to 7 days. Use only as much as you need.
  - Antibiotics to fight or prevent infection.
- You may use nonprescription drugs, such as acetaminophen, for minor pain. Avoid aspirin.

ACTIVITY
- Avoid vigorous exercise for 6 weeks after surgery.
- Do not attempt sexual relations until your surgeon determines that healing is complete.
- Resume driving 1 week after returning home.

DIET—No special diet.

CALL YOUR DOCTOR IF
- Pain, swelling, redness, drainage, or bleeding increases in the surgical area.
- You develop signs of infection including headache, muscle aches, dizziness, fever, or a general ill feeling.
- You experience new symptoms such as nausea, vomiting, constipation, or abdominal swelling.
- You have pain or difficulty with urination.
- The penile implant fails to perform properly.
- New, unexplained symptoms develop.

PENILE IMPLANT

The incision for a penile implant, which may be either semi-rigid or an inflatable prosthesis. These drawings illustrate the inflatable form only. The equipment is different for a semi-rigid prosthesis but the principles and techniques for insertion are similar for both procedures.

Cylinder tubing

After an incision has been made on the underside of the penis, the tissues on both sides of the urethra are expanded to allow placement of the implants.

Inflatable penile implant

Reservoir

Pump

Implants in place, surgical incision closed with absorbable sutures.

PEPTIC ULCER SURGERY

GENERAL INFORMATION

DEFINITION—Surgery to decrease the acid production in the stomach in order to prevent ulcer formation.

BODY PARTS INVOLVED—Esophagus, stomach, duodenum, jejunum, vagus nerves.

REASONS FOR SURGERY—Treatment of complications of peptic ulcers:
- Bleeding.
- Intolerable pain.
- Blockage of stomach contents from emptying.
- Perforation. If an ulcer perforates, the contents of the gastrointestinal tract are dumped into the abdominal cavity, causing peritonitis. This is a medical emergency requiring immediate surgery.

SURGICAL RISK INCREASES WITH
- Adults over 60.
- Chronic illness, especially pancreatitis, hepatitis, alcoholism or diabetes.
- Poor nutrition, especially vitamin and mineral deficiencies.
- Use of any drugs that irritate the stomach.
- Use of some prescription and nonprescription drugs. Inform your doctor of any drugs, medications, or vitamin and herb supplements you are using or have used in the last month.

WHAT TO EXPECT

WHO OPERATES—General surgeon.

WHERE PERFORMED—Hospital.

DIAGNOSTIC TESTS
- Before surgery: Blood and urine studies, x-ray of abdomen, endoscopy (see Glossary).
- After surgery: Blood and urine studies, x-rays of abdomen.

ANESTHESIA—General anesthesia by injection and inhalation with an airway tube placed in the windpipe.

DESCRIPTION OF OPERATION
- Any of the following procedures may be used.
- Vagotomy and pyloroplasty: The nerves that stimulate stomach-acid production are severed, and the outlet of the stomach that leads to the duodenum is enlarged.
- Gastric resection (antrectomy): The lower part of the stomach that produces acid is removed, and the remaining stomach is attached with sutures to the duodenum or the jejunum. This is usually combined with a vagotomy (cutting of the vagus nerve).
- Closure of perforated ulcer: The perforated ulcer is closed by various methods.
- Incisions that are made are closed with sutures or clips, which can usually be removed about 1 week after surgery.

POSSIBLE COMPLICATIONS
- Excessive bleeding, surgical-wound infection.
- Incisional hernia.
- Recurrence of peptic ulcer.
- Chronic diarrhea, dumping syndrome.
- Slow or poor emptying of the stomach.
- Malnutrition (lack of needed nutrients).
- Flushing, fainting or diarrhea after eating certain foods.

AVERAGE HOSPITAL STAY—3 to 7 days.

PROBABLE OUTCOME—Expect complete healing without complications. Allow about 4 to 6 weeks for recovery from surgery.

POSTOPERATIVE CARE

GENERAL MEASURES
- A hard ridge should form along the incision. As it heals, the ridge will gradually recede.
- Shower as usual. Avoid baths until the incision has completely healed. You may wash the incision gently with mild, unscented soap. After showering, replace any wet dressings with clean, dry ones.

MEDICATION
- Your doctor may prescribe:
  - Pain relievers. Don't take prescription pain medication longer than 4 to 7 days. Use only as much as you need.
  - Antibiotics to fight or prevent infection.
- You may use nonprescription drugs, such as acetaminophen, for minor pain. Do not take aspirin.

ACTIVITY
- To help recovery and aid your well-being, resume daily activities, including work, as soon as you are able.
- Resume driving about 2 weeks after returning home.

DIET—Clear liquid diet until the gastrointestinal tract functions again. Then eat a well-balanced diet to promote healing. Avoid coffee, tea, cocoa, cola drinks, alcoholic beverages and any food or spice that aggravates symptoms.

CALL YOUR DOCTOR IF

- Pain, swelling, redness, drainage, or bleeding increases in the surgical area.
- You develop signs of infection including headache, muscle aches, dizziness, fever, or a general ill feeling.
- You experience abdominal pain or swelling, constipation, nausea, vomiting, bleeding from the rectum, or black, tarry stools.
- New, unexplained symptoms develop.

PEPTIC ULCER SURGERY

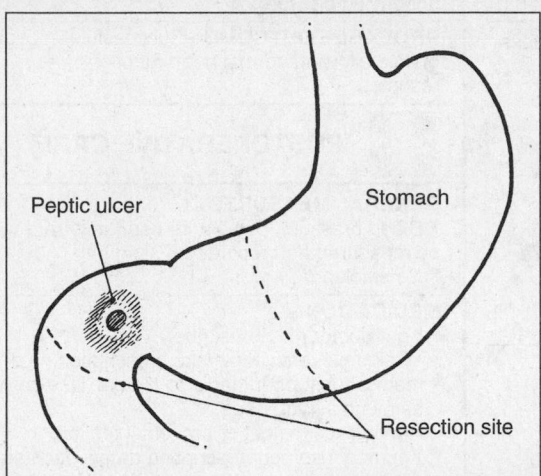

An illustration of the stomach with a peptic ulcer, the incision sites in the lower part of the stomach and the beginning portion of the duodenum.

The part of the stomach that produces acid is removed along with the part of the stomach or duodenum that has a peptic ulcer or scarring from a healed or partially healed peptic ulcer.

The remaining stomach is attached with sutures to the duodenum or sometimes to the jejunum located lower down in the small intestine.

PERICARDIOCENTESIS

GENERAL INFORMATION

DEFINITION—The needle aspiration of excess fluid from the pericardial sac.

BODY PARTS INVOLVED—Pericardium, a 2-layered membrane that surrounds the heart and the roots of the great blood vessels (aorta, pulmonary artery, pulmonary vein and vena cava).

REASONS FOR SURGERY—To remove abnormal fluid collections between the heart and the pericardium. The fluid may be there because the heart is inflamed, infected or injured (fluid may be blood).

SURGICAL RISK INCREASES WITH
- Obesity.
- Smoking.
- Excess alcohol consumption.
- Recent or chronic illness, especially chronic lung disease.
- Use of some prescription and nonprescription drugs. Inform your doctor of any drugs, medications, or vitamin and herb supplements you are using or have used in the last month.

WHAT TO EXPECT

WHO OPERATES—Cardiothoracic surgeon, cardiologist (sometimes).

WHERE PERFORMED—Hospital or outpatient surgical facility.

DIAGNOSTIC TESTS
- Before surgery: Chest x-rays, CT scan, ECG (see Glossary for both).
- During surgery: Chest x-rays.
- After surgery: Chest x-rays, fluid examination, ECG (see Glossary).

ANESTHESIA—Local anesthesia.

DESCRIPTION OF OPERATION
- Patient lies down on back with upper torso elevated about 60 degrees with arms supported by pillows.
- An I.V. is started and local anesthetic injected.
- The pericardiocentesis needle is inserted into chest wall between the left rib margin adjacent to the breastbone, usually into the space between the 5th and 6th ribs.
- The needle is advanced until fluid can be aspirated.

POSSIBLE COMPLICATIONS
- Heartbeat irregularities.
- Inadvertent organ or artery puncture (rare).
- Hemothorax (see Glossary).
- Pneumothorax (see Glossary).
- Fluid around heart recurs.

AVERAGE HOSPITAL STAY—0 to 1 day for procedure. Total time varies according to underlying disorder.

PROBABLE OUTCOME—Successful removal of fluid allowing normal heart function to resume.

POSTOPERATIVE CARE

GENERAL MEASURES
- Blood pressure, pulse and respiratory rate will be measured and recorded.
- No smoking.

MEDICATION
- Your doctor may prescribe:
  - Pain relievers. Don't take prescription pain medication longer than 4 to 7 days. Use only as much as you need.
  - Antibiotics to fight or prevent infection.
- You may use nonprescription drugs, such as acetaminophen, for minor pain. Avoid aspirin.

ACTIVITY—Avoid vigorous exercise until your doctor determines healing is complete.

DIET
- Your doctor may prescribe a special diet.
- Vitamin and mineral supplements may be prescribed.

CALL YOUR DOCTOR IF

- You experience shortness of breath or chest pain, or you feel faint.
- You become anxious.
- You develop signs of infection including headache, muscle aches, dizziness, fever, or a general ill feeling.
- New, unexplained symptoms develop.

PERICARDIOCENTESIS

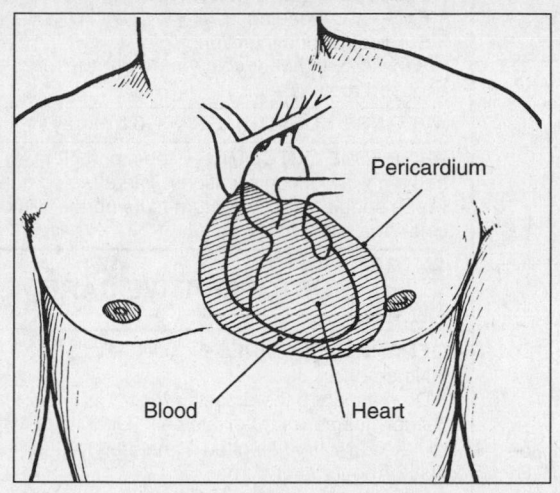

An illustration of the heart and surrounding structures.

Pericardium

Blood

Heart

The muscles of the chest are pulled aside to illustrate possible sites for the pericardiocentesis needle to be placed into the pericardium.

Pericardio-centesis sites

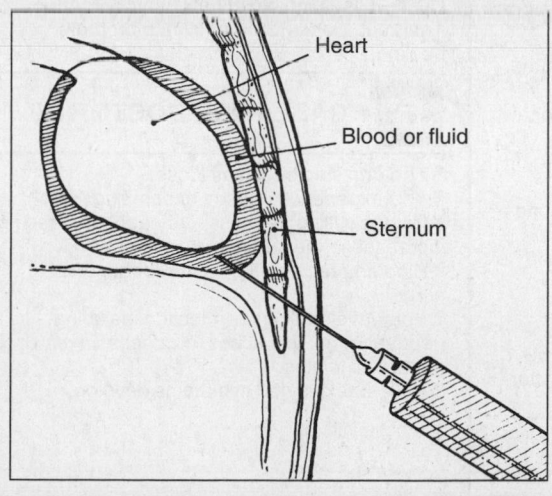

A needle attached to a syringe is advanced until the fluid can be aspirated. After fluid has been removed, the heart can function much more normally.

Heart

Blood or fluid

Sternum

PERIODONTAL SURGERY
(Pyorrhea Treatment)

 GENERAL INFORMATION

DEFINITION—Removal of infected tissue from the gums and reshaping of the bone underlying the gums.

BODY PARTS INVOLVED—Gums, surrounding bone.

REASONS FOR SURGERY—Prevention of the spread of gum infection.

SURGICAL RISK INCREASES WITH
- Adults over 60.
- Smoking.
- Excess alcohol consumption.
- Poor nutrition.
- Recent or chronic illness.
- Diabetes.
- Use of some prescription and nonprescription drugs. Inform your doctor of any drugs, medications, or vitamin and herb supplements you are using or have used in the last month.

 WHAT TO EXPECT

WHO OPERATES—Dentist or periodontist.

WHERE PERFORMED—Hospital, outpatient surgical facility, or dentist's office.

DIAGNOSTIC TESTS
- Before surgery: Blood and urine studies, x-rays of the mouth.
- After surgery: Blood studies.

ANESTHESIA
- Local anesthesia by injection.
- General anesthesia (sometimes) by injection and inhalation with an airway tube placed in the windpipe.

DESCRIPTION OF OPERATION
- The diseased periodontal tissue is carefully cut free and removed.
- The gums are lifted or flapped away from the tooth and surrounding bone.
- The diseased root surfaces are cleaned or removed.
- The bone under the gum is reshaped, if necessary.
- A special type of fabric may be sewn around a tooth to cover a crater in the bone, the gum is then sewn over the fabric. After the bone and attachment to the root regenerate, the fabric is removed using a minor surgical procedure.
- Special dressings are applied that control bleeding and hasten healing. Your dentist will remove or replace dressings 5 to 10 days after surgery.

POSSIBLE COMPLICATIONS
- Excessive bleeding.
- Surgical-wound infection.
- Sensitivity to hot or cold temperatures from exposed roots.

AVERAGE HOSPITAL STAY—0 to 1 day.

PROBABLE OUTCOME—Expect complete healing without complications. The affected gum tissue should heal and return to its normal pink color again in 2 to 3 weeks.

 POSTOPERATIVE CARE

GENERAL MEASURES
- No smoking.
- Do not disturb the dressing.
- Apply ice packs to relieve pain. Do this for 10 minutes at a time as often as needed for the first 24 hours after surgery.
- Keep your teeth free of plaque (germs, food debris and saliva). Brush your teeth and use dental floss as directed by your dentist. Mouth irrigations also help to prevent plaque.

MEDICATION
- Your dentist may prescribe:
  - Pain relievers. Don't take prescription pain medication longer than 4 to 7 days. Use only as much as you need.
  - Antibiotics to fight or prevent infection.
- You may use nonprescription drugs, such as acetaminophen, for minor pain. Avoid aspirin.

ACTIVITY
- To help recovery and aid your well-being, resume daily activities, including work, as soon as you are able.
- Avoid vigorous exercise for 3 weeks after surgery.
- Resume driving 2 days after returning home.

DIET—Clear liquid diet until healing occurs. Then eat a well-balanced diet to promote healing.

 CALL YOUR DOCTOR IF

- The dressing becomes loose.
- You experience nausea or vomiting.
- Pain, swelling, redness, drainage, or bleeding increases in the surgical area.
- Bleeding recurs 48 hours or longer after surgery.
- You develop signs of infection including headache, muscle aches, dizziness, fever, or a general ill feeling.
- New, unexplained symptoms develop.

PERIODONTAL SURGERY
(Pyorrhea Treatment)

An illustration of the mouth, gums and roots of teeth.

Gums

Roots

Periodontal tissue cut free and removed.

Special dressings are applied to control bleeding and hasten healing. These usually need to be removed or replaced 5 to 10 days after surgery.

PILONIDAL CYST REMOVAL

GENERAL INFORMATION

DEFINITION—Removal of a pilonidal cyst, a cyst that is located in area of the sacrum. (See Pilonidal Disease in Illness section.) The cyst often forms cavities, or openings to the outside, called sinuses. The cyst can also become infected, and an abscess can form.

BODY PARTS INVOLVED—Skin area over the buttocks.

REASONS FOR SURGERY—Relief of pain and prevention of the spread of infection.

SURGICAL RISK INCREASES WITH
- Obesity.
- Smoking.
- Recent or chronic illness.
- Diabetes.
- Use of some prescription and nonprescription drugs. Inform your doctor of any drugs, medications, or vitamin and herb supplements you are using or have used in the last month.

WHAT TO EXPECT

WHO OPERATES—General surgeon or proctologist.

WHERE PERFORMED—Hospital, outpatient surgical facility, doctor's office.

DIAGNOSTIC TESTS
- Before surgery: Blood and urine studies, chest x-ray, sigmoidoscopy (see Glossary).
- After surgery: Blood tests.

ANESTHESIA
- Local anesthesia by injection.
- General anesthesia by injection and inhalation with an airway tube placed in the windpipe.

DESCRIPTION OF OPERATION
- A variety of surgical treatments are available. One type is described here.
- The cyst and its cavities (also called sinuses) over the tailbone are identified with probes. An incision is made around the cyst.
- The cyst and all affected sinuses are removed.
- Bleeding is controlled with sutures or electrocauterization.
- The skin is usually left open to heal from the bottom out. This can take a period of 4 to 8 weeks.

POSSIBLE COMPLICATIONS
- Excessive bleeding.
- Surgical-wound infection.
- Slow healing.
- Recurrence of cyst.

AVERAGE HOSPITAL STAY—0 to 2 days.

PROBABLE OUTCOME—Expect complete healing without complications. Allow about 2 months for recovery from surgery.

POSTOPERATIVE CARE

GENERAL MEASURES
- Take warm baths to relieve discomfort. Do this for 15 to 20 minutes several times daily for the first week after surgery.
- Don't dry the surgical area with a towel. Drip dry or use a blow dryer after bathing.
- If the cyst is left open to heal by itself, it will drain and will require dressing changes until it is healed. Your doctor will instruct you on how to change the dressings.
- Sit on a rubber ring (available in drugstores) to relieve discomfort, if necessary.
- Avoid becoming constipated.

MEDICATION
- Your doctor may prescribe:
  - Pain relievers. Don't take prescription pain medication longer than 4 to 7 days. Use only as much as you need.
  - Stool softeners to prevent constipation.
  - Antibiotics to fight or prevent infection.
- You may use nonprescription drugs, such as acetaminophen, for minor pain. Avoid aspirin.

ACTIVITY
- To help recovery and aid your well-being, resume daily activities, including work, as soon as you are able.
- Avoid vigorous exercise for 6 weeks after surgery.
- Resume driving 1 week after returning home.
- Resume sexual relations when your doctor determines that healing is complete.

DIET—Clear liquid diet until the gastrointestinal tract functions again. Then eat a well-balanced diet to promote healing. Increase fluid intake and dietary fiber to decrease the likelihood of developing constipation.

CALL YOUR DOCTOR IF

- Pain, swelling, redness, drainage, or bleeding increases in the surgical area.
- You develop signs of infection including headache, muscle aches, dizziness, fever, or a general ill feeling.
- New, unexplained symptoms develop.

PILONIDAL CYST REMOVAL

An illustration of several sinuses that tract from the deeper cysts to the skin surface.

Tailbone

Incision site

Sinus

The cyst and all affected sinuses are identified and removed.

The skin is usually left open to heal slowly from the bottom. Some surgeons close the skin over the operative site at the time of surgery.

POPLITEAL ARTERY EMBOLECTOMY

GENERAL INFORMATION

DEFINITION—Removal of a blood clot (embolus) that has blocked blood supply to the leg and foot.

BODY PARTS INVOLVED—Blood vessel in the leg that is called the femoral artery below the groin and the popliteal artery behind the knee. The heart is the usual source of the blood clot.

REASONS FOR SURGERY—Restoration of normal blood circulation in the legs. Re-establishing blood flow can restore muscular function, prevent gangrene and enable patients to return to normal or almost normal activities.

SURGICAL RISK INCREASES WITH
- Obesity, smoking.
- Rheumatic heart disease or coronary artery disease.
- Diabetes.
- Use of some prescription and nonprescription drugs. Inform your doctor of any drugs, medications, or vitamin and herb supplements you are using or have used in the last month.

WHAT TO EXPECT

WHO OPERATES—General surgeon or vascular surgeon.

WHERE PERFORMED—Hospital.

DIAGNOSTIC TESTS
- Before surgery: Blood and urine studies, chest x-ray, ECG, arteriogram (see Glossary for both).
- During surgery: Arteriogram (see Glossary) after blood clot is removed.
- After surgery: Blood studies, heart studies, such as sonogram (see Glossary).

ANESTHESIA
- Spinal anesthesia by injection.
- General anesthesia by injection and inhalation with an airway tube placed in the windpipe.

DESCRIPTION OF OPERATION
- An incision is usually made over the artery where the clot is lodged. Sometimes, however, the incision is made in the groin.
- The blood flow is controlled and the artery is opened above the blood clot.
- A special catheter is passed into the artery beyond the blood clot. The catheter is expanded with air beyond the clot and then withdrawn, forcing the clot out of the artery.
- An anticoagulant is injected into the artery, and normal blood circulation is restored.
- The artery is closed. Muscles and connective tissue are sewn together in layers. The skin is closed with sutures or clamps, which usually can be removed about 1 week after surgery.

POSSIBLE COMPLICATIONS
- Excessive bleeding.
- Surgical-wound infection.
- Inadvertent injury to the large nerves.
- Recurrent blood clot.
- Heart problems.

AVERAGE HOSPITAL STAY—0 to 3 days.

PROBABLE OUTCOME—Expect complete healing without complications. Allow about 3 weeks for recovery from surgery.

POSTOPERATIVE CARE

GENERAL MEASURES
- A hard ridge should form along the incision. As it heals, the ridge will gradually recede.
- Shower as usual. Avoid baths until the incision has completely healed. You may wash the incision gently with mild, unscented soap. After showering, replace any wet dressings with clean, dry ones.
- Move and elevate legs often while resting in bed to decrease the likelihood of deep-vein blood clots.

MEDICATION
- Your doctor may prescribe:
  - Pain relievers. Don't take prescription pain medication longer than 4 to 7 days. Use only as much as you need.
  - Blood thinners to prevent recurrent clots.
- You may use nonprescription drugs, such as acetaminophen, for minor pain.

ACTIVITY
- Resuming daily activities, including work, as soon as you are able can help the healing process.
- Avoid vigorous exercise for 3 weeks after surgery, but start a walking exercise program as soon as your doctor recommends.
- Resume driving about 1 week after returning home.

DIET—No special diet.

CALL YOUR DOCTOR IF

- Pain, swelling, redness, drainage, or bleeding increases in the surgical area.
- You develop signs of infection including headache, muscle aches, dizziness, fever, or a general ill feeling.
- Your foot becomes cold, discolored, or numb.
- Preoperative symptoms don't improve.
- New, unexplained symptoms develop.

POPLITEAL ARTERY EMBOLECTOMY

An illustration of a clot in the popliteal artery extending behind the knee.

Clotted popliteal artery

Knee

An incision is made in the inguinal region (inside inner thigh area) and a small opening is made in the femoral artery.

Incision site

Balloon catheter

• The catheter is passed into the artery beyond the blood clot. It is expanded with air and then withdrawn, forcing the clots out of the artery.
• After the clot has been removed, muscles and connective tissues are sewn together in layers. The skin is closed with sutures or clamps.

PROSTATE GLAND REMOVAL, SUPRAPUBIC

GENERAL INFORMATION

DEFINITION—Removal of an abnormal or enlarged prostate gland through an opening in the lower abdomen.

BODY PARTS INVOLVED—Prostate gland, bladder, rectum, urethra.

REASONS FOR SURGERY
- Restoration of normal passage of urine.
- Cancer of the prostate.

SURGICAL RISK INCREASES WITH
- Adults over 60.
- Stress, smoking, obesity.
- Poor nutrition.
- Recent illness, especially upper-respiratory infection.
- Alcoholism or chronic illness.
- Diabetes.
- Use of some prescription and nonprescription drugs. Inform your doctor of any drugs, medications, or vitamin and herb supplements you are using or have used in the last month.

WHAT TO EXPECT

WHO OPERATES—Urologist.

WHERE PERFORMED—Hospital.

DIAGNOSTIC TESTS
- Before surgery: Blood and urine studies, chest x-ray, kidney function studies, intravenous pyelogram, ultrasound, cystoscopy, ECG (see Glossary for all), prostate biopsy.
- After surgery: Blood studies.

ANESTHESIA
- Spinal anesthesia by injection.
- General anesthesia by injection and inhalation with an airway tube placed in the windpipe.

DESCRIPTION OF OPERATION
- An incision is made in the lower abdomen.
- The bladder and urethra are opened, and the enlarged parts of the prostate gland cut free and removed.
- Two catheters are placed in the bladder, and a tube to drain secretions is placed next to the bladder. The urethra and bladder are closed with sutures. One of the catheters will pass through the penis, and the other will be brought out through the incision along with the drain.
- The catheters and drains will usually remain in place for several days.
- The muscles are repositioned and sewn in place. The skin is closed with sutures or clips, which usually can be removed about 1 week after surgery.

POSSIBLE COMPLICATIONS
- Excessive bleeding.
- Surgical-wound infection.
- Inability to control urinary stream.
- Impotence.
- Sterility (sometimes).

AVERAGE HOSPITAL STAY—3 to 5 days.

PROBABLE OUTCOME—Expect complete healing without complications. Allow about 6 weeks for recovery from surgery.

POSTOPERATIVE CARE

GENERAL MEASURES
- A hard ridge should form along the incision. As it heals the ridge will gradually recede.
- Shower as usual. Avoid baths until the incision has completely healed. You may wash the incision gently with mild, unscented soap. After showering, replace any wet dressings with clean, dry ones.
- Move and elevate legs often while resting in bed to decrease the likelihood of deep-vein blood clots.

MEDICATION
- Your doctor may prescribe:
  - Pain relievers. Don't take prescription pain medication longer than 4 to 7 days. Use only as much as you need.
  - Stool softeners to prevent constipation.
  - Antibiotics to fight or prevent infection.
- You may use nonprescription drugs, such as acetaminophen, for minor pain. Avoid aspirin.

ACTIVITY
- Resuming daily activities, including work, as soon as you are able can help the healing process.
- Resume driving 1 month after returning home.
- Avoid vigorous exercise for 6 weeks following surgery.
- Resume sexual relations when able.

DIET—Clear liquid diet until the gastrointestinal tract begins to function again. Then eat a well-balanced diet to promote healing. Avoid coffee, tea, cocoa, cola drinks, alcoholic beverages and any food or spice that aggravates symptoms.

CALL YOUR DOCTOR IF

- Pain, swelling, redness, or drainage increases in the surgical area.
- You experience excessive bleeding.
- You develop signs of infection including headache, muscle aches, dizziness, fever, or a general ill feeling.
- You experience constipation, abdominal swelling or pain, nausea, or vomiting.
- You have difficulty with urination.
- New, unexplained symptoms develop.

PROSTATE GLAND REMOVAL, SUPRAPUBIC

An illustration of the usual incision site for prostatectomy.

Incision site

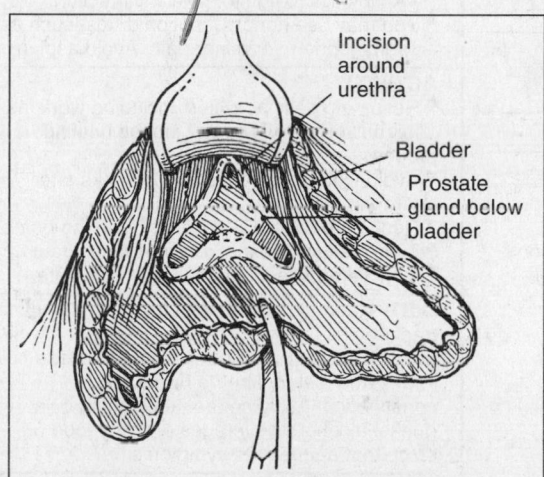

The bladder and urethra are opened and the enlarged parts of the prostate gland cut free and removed.

Incision around urethra

Bladder

Prostate gland below bladder

- Two catheters are placed in the bladder and a tube to drain secretions is placed next to the bladder. The urethra and bladder are closed with sutures.
- One of the catheters will pass through the penis and the other will be brought out through the incision along with the drain (not illustrated).

Catheter

PROSTATE GLAND REMOVAL, TRANSURETHRAL

GENERAL INFORMATION

DEFINITION—Removal of part of an enlarged prostate gland with a cystoscope, an instrument that is passed up through the urethra.

BODY PARTS INVOLVED—Penis, prostate gland, urethra, bladder.

REASONS FOR SURGERY—Restoration of normal passage of urine.

SURGICAL RISK INCREASES WITH
- Obesity, smoking.
- Poor nutrition.
- Recent or chronic illness.
- Alcoholism.
- Diabetes.
- Use of some prescription and nonprescription drugs. Inform your doctor of any drugs, medications, or vitamin and herb supplements you are using or have used in the last month.

WHAT TO EXPECT

WHO OPERATES—Urologist.

WHERE PERFORMED—Hospital.

DIAGNOSTIC TESTS
- Before surgery: Blood and urine studies, x-rays of kidneys and chest, kidney-function studies, ECG, intravenous pyelogram (IVP), ultrasound (see Glossary for all).
- After surgery: Blood studies.

ANESTHESIA
- Spinal anesthesia by injection.
- General anesthesia by injection and inhalation with an airway tube placed in the windpipe.

DESCRIPTION OF OPERATION
- A cystoscope (a thin, scope with lenses and a light at its tip) is passed up through the urethra to the prostate gland.
- The prostate gland is examined for tumors and signs of infection.
- An electrosurgical loop is inserted through the cystoscope tip and cuts away the diseased parts of the prostate gland.
- The cystoscope is removed. A catheter may be placed in the bladder for a day or two.

POSSIBLE COMPLICATIONS
- Excessive bleeding.
- Inability to control urinary stream (incontinence).
- Urinary retention.
- Impotence (sometimes).
- Sterility.
- Epididymitis.

AVERAGE HOSPITAL STAY—2 to 3 days.

PROBABLE OUTCOME—Expect complete healing without complications. Allow about 3 weeks for recovery from surgery. You may have a burning sensation when you urinate. This should get better each day, but it may take up to 6 weeks for the painful urination to completely subside.

POSTOPERATIVE CARE

GENERAL MEASURES—Move and elevate legs often while resting in bed to decrease the likelihood of deep-vein blood clots.

MEDICATION
- Your doctor may prescribe:
  - Pain relievers. Don't take prescription pain medication longer than 4 to 7 days. Use only as much as you need.
  - Stool softeners to prevent constipation.
  - Antibiotics to fight or prevent infection.
- You may use nonprescription drugs, such as acetaminophen, for minor pain. Avoid aspirin.

ACTIVITY
- Resuming daily activities, including work, as soon as you are able can help the healing process.
- Avoid vigorous exercise for 2 weeks after surgery.
- Resume driving 1 week after returning home.
- Try to resume sexual relations when your doctor determines that healing is complete.

DIET—Clear liquid diet until the gastrointestinal tract begins to function again. Then eat a well-balanced diet to promote healing. Increase fluid intake and dietary fiber to help prevent constipation. Avoid coffee, tea, cocoa, cola drinks, alcoholic beverages and any food or spice that aggravates symptoms.

CALL YOUR DOCTOR IF

- You develop signs of infection including headache, muscle aches, dizziness, fever, or a general ill feeling.
- You experience nausea, vomiting, constipation, or difficulty with urination.
- You remain impotent for longer than 3 months after surgery.
- New, unexplained symptoms develop.

PROSTATE GLAND REMOVAL, TRANSURETHRAL

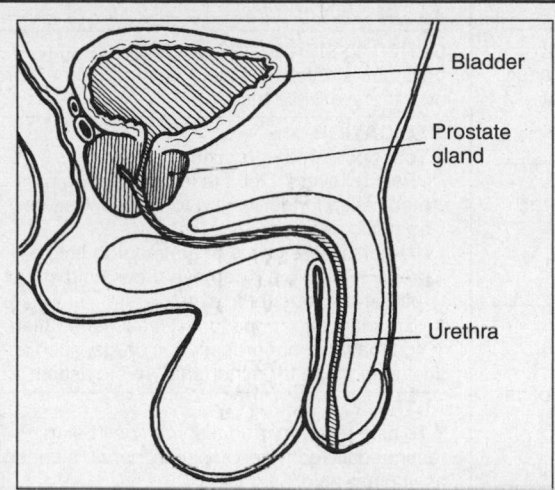

A side view of the bladder, urethra and prostate gland in the male.

Bladder

Prostate gland

Urethra

Cystoscope

Prostate gland

- The cystoscope is passed through the urethra to the segment where the prostate gland is located.
- A miniature telescope and light inside the cystoscope make the prostate gland visible through the cystoscope.

Cystoscope

Wire loop

Prostate gland

A wire loop is passed through the cystoscope tip to remove part of the diseased or enlarged prostate gland. Electrocautery is used to control bleeding.

PTERYGIUM EXCISION

GENERAL INFORMATION

DEFINITION—Removal of a pterygium, an abnormal tissue that grows from the inner edge of the sclera (white outer coat enclosing the eyeball) and extends over a portion of the cornea.

BODY PARTS INVOLVED—Eye, cornea, conjunctiva (the membrane covering the eye).

REASONS FOR SURGERY
- Restoration or protection of normal vision.
- Improved appearance.

SURGICAL RISK INCREASES WITH
- Recent or chronic illness.
- Diabetes.
- Use of some prescription and nonprescription drugs. Inform your doctor of any drugs, medications, or vitamin and herb supplements you are using or have used in the last month.

WHAT TO EXPECT

WHO OPERATES—Ophthalmologist.

WHERE PERFORMED—Hospital or outpatient surgical facility.

DIAGNOSTIC TESTS
- Before surgery: Complete eye examination.
- After surgery: Complete eye examination.

ANESTHESIA
- Local anesthesia by topical application, usually accompanied by sedation.
- Local anesthesia by injection, usually accompanied by sedation.

DESCRIPTION OF OPERATION
- An incision is made in the conjunctiva around the pterygium.
- The pterygium is cut and brought upward, clear of the cornea.
- The lower edge of the pterygium is cut free and the entire pterygium is removed.
- An autograft is fashioned from an area of the conjunctiva underneath the eyelid and is placed to cover the area from where the pterygium was removed.
- Fine sutures are used to attach the graft and to close the membrane from where the graft was taken, the sutures will dissolve and will be absorbed by the body.

POSSIBLE COMPLICATIONS
- Surgical-wound infection.
- Recurrence of the pterygium.
- Scarring.

AVERAGE HOSPITAL STAY—Usually none.

PROBABLE OUTCOME—Expect complete healing without complications. Allow about 3 weeks for recovery from surgery.

POSTOPERATIVE CARE

GENERAL MEASURES—Your doctor may prescribe a patch or shield (at night) to be worn over the eye while healing.

MEDICATION
- Your doctor may prescribe:
  - Pain relievers. Don't take prescription pain medication longer than 4 to 7 days. Use only as much as you need.
  - Antibiotic eye drops or ointment to fight or prevent infection. Keep eye drops cold in the refrigerator, but not frozen.
  - Steroidal eye drops to reduce inflammation.
- You may use nonprescription drugs, such as acetaminophen for minor pain. Avoid aspirin.

ACTIVITY
- To help recovery and aid your well-being, resume daily activities, including work, as soon as you are able.
- Avoid vigorous exercise for 3 weeks after surgery.
- Wear sunglasses with UV protection when outside to protect your eyes from the sun's rays and to help reduce the likelihood of recurrence.
- Resume driving 1 day after surgery or, if an eye patch is prescribed, after the patch is removed.

DIET—No special diet.

CALL YOUR DOCTOR IF

- Pain, swelling, redness, drainage, or bleeding increases in the eye.
- You experience difficulty with your vision.
- You develop signs of infection including headache, muscle aches, dizziness, fever, or a general ill feeling.
- New, unexplained symptoms develop.

PTERYGIUM EXCISION

An illustration of a typical pterygium extending from the edge of the eye inward to attach to the cornea.

Pterygium

- An incision is made in the conjunctiva around the pterygium.
- The pterygium is cut and brought upward clear of the cornea.

- The lower edge of the pterygium is cut free and the entire growth is removed.
- Open areas in the membrane covering the eye are closed with fine sutures that will dissolve and be absorbed by the body.

RADIOFREQUENCY ABLATION

GENERAL INFORMATION

DEFINITION—Radiofrequency ablation (RFA) is a general term for a procedure that uses radio waves to heat and destroy abnormal or dysfunctional tissue in the body. The radio waves travel through electrodes (such as needle-like probe). The tissue killed by RFA is not removed, but is gradually replaced by fibrosis and scar tissue.

BODY PARTS INVOLVED—Almost every body system and many different body parts.

REASONS FOR SURGERY
- Cancerous tumors.
- Cardiac arrhythmias (irregular and/or rapid heart rhythms).
- Enlarged prostate.
- Severe snoring and/or sleep apnea.
- Barrett's esophagus.
- Pain from soft tissue tumors, pain from spread of disease, or severe nerve pain.
- Varicose veins.
- Numerous other medical conditions.

SURGICAL RISK INCREASES WITH—Medical problems such as obesity, chronic lung or heart disease, older age, diabetes, bleeding problems, active infection, and previous RFA treatments may affect your specific risks.

WHAT TO EXPECT

WHO OPERATES—Interventional pain specialist, interventional radiologist, cardiac electrophysiologist, other specialists.

WHERE PERFORMED—Hospital or outpatient surgical facility.

DIAGNOSTIC TESTS
- Before surgery: Blood and urine studies and imaging tests depending on reason for RFA.
- After surgery: Follow up tests are usually scheduled to determine effectiveness of RFA.

ANESTHESIA—General anesthesia, local anesthesia, and/or sedative to help you relax.

DESCRIPTION OF OPERATION
- This is a general description of the procedure.
- Grounding pads are laid on the skin, usually on both thighs, so electrical current can be safely applied while the RFA is carried out.
- The area will be numbed with a local anesthetic (if the procedure is done without a general anesthetic). A very small cut is made in the skin after it is numb. The radiofrequency ablation probe is inserted into the tissue being treated using imaging guidance (ultrasound or CT) and images or pictures are shown on a screen.

- A small amount of heat will be introduced through the probe. The heat will destroy the abnormal tissue. The probe may be moved (repositioned) to destroy other areas of tissue.
- Length of time for the RFA will vary.
- After the procedure, you will be monitored for several hours in a recovery room.

POSSIBLE COMPLICATIONS
- Discomfort.
- Bruising or bleeding.
- Infection.
- Lung collapse upon insertion of the probe (when the procedure involves the lung, liver, or upper kidney).
- Blood clots or damage to heart after procedures on the heart.
- Liver abscess (small, pus-filled area).
- Damage to tissue surrounding the target area.

AVERAGE HOSPITAL STAY—0 to 2 days.

PROBABLE OUTCOME—RFA is usually a safe and effective treatment for the medical condition being treated. Complications are rare. Research is ongoing regarding the long-term efficacy and reliability of RFA therapy.

POSTOPERATIVE CARE

GENERAL MEASURES
- You may shower the day you return home.
- A low grade fever may occur for a few days.
- Be sure to keep follow up appointments with your doctor.

MEDICATION
- Your doctor may prescribe pain relievers. Use only as much as you need to be comfortable.
- You may use nonprescription pain reliever such as acetaminophen for minor pain. Ask your doctor about taking ibuprofen or aspirin.

ACTIVITY
- Resume normal activities as soon as you feel able. You will be instructed about any limits on activities (e.g., heavy lifting).
- Patients typically return to work in 1 to 3 days.

DIET—No special diet.

CALL YOUR DOCTOR IF

- Pain, swelling, redness, drainage, or bleeding increases in the treated area.
- You develop signs of infection, including headache, muscle aches, dizziness, fever, or a general ill feeling.
- Nausea or vomiting occur.
- You have shortness of breath, heart palpitations, or chest pain.
- Prescribed drugs don't control your pain.

RADIOFREQUENCY ABLATION

Grounding pads are laid on the skin, usually on both thighs, so electrical current can be safely applied while the RFA is carried out.

Grounding pad

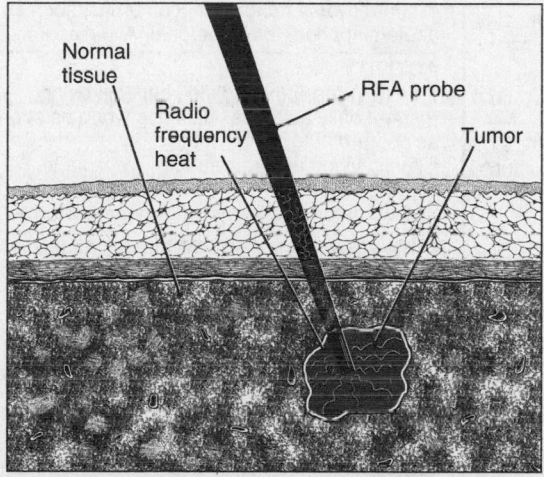

Normal tissue

Radio frequency heat

RFA probe

Tumor

A very small cut is made in the skin after it is numb. The radiofrequency ablation probe is inserted into the tumor being treated using imaging guidance (ultrasound or CT) and images or pictures are shown on a screen.

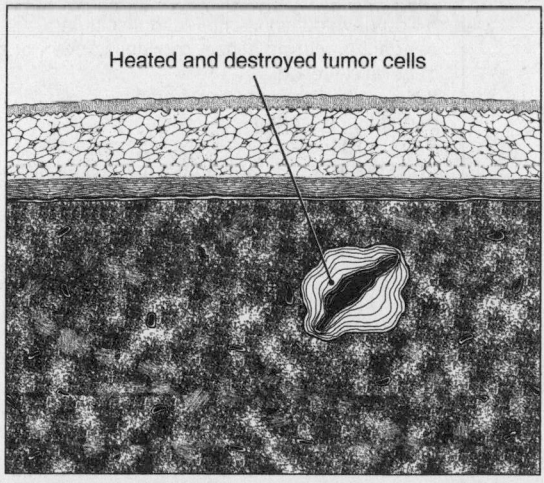

Heated and destroyed tumor cells

A small amount of heat will be introduced through the probe. The heat will destroy the abnormal tissue.

RECTAL OR COLON POLYP REMOVAL
(Polypectomy)

GENERAL INFORMATION

DEFINITION—Removal of a polyp from the membrane lining inside the rectum or colon.

BODY PARTS INVOLVED—Membrane lining of the rectum and colon.

REASONS FOR SURGERY
- Removal of a possible source of cancer.
- Removal of tissue to see if cancer is present.
- To remove the source of rectal bleeding.

SURGICAL RISK INCREASES WITH
- Obesity.
- Smoking.
- Poor nutrition.
- Recent or chronic illness.
- Diabetes.
- Use of some prescription and nonprescription drugs. Inform your doctor of any drugs, medications, or vitamin and herb supplements you are using or have used in the last month.

WHAT TO EXPECT

WHO OPERATES—General surgeon, colon-rectal surgeon, gastroenterologist, family doctor.

WHERE PERFORMED—Hospital, outpatient surgical facility, doctor's office.

DIAGNOSTIC TESTS
- Before surgery: Blood and urine studies, x-ray of lower gastrointestinal tract, sigmoidoscopy, colonoscopy (see Glossary for both).
- After surgery: Blood studies, laboratory examination of removed tissue.

ANESTHESIA—Intravenous sedative and narcotic pain killer.

DESCRIPTION OF OPERATION
- The colon is cleansed the night before by drinking various solutions.
- A colonoscope or sigmoidoscope (see Glossary for both) is inserted through the rectum into the sigmoid colon. You may feel mild cramping.
- The polyp is located and removed with a wire snare.
- Bleeding is controlled with electric current or pressure applied with gauze soaked in epinephrine (see Glossary).

POSSIBLE COMPLICATIONS
- Excessive bleeding.
- Inadvertent perforation of the colon resulting in infection.

AVERAGE HOSPITAL STAY—Usually none.

PROBABLE OUTCOME—Expect complete healing without complications. Allow 2 to 3 days for recovery from surgery. If the polyp is found to be cancerous, treatment and outcome will vary.

POSTOPERATIVE CARE

GENERAL MEASURES—Your first bowel movement may be red or maroon and may contain blood clots. If bowel movements continue to have this appearance, or if you have liquid blood in your stool, contact your doctor right away.

MEDICATION
- Your doctor may prescribe:
  - Pain relievers. Don't take prescription pain medication longer than 4 to 7 days. Use only as much as you need.
  - Stool softeners to prevent constipation.
- You may use nonprescription drugs, such as acetaminophen, to relieve pain. Avoid aspirin.

ACTIVITY
- To help recovery and aid your well-being, resume daily activities, including work, as soon as you are able.
- Avoid vigorous exercise for 4 weeks after surgery.
- Resume driving 3 days after returning home.

DIET—Clear liquid diet until the gastrointestinal tract functions again. Then eat a well-balanced diet to promote healing. Increase intake of dietary fiber and fluids to prevent constipation. Avoid coffee, tea, cocoa, cola drinks, alcoholic beverages and any food or spice that causes painful or irritating digestive symptoms.

CALL YOUR DOCTOR IF

- You develop signs of infection including headache, muscle aches, dizziness, fever, or a general ill feeling.
- You experience nausea, vomiting, constipation, abdominal swelling, or pain.
- You experience weakness, dizziness, or a rapid pulse upon standing (symptoms of internal bleeding).
- New, unexplained symptoms develop.

RECTAL OR COLON POLYP REMOVAL
(Polypectomy)

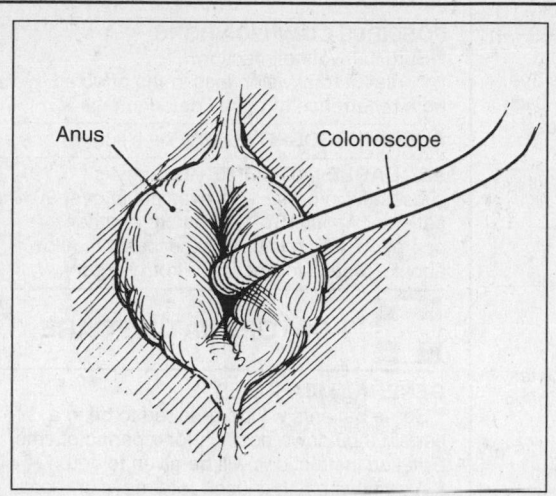

An illustration of a flexible colonoscope inserted into the anus.

Anus

Colonoscope

Polyp

- The colonoscope or sigmoidoscope is advanced to reach the sigmoid colon where polyps (when present) are usually located.
- The polyp is removed with a wire snare.

After the polyp has been removed, bleeding of the remaining stump is controlled with electric current.

RETINAL DETACHMENT REPAIR

 GENERAL INFORMATION

DEFINITION—Reattachment of a retina that has become separated from the rest of the eye. The retina is the light-sensitive area at the back of the eye. See Retinal Detachment in Illness section.

BODY PARTS INVOLVED—The eye and all its parts.

REASONS FOR SURGERY—Prevention of vision loss.

SURGICAL RISK INCREASES WITH
- Obesity, smoking, alcoholism.
- Poor nutrition.
- Recent or chronic illness, especially diabetes.
- Use of some prescription and nonprescription drugs. Inform your doctor of any drugs, medications, or vitamin and herb supplements you are using or have used in the last month.

 WHAT TO EXPECT

WHO OPERATES—Ophthalmologist.

WHERE PERFORMED—Hospital or outpatient surgical facility.

DIAGNOSTIC TESTS
- Before surgery: Complete eye examination.
- After surgery: Complete eye examination.

ANESTHESIA
- Local anesthesia by injection or topical application.
- General anesthesia by injection and inhalation with an airway tube placed in the windpipe.

DESCRIPTION OF OPERATION
- Your doctor will choose a procedure depending on severity of detachment.
- Laser photocoagulation: Tears or holes in the retina are repaired with laser beams that coagulate the eye tissue and cause it to readjust to its normal position.
- Cryopexy: The membrane lining the eye is cut. A cryosurgical probe is placed around the detached retina. The probe applies extreme cold, causing eye tissue to coagulate and to adhere to its normal position.
- Diathermy: Heat from an electric current is applied to seal a tear in the retina.
- Pneumatic retinopexy: If the tear or tears which caused the retina to detach are in the upper part of the eye, a gas can be injected into the eye to push the retina back into place. The tears can then be repaired with laser photocoagulation or cryopexy.
- Scleral buckling: If a large area of the retina is detached, it is often necessary to drain fluid from under the retina and then place a silicone band or sponge on the outside of the eye to push it against the retina.

- If a cornea transplant is required, it is performed.

POSSIBLE COMPLICATIONS
- Surgical-wound infection.
- Partial or total vision loss in the affected eye from recurrence of retinal detachment.

AVERAGE HOSPITAL STAY—Usually none.

PROBABLE OUTCOME—Surgery is successful in preserving eyesight in over 90% of patients. About 10% will require another operation, which is usually successful. Allow about 2 weeks for recovery from surgery.

 POSTOPERATIVE CARE

GENERAL MEASURES
- Some patients will be required to be in a certain face down position for a period of time. Detailed instructions will be given to you.
- A soft eye patch is used for 2 days or more. There may be some discharge from the eye. A shield is used at night to protect eye from pressure or accidental injury.
- Don't rub the eye.
- Shower as usual and wash your hair carefully. Don't let water or soap get in your eye.

MEDICATION
- Your doctor may prescribe:
  - Pain relievers. Don't take prescription pain medication longer than 4 to 7 days. Use only as much as you need.
  - Stool softeners to prevent constipation.
  - Antibiotics to fight or prevent infection.
  - Eye drops to keep the pupil dilated during healing.
- You may use nonprescription drugs, such as acetaminophen for minor pain. Avoid aspirin.

ACTIVITY
- Your doctor will advise you about specific limits on activities.
- For the first week, move your head with caution. Take slow walks.
- Avoid vigorous exercise or lifting for 6 weeks after surgery (or as advised).
- Resume driving 4 weeks after returning home.

DIET—No special diet.

 CALL YOUR DOCTOR IF

- You experience any change in vision.
- You develop constipation.
- Pain, swelling, redness, drainage, or bleeding increases in the surgical area.
- You develop signs of infection including headache, muscle aches, dizziness, fever, or a general ill feeling.
- New, unexplained symptoms develop. treatment may produce side effects.

RETINAL DETACHMENT REPAIR

- An illustration of the relationship of parts of the eye.
- Scissors cutting the sclera (the membrane lining the eye).

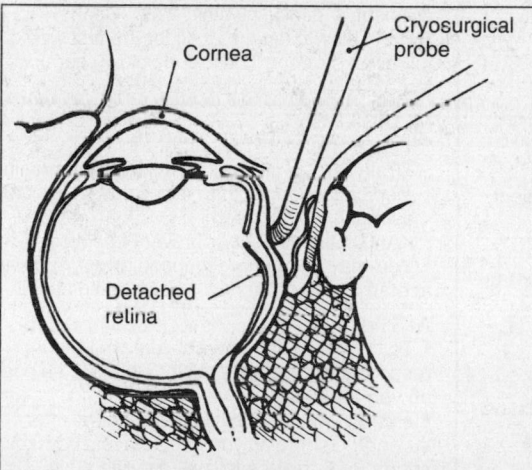

Cryosurgical probe is placed around the detached retina. The probe applies extreme cold causing eye tissue to coagulate and adhere to its normal position.

Cornea

Cryosurgical probe

Detached retina

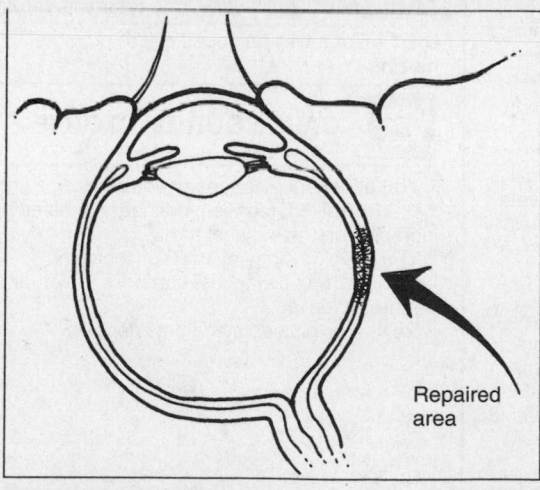

The retina returned to normal position after the detached retina has been secured in its proper position.

Repaired area

RHINOPLASTY & SEPTOPLASTY

 GENERAL INFORMATION

DEFINITION—Reconstruction of the nose (rhinoplasty) and removal of deformities of the septum (septoplasty).

BODY PARTS INVOLVED—Nose, including nasal cartilage and bone and mucous membrane of the septum.

REASONS FOR SURGERY
- Opening of blocked nasal passages.
- Improved appearance.

SURGICAL RISK INCREASES WITH
- Obesity, smoking.
- Poor nutrition.
- Excess alcohol consumption.
- Recent or chronic illness.
- Diabetes.
- Use of some prescription and nonprescription drugs. Inform your doctor of any drugs, medications, or vitamin and herb supplements you are using or have used in the last month.

 WHAT TO EXPECT

WHO OPERATES—Plastic and reconstructive surgeon or an ear, nose and throat specialist.

WHERE PERFORMED—Hospital or outpatient surgical facility.

DIAGNOSTIC TESTS
- Before surgery: Blood and urine studies, x-ray of facial bones.
- After surgery: Blood studies.

ANESTHESIA
- Local anesthesia by injection.
- General anesthesia by injection and inhalation with an airway tube placed in the windpipe.

DESCRIPTION OF OPERATION
- The nostril is held open with a speculum.
- An incision is made in the nose. To minimize visual scarring, the incision is usually made from within the nostrils, external cuts may be made if the shape of the nostrils is being changed.
- The bone or cartilage is fractured, trimmed and molded into the desired shape. If the goal is to increase the length of the nose, or to elevate the bridge, cartilage or bone from elsewhere in the body may be used as an implant. A synthetic material may also be used for the implant.
- The mucous membrane is closed with fine sutures, which usually can be removed about 10 days after surgery. Bandages are applied.
- For some procedures, petroleum-jelly-coated packing gauze or plastic splints are used to hold the septum in place during healing (up to 2 weeks).

POSSIBLE COMPLICATIONS
- Excessive bleeding.
- Excessive scarring (keloid) which can affect the contour of the nose.
- Surgical-wound infection (rare).
- Discomfort and pain caused by gauze packing.
- Recurrence of airway obstruction.

AVERAGE HOSPITAL STAY—0 to 1 day.

PROBABLE OUTCOME—Expect complete healing without complications. Allow about 3 weeks for recovery from surgery.

 POSTOPERATIVE CARE

GENERAL MEASURES
- Apply ice packs to the nose to relieve discomfort. Do this for 10 to 20 minutes at a time 4 to 8 times a day during the first 2 days after surgery.
- Swelling and discoloration around the eyes will usually diminish within 2 to 3 weeks.
- Don't blow the nose at all for the first week following surgery. Then, don't blow your nose forcefully for the next month.

MEDICATION
- Your doctor may prescribe:
  - Pain relievers. Don't take prescription pain medication longer than 4 to 7 days. Use only as much as you need.
  - Antibiotics to fight or prevent infection.
- You may use nonprescription drugs, such as acetaminophen, for minor pain. Avoid aspirin.

ACTIVITY
- To help recovery and aid your well-being, resume daily activities, including work, as soon as you are able.
- Avoid vigorous exercise for 3 weeks after surgery. Generally, you should avoid contact sports for 6 months following surgery.
- Resume driving 1 week after returning home.

DIET—Eat a well-balanced diet to promote healing.

 CALL YOUR DOCTOR IF

- You experience nausea or vomiting.
- Pain, swelling, redness, drainage, or bleeding increases in the surgical area.
- You develop signs of infection including headache, muscle aches, dizziness, fever, or a general ill feeling.
- New, unexplained symptoms develop.

RHINOPLASTY & SEPTOPLASTY

An illustration of the mouth and nose with a speculum opening one side of the nose.

Nasal septum

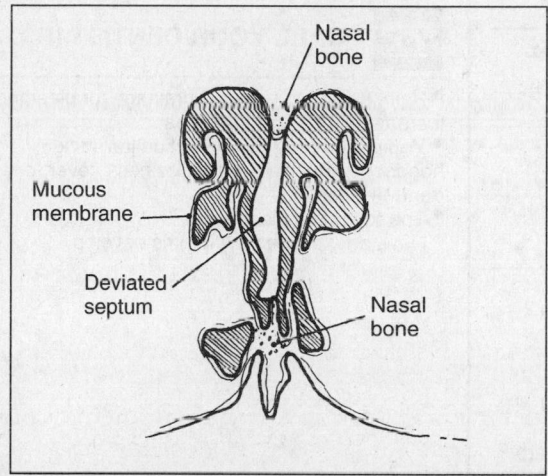

An incision is made inside the nose. The bone or cartilage is fractured, trimmed and molded into the desired shape.

Nasal bone

Mucous membrane

Deviated septum

Nasal bone

Resected septum closed with fine sutures that usually can be removed about 10 days after surgery.

Resected septum

Broken nasal bone

ROOT CANAL TREATMENT
(Endodontic Therapy)

GENERAL INFORMATION

DEFINITION—A dental procedure designed to save a tooth in which the living tissue (pulp) has died or is chronically diseased. The procedure cleans out dead or dying nerve tissue, as well as any infection, from the inside of a tooth.

BODY PARTS INVOLVED—Teeth and pulp.

REASONS FOR SURGERY—To avoid extraction of the affected tooth.

SURGICAL RISK INCREASES WITH
* Diabetes.
* Use of some prescription and nonprescription drugs. Inform your doctor of any drugs, medications, or vitamin and herb supplements you are using or have used in the last month.

WHAT TO EXPECT

WHO OPERATES—Endodontist (tooth pulp specialist), general dentist.

WHERE PERFORMED—Dentist's office.

DIAGNOSTIC TESTS
* Before surgery: X-rays.
* During surgery: X-rays.
* After surgery: X-rays.

ANESTHESIA—Local anesthetic.

DESCRIPTION OF OPERATION
* Root canal therapy is usually done in 1 to 2 appointments.
* A hole is drilled into the pulp so that any infected matter can be removed.
* The root canals are enlarged and shaped with long, fine-tipped instruments.
* Medicated cotton and a temporary filling are placed in the cavity.
* After a week, or at the next appointment, the filling is removed and the cavity is filled with special material, gutta percha, and the root is sealed.

POSSIBLE COMPLICATIONS
* Pain and swelling.
* Surgical-wound infection.
* Persistent or recurring abscess.

AVERAGE HOSPITAL STAY—Usually none.

PROBABLE OUTCOME—Expect complete healing without complications. Allow about 2 weeks for recovery from surgery. Complete healing may take several months, but there should be no symptoms or discomfort. The tooth should function as long as a normal tooth would. Teeth that undergo root canal treatment usually require a crown.

POSTOPERATIVE CARE

GENERAL MEASURES
* Use warm, salt-water rinses for mouth discomfort.
* Brush and floss teeth as usual.

MEDICATION
* Your dentist may prescribe:
  - Pain relievers. Don't take prescription pain medication longer than 2 or 3 days. Use only as much as you need.
  - Antibiotics to fight or prevent infection.
* You may use nonprescription drugs, such as ibuprofen, for minor pain. Avoid aspirin.

ACTIVITY—No restrictions.

DIET—No special diet. You may want to eat soft foods for a day or two following treatments. Avoid heavy biting.

CALL YOUR DENTIST IF

* Pain, swelling, redness, drainage, or bleeding increases in the surgical area.
* You develop signs of infection including headache, muscle aches, dizziness, fever, or a general ill feeling.
* The tooth feels loose.
* New, unexplained symptoms develop.

ROOT CANAL TREATMENT
(Endodontic Therapy)

Cavity site is identified.

Cavity is drilled and root canal is enlarged.

Canal is filled with special material to seal it off.

ROTATOR CUFF REPAIR

GENERAL INFORMATION

DEFINITION—Repair of the tendinous insertions of several shoulder muscles after they are torn by acute trauma or repeated injury. The rotator cuff is a group of muscles and tendons that form a cuff over the shoulder. They hold the arm in its "ball and socket" joint and help the shoulder to rotate.

BODY PARTS INVOLVED—Scapula (wing bone) and several of its muscles, humerus (upper arm bone).

REASONS FOR SURGERY—To alleviate or diminish pain in the shoulder and increase strength in movements requiring shoulder motion. Repair also decreases chances of shoulder dislocation.

SURGICAL RISK INCREASES WITH
- Age.
- Diabetes.
- Poor kidney function.
- High blood pressure.
- Poor nutrition.
- Chronic lung disease.
- Obesity.

WHAT TO EXPECT

WHO OPERATES—Orthopedic surgeon.

WHERE PERFORMED—Hospital.

DIAGNOSTIC TESTS
- Before surgery: Blood tests, MRI, possible arthrogram (see Glossary).
- After surgery: Possible arthrogram.

ANESTHESIA—General anesthesia.

DESCRIPTION OF OPERATION
- There are three approaches to a repair. The recommended approach will depend on the extent of the injury and the experience of the operating surgeon.
- One approach is to repair the torn cuff using an arthroscope. In this surgery small puncture sites are utilized to mobilize the torn tendons and reanchor them to the top of the humerus.
- A second approach is to assess the tear using an arthroscope and then repair the torn tendon through a mini incision.
- A third approach is the traditional open surgery through an incision extending over the shoulder joint. Again the torn tendons are mobilized and, if possible, fixed to the upper humerus using sutures or staples. Sometimes the end of the scapula (acromion) is trimmed and scar tissue is removed.
- Sometimes the tendons cannot be reattached because they have retracted too much.
- The shoulder is usually immobilized with a sling after surgery.

POSSIBLE COMPLICATIONS
- Bleeding in the joint or from the surgical site.
- Infection.
- Failure of the tendon to heal to the bone.

AVERAGE HOSPITAL STAY—Usually 0-3 days.

PROBABLE OUTCOME—Expect healing of the incision in 2-3 weeks and healing of the tendon in 8-10 weeks. Most patients experience good pain relief. Full return of shoulder function is less certain and can take 8-12 months with rehabilitation.

POSTOPERATIVE CARE

GENERAL MEASURES
- Hard ridges will form along the incisions. As they heal, the ridges will gradually recede.
- Use heat on the incision to help relieve incisional pain.
- Shower as usual. You may wash the incisions gently with mild soap. After showering, replace any dressings with a new dry dressing.

MEDICATION
- Your doctor may prescribe pain relievers. Use only as much as you need to be comfortable.
- You may use nonprescription pain relievers such as acetaminophen for minor pain. Ask your doctor if it is okay to take ibuprofen or aspirin.

ACTIVITY
- Start ambulating (walking) as soon as you are home. Avoid strenuous activity using the affected shoulder for 6 to 8 weeks.
- Shoulder rehabilitation will be prescribed by your surgeon.

DIET—No special diet.

CALL YOUR DOCTOR IF

- Pain, swelling, redness, drainage, or bleeding increases in the surgical area.
- You develop symptoms of infection including headache, muscle aches, dizziness, fever, or a general ill feeling.
- Arm becomes cold, numb, painful, or swollen.
- New unexplained symptoms develop.

ROTATOR CUFF REPAIR

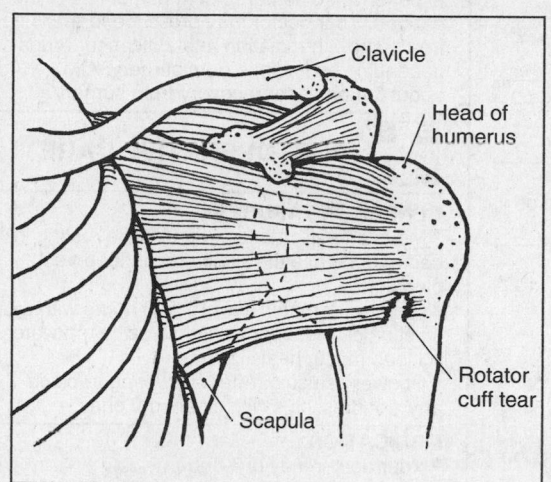

An illustration of the shoulder anatomy with a small rotator cuff tear.

Clavicle

Head of humerus

Rotator cuff tear

Scapula

The surgery can be performed open or using arthroscopy. The illustration shows an arthroscope and an instrument inserted through small puncture wounds to repair the torn cuff.

Arthroscope

Shoulder

The cuff is fixed back to the humerus with staples or sutures.

Repaired cuff

SALIVARY GLAND TUMOR REMOVAL

GENERAL INFORMATION

DEFINITION—Removal of a cancerous tumor of the salivary glands.

BODY PARTS INVOLVED—Salivary glands under the tongue (sublingual) or under the jawbone (submaxillary or parotid).

REASONS FOR SURGERY—Cancer or suspected cancer of the sublingual, parotid or submaxillary salivary glands.

SURGICAL RISK INCREASES WITH
- Adults over 60.
- Obesity.
- Smoking.
- Excess alcohol consumption.
- Poor nutrition.
- Recent or chronic illness.
- Diabetes.
- Use of some prescription and nonprescription drugs. Inform your doctor of any drugs, medications, or vitamin and herb supplements you are using or have used in the last month.

WHAT TO EXPECT

WHO OPERATES—Ear, nose and throat specialist (otolaryngologist) or general surgeon.

WHERE PERFORMED—Hospital.

DIAGNOSTIC TESTS
- Before surgery: Blood and urine studies, x-rays of the head, neck, upper gastrointestinal tract and chest.
- After surgery: Blood studies.

ANESTHESIA—General anesthesia by injection and inhalation with an airway tube placed in the windpipe.

DESCRIPTION OF OPERATION
- Incisions are made in the skin over the tumor.
- The tumor is isolated, cut free and removed.
- The tissue is examined to determine if the tumor is benign or cancerous.
- If the tumor is benign, the skin over the tumor is closed with several layers of fine sutures.
- A plastic drain tube may be placed in the incision and left for several days.
- If the tumor is cancerous, a radical neck dissection (see in Surgery section) is usually performed.

POSSIBLE COMPLICATIONS
- Excessive bleeding.
- Surgical-wound infection.
- Facial nerve injury.
- Fistula (see Glossary) from salivary gland.

AVERAGE HOSPITAL STAY—1 to 2 days.

PROBABLE OUTCOME—Expect complete healing without complications. You may experience some permanent numbness of the earlobe. Your doctor may prescribe further treatment with radiation and anticancer drugs depending on findings from surgery. Allow about 3 months for recovery from surgery.

POSTOPERATIVE CARE

GENERAL MEASURES
- Move and elevate legs often while resting in bed to decrease the likelihood of deep-vein blood clots.
- Rinse your mouth every 2 to 3 hours with a solution of 1 teaspoon salt in 8 oz. warm water. A clean mouth heals faster.
- Shower as usual. After showering, replace any wet dressings with clean, dry ones.

MEDICATION
- Your doctor may prescribe:
  - Pain relievers. Don't take prescription pain medication longer than 4 to 7 days. Use only as much as you need.
  - Stool softeners to prevent constipation.
  - Antibiotics to fight or prevent infection.
- You may use nonprescription drugs, such as acetaminophen, for minor pain. Avoid aspirin.

ACTIVITY
- To help recovery and aid your well-being, resume daily activities, including work, as soon as you are able.
- Avoid vigorous exercise for 3 weeks after surgery.

DIET—Clear liquid diet until the gastrointestinal tract functions again. Then eat a well-balanced diet to promote healing.

CALL YOUR DOCTOR IF

- Pain, swelling, redness, drainage, or bleeding increases in the surgical area.
- You develop symptoms of infection including headache, muscle aches, dizziness, fever, or a general ill feeling.
- You experience nausea, vomiting, or constipation.
- New, unexplained symptoms develop.

SALIVARY GLAND TUMOR REMOVAL

An illustration of the submandibular area with the dotted line indicating the incision site for submandibular gland removal.

Incision site

Incisions are made through the skin and tissues under the skin to expose the tumor.

Tumor

Submandibular gland

The tumor is isolated, cut free and scooped out with a finger or surgical instrument.

SEBACEOUS CYST REMOVAL
(Epidermoid Cyst Removal)

 GENERAL INFORMATION

DEFINITION—Removal of benign sebaceous cysts, sometimes called epidermoid cysts.

BODY PARTS INVOLVED—Sebaceous cysts, usually occurring on the skin of the trunk, face, scalp, neck, and often appear behind the ear.

REASONS FOR SURGERY
- Prevention of infections.
- Improved appearance.

SURGICAL RISK INCREASES WITH
- Any bleeding disorder.
- Diabetes.
- Use of some prescription and nonprescription drugs. Inform your doctor of any drugs, medications, or vitamin and herb supplements you are using or have used in the last month.

 WHAT TO EXPECT

WHO OPERATES—Family doctor, general surgeon, or dermatologist.

WHERE PERFORMED—Doctor's office or outpatient surgical facility.

DIAGNOSTIC TESTS
- Before surgery: Usually none.
- After surgery: Laboratory examination of removed tissue.

ANESTHESIA—Local anesthesia by injection.

DESCRIPTION OF OPERATION
- An incision is made over the cyst, with care taken not to rupture its confining wall. Leakage from the cyst can cause inflammation and delayed healing.
- The cyst and its contents are removed intact.
- The skin is closed with sutures or clips, which usually can be removed about 1 week after surgery.

POSSIBLE COMPLICATIONS
- Excessive bleeding.
- Surgical-wound infection.
- Recurrence of the cyst, if the cyst wall is not completely removed.

AVERAGE HOSPITAL STAY—Usually none.

PROBABLE OUTCOME—Expect complete healing without complications. Allow about 2 to 3 weeks for healing to be fairly complete.

 POSTOPERATIVE CARE

GENERAL MEASURES
- If the wound bleeds during the first 24 hours after surgery, press a clean tissue or cloth to it for 10 minutes.
- A hard ridge should form along the incision. As it heals, the ridge will gradually recede.
- Shower as usual. Avoid baths until the incision has completely healed. You may wash the incision gently with mild, unscented soap. After showering, replace any wet dressings with clean, dry ones.
- Keep the wound dry with a bandage for the first 2 days after surgery. If a bandage gets wet, change it promptly.
- Apply nonprescription antibiotic ointment to the wound before applying bandages.

MEDICATION
- Your doctor may prescribe antibiotics to fight or prevent infection.
- You may use nonprescription drugs, such as acetaminophen, for minor pain. Avoid aspirin.

ACTIVITY—Usually no limits unless advised by your doctor..

DIET—No special diet.

 CALL YOUR DOCTOR IF

- Pain, swelling, redness, drainage, or bleeding increases in the surgical area.
- You develop symptoms of infection including headache, muscle aches, dizziness, fever, or a general ill feeling.

SEBACEOUS CYST REMOVAL
(Epidermoid Cyst Removal)

An illustration of a typical sebaceous cyst. In this case, on the side of the face.

Sebaceous cyst

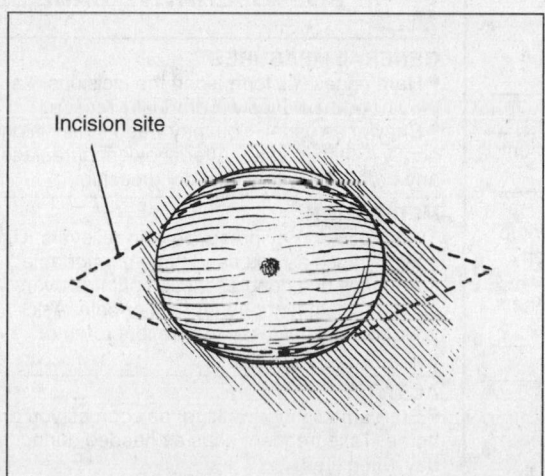

An incision is made over the cyst with care taken not to rupture its capsule (soft tissue lining the surface of the cyst).

Incision site

The cyst and its contents are removed intact.

SENTINEL NODE BIOPSY

 GENERAL INFORMATION

DEFINITION—Removal of one or more lymph nodes usually in the axilla (armpit) to assess the possible spread of cancer. This is most frequently done with breast cancer but is also done with melanoma and several other solid cancers. The sentinel node is the lymph node where the cancer cells are most likely to go.

BODY PARTS INVOLVED—Axillary lymph nodes. Occasionally groin, chest, or intraabdominal lymph nodes.

REASONS FOR SURGERY—To identify any spread of cancer cells which assists in staging (describing the extent of cancer) and treating the disease.

SURGICAL RISK INCREASES WITH
- Age.
- Diabetes.
- Obesity.

 WHAT TO EXPECT

WHO OPERATES—General surgeon.

WHERE PERFORMED—Hospital or outpatient surgical center.

DIAGNOSTIC TESTS
- Before surgery: Only those needed to workup primary cancer. EKG (see Glossary) in elderly patients or previous history of heart disease.
- After surgery: Laboratory examination of the removed node(s).

ANESTHESIA—General anesthesia.

DESCRIPTION OF OPERATION
- The sentinel node can be identified by a radioactive marker or with a blue dye. Frequently both methods are employed to increase the accuracy.
- Prior to surgery a radioactive substance is injected around the tumor or the area where the tumor was removed. In the breast it is sometimes injected around the nipple. A scan may be done to track the progress of the radioactive material.
- After general anesthesia, a blue dye is injected and an incision is made in the nodal area of concern. A probe is used to track and locate a node which has collected the greatest amount of radioactive substance and the blue dye is tracked in addition, usually to the same one or few nodes.

- The identified node(s) are removed and sent for immediate review by the pathologist. If no cancer cells are seen, the wound is closed. If cancer cells are detected, the rest of the lymph nodes in the area are also removed and examined routinely over the next day or two. A drain may be left if all of the nodes are removed.

POSSIBLE COMPLICATIONS
- Prolonged drainage of serum in the area of surgery.
- Infection of the surgical site.
- Numbness in the surrounding region or possible nerve damage.
- Swelling of the extremity.

AVERAGE HOSPITAL STAY—Usually performed as an outpatient.

PROBABLE OUTCOME—Expect full recovery in 3-4 weeks.

 POSTOPERATIVE CARE

GENERAL MEASURES
- Hard ridges will form along the incisions. As they heal, the ridges will gradually recede.
- Shower as usual. You may wash the incisions gently with mild soap. After showering, replace any dressings with a new dry dressing.

MEDICATION
- Your doctor may prescribe pain relievers. Use only as much as you need to be comfortable.
- You may use nonprescription pain relievers such as acetaminophen for minor pain. Ask your doctor if it is okay to take ibuprofen or aspirin.

ACTIVITY
- Start ambulating (walking) as soon as you are home. Take frequent naps as needed during the day when tired.
- You may swim once all sutures are out.
- Resume sexual relations when comfortable and when advised by your surgeon.

DIET—No special diet.

 CALL YOUR DOCTOR IF

- Pain, swelling, redness, drainage, or bleeding increases in the surgical area.
- You develop symptoms of infection including headache, muscle aches, dizziness, fever, or a general ill feeling.
- Arm becomes cold, numb, painful, or swollen.
- New unexplained symptoms develop.

SENTINEL NODE BIOPSY

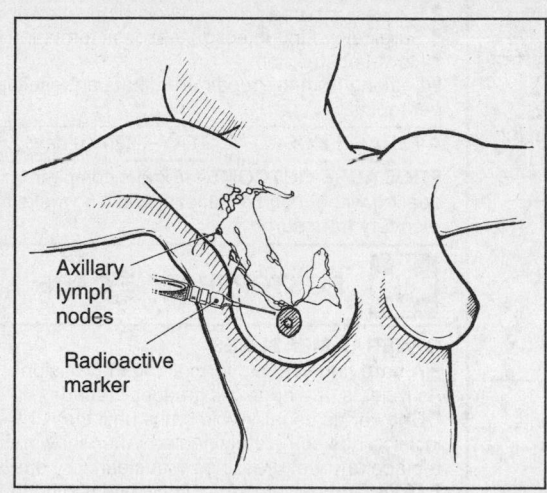

Blue dye and/or a radioactive marker are injected near the tumor or around the areola.

Axillary lymph nodes

Radioactive marker

A probe similar to a Geiger counter is used to locate lymph nodes that take up the radioactive marker.

Probe

Axilla

The lymph node(s) containing radioactive marker and/or blue dye is carefully dissected free from the surrounding tissue and examined for cancer cells.

Sentinel node

SIGMOID COLON REMOVAL
(Colectomy)

GENERAL INFORMATION

DEFINITION—Removal of part or all of the sigmoid colon.

BODY PARTS INVOLVED—Sigmoid colon, the part of the large intestine (colon) that extends from the descending colon to the rectum.

REASONS FOR SURGERY
- Diverticulitis with bleeding or infection.
- Cancer or precancerous polyps.
- Volvulus (see Glossary).
- Colon stricture.
- Colovaginal fistula.
- Prolapse of rectum.

SURGICAL RISK INCREASES WITH
- Adults over 60 years, newborns, and infants.
- Obesity or smoking.
- Poor nutrition.
- Excess alcohol consumption.
- Chronic illness or recent illness such as acute, recurrent diverticulitis.
- Diabetes.
- Use of some prescription and nonprescription drugs. Inform your doctor of any drugs, medications, or vitamin and herb supplements you are using or have used in the last month.

WHAT TO EXPECT

WHO OPERATES—General surgeon.

WHERE PERFORMED—Hospital.

DIAGNOSTIC TESTS
- Before surgery: Blood and urine studies, x-rays of upper and lower gastrointestinal tract, ECG, endoscopy, proctoscopy, colonoscopy (see Glossary for all).
- After surgery: Blood studies.

ANESTHESIA—General anesthesia by injection and inhalation with an airway tube placed in the windpipe.

DESCRIPTION OF OPERATION
- An incision is made in the abdomen, and the abdominal muscles are opened.
- The sigmoid colon is isolated and clamps are placed at each end.
- All of the diseased sigmoid colon is cut free and removed. The two healthy ends are brought back together and joined.
- The abdominal contents are replaced into the abdomen, and the muscles are closed. The skin is closed with sutures or skin clips, which usually can be removed about 1 week after surgery.
- If surgery is performed to treat infection or tumor, a temporary colostomy (see Surgery section) may be necessary.

POSSIBLE COMPLICATIONS
- Excessive bleeding, deep-vein blood clots.
- Surgical-wound infection, abscess formation.
- Bowel obstruction.
- Leaking from the repair area that can result in peritonitis.

AVERAGE HOSPITAL STAY—7 to 10 days.

PROBABLE OUTCOME—Expect complete healing without complications. Allow 6 weeks for recovery from surgery.

POSTOPERATIVE CARE

GENERAL MEASURES
- A hard ridge should form along the incision. As it heals, the ridge will gradually recede.
- Shower as usual. Avoid baths until the incision has completely healed. After showering, replace any wet dressings with clean, dry ones.
- Move and elevate legs often while resting in bed to help decrease the likelihood of deep-vein clots.

MEDICATION
- Your doctor may prescribe:
  - Pain relievers. Don't take prescription pain medication longer than 4 to 7 days. Use only as much as you need.
  - Stool softeners to prevent constipation.
  - Antibiotics to fight or prevent infection.
- You may use nonprescription drugs, such as acetaminophen, for minor pain. Avoid aspirin.

ACTIVITY
- Resume daily activities slowly as you recover. Do not overexert yourself.
- Avoid heavy lifting or vigorous exercise for 6 weeks after surgery.
- Resume driving 3 weeks after returning home.
- Resume sexual relations when able.

DIET—Nasogastric suction is used initially, followed by clear liquid diet until the gastrointestinal tract functions again. Then, eat a well-balanced diet to promote healing.

CALL YOUR DOCTOR IF

- You experience nausea, vomiting, abdominal cramps, or bloating.
- Pain, swelling, redness, drainage, or bleeding increases in the surgical area.
- You develop symptoms of infection including headache, muscle aches, dizziness, fever, or a general ill feeling.
- New, unexplained symptoms develop.

SIGMOID COLON REMOVAL
(Colectomy)

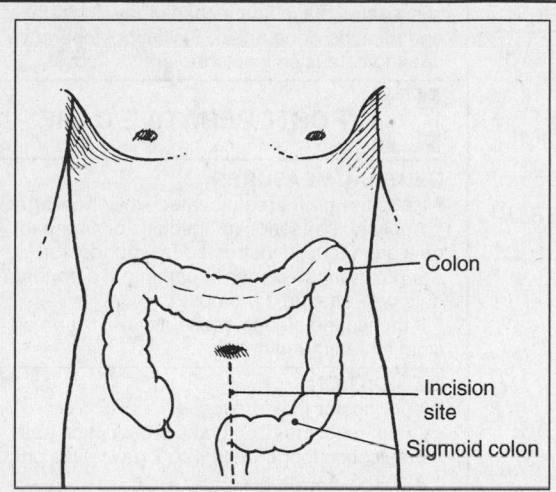

An illustration of the large intestine, sigmoid colon and the usual incision site for this surgical procedure.

Colon

Incision site

Sigmoid colon

- The sigmoid colon is isolated and clamps are placed at each end.
- All of the diseased sigmoid colon is cut free and removed.

Sigmoid colon

Cancerous tumor

The two healthy ends of the colon are repositioned and joined whenever possible.

Anus

SKIN GRAFT

GENERAL INFORMATION

DEFINITION—Taking skin from one area of the body and attaching it to another area where no skin exists.

BODY PARTS INVOLVED—Skin (donor sites and recipient sites).

REASONS FOR SURGERY—Extensive wounds, burns, or certain surgeries may require skin grafts for healing to occur.

SURGICAL RISK INCREASES WITH
- Adults over 60.
- Newborns and infants.
- Obesity, smoking.
- Poor nutrition.
- Anemia.
- Recent or chronic illness.
- Diabetes.
- Use of some prescription and nonprescription drugs. Inform your doctor of any drugs, medications, or vitamin and herb supplements you are using or have used in the last month.

WHAT TO EXPECT

WHO OPERATES—General surgeon or plastic and reconstructive surgeon.

WHERE PERFORMED—Hospital, outpatient surgical facility, or emergency room (rarely).

DIAGNOSTIC TESTS
- Before surgery: Blood and urine studies.
- After surgery: Blood studies.

ANESTHESIA
- Local anesthesia by injection.
- General anesthesia by injection and inhalation with an airway tube placed in the windpipe.

DESCRIPTION OF OPERATION
- Skin is removed from a donor site. The donor site is covered with gauze.
- Debris is cleared from the recipient site.
- The skin from the donor site is placed on the recipient site and fastened at each corner with sutures. Bandages are applied. New blood vessels begin growing from the recipient area into the transplanted skin within 36 hours.

POSSIBLE COMPLICATIONS
- Excessive bleeding.
- Surgical-wound infection.
- Collection of serum under recipient site that prevents growth of new blood vessels.
- Loss of grafted skin.

AVERAGE HOSPITAL STAY—2 to 12 days, depending on extent of surgery.

PROBABLE OUTCOME—Allow about 6 weeks for recovery from surgery. Most skin grafts are successful, but in some cases they don't "take" and must be done again. Skillful postoperative nursing care is critical to the graft's success.

POSTOPERATIVE CARE

GENERAL MEASURES
- Keep the graft area elevated while healing.
- Apply nonprescription antibiotic ointment to new bandages, if instructed by your doctor. Keep bandages dry while bathing. If a bandage gets wet, change it promptly.
- If the wound bleeds, press a clean tissue or cloth to it for 10 minutes.

MEDICATION
- Your doctor may prescribe:
  - Pain relievers. Don't take prescription pain medication longer than 4 to 7 days. Use only as much as you need.
  - Antibiotics to fight or prevent infection.
- You may use nonprescription drugs, such as acetaminophen, for minor pain. Avoid aspirin.

ACTIVITY
- Minimize movement of the graft site until healing is complete.
- Avoid vigorous exercise for 6 weeks following surgery (or as advised).
- Resume driving 1 week after returning home.

DIET—No special diet.

CALL YOUR DOCTOR IF

- You have pain, swelling, redness, drainage, bleeding, or odor in the surgical area.
- You develop symptoms of infection including headache, muscle aches, dizziness, fever, or a general ill feeling.
- You have persistent weakness.
- Your dressings accidentally get wet.
- New, unexplained symptoms develop.

SKIN GRAFT

Donor skin

A thin layer of skin to be used for grafting is removed with a dermatome (skin cutting instrument).

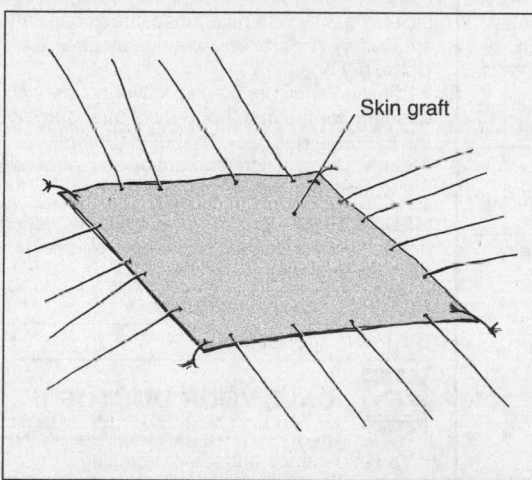

Skin graft

After skin has been removed from donor site, it is placed over the recipient site and fastened to normal skin around the periphery.

Pressure bandages are applied over the skin graft. The new blood vessels begin growing from the recipient area into the transplanted skin within 36 hours.

SKIN LESION REMOVAL

 GENERAL INFORMATION

DEFINITION—Removal or ablation of any benign or cancerous lesion on the skin.

BODY PARTS INVOLVED—Abnormal growth on the skin. The most common are warts, moles, skin cancers, molluscum contagiosum, or actinic keratosis.

REASONS FOR SURGERY
- Diagnosis of the abnormal growth.
- Removal of any abnormality suspected to be cancerous.
- Concern about appearance.
- Irritation of the lesion due to clothing.

SURGICAL RISK INCREASES WITH
- Adults over 60.
- Obesity, poor nutrition, anemia.
- Recent or chronic illness, diabetes.
- Use of some prescription and nonprescription drugs. Inform your doctor of any drugs, medications, or vitamin and herb supplements you are using or have used in the last month.

 WHAT TO EXPECT

WHO OPERATES—Family doctor, dermatologist, general surgeon, or plastic and reconstructive surgeon.

WHERE PERFORMED—Hospital, emergency room, doctor's office, or outpatient surgical facility.

DIAGNOSTIC TESTS
- Before surgery: Blood and urine studies.
- After surgery: Laboratory examination of removed tissue.

ANESTHESIA
- Local anesthesia by injection.
- General anesthesia by injection and inhalation with an airway tube placed in the windpipe (for large excisions, skin grafts, or for procedures on young children).

DESCRIPTION OF OPERATION
- There are different techniques to remove or ablate abnormal growths from the skin.
- Scraping the abnormality away (curettement).
- Cutting with scissors, especially if the lesion is on a stalk.
- Freezing (cryotherapy) warts and benign superficial keratoses.
- Using heat (electrosurgery).
- Incising the skin with a cold scalpel, removing the lesion and sewing the skin edges together.
- The technique chosen depends on the nature of the lesion and the condition of the patient. If sutures or clips are used to close the wound, they can usually be removed about 1 week after surgery.
- Skin grafting is sometimes required.

POSSIBLE COMPLICATIONS
- Excessive bleeding.
- Surgical-wound infection.
- Recurrent skin cancer.
- Excessive scarring (keloid).

AVERAGE HOSPITAL STAY—None.

PROBABLE OUTCOME—Expect complete healing without complications. Allow about 2 weeks for recovery from surgery.

 POSTOPERATIVE CARE

GENERAL MEASURES
- If the wound bleeds during the first 24 hours after surgery, press a clean tissue or cloth to it for 10 minutes.
- If an incision was made, a hard ridge should form along the incision. As it heals, the ridge will gradually recede.
- Shower as usual. Avoid baths until the wound has completely healed. You may wash the incision gently with mild, unscented soap. After showering, replace any wet dressings with clean, dry ones.
- Between showers, keep the wound dry with a bandage for the first 2 or 3 days after surgery. If the bandage gets wet, change it promptly.
- Apply a nonprescription antibiotic ointment to the wound before applying bandages.

MEDICATION—You may use nonprescription drugs, such as acetaminophen, to relieve minor pain. Avoid aspirin.

ACTIVITY—Usually, no limits.

DIET—No special diet.

 CALL YOUR DOCTOR IF

- You experience nausea or vomiting.
- Pain, swelling, redness, drainage, or bleeding increases in the surgical area.
- You develop symptoms of infection including headache, muscle aches, dizziness, fever, or a general ill feeling.

SKIN LESION REMOVAL

An illustration of a skin lesion on the neck to be removed surgically.

Lesion

An incision is made around the lesion in an elllpse for easier closure.

The skin is closed and a bandage has been applied.

SMALL-BOWEL RESECTION

GENERAL INFORMATION

DEFINITION—Removal of diseased, injured, or abnormal section of the small bowel (small intestine).

BODY PARTS INVOLVED—Small intestine, including the mesentery (blood supply) around it.

REASONS FOR SURGERY
- Tumor, gangrene, narrowing or obstruction in the small intestine.
- Trauma, such as from a wound.

SURGICAL RISK INCREASES WITH
- Adults over 60.
- Obesity.
- Smoking.
- Poor nutrition.
- Previous abdominal surgery.
- Recent or chronic illness.
- Diabetes.
- Use of some prescription and nonprescription drugs. Inform your doctor of any drugs, medications, or vitamin and herb supplements you are using or have used in the last month.

WHAT TO EXPECT

WHO OPERATES—General surgeon.

WHERE PERFORMED—Hospital.

DIAGNOSTIC TESTS
- Before surgery: Blood and urine studies, x-rays of chest and gastrointestinal tract, CT, MRI, colonoscopy (see Glossary for all).
- After surgery: Blood studies.

ANESTHESIA
- Spinal anesthesia by injection.
- General anesthesia by injection and inhalation with an airway tube placed in the windpipe.

DESCRIPTION OF OPERATION
- Operative procedures will vary depending on the cause.
- An incision is made in the abdomen.
- The muscles are separated or cut, and the abdominal cavity is entered.
- The intestine is examined for disease.
- The small intestine is clamped above and below the diseased section. The diseased section between the clamps is cut free and removed.
- The two open ends of the remaining small bowel are fastened together with sutures or staples. Occasionally, a temporary ileostomy (see Surgery section) is necessary.
- The peritoneum and muscles are closed with sutures. The skin is closed with sutures or clips, which usually can be removed about 1 week after surgery.

POSSIBLE COMPLICATIONS
- Excessive bleeding.
- Deep-vein blood clots.
- Abscess formation.
- Surgical-wound infection.
- Leak where bowel is put back together.
- Recurrence of intestinal obstructions caused by adhesions.

AVERAGE HOSPITAL STAY—7 to 10 days.

PROBABLE OUTCOME—Expect complete healing of surgical wound. Allow about 6 weeks for recovery from surgery.

POSTOPERATIVE CARE

GENERAL MEASURES
- A hard ridge should form along the incision. As it heals, the ridge will gradually recede.
- Shower as usual. Avoid baths until the incision has completely healed. You may wash the incision gently with mild, unscented soap. After showering, replace any wet dressings with clean, dry ones.
- Move and elevate legs often while resting in bed to decrease the likelihood of deep-vein blood clots.

MEDICATION
- Your doctor may prescribe:
  - Pain relievers. Don't take prescription pain medication longer than 4 to 7 days. Use only as much as you need.
  - Stool softeners to prevent constipation.
  - Antibiotics to fight or prevent infection.
- You may use nonprescription drugs, such as acetaminophen, for minor pain. Avoid aspirin.

ACTIVITY
- Resume daily activities slowly as you recover. Do not overexert yourself.
- Avoid vigorous exercise for 6 weeks after surgery.
- Resume driving 3 weeks after returning home.
- Resume sexual relations when you feel able to.

DIET—Intravenous feeding with nasogastric suctioning for several days, then return slowly to a diet your doctor will prescribe.

CALL YOUR DOCTOR IF

- Pain, swelling, redness, drainage, or bleeding increases in the surgical area.
- You develop symptoms of infection including headache, muscle aches, dizziness, fever, or a general ill feeling.
- You experience nausea, vomiting, abdominal swelling, constipation, or bloody or tarry stools.
- New, unexplained symptoms develop.

SMALL-BOWEL RESECTION

An illustration of a typical incision site for small bowel removal.

Incision site

Small bowel

- After the abdominal muscles are separated, the abdominal cavity is entered and the intestinal tract is examined for disease.
- The small intestine is clamped above and below the diseased section. The diseased section between the clamps is cut free and removed.

The 2 open ends of the remaining small bowel are fastened together with sutures or staples.

Stapler

SPINAL TAP
(Lumbar Puncture)

 GENERAL INFORMATION

DEFINITION—Removal of spinal fluid from the spinal canal, either for laboratory analysis or prior to surgery with spinal anesthesia.

BODY PARTS INVOLVED—Skin, muscles, covering of spinal cord (meninges), vertebral column.

REASONS FOR SURGERY
- Diagnosis of disorders of the central nervous system that may involve the brain, spinal cord, or their coverings.
- Injection of spinal anesthesia.
- Myelogram (see Glossary).

SURGICAL RISK INCREASES WITH
- Recent or chronic illness.
- Alcoholism.
- Increased intracranial pressure due to any cause.
- Central nervous system infection.
- Severe arthritis in spine.
- Diabetes.
- Use of some prescription and nonprescription drugs. Inform your doctor of any drugs, medications, or vitamin and herb supplements you are using or have used in the last month.

 WHAT TO EXPECT

WHO OPERATES—General surgeon, family doctor, anesthesiologist, neurologist, neurosurgeon, or internist.

WHERE PERFORMED—Hospital, outpatient surgical facility, or emergency room.

DIAGNOSTIC TESTS
- Before surgery: Blood and urine studies.
- During surgery: Pressure of spinal fluid measured with a manometer (see Glossary).
- After surgery: Laboratory examination of removed fluid.

ANESTHESIA—Local anesthesia by injection.

DESCRIPTION OF OPERATION
- The patient is positioned on his side with the knees drawn as close to the chest as possible.
- A hollow needle is inserted in the back between the 2nd and 3rd lumbar vertebrae.
- The spinal canal is penetrated with the needle. Fluid pressure is measured and then fluid is removed.
- The surgical wound will heal by itself.

POSSIBLE COMPLICATIONS
- Surgical wound infection.
- Headaches (common during the first 24 hours after the procedure).
- Meningitis (rare).

AVERAGE HOSPITAL STAY—Usually 6 to 24 hours in the surgical facility.

PROBABLE OUTCOME—Expect complete healing without complications.

 POSTOPERATIVE CARE

GENERAL MEASURES—Moving the head and neck as little as possible for 12 hours after surgery helps prevent headache. Resume activity slowly.

MEDICATION
- Your doctor may prescribe pain relievers. Don't take prescription pain medication longer than 4 to 7 days. Use only as much as you need.
- You may use nonprescription drugs, such as acetaminophen, for minor pain. Avoid aspirin.

ACTIVITY
- Avoid vigorous exercise for 2 weeks after surgery.
- Resume driving 3 days after returning home.

DIET—No special diet. Increase fluid intake to help prevent post-spinal-tap headaches.

 CALL YOUR DOCTOR IF

- Pain, swelling, redness, drainage, or bleeding increases in the needle insertion area.
- You develop symptoms of infection including headache, muscle aches, dizziness, fever, or a general ill feeling.
- You experience nausea or vomiting.
- You develop pain or stiffness in your neck.
- New, unexplained symptoms develop.

SPINAL TAP
(Lumbar Puncture)

An illustration of a typical needle insertion site and the mid-spine.

Needle insertion site

The needle is inserted between sinus processes of the bone into the cavity of the spinal canal, which surrounds the spine and is filled with fluid.

The spinal canal is penetrated with the needle. The fluid pressure is measured, then fluid is removed for laboratory examination.

SPLEEN REMOVAL
(Splenectomy)

GENERAL INFORMATION

DEFINITION—Removal of the spleen.

BODY PARTS INVOLVED—The spleen, a large organ on the left side of the upper abdominal cavity next to the stomach.

REASONS FOR SURGERY
- Injury to the spleen causing rupture and bleeding.
- Various blood diseases, including spherocytosis, thrombocytopenia or lymphatic leukemia (see Glossary for all).
- Splenic-vein thrombosis caused by esophageal varices (see Glossary).
- Benign or cancerous tumors.

SURGICAL RISK INCREASES WITH
- Adults over 60.
- Newborns and infants.
- Obesity.
- Smoking.
- Excess alcohol consumption.
- Poor nutrition.
- Recent or chronic illness.
- Diabetes.
- Use of some prescription and nonprescription drugs. Inform your doctor of any drugs, medications, or vitamin and herb supplements you are using or have used in the last month.

WHAT TO EXPECT

WHO OPERATES—General surgeon.

WHERE PERFORMED—Hospital.

DIAGNOSTIC TESTS
- Before surgery: Blood and urine studies, x-rays of abdomen, CT scan (see Glossary).
- After surgery: Blood studies.

ANESTHESIA—General anesthesia by injection and inhalation with an airway tube placed in the windpipe.

DESCRIPTION OF OPERATION
- An incision is made in the abdomen.
- The spleen is located and isolated.
- Blood vessels to the spleen are cut and tied off.
- The spleen is rotated and removed from its bed where it is attached to the coverings of the stomach, kidney and diaphragm (see Glossary).
- If the spleen has been ruptured, the abdomen is explored to identify any other injured organs or blood vessels. Other surgeries may be performed at this time.
- The muscles are closed in layers. The skin is closed with sutures or skin clips, which usually can be removed in about 1 week.

POSSIBLE COMPLICATIONS
- Excessive bleeding.
- Infection, especially in young children.
- Incisional hernia.
- Atelectasis (see Glossary).
- Pancreatitis (see Glossary).
- Deep-vein blood clots.
- Pneumonia.

AVERAGE HOSPITAL STAY—3 to 5 days.

PROBABLE OUTCOME—Expect complete healing without complications. Allow about 4 weeks for recovery from surgery.

POSTOPERATIVE CARE

GENERAL MEASURES
- A hard ridge should form along the incision. As it heals, the ridge will gradually recede.
- Shower as usual. Avoid baths until the incision has completely healed. You may wash the incision gently with mild, unscented soap. After showering, replace any wet dressings with clean, dry ones.

MEDICATION
- Your doctor may prescribe:
  - Pain relievers. Don't take prescription pain medication longer than 4 to 7 days. Use only as much as you need.
  - Antibiotics to fight or prevent infection.
  - Stool softeners to prevent constipation.
  - Pneumonia vaccinations.
- You may use nonprescription drugs, such as acetaminophen, for minor pain. Avoid aspirin.

ACTIVITY
- Resume daily activities slowly as you recover. Do not overexert yourself.
- Avoid vigorous exercise for 6 weeks after surgery.
- Resume sexual relations when your doctor determines that healing is complete.
- Resume driving 4 weeks after returning home.

DIET—Clear liquid diet until the gastrointestinal tract functions again. Then eat a well-balanced diet to promote healing. Increase dietary fiber and fluid intake to help prevent constipation.

CALL YOUR DOCTOR IF

- You develop symptoms of infection including headache, muscle aches, dizziness, fever, or a general ill feeling.
- Pain, swelling, redness, drainage, or bleeding increases in the surgical area.
- New, unexplained symptoms develop.

SPLEEN REMOVAL
(Splenectomy)

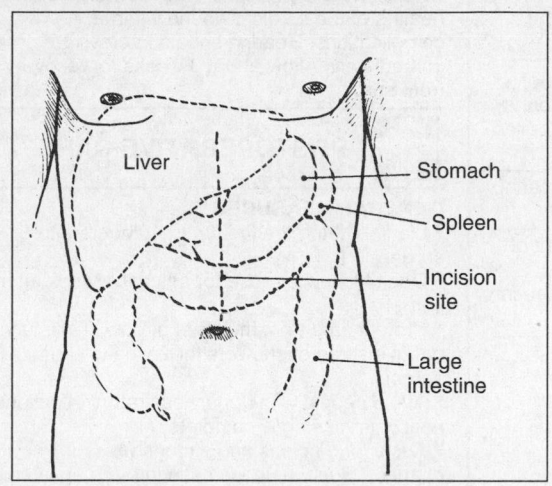

An illustration of the spleen, other internal organs and the usual incision site for a spleen removal. An alternate incision is under the left rib cage.

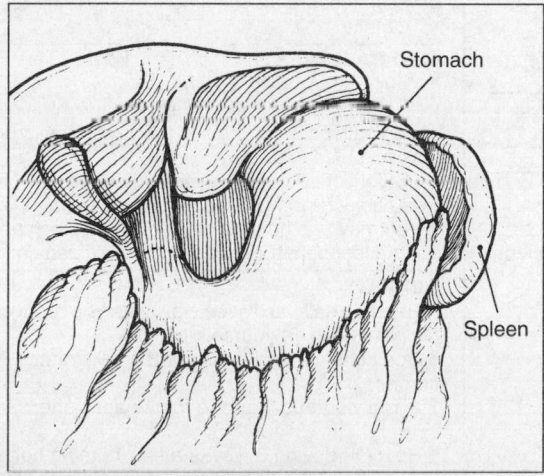

The spleen is rotated and removed from its bed where it's attached to the coverings of the stomach, kidney and diaphragm.

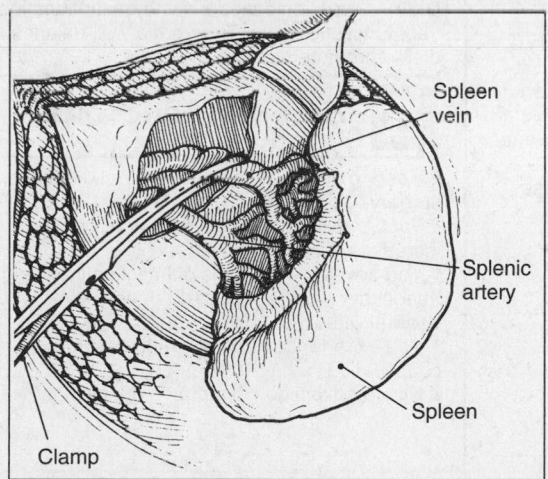

Blood vessels that supply the spleen are clamped and tied and the spleen is removed.

STAPES REMOVAL
(Stapedectomy)

GENERAL INFORMATION

DEFINITION—Removal of the stapes, one of the bones in the middle ear that transmit sound waves to the inner ear. The stapes is also called the stirrup.

BODY PARTS INVOLVED—External ear canal, eardrum, middle ear, stapes.

REASONS FOR SURGERY—Improvement of hearing ability or prevention of continued hearing loss, usually due to otosclerosis (see in Illness section).

SURGICAL RISK INCREASES WITH
- Obesity.
- Smoking.
- Poor nutrition.
- Recent or chronic illness.
- Diabetes.
- Use of some prescription and nonprescription drugs. Inform your doctor of any drugs, medications, or vitamin and herb supplements you are using or have used in the last month.

WHAT TO EXPECT

WHO OPERATES—Ear, nose and throat specialist (otolaryngologist).

WHERE PERFORMED—Hospital or outpatient surgical facility.

DIAGNOSTIC TESTS
- Before surgery: Blood and urine studies, hearing tests.
- After surgery: Hearing tests.

ANESTHESIA—General anesthesia by injection and inhalation with an airway tube placed in the windpipe.

DESCRIPTION OF OPERATION
- If both ears are affected, surgery is usually done on separate occasions.
- The operating microscope is positioned, and an incision is made in the middle ear.
- The small bones in the ear are identified, and the stapes is isolated and removed.
- Sometimes, a prosthesis made of stainless steel wire and cellulose sponge is inserted to replace the stapes.
- Blood and fluid are suctioned gently from the ear.
- The wound is closed with fine sutures, which can usually be removed about 1 week after surgery.

POSSIBLE COMPLICATIONS
- Excessive bleeding.
- Surgical-wound infection.

AVERAGE HOSPITAL STAY—3 to 5 days.

PROBABLE OUTCOME—Expect complete healing of the surgical wound without complications. Hearing should improve immediately. Allow about 3 weeks for recovery from surgery.

POSTOPERATIVE CARE

GENERAL MEASURES
- Lie flat during the first 24 to 48 hours after surgery.
- Don't blow your nose for at least 1 week after surgery.
- Protect ears from moisture or cold. Take tub baths instead of showers for 2 weeks after surgery.
- Avoid people with upper-respiratory infections until your healing is complete.
- Avoid loud noises and sudden pressure changes, such as those caused by flying in non-pressurized aircraft or scuba diving, for the rest of your life.

MEDICATION
- Your doctor may prescribe:
  - Pain relievers. Don't take prescription pain medication longer than 4 to 7 days. Use only as much as you need.
  - Stool softeners to prevent constipation.
  - Antibiotics to fight or prevent infection.
- You may use nonprescription drugs, such as acetaminophen, for minor pain. Avoid aspirin.

ACTIVITY
- Resume daily activities slowly as you recover. Do not overexert yourself.
- Don't strain, bend, or lift for 3 weeks after surgery.
- Avoid vigorous exercise for 6 weeks after surgery.
- Resume driving 3 weeks after returning home.

DIET—Clear liquid diet until the gastrointestinal tract functions again. Then eat a well-balanced diet to promote healing.

CALL YOUR DOCTOR IF

- Hearing does not improve within 2 days after surgery.
- Pain, swelling, redness, drainage, or bleeding increases in the surgical area.
- You develop symptoms of infection including headache, muscle aches, dizziness, fever, or a general ill feeling.
- You experience nausea, vomiting, or constipation.
- New, unexplained symptoms develop.

STAPES REMOVAL
(Stapedectomy)

An illustration of the outer ear, middle ear and the stapes (one of the bones in the middle ear that transmits sound waves to the inner ear). The stapes is also called the stirrup.

Middle ear

Stapes

Appearance of the middle ear structure as seen through an operating microscope. Small bones in the ear are identified and the stapes is isolated and removed.

Stapes with defect

Sometimes a prosthesis made of stainless steel wire and cellulose sponge is inserted to replace the defective stapes.

Prosthesis

STEM CELL TRANSPLANT

GENERAL INFORMATION

DEFINITION—Transplantation of stem cells (see Glossary) from a donor for introduction into the bloodstream of a recipient. The donor may be a different person than the recipient (allogenic transplant), or may be the same person as the recipient (autologous transplant). The topic of stem cell transplantation is a very complicated one and the information contained herein provides only an overview of the subject. Consult your doctor for additional information.

BODY PARTS INVOLVED—The subclavian vein or internal jugular vein of the donor and the recipient.

REASONS FOR SURGERY
- Replacement of stem cells which have become weakened or been destroyed due to causes such as:
  - Acute leukemia or aplastic anemia.
  - Multiple myeloma.
  - High dose chemotherapy for treatment of cancer.

SURGICAL RISK INCREASES WITH
- Both donor and recipient:
  - Obesity, smoking, poor nutrition.
  - Recent or chronic illness, diabetes.
  - Use of some prescription and nonprescription drugs. Inform your doctor of any drugs, medications, or vitamin and herb supplements you are using or have used in the last month.

WHAT TO EXPECT

WHO OPERATES—Specially trained oncologist or hematologist. Catheter in vein is placed by surgeon or anesthesiologist.

WHERE PERFORMED—Hospital or outpatient surgical facility.

DIAGNOSTIC TESTS
- Before surgery: Blood studies of both donor and recipient.
- After surgery: Blood studies in recipient to determine success of transplant.

ANESTHESIA—Local anesthetic for catheter placement.

DESCRIPTION OF OPERATION
- Before surgery, the donor is examined for communicable diseases.
- Stem cells are usually removed through venous access lines which are placed in surgery under local anesthesia and heavy sedation.
- The stem cells are filtered and then injected into the recipient's vein.

POSSIBLE COMPLICATIONS
- Donor: None expected.
- Recipient:
  - Rejection of transplanted stem cells.
  - Uncontrolled infections.
  - Bleeding problems.
  - Anemia.
  - If the transplant is autologous (from oneself), there is a possibility of receiving cancer cells back in the new marrow, especially in leukemia.

AVERAGE HOSPITAL STAY
- Donor: Outpatient.
- Recipient: Varies from outpatient to several months.

PROBABLE OUTCOME
- Donor: Expect complete healing without complications.
- Recipient: Survival rate depends on disease process involved.

POSTOPERATIVE CARE

GENERAL MEASURES—The recipient should be isolated from attendants, family, and visitors to protect the recipient from infection.

MEDICATION—
- Donor may be prescribed:
  - Pain relievers. Don't take prescription pain medication longer than 4 to 7 days. Use only as much as you need.
  - Antibiotics to fight or prevent infection.
  - You may use nonprescription drugs, such as acetaminophen, for minor pain. Avoid aspirin.
- Recipient may be prescribed:
  - Immunosuppressant drugs to prevent rejection of bone marrow.
  - Antibiotics to fight or prevent infection.

ACTIVITY—For both donor and recipient:
- Resume daily activities as you are able.
- Avoid vigorous exercise for 6 weeks after surgery or as advised by doctor.

DIET—Eat a well-balanced diet to promote healing.

CALL YOUR DOCTOR IF

- For both donor and recipient:
  - You experience nausea or vomiting, or develop a rash or flushing.
  - You develop symptoms of infection including headache, muscle aches, dizziness, fever, or a general ill feeling.
  - You experience bleeding from your gums or other unusual bleeding.
  - New, unexplained symptoms develop.

STEM CELL TRANSPLANT

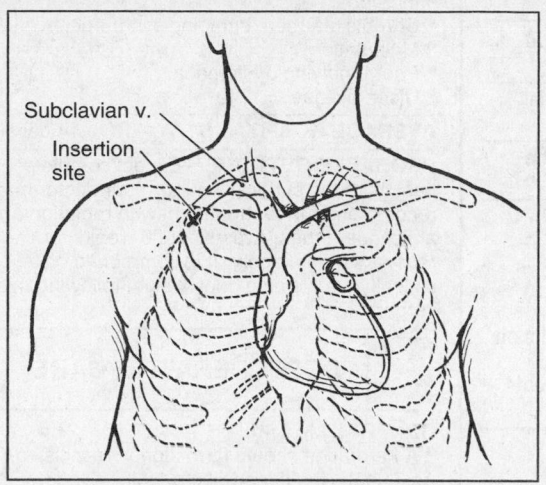

Illustration showing anatomy of region catheter is usually placed.

Subclavian v.

Insertion site

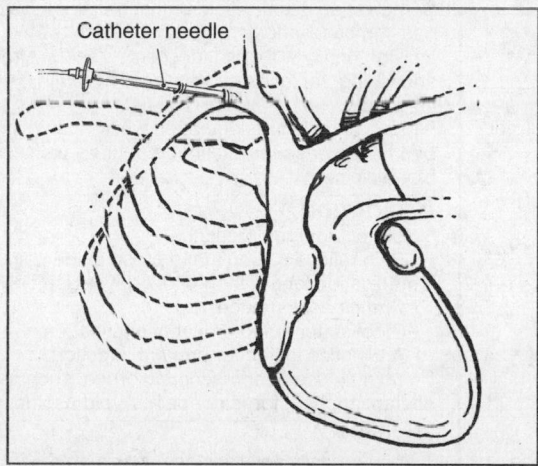

Catheter needle

The subclavian vein is punctured with a needle and a soft plastic catheter is threaded into the vein.

The catheter is used to withdraw blood for stem cells and replace unused portions of the blood.

Central catheter

STOMACH CANCER SURGERY

 GENERAL INFORMATION

DEFINITION—Removal of cancerous tissue (gastric carcinoma) in the stomach.

BODY PARTS INVOLVED—Stomach, small intestine, esophagus (sometimes).

REASONS FOR SURGERY—Cancer of the stomach.

SURGICAL RISK INCREASES WITH
- Adults over 60.
- Obesity, poor nutrition, smoking.
- Alcoholism.
- Recent or chronic illness, diabetes.
- Use of some prescription and nonprescription drugs. Inform your doctor of any drugs, medications, or vitamin and herb supplements you are using or have used in the last month.

 WHAT TO EXPECT

WHO OPERATES—General surgeon.

WHERE PERFORMED—Hospital.

DIAGNOSTIC TESTS
- Before surgery: X-rays of gastrointestinal tract and chest, blood and urine studies, ECG, endoscopy, CT scan (see Glossary for all).
- During surgery: Laboratory examination of removed tissue by frozen section (see Glossary).
- After surgery: Blood studies, laboratory examination of removed tissue.

ANESTHESIA—General anesthesia by injection and inhalation with an airway tube placed in the windpipe.

DESCRIPTION OF OPERATION
- An incision is made below the ribs.
- Abdominal muscles are cut or retracted, the peritoneum is opened and the stomach is isolated.
- Usually, the entire stomach is removed. The esophagus is attached to a pouch made of small intestine, to create a new "stomach." The nearby lymph nodes and omentum (see Glossary) are removed; sometimes the spleen is also removed.
- If any stomach is left, the remaining stump of stomach is joined to a loop of small intestine (usually the jejunum) for normal digestive flow.
- The peritoneum is closed and the muscles are sewn together. The skin is closed with sutures or clips, which usually can be removed about 10 days after surgery.

POSSIBLE COMPLICATIONS
- Excessive bleeding; surgical-wound infection.
- Incisional hernia.
- Chronic diarrhea, dumping syndrome.
- Malnutrition.
- Poor emptying of stomach.
- Ulcer disease.

AVERAGE HOSPITAL STAY—10 to 14 days.

PROBABLE OUTCOME—Expect complete healing of the surgical wound. Your doctor may recommend further treatment with radiation and anticancer drugs. Allow about 6 weeks for recovery from surgery. It is common to have difficulty maintaining body weight following this surgery.

 POSTOPERATIVE CARE

GENERAL MEASURES
- A hard ridge should form along the incision. As it heals, the ridge will gradually recede.
- Shower as usual. Avoid baths until the incision has completely healed. You may wash the incision gently with mild, unscented soap. After showering, replace any wet dressings with clean, dry ones.
- Move and elevate legs often while resting in bed to decrease the likelihood of deep-vein blood clots.

MEDICATION
- Your doctor may prescribe:
  - Pain relievers. Don't take prescription pain medication longer than 4 to 7 days. Use only as much as you need.
  - Stool softeners to prevent constipation.
  - Antibiotics to fight or prevent infection.
- You may use nonprescription drugs, such as acetaminophen, for minor pain. Avoid aspirin.

ACTIVITY
- Resume daily activities as you are able.
- Resume driving 3 to 4 weeks after returning home.
- Avoid vigorous exercise for 6 weeks after surgery.
- Resume sexual relations when you feel able.

DIET—Your doctor will prescribe a diet.

 CALL YOUR DOCTOR IF

- Pain, swelling, redness, drainage, or bleeding increases in the surgical area.
- You develop symptoms of infection including headache, muscle aches, dizziness, fever, or a general ill feeling.
- You experience constipation, abdominal swelling, nausea, or vomiting.
- New, unexplained symptoms develop.

STOMACH CANCER SURGERY

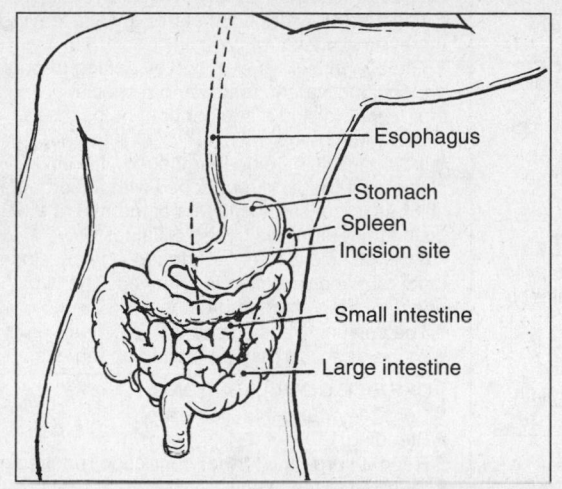

An illustration of the digestive system which shows the esophagus, stomach, spleen, large and small intestines, and a typical incision site for stomach cancer surgery.

Esophagus

Stomach

Spleen

Incision site

Small intestine

Large intestine

Esophagus

Incision sites

- The abdominal muscles are cut and retracted, the peritoneum is opened and the stomach is isolated (not shown).
- Incisions are made in the lower part of the esophagus and the top of the small intestine, and the entire stomach is removed.

Esophagus

Small intestine

- The esophagus is attached to a pouch made of small intestine, to create a new "stomach."
- Not shown: The peritoneum is closed and the muscles are sewn together. The skin is closed with sutures or clips which usually can be removed about 10 days after surgery.

STRABISMUS SURGERY
(Crossed Eyes Surgery)

 GENERAL INFORMATION

DEFINITION—Surgery to strengthen or weaken the muscles that regulate movement of the eyeball (see Strabismus in Illness section). The surgery will vary with the extent of the deviation of the movement, and may require more than one operation.

BODY PARTS INVOLVED—Eyes.

REASONS FOR SURGERY—Realign the eyes to restore single binocular vision and a balance in the appearance of the eyes. The procedure is usually performed in children while the eye is still developing to save vision in the affected eye. In adults, the surgery is for reconstruction reasons only.

SURGICAL RISK INCREASES WITH
- Poor nutrition.
- Recent or chronic illness.
- Diabetes.
- Use of some prescription and nonprescription drugs. Inform your doctor of any drugs, medications, or vitamin and herb supplements you are using or have used in the last month.

 WHAT TO EXPECT

WHO OPERATES—Ophthalmologist.

WHERE PERFORMED—Hospital, outpatient surgical facility.

DIAGNOSTIC TESTS
- Before surgery: Special eye examinations to determine the amount of deviation. Tests performed will depend on the age of the patient, usually an older child or an adult can cooperate with instructions for visual testing, while an infant cannot.
- After surgery: Eye examinations may be repeated as necessary.

ANESTHESIA—General anesthesia by injection and inhalation with an airway tube placed in the windpipe.

DESCRIPTION OF OPERATION
- The head is wrapped in sterile towels, leaving the eyes exposed.
- The eye muscle is exposed by cutting through the conjunctiva and fascia and a special instrument (called a squint hook) holds the whole width of the muscle.
- If the muscle is to be lengthened, it is cut close to its root and reattached with absorbable stitches to the surface layers of the eye at a distance determined by the initial tests.
- If the muscle is to be shortened, it is cut close to its root and a section is removed. The two ends are then stitched together.
- The conjunctiva is closed with stitches.
- A pad or shade may be placed on the eye.

POSSIBLE COMPLICATIONS
- Surgical-wound infection (rare).
- Bleeding.
- Repeat surgery if further correction required.
- Swelling of the eyelid.

AVERAGE HOSPITAL STAY—Usually none.

PROBABLE OUTCOME—Expect complete healing and improved appearance without complications. Allow about 2 weeks for recovery from surgery.

 POSTOPERATIVE CARE

GENERAL MEASURES—Avoid getting the eye wet until your doctor indicates it is safe to do so.

MEDICATION
- Your doctor may prescribe:
  - Pain relievers.
  - Antibiotic drops to fight or prevent infection.
  - Steroidal eye drops or ointment to relieve inflammation. Keep both types of eye drops cold in the refrigerator, but not frozen.
- You may use nonprescription drugs, such as acetaminophen, for minor pain. Avoid aspirin.

ACTIVITY
- Rest until the effects of the anesthesia wear off. The eye may water and be sensitive to light at first.
- Most normal activities can be resumed in about a week. Avoid swimming for 10 days.

DIET—No special diet.

 CALL YOUR DOCTOR IF

- Pain, swelling, redness, drainage, or bleeding increases in the surgical area.
- You develop symptoms of infection including headache, muscle aches, dizziness, fever, or a general ill feeling.
- New, unexplained symptoms develop.

STRABISMUS SURGERY
(Crossed Eyes Surgery)

An infant's left eye demonstrates an external deviation.

The eye muscle is surgically exposed and cut.

Muscle reattached

Muscle stump

A.

A. Muscle lengthening.

B.

B. Muscle shortening.

STRESS INCONTINENCE OPERATIONS

 GENERAL INFORMATION

DEFINITION—Operations to relieve uncontrolled leakage of urine from the bladder.

BODY PARTS INVOLVED—Abdominal cavity, bladder, urethra, and vagina.

REASONS FOR SURGERY—To improve quality of life in women who leak urine either spontaneously or with stress (such as when lifting or coughing), and to prevent excoriation (red, sore skin) and breakdown of the skin of the perineum.

SURGICAL RISK INCREASES WITH
- Age.
- Diabetes.
- Poor kidney function.
- High blood pressure.
- Poor nutrition.
- Chronic lung disease.
- Obesity.

 WHAT TO EXPECT

WHO OPERATES—Urologist or gynecologist.

WHERE PERFORMED—Hospital.

DIAGNOSTIC TESTS
- Before surgery: Blood tests and cystogram (see Glossary).
- After surgery: Blood tests (sometimes).

ANESTHESIA—General anesthesia or spinal anesthesia.

DESCRIPTION OF OPERATION
- There are multiple operations that have been designed to control incontinence. Most are variations of ways to alter the angle that the urethra exits the bladder. Advancing age and vaginal deliveries cause relaxation of the perineal muscles (those between the urethral opening and the rectum), causing the urethra to exit the bladder at a more obtuse angle, making it difficult for the sphincter to completely control the flow urine.
- The simplest operation to change the angle of the urethra is called an anterior repair. This is done through the vagina, tightening the anterior wall by pulling the side walls in for support.
- More complex operations involve incisions in the lower abdomen to create a sling with sutures to pull the urethra forward. These involve more extensive surgery and recovery but tend to also be more successful and durable than the simple operations. Your doctor will help you decide which operation is best for your individual situation.
- A catheter is left in the bladder for 1-2 weeks after the operation.

POSSIBLE COMPLICATIONS
- Bleeding.
- Infection.
- Urinary retention (unable to void).

AVERAGE HOSPITAL STAY—Usually 2 to 5 days depending on the type of operation.

PROBABLE OUTCOME—Expect full recovery in 6-8 weeks with some difficulty voiding initially. Most patients have much improvement in continence which may again deteriorate with time.

 POSTOPERATIVE CARE

GENERAL MEASURES
- Hard ridges will form along the incisions. As they heal, the ridges will gradually recede.
- Use heat on the incision to help relieve incisional pain.
- Shower as usual. You may wash the incisions gently with mild soap. After showering, replace any dressings with a new dry dressing.

MEDICATION
- Your doctor may prescribe pain relievers. Use only as much as you need to be comfortable.
- You may use nonprescription pain relievers such as acetaminophen for minor pain. Ask your doctor if it is okay to take ibuprofen or aspirin.

ACTIVITY
- Start ambulating (walking) as soon as you are home. Take frequent naps as needed during the day when tired. Avoid strenuous activity for 6 to 8 weeks (or as advised).
- You may swim once all sutures are out.
- Resume sexual relations when comfortable and when advised by your surgeon.

DIET—No special diet.

 CALL YOUR DOCTOR IF

- Pain, swelling, redness, drainage, or bleeding increases in the surgical area.
- You develop symptoms of infection including headache, muscle aches, dizziness, fever, or a general ill feeling.
- You develop nausea and vomiting.
- Prolonged constipation occurs.
- You have urinary frequency, burning, or urinary retention.
- New unexplained symptoms develop.

STRESS INCONTINENCE OPERATIONS

A cross sectional view of the bladder and surrounding structures.

Uterus
Bladder
Rectus muscles
Pubic bone
Bladder neck
Urethra
Vagina

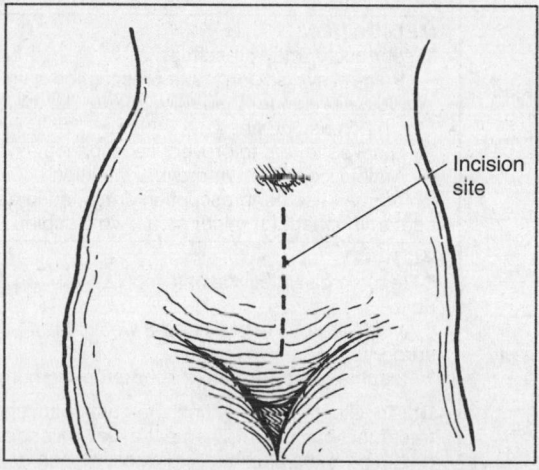

An incision is made through the skin and muscles of the lower abdomen either vertical (as shown) or transverse.

Incision site

A sling is constructed to change the angle of the urethra as it exits the bladder (bladder neck).

Bladder
Sling
Bladder neck

SYMPATHECTOMY, CERVICODORSAL

GENERAL INFORMATION

DEFINITION—Interruption of the sympathetic nerve chain at the base of the neck near the spine.

BODY PARTS INVOLVED—Cervicodorsal sympathetic nerves (part of the autonomic nervous system) that control contraction and expansion of small arteries in the arms, lungs, upper ribs.

REASONS FOR SURGERY
- Relieve post-traumatic pain complex.
- Restoration of normal blood supply to the arms. Removing part of the sympathetic nervous system stops spasms in the blood vessels that can cause or aggravate decreased circulation.

SURGICAL RISK INCREASES WITH
- Obesity, smoking, alcoholism.
- Recent or chronic illness.
- Atherosclerosis.
- Diabetes.
- Use of some prescription and nonprescription drugs. Inform your doctor of any drugs, medications, or vitamin and herb supplements you are using or have used in the last month.

WHAT TO EXPECT

WHO OPERATES—General surgeon, neurosurgeon, or vascular surgeon.

WHERE PERFORMED—Hospital.

DIAGNOSTIC TESTS
- Before surgery: Blood and urine studies, x-ray of chest, ECG (see Glossary), diagnostic sympathetic nerve block.
- After surgery: Blood studies, x-rays of chest.

ANESTHESIA—General anesthesia by injection and inhalation with an airway tube placed in the windpipe.

DESCRIPTION OF OPERATION
- An incision is made in the armpit.
- The muscles are divided, and part of the 3rd rib is removed.
- One lung is allowed to collapse temporarily to allow easier entry into the chest cavity.
- The cervical and dorsal sympathetic nerve chains are identified and divided.
- The lung is reexpanded. The muscles and skin edges are closed with sutures or clips, which usually can be removed about 1 week after surgery.
- This procedure can now be done via a thoracoscope (an optical instrument with a lighted tip).

POSSIBLE COMPLICATIONS
- Excessive bleeding.
- Surgical-wound infection.
- Inadvertent injury to lung tissue or lung collapse.

AVERAGE HOSPITAL STAY—1 to 3 days.

PROBABLE OUTCOME—Expect complete healing without complications. Circulation will improve in 3 to 4 days. Allow about 4 weeks for recovery from surgery.

POSTOPERATIVE CARE

GENERAL MEASURES
- Don't smoke.
- A hard ridge should form along the incision. As it heals, the ridge will gradually recede.
- Bathe and shower as usual. You may wash the incision gently with mild, unscented soap.
- Move and elevate legs often while resting in bed to decrease the likelihood of deep-vein blood clots.

MEDICATION
- Your doctor may prescribe:
  - Pain relievers. Don't take prescription pain medication longer than 4 to 7 days. Use only as much as you need.
  - Stool softeners to prevent constipation.
  - Antibiotics to fight or prevent infection.
- You may use nonprescription drugs, such as acetaminophen, for minor pain. Avoid aspirin.

ACTIVITY
- Resume daily activities as soon as you are able.
- Avoid vigorous exercise for 6 weeks after surgery.
- Resume driving 2 weeks after returning home.

DIET—Clear liquid diet until the gastrointestinal tract functions again. Then eat a well-balanced diet to promote healing. After recovery, eat a low-fat, low-salt diet (see diets in Appendix).

CALL YOUR DOCTOR IF

- Pain, swelling, redness, drainage, or bleeding increases in the surgical area.
- You develop symptoms of infection including headache, muscle aches, dizziness, fever, or a general ill feeling.
- You experience constipation, abdominal swelling, nausea, or vomiting.
- You experience coldness, discoloration, or numbness in the hand.
- You develop a cough, shortness of breath, or chest pain.
- New, unexplained symptoms develop.

SYMPATHECTOMY, CERVICODORSAL

An illustration of the usual incision site for a cervicodorsal sympathectomy.

Incision site

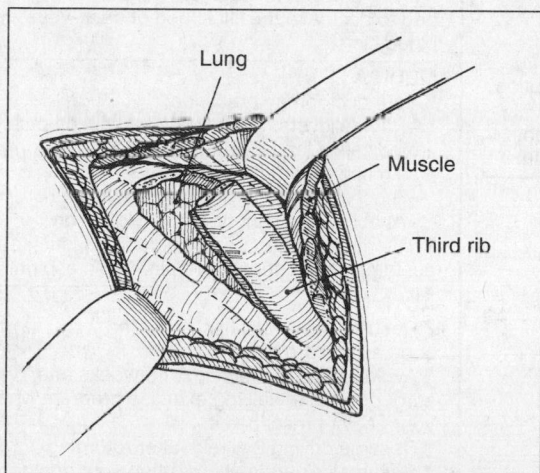

Lung

Muscle

Third rib

Muscles attached to ribs are divided and part of the 3rd rib is removed. One portion of the lung is allowed to temporarily collapse to allow easier entry into the chest cavity.

● The cervical and dorsal sympathetic nerve chains are identified and divided.
● Following the operation, the ribs are reconstructed and held in place with heavy sutures. The lung is reexpanded and the muscles and skin edges are closed with sutures or clips (not illustrated).

SYMPATHECTOMY, LUMBAR

GENERAL INFORMATION

DEFINITION—Removing a section of the sympathetic nerves located near the spinal cord in the lower back.

BODY PARTS INVOLVED—The lumbar sympathetic nerves (part of the autonomic nervous system) that control contraction and expansion of small arteries in the legs.

REASONS FOR SURGERY
- Improve blood flow to the legs. Removing part of the sympathetic nervous system stops spasms in the blood vessels that can cause or aggravate decreased blood flow and cause severe pain.
- Relieve symptoms of reflex sympathetic dystrophy.
- Nonhealing ulcers in legs or feet.

SURGICAL RISK INCREASES WITH
- Obesity, smoking.
- Recent or chronic illness.
- Atherosclerosis.
- Diabetes.
- Use of some prescription and nonprescription drugs. Inform your doctor of any drugs, medications, or vitamin and herb supplements you are using or have used in the last month.

WHAT TO EXPECT

WHO OPERATES—General surgeon, neurosurgeon or vascular surgeon.

WHERE PERFORMED—Hospital.

DIAGNOSTIC TESTS
- Before surgery: Blood and urine studies, lumbar sympathetic nerve block.
- After surgery: Blood studies.

ANESTHESIA—General anesthesia by injection and inhalation with an airway tube placed in the windpipe.

DESCRIPTION OF OPERATION
- A short, horizontal incision is made on the abdomen slightly above and to the side of the navel. The muscles are separated.
- The lumbar sympathetic chain of nerves is located, cut free, and a short segment is removed.
- The muscles are sewn together with large sutures.
- The skin is closed with sutures or clips, which usually can be removed about 1 week after surgery.

POSSIBLE COMPLICATIONS
- Excessive bleeding.
- Surgical-wound infection.
- Incisional hernia (rare).
- Inadvertent injury to the ureter (rare).

- May result in impotence.
- Incomplete resection of nerves due to accessory fibers.

AVERAGE HOSPITAL STAY—3 to 5 days.

PROBABLE OUTCOME—Expect complete healing without complications. Circulation will improve in 3 to 4 days. Allow about 4 weeks for recovery from surgery.

POSTOPERATIVE CARE

GENERAL MEASURES
- Don't smoke.
- A hard ridge should form along the incision. As it heals, the ridge will gradually recede.
- Shower as usual. Avoid baths until the incision has completely healed. You may wash the incision gently with mild, unscented soap. After showering, replace any wet dressings with clean, dry ones.
- Move and elevate legs often while resting in bed to decrease the likelihood of deep-vein blood clots.

MEDICATION
- Your doctor may prescribe:
  - Pain relievers. Don't take prescription pain medication longer than 4 to 7 days. Use only as much as you need.
  - Stool softeners to prevent constipation.
  - Antibiotics to fight or prevent infection.
- You may use nonprescription drugs, such as acetaminophen, for minor pain. Avoid aspirin.

ACTIVITY
- Resume daily activities, including work, as soon as you are able.
- Avoid vigorous exercise for 6 weeks after surgery. Start a walking exercise program when your doctor prescribes it.
- Resume driving 2 weeks after returning home.
- Resume sexual relations when your doctor determines that healing is complete.

DIET—Clear liquid diet until the gastrointestinal tract functions again. Then eat a well-balanced diet to promote healing.

CALL YOUR DOCTOR IF

- Pain, swelling, redness, drainage, or bleeding increases in the surgical area.
- You develop symptoms of infection including headache, muscle aches, dizziness, fever, or a general ill feeling.
- You experience constipation, abdominal swelling, nausea, or vomiting.
- Your foot becomes cold, discolored, or numb.
- New, unexplained symptoms develop.

SYMPATHECTOMY, LUMBAR

An illustration of a typical incision site to allow access to the sympathetic chain.

Muscles overlying the spine are separated.

The lumbar sympathetic chain of nerves is located, cut free and removed.

TEAR DUCT, OPENING OF

GENERAL INFORMATION

DEFINITION—Opening of tear ducts (also called lacrimal ducts) in the corners of the eyes closer to the nose. They may be blocked by infection or foreign material, or may be incompletely open in newborns. This is a common problem, affecting 6% of newborns. In 90% of these cases, however, the ducts open spontaneously by 1 year of age.

BODY PARTS INVOLVED—Tear glands and tear ducts, usually in newborns, infants, or young children.

REASONS FOR SURGERY—Infection or complete blockage that does not respond to simple treatment.

SURGICAL RISK INCREASES WITH
* Obesity.
* Poor nutrition.
* Recent or chronic illness.
* Diabetes.
* Use of some prescription and nonprescription drugs. Inform your doctor of any drugs, medications, or vitamin and herb supplements your child is using or has used in the last month.

WHAT TO EXPECT

WHO OPERATES—Ophthalmologist or pediatric surgeon.

WHERE PERFORMED—Hospital or outpatient surgical facility.

DIAGNOSTIC TESTS
* Before surgery: Blood and urine studies.
* After surgery: Blood studies.

ANESTHESIA
* Local anesthesia by injection or topical application (sometimes).
* General anesthesia by injection and inhalation with an airway tube placed in the windpipe.

DESCRIPTION OF OPERATION
* The tear duct is expanded, probed and irrigated until fluid flows freely through it. The procedure is repeated on the other tear duct.
* Sutures are not needed. Bleeding should not be a problem.

POSSIBLE COMPLICATIONS—Surgical-wound infection.

AVERAGE HOSPITAL STAY—0 to 1 day.

PROBABLE OUTCOME—Expect complete healing without complications. Allow about 10 days for recovery from surgery.

POSTOPERATIVE CARE

GENERAL MEASURES
* Bathe your child as usual.
* Use a warm compress to relieve pain in the surgical area.

MEDICATION
* Your doctor may prescribe antibiotic eye drops or ointment to fight or prevent infection. Keep eye drops cold, but not frozen, in the refrigerator.
* You may give your child nonprescription drugs, such as acetaminophen, for minor pain. Avoid giving aspirin.

ACTIVITY—Have your child avoid vigorous exercise for 1 week after surgery.

DIET—No special diet.

CALL YOUR DOCTOR IF

* Your child experiences nausea or vomiting.
* Your child has increased pain, swelling, redness, or drainage in the surgical area.
* Your child develops symptoms of infection including headache, muscle aches, dizziness, fever, or a general ill feeling.
* New, unexplained symptoms develop.

TEAR DUCT, OPENING OF

An illustration of tear glands, tear duct and other parts of the eye.

The blocked tear duct is identified.

The blocked duct is expanded, probed and irrigated until fluid freely flows through it.

TENDON REPAIR

GENERAL INFORMATION

DEFINITION—Reattaching tendons (see Glossary) to their connective tissue, or sewing sections of cut or torn tendons together.

BODY PARTS INVOLVED—Injured tendons, most frequently in the hand, foot, ankle, wrist, shoulder, hip, knee and elbow.

REASONS FOR SURGERY—Restoration of normal function of joints or tissue surrounding tendons.

SURGICAL RISK INCREASES WITH
- Adults over 60.
- Obesity, smoking, alcoholism.
- Poor nutrition.
- Recent or chronic illness.
- Diabetes.
- Use of some prescription and nonprescription drugs. Inform your doctor of any drugs, medications, or vitamin and herb supplements you are using or have used in the last month.

WHAT TO EXPECT

WHO OPERATES—Orthopedic surgeon, hand surgeon, or general surgeon.

WHERE PERFORMED—Hospital, outpatient surgical facility, or emergency room.

DIAGNOSTIC TESTS
- Before surgery: Blood and urine studies, x-ray of the injured part.
- After surgery: Blood studies.

ANESTHESIA
- Local anesthesia by injection.
- Spinal anesthesia by injection.
- General anesthesia by injection and inhalation with an airway tube placed in the windpipe.

DESCRIPTION OF OPERATION
- An incision is made over the injured tendon.
- The severed ends of the tendon are located and sewn together. If the tendon has been destroyed, a tendon graft may be required to bridge the gap.
- If necessary, tendons are reattached to surrounding connective tissue.
- The surgical area is examined for injuries to nerves and blood vessels.
- The skin is closed with sutures, which usually can be removed about 10 days after surgery.
- Usually, the injured part is kept rigid with a splint or plaster cast.

POSSIBLE COMPLICATIONS
- Excessive bleeding.
- Surgical-wound infection.
- Partial loss of function in joint served by the injured tendon(s).
- Repeat rupture of tendon.

AVERAGE HOSPITAL STAY—0 to 1 day.

PROBABLE OUTCOME—Expect complete healing without complications. Allow about 3 to 6 months for recovery from surgery.

POSTOPERATIVE CARE

GENERAL MEASURES
- If the wound bleeds during the first 24 hours after surgery, press a clean tissue or cloth to it for 10 minutes.
- A hard ridge should form along the incision. As it heals, the ridge will gradually recede.
- Shower as usual after the splint is removed. Avoid baths until the incision has completely healed.
- Between showers, keep the wound dry with a bandage for the first 2 or 3 days after the splint is removed. If a bandage gets wet, change it promptly.

MEDICATION
- Your doctor may prescribe:
  - Pain relievers. Don't take prescription pain medication longer than 4 to 7 days. Use only as much as you need.
  - Antibiotics to fight or prevent infection.
- You may use nonprescription drugs, such as acetaminophen, for minor pain. Avoid aspirin.

ACTIVITY
- Resume daily activities as advised by your doctor.
- Avoid vigorous exercise for 6 weeks after surgery.
- Your doctor may refer you to a physical therapist who will help you strengthen and rehabilitate the limb.
- Ask your doctor when you may resume driving; will vary depending upon area repaired.

DIET—No special diet.

CALL YOUR DOCTOR IF

- Pain, swelling, redness, drainage, or bleeding increases in the surgical area.
- Skin below a cast becomes cold, discolored, or numb.
- You develop symptoms of infection including headache, muscle aches, dizziness, fever, or a general ill feeling.
- You experience nausea or vomiting.
- New, unexplained symptoms develop.

TENDON REPAIR

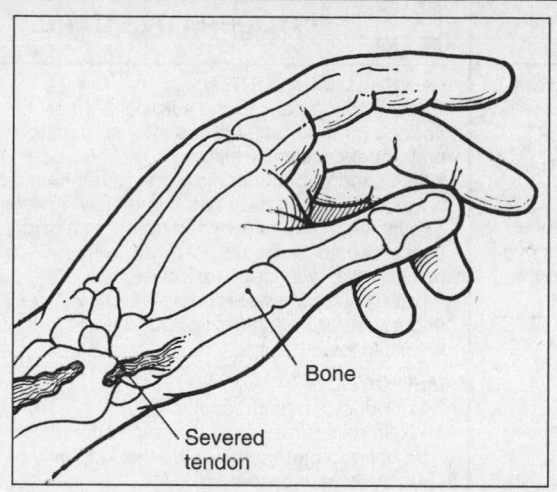

An illustration of a typical severed tendon in the wrist.

Bone

Severed tendon

Severed ends of a tendon are located and sewn together.

If necessary, tendons are reattached to surrounding connective tissue.

TESTICLE FIXATION
(Orchiopexy)

 GENERAL INFORMATION

DEFINITION—Fastening an undescended or twisted testicle in its normal position.

BODY PARTS INVOLVED—Scrotum, testicle, vas deferens, blood vessels and nerves in the scrotum.

REASONS FOR SURGERY—Placement of an undescended testicle in its normal position, or correction of a twisted testicle. Usually done before a boy is age 5.

SURGICAL RISK INCREASES WITH
- Congenital disorders.
- Chronic illness.
- Diabetes.
- Use of some prescription and nonprescription drugs. Inform your doctor of any drugs, medications, or vitamin and herb supplements your child is using or has used in the last month.

 WHAT TO EXPECT

WHO OPERATES—Urologist or general surgeon.

WHERE PERFORMED—Hospital.

DIAGNOSTIC TESTS
- Before surgery: Blood and urine studies, ultrasound (see Glossary).
- After surgery: Blood studies.

ANESTHESIA
- Spinal anesthesia by injection.
- Local anesthesia by injection.

DESCRIPTION OF OPERATION
- An incision is made in the scrotum or groin area.
- The blood supply and nerves leading to the testicle are located and carefully preserved.
- If the testicle has not descended from the abdomen, the surgeon reaches into the inguinal canal with special instruments and gently pulls it down.
- The testicle and its blood supply and nerves are pulled to the bottom of the scrotum and sewn in place.
- The skin is closed with sutures that will be absorbed by the body.

POSSIBLE COMPLICATIONS
- Excessive bleeding.
- Surgical-wound infection.
- Damage to blood supply to the testicle, death of the testicle.

AVERAGE HOSPITAL STAY—0 to 2 days.

PROBABLE OUTCOME—Expect complete healing without complications. Allow about 3 weeks for recovery from surgery.

 POSTOPERATIVE CARE

GENERAL MEASURES
- Apply an ice pack to the surgical area as needed for the first 24 hours after surgery to prevent excessive swelling.
- Use sponge baths or showers, rather than tub baths, until the incision has completely healed. The incision may be washed gently with mild, unscented soap. Replace any dressings which become wet with clean, dry ones.
- Have your child wear 2 pairs of jockey type underwear or an athletic supporter for 4 to 6 weeks following surgery.

MEDICATION
- Your doctor may prescribe:
  - Pain relievers. Pain medication should not be used longer than 4 to 7 days. Use only as much as your child need.
  - Stool softeners to prevent constipation.
  - Antibiotics to fight or prevent infection.
- You may give your child nonprescription drugs, such as acetaminophen, for minor pain. Avoid aspirin.

ACTIVITY
- Resume daily activities as soon as advised by doctor.
- Avoid vigorous exercise for 6 weeks.

DIET—Eat a well-balanced diet to promote healing. Increase dietary fiber and fluid intake to help prevent constipation.

 CALL YOUR DOCTOR IF

- Your child experiences nausea or vomiting.
- Your child has discomfort or difficulty with urination.
- Pain, swelling, redness, drainage, or bleeding increases in the surgical area.
- Your child develops symptoms of infection including headache, muscle aches, dizziness, fever, or a general ill feeling.

TESTICLE FIXATION
(Orchiopexy)

An illustration of an undescended testicle on the patient's left side and a typical incision site into the scrotum.

Undescended testicle

Incision

- The blood supply and nerves leading to the testicle are carefully preserved.
- The surgeon reaches into the inguinal canal with special instruments and gently pulls the testicle down into the scrotum.

Testicle

The testicle, its blood supply and nerves are pulled to the bottom of the scrotum and sewn into place.

Scrotum

TESTICLE REMOVAL
(Orchiectomy)

GENERAL INFORMATION

DEFINITION—Removal of one of the testicles (orchiectomy).

BODY PARTS INVOLVED—Scrotum, testicle, vas deferens, blood vessels and nerves in the scrotum.

REASONS FOR SURGERY
- Cancer or gangrene of the testicle.
- Prostate cancer.
- Undescended testicle.

SURGICAL RISK INCREASES WITH
- Adults over 60.
- Smoking.
- Recent or chronic illness.
- Diabetes.
- Use of some prescription and nonprescription drugs. Inform your doctor of any drugs, medications, or vitamin and herb supplements you are using or have used in the last month.

WHAT TO EXPECT

WHO OPERATES—Urologist or general surgeon.

WHERE PERFORMED—Hospital.

DIAGNOSTIC TESTS
- Before surgery: Blood and urine studies, x-rays, CT scan, ultrasound, ECG (see Glossary for all).
- After surgery: Blood studies, laboratory studies of the removed testicle.

ANESTHESIA
- Local anesthesia by injection.
- Spinal anesthesia by injection.
- General anesthesia by injection and inhalation with an airway tube placed in the windpipe.

DESCRIPTION OF OPERATION
- An incision is made in the inguinal region or scrotum. The blood supply and nerves leading to the testicle are located and cut free.
- The testicle is cut free from surrounding tissue and removed.
- The skin is closed with sutures that will be absorbed by the body.

POSSIBLE COMPLICATIONS
- Excessive bleeding.
- Surgical-wound infection.
- Urinary retention.

AVERAGE HOSPITAL STAY—0 to 2 days.

PROBABLE OUTCOME—Expect complete healing without complications. Allow about 3 weeks for recovery from surgery. Removal of one testicle should not interfere with normal sexual function or the ability to have children.

POSTOPERATIVE CARE

GENERAL MEASURES
- Apply an ice pack to the surgical area as needed for the first 24 hours after surgery to prevent excessive swelling.
- Shower as usual. Avoid baths until the incision has completely healed. You may wash the incision gently with mild, unscented soap. After bathing, replace any wet dressings with clean, dry ones.
- Wear an athletic supporter for 4 to 6 weeks.

MEDICATION
- Your doctor may prescribe:
  - Pain relievers. Don't take prescription pain medication longer than 4 to 7 days. Use only as much as you need.
  - Stool softeners to prevent constipation.
  - Antibiotics to fight or prevent infection.
- You may use nonprescription drugs, such as acetaminophen, for minor pain. Avoid aspirin.

ACTIVITY
- To help recovery and aid your well-being, resume daily activities, including work, as soon as you are able.
- Avoid vigorous exercise for 6 weeks after surgery.
- Resume driving 2 weeks after returning home.
- Resume sexual relations when your doctor determines that healing is complete.

DIET—Clear liquid diet until the gastrointestinal tract functions again. Then eat a well-balanced diet to promote healing.

CALL YOUR DOCTOR IF

- You experience nausea, vomiting, or problems with urination.
- Pain, swelling, redness, drainage, or bleeding increases in the surgical area.
- You develop symptoms of infection including headache, muscle aches, dizziness, fever, or a general ill feeling.
- New, unexplained symptoms develop.

TESTICLE REMOVAL
(Orchiectomy)

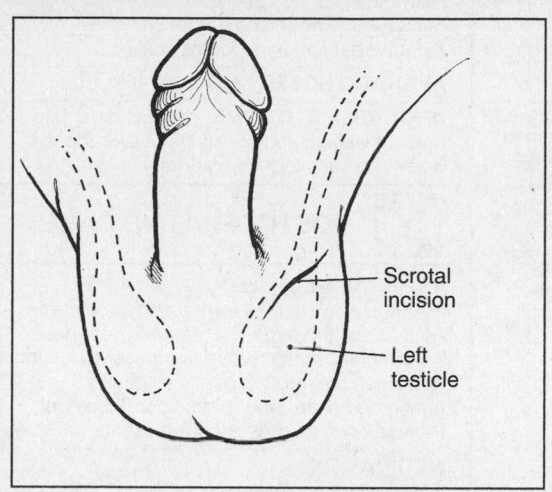

Scrotal incision

Left testicle

- An illustration of the penis, scrotum, testicle and incision site for removal of a testicle.
- Sometimes the incision for this operation is made higher up in the groin.
- Usually the incision is made in the scrotum.

Testicle

The blood supply, vas deferens (carries sperm for testicle) and nerves leading to the testicle are located and cut free. The testicle is then cut free from surrounding tissue.

- The excised testicle is removed.
- The skin is closed with sutures that will be absorbed by the body.

THYROGLOSSAL DUCT & CYST REMOVAL

GENERAL INFORMATION

DEFINITION—Removal of a thyroglossal duct that has a cyst. The cyst results from remnants of the thyroid gland that do not descend normally during early fetal development. The cyst usually appears during childhood, attached to the hyoid bone by the duct. The duct then passes upward to its origin at the base of the tongue. Surgery is usually performed when the patient is between 6 and 10 years old.

BODY PARTS INVOLVED—Thyroglossal cyst, remnants of the thyroglossal duct, hyoid bone.

REASONS FOR SURGERY
- Prevention of infections.
- Relief of pressure on the airway that causes difficulty in breathing or swallowing.

SURGICAL RISK INCREASES WITH
- Obesity.
- Poor nutrition.
- Recent or chronic illness.
- Other congenital disorders.
- Diabetes.
- Use of some prescription and nonprescription drugs. Inform your doctor of any drugs, medications, or vitamin and herb supplements you are using or have used in the last month.

WHAT TO EXPECT

WHO OPERATES—General surgeon or ear, nose and throat specialist (otolaryngologist).

WHERE PERFORMED—Hospital.

DIAGNOSTIC TESTS
- Before surgery: Blood and urine studies, ultrasound, CT scan (see Glossary).
- After surgery: Blood studies.

ANESTHESIA—General anesthesia by injection and inhalation with an airway tube placed in the windpipe.

DESCRIPTION OF OPERATION
- An incision is made in the neck over the thyroglossal cyst.
- The cyst is cut free of muscle and connective tissue. The part of the hyoid bone to which the cyst is attached is cut, and the cyst and bone are removed.
- The thyroglossal duct is located, tied, cut and removed.
- The neck muscles are closed with fine sutures.
- The skin is closed with either sutures or clips, which usually can be removed about 4 to 7 days after surgery.

POSSIBLE COMPLICATIONS
- Excessive bleeding.
- Surgical-wound infection.
- Injury to surrounding nerves.
- Inadvertent injury to larynx (rare).

AVERAGE HOSPITAL STAY—0 to 1 day.

PROBABLE OUTCOME—Expect complete healing without complications. Allow about 6 weeks for recovery from surgery.

POSTOPERATIVE CARE

GENERAL MEASURES
- A hard ridge should form along the incision. As it heals, the ridge will gradually recede.
- Your child should bathe or shower as usual, and wash the incision gently with mild, unscented soap. After bathing or showering, replace any wet dressings with clean, dry ones.

MEDICATION
- Your doctor may prescribe:
  - Pain relievers. Don't give your child prescription pain medication longer than 4 to 7 days. Use only as much as needed.
  - Antibiotics to fight or prevent infection.
- You may give your child nonprescription drugs, such as acetaminophen, for minor pain. Avoid aspirin.

ACTIVITY
- Return to normal activity as soon as possible to promote healing.
- Avoid vigorous exercise for 3 weeks after surgery.

DIET—Clear liquid diet until the gastrointestinal tract functions again. Then provide a well-balanced diet to promote healing.

CALL YOUR DOCTOR IF

- Pain, swelling, redness, drainage, or bleeding increases in the surgical area.
- Your child experiences nausea or vomiting.
- Your child develops symptoms of infection including headache, muscle aches, dizziness, fever, or a general ill feeling.
- Your child develops hoarseness that doesn't go away within 2 weeks after surgery.
- Your child experiences difficulty in breathing or has a harsh vibrating sound when breathing.
- New, unexplained symptoms develop.

THYROGLOSSAL DUCT & CYST REMOVAL

An illustration of the tongue, thyroglossal duct, hyoid bone and a cyst in the thyroglossal duct.

Tongue

Thyroglossal duct

Hyoid bone

Cyst

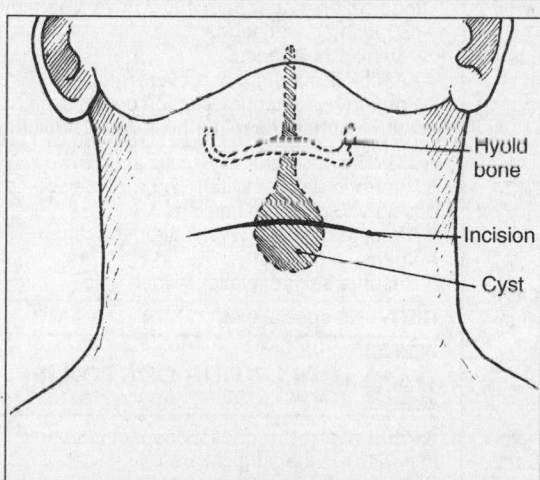

The skin is incised directly over the cyst.

Hyoid bone

Incision

Cyst

- The cyst is cut free of muscle, connective tissue and part of the hyoid bone to which the cyst is attached. The cyst and bone are removed.
- Muscles and connective tissue are returned to their normal positions (not illustrated).

Cyst

THYROID GLAND REMOVAL
(Thyroidectomy)

 GENERAL INFORMATION

DEFINITION—Removal of part or all of the thyroid gland.

BODY PARTS INVOLVED—Thyroid gland, the organ in the neck below the Adam's apple that controls the body's metabolism; lymph nodes in the neck.

REASONS FOR SURGERY
- Hyperthyroidism.
- Benign or cancerous tumors of the thyroid.
- Goiter (see Glossary).

SURGICAL RISK INCREASES WITH
- Adults over 60.
- Obesity; poor nutrition.
- Smoking.
- Untreated hyperthyroidism (see Glossary).
- Diabetes.
- Use of some prescription and nonprescription drugs. Inform your doctor of any drugs, medications, or vitamin and herb supplements you are using or have used in the last month.

 WHAT TO EXPECT

WHO OPERATES—General surgeon.

WHERE PERFORMED—Hospital.

DIAGNOSTIC TESTS
- Before surgery: Blood studies; ultrasound; CT scan; needle biopsy; radioactive-iodine uptake and scan (see Glossary for all).
- After surgery: Blood studies.

ANESTHESIA—General anesthesia by injection and inhalation with an airway tube placed in the windpipe.

DESCRIPTION OF OPERATION
- An incision is made in the neck following natural skin lines.
- Neck muscles are cut or retracted.
- Blood supply to the thyroid gland is clamped.
- The thyroid gland is cut free and removed, and a drain is left in place. In certain cases, some normal thyroid gland tissue is left intact.
- If cancer is present, some lymph nodes may be removed around the thyroid.
- The muscles are closed and the skin is closed with sutures or clips, which can usually be removed in 2 to 10 days after surgery.

POSSIBLE COMPLICATIONS
- Hoarseness or loss of voice, if vocal-cord nerves are damaged during surgery.
- Hypothyroidism (see Glossary).
- Hypoparathyroidism (see Glossary).
- Excessive bleeding.
- Surgical-wound infection.

AVERAGE HOSPITAL STAY—0 to 3 days.

PROBABLE OUTCOME—Underlying problem cured in most patients. Cancer that is present but has not spread may require radiation treatment. Allow about 6 weeks for recovery from surgery.

 POSTOPERATIVE CARE

GENERAL MEASURES
- A hard ridge should form along the incision. As it heals, the ridge will gradually recede.
- Shower as usual. You may wash the incision gently with mild, unscented soap. After showering, replace any wet dressings with clean, dry ones.

MEDICATION
- Your doctor may prescribe:
  - Pain relievers. Don't take prescription pain medication longer than 4 to 7 days. Use only as much as you need.
  - Thyroid hormones.
  - Antibiotics to fight or prevent infection.
- You may use nonprescription drugs, such as acetaminophen, for minor pain. Avoid aspirin.

ACTIVITY
- Return to daily activities and work as soon as possible to promote healing.
- Resume driving 2 weeks after you return home.
- Resume sexual relations when able.

DIET—No special diet.

 CALL YOUR DOCTOR IF

- Pain, swelling, redness, drainage, or bleeding increases in the surgical area.
- You develop symptoms of infection including headache, muscle aches, dizziness, fever, or a general ill feeling.
- You develop symptoms of hypothyroidism, including excessive weakness, fatigue, intolerance to cold, menstrual irregularities, constipation, or dry and coarse skin and hair.
- You develop symptoms of hypoparathyroidism (see Glossary) including dry hair, brittle fingernails, dry or scaly skin, or irregular heartbeat.
- New, unexplained symptoms develop.

THYROID GLAND REMOVAL
(Thyroidectomy)

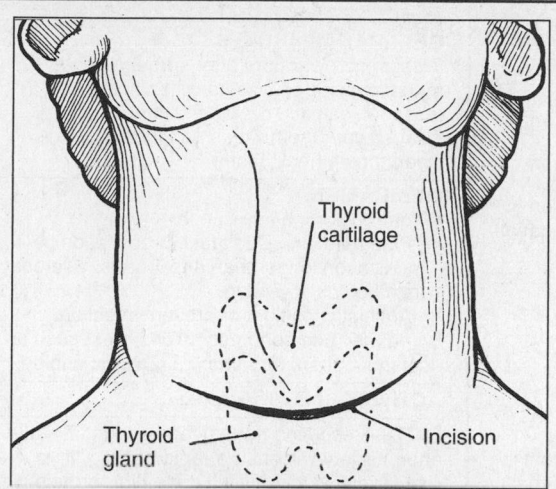

An illustration of structures in the neck and the typical incision site for thyroid gland removal.

Thyroid cartilage

Thyroid gland

Incision

Muscles and connective tissue are retracted revealing the thyroid gland.

Thyroid gland

Thyroid gland

- The blood supply to the thyroid gland is clamped and all or part of the gland is cut free and removed.
- The remaining tissue is replaced in its normal position. The skin is closed with sutures or clips (not illustrated).

TONGUE, CHEEK, OR GUM BIOPSY

 GENERAL INFORMATION

DEFINITION—Removal of tissue from the oral cavity.

BODY PARTS INVOLVED—Tongue, cheek, gums, roof of mouth, salivary glands under the tongue.

REASONS FOR SURGERY—Usually performed to determine if any unusual lesion in the mouth is cancerous. Laboratory examination of the removed tissue aids in diagnosis.

SURGICAL RISK INCREASES WITH
- Adults over 60.
- Smoking.
- Excess alcohol consumption.
- Diabetes.
- Use of some prescription and nonprescription drugs. Inform your doctor of any drugs, medications, or vitamin and herb supplements you are using or have used in the last month.

 WHAT TO EXPECT

WHO OPERATES—Dentist; oral surgeon; general surgeon; or ear, nose and throat specialist.

WHERE PERFORMED—Hospital, outpatient surgical facility, or a medical office.

DIAGNOSTIC TESTS
- Before surgery: Blood and urine studies, CT scan, MRI (see Glossary for both).
- After surgery: Laboratory examination of removed tissue.

ANESTHESIA
- Local anesthesia by injection.
- General anesthesia (sometimes) by injection and inhalation with an airway tube placed in the windpipe.

DESCRIPTION OF OPERATION
- The area where the tissue is to be gathered is numbed with a local anesthetic.
- Abnormal tissue and a small amount of healthy surrounding tissue is removed.
- Small stitches may be needed to close the incision. These usually can be removed in 3 to 5 days after surgery.

POSSIBLE COMPLICATIONS
- Excessive bleeding.
- Surgical-wound infection.

AVERAGE HOSPITAL STAY—None.

PROBABLE OUTCOME—Tissue obtained successfully without complications in virtually all cases. Allow about 2 weeks for recovery from surgery.

 POSTOPERATIVE CARE

GENERAL MEASURES
- Beginning 24 hours after surgery, rinse your mouth every 1 or 2 hours with a solution of 1/2 teaspoon salt in 8 oz. warm water.
- Brush your teeth with a soft toothbrush. A clean mouth heals faster.

MEDICATION
- Your doctor may prescribe:
  - Pain relievers. Don't take prescription pain medication longer than 4 to 7 days. Use only as much as you need.
  - Antibiotics to fight or prevent infection.
- You may use nonprescription drugs, such as acetaminophen, for minor pain. Avoid aspirin.

ACTIVITY—No restrictions.

DIET—Resuming normal food and fluid intake after surgery will ensure rapid healing. If your regular diet is too difficult, try a high-protein liquid diet for 2 or 3 days.

 CALL YOUR DOCTOR IF

- Pain, swelling, redness, drainage, or bleeding increases in the surgical area.
- You develop symptoms of infection including headache, muscle aches, dizziness, fever, or a general ill feeling.
- New, unexplained symptoms develop.

TONGUE, CHEEK, OR GUM BIOPSY

An illustration of the roof of the mouth, gums, teeth and tongue.

Roof of mouth

Gums

Tongue

The abnormal tissue on the edge of the tongue illustrated here.

Abnormal tissue on tongue

- After injecting a local anesthetic, the abnormal tissue and a small amount of healthy surrounding tissue is removed.
- Small stitches may be needed to close the incision. If so, they usually can be removed in 3 to 5 days after surgery (not illustrated).

TONSIL & ADENOID REMOVAL
(Tonsillectomy & Adenoidectomy)

GENERAL INFORMATION

DEFINITION—Removal of the tonsils and adenoids.

BODY PARTS INVOLVED—Tonsils, adenoids, opening from the nose into the throat, back of the throat.

REASONS FOR SURGERY
- In tonsils:
  - More than 5 attacks of tonsillitis in 1 year.
  - Peritonsillar abscess (see Glossary).
- In adenoids:
  - Obstruction of air through the nose.
  - Infections in the middle ear.

SURGICAL RISK INCREASES WITH
- Obesity, smoking.
- Poor nutrition.
- Recent or chronic illness.
- Diabetes.
- Use of some prescription and nonprescription drugs. Inform your doctor of any drugs, medications, or vitamin and herb supplements you are using or have used in the last month.

WHAT TO EXPECT

WHO OPERATES—Ear, nose and throat specialist or general surgeon.

WHERE PERFORMED—Hospital or outpatient surgical facility.

DIAGNOSTIC TESTS
- Before surgery: Blood and urine studies.
- After surgery: Laboratory examination of removed tissue, blood studies.

ANESTHESIA—General anesthesia by injection and inhalation with an airway tube placed in the windpipe.

DESCRIPTION OF OPERATION
- Several techniques are available, one is described here.
- The mouth is held open to expose the tonsils.
- The tonsils are grasped with clamps and pulled toward the middle of the mouth. The tonsils are cut free of surrounding membrane and removed.
- Bleeding is controlled by pressure, sutures or clamps and ties, or with use of electrocautery (see Glossary).
- The adenoids are located and removed with a special instrument.

POSSIBLE COMPLICATIONS
- Excessive bleeding, sometimes requiring another operation.
- Adenoid-tissue regrowth.
- Nausea and dehydration.

AVERAGE HOSPITAL STAY—0 to 2 days.

PROBABLE OUTCOME—Expect complete healing without complications. You will experience moderate nasal congestion and drainage, a sore throat and earaches for a few days after surgery. Allow about 3 weeks for recovery from surgery. During this time, avoid becoming hot, tired, or excited.

POSTOPERATIVE CARE

GENERAL MEASURES
- Bathe or shower as usual.
- Use ice packs or popsicles to relieve pain.
- Minimize talking in the first 2 to 3 days following surgery.
- Try not to cough, clear the throat, cry, or sing for 1 week after surgery.
- The pain in your throat may worsen before it improves.
- You may notice a bad odor from the nose or mouth during healing. This will diminish in 1 to 2 weeks.

MEDICATION
- Your doctor may prescribe:
  - Pain relievers. Don't take prescription pain medication longer than 4 to 7 days. Use only as much as you need.
  - Stool softeners to prevent constipation.
  - Antibiotics to fight or prevent infection.
- You may use nonprescription drugs, such as acetaminophen, for minor pain. Avoid aspirin.

ACTIVITY
- Rest in bed for 2 to 3 days, then resume normal activities slowly to promote healing.
- Avoid vigorous exercise for 6 weeks after surgery.

DIET—Begin with a clear, liquid diet following surgery. Sucking on ice chips or eating popsicles may help to numb the throat and relieve pain. Avoid steamy, hot, crunchy, spicy, or hard-to-digest foods. Eat soft foods, such as gelatin and custard, for 3 to 4 days after surgery. Gradually return to a normal diet.

CALL YOUR DOCTOR IF

- You experience nausea or vomiting.
- Pain, swelling, redness, drainage, or bleeding increases in the surgical area.
- You experience coughing, spitting, or vomiting of blood.
- You develop symptoms of infection including headache, muscle aches, dizziness, fever, or a general ill feeling.
- New, unexplained symptoms develop.

TONSIL & ADENOID REMOVAL
(Tonsillectomy & Adenoidectomy)

An illustration of the roof of the mouth, tongue (pushed downward by a retractor), the soft and hard palate, and tonsils.

Soft palate

Tonsil

The tonsils are grasped with clamps and pulled toward the middle of the mouth. The tonsils are cut free of surrounding membrane and tension is applied to the base of the tonsil.

Tonsil

- The base of the tonsil is generally reached with a wire snare that cuts through the tonsil allowing easy removal.
- Bleeding is controlled by pressure sutures, electrocautery, or clamps and ties.
- Frequently, the adenoids will be removed at the same time (not shown in this illustration). Adenoids are tissues similar anatomically to tonsillar tissue and are located in the back of the throat up behind the hard palate toward the rear opening into the nose.

Tonsil

TOOTH EXTRACTION

GENERAL INFORMATION

DEFINITION—Removal (extraction) of a tooth.

BODY PARTS INVOLVED—Teeth, gums, bones in jaw.

REASONS FOR SURGERY
- Routine removals:
  - Loss of supporting tissue, bone, or gums.
  - Infection of the nerve in the tooth.
  - Fractured teeth that cannot be restored.
- Impacted-tooth removals:
  - Infection and pain around the lower wisdom teeth.
  - Pain upon closing the jaws.
  - Destruction or erosion of nearby teeth and bone due to growth of surrounding tissue.
  - Lack of space for normal tooth growth.

SURGICAL RISK INCREASES WITH
- Smoking.
- Poor nutrition.
- Diabetes.
- Use of some prescription and nonprescription drugs. Inform your doctor of any drugs, medications, or vitamin and herb supplements you are using or have used in the last month.

WHAT TO EXPECT

WHO OPERATES—Dentist or oral surgeon.

WHERE PERFORMED—Hospital, outpatient surgical facility, or dentist's office.

DIAGNOSTIC TESTS
- Before surgery: Blood and urine studies, x-ray of mouth.

ANESTHESIA
- Local anesthesia by injection.
- General anesthesia by injection and inhalation with an airway tube placed in the windpipe.

DESCRIPTION OF OPERATION
- For impacted teeth, the gum is incised over the tooth to be removed.
- For all extractions, the tooth is grasped with special instruments, rotated and elevated from the surrounding gum and bone.
- A gauze sponge is packed into the space left by the extracted tooth.
- Sometimes, sutures are used to close the gum edges. They usually come out by themselves, but may need removal in 3 or 4 days after surgery.

POSSIBLE COMPLICATIONS
- Excessive bleeding.
- Surgical-wound infection.
- Dry sockets (see Glossary).

AVERAGE HOSPITAL STAY—Usually none.

PROBABLE OUTCOME—Expect complete healing without complications. Allow about 3 weeks for recovery from surgery.

POSTOPERATIVE CARE

GENERAL MEASURES
- Do not smoke or use drinking straws for the next 24 hours.
- Keep your mouth closed firmly on the gauze sponge. Don't spit.
- Change the gauze sponge about every 30 minutes if it becomes soaked with blood. If not, leave it in place for about 3 to 4 hours after surgery.
- Use ice to relieve pain. Apply an ice pack for 10 minutes at a time every hour for 12 hours after surgery.
- Beginning 24 hours after surgery, rinse your mouth gently as needed with a solution of 1/2 teaspoon of salt in 8 oz. lukewarm water.

MEDICATION
- Your doctor or dentist may prescribe:
  - Pain relievers. Don't take prescription pain medication longer than 4 to 7 days. Use only as much as you need.
  - Antibiotics to fight or prevent infection.
- You may use nonprescription drugs, such as acetaminophen, for minor pain. Avoid aspirin.

ACTIVITY—Rest quietly at home for 24 hours after surgery, then resume limited activity for 1 or 2 days. Then, no restrictions.

DIET—Soft or liquid diet (See Appendix) for 24 hours after surgery. Do not drink alcoholic beverages during this time.

CALL YOUR DENTIST IF

- You experience nausea or vomiting.
- Medication does not relieve pain.
- Sutures drop out during the first 48 hours after surgery.
- Excessive bleeding (one gauze sponge becoming deep red in 10 to 15 minutes) continues for more than 4 hours after surgery.
- Pain, swelling, redness, or drainage increases in the surgical area.
- You develop symptoms of infection including headache, muscle aches, dizziness, fever, or a general ill feeling.
- New, unexplained symptoms develop.

TOOTH EXTRACTION

A bony impacted tooth.

The gum is incised over the tooth to be removed.

Tooth to be extracted is grasped with special instruments, rotated and elevated from the gum and bone. If sutures are used to close the surgical site, they may need removal 3 to 4 days after surgery.

TOOTH REPLANTATION

GENERAL INFORMATION

DEFINITION—Replanting a tooth that has been knocked out of its normal position. Best results are obtained when the tooth is replanted within 2 hours after injury.

BODY PARTS INVOLVED—Mouth, teeth, gums.

REASONS FOR SURGERY—Prevention of permanent loss of a tooth.

SURGICAL RISK INCREASES WITH
* Smoking, poor nutrition.
* Recent or chronic illness.
* Poor dental hygiene or gum disease.
* Diabetes.
* Use of some prescription and nonprescription drugs. Inform your doctor of any drugs, medications, or vitamin and herb supplements you are using or have used in the last month.

WHAT TO EXPECT

WHO OPERATES—Oral surgeon or dentist.

WHERE PERFORMED—Hospital, oral surgeon's or dentist's office, outpatient surgical facility, doctor's office, or emergency room.

DIAGNOSTIC TESTS—Before surgery: Usually none, because of the need for immediate surgery.

ANESTHESIA—Local anesthesia by injection.

DESCRIPTION OF OPERATION
* If you or your child has a tooth knocked out, try to find the tooth, wash it and replace it in the socket as quickly as possible. Go to your dentist as soon as possible.
* If you cannot replace the tooth in its socket, wash it and keep it wet. Go to your dentist immediately.
* Usually the root canal nerve of the tooth is removed and filled with plastic material before the tooth is reinserted. Some dentists simply place the tooth back into the socket immediately.
* The replanted tooth is anchored to neighboring teeth with wire or plastic.

POSSIBLE COMPLICATIONS
* Excessive bleeding.
* Surgical-wound infection.
* Rejection of tooth (rare if surgery is performed within 2 hours after injury).

AVERAGE HOSPITAL STAY—0 to 1 day.

PROBABLE OUTCOME—Expect complete healing without complications. Allow about 4 weeks for recovery from surgery. The tooth often appears normal. If it darkens, a plastic dental veneer can be applied to make it cosmetically acceptable.

POSTOPERATIVE CARE

GENERAL MEASURES
* Do not rinse your mouth, spit, smoke, or use drinking straws for 24 hours after surgery.
* Beginning 24 hours after surgery, rinse your mouth with a solution of 1/2 teaspoon salt in 8 oz. of lukewarm water every 1 or 2 hours.
* Brush your teeth with a soft toothbrush in the area not affected by surgery. A clean mouth heals faster.
* Do not bite down on the affected tooth until healing is complete.

MEDICATION
* Your doctor or dentist may prescribe:
  - Pain relievers. Don't take prescription pain medication longer than 4 to 7 days. Use only as much as you need.
  - Antibiotics to fight or prevent infection.
* You may use nonprescription drugs, such as acetaminophen, for minor pain. Avoid aspirin.

ACTIVITY—Avoid vigorous exercise for 6 weeks after surgery.

DIET—Resuming your normal food and fluid intake will promote more rapid healing. If your regular diet is too difficult, try a high-protein liquid diet for 2 or 3 days. Avoid alcoholic beverages until healing is complete.

CALL YOUR DENTIST IF

* Pain, swelling, redness, drainage, or bleeding increases in the surgical area.
* You develop symptoms of infection including headache, muscle aches, dizziness, fever, or a general ill feeling.
* You experience nausea or vomiting.
* New, unexplained symptoms develop.

TOOTH REPLANTATION

An illustration of teeth, gums and a socket left by a missing tooth.

Reinserted tooth

The root canal nerve of the tooth is removed and filled with plastic material before the tooth is reinserted.

The replanted tooth is anchored to neighboring teeth with wire or plastic.

TOOTH TRANSPLANTATION

 ## GENERAL INFORMATION

DEFINITION—Replacement of an injured or diseased first or second molar with a third molar (wisdom tooth).

BODY PARTS INVOLVED—Mouth, teeth, gums.

REASONS FOR SURGERY—Restoration of normal tooth function.

SURGICAL RISK INCREASES WITH
- Recent or chronic illness.
- Smoking.
- Diabetes.
- Use of some prescription and nonprescription drugs. Inform your doctor of any drugs, medications, or vitamin and herb supplements you are using or have used in the last month.

 ## WHAT TO EXPECT

WHO OPERATES—Dentist or oral surgeon.

WHERE PERFORMED—Dentist's or oral surgeon's office, outpatient surgical facility, or hospital.

DIAGNOSTIC TESTS
- Before surgery: Blood and urine studies.
- After surgery: Blood studies.

ANESTHESIA
- Local anesthesia by injection.
- General anesthesia (sometimes) by injection and inhalation, with an airway tube placed in the windpipe.

DESCRIPTION OF OPERATION
- A wisdom tooth is pulled.
- Sometimes, the root of the pulled tooth may be shortened for better fit.
- The socket where the tooth will be transplanted is enlarged.
- The wisdom tooth is inserted in the socket and secured to neighboring teeth. This provides support during healing.

POSSIBLE COMPLICATIONS
- Excessive bleeding.
- Surgical-wound infection.
- Rejection of transplanted tooth (rare).

AVERAGE HOSPITAL STAY—0 to 1 day.

PROBABLE OUTCOME—Expect complete healing without complications. Allow about 1 month for recovery from surgery.

 ## POSTOPERATIVE CARE

GENERAL MEASURES
- Do not rinse your mouth, spit, smoke, or use drinking straws for 24 hours after surgery.
- Beginning 24 hours after surgery, rinse your mouth with a solution of 1/2 teaspoon salt in 8 oz. lukewarm water every 1 or 2 hours.
- Brush your teeth with a soft toothbrush in the area of the mouth not affected by surgery. A clean mouth heals faster.
- Do not bite down on the affected tooth until healing is complete.

MEDICATION
- Your doctor or dentist may prescribe:
  - Pain relievers. Don't take prescription pain medication longer than 4 to 7 days. Use only as much as you need.
  - Antibiotics to fight or prevent infection.
- You may use nonprescription drugs, such as acetaminophen, for minor pain. Avoid aspirin.

ACTIVITY—Avoid vigorous exercise for 3 weeks after surgery.

DIET—Resuming your normal food and fluid intake will promote more rapid healing. If you find that your regular diet is too difficult, try a high-protein liquid diet (see Appendix) for 2 or 3 days. Avoid alcoholic beverages until healing is complete.

 ## CALL YOUR DENTIST IF

- Pain, swelling, redness, drainage, or bleeding increases in the surgical area.
- You develop symptoms of infection including headache, muscle aches, dizziness, fever, or a general ill feeling.
- You experience nausea and vomiting.
- New, unexplained symptoms develop.

TOOTH TRANSPLANTATION

Shown here are the gums, bones and lower teeth, with forceps grasping the tooth to be transplanted.

Gum incision

Bone

The socket where the tooth will be transplanted is enlarged.

In this example, the wisdom tooth, having been removed, is inserted in the socket and secured to neighboring teeth to provide support during healing.

TRACHEOSTOMY

GENERAL INFORMATION

DEFINITION—Creation of an opening in the windpipe (trachea) that will function as an airway either temporarily or permanently. The opening bypasses obstructions that prevent air from being inhaled or exhaled.

BODY PARTS INVOLVED—Windpipe, muscles, blood vessels, and nerves in the neck.

REASONS FOR SURGERY
- Restoration of normal breathing.
- Control of secretions from the nose and throat, particularly in patients who are unconscious.
- Creation of an open airway in patients who require prolonged breathing assistance.
- Creation of an airway in patients whose larynx is removed.

SURGICAL RISK INCREASES WITH
- Newborns and infants.
- Adults over 75.
- Obesity, smoking, poor nutrition.
- Recent illness, especially upper-respiratory infection.
- Alcoholism or chronic illness.
- Diabetes.
- Use of some prescription and nonprescription drugs. Inform your doctor of any drugs, medications, or vitamin and herb supplements you are using or have used in the last month.

WHAT TO EXPECT

WHO OPERATES—Ear, nose and throat specialist or general surgeon.

WHERE PERFORMED—Hospital, outpatient surgical facility, or emergency room.

DIAGNOSTIC TESTS—Blood and urine studies and x-rays of chest before and after surgery if necessary.

ANESTHESIA
- Local anesthesia (in emergencies) by injection.
- General anesthesia (when time allows) by injection and inhalation with an airway tube placed in the windpipe.

DESCRIPTION OF OPERATION
- An incision is made in the neck. The muscles and connective tissue around the windpipe are divided.
- A section at the front of the windpipe is cut free and removed or a flap is created.
- A tracheostomy tube is fitted into the opening in the windpipe to function as an airway. The patient will breathe through this tube as long as it is in place. Supplemental oxygen and mechanical assisted breathing can be supplied if necessary.

- The skin is closed around the tube with sutures or clips, which usually can be removed about 1 week after surgery.

POSSIBLE COMPLICATIONS
- Excessive bleeding.
- Surgical-wound infection.
- Inadvertent damage to the vocal cords, vocal-cord nerves, or esophagus.
- Scarring of trachea which causes stricture (see Glossary).

AVERAGE HOSPITAL STAY—1 to 3 days, depending on underlying condition.

PROBABLE OUTCOME—Expect complete healing without complications. Allow about 2 weeks for recovery from surgery.

POSTOPERATIVE CARE

GENERAL MEASURES
- Keep the surgical area clean. Cleanse daily with mild, unscented soap and water or with hydrogen peroxide. After cleansing, replace the dressing with a clean, dry one.
- Consult a speech therapist if recommended by your doctor.

MEDICATION
- Your doctor may prescribe:
  - Pain relievers. Don't take prescription pain medication longer than 4 to 7 days. Use only as much as you need.
  - Antibiotics to fight or prevent infection.
- You may use nonprescription drugs, such as acetaminophen, for minor pain. Avoid aspirin.

ACTIVITY
- Return to daily activities and work as soon as possible to promote healing.
- Avoid vigorous exercise for 6 weeks after surgery.

DIET—Your doctor will recommend a diet.

CALL YOUR DOCTOR IF

- Pain, swelling, redness, drainage, or bleeding increases in the surgical area.
- You develop symptoms of infection including headache, muscle aches, dizziness, fever, or a general ill feeling.
- You experience nausea or vomiting.
- Speech difficulties persist after a temporary tracheostomy tube has been removed.
- New, unexplained symptoms develop.

TRACHEOSTOMY

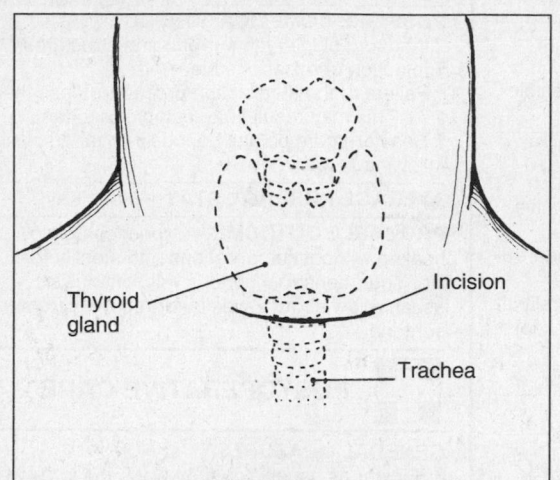

An illustration of structures in the neck and the usual incision site through the skin.

Thyroid gland

Incision

Trachea

A section at the front of the windpipe is incised and widened.

A tracheostomy tube is fitted into the opening in the windpipe to function as an airway. As long as the tracheostomy tube is in place and open, the patient will breathe through it instead of through the mouth or nose.

TUBAL LIGATION

GENERAL INFORMATION

DEFINITION—A method of sterilization that involves blocking the Fallopian tubes in such a way that the ovum (egg) becomes inaccessible for fertilization.

BODY PARTS INVOLVED—Fallopian tubes.

REASONS FOR SURGERY—Prevention of unwanted pregnancy. It is important to receive professional counseling before deciding to undergo this surgery. Sterilization is considered a permanent form of birth control. In some cases, it can be surgically reversed, generally at a considerable cost and with increased risk for subsequent pregnancies (e.g., ectopic pregnancy).

SURGICAL RISK INCREASES WITH
- Obesity, smoking, poor nutrition.
- Recent or chronic illness, diabetes.
- Use of some prescription and nonprescription drugs. Inform your doctor of any drugs, medications, or vitamin and herb supplements you are using or have used in the last month.

WHAT TO EXPECT

WHO OPERATES—Obstetrician-gynecologist or general surgeon.

WHERE PERFORMED—Hospital or outpatient surgical facility.

DIAGNOSTIC TESTS
- Before surgery: Blood and urine studies.
- After surgery: Blood studies.

ANESTHESIA
- Local anesthesia by injection.
- Spinal anesthesia by injection.
- General anesthesia by injection and inhalation with an airway tube placed in the windpipe.

DESCRIPTION OF OPERATION
- One of several techniques is used to expose the Fallopian tubes for surgery. The most common is laparoscopy, which involves two small incisions, and the use of a scope instrument with a fiberoptic light.
- Other methods used are:
  - Minilaparotomy, which involves a vaginal approach and an incision just at or above the pubic hairline.
  - Laparotomy, which requires a standard surgical incision through the abdomen.
  - Posterior colpotomy (rare) which utilizes an approach through the rear of the vagina.
- Once the Fallopian tubes are exposed, a small section of each tube is cut free and removed. The severed ends are tied (ligated) or blocked completely by coagulation using an electric current. In some cases, the tubes are clamped using a clip or band.

- The skin is closed with sutures or clips, which can usually be removed 1 week after surgery.

POSSIBLE COMPLICATIONS
- Inadvertent injury to surrounding structures.
- Infection or excessive bleeding.
- Failure of the sterilization procedure (less than 1%). This may result in an ectopic pregnancy.
- Heavier, more painful periods or ovarian cysts following surgery.

AVERAGE HOSPITAL STAY—0 to 1 day.

PROBABLE OUTCOME—Expect complete healing without complications and sterility for life. Your menstrual periods will continue as usual. Allow about 2 weeks for recovery from surgery.

POSTOPERATIVE CARE

GENERAL MEASURES
- Shower as usual. You may wash the incision gently with mild, unscented soap.
- Use another method of birth control until the next menstrual period in case ovulation has already occurred.

MEDICATION
- Your doctor may prescribe:
  - Pain relievers. Don't take prescription pain medication longer than 4 to 7 days. Use only as much as you need.
  - Stool softeners to prevent constipation.
  - Antibiotics to fight or prevent infection.
- You may use nonprescription drugs, such as acetaminophen, for minor pain. Avoid aspirin.

ACTIVITY
- Return to daily activities and work as soon as possible to promote healing.
- Avoid vigorous exercise for 2 weeks after surgery.
- Resume driving 3 days after returning home.
- Resume sexual relations when your doctor has determined that healing is complete.

DIET—Clear liquid diet until the gastrointestinal tract functions again. Then eat a well-balanced diet to promote healing.

CALL YOUR DOCTOR IF

- Pain, swelling, redness, drainage, or bleeding increases in the surgical area.
- You develop symptoms of infection including headache, muscle aches, dizziness, fever, or a general ill feeling.
- You experience nausea, vomiting, constipation, or abdominal swelling.
- New, unexplained symptoms develop.

TUBAL LIGATION

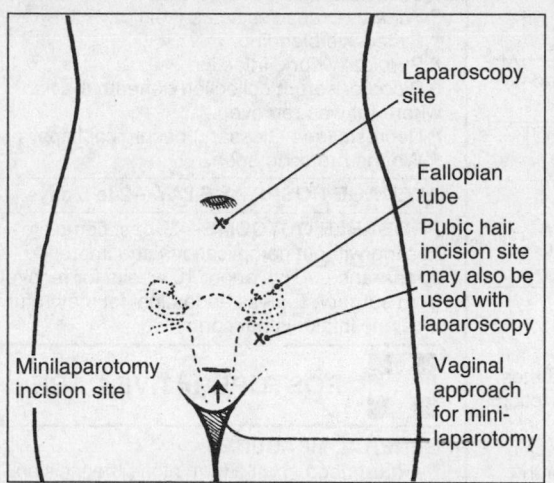

An illustration of structures of the female abdomen and pelvis showing 3 possible sites for a tubal ligation. One is a laparoscopy site; the other a vaginal approach; the third an incision at about the top of the pubic hairline.

Laparoscopy site

Fallopian tube

Pubic hair incision site may also be used with laparoscopy

Vaginal approach for mini-laparotomy

Minilaparotomy incision site

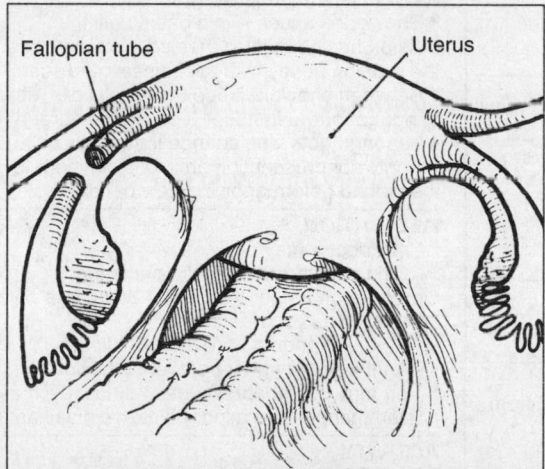

Fallopian tube

Uterus

Once the fallopian tubes are exposed, a small section of each tube is cut free and removed.

The severed ends are tied.

TUMMY TUCK
(Abdominoplasty)

GENERAL INFORMATION

DEFINITION—Removal of excess skin and fat from the abdomen.

BODY PARTS INVOLVED—Fat between skin and muscles in abdomen, skin.

REASONS FOR SURGERY
- Improved appearance.
- Reduce incidence of fungal infections in overlapping tissue.

SURGICAL RISK INCREASES WITH
- Smoking, alcoholism, poor nutrition.
- Previous abdominal surgery.
- Recent or chronic illness, especially diabetes.
- Use of some prescription and nonprescription drugs. Inform your doctor of any drugs, medications, or vitamin and herb supplements you are using or have used in the last month.

WHAT TO EXPECT

WHO OPERATES—Plastic and reconstructive surgeon.

WHERE PERFORMED—Hospital or special surgical facility.

DIAGNOSTIC TESTS
- Before surgery: Blood and urine studies.
- After surgery: Blood studies.

ANESTHESIA—General anesthesia by injection and inhalation with an airway tube placed in the windpipe.

DESCRIPTION OF OPERATION
- A large, elliptical incision, usually running from hip to hip, is made in the abdomen. Another incision is usually made around the navel so that it can be moved to a new position after the excess skin has been removed.
- Excessive skin and the underlying apron of excess fat are cut free and removed. Liposuction may also be performed to remove some of the excess fat.
- The navel is reattached in its new location.
- Drains are left under the operative site to prevent accumulation of blood and fluid from tissue drainage.
- Both edges of the skin are gently stretched and carefully sewn together with sutures. Bandages and a firm, elastic dressing similar to a girdle may be placed over the abdomen and buttocks to help hold the stitches together while healing takes place.
- Sutures can usually be removed in 10 to 14 days.

POSSIBLE COMPLICATIONS
- Wide or excessive scars (keloid).
- Excessive bleeding.
- Surgical-wound infection.
- Blood or serum collection beneath the flap where fat was removed.
- Necrosis (see Glossary) of surgical flaps.
- Wound breaking open.

AVERAGE HOSPITAL STAY—2 to 5 days.

PROBABLE OUTCOME—Expect complete healing without complications and improved appearance. Allow about 10 weeks for recovery from surgery. Excess abdominal fat may return if caloric intake is not controlled.

POSTOPERATIVE CARE

GENERAL MEASURES
- A hard ridge should form along the incision. As it heals, the ridge will gradually recede.
- Shower as usual. Avoid baths until the incision has completely healed. You may wash the incision gently with mild, unscented soap.
- Between showers, keep the wound dry with a bandage for the first 2 or 3 days after surgery. If a bandage gets wet, change it promptly.
- Apply nonprescription antibiotic ointment to the wound before applying new bandages.

MEDICATION
- Your doctor may prescribe:
  - Pain relievers. Don't take prescription pain medication longer than 4 to 7 days. Use only as much as you need.
  - Stool softeners to prevent constipation.
  - Antibiotics to fight or prevent infection.
- You may use nonprescription drugs, such as acetaminophen, for minor pain. Avoid aspirin.

ACTIVITY
- To help recovery and aid your well-being, resume daily activities, including work, as soon as you are able.
- Resume sexual relations when able.
- Exercise will help maintain improved appearance. Consult your doctor about an exercise program after recovery.

DIET—No special diet, but diet must be controlled to maintain improved appearance.

CALL YOUR DOCTOR IF

- Pain, swelling, redness, drainage, or bleeding increases in the surgical area.
- You develop symptoms of infection including headache, muscle aches, dizziness, fever, or a general ill feeling.
- You experience nausea, vomiting, constipation, or abdominal swelling.
- New, unexplained symptoms develop.

TUMMY TUCK
(Abdominoplasty)

An illustration of typical distribution of excess skin and fat in the lower abdomen.

Undermining

Resection

- A large elliptical incision is made in the lower abdomen.
- The skin is separated from underlying tissues (called undermining).
- Excessive skin and the underlying apron of excess fat are cut and removed.

- Drains are usually left under the operative site to prevent accumulation of blood and fluid from tissue drainage.
- Both edges of the skin are gently stretched and carefully sewn together with sutures, which can usually be removed in 10 to 14 days.

TYMPANOPLASTY

GENERAL INFORMATION

DEFINITION—Repair, removal or bypass of an obstruction or defect in the middle ear that prevents sound waves from reaching the inner ear. This is called conductive hearing loss, which can be total or partial. Usually, it is caused by chronic infection in the middle ear.

BODY PARTS INVOLVED—Eardrum (tympanic membrane), middle ear cavity, skin separating middle ear from inner ear, inner ear.

REASONS FOR SURGERY—Restoration of, or improvement in, hearing ability.

SURGICAL RISK INCREASES WITH
- Recent or chronic illness.
- Diabetes.
- Use of some prescription and nonprescription drugs. Inform your doctor of any drugs, medications, or vitamin and herb supplements you are using or have used in the last month.

WHAT TO EXPECT

WHO OPERATES—Ear, nose and throat specialist (otolaryngologist).

WHERE PERFORMED—Hospital.

DIAGNOSTIC TESTS
- Before surgery: Blood and urine studies, hearing tests.
- After surgery: Hearing tests.

ANESTHESIA—General anesthesia by injection and inhalation with an airway tube placed in the windpipe.

DESCRIPTION OF OPERATION
- An instrument called an ear speculum is placed in the external ear canal, and the operating microscope is positioned.
- The middle ear is entered through an incision in the eardrum.
- Depending on the type of defect, one of the following procedures is performed:
  - Repair of a defect in the eardrum.
  - Closure of the defect in the eardrum with a graft.
  - Fenestration, which is the creation of a new opening into a part of the inner ear. This method is used to treat otosclerosis (see Illness section).

POSSIBLE COMPLICATIONS
- Excessive bleeding.
- Surgical-wound infection.
- Recurrence of hole in the eardrum.

AVERAGE HOSPITAL STAY—0 to 2 days.

PROBABLE OUTCOME—Expect complete healing without complications. Hearing should improve noticeably. Allow about 6 weeks for recovery from surgery.

POSTOPERATIVE CARE

GENERAL MEASURES
- Bathe or shower as usual, but be sure to keep the ear dry until your doctor advises otherwise.
- Sleep with your head elevated (e.g., on pillows) for the first week.
- Eye glasses may be worn after dressings are removed. Cover incision with a bandage if frames rub on it.

MEDICATION
- Your doctor may prescribe:
  - Pain relievers. Don't take prescription pain medication longer than 4 to 7 days. Use only as much as you need.
  - Antibiotics to fight or prevent infection.
- You may use nonprescription drugs, such as acetaminophen, for minor pain. Avoid aspirin.

ACTIVITY
- Dizziness often occurs for a few days as hearing and balance are closely associated. Be cautious when resuming daily activities.
- After surgery, avoid bending over or heavy lifting for 2 weeks and vigorous exercise for 4 weeks.
- Resume driving about 2 weeks after surgery (or as advised).
- No swimming until your doctor advises that it is all right to do so.

DIET—A liquid diet may be prescribed the first day after surgery, then no special diet.

CALL YOUR DOCTOR IF

- Pain, swelling, redness, drainage, or bleeding increases in the surgical area.
- You develop symptoms of infection including headache, muscle aches, dizziness, fever, or a general ill feeling.

TYMPANOPLASTY

External ear

Speculum

Eardrum (tympanic membrane)

An illustration of the external ear with a speculum in place showing the appearance of the eardrum through the ear speculum.

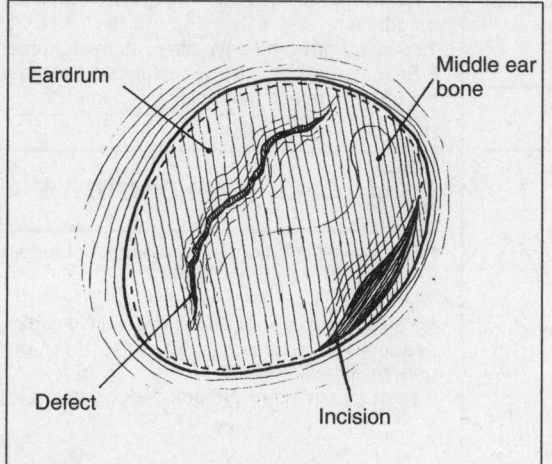

Eardrum

Middle ear bone

Defect

Incision

The middle ear is entered through an incision in the eardrum.

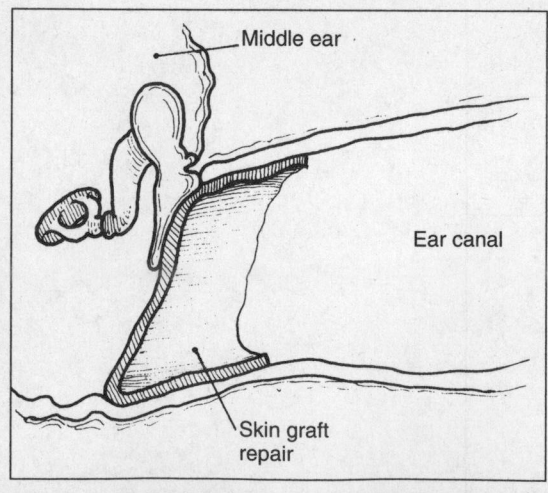

Middle ear

Ear canal

Skin graft repair

A graft repair of the defect once again seals off the middle and inner ear from air and debris in the ear canal.

URETHRAL CARUNCLE REMOVAL

GENERAL INFORMATION

DEFINITION—Removal of a urethral caruncle, a small benign tumor that develops at the opening of the female urethra.

BODY PARTS INVOLVED—Urethra, vagina (route for surgery).

REASONS FOR SURGERY—Treatment of excessive bleeding or discomfort.

SURGICAL RISK INCREASES WITH
- Adults over 60.
- Obesity, smoking.
- Poor nutrition.
- Recent or chronic illness.
- Alcoholism.
- Diabetes.
- Use of some prescription and nonprescription drugs. Inform your doctor of any drugs, medications, or vitamin and herb supplements you are using or have used in the last month.

WHAT TO EXPECT

WHO OPERATES—Urologist or obstetrician-gynecologist.

WHERE PERFORMED—Hospital, outpatient surgical facility, or doctor's office.

DIAGNOSTIC TESTS
- Before surgery: Pap smear (see Glossary), pelvic examination, blood and urine studies.
- After surgery: Pelvic examination.

ANESTHESIA—Local anesthesia by injection and topical application.

DESCRIPTION OF OPERATION
- The vagina is held open with a speculum. The caruncle is located, cleansed and anesthetized with local anesthesia.
- The caruncle is then removed with electrocauterization or a scalpel.
- Bleeding is controlled with pressure or electrocauterization.

POSSIBLE COMPLICATIONS
- Excessive bleeding.
- Surgical-wound infection.

AVERAGE HOSPITAL STAY—Usually none.

PROBABLE OUTCOME—Expect complete healing without complications. Allow about 2 weeks for recovery from surgery.

POSTOPERATIVE CARE

GENERAL MEASURES
- Bathe or shower as usual. Wash the vaginal area gently with mild, unscented soap and water after urination.
- Use a warm compress in the genital area to relieve surgical-wound pain.

MEDICATION
- Your doctor may prescribe:
  - Pain relievers. Don't take prescription pain medication longer than 4 to 7 days. Use only as much as you need.
  - Antibiotics to fight or prevent infection.
- You may use nonprescription drugs, such as acetaminophen, for minor pain. Avoid aspirin.

ACTIVITY
- To help recovery and aid your well-being, resume daily activities, including work, as soon as you are able.
- Avoid vigorous exercise for 2 weeks after surgery.
- Resume driving 3 days after returning home.
- Sexual relations may be resumed when your doctor determines that healing is complete.

DIET—No special diet.

CALL YOUR DOCTOR IF

- Pain, swelling, redness, drainage, or bleeding increases in the surgical area.
- Urination is painful or difficult.
- You develop symptoms of infection including headache, muscle aches, dizziness, fever, or a general ill feeling.
- New, unexplained symptoms develop.

URETHRAL CARUNCLE REMOVAL

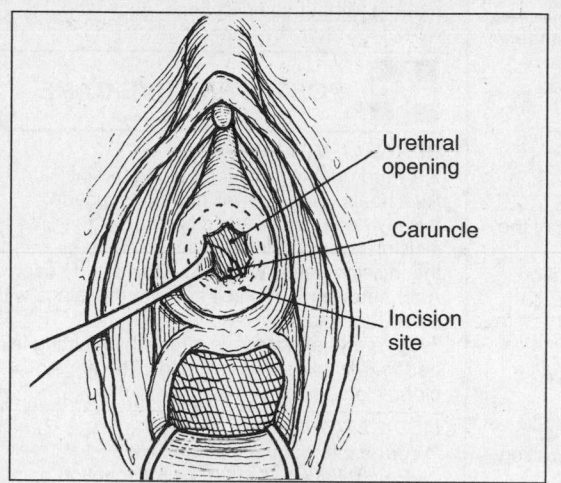

View of the vagina, held open with a speculum, showing the caruncle to be removed and the usual incision site.

Urethral opening

Caruncle

Incision site

Caruncle is removed with electrocauterization or by cutting with a scalpel.

Caruncle excised

After repair, a catheter may be left inside the bladder until healing begins.

Catheter

VAGOTOMY

GENERAL INFORMATION

DEFINITION—Disconnecting branches of the vagus nerve to slow acid production in the stomach. Usually, this surgery is performed before other surgeries such as gastroenterostomy (see in Surgery section).

BODY PARTS INVOLVED—Stomach, branches of the vagus nerve.

REASONS FOR SURGERY—Treatment of the complications of peptic ulcers such as obstruction of digestive flow, ulcer perforation, bleeding of an ulcer, or intolerable pain.

SURGICAL RISK INCREASES WITH
• Obesity or smoking.
• Poor nutrition.
• Recent or chronic illness.
• Diabetes.
• Use of some prescription and nonprescription drugs. Inform your doctor of any drugs, medications, or vitamin and herb supplements you are using or have used in the last month.

WHAT TO EXPECT

WHO OPERATES—General surgeon.

WHERE PERFORMED—Hospital.

DIAGNOSTIC TESTS
• Before surgery: Blood and urine studies, x-ray of gastrointestinal tract, gastroscopy, gastroduodenoscopy, ECG (see Glossary).
• After surgery: Blood studies, tissue studies.

ANESTHESIA—General anesthesia by injection and inhalation with an airway tube placed in the windpipe.

DESCRIPTION OF OPERATION
• An incision is made in the abdomen, and the abdominal muscles are separated.
• The vagus nerve is identified, and the branches that control stomach-acid production are isolated, divided and clipped. Segments of the vagus nerve are removed for laboratory study.
• The abdominal muscles are sewn together in layers. The skin is closed with sutures or clips, which usually can be removed about 7 to 10 days after surgery.

POSSIBLE COMPLICATIONS
• Excessive bleeding.
• Surgical-wound infection.
• Incisional hernia.
• Dumping syndrome.
• Diarrhea.
• A sensation of flushing or fainting after eating some foods.
• Recurrent ulcer due to incomplete vagotomy.

AVERAGE HOSPITAL STAY—3 to 5 days.

PROBABLE OUTCOME—Expect complete healing without complications. Allow about 6 weeks for recovery from surgery.

POSTOPERATIVE CARE

GENERAL MEASURES
• A hard ridge should form along the incision. As it heals, the ridge will gradually recede.
• Shower as usual. Avoid baths until the incision has completely healed. You may wash the incision gently with mild, unscented soap. After showering, replace any wet dressings with clean, dry ones.
• Move and elevate legs often while resting in bed to decrease the likelihood of deep-vein blood clots.

MEDICATION
• Your doctor may prescribe:
  - Pain relievers. Don't take prescription pain medication longer than 4 to 7 days. Use only as much as you need.
  - Stool softeners to prevent constipation.
  - Antibiotics to fight or prevent infection.
• You may use nonprescription drugs, such as acetaminophen and antacids, for minor pain. Avoid aspirin and other nonsteroidal anti-inflammatory drugs because they can irritate the lining of the stomach.

ACTIVITY
• Return to daily activities and work as soon as possible to promote healing.
• Avoid vigorous exercise for 6 weeks after surgery.
• Resume driving 2 weeks after returning home.

DIET—Nasogastric suctioning is required for 3-4 days, followed by clear liquid diet until the gastrointestinal tract functions again. Then eat a well-balanced diet to promote healing. Avoid coffee, tea, cocoa, cola drinks, alcoholic beverages and any food or spice that aggravates ulcer symptoms.

CALL YOUR DOCTOR IF

• Pain, swelling, redness, drainage, or bleeding increases in the surgical area.
• You develop symptoms of infection including headache, muscle aches, dizziness, fever, or a general ill feeling.
• You experience nausea, vomiting, constipation, diarrhea, black tarry stools, or abdominal swelling.
• New, unexplained symptoms develop.

VAGOTOMY

An illustration of the esophagus, stomach, rib cage and a typical incision site.

Esophagus

Incision site

Stomach

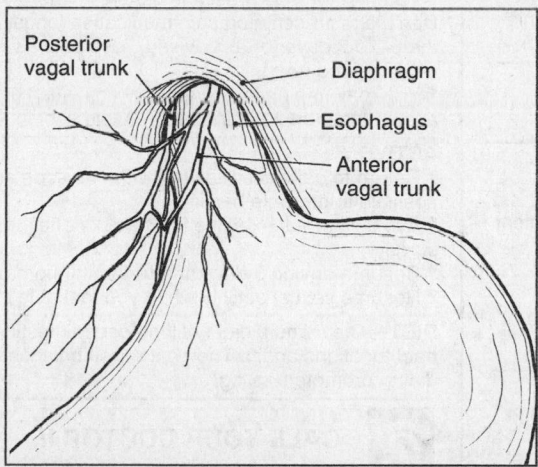

The vagus nerve is identified.

Posterior vagal trunk

Diaphragm

Esophagus

Anterior vagal trunk

- The branches that control stomach acid production are isolated, divided and clipped.
- The overlying muscles and skin are repaired with sutures or clips (not illustrated).

VARICOCELE REMOVAL
(Varicocelectomy)

 GENERAL INFORMATION

DEFINITION—Removal of a varicocele, a swelling in the scrotum caused by veins that have become distended and twisted.

BODY PARTS INVOLVED—Scrotum and its contents (usually the left testis), varicocele.

REASONS FOR SURGERY
- Relief of discomfort in the scrotum.
- Reduced congestion of the venous system around the testicles.
- Improved quality and quantity of sperm production (sometimes).

SURGICAL RISK INCREASES WITH
- Recent or chronic illness.
- Obesity.
- Diabetes.
- Use of some prescription and nonprescription drugs. Inform your doctor of any drugs, medications, or vitamin and herb supplements you are using or have used in the last month.

 WHAT TO EXPECT

WHO OPERATES—General surgeon or urologist.

WHERE PERFORMED—Hospital or outpatient surgical facility.

DIAGNOSTIC TESTS
- Before surgery: Blood and urine studies, ultrasound (see Glossary).
- After surgery: Blood studies.

ANESTHESIA
- Local anesthesia by injection.
- Spinal anesthesia by injection.

DESCRIPTION OF OPERATION
- An incision is made in the scrotum.
- The spermatic cord is identified.
- Abnormal veins are cut and tied. The twisted, dilated vein (or veins) that form the varicocele are cut free and removed. The artery and normal-appearing veins are protected.
- The skin is closed with sutures that will be absorbed by the body.
- A snug bandage is placed over the incision.

POSSIBLE COMPLICATIONS
- Excessive bleeding.
- Surgical-wound infection.
- Difficulty with urination.
- Inadvertent injury to the spermatic cord.

AVERAGE HOSPITAL STAY—0 to 1 day.

PROBABLE OUTCOME—Expect complete healing without complications. Allow about 1 week for recovery from surgery.

 POSTOPERATIVE CARE

GENERAL MEASURES
- A hard ridge should form along the incision. As it heals, the ridge will gradually recede.
- Lie down as much as possible for the first day or two.
- Apply ice packs to the surgical area to relieve discomfort immediately after surgery. After 24 hours, use heat to relieve pain if it helps.
- Shower as usual. Avoid baths until the incision has completely healed. You may wash the incision gently with mild, unscented soap. After you finish showering, replace any wet dressings with clean, dry ones.
- Wear an athletic supporter or two pairs of jockey shorts for support for 2 months after surgery.

MEDICATION
- Your doctor may prescribe pain relievers. Don't take prescription pain medication longer than 4 to 7 days (or as advised). Use only as much as you need.
- You may use nonprescription drugs, such as acetaminophen, for minor pain. Avoid aspirin.

ACTIVITY
- Return to daily activities and work as soon as possible to promote healing.
- Avoid vigorous exercise for 6 weeks after surgery.
- Resume driving 3 days after returning home.
- Resume sexual activity when you feel able to.

DIET—Clear liquid diet until the gastrointestinal tract functions again. Then eat a well-balanced diet to promote healing.

 CALL YOUR DOCTOR IF

- You experience excessive bleeding.
- You have discomfort with urination.
- You develop nausea or vomiting.
- Pain, swelling, redness, or drainage increases in the surgical area.
- You develop symptoms of infection including headache, muscle aches, dizziness, fever, or a general ill feeling.
- New, unexplained symptoms develop.

VARICOCELE REMOVAL
(Varicocelectomy)

An illustration of the penis, scrotum, spermatic cord, testicle and a typical incision site.

Spermatic cord

Incision site

Testicle

The open cord revealing the abnormal veins.

Abnormal veins

- Abnormal veins are cut and tied. The twisted, dilated vein (or veins) that form the varicocele are cut free and removed.
- The skin is closed with sutures that will be absorbed by the body (not illustrated).

VARICOSE VEIN REMOVAL

GENERAL INFORMATION

DEFINITION—Removal of varicose veins, which are veins in the leg that have become abnormally swollen or dilated.

BODY PARTS INVOLVED—Diseased veins in the legs, usually in the greater and lesser saphenous veins.

REASONS FOR SURGERY
- Improvement of appearance.
- Relief of pain or pressure symptoms.
- Treatment of recurrent superficial phlebitis (see Glossary).
- Help heal venous statis ulcers (see Glossary).

SURGICAL RISK INCREASES WITH
- Obesity, smoking, poor nutrition.
- Excess alcohol consumption.
- Adults over 60.
- History of phlebitis (blood clots), diabetes.
- Use of some prescription and nonprescription drugs. Inform your doctor of any drugs, medications, or vitamin and herb supplements you are using or have used in the last month.

WHAT TO EXPECT

WHO OPERATES—Vascular or general surgeon, plastic surgeon.

WHERE PERFORMED—Outpatient surgical facility or hospital.

DIAGNOSTIC TESTS
- Before surgery: Blood and urine studies, chest x-ray, ultrasound, ECG, doppler venous studies (see Glossary for all).
- After surgery: Blood studies.

ANESTHESIA
- Local anesthesia by injection.
- Spinal anesthesia by injection.
- General anesthesia by injection and inhalation with an airway tube placed in the windpipe.

DESCRIPTION OF OPERATION
- An incision is made over the top of the saphenous-femoral vein system (see Glossary).
- The large, diseased veins are identified. The upper and lower ends of each diseased vein are cut and tied. A thin wire instrument is passed through the vein, beginning at the ankle and extending upward through the inside of the vein, the wire is used to strip (remove) the entire vein.
- After the main veins have been removed, smaller veins are identified, incisions are made and the smaller veins are tied individually and removed.
- The skin is closed with sutures, which usually can be removed about 1 week after surgery.
- The legs are wrapped snugly in elastic bandages.

POSSIBLE COMPLICATIONS
- Excessive bleeding, surgical-wound infection.
- Inadvertent injury to nearby arteries or nerves.
- Deep-vein blood clots (rare).
- Recurrence of varicose veins.

AVERAGE HOSPITAL STAY—0 to 2 days.

PROBABLE OUTCOME—Expect complete healing without complications. Allow about 6 weeks for recovery from surgery.

POSTOPERATIVE CARE

GENERAL MEASURES
- A hard ridge should form along the incision. As it heals, the ridge will gradually recede.
- Avoid showering or bathing. Take sponge baths until your doctor advises that it is all right to get the surgical area wet.
- Keep your legs elevated whenever possible. Raise the foot of your bed and use foot rests when sitting.
- Move and elevate legs often while resting in bed to decrease the likelihood of deep-vein blood clots. Wear elastic compression stockings for 4-6 weeks.

MEDICATION
- Your doctor may prescribe:
  - Pain relievers. Don't take prescription pain medication longer than 4 to 7 days. Use only as much as you need.
  - Stool softener laxatives.
  - Antibiotics to fight or prevent infection.
- You may use nonprescription drugs, such as acetaminophen, for minor pain. Avoid aspirin.

ACTIVITY
- To help recovery and aid your well-being, resume daily activities as soon as you are able.
- Avoid vigorous exercise for 6 weeks after surgery.
- Resume driving 3 weeks after returning home.
- Resume sexual relations when able.

DIET—Clear liquid diet until the gastrointestinal tract functions again. Then eat a well-balanced diet to promote healing. Increase dietary fiber and fluid intake to help prevent constipation.

CALL YOUR DOCTOR IF

- Pain, swelling, redness, drainage, or bleeding increases in the surgical area.
- Your foot becomes cold, numb, or discolored.
- You develop symptoms of infection including headache, muscle aches, dizziness, fever, or a general ill feeling.
- New, unexplained symptoms develop.

VARICOSE VEIN REMOVAL

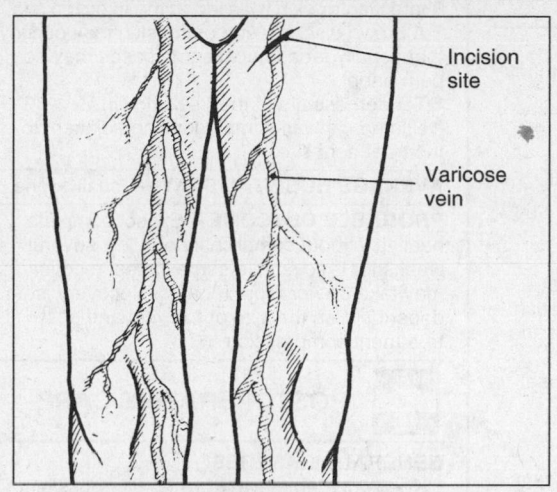

Incision
site

Varicose
vein

An illustration of diseased veins in the legs, usually the greater and lesser saphenous veins.

- The large diseased veins are identified.
- The upper and lower ends of each diseased vein are cut and tied and a thin wire instrument is passed through the inside of the vein, the wire is used to strip (remove) the entire vein (see lower illustration).

- After the main veins have been removed, smaller veins are identified, incisions are made into the skin and smaller veins are tied individually and removed.
- After surgery, the legs are wrapped snugly in elastic bandages.

VARICOSE VEIN SCLEROTHERAPY

GENERAL INFORMATION

DEFINITION—Use of a special injected chemical solution to collapse veins so that they no longer carry blood.

BODY PARTS INVOLVED—Veins in the legs, usually on the backs of the calves or on the insides of the leg. Spider veins (superficial, small veins in skin) usually form a linear, discrete or grouped pattern.

REASONS FOR SURGERY
- To relieve symptoms of varicose veins (swelling, distortion, or twisting of a vein) such as pain, aching, fatigue, or swelling of feet and ankles.
- As a follow-up treatment following varicose vein removal (see in Surgery section).
- As an early treatment to prevent the development of larger varicose veins.
- To improve cosmetic appearance of the legs.

SURGICAL RISK INCREASES WITH
- Obesity, smoking.
- Excess alcohol consumption.
- Adults over 60.
- History of thrombophlebitis, deep-vein thrombosis, or pulmonary embolism.
- Diabetes.
- Use of some prescription and nonprescription drugs. Inform your doctor of any drugs, medications, or vitamin and herb supplements you are using or have used in the last month.

WHAT TO EXPECT

WHO OPERATES—General surgeon, family doctor, dermatologist, vascular surgeon, or plastic surgeon.

WHERE PERFORMED—Outpatient surgical facility or doctor's office.

DIAGNOSTIC TESTS
- Before surgery: Normally a physical examination is sufficient, but your doctor may perform a tourniquet test to evaluate the problem or special x-rays (venography).
- After surgery: None expected.

ANESTHESIA—None required.

DESCRIPTION OF OPERATION
- A special solution (called a sclerosant) is injected into the vein or veins. This causes inflammation in the lining of the vein, and eventual fibrosis (scar tissue formation), which leads to the vein's obliteration. The blood is forced to reroute itself through healthier veins. Complete treatment may take several injections.
- After injection, firm pressure is applied so that the walls of the vein are pressed together.
- In some cases, a compression bandage may be required.

POSSIBLE COMPLICATIONS
- Varicose veins may recur.
- Infection or skin reaction at the injection site.
- A brown discoloration of the skin may occur that usually fades but in some cases may be permanent.
- Tenderness along the treated vein.
- Dilated capillaries may develop adjacent to the treatment site.

AVERAGE HOSPITAL STAY—Usually none.

PROBABLE OUTCOME—Expect complete healing without complications. Allow several weeks for recovery, in some cases, recovery may take one or more months. Recovery is dependent on the size of the vein and post-treatment compression.

POSTOPERATIVE CARE

GENERAL MEASURES
- Keep your leg elevated whenever possible. Use a foot rest when sitting.
- Bathe or shower as usual.

MEDICATION—Usually none required. You may use nonprescription drugs, such as acetaminophen, for minor pain. Avoid aspirin.

ACTIVITY
- Most activities can be resumed immediately.
- Walk as often as you can to help circulation in the legs.

DIET—No special diet.

CALL YOUR DOCTOR IF

- Pain, swelling, or redness occurs in the treated area.
- Your foot becomes cold, numb, or discolored.
- You develop symptoms of infection including headache, muscle aches, dizziness, fever, or a general ill feeling.
- New, unexplained symptoms develop.

VARICOSE VEIN SCLEROTHERAPY

Leg is prepared and positioned for treatment.

A special solution is injected into a vein.

Bandage

In severe cases, a compression bandage may be required.

VASECTOMY

GENERAL INFORMATION

DEFINITION—A method of sterilization that involves cutting and tying the vas deferens (sperm channels inside the scrotum). The surgery stops the flow of sperm and provides a safe, effective form of birth control without affecting sexual desire or ability.

BODY PARTS INVOLVED—Scrotum, vas deferens.

REASONS FOR SURGERY
- Voluntary sterilization.
- Recurrent epididymitis (see Glossary) when caused by chronic prostate infection.

SURGICAL RISK INCREASES WITH
- Recent or chronic illness, diabetes.
- Use of some prescription and nonprescription drugs. Inform your doctor of any drugs, medications, or vitamin and herb supplements you are using or have used in the last month.

WHAT TO EXPECT

WHO OPERATES—General surgeon, family doctor, or urologist.

WHERE PERFORMED—Doctor's office, outpatient surgical facility, or hospital.

DIAGNOSTIC TESTS
- Before surgery: None required.
- After surgery: Sperm studies, at least twice during 10 weeks after surgery.

ANESTHESIA—Local anesthesia by injection.

DESCRIPTION OF OPERATION
- The scrotum is shaved at home before surgery.
- Incisions are made on both sides of the scrotum. The vas deferens is identified, tied in two places and cut between the ties.
- The divided vas deferens is returned to the scrotum.
- The edges of incised skin are reconstructed with fine sutures, which usually fall out in about 7 days.
- Another method for vasectomy is called the no-scalpel technique. It requires 2 specialized instruments and avoids the usual surgical incisions. It requires no sutures to close the surgical site, and may result in fewer complications. Some men may not be appropriate candidates for this type of surgery because of differences in scrotal anatomy.

POSSIBLE COMPLICATIONS
- Collection of blood in scrotum.
- Excessive bleeding, surgical-wound infection.
- Epididymitis (see Glossary).
- Sperm granuloma (benign lump in the surgical area).
- Small possibility of reestablishing fertility.

- Pregnancy may still occur in about 1% of cases (often as a result of unprotected intercourse too soon after the procedure).

AVERAGE HOSPITAL STAY—Usually none.

PROBABLE OUTCOME—Expect sterility without complications. You may have up to 30 ejaculations before sperm completely disappears from semen. Allow 2 to 3 days for full recovery from surgery.

POSTOPERATIVE CARE

GENERAL MEASURES
- Return home immediately. Rest in bed for 24 hours. Apply ice bags to both sides of the scrotum for 20 minutes out of each hour for the first 6 to 8 hours.
- Hard ridges should form along the incisions. As they heal, the ridges will gradually recede.
- Shower as usual. Avoid baths for 24 to 48 hours after surgery. You may wash the incisions gently with mild, unscented soap. After showering, replace any wet dressings with clean, dry ones.
- Between showers, keep the incisions clean and dry.
- Wear scrotal support or two pairs of jockey shorts for 4 to 6 weeks after surgery.

MEDICATION
- Your doctor may prescribe:
  - Pain relievers. Don't take prescription pain medication longer than 4 to 7 days. Use only as much as you need.
  - Antibiotics to fight or prevent infection.
- You may use nonprescription drugs, such as acetaminophen, for minor pain. Avoid aspirin.

ACTIVITY
- Return to daily activities and work as soon as possible (usually 2 to 3 days after surgery).
- Avoid strenuous activity for 5 to 7 days following surgery. Don't swim until the incisions have completely healed.
- Resume sexual relations when able, as soon as 1 week after surgery. Use birth-control measures until laboratory studies confirm sterility (about 12 weeks).

DIET—No special diet.

CALL YOUR DOCTOR IF

- Pain, swelling, redness, drainage, or bleeding increases in the surgical area.
- You develop symptoms of infection including headache, muscle aches, dizziness, fever, or a general ill feeling.
- New, unexplained symptoms develop.

VASECTOMY

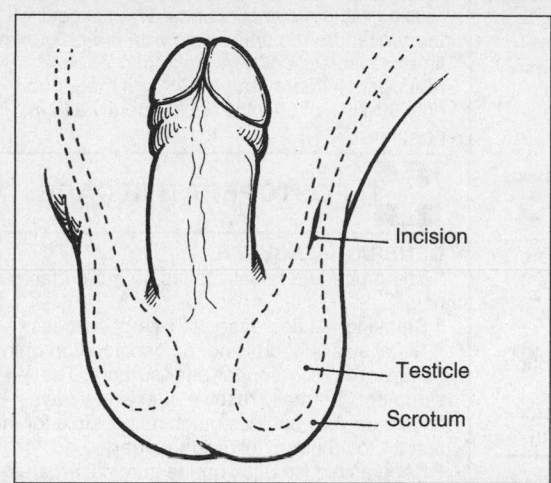

The penis, scrotum and testicles showing a typical incision site for a vasectomy.

Incision

Testicle

Scrotum

The vas deferens is identified, tied in 2 places and cut between the ties.

Vas deferens

The divided vas deferens is returned to the scrotum and the edges of incised skin are reconstructed with fine sutures that usually fall out in about 7 days (not illustrated).

VASECTOMY REVERSAL

GENERAL INFORMATION

DEFINITION—A procedure to restore the flow of sperm through the vas deferens (the tubes that carry the sperm from the testicle to the urethra). There are two types of vasectomy reversal: a vasovasostomy and a vasoepididymostomy.

BODY PARTS INVOLVED—Scrotum, vas deferens.

REASONS FOR SURGERY—Restores male reproduction ability (fertility).

SURGICAL RISK INCREASES WITH
• Diabetes.
• Use of some prescription and nonprescription drugs. Inform your doctor of any drugs, medications, or vitamin and herb supplements you are using or have used in the last month.

WHAT TO EXPECT

WHO OPERATES—Urologist.

WHERE PERFORMED—Doctor's office, outpatient surgical facility, or a hospital.

DIAGNOSTIC TESTS—Usually none. For men over 40, an ECG (see Glossary) may be performed.

ANESTHESIA
• Local anesthesia by injection.
• Regional anesthesia by injection.
• General anesthesia by injection and inhalation with an airway tube placed in the windpipe.

DESCRIPTION OF OPERATION
• The area around the scrotum is anesthetized.
• The previously cut ends of the vas deferens are located and trimmed back to normal tissue.
• The ends are then sewn back together with very fine sutures.
• When too much scarring or inflammation has occurred in the epididymis, sperm can be blocked from getting to the vas deferens. If this blockage has occurred, connecting the two ends of the vas deferens will not prove successful, and bypassing the blockage via a vasoepididymostomy must be performed.
• A vasoepididymostomy is performed by connecting the vas deferens directly to the epididymis.

POSSIBLE COMPLICATIONS
• Infection.
• Scrotal hematoma (black and blue bruised scrotum).
• Scarring where the ends are connected, causing continued blockage.
• Epididymitis (see Glossary).
• Urinary retention.

AVERAGE HOSPITAL STAY—0 to 1 day.

PROBABLE OUTCOME—Expect complete healing without complications. The success of the procedure depends largely on the amount of time elapsed since the vasectomy. Sperm reappears in more than 80-95% of men, but only 50-75% of couples subsequently achieve pregnancy.

POSTOPERATIVE CARE

GENERAL MEASURES
• The procedure usually takes no more than 5 hours.
• Smoking will decrease the rate of success.
• Slight swelling, bruising, or discoloration of the scrotal area may appear after surgery. These symptoms normally resolve after a few days.
• Rest on your back as much as possible for the first 24 to 48 hours following surgery.
• Keep a cold ice pack on the surgical area as much as possible for the first 24 to 48 hours following surgery to help reduce swelling and bruising.

MEDICATION
• Your doctor may prescribe:
  - Pain relievers. Don't take prescription pain medication longer than 4 to 7 days. Use only as much as you need.
  - Antibiotics to fight or prevent infection.
• You may use nonprescription drugs, such as acetaminophen, for minor pain. Avoid aspirin.

ACTIVITY
• Avoid vigorous physical activity for 4 weeks after the surgery.
• Resume sexual activity 3 weeks after the surgery.

DIET—No special diet.

CALL YOUR DOCTOR IF

• Pain, swelling, redness, or other abnormal symptoms appear in the surgical area.
• You develop symptoms of infection including headache, muscle aches, dizziness, fever, or a general ill feeling.
• New, unexplained symptoms develop.

VASECTOMY REVERSAL

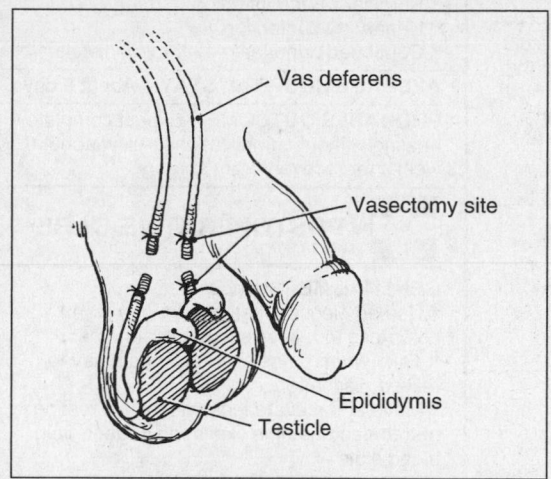

An illustration showing the site of a previous vasectomy. The vas deferens has previously been cut and tied to prevent the flow of sperm from the testicles to the urethra.

Vas deferens

Vasectomy site

Epididymis

Testicle

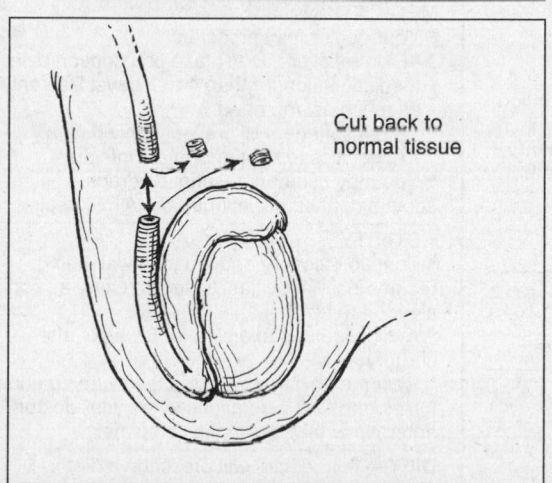

The previously cut ends of the vas deferens have been located and trimmed back to reveal normal tissue.

Cut back to normal tissue

The ends are sewn back together with very fine sutures.

End sewn back

VESICOVAGINAL FISTULA REPAIR

GENERAL INFORMATION

DEFINITION—Repair of a vesicovaginal fistula, an abnormal tract between the bladder and the vagina that usually results from tearing in childbirth, as a complication of cervical uterine surgery (e.g., vaginal hysterectomy), or as a complication of cervical cancer (particularly when radiation therapy is used).

BODY PARTS INVOLVED—Vagina and bladder.

REASONS FOR SURGERY
- Control of urine flow from the bladder.
- Prevention of vaginal and urinary tract infections.

SURGICAL RISK INCREASES WITH
- Adults over 60.
- Obesity or smoking.
- Poor nutrition.
- Recent or chronic illness.
- Alcoholism.
- Previous pelvic surgery.
- Diabetes.
- Use of some prescription and nonprescription drugs. Inform your doctor of any drugs, medications, or vitamin and herb supplements you are using or have used in the last month.

WHAT TO EXPECT

WHO OPERATES—Obstetrician-gynecologist, urologist, or general surgeon.

WHERE PERFORMED—Hospital.

DIAGNOSTIC TESTS
- Before surgery: Blood and urine studies, pelvic exam, cystoscopy (see Glossary) with biopsy (sometimes).
- After surgery: Blood studies, laboratory examination of removed tissue.

ANESTHESIA
- Spinal anesthesia by injection.
- General anesthesia by injection and inhalation with an airway tube placed in the windpipe.

DESCRIPTION OF OPERATION
- A speculum is used to hold the vagina open.
- Scar tissue around the fistula is cut free and removed. This tissue is often sent to the laboratory for examination.
- Healthy tissue is interposed between the 2 layers of the fistula.
- The bladder wall and vaginal wall are closed with sutures that will be absorbed by the body.
- The bladder is filled with sterile water to search for leaks. If leaks exist, further repairs are made. If no leaks are found, a catheter is placed in the bladder.
- The catheter usually can be removed about 5 to 7 days after surgery.

POSSIBLE COMPLICATIONS
- Excessive bleeding.
- Surgical-wound infection.
- Urinary tract infection.
- Continued urine leakage through fistula.

AVERAGE HOSPITAL STAY—About 6 days.

PROBABLE OUTCOME—Expect complete healing without complications. Allow about 6 weeks for recovery from surgery.

POSTOPERATIVE CARE

GENERAL MEASURES
- Use an electric heating pad, or a warm compress to relieve surgical-wound pain.
- Take warm baths several times a day to relieve discomfort.
- Move and elevate legs often while resting in bed to decrease the likelihood of deep-vein blood clots.

MEDICATION
- Your doctor may prescribe:
  - Pain relievers. Don't take prescription pain medication longer than 4 to 7 days. Use only as much as you need.
  - Stool softeners to prevent constipation.
  - Antibiotics to fight or prevent infection.
- You may use nonprescription drugs, such as acetaminophen, for minor pain. Avoid aspirin.

ACTIVITY
- To help recovery and aid your well-being, resume daily activities, including work, as soon as you are able.
- Avoid vigorous exercise for 6 weeks after surgery.
- Resume driving 3 weeks after returning home.
- Resume sexual relations when your doctor determines that healing is complete.

DIET—Your doctor will prescribe a diet.

CALL YOUR DOCTOR IF

- Pain, swelling, redness, drainage, or bleeding increases in the surgical area.
- You develop symptoms of infection including headache, muscle aches, dizziness, fever, or a general ill feeling.
- You experience nausea, vomiting, or constipation.
- You develop urinary frequency or stinging or burning on urination.
- New, unexplained symptoms develop.

VESICOVAGINAL FISTULA REPAIR

Urethra opening

Vagina

Fistula

The vagina with a retractor in place to expose the fistula, an abnormal tract between the bladder and the vagina that usually results from tearing in childbirth, as a complication of cervical uterine surgery (e.g., vaginal hysterectomy), or as a complication of cervical cancer (particularly when radiation therapy is used).

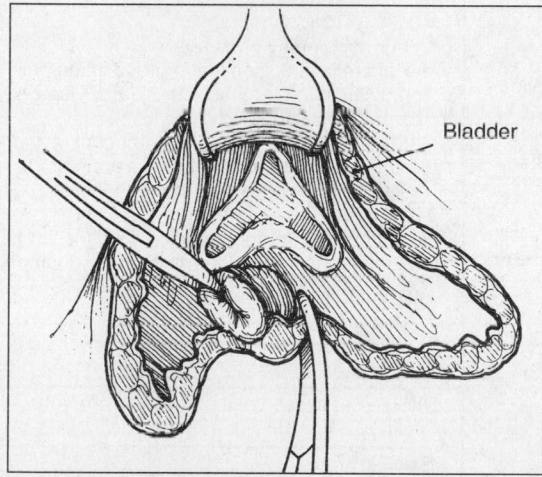

Bladder

* Scar tissue around the fistula is cut free and removed. Healthy tissue is interposed between the 2 layers of the fistula.
* The bladder wall and vaginal wall are both closed with absorbable sutures.

Catheter

The bladder is filled with sterile water to search for leaks. If leaks exist, further repairs are made. If no leaks are found, a catheter is placed in the bladder and the opening closed with sutures.

VITRECTOMY

GENERAL INFORMATION

DEFINITION—Removal of fluid from the eyeball that has clouded and blocked light from reaching the retina, causing loss of vision. A chemical solution is injected to replace the removed fluid.

BODY PARTS INVOLVED—Eye and all its parts.

REASONS FOR SURGERY—Restoration of normal vision or prevention of continued vision loss resulting from disease that blocks light from reaching the retina. These include—bleeding, injury, or infection inside the eyeball; diabetes; sickle-cell disease; complications of cataract surgery; or glaucoma.

SURGICAL RISK INCREASES WITH
- Adults over 60.
- Obesity or smoking.
- Poor nutrition.
- Recent or chronic illness.
- Alcoholism.
- Diabetes.
- Use of some prescription and nonprescription drugs. Inform your doctor of any drugs, medications, or vitamin and herb supplements you are using or have used in the last month.

WHAT TO EXPECT

WHO OPERATES—Ophthalmologist.

WHERE PERFORMED—Hospital.

DIAGNOSTIC TESTS
- Before surgery: Eye examination, blood and urine studies.
- After surgery: Eye examination.

ANESTHESIA
- Local anesthesia by injection.
- General anesthesia by injection and inhalation with an airway tube placed in the windpipe.

DESCRIPTION OF OPERATION
- A small instrument is inserted behind the cornea. The instrument is used to cut free and remove the clouded vitreous fluid and scar tissue.
- This surgery often causes a retinal detachment. Usually this is corrected by injecting gas into the vitreous cavity.
- A chemical solution that promotes healing and stimulates normal vitreous fluid production is injected.
- If sutures are needed to close the surgical wound, they may be absorbed by the body or may need to be removed in 4 to 6 days.

POSSIBLE COMPLICATIONS
- Surgical-wound infection in the eye.
- Recurrent retinal detachment.

AVERAGE HOSPITAL STAY—Usually none.

PROBABLE OUTCOME—Expect complete healing without complications. Allow about 6 weeks for recovery from surgery. Vision will greatly improve by then.

POSTOPERATIVE CARE

GENERAL MEASURES
- Specific instructions will be provided by your doctor. Follow up care can vary depending on the extent of the procedure.
- Wear the eye patch and eye shield as prescribed.
- You may read or watch television.
- Don't lift heavy objects, bend over, or strain with bowel movements until your doctor determines that healing is complete.

MEDICATION
- Your doctor may prescribe:
  - Pain relievers. Don't take prescription pain medication longer than 4 to 7 days. Use only as much as you need.
  - Stool softeners to help prevent constipation.
  - Antibiotic eye drops to fight or prevent infection. Keep eye drops cold in the refrigerator, do not freeze.
- You may use nonprescription drugs, such as acetaminophen, for minor pain. Avoid aspirin.

ACTIVITY
- Wear sunglasses when outdoors.
- Avoid vigorous exercise until doctor gives approval.

DIET—Eat a well-balanced diet to promote healing.

CALL YOUR DOCTOR IF

- Pain, swelling, redness, drainage, or bleeding increases in the surgical area.
- You develop symptoms of infection including headache, muscle aches, dizziness, fever, or a general ill feeling.
- You experience nausea, vomiting, or constipation.
- New, unexplained symptoms develop.

VITRECTOMY

An instrument is used to make a small incision just outside the cornea.

- The vitreous fluid is drained and any scar tissue is removed.
- Occasionally gas is injected into the vitreous cavity to help prevent the complication of retinal detachment.

The incision is closed with sutures. These sutures may spontaneously absorb or may need to be removed in 4 to 6 days.

Appendix

Diets

General Topics

Websites for Health & Medical Information

ADULT DIET, STANDARD

PURPOSE:
This diet is designed to promote optimum health through good nutrition. It is to be used for those individuals requiring no special dietary modification or restrictions.

DESCRIPTION:
The United States Department of Agriculture provides Dietary Guidelines for the general public to eat more healthfully. Individuals with a chronic health condition, those who want to lose weight or athletes with special needs should consult a health care provider and/or dietitian to determine what type of diet plan is appropriate for them.

The website—www.choosemyplate.gov—will help you choose the foods and amounts that are right for you (one specific diet doesn't fit all individuals) and your activity levels (30 minutes of daily exercise is recommended).

BASIC INFORMATION:
Food groups to choose from:
● **Grains:** Bread, pasta, oatmeal, breakfast cereals, tortillas, and grits are examples of grain products. Grains are divided into 2 subgroups: Whole grains contain the entire grain kernel—the bran, germ, and endosperm; refined grains have been milled, a process that removes the bran and germ.
● **Milk, Yogurt, Cheese:** All fluid milk products and many foods made from milk are considered part of this food group. Foods made from milk that retain their calcium content are part of the group, while foods made from milk that have little to no calcium, such as cream cheese, cream, and butter, are not. Most milk group choices should be fat-free or low-fat.
● **Vegetables:** Any vegetable or 100% vegetable juice counts as a member of the vegetable group. Vegetables may be raw or cooked; fresh, frozen, canned, or dried/dehydrated; and may be whole, cut-up, or mashed.
● **Fruits:** Fruit or 100% fruit juice counts as part of the fruit group. Fruits may be fresh, canned, frozen, or dried, and may be whole, cut-up, or pureed.
● **Meat, Poultry, Fish, Dry Beans, Peas, Eggs, Nuts:** Meat and poultry choices should be lean or low-fat. Fish, nuts, and seeds contain healthy oils, so choose these foods frequently instead of meat or poultry. Eat fish or seafood at least twice a week (for a total of 8 ounces).
● **Fats and Oils:** Solid fats include butter, stick margarine, shortening, and lard. Oils are fats that are liquid at room temperature, like the vegetable oils used in cooking.
● **Sugar and Salt:** Choose and prepare foods with little added sugars and salt (sodium). Read food labels and avoid products high in sugar and sodium. Limit salt intake to less than 2,300 mg (one teaspoon) daily, or if over age 51, limit salt to 1,500 mg daily (3/4 of a teaspoon).

NUTRITIONAL ADEQUACY:
This diet should be adequate in all nutrients. Choose nutrient-rich foods that offer beneficial nutrients and fewer calories. Choose fruits and vegetables, whole grains, lean meats, beans and nuts, and low-fat and fat-free dairy foods more often.

TWO SAMPLE MENUS
(for someone on a 2,000 calories-per-day diet)

BREAKFAST: 1 1/2 cups oat bran flakes with 4 ounces fat-free milk; a medium-sized banana; drink may be coffee or tea (without any added sugar or cream).
LUNCH: 1 small whole wheat bagel topped with 2 ounces lean turkey breast lunch meat, 2 romaine lettuce leaves, 1 tomato slice and reduced-fat dressing; 10 baby carrots
DINNER: 3 ounces broiled lean beef steak with herbal seasoning; 1 large sweet potato with 2 teaspoons low fat margarine; 1/2 cup cooked broccoli; beverage is 8 ounce glass of fat-free milk
3 SNACKS: 1/2 cup natural applesauce; 1/3 cup almonds
          1 cup nonfat pudding
          1 cup low-fat frozen yogurt; 1 medium-sized peach

BREAKFAST: 1 cup of oatmeal; 1 cup of low-fat yogurt; 1/2 cup of berries; drink may be coffee or tea (without any added sugar or cream).
LUNCH: Fill 2 whole wheat tortillas with 1 ounce cooked chicken breast, 1/4 cup refried beans, 1/4 cup onion and tomato, 2 tablespoons light, shredded cheese, and 1/4 cup romaine lettuce
DINNER: 1 1/2 cups cooked whole wheat pasta; 1/2 cup low fat pasta sauce, 1/2 cup cooked mushrooms, 1/4 cup cooked onions and 2 ounces cooked extra lean ground turkey breast; beverage is 8 ounce glass of fat-free milk.
3 SNACKS: A medium-sized banana
          1/4 cup unsalted peanuts, a medium-sized apple
          6 ounces fat-free yogurt; 1 cup grapes

ALLERGY/FOOD SENSITIVITY DIET
(continued on next page)

PURPOSE:
The diet is individually tailored to omit those foods that cause an immediate or delayed allergic reaction.

DESCRIPTION:
The diet may be recommended once a recognized relationship has been established between a particular food or foods and a symptomatic reaction. Common signs and symptoms of food allergies include skin reactions (itching, erythema, hives, eczema, edema) or reactions of the gastrointestinal tract (vomiting, diarrhea, abdominal pain). Systemic anaphylactic reactions could include sneezing, wheezing, conjunctivitis, palpitations, cardiac arrhythmia, shock, or collapse. Reactions can be immediate or take up to 72 hours to appear.

BASIC INFORMATION:
This information describes some of the more common food allergies (wheat, eggs, milk, corn). Other food allergens include: Seafood, nuts, legumes, chocolate, caffeine, citrus fruit, strawberries, beef, white potatoes, pork, chicken, oatmeal, rye, mustard, garlic, tomatoes, and cucumbers. The wheat-, egg-, corn-, and milk-free diets commonly use an "elimination" approach to assess potential food allergens and intolerances. Elimination diets must be planned carefully and monitored regularly.

NUTRITIONAL ADEQUACY:
If planned carefully, allergy diets are generally adequate in all nutrients. The exception would be the milk-free diet, which is inadequate in calcium and possibly vitamin D and will likely require supplementation. The elimination diets can be deficient in calories, carbohydrates, vitamins, and minerals; therefore, long-term use is not advised, and monitoring of nutritional sufficiency is essential. NOTE: These diets should be utilized under the prescription and careful guidance of a health care provider and/or dietitian.

COMMON FOOD ALLERGENS

WHEAT SENSITIVITY
Avoid foods containing wheat and wheat products. These include:
- **Milk/Dairy:** Flavored milk drinks: malted milk, chocolate milk, Ovaltine.
- **Meat/Meat Substitutes:** Meat loaf, croquettes; meats, fish, and poultry, breaded or prepared with wheat flour; hot dogs, sausage, luncheon meats; canned meat dishes with sauce; casseroles made with wheat-based ingredients.
- **Breads and Grains:** All dry or cooked wheat cereals, wheat germ, wheat bran; graham flour; all commercial breads, crackers, muffins, and biscuits (unless 100% rye), soy, corn, or specifically labeled "wheat-free"; French toast, waffles, pancakes; flour tortillas; pasta, except those specifically labeled "wheat-free."
- **Fruits and Vegetables:** Breaded, fried vegetables; scalloped tomatoes.
- **Desserts/Sweets:** All commercial cookies, cakes, pies, doughnuts, pastries; commercial pie fillings, custards, puddings thickened with wheat flour; commercial ice cream, ice cream cones; prepared cake and cookie mixes.
- **Beverages:** Coffee substitutes, flavored instant coffee mixes; instant coffee (unless 100% coffee); beer, gin, whiskey.
- **Miscellaneous:** Pretzels, seasoned potato and corn chips; cream soups; cream cheese dips, salad dressings (thickened with wheat); commercially prepared baked beans; soy sauce; commercially prepared gravies and sauces (usually thickened with wheat flour).

EGG SENSITIVITY
Avoid foods containing whole eggs, egg whites, or egg yolk. These include:
- **Milk/Dairy:** Eggnog, Ovaltine, malted milk.
- **Meat/Meat Substitutes:** Meatloaf, meat balls, croquettes; breaded or batter-dipped meat, fish, poultry; egg substitutes containing eggs or egg whites; soufflé, quiche.
- **Breads and Grains:** Breads and rolls with glazed crust; muffins, sweet rolls, doughnuts; French toast, pancakes, waffles; some commercial cake, cookie, muffin mixes; egg noodles.
- **Fruits and Vegetables:** Batter-dipped fruits or vegetables; fruit fritters.
- **Desserts/Sweets:** Cream pies; meringues, custards; french ice cream; commercially prepared cookies and cakes; candies made with almond paste or egg whites (such as divinity or commercially prepared chocolate-covered peppermint candies), cream, chocolate, fondant, marshmallow; macaroons.

ALLERGY/FOOD SENSITIVITY DIET
(continued from previous page)

MILK SENSITIVITY
Avoid all products containing milk. These include:
- Milk/Dairy: Cow's milk in all forms: fresh, dry, evaporated, condensed, buttermilk; chocolate milk, cocoa, milkshakes, malted milk, eggnog; Ovaltine; flavored instant coffee mixes; yogurt; whey.
- Meat/Meat Substitutes: Meatloaf, cold cuts, hot dogs/sausages; creamed meats, fish, poultry; scrambled eggs, quiche, souffles; all cheeses.
- Breads and Grains: Commercial breads or rolls made with milk; muffins, pancakes, French toast, waffles; prepared mixes made with milk or milk products; macaroni and cheese; pasta in cream sauce.
- Fruits and Vegetables: Mashed, scalloped, au gratin potatoes; vegetables with cheese or cream sauce.
- Desserts/Sweets: Custards, puddings; cream pies; ice cream, sherbet, frozen yogurt; candies made with chocolate, caramel, or milk ingredients; cakes and cookies made with milk or milk ingredients; whipped cream.
- Beverages: All milk-based beverages as noted above.
- Miscellaneous: Butter, margarine; sour cream; milk gravy, cream sauces, cheese sauce; salad dressings made with milk or milk-based ingredients; egg substitutes made with milk-based ingredients; Simplesse.

CORN SENSITIVITY
Avoid food containing corn, corn syrup, and cornstarch. This includes:
- **Milk/Dairy:** Chocolate milk, milkshakes, milk substitutes, cheese spreads, soy milk.
- **Meat/Meat Substitutes:** Bacon, ham, cold cuts, sausage, enchiladas, tacos, tostados, tamales, commercial entrees except those specifically labeled corn-free, commercial peanut butter.
- **Breads and Grains:** Cornbread, muffins, or rolls; English muffins, corn chips, corn tortillas, graham crackers, hominy, grits, packaged mixes of all types, corn fritters, pizza crust sprinkled with cornmeal, Cheerios, Corn Chex, Toasties, presweetened ready-to-eat cereals.
- **Fruits and Vegetables:** Sweetened fruit juice and juice products; fruits canned in heavy syrup, fruit desserts thickened with cornstarch, Harvard beets, corn, mixed vegetables, succotash, potatoes fried in corn oil, polenta.
- **Desserts/Sweets:** Cakes, candied fruits, cream pie, ice cream, pastries, sherbet.
- **Beverages:** Carbonated beverages containing corn syrup, presweetened ice tea, sweetened fruit punch, ale, beer, malted beverages, whiskey, gin.
- **Miscellaneous:** All commercial soups, homemade soup thickened with cornstarch, cane sugar, corn syrup, imitation maple syrup, Karo syrup, confectioner's (powdered) sugar, jam, jelly, and preserves, corn oil, corn oil margarine, baking powder, corn starch, chewing gum, distilled vinegar, MSG (monosodium glutamate), popcorn, yeast.

WHEAT-FREE, EGG-FREE, MILK-FREE, CORN-FREE DIET — SAMPLE MENU	
Suggested Meal Plan	Suggested Foods and Beverages
BREAKFAST	
Citrus fruit or juice	orange juice (1/2 cup)
Cereal	Rice Chex cereal (1 cup) with rice milk (3/4 cup)
Meat/meat substitute	peanut butter (no added corn syrup) (1 Tbsp)
Bread and spread	rice cakes (2)
Beverage	coffee
LUNCH (can be noon or evening meal)	
Meat/meat substitute	lean beef patty (no fillers) (3 oz)
Potato/potato substitute	baked potato (1)
Bread	Rye-Krisp crackers (4)
Vegetable and/or salad	tossed salad (1 cup)/vinegar/olive oil (2 Tbsp)
Dessert	apple (1)
Beverage	iced tea
DINNER (can be evening or noon meal)	
Soup or juice	turkey rice soup (1 cup)
Meat/meat substitute	baked boneless, skinless chicken (3 oz)
Potato/potato substitute	rice (1/2 cup)
Vegetable and/or salad	green beans (1/2 cup)
Bread and spread	slice 100% rye bread
Dessert	gelatin dessert (1/2 cup)
Beverage	coffee
SNACK	
Fruit or juice	fresh strawberries (1 cup)
Bread	rice cakes (2)

BLAND DIET
(continued on next page)

PURPOSE:
This diet is designed to provide adequate nutrition during treatment of inflammatory or ulcerative conditions of the esophagus, stomach, and intestines. It is intended to decrease irritation of the mucosa, aid in physical comfort, and provide increased dietary variety as individual tolerance improves.

DESCRIPTION:
The basic food groups are used for planning nutritionally adequate meals. The diet may vary due to individual food intolerances and the patient's lifestyle. Active mucosal irritants are avoided. These include caffeine, coffee, decaffeinated coffee, tea, cocoa, carbonated beverages containing caffeine, alcohol, chocolate, pepper, chili powder, and any other foods that cause individual discomfort. Some patients find acid fruits and fruit juices too irritating for regular use. Most foods stimulate gastric secretions and are therefore not useful as buffers to gastric acid. Three to five small moderate meals per day are recommended, if tolerable. Avoid bedtime snacks, which can stimulate acid production during the night.

BASIC INFORMATION:
There is no scientific evidence that foods other than those listed above will contribute to the formation or continuation of ulcerative disease.

NUTRITIONAL ADEQUACY:
The bland diet will meet the requirements for all essential nutrients. Food intolerances or habits that limit variety and quantity of food selection may cause some nutrient deficiencies. Patients on this diet will need to be individually assessed to determine if nutritional supplements are necessary. Chronic or severe blood loss may lead to iron deficiency.

FOOD LISTS

Food Group	Foods Allowed	Foods to Avoid
Milk & Dairy	Milk (whole, low fat or fat-free), dry or instant milk, evaporated milk, buttermilk or yogurt.	Chocolate milk or cocoa.
Meats & Meat Substitutes	Lean and tender meats with visible fat removed; beef, veal, lamb, fresh pork (cook medium to well done). Poultry; fresh, frozen or canned fish or shellfish; organ meats—liver and sweetbreads; eggs, cottage cheese, cheese.	Fried or smoked meats, processed ham, sausage, spiced or highly seasoned meats, fried eggs.
Breads & Grains	Enriched breads, cooked or ready-to-eat cereals, tortillas, rolls, melba toast, English muffins, rusks, saltines, zwieback, crackers, pasta, rice.	Fried tortillas, fry bread.
Fruits & Vegetables	All fruits, juices, and vegetables as tolerated; baked (without skin), boiled, mashed, diced, or creamed potatoes, yams.	Raw fruits and vegetables, citrus fruits, mild or hot peppers, gas-forming vegetables, fried potatoes, hash brown potatoes.
Desserts & Sweets	Custard, vanilla or fruit-flavored puddings, tapioca pudding, sherbet, ice cream, frozen yogurt, or ice milk (except chocolate and peppermint), fruit ices, flavored and plain gelatin, plain or iced cakes, sponge cake, angel food or pound cake, cookies without chocolate or peppermint, sugar, jam, jelly, honey, syrup.	Any foods containing chocolate, cocoa, or other seasonings not allowed.

BLAND DIET
(continued from previous page)

Food Group	Foods Allowed	Foods to Avoid
Beverages	Decaffeinated tea, juices as tolerated, carbonated beverages as tolerated, sports drinks as tolerated.	Coffee, tea or other drinks that contain caffeine; decaffeinated coffee; chocolate drinks; alcoholic beverages.
Miscellaneous	Salt, lemon and lime juice, vanilla and other extracts and flavorings, sage, cinnamon, thyme, mace, all-spice, paprika, vinegar, prepared mustard.	Pepper, chili powder, cocoa, or chocolate.

SAMPLE MENU

	Suggested Meal Plan	Suggested Foods and Beverages
BREAKFAST		
	Fruit juice	apricot nectar (1/2 cup)
	Cereal with milk	oatmeal (1/2 cup)
	Meat/meat substitute	soft cooked egg (1)
	Bread and spread	slice of toast, margarine (1 tsp)
	Beverage	low-fat milk (1 cup), decaffeinated tea
LUNCH (noon or evening meal)		
	Meat/meat substitute	meat loaf (3 oz), no gravy
	Vegetable	green beans (1/2 cup)
		cooked carrots (1/2 cup)
	Potato/potato substitute	whipped potatoes (1/2 cup)
	Dessert	lemon sponge pudding (1/2 cup)
	Bread and spread	dinner roll (1), margarine (1 tsp)
	Beverage	low-fat (1%) milk (1 cup)
DINNER (noon or evening meal)		
	Soup or juice	vegetable bean soup (1 cup)
	Meat/meat substitute	baked chicken (3 oz)
	Potato/potato substitute	noodles (1/2 cup)
	Vegetable	green peas (1/2 cup)
	Dessert	applesauce (1/2 cup)
	Bread and spread	slice of bread, margarine (1 tsp)
	Beverage	low-fat (1%) milk, decaffeinated tea

GLUTEN-RESTRICTED DIET
(continued on next page)

PURPOSE:
This diet is designed to eliminate the protein gluten found in barley, buckwheat, bulgur, millet, oats, quinoa, rye, spelt, triticale, wheat germ, wheat, or their derivatives for individuals with gluten-sensitive enteropathy or celiac sprue and dermatitis herpetiformis. The gliadin component of gluten is believed to be the trigger for intolerance; however, there are many components to the wheat molecule that may cause intolerance.

DESCRIPTION:
The USDA Dietary Guidelines are used as the basis for meal planning. All protein sources are acceptable except those containing gluten. Products made from the flours or starches of arrowroot, corn, potato, rice, and soybean replace products made from wheat, rye, oats, and barley and those cereals and grains listed above.

Tips on Reading Labels: Those from wheat, rye, oat, or barley sources must be excluded from the diet. Only those from arrowroot, corn, potato, soy, or tapioca are permitted. Specific ingredient information may be obtained from manufacturers or the Celiac Sprue Association, PO Box 31700, Omaha, NE 68131; (877) 272-4272; website: www.csaceliacs.org. Gluten-free products are available from certain stores. Ask your pharmacist about your medications; some drugs contain gluten.

BASIC INFORMATION:
The following ingredients contain gluten and are frequently listed on product labels.
- Flour or Cereal Products
- Hydrolyzed Vegetable Protein (HVP) or Texturized Vegetable Protein (TVP)
- Malt or Malt Flavoring
- Modified Starch or Modified Food Starch
- Monosodium Glutamate
- Soy Sauce or Soy Sauce Solids
- Starch
- Vegetable Protein
- Vegetable Gum

NUTRITIONAL ADEQUACY:
This diet should be adequate in all nutrients. An added effort will need to be made to ensure adequate fiber.

FOOD LISTS

Food Group	Foods Allowed	Foods to Avoid
Milk & Dairy	All except items listed to avoid.	Chocolate milk with cereal addition; malted milk; instant milk drinks; cocoa mix; non-dairy cream substitutes; processed cheese, cheese foods, and spreads from a gluten source.
Meat & Meat Substitutes	All unprocessed meats, poultry, fish, eggs, dried beans, legumes, nuts, peanut butter, or soybeans.	Any prepared with stabilizers or fillers such as frankfurters, luncheon meats, sandwich spreads, sausages, and canned meats; breaded fish, poultry, or meats; any meats containing vegetable protein.
Breads & Grains	Cornflakes; cornmeal; hominy; rice; puffed rice; grits; Cream of Rice; or Rice Krispies. Food items made from rice, corn, or soybean flours or gluten-free wheat starch, arrowroot, or tapioca. Homemade broth, vegetable, or cream soups made with allowed ingredients.	All products made from barley; buckwheat; bulgur; millet; oats; quinoa; rye; spelt; triticale; wheat germ or wheat; cereals containing malt flavorings; prepared mixes (cake, cookie, bread, biscuit, muffin, pancake, or waffle).
Fruits & Vegetables	All except items listed to avoid.	Any thickened or prepared. Any creamed or breaded vegetables.

GLUTEN-RESTRICTED DIET
(continued from previous page)

FOOD LISTS (continued)

Food Group	Foods Allowed	Foods to Avoid
Desserts & Sweets	Ices; homemade ice-cream; custard; junket; rice pudding; tapioca; gelatin; cakes, cookies, and pastries prepared with gluten-free wheat starch; syrup; jelly; jam; hard candies; molasses; plain chocolate candies; marshmallows.	All others unless labeled gluten-free. Read labels.
Beverages	Carbonated beverages, fruit juices, tea, coffee, decaffeinated coffee to which no wheat flour was added, sports beverages.	Postum, Ovaltine, ale, beer, root beer.
Miscellaneous	Herbs. spices, pickles,. vinegar, popcorn, potato chips, homemade broth. vegetable or cream soup made with allowed ingredients, jelly, jam, honey, corn syrup, butter or margarine.	Commercial salad dressings except pure mayonnaise, chip dips, some catsup, chili sauce, soy sauce, steak sauce, mustard, horseradish, sauces and gravies with gluten sources, some dry seasoning mixes, pickles, distilled white vinegar, stabilizers, some chewing gum, malt or malt flavoring unless derived from corn, baking powder.

SAMPLE MENU

Suggested Meal Plan	Suggested Foods and Beverages
BREAKFAST	
Fruit juice	apricot nectar (1/2 cup)
Cereal	cream of rice (1 cup)
Meat/meat substitute	poached egg (1)
Bread and spread	rice cake (1)/margarine (1 tsp)
Milk/beverage	1% milk (1 cup); coffee or tea
LUNCH (noon or evening meal)	
Meat/meat substitute	beef patty (no fillers) (3 oz)
Potato/potato substitute	mashed potato (1/2 cup)
Vegetable and/or salad salad dressing (1 Tbsp)	frozen peas (1/2 cup), lettuce/tomato salad (1 cup)
Bread and spread	slice gluten-free bread/margarine (1 tsp)
Dessert	fresh apple (1)
Beverage	coffee or tea
DINNER (noon or evening meal)	
Soup or juice	tomato juice (1/2 cup)
Meat/meat substitute	baked chicken (3 oz)
Potato/potato substitute/	rice (1/2 cup)
Vegetable and/or salad	spinach (1/2 cup)
Bread and spread	corn tortilla (1)
Dessert	rice pudding (1/2 cup)
Milk/beverage	1% milk (1 cup), coffee or tea

HIGH-FIBER DIET
(continued on next page)

PURPOSE:
This diet is designed to emphasize foods rich in dietary fiber as a part of preventive and/or therapeutic nutrition. High-fiber diets may be used in the treatment of irritable bowel syndrome, uncomplicated diverticulosis, and constipation. They may also play a role in lowering chronic disease risk such as coronary artery disease, diabetes, and certain types of cancer.

DESCRIPTION:
The high-fiber diet is based on the USDA Dietary Guidelines with an emphasis on fiber-rich foods such as fruits, legumes, vegetables, whole-grain breads, and high-fiber cereals. The Daily Reference Value for fiber is 25 gm (based on 2000 calorie-per-day diet). A maximum of 50 gm of fiber per day is suggested.

BASIC INFORMATION:
Dietary fiber is the component found in many foods that cannot be digested by the enzymes in the intestinal tract. Adequate fluid intake is important when following a high-fiber diet due to the water binding capacity of fiber. Fiber should be increased in the diet slowly to avoid unpleasant side effects (gas, abdominal bloating, cramps). Unprocessed wheat bran can increase fiber intake. Its intake should be increased slowly. It can be added to milk, cereal, yogurt, and other recipes and mixes. Dietary fiber can be divided into two separate categories: water-insoluble fiber and water-soluble fiber.

Water-Insoluble Fiber:
Water-insoluble components such as cellulose, hemicellulose, and lignin remain essentially unchanged during digestion. Foods containing water-insoluble fiber include the following: fruits, vegetables, cereals, and whole-grain products. Research suggests that insoluble fiber may be beneficial in the prevention and/or treatment of constipation and diverticular disease and may decrease the risk of colon cancer.

Water-Soluble Fiber:
Water-soluble fiber such as gum, pectin, and mucilages does dissolve in water and is found in oats, beans, barley, and some fruits and vegetables. Some studies show that this type of fiber may improve blood glucose and cholesterol levels and appetite regulation.

NUTRITIONAL ADEQUACY:
The high-fiber diet is adequate in all nutrients. Some studies indicate that excessive consumption of some high-fiber foods may bind and decrease the absorption of the following minerals: calcium, copper, iron, magnesium, selenium, and zinc. However, it is believed that with a varied, well-balanced diet, mineral or nutrient imbalances are unlikely to happen in those consuming a high-fiber diet.

DIETARY FIBER CONTENT OF FOODS IN COMMONLY SERVED PORTIONS
FOOD GROUP

(gm = gram)	Breads (1 slice)	Cereals (1 oz.)	Pasta (1 cup)	Rice (1/2 cup)	Legumes (1/2 cup)
1 gm or less	bagel, white French	Rice-Krispies, Special K, cornflakes		white	
1-1.9 gm	whole-wheat flour tortilla	oatmeal, Nutri-Grain, Cheerios	macaroni, spaghetti	brown	
2-2.9 gm	bran muffin	Wheaties, Shredded-Wheat, Total			
3-3.9 gm	corn tortilla	Cream of Wheat, Honey-Bran	whole-wheat spaghetti		lentils
4-4.9 gm		Bran Chex, 40% Bran-Flakes, Raisin Bran			lima beans, dried peas
5-5.9 gm		Corn Bran			
6 gm or more		All-Bran, Bran Buds, 100% Bran			kidney beans, baked beans, navy beans

HIGH-FIBER DIET
(continued from previous page)

DIETARY FIBER CONTENT OF FOODS IN COMMONLY SERVED PORTIONS (continued)
FOOD GROUP

(gm = gram)	Vegetables (1/2 cup)	Fruits 1 (medium unless stated)
1 gm or less	cucumber, lettuce (1 cup) green pepper, mushrooms, onions	grapes (20), watermelon (1 cup) plums
1-1.9 gm	asparagus, green beans, cabbage, potato (no skin), celery, cauliflower, sweet potato	apricots (3), grapefruit (1/2), peach with skin, pineapple (1/2 cup)
2-2.9 gm	broccoli, spinach, Brussels sprouts, carrots, corn, potato (with skin)	apple without skin, banana, orange
3-3.9 gm	peas	apple with skin, pear with skin, raspberries (1/2 cup)
4-4.9 gm		
5-5.9 gm		
6 gm or more		

SAMPLE MENU

	Suggested Meal Plan	Suggested Foods and Beverages
BREAKFAST	Fruit juice	prune juice (1/2 cup)
	Cereal	All Bran cereal (1/2 cup)
	Meat/meat substitute	poached egg (1)
	Bread and spread	slice whole grain toast & tsp margarine
	Beverage	1% milk (1 cup) & coffee or tea
LUNCH (can be noon or evening meal)		
	Meat/meat substitute	meat loaf (3 oz)
	Potato/potato substitute	baked potato (1)
	Vegetable and/or salad	lima beans (1/2 cup), tossed salad (1 cup), dressing (1 Tbsp)
	Bread and spread	slice rye bread & margarine (1 tsp)
	Dessert	fig cookies (4)
	Beverage	coffee or tea
DINNER (can be evening or noon meal)		
	Soup or juice	lentil soup (1/2 cup)
	Meat/meat substitute	baked chicken (3 oz)
	Vegetable and/or salad	banana squash (1/2 cup), tossed salad (1 cup), dressing (1 Tbsp)
	Bread and spread	slice rye bread & margarine (1 tsp)
	Dessert	baked apple with cinnamon
	Beverage	1% milk (1 cup), coffee or tea

LACTOSE INTOLERANCE DIET
(continued on next page)

PURPOSE:
This diet is designed to minimize gastrointestinal (GI) disturbances such as abdominal cramps, bloating, flatulence, increased GI motility, and diarrhea associated with ingestion of the carbohydrate lactose.

DESCRIPTION:
This diet is individualized to provide the appropriate amount of lactose that a lactose-intolerant individual may tolerate. Milk and milk products, including whey and milk solids, are limited.

BASIC INFORMATION:
Current research indicates that most lactose-intolerant individuals can consume 15–30 grams of lactose per day (about 2 cups milk) without experiencing severe symptoms. Tolerance level is highly individualized. There are a number of commercial products that will break down lactose (milk sugar), allowing more flexibility in the diet.

NUTRITIONAL ADEQUACY:
This diet may provide adequate amounts of essential nutrients based on the use of lactose-reduced food choices. If lactose-reduced foods are not included, the diet may be deficient in calcium, vitamin D, or riboflavin.

FOOD LISTS

Food Group	Foods Allowed	Foods to Avoid
Milk & Dairy	Milk substitutes and non-dairy products. Milk treated with lactose reducing enzymes, soy milk, as tolerated, buttermilk, acidophilus milk, yogurt.	Milk or milk products in excess of allowed amounts. Avoid or decrease intake with development of intolerance.
Meats & Meat Substitutes	Any meat, fish, and poultry, except those listed to avoid; peanut butter; kosher hot dogs; dried beans; eggs. Cheeses as tolerated: blue, brick, Swiss, Camembert, cheddar, Colby, mozzarella, muenster, provolone.	All other cheese and cheese products, creamed meats, luncheon meats, hot dogs, other processed meats with added lactose, breaded meats, fish or poultry, casseroles and egg dishes made with milk or foods to avoid.
Breads & Grains	Breads, cereals, crackers, quick breads such as muffins, biscuits, etc., in moderation if made with milk, rice, pasta, no lactose cereals.	Excessive use of commercial products with added milk or lactose, milk or cream-based soups or pasta, cooked or dry cereal with milk, French toast, macaroni and cheese.
Fruits & Vegetables	Any fresh, canned, or frozen.	Fruit juice products containing lactose and dietetic fruits with added lactose; creamed vegetables or vegetables in cheese sauce; mashed, au gratin, scalloped potatoes.
Desserts & Sweets	Sugar, honey, jelly, jams, plain sugar candies such as gumdrops, jelly beans, marshmallows, angel food cake, fruit ices, gelatin, commercial mixes or baked products containing milk in moderation, non-dairy frozen desserts, 1 serving milk chocolate per day.	Cream candies, tablet candies containing lactose, cream pies, products with cream fillings, cream cheese or sour cream, commercial puddings, artificial sweeteners containing lactose, toffee, caramels.
Beverages	Coffee, tea, carbonated beverages, cereal beverages, sports drinks, alcoholic beverages (if allowed by doctor), Isomil, Pregestimil, ProSobee, Ensure.	Cocoa, Ovaltine, cocoa malt, cocoa mixes, beverages containing cream, flavored instant coffee mixes.

LACTOSE INTOLERANCE DIET
(continued from previous page)

FOOD LISTS (continued)

Food Groups	Foods Allowed	Foods to Avoid
Miscellaneous	Condiments, pure flavorings, popcorn, nuts, salt, vinegar, spices, lactate, lactic acid, lactalbumin, citric acid, MSG, margarine, butter, bacon, lard, mayonnaise, vegetable oils, vegetable shortenings, most oil-based commercial salad dressings, non-dairy whipped cream, broth-type soups.	Cream sauces, milk gravies, gum, ascorbic acid tablets, spice blends with lactose added, milk or cream soups, whey, salad dressing with added milk or cheese not allowed, sour cream (alone or in spreads and dips), cream cheese and spreads, whipped cream

SAMPLE MENU

Suggested Meal Plan	Suggested Foods and Beverages
BREAKFAST	
Fruit juice	orange juice w/calcium (1 cup)
Cereal	shredded wheat (1/2 cup)
Meat/meat substitute	soft cooked egg (1)
Bread and spread	slice wheat toast with margarine (1 tsp)
Milk	lactose-free, low fat milk (1 cup)
Beverage	coffee or tea
LUNCH (can be noon or evening meal)	
Meat/meat substitute	baked chicken (3 oz)
Potato/potato substitute	brown rice (1/2 cup)
Vegetable	spinach (1/2 cup),
Salad	lettuce & tomato salad (1 cup).salad dressing (1 Tbsp)
Bread and spread	slice wheat bread with margarine (1 tsp)
Dessert	angel food cake (1 slice), strawberries (1/2 cup)
Beverage	coffee or tea
DINNER (can be evening or noon meal)	
Soup or juice	apple juice (1/2 cup)
Meat/meat substitute	lean roast beef (3 oz)
Vegetable	cooked carrots (1/2 cup)
Salad	three-bean salad (1/2 cup)
Bread and spread	dinner roll (1) with margarine (1 tsp)
Dessert	fruit sorbet (1/2 cup)
Beverage	coffee or tea

LOW-FAT/LOW-CHOLESTEROL DIET
(continued on next page)

PURPOSE:
The low-fat/low-cholesterol diets are designed to improve serum lipid profiles for the treatment and prevention of coronary heart disease (CHD).

DESCRIPTION:
Foods high in total fat, saturated fat, and cholesterol are controlled. Total cholesterol intake is restricted. Limited amounts of monounsaturated and polyunsaturated fats are used as replacements for saturated fats. Calories need to be adjusted to achieve or maintain desired body weight. Lean meat, fish, skinless poultry, and non- or low-fat dairy products are included as well as plant sources of protein such as legumes, dried beans, and dried peas. High-fat meats and poultry, organ meats, egg yolks, and cheese are limited. Foods high in complex carbohydrates and fiber such as fruits, vegetables, whole-grain products, and legumes are emphasized.

BASIC INFORMATION:
The National Cholesterol Education Program (NCEP) guidelines indicate that a serum total cholesterol should be measured in all adults over the age of 20 at least once every 5 years. Total cholesterol levels below 200 mg/dL are classified as "desirable blood cholesterol," those 200–239 mg/dL as "borderline high cholesterol," and those 240 mg/dL and over as "high blood cholesterol." Serum (blood-level) high-density lipoprotein cholesterol (HDL-C) of at least 40 mg/dL for men and 50 mg/dL for women is desirable. Elevated total serum cholesterol should be confirmed by repeat testing per your health care provider's recommendation.

Dietary treatment is the primary treatment for elevated serum cholesterol. The goals of therapy are to reduce serum cholesterol to less than 200 mg/dL and low-density lipoprotein (LDL) to less than 130 mg/dL. Another goal of therapy is to maintain a nutritionally adequate eating pattern.

Recommendations for an eating plan

Nutrient	Recommended Intake
Total fat	25% to 35%% of total calories
Saturated fat	Less than 7% of total calories
Polyunsaturated fat	Up to 10% of total calories
Monounsaturated fat	Up to 20% of total calories
Carbohydrates	At least 50% to 60% of total calories
Protein	Approximately 15% of total calories
Cholesterol	Less than 200 mg
Total calories	To achieve and maintain desirable weight

After starting the diet plan, patients should be checked at 4 to 6 weeks and then 3 months for cholesterol levels and diet adherence. It usually takes 6 months for results. Drug therapy may be recommended if cholesterol levels are still high.

Cholesterol is found only in animal products. Saturated fats are often solid at room temperature and are usually found in animal products such as meats, poultry, butter, cheese, and ice cream. Plant sources of saturated fats include palm oil, palm kernel oil, and coconut oil. Monounsaturated fats are found in products such as olive oil, peanuts, flaxseed oil, and canola (rapeseed) oil. Polyunsaturated fats are usually liquid at room temperature and are found in safflower, sunflower, corn, soybean and cottonseed oils; seeds; and certain nuts.

Along with cholesterol testing, all adults should be evaluated for other CHD risk factors such as hypertension, smoking, diabetes, and obesity.

LOW-FAT/LOW-CHOLESTEROL DIET
(continued on next page)

FOOD LISTS

Food Group	Foods Allowed	Foods to Avoid
Milk & Dairy	Fat-free or 1% fat milk (liquid, powdered, or evaporated), fat-free or low-fat yogurt, fat-free or low-fat cottage cheese, fat-free or low-fat cheese, fat-free sour cream, and fat-free cream cheese.	Whole milk (over 3% fat) (liquid, evaporated, or condensed), 2% milk, cream; half-and-half, imitation milk products, most nondairy creamers, whipped toppings, whole milk yogurt, regular cottage cheese (4% fat), natural cheeses made from whole milk (cheddar, Swiss, blue, Camembert, etc.), low-fat or regular cream cheese, low-fat or regular sour cream, low-fat sour cream.
Meat & Meat Substitutes	Cooked dried beans, split peas, lentils, pinto beans, poultry without the skin, fish, tuna packed in water, lean beef (extra lean ground beef, eye of round, sirloin, round tip, round, top round, tenderloin, top loin), lean pork (tenderloin, leg, shoulder), lamb (arm, leg, loin, rib), luncheon meats (1 gram of fat or less per ounce), egg whites (2 egg whites will equal 1 whole egg), low-cholesterol egg substitutes.	Fried meats or meat substitutes; fatty cuts of beef, pork, or lamb; goose; duck; liver, kidney, brains, or other organ meats; sausages; bacon; regular luncheon meats; peanut butter (except as allowed under Miscellaneous); or egg yolks beyond allowed.
Breads & Grains	Whole-grain breads (oatmeal, whole wheat, rye, bran, multigrains, etc.) English muffins, bagels, pita bread, rice, pasta, homemade baked goods low in fat, low-fat crackers (rice cakes, popcorn cakes, Rye Krisp, Melba toast, pretzels, breadsticks), or hot or cold cereals (with 1 to 2 grams of fat or less per serving).	High-fat baked goods (pies, cakes, doughnuts, croissants, pastries, biscuits); fry bread; high-fat crackers; egg noodles; granola type cereals; cereals with more than 2 grams of fat per serving; pasta and rice prepared with cream, butter, and cheese sauces.
Fruits & Vegetables	Any fresh, frozen, canned, or dried.	Vegetables prepared in butter, cream, and other sauces; fried vegetables, coconuts, avocados, and olives, except as allowed under Miscellaneous.
Desserts & Sweets	Sugar, jelly, jam, honey, molasses, low-fat or fat-free frozen desserts (such as sherbet, sorbet, ices, fat-free frozen yogurt, and Popsicles), angel food cake, low-fat or fat-free cakes and cookies (such as vanilla wafers, graham crackers, ginger snaps [and others with less than 2 grams of fat per serving]), baking cocoa, low-fat or fat-free candy (such as jelly beans or hard candy), low-fat or fat-free puddings, gelatin desserts.	Ice cream; high-fat cakes, pies, and cookies (most commercially made); chocolate; puddings made with whole milk; and nut candies.
Beverages	Juices, tea, coffee, decaffeinated coffee, carbonated drinks, and most alcoholic beverages. (if allowed by doctor)	Milkshakes; ice cream floats; eggnog; and alcoholic beverages containing milk, cream, and coconut.

LOW-FAT/LOW-CHOLESTEROL DIET
(continued from previous page)

FOOD LISTS (continued)

Food Group	Foods Allowed	Foods to Avoid
Miscellaneous	Limit fat based on total number of calories consumed. Generally no more than 6 to 8 servings/day of added fat such as margarine and salad dressing should be eaten; overweight, sedentary, or elderly individuals may need less. Unsaturated vegetable oils (corn, olive, canola, flaxseed, safflower, sesame, soybean, or sunflower), margarine or shortening made from unsaturated vegetable oils, salad dressings and mayonnaise made from unsaturated oils (1 Tbsp), diet margarine (2 tsp), olives (10 small or 5 large), avocado (1/8 medium or 2 Tbsp), seeds and nuts (1 Tbsp seeds, 6 almonds, 20 small peanuts), peanut butter (2 tsp); vegetable oil sprays; fat-free mayonnaise and salad dressings; fat-free sour cream; herbs, spices, pepper, and salt substitute (with doctor's approval); mustard; catsup; vinegar; lemon and lime juice; fat-free sauces; cream sauces made with allowed ingredients.	Butter, coconut oil, palm oil, palm kernel oil, lard, bacon fat, salad dressings made with egg yolk, fried snack foods (potato chips, cheese curls, tortilla chips), regular cream sauces.

SAMPLE MENU

	Suggested Meal Plan	Suggested Foods and Beverages
BREAKFAST		
	Citrus fruit or juice	grapefruit half
	Cereal	bran flakes (1/2 cup)
	Meat/meat substitute	low-cholesterol egg substitute (1/4 cup)
	Bread and spread	2 slices whole wheat toast with jelly (1 tsp)
	Beverage	1% milk (1 cup), coffee
LUNCH (can be noon or evening meal)		
	Meat/meat substitute	baked chicken breast (3 oz)
	Potato/potato substitute	sweet potato (1/2 cup)
	Vegetable and/or salad	fat-free green beans (1/2 cup)
		garden salad (1 cup) with low-fat dressing (2 Tbsp)
	Bread and spread	whole wheat rolls (2) with honey (2 tsp)
	Dessert	strawberries (1 cup)
	Beverage	iced tea
DINNER (can be evening or noon meal)		
	Soup or juice	vegetable juice (1/2 cup)
	Meat/meat substitute	fat-free meatballs (3 oz) in spaghetti sauce (1/2 cup)
	Potato/substitute	spaghetti (1/2 cup)
	Vegetable and/or salad	fat-free broccoli (1/2 cup)
		spinach salad (1 cup) with low-fat dressing (2 Tbsp)
	Bread and spread	slice Italian bread with margarine (1 tsp)
	Dessert	fruit sorbet (1/2 cup)
	Beverage	1% milk (1 cup), coffee or tea

LOW-SALT DIET
(continued on next page)

PURPOSE:
Sodium-controlled diets are used to reduce blood pressure in salt-sensitive hypertension and to promote the loss of excess fluids in edema due to cardiovascular or renal disease and in ascites due to hepatic disease. Sodium-controlled diets may also enhance the action of some medications. Over 90% of sodium in an average diet is in the form of salt, so the diet may be termed salt-restricted.

DESCRIPTION: 1.5–2.3 Gram Sodium (65–100 mEq Na)
This level of sodium is used for low salt, low sodium, salt-free, and no salt diet prescriptions. Foods high in sodium content are omitted. One-fourth teaspoon of salt is allowed in the preparation of food or may be used at the table. Because sodium is widely distributed in foods, portions and number of servings are restricted according to the sodium content.

BASIC INFORMATION:
Salt substitutes should be approved by your health care provider. Salt-free herbs and spices may be used freely. Carefully reading labels is important, as some salt-replacement seasonings contain sodium chloride. "Light" salts, which are a mixture of potassium chloride and sodium chloride, are also limited on sodium-controlled diets.

Approximately 75% of the sodium Americans consume is added to foods during processing or preparation. The following list will help you interpret sodium information on food labels:
- Sodium Free—5 mg or less of sodium per serving.
- Very Low Sodium—35 mg or less of sodium per serving.
- Low Sodium—140 mg or less of sodium per serving.
- Reduced Sodium—25% less sodium per standard serving than the regular product.
- Light in sodium—50% less sodium per standard serving than the regular product.
- No Added Salt or Unsalted—no salt is added during processing.

Water Supply
Water supplies vary in natural sodium content. Up to 25% of dietary sodium may come from drinking water. For the sodium content in your water supply, call your city's water department. Water softeners may add large amounts of sodium to the water. The sodium content of softened water ranges between 7 and 220 milligrams per quart. The company that installed your softener can provide sodium level information. Distilled drinking water may be used for cooking and drinking when water supplies contain more than 120 mg sodium per liter and the diet is below 2 grams.

Recommended Intake
The estimated average daily intake of sodium in the American diet ranges from 3.5 to 6.0 grams per day. The American Heart Association and the National Heart, Lung, and Blood Institute recommend that daily sodium intake should not exceed 2.4 grams (2400 milligrams) for healthy adults.

Hypertension (High Blood Pressure)
Although salt/sodium restriction is frequently used in the prevention and treatment of hypertension, not all persons respond equally to this restriction. African Americans, the elderly, and hypertensive adults are more sensitive to dietary sodium than other population groups. Changing lifestyle or diet will often result in a reduction in drug requirements and thereby decrease costs and adverse reactions.
Treatment for hypertension is not limited to taking medicines and the control of sodium intake.
Lifestyle and dietary treatments also play a role:
- Weight reduction, even if modest.
- Increased physical activity.
- Avoidance of tobacco.
- Moderation of alcohol intake.
- Stress management.
- Maintenance of adequate potassium, magnesium, and calcium intakes.

NUTRITIONAL ADEQUACY:
The 2.3–gram sodium-controlled diet is designed to provide adequate nutrients to meet the needs of healthy adults.

LOW-SALT DIET
(continued on next page)

FOOD LISTS

Food Group	Foods Allowed	Foods to Avoid
Milk & Dairy	Any milk—white, low-fat, fat-free, chocolate and cocoa; yogurt; natural cheese (limit 1 oz per day), low-sodium cheese and cottage cheese.	Buttermilk, malted milk, instant cocoa or milk mixes, processed cheese.
Meats & Meat Substitutes	Fresh or fresh frozen: beef, lamb, pork, veal, and game; chicken, turkey, Cornish hen, or other poultry; any fresh-water or fresh-frozen unbreaded fish and shellfish; low-sodium canned tuna or salmon; low-sodium peanut butter; eggs; dried beans and peas; unsalted nuts.	Any meat, fish, or poultry that is smoked, cured, salted, or canned such as bacon, dried beef, corned beef, cold cuts or luncheon meat, ham, turkey ham, hot dogs, sausages, sardines, anchovies, pickled items (herring, meats, or eggs), koshered meats and poultry, imitation crab, frozen/boxed entrees with more than 500 mg sodium per serving, salted nuts or peanut butter.
Breads & Grains	Enriched white, wheat, rye, and pumpernickel bread; hard rolls, bagels, English muffins, cooked cereal without salt; dry low-sodium cereals; unsalted crackers and bread-sticks; corn or flour tortillas; biscuits, muffins, cornbread, pancakes, and waffles all made with low-sodium baking powder; low-sodium or home-made bread crumbs; rice, noodles, barley, spaghetti, macaroni, other pastas; homemade bread stuffing.	Breads and rolls with salted tops; quick breads; instant hot cereals; dry cereals with added salt; crackers with salted tops; pancakes, waffles, muffins, biscuits, and cornbread with salt, baking powder, self-rising flour or instant mixes; regular bread crumbs or cracker crumbs; commercial stuffing
Fruits & Vegetables	Fresh, frozen, and low-sodium canned vegetables; regular canned, drained vegetables (limit to 1/2 cup serving per day); unsalted tomato sauce, low-sodium vegetable juice; sauerkraut, salt-free potato chips. All fruits and juices.	Regular canned vegetables (over 1/2 cup per day); vegetable juices; sauerkraut; pickled vegetables and others prepared in brine; instant potato products with added salt, and salted prunes (saladitos).
Desserts & Sweets	Any sweets such as sugar, honey, jam, jelly, syrup, marmalade, hard candy; limit regular baked products (cake, pie, cookies) to 1 serving a day.	More than 1 serving a day of regular baked products.
Beverages	Coffee, tea, soft drinks with less than 35 mg sodium per serving; alcoholic beverages (if your health care provider approves).	Commercially softened water as a beverage or in food preparation.

LOW-SALT DIET
(continued from previous page)

Food Group	Foods Allowed	Foods to Avoid
Miscellaneous	Limit added salt to 1/4 teaspoon per day, may be used in cooking or at the table; limit to 3 tsp salted butter or margarine per day; salt-free butter or margarine; vegetable oils, shortening, and mayonnaise; salt-free salad dressings; salt substitute (with health care provider's approval); pepper, herbs, and spices; flavorings; vinegar and lemon or lime juice; salt-free seasonings; low-sodium condiments such as catsup, chili sauce, and mustard; fresh-ground horseradish; homemade or salt-free soups; low-sodium baking powder; unsalted snacks such as nuts, seeds, pretzels, chips, and popcorn.	Added salt in excess of 1/4 tsp per day; light-salt; garlic salt, celery salt, onion salt, and seasoned salt; sea salt, rock salt, and kosher salt; seasonings containing salt and sodium compounds; monosodium glutamate (MSG, Accent); regular catsup, chili sauce, mustard, pickles, relishes, olives, and horse-radish; Kitchen Bouquet; gravy and sauce mixes; barbecue sauce, soy and teriyaki sauce; Worcestershire and steak sauce; salted snack foods such as nuts, seeds, pretzels, chips, and popcorn; commercially prepared convenience foods; regular canned or dried soups.

SAMPLE MENU
(approximately 1,500 mg salt; 4,700 mg potassium)

Suggested Meal Plan	Suggested Foods and Beverages
BREAKFAST	
Fruit or fruit juice	orange juice (6 oz), cantaloupe (1/2 cup)
Cereal	shredded wheat cereal (1 cup)
Bread and spread	slice white toast, unsalted margarine (1 tsp)
Beverage	1% milk (1 cup), coffee or tea (no sugar or cream)
LUNCH (can be noon or evening meal)	
Meat/meat substitute	turkey (2 oz in a sandwich) Swiss cheese (1 oz)
Vegetable or salad	tomato slice (1) and lettuce leaves (2), baby carrots (8)
Bread and spread	2 slices whole-wheat bread, mayonnaise (1 Tbsp)
Dessert	fig bar cookies (2)
Beverage	coffee or tea (no sugar or cream)
DINNER (can be evening or noon meal)	
Meat/meat substitute	baked salmon (3 oz)
Potato/potato substitute	long grain brown rice (1/2 cup)
Vegetable and/or salad	tossed salad (1 1/2 cups), oil and vinegar dressing (2 Tbsp) asparagus spears (6)
Bread and spread	whole wheat dinner roll (1 medium), unsalted margarine (1 tsp)
Dessert	slice angel food cake, strawberries (1/2 cup), whipped cream (2 Tbsp)
Beverage	coffee or tea (no sugar or cream)
SNACK	Fruit: banana (1 medium)
Meat/meat substitute	unsalted dry roasted almonds (1/4 cup)

WEIGHT REDUCTION DIET
(continued on next page)

PURPOSE:
This is a simple "exchange list" diet for individuals who want to lose weight. The goal of diet therapy is to reduce caloric intake to a level that can be safely and comfortably tolerated. Usually diets that provide 1,200 to 1,500 calories a day are acceptable for most people. However, you and your health care provider should determine the appropriate amount of calories required for your weight, height, activity level, and general health. The example shown is for a 1,400 calories per day menu. It may be modified by adding more food portions.

DESCRIPTION:
Plan your breakfast, lunch, and dinner meals by selecting items from the appropriate food list. This sample diet allows you one fruit portion, one starch, and one milk for breakfast. You may choose cereal with banana and milk. Coffee or tea is a "free" item. Amounts of each portion are indicated in each food list. Portions can be interchanged among breakfast, lunch, and dinner as long as the total for the day doesn't exceed those indicated. For example, you can eat all your fruits for breakfast if desired, but don't exceed four portions for the day.

SUGGESTED MEAL PLANS FOR APPROXIMATELY 1,400 CALORIES PER DAY DIET
DAILY PORTIONS FROM FOOD LISTS
(See lists below and following page)

BREAKFAST	LUNCH	DINNER	SNACK
1 Fruit	2 Meats	3 Meats	1 Starch
2 Starches/Bread	1 Vegetable	1 Fat	1 Fruit
1 Milk	1 Fat	2 Starches/bread	1 Milk
	2 Starches/bread	1 Vegetable	
	1 Fruit	1 Fruit	
	(raw vegetable	(raw vegetable	
	as desired)	as desired)	

FRUIT LIST (60 calories, 15 grams carbohydrates):
(A portion is 1 small piece or 1/2 cup unless listed)

Apples (juice or sauce)	Fruit cocktail	Plums (2)
Apricots (4)	Grapefruit or juice	Prunes (3)
Apricots, dried (7 halves)	Grapes (15)	Prune Juice (1/4 cup)
Banana (1/2)	Grape juice	Raspberries (1 cup)
Blackberries (3/4 cup)	Lemon	Raisins (2 Tbsp)
Blueberries (3/4 cup)	Orange/orange Juice	Rhubarb
Cantaloupe (1/3)	Peach	Strawberries (10)
Cherries (12 or 1/2 cup)	Pear	Tangerine
Dates (2)	Pineapple (3/4 cup fresh)	Watermelon (1 cup)

VEGETABLE LIST (25 calories, 5 grams carbohydrates, 2 grams protein):
(A portion is 1 cup raw or 1/2 cup cooked)

Artichoke	Celery	Peppers
Asparagus	Cucumber	Peas
Beans	Eggplant	Pumpkin
(green, wax, or sprouts)	Endive	Radish
Beets	Mixed vegetables	Rutabaga
Broccoli	Mushrooms	Spinach
Brussels sprouts	Okra	Squash
Cabbage or sauerkraut	Onions	Tomato
Cauliflower	Parsnips	Turnips
Carrot		

Note: Some vegetables are shown in the Starch List.

WEIGHT REDUCTION DIET
(continued from previous page)

STARCH LIST (80 calories, 15 grams carbohydrates, 2–3 grams protein, 1–2 grams fat):
(A portion is 1/4 cup or as listed)

Angel food cake (1 oz)
Bagel (small or 1 oz)
Beans, canned (1/3 cup)
Biscuit (2 1/2 inch size, 1)
Bread (1 slice)
Bun (1/2)
Cereal (3/4 cup, dry;
  1/2 cup, hot)
Corn (1/2 cup)
Cookies (fat-free, 1 or 2
  small)

Cornbread (2-inch cube)
Cornstarch (2 Tbsp)
English muffin (1/2)
Gelatin (1/2 cup)
Graham crackers (2)
Lentils, canned (1/3 cup)
Matzo crackers (3/4 oz)
Pancake (4-inch size, 1)
Pasta (1/2 cup)
Pita bread (6 inch size, 1/2)

Popcorn, fat-free (3 cups)
Potato, white (1/2 cup)
Potato, sweet (1/3 cup)
Pretzels (5 small)
Rice (1/3 cup)
Rice cakes (2)
Saltines (6)
Taco shell (1)
Tortilla (6–inch, 1)

MEAT OR MEAT SUBSTITUTE LIST (55–70 calories, 7 grams protein, 3–5 grams fat):
(A portion is 1 ounce or 1/4 cup or as listed)

Beef (lean cuts)
Cheese (fat-free milk types)
Cold cuts or frankfurters
  (95% fat-free)
Cottage cheese (1/3 cup)

Eggs (3 per week)
Fish (all types)
Lamb (leg, roasted)
Peanut butter (1 Tbsp)
Poultry (no skin)

Pork (chops, ham, roast)
Shellfish
Soybeans, cooked (1/3 cup)
Veal

FAT LIST (45 calories, 5 grams fat):
(Use fat-free or low-fat products when they are available)

Bacon, crisp (1 slice)
Cheese, cream* (1 Tbsp)
Coconut (2 Tbsp)
Cream, light (2 Tbsp)

Gravy (2 Tbsp)
Margarine* (1 teaspoon)
Mayonnaise* (1 teaspoon)
Nuts (6 to 10)

Oils (1 teaspoon)
Olives (5 large)
Salad dressings* (1 Tbsp)
Seeds (1 Tbsp)

* Portion amounts may be increased if using fat-free products (e.g., mayonnaise, 2 Tbsp)

MILK LIST (80 calories, 12 grams carbohydrates, 8 grams protein):
Fat-free milk (1 cup)
Yogurt (1 cup plain, fat-free, unsweetened,
  except with sugar substitute)

FREE ITEMS: (You may have these as desired)
Beverages—coffee, tea, sugar-free beverages
Pickles, except sweet pickles
Bouillon and consommés
All spices, herbs, flavorings, and
  artificial sweeteners
Catsup, mustard, soy sauce, vinegar
Worcestershire sauce
Sugar-free gelatin

Raw salad greens—lettuce, parsley,
  romaine, spinach, watercress, endive,
  escarole, cabbage, Chinese cabbage,
  other greens
Nonstick pan spray
Lemon or lime juice
Sugar substitutes

ADDITIONAL INFORMATION:
- Purchase fruits fresh, fresh-frozen, canned unsweetened, or in natural juices. All juices should be unsweetened.
- Vegetable and fruit portions are for the edible amounts of the item.
- Allowed amounts of meats are after cooking; amounts shown are for edible parts only (excluding bones). Be sure to trim all extra fat away from meat before cooking. Remove skin from all poultry. Roasting, grilling, or broiling of meats is preferred.
- If salt intake is limited, avoid foods high in sodium (e.g., pickles) and don't use salt at the table.
- Even though the diet should meet your nutritional needs, a vitamin and mineral supplement may be recommended by your health care provider.
- Everyone on a diet will experience an occasional setback. This doesn't mean failure. Long-term success is still possible.
- Combine your diet with eating behavior modification and exercise to help you maintain the weight loss.

WEIGHT CONTROL SUGGESTIONS

Weight control diets are designed to provide a specific calorie level calculated to meet an individual's requirement to attain optimal body weight. An exercise program is also highly recommended. Weight loss of 1–2 pounds per week is generally optimal.

Weight loss diets of greater than 1,200 calories per day are generally adequate in all nutrients (except possibly, iron) as long as the diet is planned to include a variety of foods from all food groups.

BEHAVIORAL STRATEGIES IN MANAGEMENT OF WEIGHT CONTROL

Individuals seeking to make a lifetime commitment to improve their eating and exercise habits can succeed at long-term weight loss. Most of the successful long-term weight-loss programs include several components: behavior modification; exercise; nutrition; social support; and cognitive changes, including goal setting, assertiveness training, and coping with mistakes and motivation. Emphasis should be placed on slow, progressive weight loss of approximately 1/2 to 2 pounds per week.

The following is a list of behavior modification techniques that can be used to promote healthy eating, lifestyle and, in turn, weight loss.

BEHAVIOR MODIFICATION TECHNIQUES:

- Evaluate what behaviors, activities, or feelings trigger eating.
- Don't use food as a reward for desired behavior.
- Drink plenty of non-caloric fluids, including water, daily.
- Change usual eating-places; avoid eating while involved in other activities.
- Make an effort to eat breakfast and small, frequent meals.
- Eat fresh fruits and raw vegetables at least four times daily.
- Exercise along with television exercise programs or during commercials when watching television.
- Eat slowly, putting your utensil down between bites.
- Weight should be checked on a weekly basis only.
- Remove high-calorie, low-nutrient foods from cupboards.
- Keep busy so the focus is not on food.
- Shop from a healthy food list and not when hungry.
- Leave the table soon after eating and don't feel a need to finish everything.
- Trim visible fat off meat and skin off poultry.
- Place a photo of a thinner you on the mirror.
- Plan ahead, especially when attending social events.
- Keep records of intake and/or weight loss progress.
- When weight drops, give away clothes that no longer fit.
- Break the habit of nibbling while cooking or cleaning up from meals.
- Try fat-free, low-fat, and low-calorie food items.

BREAST SELF-EXAMINATION

FINDING BREAST CANCER EARLY
* There have been many advances made in diagnosing and treating breast cancer. More and more women are surviving the disease. In many cases, breast cancers found early and treated promptly have a better chance for a cure.
* Tools to detect breast cancer include exams by a medical professional, mammography, ultrasound, and breast self-examination (BSE). BSE has come under some debate about how effective it is. Studies have shown that there is no difference in the number of lives saved among women who did perform a BSE and those who did not. In addition, they have found that BSE may increase unneeded biopsies and anxiety.
* Per the American Cancer Society, BSE is an option for women starting in their 20s. BSE can help a woman under age 40 learn what her breasts feel like under normal conditions. If a lump or other change is discovered, she can see her health care provider about it. Exams by a medical professional and mammography should have the most emphasis in early detection of breast cancer.
* Products have been approved by the Food & Drug Administration (FDA) to help women perform monthly breast self-examinations. They may help make the exams easier for some women. Ask your health care provider about their use.

WHEN TO EXAMINE YOUR BREASTS
* Follow the same procedure once a month a few days to about a week after your period ends, when your breasts are usually not tender or swollen. Breast tissue in adult women changes throughout the month as it responds to hormone levels occurring during the menstrual cycle. Some women have normally lumpy breasts, but they can still learn the pattern of the lumps and should be able to detect new or unusual lumps.
* After menopause, check your breasts on the same day of each month. After a hysterectomy, ask your health care provider about the best time of the month.

BREAST EXAM WHILE LYING DOWN ON YOUR BACK
* To examine your right breast, put a pillow or folded towel under your right shoulder. Place your right hand under your head—this distributes breast tissue more evenly on the chest.
* Use the finger pads of the three middle fingers of your left hand. Press gently and firmly. A ridge of firm tissue in the lower curve of each breast is normal. Then move around the breast in 1) a circular pattern, 2) up and down line, or 3) in a wedge pattern. Always use the same pattern each month. Now repeat the procedure on your left breast with a pillow under your left shoulder and the left hand under your head. Notice how your breast structure feels.
* Check the area under each arm (with your elbow slightly bent). The lymph glands are in this area. They may become swollen if you are sick. If you feel a small lump that moves freely, check it daily for a few days. If it doesn't go away, call your health care provider.
* Any discharge from the nipple, clear or bloody, should be reported to your health care provider.

BREAST EXAM IN THE SHOWER
Examine your breasts during a shower (hands glide easier over wet skin). With the fingers flat, move the hand gently over every part of each breast. Use your right hand to examine the left breast, left hand for the right breast. Check for any lump, hard knot, or thickening.

BREAST EXAM IN FRONT OF A MIRROR
Inspect your breasts with arms at your sides. Next, raise your arms high overhead. Look for any changes in each breast (swelling, dimpling, or changes in the nipple).

SIGNS OF POSSIBLE PROBLEMS IN YOUR BREASTS
* Lumps, hard knots, or thickening in the breast.
* Unusual swelling, warmth, redness, or darkening that does not go away.
* Change in the size or shape of your breast.
* Dimpling or puckering of the skin.
* Itchy, scaly, sore, or rash on the nipple.
* Pulling in of the nipple or other parts of the breast.
* Nipple discharge that starts suddenly.
* Pain in one spot that does not vary or change with your monthly cycle.

WHAT TO DO
* It is important to see your health care provider as soon as possible if you find any suspicious changes in your breasts. Don't be frightened. Most breast lumps or changes are not cancer.
* Remember that a monthly breast exam is not a substitute for the other two critical parts of the guidelines for early breast cancer detection. The American Cancer Society recommends an annual mammogram after age 40, and an exam by a medical professional every three years for women ages 20–39, and annually for women over age 40. Ask your health care provider about when you should schedule a mammogram and a breast exam.
* To learn more: American Cancer Society, 1599 Clifton Rd., Atlanta, GA 30329, (800) ACS-2345; website: www.cancer.org or National Cancer Institute, (800) 4-CANCER; website: www.nci.nih.gov.

CONDOM USAGE
(continued on next page)

 GENERAL INFORMATION

WHO SHOULD USE A CONDOM?
- Condoms are used for both birth control and reducing the risk of disease. Some people think that other forms of birth control will also protect them against disease. This is not true. Even if you use another form of birth control, you need a condom to help reduce the risk of getting STDs (sexually transmitted diseases) including the human immunodeficiency virus (HIV) infection.
- Condoms do not make sex 100% safe, but, if properly used, they can reduce the chance of contracting STDs. This can mean protection not only for you and your partner, but also for any children you may have in the future.

CHOOSING A CONDOM
Read the label and look for the following:
- The condoms should be made of latex (rubber) or made of polyurethane.
- It should say that the condoms are to prevent disease, and if used properly, latex condoms help reduce risk of HIV transmission and many other STDs. If the package doesn't say anything about preventing disease, the condoms may not provide the protection you need. Novelty condoms, for example, will not be labeled for either disease- or pregnancy-prevention. Condoms that don't cover the entire penis are not labeled for disease prevention and should not be used for this purpose. For proper protection, a condom must unroll to cover the entire penis.
- Check the expiration date (EXP followed by date). The condom should not be purchased or used after that date.
- Condoms are available in many stores and from vending machines. If buying condoms from vending machines, check for proper labeling. Do not buy condoms from a vending machine located where it may be subject to extreme temperatures or direct sunlight.
- Condoms should be stored in a cool, dry place out of direct sunlight. Closets or drawers usually make good storage places. Condoms should not be kept in a pocket, wallet, or purse for more than a few hours at a time because they may be exposed to extreme temperatures.

HOW TO USE A CONDOM
- When opening a condom, handle the package gently. Don't use teeth, sharp fingernails, scissors, or other sharp instruments. These may damage the condom. Make sure you can see what you're doing!
- After you open the package, inspect the condom. If the material sticks to itself or is gummy, the condom is no good. Check the condom top for other obvious damage such as brittleness, tears, and holes. Do not unroll the condom to check it; this could damage it.
- Use a new condom at the beginning of every sexual act (vaginal or anal intercourse and oral sex).
- Put the condom on as soon as the penis is erect and before any contact is made between the penis and any part of the partner's body. Don't delay condom use. Studies have shown that while pre-ejaculatory fluid is not semen, it does contain HIV.
- If the condom does not have a reservoir tip, pinch the tip enough to leave a half-inch space for semen to collect. Make sure to squeeze out any air in the tip to help keep the condom from breaking.
- While holding the condom by the rim (and pinching the half-inch tip, if needed), place the condom on top of the penis. Then, continuing to hold it by the rim, unroll it all the way to the base of the penis. If you are using water-based lubricant, you can put more on the outside of the condom.
- If you feel the condom break, stop right away, withdraw, and put on a new condom.
- After ejaculation and before the penis gets soft, grip the rim of the condom and carefully withdraw.
- To remove the condom, gently pull it off the penis, being careful the semen doesn't spill out.
- Wrap the used condom in a tissue and throw it in the trash. Because condoms may cause problems in sewers, don't flush them down the toilet. Then wash your hands with soap and warm water.

PRECAUTION
Condoms provide good protection for vaginal and oral sex (where the penis is in contact with the mouth). The protection they give for anal sex is questionable. The Surgeon General of the Public Health Service has said, "Condoms provide some protection, but anal intercourse is simply too dangerous a practice." Condoms may be more likely to break during anal intercourse than during other types of sex. This is due to the greater amount of friction and other stresses involved. Even if the condom doesn't break, anal intercourse is very risky because it can cause rectal tissue to tear and bleed. This allows disease germs to pass more easily from one partner to another.

CONDOM USAGE
(continued from previous page)

SPERMICIDES

Spermicides (gels, creams, foams, or films), which kill sperm, are used for birth control, either alone or with barrier contraceptives such as the diaphragm or cervical cap. A spermicide called nonoxynol 9 has been widely used with condoms to supposedly help reduce the risk of STD transmission. Studies now show that nonoxynol 9 does not reduce the risk of transmission of the human immunodeficiency virus (HIV) or other STDs during intercourse. Some condoms come with nonoxynol-9 already added but they are not recommended for prevention of STDs. The best STD and HIV barrier is a latex condom without nonoxynol-9. Nevertheless, a condom that is lubricated with nonoxynol-9 is safer than unprotected sex with no condom at all. Condom packages are required to be labeled with the expiration date of the spermicide, and they should not be used after that date. In females, frequent use of spermicides containing nonoxynol 9 can cause vaginal irritation and lesions (sores), which may actually increase the possibility of transmitting an STD from an infected partner.

LUBRICANTS

Lubricants may help prevent condoms from breaking during use. They may prevent irritation that might increase the chance of infection. Some condoms come lubricated with dry silicone, jelly, or cream, or you can add water-based lubricants specifically made for this purpose (for example, K-Y Lubricating Jelly). If you use a separate lubricant, never use a product that contains oils, fats, or greases such as a petroleum-based jelly (for example, Vaseline), baby oil or lotion, hand or body lotion, cooking shortening, or oily cosmetics such as cold creams. These can seriously weaken latex, causing a condom to tear easily. If you use a spermicide, you do not necessarily need to use a lubricant because some spermicide acts as a lubricant.

TO LEARN MORE

Centers for Disease Control and Prevention STD Hotline (800) 227-8922; website: www.cdc.gov/std.

EXERCISE & PHYSICAL FITNESS BENEFITS

 GENERAL INFORMATION

DESCRIPTION
Exercise is a part of a healthy lifestyle at any age. It helps you feel and look better, aids in weight loss, and can lower the risk for many common diseases. Exercise can be fun—even though it may not seem fun at first. Talk to your health care provider about exercising. People who have not been active, have health problems, are pregnant, or elderly may need special advice.

REASONS PEOPLE GIVE FOR NOT EXERCISING
People have many reasons for not exercising. Look for ways to overcome the ones that affect you.
* Not enough time or exercising is inconvenient: Find available time slots. Take exercise breaks at work. Walk for 10 to 15 minutes at a time.
* Lack of energy: Plan exercise time during the day or week when you do feel more energetic. Convince yourself that exercise will actually boost your energy level.
* It is not enjoyable, or it is boring: Watch television while you exercise. Do gardening or mow the lawn. Exercise with a friend. Join an exercise class.
* Fear of injury, or have had a recent injury: Learn how to warm up and cool down. Wear proper shoes for the activity. Pick activities that have little risk.
* Lack of confidence in being able to exercise: Exercise with friends who have the same skill level. Take a class to learn a new skill. Walking is the easiest exercise.
* Not able to maintain an exercise routine due to travel for work or other conflicting schedules: Walk in hotel halls and take stairs instead of elevators. Pack stretch bands and jump rope and use them in your room. Pick places to stay with pools or fitness rooms.
* Family or friends are not supportive or encouraging: Ask your family for support. Invite family or friends to exercise with you. Join a fitness class or hiking club.
* No place to walk nearby, such as a park or sidewalks, or the weather is bad: Always have activities that you can do indoors. Exercise to a video-tape. Walk in the mall. Ride an exercise bike.
* Family obligations take too much time: Exercise with the kids, such as walking or swimming. Plan on exercising when kids are at school, playing, or sleeping.

WHAT TO DO TO GET STARTED
* Plan on making exercise or physical activity a part of your everyday life. Do things you enjoy. Many people are getting their exercise doing things such as biking, skiing and tennis. Others prefer less active recreation such as walking, gardening, or golf.
* Children and adults should try to get at least 30 to 60 minutes of exercise a day. You can break this into shorter periods of 10 or 15 minutes during the day.

PARTS OF AN EXERCISE PLAN
* Endurance: Find an activity that makes you breathe harder, on most or all days of the week. That's called "endurance activity," because it builds your stamina.
* Muscle strength: Lack of use lets muscles waste away. Start lifting weights and increase the weight slowly. This will build bone mass and help avoid osteoporosis.
* Balance: Do things to help your balance. Stand on one foot, then the other, without holding onto anything for support. Walk heel-to-toe (the toes of the foot in back should almost touch the heel of the foot in front when you walk this way).
* Stretching: It won't build endurance or muscles, but keeps you limber and flexible, and reduces injuries.

SUGGESTIONS FOR BEING ACTIVE
* Walk, cycle, jog, or skate to work, school, stores, etc. Walk during breaks at work. Keep a comfortable pair of shoes handy in your office or car.
* Park the car farther away from where you want to go.
* Take the stairs instead of the elevator.
* Play actively with children or pets.
* Garden at home, or do home repair work.
* Exercise while watching television. Ride an exercise bike, walk in place, lift weights, or stretch.

CAUTIONS
* Don't overdo the activity. Listen to your body. A few muscle aches are to be expected, but not pain.
* Start off a new routine at an easy pace. Then increase your time and effort. If you can talk without any trouble at all, your activity is probably too easy. If you can't talk at all, it's too hard.
* Use the correct equipment, especially shoes.
* Take 3 to 5 minutes to warm up (e.g., start a walk at a slow pace, and then increase to a brisk pace).
* Be aware of any warning signs of heart problems: Severe sweating, chest and arm pain, and dizziness.
* Drink plenty of water to replace any lost fluids.

KEGEL EXERCISES
(Pelvic Floor Exercises)

 GENERAL INFORMATION

DESCRIPTION
* Life's events can weaken pelvic muscles. Pregnancy, childbirth, and being overweight can do it. Luckily, when these muscles get weak, you can help make them strong again.
* Pelvic floor muscles are just like other muscles. Exercise can make them stronger. Women with bladder control problems can regain control through Kegel exercises (pelvic floor exercises).

THE PELVIC MUSCLES
* Exercising your pelvic floor muscles for just 5 minutes, three times a day can make a big difference to your bladder control. Exercise strengthens muscles that hold the bladder and many other organs in place.
* The part of your body including your hip bones is the pelvic area. At the bottom of the pelvis, several layers of muscle stretch between your legs. The muscles attach to the front, back, and sides of the pelvis bone.
* Two pelvic muscles do most of the work. The biggest one stretches like a hammock. The other is shaped like a triangle. These muscles prevent leaking of urine and stool.
* You can make these pelvic floor muscles stronger with a few minutes of exercise every day.

DOING THE EXERCISES
* Find the right muscles. This is very important. Your doctor, nurse, or physical therapist will help make sure you are doing the exercises the right way.
* You should tighten the two major muscles that stretch across your pelvic floor. They are the "hammock" muscle and the "triangle" muscle. Here are three methods to check for the correct muscles.
    1. Try to stop the flow of urine when you are sitting on the toilet. If you can do it, you are using the right muscles.
    2. Imagine that you are trying to stop passing gas. Squeeze the muscles you would use. If you sense a "pulling" feeling, those are the right muscles for pelvic exercises.
    3. Lie down and put your finger inside your vagina. Squeeze as if you were trying to stop urine from coming out. If you feel tightness on your finger, you are squeezing the right pelvic muscle.
* Don't squeeze other muscles at the same time. Be careful not to tighten your stomach, legs, or other muscles. Squeezing the wrong muscles can put more pressure on your bladder control muscles. Just squeeze the pelvic muscle. Don't hold your breath.
* Repeat, but don't overdo it. At first, find a quiet spot to practice—your bathroom or bedroom—so you can concentrate. Lie on the floor. Pull in the pelvic muscles and hold for a count of 3. Then relax for a count of 3. Work up to 10 to 15 repeats each time you exercise. Healthy sphincter muscles can keep the urethra closed.
* Do your pelvic exercises at least three times a day. Every day, use three positions: lying down, sitting, and standing. You can exercise while lying on the floor, sitting at a desk, or standing in the kitchen. Using all three positions makes the muscles strongest.
* Be patient. Don't give up. It's just 5 minutes, three times a day. You may not feel your bladder control improve until after 3 to 6 weeks. Still, most women do notice an improvement after a few weeks.
* Exercise aids. You can also exercise by using special weights or biofeedback. Ask your health care provider about these exercise aids.

HOLD THE SQUEEZE UNTIL AFTER THE SNEEZE
* You can protect your pelvic muscles from more damage by bracing yourself.
* Think ahead just before sneezing, lifting, or jumping. Sudden pressure from such actions can hurt those pelvic muscles. Squeeze your pelvic muscles tightly and hold on until after you sneeze, lift, or jump.
* After you train yourself to tighten the pelvic muscles for these moments, you will have fewer accidents.

POINTS TO REMEMBER
* Weak pelvic muscles often cause bladder control problems.
* Daily exercises can strengthen pelvic muscles.
* These exercises often improve bladder control.
* Ask your health care provider or nurse if you are squeezing the right muscles.
* Tighten your pelvic muscles before sneezing, lifting, or jumping. This can prevent pelvic muscle damage.

R.I.C.E. THERAPY

GENERAL INFORMATION

R.I.C.E. is an acronym (a word coined from first letters) for the most important elements—rest, ice, compression and elevation—in first aid for many injuries. This acronym appears in medical information in reference to athletic injuries. Use the word R.I.C.E. to jog your memory if you have injuries, such as contusions, sprains, strains, dislocations, or uncomplicated fractures.

REST
Stop using the injured part, and rest it (for about 48 hours) as soon as you realize an injury has taken place. Continued exercise or other activity could cause further injury, delay healing, increase pain, and risk bleeding. Use crutches to avoid bearing weight on injuries of the foot, ankle, knee, or leg. Use splints for injuries of the hand, wrist, elbow or arm. After medical care, the injured part may require immobilization with splints or a cast to keep the area at rest until it heals.

ICE
Ice helps stop internal bleeding from injured blood vessels. Sudden cold causes small blood vessels to contract. This contraction of blood vessels decreases the amount of blood that can collect around the wound. The more blood that collects, the longer the healing time. Ice can be safely applied in several ways using the following instructions:
* For injury to a small area, such as a finger, toe, foot, or wrist, immerse the injured area in a bucket of ice water. Use ice cubes to keep the water cold, as ice dissolves.
* For injury to a larger area, use ice packs. Avoid placing ice directly on the skin. Before applying the ice, place a towel, cloth, or one or two layers of an elasticized compression bandage (Ace bandage) on the skin to be iced. To make the ice pack, put ice chips or ice cubes in a plastic bag, or wrap them in a thin towel. Place the ice pack over the cloth. The pack may sit directly on the injured part, or it may be wrapped in place.
* Ice the injured area for about 20 minutes at a time.
* Repeat the icing four to eight times a day, while following the instructions below for compression and elevation. After 48 to 72 hours, you may add heat as a treatment. Or you might try both. Alternate five minutes of hot water with five minutes of ice water. Continue to ice the injured area until it is healed.

COMPRESSION
Compression decreases swelling by slowing the bleeding and limiting the accumulation of blood near the injured site. Without compression, fluid from adjacent normal tissues seeps into the injury area. The more blood and fluid that accumulate around an injury, the slower the healing. The following are instructions for safely applying compression to an injury:
* Use an elasticized bandage (Ace bandage) for compression, if possible. If you do not have one available, any kind of cloth will suffice for a short time. Wrap the injured part firmly, wrapping over the ice also. Begin wrapping below the injury site, and extend above the injury site.
* Be careful not to compress the area so tightly that the blood supply is impaired. Signs of deprived blood supply include pain, numbness, cramping, and blue or dusky colored nails. Remove the compression bandage immediately if any of these symptoms appear. Leave the bandage off until all signs of impaired circulation disappear. Then rewrap the area—less tightly this time.

ELEVATION
Elevating the injured part to, or above, the level of the heart is another way to decrease swelling and pain at the injury site. Elevate the iced, compressed area in whatever way is most convenient. Prop an injured leg on solid objects or pillows. Elevate an injured arm by lying down and placing pillows under the arm or placing them on the chest with the arm folded across. The whole upper part of the body may be elevated gently with pillows or a reclining chair or by raising the head of the bed on blocks.

SAFE USE OF MEDICINE

LIST FOR SAFER DRUG USE
These suggestions for wise, safe use of medicine apply to all medicines.

INFORMATION YOU SHOULD PROVIDE
Always give the information listed in 1 and 2 below to your doctor, dentist, or other health care provider so that they can prescribe drugs properly:

1. Your medical history: Tell the important facts of your medical history dealing with drugs. Include allergic reactions, side effects, or adverse reactions you have experienced in the past. Describe the allergic problems you have such as hay fever, asthma, eye watering and itching, throat irritation, and reactions to food. People who have allergies to common substances are more likely to develop side effects or adverse reactions to drugs.

2. Drugs you are taking now: List all prescription and nonprescription drugs. Don't forget common ones such as laxatives; herbal, vitamin, or mineral supplements; skin, rectal, vaginal drugs; antacids; antihistamines; cold and cough remedies; aspirin and aspirin-containing pain pills; motion sickness remedies; weight-loss aids; salt and sugar substitutes; caffeine (in coffee, tea, cola drinks, and cocoa); oral contraceptives; sleeping pills; or "tonics."

INFORMATION TO KNOW BEFORE TAKING A DRUG
- Generic names and brand names of all the drugs you take. Write them down to help you remember. If a drug is a mixture of two or more generic ingredients, learn the names of each.
- Uses for each drug you take.
- How to take each drug—for example, with or without water, or with or without food.
- When to take it.
- What to do if you forget a dose.
- How each drug works in your body.
- Time lapse before drug works.
- Symptoms and treatment of overdose.
- Possible adverse reactions and side effects and what to do if they occur.
- Interactions with other drugs and other substances such as alcohol, food, beverages, cocaine, marijuana, and tobacco. When mixed, they can sometimes cause serious interactions.
- Know all warnings and precautions that apply to special circumstances, such as the following:

    1. Reasons (called contraindications) not to take the drug in the presence of some medical conditions.

    2. Special considerations for elderly patients, pregnant or breast-feeding women, infants, and children.

    3. Information about long-term use, exposure to sun and sunlight, driving, piloting aircraft, hazardous work, or flying in airplanes.

    4. Instructions before discontinuing the drug.

OTHER SAFETY TIPS
- Before taking any prescribed drug, discuss plans with the doctor that you may have for elective surgery, pregnancy, and breast-feeding.
- Don't hesitate to ask questions about a drug. We will be able to provide more information if we are familiar with you and your past medical history, especially regarding drugs.
- Never take a drug in the dark! It is always possible to take the wrong one. Recheck the label before each drug use.
- Notify our office about any new or unexpected symptoms you develop while taking a drug. You may need to change drugs or have a dose adjustment.
- Store all drugs out of children's reach. Keep drugs in a cool, dry place, such as a kitchen cabinet or bedroom. Avoid medicine cabinets in bathrooms—they get too moist and warm at times. Keep drugs in their original containers, tightly closed. Don't remove the labels! If directions call for refrigeration, keep the drug cool, but don't freeze it.
- Don't save leftover drugs to use later. Discard them on or before the expiration date shown on the label.
- Do not flush old drugs down the toilet or dispose in a drain. Doing so may result in traces of the drug seeping into the water supply. Throw the drugs in the trash, packaged in childproof containers and/or sealed plastic bags (out of the reach of children and pets). Another option is to check if local household hazardous-waste collection programs—where you're supposed to take motor oil and batteries—accept expired drugs.
- Don't take any drug prescribed for someone else.
- Prior to any surgery (including oral surgery or simple dental procedures), tell the doctor or dentist about all drugs you take or have taken in the past few weeks.
- If you become pregnant while taking any drug, tell your health care provider right away. Avoid all drugs when you are pregnant, if possible.

SKIN SELF-EXAMINATION

GENERAL INFORMATION

Skin self-exam means checking your own skin regularly for any abnormal growths or unusual changes. This helps you detect and treat skin cancer (or other skin abnormalities) as early as possible. Two types of skin cancer (basal cell carcinoma and squamous cell carcinoma) are almost always cured once correctly diagnosed. With melanoma (the most serious type of skin cancer), early diagnosis is essential to start treatment before it spreads.

The National Cancer Institute (NCI) and the American Academy of Dermatology (AAD) recommend that people should perform a skin self-exam once a month. It may take about 10 to 15 minutes. Along with your self-exam, always practice sun-protection care by using a sunscreen (SPF of 30 or higher) with both UVA and UVB protection. Wear protective clothing, and limit exposure time to the sun.

Get to know your skin, so you know what is normal for you. The first time you do the self-examination, locate all moles, warts, birthmarks, scars, spots, bumps, lumps, or other skin markings. It may be difficult to remember the color, shape, and size of each, so you may want to write down the information or draw a sketch of each area and abnormality.

HOW THE TEST IS PERFORMED
- The easiest time to do the exam may be after you take a bath or shower. Women may wish to perform their skin self-exam at the same time that they perform their monthly breast self-exam.
- Ideally, the room should have a full-length mirror and bright lights so that you can see your entire body well. Use a hand-held mirror also. It is very important to be able to examine all areas of your skin, including hard-to-see areas, such as the genitals, buttocks, scalp, and back.

WHEN YOU ARE PERFORMING THE TEST, LOOK FOR:
- New skin markings (e.g., moles, blemishes, colorations, bumps).
- Moles that have changed their size, texture, color, or shape.
- Moles or lesions that won't heal or that continue to bleed.
- Moles with ragged edges, differences in colors, or lack of symmetry.
- Observe and examine your entire body, both front and back, in the mirror.
- Check under your arms and both sides of each arm.
- Examine your forearms after bending your arms at the elbows, and then look at the palms of your hands and underneath your upper arms.
- Look at the front and back of both legs.
- Look at your buttocks and between your buttocks.
- Examine your genital area.
- Observe your face, neck, back of neck, and scalp. It is best to use both a hand mirror and full-length mirror, along with a comb, to see areas of your scalp.
- Look at your feet, including the soles and the space between your toes.
- Have a partner, friend, or relative help by examining hard-to-see areas. You may want to them to take photographs of your body (or certain moles) every six months to one year. Sometimes it is difficult to tell if a mole has grown or changed, or a new one has developed, and a photo may help.

STRESS, HOW TO COPE

GENERAL INFORMATION

CAUSES OF STRESS
• There are numerous ways to reduce stress in your life; the correct answer is finding what works for you. A certain amount of stress is not always bad. It varies from person to person how much stress one can handle easily. Sometimes, stress can push us on to greater achievement. But excessive stress or chronic stress can be self-defeating. Many health professionals believe that stress has a role in almost any disorder. Stress can complicate an illness by preventing normal recovery, prolonging pain, and adding to disability.
• Reducing stress could be as simple has adding exercise to your daily routine or making new friends. To make the most of your life, limit your stress, and for that stress that you cannot avoid, learn to manage it.

TIPS FOR COPING
Here are some tips that may help you reduce stress:
• Learn a meditation technique and practice it regularly—daily if possible. There are many methods available. Most of them include "tuning in to" and giving complete attention to a word, sound, sentence, or concept that you silently repeat to yourself. Don't try to banish other thoughts that enter your mind during your period of concentration, but don't focus on them enough to stop you from meditating. The purpose of meditation is to empty your mind of all disturbing thoughts for a given period of time to aid in mental relaxation. Mental relaxation, in turn, will help reduce stress.
• Take a short period of time away from any stressful situation you meet up with during a day. Practice a muscle-tensing and muscle-relaxing technique. Close your eyes. Take a series of deep breaths. Then start with the muscle groups in your face. Consciously tense them and hold the tension for a few seconds. Then consciously relax them. Continue through all major muscle groups in the body: neck, shoulders, hands, abdomen, back, and legs. You can use this technique to help you relax quickly any time you need to.
• Begin an exercise program. People who are physically fit are less likely to suffer the negative effects of stress, anxiety, or depression. One form of exercise is yoga. Yoga involves both stretching exercises and deep breathing techniques. However, any form of exercise is helpful in reducing the affects of stress on the body.
• Humor is another way of dealing with stress. Having the ability to find humor in a stressful situation and being able to laugh about it releases all the tension that is building inside. Even if the situation cannot be made light of, think of something else that will make you laugh.
• Healthy lifestyle changes can reduce the level of stress. A few suggestions include reducing caffeine intake, making new friends, eating healthy, and avoiding alcohol. Healthy lifestyle changes can help manage the stress as well as improve your overall well being.
• Get enough sleep. Avoid taking your problems to bed with you. At the end of the day, spend a few minutes going back over your entire day's experiences, event by event, as if you're replaying a tape. Release all negative emotions you have built up (anger, feelings of insecurity or anxiety). Relish all good energy or emotion (loving thoughts, praise, feeling good about your work or yourself). Reach a decision about undone events, and release mental or muscular tension. Now you're ready for a relaxing and emotionally healing sleep.
• Avoid self-medication or escape. Alcohol or other drugs of abuse can mask stress. They don't help deal with the problem.
• Set realistic goals for yourself. Reduce the number of events going on in your life and you may reduce the feeling of being overloaded.
• Don't overwhelm yourself by fretting about your entire workload. Handle each task as it comes, or selectively deal with matters in some priority.
• Do something for others to help get your mind off yourself.
• Avoid extreme reactions. Think about disliking something rather than hating it. Be a little nervous, not anxious. Don't be full of rage when anger will do the job. Don't be depressed when you can just be sad.
• Try to be positive. Give yourself messages as to how well you can cope rather than how horrible everything is going to be.
• Keep a stress diary. Write down stressful events, how they made you feel, what caused the event, and how you coped. On a scale of 0 (very relaxed) to 10 (extremely stressed), put down a number for your stress level.
• Research has shown that cognitive-behavioral therapy can be effective in reducing stress. Ask your health care provider about this option.

TESTICULAR SELF-EXAMINATION

 GENERAL INFORMATION

This is an exam of the testicles to look for lumps that may be testicular cancer. The testicles are the male reproductive organs, and produce sperm and the hormone testosterone. They are located in the scrotum under the penis.

The exam should be performed on a monthly basis, especially if you have a family history of this cancer, have had a previous testicular tumor, or have an undescended testicle.

NORMAL TESTICLES
Each testicle should feel firm but not rock hard. One testicle may or may not be lower or slightly larger than the other. Normal testicles contain blood vessels and other structures that can make the exam confusing. Performing the self-exam monthly allows you to become familiar with your normal anatomy. Then, if you notice any changes from the previous exam, this will alert you to contact your health care provider. Always ask you health care provider if you have any doubts or questions.

HOW THE TEST IS PERFORMED
• Perform this test during or after a shower. This way, the scrotal skin is warm and relaxed. The test is best done while standing.

1. Gently feel your scrotal sac to locate a testicle.

2. Firmly, but gently roll the testicle between the thumb and fingers of both hands to examine the entire surface. Feel the testicle for lumps, swellings, or other changes in consistency.

3. Repeat the procedure with the other testicle.

• Examine the epididymis for lumps. This is a rope-like cord that is located behind each testicle. This area is fairly tender, so be cautious with your touch.

• Examine the spermatic cord for lumps. This is the sperm-carrying tube that extends from the epididymis of each testicle.

ABNORMAL FINDINGS
A lump, swelling, or other change on the testicle, epididymis, or spermatic cord may be the first sign of testicular cancer. Therefore, if you find a lump, see a health care provider right away. Keep in mind that some cases of testicular cancer do not show symptoms until they reach an advanced stage.

CALL YOUR HEALTH CARE PROVIDER IF:
• You find a small hard lump (like a pea), have an enlarged testicle, or notice any other differences from your last self-exam.

• You can't find one or both testicles. The testicles may not have descended properly in the scrotum.

• There is a soft collection of thin tubes above the testicle. It may be a collection of dilated veins (varicocele).

• There is pain or swelling in the scrotum. It may be an infection or a fluid-filled sac (hydrocele) causing blockage of blood flow to the area.

• Acute pain in the scrotum or testicle is a surgical emergency. If you experience acute pain in the scrotum or testicle, seek immediate medical help.

Websites & Other Resources for Information on Specific Health Problems & Medical Disorders

The following list provides names of organizations and support groups that offer medical information and assistance by telephone, mail or the internet. Toll-free numbers use prefixes of 800, 888, 877, 866, and 855.

If you are unable to find a listing for your disorder or problem, call the National Health Information Center at (800) 336-4797; website www.health.gov/nhic or the National Organization for Rare Disorders information line, (800) 999-6673; website www.raredisorders.org.

Acne Rosacea
National Rosacea Society
196 James St.
Barrington, IL 60010
(888) 662-5874
www.rosacea.org

Aging
National Council on the Aging
1901 L. St. NW, 4th floor
Washington, DC 20036
(800) 677-1116
www.ncoa.org

AIDS
HIV/AIDS Information Resources
P.O. Box 6303
Rockville, MD 20849
(800) 448-0440
www.aidsinfo.nih.gov

Alcoholism
Alcoholics Anonymous
A.A. World Services, Inc. 11th floor
475 Riverside Drive at West 120th St.
New York, NY 10163
(212) 870-3400
www.aa.org

National Council on Alcoholism
20 Exchange Place, Suite 2902
New York, NY 10115
(800) 622-2255
www.ncadd.org

Allergies
American Academy of Allergy & Immunology
555 E. Wells St., Suite 1100
Milwaukee, WI 53202
(800) 822-2762
www.aaaai.org

Alopecia Areata
National Alopecia Areata Foundation
14 Mitchell Boulevard
San Rafael, CA 94903
(415) 472-3780
www.naaf.org

Alzheimer's
Alzheimer's Association
225 N. Michigan Ave., Fl.17
Chicago, IL 60601
(800) 272-3900
www.alz.org

Amyotrophic Lateral Sclerosis
Amyotrophic Lateral Sclerosis Association
1275 K Street NW, Suite 1050
Washington, DC 20005
(800) 792-4747
www.alsa.org

Anorexia Nervosa
Anorexia Nervosa & Related Eating Disorders
P.O. Box 5102
Eugene, OR 97405
(503) 344-1144
www.anred.com

Anxiety
Anxiety Disorders Association of America
8730 Georgia Ave., Suite 600
Silver Spring, MD 20910
(240) 485-1001
www.adaa.org

National Institute of Mental Health (NIMH)
6001 Executive Blvd., Rm 8184,
MSC 9663
Bethesda, MD 20892
(866) 615-6464
www.nimh.nih.gov

Arthritis
Arthritis Foundation
P.O. Box 7669
Atlanta, GA 30357
(800) 283-7800
www.arthritis.org

Asbestosis
American Lung Association
1301 Pennsylvania Ave. NW, Suite 800
Washington, DC 20004
(800) 548-8252
www.lungusa.org

Asthma
Asthma & Allergy Foundation of America
8201 Corporate Drive Suite 1000
Landover, MD 20785
(800) 727-8462
www.aafa.org

National Jewish Medical & Research
   Center - Lung Line
1400 Jackson St.
Denver, CO 80206
(800) 222-5864
www.nationaljewish.org

Atelectasis—See Lung Disorders

Atherosclerosis—See Heart Disorders

Atrial Fibrillation—See Heart Disorders

Autism
Autism Society of America
4340 East-West Hwy, Suite 350
Bethesda, MD 20814
(800) 328-8476
www.autsim-society.org

Bed Wetting
American Academy of Pediatrics
141 Northwest Point Blvd.
Elk Grove Village, IL 60007
(847) 434-4000
www.aap.org

Birth Control & Family Planning
Planned Parenthood Federation of America
434 West 33rd Street.
New York, NY 10001
(212) 541-7800
www.plannedparenthood.org

Birth Defects
March of Dimes
1275 Mamaroneck Ave.
White Plains, NY 10605
(888) 663-4637
www.marchofdimes.com

Blindness
American Council of the Blind
2200 Wilson Boulevard, Suite 650
Arlington, VA 22201
(800) 424-8666
www.acb.org

American Foundation for the Blind (AFB)
2 Penn Plaza, Suite 1102
New York, NY 10121
(800) 232-5463
www.afb.org

Brain Tumor
American Brain Tumor Association
8550 W. Bryn Mawr Ave., Ste. 550
Chicago, IL 60631
(800) 886-2282
www.abta.org

Brain Disorders
Brain Research Foundation
111 West Washington Street, Suite 1710
Chicago, IL 60602
(312) 759-5150
www.brainresearchfdn.org

Breast Cancer
Y-ME National Breast Cancer Organization
135 S. LaSalle St. Suite 2000
Chicago, IL 60603
(800) 221-2141
www.y-me.org

Bronchiectasis—See Lung Disorders

Bronchitis—See Lung Disorders

Bulimia—See Eating Disorders

Cancer
American Cancer Society
250 Williams St. NW
Atlanta, GA 30303
(800) 227-2345
www.cancer.org

National Cancer Institute
6116 Executive Blvd., Suite 300
Bethesda, MD 20892
(800) 422-6237
www.cancer.gov

Celiac Disease
Celiac Disease Foundation
13251 Ventura Blvd., Suite 1
Studio City, CA 91604
(818) 990-2354
www.celiac.org

Celiac Sprue Association
1941 S. 42nd St. Suite 522
Omaha, NE 68105
(877) 272-4272
www.csaceliacs.org

Cerebral Palsy
United Cerebral Palsy Association
1825 K Street NW, Suite 600
Washington, DC 20006
(800) 872-5827
www.ucp.org

Cholecystitis or Cholangitis—See
Digestive Diseases

Chronic Fatigue Syndrome
Chronic Fatigue and Immune Dysfunction
    Syndrome (CFIDS) Association
P.O. Box 220398
Charlotte, NC 28222
(704) 365-2343
www.cfids.org

**Chronic Obstructive Pulmonary
Disease**—See Lung Disorders

Cirrhosis of the Liver—See Liver
Disorders

Colitis, Ulcerative
Crohn's & Colitis Foundation of America
386 Park Ave. South, 17th Floor
New York, NY 10016
(800) 932-2423
www.ccfa.org

Cor Pulmonale—See Heart Disorders

Coronary Artery Disease—See Heart
Disorders

Crohn's Disease
Crohn's & Colitis Foundation of America
386 Park Ave. South, 17th Floor
New York, NY 10016
(800) 932-2423
www.ccfa.org

Cystic Fibrosis
Cystic Fibrosis Foundation
6931 Arlington Rd.
Bethesda, MD 20814
(800) 344-4823
www.cff.org

Dementia—See Alzheimer's Disease

Dental Problems
American Dental Association
211 E. Chicago Ave.
Chicago, IL 60611
(312) 440-2500
www.ada.org

Depression
National Institute of Mental Health (NIMH)
6001 Executive Blvd., Rm 8184, MSC 9663
Bethesda, MD 20892
(866) 615-6464
www.nimh.nih.gov

Diabetes
American Diabetes Association
National Call Center
1701 North Beauregard St.
Alexandria, VA 22311
(800) 342-2383
www.diabetes.org

Digestive Diseases
National Digestive Diseases
    Information Clearinghouse
2 Information Way
Bethesda, MD 20892
(800) 891-5389
www.digestive.niddk.nih.gov

Diverticular Disease—See Digestive
Diseases

Domestic Violence
National Domestic Violence Hotline
(800) 799-7233
www.ndvh.org

National Coalition Against Domestic
    Violence
One Broadway, Suite B210
Denver, CO 80203
(303) 839-1852
www.ncadv.org

Down Syndrome
National Down Syndrome Congress
30 Mansell Court, Suite 108
Roswell, GA 30076
(800) 232-6372
www.ndscenter.org

National Down Syndrome Society
666 Broadway
New York, NY 10012
(800) 221-4602
www.ndss.org

Drug Abuse
Cocaine Abuse Hotline
(800) 262-2463

National Institute on Drug Abuse
6001 Executive Blvd., Rm 5213
Bethesda, MD 20892
(301) 443-1124
www.drugabuse.gov

Eating Disorders
Anorexia Nervosa & Related Eating
  Disorders
P.O. Box 5102
Eugene, OR 97405
(503) 344-1144
www.anred.com

National Eating Disorders Association
165 West 46th St.
New York, NY 10036
(800) 931-2237
www.nationaleatingdisorders.org

Eczema
National Eczema Association
4460 Redwood Hwy, Suite 16-D
San Rafael, CA 94903
(800) 818-7546
www.nationaleczema.org

**Endocrine Disorders (Thyroid, Pituitary,
Parathyroid, Sex Glands, Adrenals)**
National Endocrine & Metabolic Diseases
  Information Service
6 Information Way
Bethesda, MD 20892
(888) 828-0904
endocrine.niddk.nih.gov

Endometriosis
Endometriosis Association
8585 N. 76 Pl.
Milwaukee, WI 53223
(800) 992-3636
www.endometriosisassn.org

Fertility Problems
Fertility Research Foundation
877 Park Ave.
New York, NY 10021
(212) 744-5500
www.frfbaby.com

National Infertility Association
1760 Old Meadow Rd., Suite 500
McLean, VA 22102
(703) 556-7172
www.resolve.org

Fibromyalgia
National Fibromyalgia Association
2121 S. Towne Centre Place, Suite 300
Anaheim, CA 92806
(714) 921-0150
www.fmaware.org

Food Allergy
Food Allergy & Anaphylaxis Network
11781 Lee Jackson Hwy., Suite 160
Fairfax, VA 22033
(800) 929-4040
www.foodallergy.org

Foot Disorders
American Podiatry Association
9312 Old Georgetown Rd.
Bethesda, MD 20814
(800) 366-8227
www.apma.org

Gallstones—See Digestive Diseases

Glaucoma
Glaucoma Foundation
80 Maiden Lane, Suite 700
New York, NY 10038
(212) 285-0080
www.glaucomafoundation.org

Glaucoma Research Foundation
251 Post St., Suite 600
San Francisco, CA 94108
(800) 826-6693
www.glaucoma.org

Gonorrhea—See Sexually Transmitted
Diseases

Guillain-Barré
Guillain-Barré Syndrome Foundation
The Holly Building
104 1/2 Forrest Ave.
Narberth, PA 19072
(610) 667-0131
www.gbs-cidp.org

Head Injury
Brain Injury Association
1608 Spring Hill Rd., Suite 110
Vienna, VA 22182
(800) 444-6443
www.biausa.org

Headache
National Headache Foundation
820 N. Orleans, Suite 217
Chicago, IL 60610
(312) 274-2650
www.headaches.org

Hearing Disorders
National Association of the Deaf
8630 Fenton St., Suite 820
Silver Spring, MD 20910
(301) 587-1788
www.nad.org

American Speech-Language-Hearing
  Association
2200 Research Blvd.
Rockville, MD 20850
(800) 638-8255
www.asha.org

International Hearing Society
16880 Middlebelt Rd.
Livonia, MI 48154
(800) 521-5247
www.ihsinfo.org

Heart Disorders
American Heart Association
7272 Greenville Ave.
Dallas, TX 75231
(800) 242-8721
www.americanheart.org

National Heart, Lung & Blood Institute
P.O. Box 30105
Bethesda, MD 20824
(301) 592-8573
www.nhlbi.nih.gov

Hemophilia
National Hemophilia Foundation
116 W. 32 St., 11 Floor
New York, NY 10001
(800) 424-2634
www.hemophilia.org

Herpes
American Social Health Association
P.O. Box 13827
Research Triangle Park, NC 27709
(919) 361-8400
www.ashastd.org

HIV—See AIDS

Hypertension—See Heart Disorders

Immunodeficiency Disease
Immune Deficiency Foundation
40 W. Chesapeake Ave., Suite 308
Towson, MD 21204
(800) 296-4433
www.primaryimmune.org

Impotence, Male Sexual
American Foundation for Urologic Disease
1000 Corporate Blvd., Suite 410
Linthicum, MD 21090
(800) 828-7866
www.urologyhealth.org

Incontinence
National Association for Continence
P.O. Box 1019
Charleston, SC 29402
(800) 252-3337
www.nafc.org

Simon Foundation for Continence
P.O. Box 815
Wilmette, IL 60091
(800) 237-4666
www.simonfoundation.org

Irritable Bowel Syndrome
Crohn's & Colitis Foundation of America
386 Park Ave. S., 17th Flr.
New York, NY 10016
(800) 932-2423
www.ccfa.org

Kidney Disorders
American Kidney Fund
6110 Executive Blvd., Suite 1010
Rockville, MD 20852
(866) 300-2900
www.kidneyfund.org

National Kidney Foundation
30 E. 33rd St.
New York, NY 10016
(800) 622-9010
www.kidney.org

Lead Poisoning
Environmental Protection Agency (EPA)
1200 Pennsylvania Ave., NW
Mail Code 7404T
Washington, DC 20460
(800) 424-5323
www.epa.gov/lead/

Leukemia
Leukemia & Lymphoma Society
1311 Mamaroneck Ave., Suite 310
White Plains, NY 10605
(800) 955-4572
www.lls.org

Lice
National Pediculosis Association
1005 Boylston Street, Suite 343
Needham, MA 02461
(617) 905-0176
www.headlice.org

Liver Disorders
American Liver Foundation
39 Broadway, Suite 2700
New York, NY 10006
(800) 465-4837
www.liverfoundation.org

Lung Disorders
American Lung Association
1301 Pennsylvania Ave. NW, Suite 800
Washington, DC 20004
(800) 548-8252
www.lungusa.org

National Heart, Lung & Blood Institute
P.O. Box 30105
Bethesda, MD 20824
(301) 592-8573
www.nhlbi.nih.gov

Lupus
Lupus Foundation of America, Inc.
2000 L St., NW, Suite 410
Washington, DC 20036
(800) 558-0121
www.lupus.org

Lyme Disease
American Lyme Disease Foundation, Inc.
P.O. Box 466
Lyme, CT 06371
www.aldf.com

Lyme Disease Foundation
P.O. Box 332
Tolland, CT 06084
(800) 886-5963
www.lyme.org

Marfan Syndrome
National Marfan Foundation
22 Manhasset Ave.
Port Washington, NY 11050
(800) 862-7326
www.marfan.org

Medical Identification
Medic Alert Foundation International
2323 Colorado Ave.
Turlock, CA 95382
(888) 633-4298
www.medicalalert.org

Menopause
National Institute on Aging
Building 31, Room 5C27
31 Center Dr., MSC 2292
Bethesda, MD 20892
(800) 222-2225
www.nia.nih.gov

North American Menopause Society
5900 Landerbrook Drive, Suite 390
Mayfield Heights, OH 44124
(440) 442-7550
www.menopause.org

Mental Health
Mental Health America
2000 N. Beauregard St., 6th Floor
Alexandria, VA 22311
(800) 969-6642
www.nmha.org

National Institute of Mental Health
6001 Executive Blvd., Rm 8184 MSC 9663
Bethesda, MD 20892.
(866) 615-6464
www.nimh.nih.gov

Movement Disorders
We Move
5731 Mosholu Avenue.
Bronx, NY 10471
(347) 843-6132
www.wemove.org

Multiple Sclerosis
National Multiple Sclerosis Society
733 3rd Ave.
New York, NY 10017
(800) 344-4867
www.nmss.org

Multiple Sclerosis Association
706 Haddonfield Rd.
Cherry Hill, NJ 08002
(856) 488-4500
www.msaa.com

Muscular Dystrophy
Muscular Dystrophy Association
3300 E. Sunrise Dr.
Tucson, AZ 85718
(800) 572-1717
www.mdausa.org

Myasthenia Gravis
Myasthenia Gravis Foundation
355 Lexington Avenue, 15th Floor
New York, New York 10017
(800) 541-5454
www.myasthenia.org

Myocarditis—See Heart Disorders

Narcolepsy
Narcolepsy Network
P.O. Box 294
Pleasantville, NY 10570
(888) 292-6522
www.nacolepsynetwork.org

Nephrosis—See Kidney Disorders

Nutrition & Dietetics
National Center for Nutrition & Dietetics
120 S. Riverside Plaza, Suite 2000
Chicago, IL 60606
(312) 899-0040
www.eatright.org

Department of Agriculture
U.S. Department of Agriculture
1400 Independence Ave, SW
Washington, DC 20250
(888) 674-6854
www.fsis.usda.gov

Obesity
American Obesity Treatment Association
217 Anderson Court, Suite 1
Dothan, AL 36303
(334) 651-0821
www.americanobesity.org

Obsessive-Compulsive Disorder
Obsessive-Compulsive Foundation, Inc.
112 Water Street, Suite 501
Boston, MA 02109
(617) 973-5801
www.ocfoundation.org

Osteoporosis
National Osteoporosis Foundation
1150 17th Street NW
Washington, DC 20036
(800) 223-9994
www.nof.org

Otosclerosis—See Hearing Problems

Pancreatitis—See Digestive Diseases

Parkinson's Disease
American Parkinson Disease Association
135 Parkinson Ave.
Staten Island, NY 10305
(800) 223-2732
www.apdaparkinson.org

National Parkinson Foundation
1501 N.W. 9th Ave/Bob Hope Road
Miami, FL 33136
(800) 473-4636
www.parkinson.org

Pericarditis, Acute—See Heart Disorders

Phobias
Anxiety Disorders Association of America
8730 Georgia Ave., Suite 600
Silver Spring, MD 20910
(240) 485-1001
www.adaa.org

Pneumonia—See Lung Disorders

**Polymyalgia Rheumatica or Temporal
   Arteritis**—See Arthritis

Polymyositis—See Muscular Dystrophy

Porphyria
American Porphyria Foundation
4900 Woodway, Suite 780
Houston, TX 77056
(713) 266-9617
www.porphyriafoundation.com

Premenstrual Syndrome
Women's Health
8270 Willow Oaks Corporate Dr., Suite 101
Fairfax, VA 22031
(800) 994-9662
www.womenshealth.gov

Psoriasis
National Psoriasis Foundation
6600 SW 92 Ave., Suite 300
Portland, OR 97223
(800) 723-9166
www.psoriasis.org

Rape Crisis Syndrome
National Sexual Assault Hotline
(800) 656-4673
(connects callers to a nearby rape crisis
    center)
www.rainn.org

Women Organized Against Rape
1617 JFK Boulevard, Suite 1100
Philadelphia, PA 19103
(215) 985 3333
www.woar.org

Rare Disorders
National Organization for Rare Disorders
55 Kenosia Ave., P.O. Box 1968
Danbury, CT 06813
(800) 999-6673
www.raredisorders.org

Raynaud's
Raynaud's Association
94 Mercier Ave.
Hartsdale, NY 10530
(800) 280-8055
www.raynauds.org

Reflex Sympathetic Dystrophy Syndrome
Reflex Sympathetic Dystrophy Syndrome
    Association
P.O. Box 502
Milford, CT 06460
(877) 662-7737
www.rsds.org

Renal Failure—See Kidney Disorders

Reye's Syndrome
National Reye's Syndrome Foundation
426 N. Lewis, P.O. Box 829
Bryan, OH 43506
(800) 233-7393
www.reyessyndrome.org

Rheumatic Fever—See Heart Disorders

Scleroderma
Scleroderma Foundation
300 Rosewood Dr. Suite 105
Danvers, MA 01923
(800) 722-4673
www.scleroderma.org

Scoliosis
Scoliosis Association, Inc.
P.O. Box 811705
Boca Raton, FL 33481
(800) 800-0669
www.scoliosis-assoc.org

National Scoliosis Foundation
5 Cabot Pl.
Stoughton, MA 02072
(800) 673-6922
www.scoliosis.org

Seizure Disorders
Epilepsy Foundation of America
8301 Professional Place
Landover, MD 20785
(800) 332-1000
www.efa.org

Sexually Transmitted Diseases
American Social Health Association
P.O. Box 13827
Research Triangle Park, NC 27709
(919) 361-8400
www.ashastd.org

Sickle Cell Disease
Sickle Cell Disease Association of America
231 E. Baltimore Street, Suite 800
Baltimore, MD 21202
(800) 421-8453
www.sicklecelldisease.org

Silicosis—See Lung Disorders

Sjögren's Syndrome
Sjögren's Syndrome Foundation
6707 Democracy Boulevard Suite 325
Bethesda, MD 20817
(800) 475-6473
www.sjogrens.org

Skin Cancer
Skin Cancer Foundation
149 Madison Avenue
New York, NY 10016
(212) 725-5176
www.skincancer.org

Skin Disorders
American Academy of Dermatology
P.O. Box 4014
Schaumber, IL 60168
(847) 240-1280
www.aad.org

Sleep Disorders
National Sleep Foundation
1010 N. Glebe Rd., Suite 310
Arlington, VA 22201
(703) 243-1697
www.sleepfoundation.org

Stroke
National Stroke Association
9707 E. Easter Lane, Suite B
Englewood, CO 80112
(800) 787-6537
www.stroke.org

American Heart Association
7272 Greenville Ave.
Dallas, TX 75231
(800) 242-8721
www.americanheart.org

Syphilis—See Sexually Transmitted
Diseases

Tay-Sachs Disease
National Tay-Sachs and Allied Disease
   Association
2001 Beacon St., Suite 204
Brighton, MA 02135l
(800) 906-8723
www.ntsad.org

Thyroid Disorders
American Thyroid Association
6066 Leesburg Pike, Suite 550
Falls Church, VA 22041
(800) 849-7643
www.thyroid.org

Tinnitus
American Tinnitus Association
P.O. Box 5
Portland, OR 97207
(800) 634-8978
www.ata.org

Tooth Problems
American Dental Association
211 E. Chicago Ave.
Chicago, IL 60611
(312) 440-2500
www.ada.org

Travel & Health
Centers for Disease Control and Prevention
1600 Clifton Rd.
Atlanta, GA 30333
(877) 394-8747
www.cdc.gov/travel

Tuberculosis—See Lung Disorders

Tumors, Malignant—See Cancer

Ulcer, Peptic—See Digestive Diseases

Urinary Calculi—See Kidney Disorders

Vision
American Council of the Blind
2200 Wilson Boulevard, Suite 650
Arlington, VA 22201
(800) 424-8666
www.acb.org

Lighthouse International
111 E. 59 St.
New York, NY 10022
(800) 829-0500
www.lighthouse.org

National Eye Institute
31 Center Drive MSC 2510
Bethesda, MD 20892
(301) 496-5248
www.nei.nih.gov

Wilms' Tumor—See Cancer

Websites for
General Health & Medical Information

This is a selected list of websites that provide general medical and health information. There are also many others (sponsored by different types of organizations) that are useful for valid and quality medical information, patient education materials, and helpful ideas for managing your health.

People looking for health and medical information have many choices on the World Wide Web. It is important to know the source and if it is reliable. Look at the web page address (also called the URL or Unifrom Resource Locator). The following types of addresses often have excellent websites:

1. Addresses that end in .gov are provided by the U.S. government.
2. Addresses that end in .org are normally provided by nonprofit organizations, such as the American Heart Association.
3. Addresses ending in .edu are provided by educational institutions such as universities or colleges.

Websites that advertise products (e.g., .com) can be good sources for medical information also, but should be read with some caution. It is often helpful to compare several different web resources on the same topic.

Information on the Web is not a substitute for your health care provider's instructions and advice. It can not replace the knowledge and experience that your health care provider can share with you.

American Dental Association
www.ada.org/public//index.aspx
The American Dental Association provides information on topics about your teeth and oral health (such as Anxiety about dental visits).

Centers for Disease Control (CDC) Division of Sexually Transmitted Diseases (STD)
www.cdc.gov/std/
Provides information on specific diseases. A good starting point for reliable STD facts.

Family Doctor
www.familydoctor.org
The American Academy of Family Physicians provides information for general educational purposes for the whole family. All of the information has been written and reviewed by physicians and patient education professionals.

Healthfinder
www.healthfinder.gov
The U.S. Department of Health & Human services along with other federal agencies designed this web site as a gateway to consumer health information. It provides access to selected online publications, clearinghouses, databases, web sites, and support and self-help groups. It also links to government agencies and not-for-profit organizations that produce reliable information for the public.

Kids Health
www.kidshealth.org
Provides doctor-approved, up-to-date and accurate health information about children from before birth through adolescents.

Mayo Clinic
www.mayoclinic.com
Sponsored by the Mayo Clinic, this site offers general information about health and medical topics. New information is added daily

Medlineplus
www.medlineplus.gov
A web site established by the U.S. National Library of Medicine, the world's largest biomedical library and creator of the Medline database. An alphabetical list of medical and health topics consists of hundreds of specific diseases, conditions and wellness issues. Health information in Spanish is also included.

National Cancer Institute
www.cancer.gov
A source of current cancer information for patients and anyone interested in learning more about cancer.

National Health Information Center
www.health.gov/nhic
This site is run by the U.S. Department of Health and Human Services. It provides links to many organizations that have information about specific medical topics.

National Women's Health Information Center (NWHIC) www.womanshealth.gov
A project of the Office on Women's Health in the U.S. Department of Health and Human Services (HHS). NWHIC is a gateway to women's health information resources that allows visitors to read and download a wide variety of materials developed by federal government agencies, and private sector resources.

Glossary

Introduction to the Glossary

The glossary contains brief definitions and/or descriptions of medical-related words and terminology. This includes easy-to-understand explanations about medical tests and medical abbreviations that are used throughout the book.

In addition, the glossary provides a brief description of some rare illnesses and disorders that are not covered in the other sections due to lack of space.

A

Abdominal Aorta—Section of the aorta that passes through the abdomen to supply blood to the lower part of the body.

Abscess—Swollen, inflamed, tender area of infection containing pus.

Accident Proneness—Tendency of some persons to have more accidents than normal. It may be due to a risk factor such as poor vision, but unconscious factors are often the cause.

Acetaminophen—Nonprescription medication used to relieve minor pain and to reduce fever. Its analgesic effects are similar to aspirin, but it does not reduce inflammation or swelling. It is less irritating to the stomach than aspirin.

Achalasia—Condition of the esophagus that disrupts normal swallowing.

Acquired Immune Deficiency Syndrome, Acquired Immunodeficiency Syndrome, AIDS—A disease of the human immune system that is caused by infection with HIV (human immunodeficiency virus).

Acupuncture—Method of anesthesia and treatment of pain developed by the Chinese. Needles are inserted through the skin to stimulate precise areas.

Acute—Beginning suddenly; also severe, but of short duration.

Addiction—Intense craving for substances such as alcohol, tobacco or narcotics, or a compulsive behavior such as gambling.

Adenoids—Infection-fighting tissue (part of the lymphatic system) in the upper throat, near the tonsils.

Adenoids, Enlarged—Adenoids that have swollen and impaired speech.

Adenovirus—Group of viruses that cause certain respiratory and eye infections.

Adhesions—Small strands of fibrous tissue that cause organs in the abdomen and pelvis to cling together abnormally, creating a risk of intestinal obstruction.

Adolescence—Time of life from the beginning of puberty until maturity.

Adrenal Glands—Two glands attached to the kidneys. Each has an outer layer (cortex) that produces steroid hormones and an inner layer (medulla) that produces adrenalin.

Adrenalin—Hormone produced by the adrenal glands that increases heart rate and prepares the body for crisis. Also called epinephrine.

Aging—The normal process of gradual physical and mental decline.

AIDS—See *Acquired Immune Deficiency Syndrome*.

Airways—Tubular passages that air passes through to the lungs: the trachea (windpipe), bronchi and bronchioles.

Alcoholic Cirrhosis—Widespread destruction of normal liver tissue caused by excessive intake of alcohol.

Alveoli—Lung cells at ends of the airways where oxygen enters the blood and waste gases leave the blood.

Ambulatory Medical Center—A health-care facility for patients who do not require prolonged bed rest or hospitalization.

Amniocentesis—The extraction and examination of a small amount of amniotic fluid in order to determine genetic and other disorders in the unborn child.

Amniotic Sac—The thin, transparent membrane filled with fluid in which the fetus lives until born.

Amphetamine Drugs—Habit-forming drugs that stimulate the brain and central nervous system, increase blood pressure, reduce nasal stuffiness or suppress appetite.

Amyloid Deposits—Abnormal protein material deposited in tissues, usually caused by diseases. These deposits cause impairment of certain organs.

Analgesics—Medications that relieve pain.

Anemia—Condition in which red blood cells or hemoglobin (oxygen-carrying substance in blood) is inadequate.

Anesthesia, General—Causing temporary loss of consciousness and inability to feel pain by use of inhaled gases or injected anesthetics.

Anesthesia, Local (Nerve Block)—Injection of the local anesthetic near the nerves of the surgical area.

Anesthesia, Local—Temporary prevention of pain by injecting medication (local anesthetic).

Aneurysm—Abnormal swelling or ballooning of a blood vessel.

Angina—Pain or pressure beneath the breastbone caused by inadequate blood supply to the heart.

Angiogram, Angiography—Study of arteries and veins by injecting material into them that x-rays can outline.

Anoscopy—Visual examination of the anus by means of a short tube called an anoscope, an optical instrument with lenses and a lighted tip.

Antacid—Medicine taken orally that reduces or neutralizes stomach acid.

Anti-inflammatory Drugs—Medications used to control inflammation not caused by infection.

Anti-arrhythmics—Medications used to treat heartbeat irregularities (arrhythmias).

Antibiotics—Medications that attack germs and fight infection.

Antibiotics, Cephalosporin—Class of antibiotics related to penicillin, capable of destroying more kinds of germs than penicillin.

Antibiotics, Erythromycin—Class of antibiotics that destroys germs similar to those destroyed by penicillin. Often used to treat infections in patients who are allergic to penicillin.

Antibodies—Proteins created in blood and body tissue by the immune system to neutralize or destroy sources of disease.

Anticancer Drugs—Medications that weaken or destroy cancerous tissues without harming healthy tissues.

Anticholinergic Drugs—Medications that reduce nerve impulses in the parasympathetic nervous system. They control some activities of the gastrointestinal system, heart, bladder and other organs.

Anticoagulants—Medications that slow or delay blood clotting.

Anticonvulsants—Medications that control seizures (convulsions), pain or conditions in which the brain or nerves are overly sensitive.

Antidepressants—Medications that help control depression.

Antiemetic Drugs—Medications that prevent or stop nausea and vomiting.

Antifungal Drugs—Medications used to treat fungus diseases.

Antigens—Germs or other sources of disease that antibodies (produced by the immune system) neutralize or destroy.

Antihelmintic Drugs—Medications used to treat worms in the intestines.

Antihistamines—Medications used to treat allergies.

Antihyperlipidemic Drugs—Medications that reduce fat (cholesterol) in the blood. They help prevent blood-vessel disease.

Antihypertensives—Medications used to reduce blood pressure.

Antimalarial Drugs—Medications used to prevent or treat malaria.

Antimetabolite Drugs—Medications that are used to treat some cancers and autoimmune diseases.

Antimicrobial Drugs—Same as Antibiotics.

Antinuclear Antibody—Substance that appears in the blood, indicating presence of an autoimmune disease.

Antiparkinsonian Drugs—Medications used to treat Parkinson's disease.

Antiprotozoal Drugs—Medications used in treatment of single-celled parasites (protozoa).

Antipruritic Drugs—Medications that reduce itching.

Antispasmodic Drugs—Medications that improve digestion and relieve intestinal cramps.

Antistreptococcal Titer—Blood test that measures body's response to infection by streptococcal bacteria.

Antithyroid Drugs—Medications used to counter the effects of an overactive thyroid gland.

Antiviral Drugs—Medications used to treat infections caused by viruses.

Anus—A muscular band at the end of the rectum that opens and expands to allow passage of feces.

Anus, Imperforate—Congenital abnormality of newborn infants in which the anus cannot pass feces.

Anxiety—Uncomfortable feeling that something unpleasant or dangerous will happen.

Aorta—Body's largest blood vessel, arising from the top of the heart. It carries blood from the heart to all parts of the body.

Aphrodisiac—Substance claimed to increase sexual arousal or pleasure.

Appendage—Body part that has a minor role (or no role at all) in normal body function. For example, the appendix is an appendage to the colon that seems to have no function.

Arteriogram, Arteriography—Studying arteries by injecting material into them that x-rays can outline.

Arteriosclerosis—Hardening of the arteries.

Arterial Doppler Studies—Measurement of blood flow through the arteries by means of doppler ultrasound.

Artery—Blood vessels that carry blood from the heart to the body.

Arthrograms—X-rays of the joints taken with an arthroscope.

Arthroscope—Slender optical instrument with a lighted tip that allows direct visual examination of some joints. It can also be used to correct some defects in joints.

Artificial Limbs—Mechanical substitutions for amputated arms or legs.

Ascending Colon—First part of the large colon (intestine) extending from the lower end of the small intestine.

Aspiration—1) Removal of accumulated pus or fluid with a needle. 2) Accidental inhalation of objects or fluids into the lungs.

Astigmatism—Visual impairment caused by abnormal eye shape.

Asymmetrical—Uneven in size, shape or position.

Atelectasis—Collapse of the expanded lung.

Atriums—Small chambers in the heart that pump blood into the ventricles. Also called auricles.

Atropine—Medication used to treat diseases of the eye, heart, gastrointestinal system and nervous system.

Audiogram, Audiometry—Test of hearing ability.

Autism—Mental illness of children in which they seem unaware of their surroundings.

Autoimmune Assays (ANA Tests)—Blood tests to identify autoimmune disease.

Autoimmune Disorder—Disease in which the immune system produces antibodies that attack the body's own tissues.

Autoimmune, Autoimmunity—Disease in which a person's immune system attacks its own tissues.

Autonomic Nervous System—Part of the nervous system that controls organs that function involuntarily, such as the heart, lungs, digestive system and blood vessels.

B

Bacteria—One-celled micro-organisms that can sometimes cause disease.

Balloon Angioplasty—Treatment for obstructed arteries, especially those supplying blood to the heart and brain. A small uninflated balloon is passed up the artery to the obstruction, and then expanded to release the obstruction.

Barium Enema—See *Barium X-Rays*.

Barium X-Rays—Examining the gastrointestinal system by filling it with a barium solution that is detected by x-rays. Common barium tests are the barium swallow (upper GI series) and the barium enema (lower GI series).

Bartholin's Glands—Small glands in the lips of the vagina that secrete a lubricating fluid, especially during sexual arousal.

Behavior Therapy—Psychotherapy that focuses on ways to change the undesired behavior.

Belladonna—Medication derived from a plant used to treat some diseases of the gastrointestinal system. It is similar to atropine.

Benign—1) Tumor or growth that is neither cancerous nor located where it might impair normal function. 2) Harmless.

Beta-Adrenergic Blockers (Beta-Blockers)—Medications that reduce heart or blood-vessel overactivity to improve blood circulation. Also used to prevent migraine headaches, high blood pressure and angina.

Bile Duct—A small tube that allows bile to pass from the gallbladder into the intestines.

Bile—A digestive juice produced in the liver and stored in the gallbladder. Bile empties into the small intestine for digestive processes.

Biliary Cirrhosis—Cirrhosis of the liver due to inflammation or obstruction of the bile ducts.

Bilirubin—A yellowish, red-blood-cell waste product in bile that the blood carries to the liver. It contributes to urine's yellowish color and can cause jaundice if it builds up in the blood.

Biopsy—Removal of a small amount of tissue or cells (such as fluid from a cyst) for laboratory examination that aids in diagnosis. The tissue sample may be removed by a variety of methods depending on the site to be biopsied.

Biopsy Needle—Instrument often used to perform a biopsy.

Biopsy, Skin—Removal of a sample of skin tissue for laboratory examination that aids in diagnosis. Skin biopsy is often required to confirm a clinical (visual) diagnosis. Removal techniques include shave excision, punch excision and elliptical excision.

Birth Canal—Passageway through the cervix and the vagina through which the baby passes during childbirth.

Bladder—An organ that holds fluids such as urine (urinary bladder) or bile (gallbladder).

Blood Cells, Red—Microscopic cells in the blood that carry oxygen to tissues of the body. One drop of blood contains about 200 million red cells.

Blood Cells, White—Microscopic cells in the blood that help fight infection by destroying germs. One drop of blood contains about 400,000 white cells.

Blood Chemistries—Tests that measure chemicals in the blood.

Blood Count—Counting red and white blood cells to aid in diagnosis of many diseases.

Blood Platelets—See *Platelet Count*.

Blood Studies—Examination of a blood sample to measure white blood cells, red blood cells, hemoglobin, hematocrit and chemical substances. See *Blood Chemistries*.

Blood Vessels—Arteries, veins and capillaries; the tubes in which blood circulates through the body.

Bone Bank—Facility where human bone is stored and made available for transplantation.

Bone Scan—Method of studying the bone structure or function by injecting into the bloodstream a medication that can be detected by a special scanning camera.

Bone Spurs—Abnormal and sometimes painful protrusions of bone with sharp points near joints or tendons.

Bronchial Tubes (Bronchi)—Hollow air passageways that branch from the windpipe (trachea) into the lungs. They carry oxygen into the lungs and pass waste gases (mostly carbon dioxide) out of the body.

Bronchioles—Small air passageways that serve the same purpose as bronchial tubes. Bronchioles are the smallest parts of the respiratory system.

Bronchodilator Drugs—Medications used to treat diseases of the bronchi that cause shortness of breath, such as asthma. The medicines help constricted tubes to relax.

Bronchogram—Diagnosing lung diseases by placing a material in the lung that x-rays can outline.

Bronchoscope, Bronchoscopy—An optical instrument with a lighted tip that is passed into the windpipe, then into the bronchi.

Bruising—Discoloration under the skin caused by injury or bleeding.

C

Calcification—A process in which calcium from the blood is deposited abnormally into tissues due to injury, infection or aging. Often it is part of healing and not a sign of active disease.

Calcium-Channel Blocker Drugs—Medication used to treat angina, hypertension, and heartbeat irregularities.

Cancerous Growths—Extensions of cancerous tissues that invade nearby healthy tissues.

Cancers—Destructive tumors that can arise in almost all parts of the body. Cancer can destroy nearby healthy tissue and may spread to distant organs.

Capillaries—Microscopic vessels that supply all body cells and tissues with blood.

Carbohydrates, Complex—Starches, sugars, cellulose and gums. Complex carbohydrates are those contained in whole grains, fresh fruits and fresh vegetables. These are considered more nutritious than simple carbohydrates.

Carbohydrates, Simple—Refined carbohydrates (sugars) that have lower molecular weights than complex carbohydrates. They produce a quick rise in blood-sugar levels. Most nutrition counselors recommend that daily diets contain minimal amounts of refined sugars. So-called "junk foods" are frequently very high in simple carbohydrates.

Cardiac Catheter—A slender tube that is inserted into an artery or vein and then passed into the heart. It is used to examine the heart and nearby blood vessels by injecting material into the heart that x-rays can detect.

Cardiac Catheterization—Studying heart function with a cardiac catheter.

Cardiac Monitoring—See *ECG*.

Cardiac Output—The volume of blood ejected from the left side of the heart in a one minute period.

Cardiopulmonary Resuscitation (CPR)—Emergency treatment for a patient whose heart has stopped (cardiac arrest).

Cardiovascular—Relating to the heart and blood vessels.

Cardiovascular Surgeon—Doctor specially trained to operate on the heart and blood vessels.

Cardiovascular System—System that supplies the body with blood. It consists of the heart and blood vessels (arteries, capillaries, veins).

Carotid Arteries—Large arteries that supply much of the blood to the brain.

Cartilage—Rubbery, dense connective tissue that permits smooth movement of joints. It also helps shape flexible parts of the nose and external ear.

Caruncle—Small, red protrusion of tissue near a body opening. The most common caruncles arise from the urethra or cervix.

CAT Scan—See *CT Scan*.

Catheter—A hollow tube used to introduce fluids into the body or to drain fluids away.

Catheterization—Any procedure in which a small flexible tube is inserted into the body for the purpose of withdrawing or introducing substances. It most often involves the passage of a small catheter through a vein in the arm or leg or the neck and into the heart for securing blood samples or to detect problems.

Caudal Anesthesia—Form of local (low-spinal) anesthesia used to reduce pain during childbirth and surgery on pelvic areas.

Cauterant—Chemical used to destroy abnormal or diseased cells on the skin.

Cauterization—Destruction of tissue by burning or searing it with a red-hot instrument, caustic chemicals or electricity.

Cautery—Destroying small areas of diseased tissue by burning with an electric needle or laser beam, freezing with low-temperature instruments or using a chemical that destroys tissue.

Cecum—The part of the intestinal tract at the beginning of the large colon (intestine).

Central Nervous System—System that controls the body's voluntary acts. It consists of the brain and spinal cord.

Cervical Spine—Bones in the neck at the top of the spinal column.

Cervix—Lower third of the uterus, which protrudes into the vagina.

Cesarean Section—Delivery of a baby through incisions in the mother's abdomen and uterus. It is performed when normal vaginal delivery would be dangerous for the mother or baby.

Chancre—Hard, slightly ulcerated, painless lesion that forms where syphilis enters the body, usually on the genital lips.

Chemocautery—Destruction of abnormal tissue by means of acids, caustics or poisons.

Chemotherapy—Treatment of cancer by injecting medications that kill cancer cells without harming healthy tissue. It is used to treat cancers that cannot be completely cured or treated with surgery or radiation.

Chiggers—Small red biting insects. Also called "red bugs."

Child—Person in the first 10 years of life.

Chiropractor—Practitioner of chiropractic treatment of disease, which involves massage and manipulations to restore normal body functions.

Chokes—Severe breathing difficulty experienced by scuba divers and others who go from high to normal air pressure too rapidly. Bubbles of nitrogen develop in the blood stream and obstruct blood supply to vital organs, sometimes resulting in severe injury or death.

Cholangiogram, Cholangiography—X-ray procedures to diagnose diseases of the bile system (liver, gallbladder, bile ducts). Special medications are used to make the bile system visible on x-rays.

Cholecystectomy—Surgical removal of the gallbladder.

Cholecystography—An x-ray of the gallbladder.

Cholera—Acute, severe, infectious disease causing extreme diarrhea and dehydration.

Choroiditis—Inflammation of the part of the eye that supports the retina and supplies blood to it.

Chromosome—Structures inside the nucleus of living cells that contain hereditary information. Defects in chromosomes cause many birth defects and inherited diseases.

Chronic—Long-term, continuing. Chronic illnesses are usually not curable, but they can often be prevented from worsening. Symptoms usually can be controlled.

Cinematography—Form of motion-picture photography used to record a fast-moving series of x-ray images.

Circulatory System—The system that provides blood to the body, consisting of the heart, arteries, veins and lymphatic system.

Cirrhosis—Chronic scarring of the liver, leading to loss of normal liver function.

Clinician—Health-care professional who has direct contact with patients. The word literally means "someone who is at the patient's bedside."

Clips—See *Skin Clips*.

Clot Retraction Test—Measurement of the time necessary for a tube of blood to form a clot. Abnormal results often indicate a defect in blood platelets, cells important in blood coagulation.

Clotting—Activity of the blood and blood vessels that cause blood to form a jellylike clot, usually near an injury. Clotting helps stop bleeding. The body's clotting mechanism is slowed or reduced ("thinning the blood") with anticoagulants to treat certain diseases.

Coagulation—Same as *Clotting*.

Cocaine—Medication applied directly to mucous membranes to control pain in the nose and throat. Used illegally as a mind-altering drug, it is addicting and dangerous.

Cognitive Therapy—Psychotherapy that is based on the idea that the way we think about the world and ourselves affects our emotions and behavior.

Colic, Colicky—A pain that recurs in a regular pattern every few seconds or minutes.

Collagen—A gelatinous protein from which body tissues are formed.

Colon—The last major portion of the gastrointestinal tract, where waste material is formed into feces and held for elimination. It is also known as the large intestine.

Colonoscope, Colonoscopy—Method of diagnosing diseases of the colon by visual examination of the inside of the colon through a flexible colonoscope, a fiber-optic instrument with a lighted tip.

Color-Blindness—Inability to recognize red and green, which appear to be gray. It is usually hereditary.

Colposcopy—Visual examination of the cervix by means of a colposcope, a slender optical instrument with a lighted tip.

Combined Immunodeficiency Disease—Serious inherited disease in which the immune system of infants is unable to defend against disease.

Complication—Undesirable event during disease or treatment that causes further symptoms and delay in recovery.

Compress—Cloth, sometimes soaked in warm water or coated with medication. It is applied to the skin to relieve discomfort.

Compression—Applying pressure to the surface of the body, usually to stop bleeding.

Compulsion, Compulsive—Intense, irrational urge to perform some action.

Condom—A thin sheath, usually of latex, applied to the penis before sexual intercourse. It is used to help prevent disease of the genitals and as a contraceptive.

Congenital—Abnormality of the body, present at birth, usually meaning a defect. Congenital defects may be inherited or caused by conditions occurring while the fetus grows in the uterus.

Congenital Hypoplastic Anemia—See *Hypoplastic Anemia*.

Conization of the Cervix—Removal of a cone of tissue from the cervix. Laboratory examination of the removed tissue identifies possible cancer.

Conjunctiva—The mucous membrane lining the outermost surface of the eye (white of the eye).

Connective Tissue—Body's supporting framework of tissue consisting of strands of collagen, elastic fibers and simple cells.

Contact Lenses—Small plastic lenses worn on the eyes to correct nearsightedness, farsightedness or astigmatism.

Contagious—Disease or condition that spreads from one person to another.

Convalescence—Recovery from an illness or surgery.

Copious—Large in amount.

Cornea—Clear thickened surface of the eye through which light passes. It has no blood supply and can be transplanted without danger of rejection.

Coronary—Referring to the blood vessels supplying the heart. Sometimes, it refers to a heart attack resulting from coronary-artery obstruction.

Coronary-Care Unit (CCU)—Area of a hospital equipped to care for patients who have suffered a heart attack or other life-threatening heart conditions.

Cortisone Drugs—Medications similar to natural hormones produced by the central core of the adrenal glands.

Cosmetic Surgery—Surgery to improve appearance.

Coxsackie Viruses—Group of viruses causing infections such as poliomyelitis, aseptic meningitis, herpangina and myocarditis.

CPR—See *Cardiopulmonary Resuscitation*.

Cranium—Bones that make up the skull.

Cryosurgery—Destruction of abnormal tissue by applying freezing temperatures, usually with liquid nitrogen.

Cryotherapy—The use of cold (below -200°F) temperatures in treatment.

CT Scan, CAT Scan (Computerized Axial Tomography)—A computerized x-ray procedure that provides exceptionally clear images of parts of the body. It aids in diagnosis of diseases that cannot be diagnosed by ordinary x-ray methods.

Culdocentesis—Piercing of the space deep in the vagina under the cervix, to obtain fluid. Laboratory examination of the removed fluid aids in diagnosis of ectopic pregnancy and other disorders.

Culdoscopy—Visual examination of the female pelvic organs using a slender instrument brought into the pelvic cavity by penetrating through the space deep in the vagina under the cervix.

Culture—Identification of bacteria, fungi and viruses. Material (pus, blood or urine) from an infected area is collected, placed on nutrient material, and kept warm (usually in an incubator) until the infecting agent has grown. The resulting growth is examined with a microscope.

Curettage—Scraping process frequently used to obtain tissue from the lining of the uterus for laboratory examination that aids in diagnosis.

Curette—Instrument with a sharp end used to scrape tissue from the inner lining of the uterus and to scrape away skin lesions.

Cyst—Sac or cavity filled with fluid or diseased matter.

Cyst Aspiration—Removal of cyst contents for examination, or drainage for relief of symptoms.

Cystogram—An x-ray of the urinary bladder that is obtained by injecting a solution visible on x-rays into the bladder.

Cystoscopy—Visual examination of the inside of the urinary bladder by means of a cystoscope, a slender optical instrument with a lighted tip.

Cystourethroscope, Cystourethroscopy—An instrument used for examination of the posterior urethra and bladder.

Cytotoxic Drugs—Medications used to destroy cancerous cells with minimal harm to healthy cells.

D

DC Cardioversion—The restoration of normal rhythm of the heart by a brief electrical shock via two metal plates placed on the wall of the chest.

D & C—Same as *Dilatation and Curettage*.

Debilitating—Causing a general weakening or deterioration in health.

Defibrillation, Cardiac—Applying an electric current to the chest over the heart to interrupt fibrillation, a disturbance of heartbeat.

Dehydration—Loss of essential fluids from the tissues and blood of the body.

Dependence—Condition in which a person requires substances such as narcotics or alcohol to remain comfortable. If the substances are not used, withdrawal symptoms develop.

Dermatome—Area of the skin to which feeling (sensation) is provided by a nerve to the spinal cord.

Descending Colon—The part of the colon in the left side of the abdomen that stores feces until they are passed from the body.

Desensitization—1) Reduction or prevention of allergic (hypersensitivity) reactions by administration of graded doses of allergen. 2) Treatment for phobias and other psychological disorders. A patient gradually increases the exposure to the source of fear while simultaneously learning to relax.

Diabetic Retinopathy—Degeneration of the retina that develops in patients with diabetes mellitus. It may cause vision impairment or blindness.

Diagnosis—Identifying disease. A complete diagnosis names the part of the body affected, the disease process (such as inflammation, cancer or allergy) and the cause of disease.

Dialysis—Removal of natural wastes from the bloodstream. It is used to treat patients with kidney failure.

Diaphragm—Thin, broad sheet of muscle separating the chest cavity from the abdominal cavity.

Diathermy—Treatment in which mild heat is generated within the body by high-frequency radio waves.

Digestive System—Organs in which food is processed for absorption into the blood stream. The major digestive organs are the mouth, esophagus, stomach, duodenum, small bowel (small intestine), colon (large intestine), and rectum. The liver, gallbladder and pancreas are also considered parts of the digestive system.

Digitalis—A drug used to treat congestive heart failure and some other heart diseases.

Dilatation and Curettage—A gynecological treatment or diagnostic procedure that involves the stretching (dilatation) of the cervix so that a spoon-shaped instrument (curet) can be inserted into the uterus to scrape away the lining (endometrium). The scrapings may be examined under a microscope to assess the condition of the uterus.

Dilate, Dilation, Dilatation—To widen, expand or open up.

Dilator—Instrument used to widen organs that have narrowed because of disease.

Discolored Teeth—A yellowish-brown discoloration of the teeth frequently occurring in infants whose mothers took tetracycline while pregnant. Children may also be affected if they take tetracycline before they have their permanent teeth.

Discomfort—Unpleasant physical or mental sensation.

Disease—Adverse change in health; sickness or ailment. A disease can be defined by the body part involved (for example, the heart or liver), by the abnormality present (cancer, infection, allergy, degeneration, etc.) or by its cause (bacteria, poisons, injury, etc.).

Disc—Same as *Intervertebral Disc.*

Disorder—Same as *Disease.*

Diuretics—Medications that force the kidneys to excrete more urine, sodium and potassium than normal, which helps eliminate excessive body fluid.

Diverticulum—Small pouch or sac that develops in the wall of tubular organs such as the esophagus or colon.

Dizziness—Sensation of faintness, lightheadedness or spinning (vertigo).

Donor—Person who gives to someone else. In transplantation surgery, the donor gives up an organ (such as a kidney) to be transplanted into the recipient.

Doppler Ultrasound—See *Ultrasound*; this is one of several methods of ultrasound.

Doppler Venous Studies—Measurement of blood flow through the veins by means of doppler ultrasound.

Dormant—Sleeping or inactive state of living things. Also, an inactive state of a disease.

Drainage—Passage of fluids out of the body through an opening or incision.

Dry Socket—A tooth socket in which after extraction a blood clot fails to form; a condition marked by pain associated with the occurrence of a dry socket.

Ductus Arteriosus—Small blood vessel connecting the aorta and the pulmonary artery, which is the main artery to the lung. The vessel is open during the time the fetus is in the uterus, but normally closes at birth.

Duodenum—First 12 inches of the small intestine.

Dupuytren's Contracture—Chronic condition in which scar tissue forms in the palms. In severe cases, it can impair use of the fingers.

Dwarfism—Condition of being undersized for one's age. It may be due to endocrine disorders, malnutrition or an inherited defect.

Dyspnea—Difficult or painful breathing.

E

Ear Canal—Passageway extending from the outer ear inward to the eardrum.

Ear, Nose and Throat (ENT) Specialist—A physician specially trained to treat diseases of the ears, nose and throat.

ECG (Electrocardiography)—Method of diagnosing heart diseases by measuring electrical activity of the heart with an electrocardiograph. The record produced is called an electrocardiogram.

Echocardiogram, Echocardiography—Studying the heart by examining sound waves created by an instrument placed on the chest. The waves reflected from the heart form an image (echocardiogram) on a monitor, aiding in diagnosis of heart diseases.

Echography—The use of ultrasound as a diagnostic aid.

Eclampsia—Convulsions or coma late in pregnancy in an individual affected with preeclampsia.

Ectopic Pregnancy—A gestation which occurs elsewhere than in the uterus, usually in a Fallopian tube or the peritoneal cavity.

Edema—Accumulation of fluid under the skin, in the lungs or elsewhere.

EEG (Electroencephalography)—Studying the brain by measuring electric activity ("brain waves") with an electroencephalograph. The record produced is the electroencephalogram.

EKG—See *ECG*.

Electrocardiography—See *ECG*.

Electrocautery—Destruction of tissue by heat applied with a controlled electric current.

Electroencephalography—See *EEG*.

Electrolyte—A chemical that is dissolved in the blood and all other body fluids. Electrolytes play an essential role in all body functions. The major electrolytes are: sodium, potassium, chloride, calcium, phosphorus, magnesium and carbon dioxide. Electrolytes come from food. They are regulated mostly by the kidneys and lungs.

Electrolyte Measurement—Laboratory test on blood or urine to identify and measure the electrolytes present.

Electrolyte Supplements—Electrolytes taken to correct or to prevent body-fluid or electrolyte imbalance.

Electromyography—Studying nerve and muscle disorders by recording electrical activity of muscles with an electromyograph. The record produced is the electromyogram.

Electroneuronography—A diagnostic procedure in which the nerve of a muscle under study is stimulated by application of an electric current.

Endemic—Disease that is constantly present in a community or group of people. Endemic disease may affect only a few people at any one time.

Endocrine System—System of organs that secrete hormones into the blood to regulate basic functions of cells and tissues. The endocrine organs are the anterior and posterior pituitary glands, thyroid and parathyroid glands, pancreas, adrenal glands, ovaries (in women) and testicles (in men).

Endocrinologist—Doctor specially trained in diagnosis and treatment of endocrine disorders.

Endometritis—Inflammation of the endometrium.

Endometrium—The mucous membrane lining of the uterus.

Endoscopy—Method of diagnosing diseases in hollow organs. An endoscope (an optical instrument with a lighted tip) is inserted into the organ, which allows visual examination of the cavity. Used in the abdomen, pelvis, lumen of the bronchial tubes or intestines.

Endotracheal Tube—Tube temporarily placed in the trachea (windpipe) of patients who are unable to breathe normally because of disease or surgery.

Enteric—Relating to the small intestine. Enteric-coated medicine is coated with a hard shell that dissolves when it reaches the small intestine.

Enteroscopy—Examination of the inside of the intestines with an endoscope, an optical instrument.

Enterostomy—Surgically created artificial opening for elimination of feces.

Enterostomy Nurse, Enterostomy Specialist—a professional who teaches patients how to care for an enterostomy.

Enzymes—Proteins manufactured by the body that regulate the rate of essential life processes (metabolism).

Epididymis—A system of ducts at the rear of the testes which holds sperm during maturation.

Epididymitis—Inflammation of the epididymis.

Epinephrine—Same as *Adrenalin*.

Episcleritis—Inflammation of tissues on the sclera (the white of the eye).

Epithelial Horn—Thick, rough lesion protruding from the skin. It may become cancerous if not removed.

Equine Virus—Virus that causes a serious form of encephalitis in horses and humans.

Ergot—Medication derived from a fungus that grows on rye plant. It is used to treat migraine headache and to increase strength of uterine contractions during and immediately after childbirth.

Esophageal Varices—Enlarged veins on the lining of the esophagus. They are subject to severe bleeding and often appear in patients with severe liver disease.

Esophagogram, Esophagoscopy—Method of diagnosing diseases of the esophagus by means of an esophagoscope, an optical instrument with lenses and a lighted tip.

Esophagus—Muscular tube connecting the throat and stomach.

Estrogen—Female sex hormone, primarily secreted by the ovaries. It can also be produced synthetically for use in estrogen replacement therapy.

Estrogen Receptor Value—Used in the study of breast-cancer cells to determine the best treatment.

Etiology—Cause or causes of a disease.

Eustachian Tubes—Slender passages between the throat and the middle ear that maintain normal air pressure in the middle ear.

Excise—To remove by cutting out.

Exploratory Laparotomy—Diagnosing abdominal disease by surgically opening the abdomen and examining its contents.

Extremities—Arms and legs.

Eye Bank—Facility where living corneas are stored and made available for transplantation.

Eyes, Crossed—Condition in which muscles controlling the eyes are unbalanced. The eyes point in different directions. Also called squint or strabismus.

F

Fallopian Tubes—Organs of the female reproductive tract through which an egg (ovum) passes from the ovary to the uterus. Tying these tubes (tubal ligation) accomplishes sterility.

Familial Polyposis—Inherited condition in which the lining of the intestines contains many polyps, some of which may become cancerous.

Family History—Information about illnesses that tend to occur within a family. This information is used to determine the likelihood of diseases occurring in other members of the family.

Farsightedness—Same as *Hypermetropia*.

Fascia—Sheet or band of tough, fibrous tissue that covers muscles and other body organs.

Fecal—Relating to feces, waste products eliminated through the lower intestinal tract.

Fecal-Oral—Pathway by which some fecal germs gain entry into the bloodstream. Sewage in drinking water, hand-to-mouth transmission after bowel movements or sexual contact can cause infection.

Feces—Body waste formed of undigested food that has passed through the gastrointestinal system to the colon. Feces are and stored in the colon until eliminated.

Fetal Monitoring—Measuring the heart rate of the fetus during labor.

Fetal-Scalp Electrodes—Fine wires attached to the scalp of a fetus to measure heart rate and rhythm during labor.

Fetal-Scalp Monitoring—Measuring the well-being of the fetus during labor by obtaining blood from the scalp or by measuring the heart rate of the fetus or contraction strength of the uterus.

Fever—Above-normal body temperature. Normal mouth temperature is 98.6°F (37°C). Normal rectal temperature is 99.6°F (37.6°C).

Fiber Optics—System of transmitting light and images through thread-like strands of glass. Fiber-optic instruments make some examinations and surgical procedures simple, safe and effective.

Fiber—A non-nutritious ingredient of many complex carbohydrates. Fiber increases bulk in the diet. Many nutritionists recommend including ample fiber in the diet. Experimental studies and clinical studies show that people who eat high-fiber diets are less likely to develop colon cancer, diverticulitis, atherosclerosis and gallbladder disease.

Fibrin—Protein formed by the action of blood clotting on fibrinogen.

Fibrinogen—Protein in the blood needed for blood clotting.

Fibrositis—Inflammatory conditions affecting connective tissue of muscles, joints, ligaments and tendons.

Fine Needle Biopsy—The use of a fine needle to remove cells or fluid from the body for microscopic laboratory examination.

First Molars—First permanent flat teeth, used for grinding food, which appear at about age 6 to 7.

Fissure—Break in the skin or inner lining of organs.

Fistula—Abnormal passage between two organs or between the body and the outside.

Flank—Area on the side of the body below the ribs and above the hip.

Fleas—Tiny biting insects. Most cause minor skin irritation; some carry and transmit serious diseases such as plague and typhus.

Flooding—A drastic form of psychotherapy used for treatment of phobias. A patient is suddenly confronted with the feared object or placed in the feared situation with no chance of escape. Having experienced the phobia at its fullest intensity, a person comes to realize that the dreaded thing is not dangerous.

Only a competent therapist should subject a phobic person to flooding.

Fluorescein-Dye Test—Method of diagnosis using fluorescein, a dye, to study tissues and germs. When these dyed tissues are exposed to ultraviolet light, they glow. Substances to which the dye does not cling do not glow.

Fluorescent Antibody Studies—Tests used to study some allergic and infectious conditions. When antibodies created by these conditions are present in the blood, they can be made to glow by using a dye and a microscope with ultraviolet light.

Fluoroscopy—Method of x-ray diagnosis in which moving organs (such as the heart or intestinal tract) can be studied in action.

Foley Catheter—Slender, flexible tube used to drain urine from the bladder of patients who are unable to urinate normally.

Forceps—Instrument with two blades and handles. It is used to grasp tissue, body parts or sterile materials. Also used to deliver babies when progress of labor is slow.

Fracture—Break; usually used to refer to a bone or tooth.

Frei Test—Test used to make a precise diagnosis of lymphogranuloma, a sexually transmitted disease.

Friedreich's Ataxia—Rare, inherited nervous-system disease that causes loss of balance and coordination, awkward walking, speech difficulty and tremors.

Frozen Section—A study in a pathology laboratory of fresh tissue that was removed during surgery. The purpose is to determine if a suspicious area is or is not cancerous.

Fungus—Mold or yeast that may infect skin, internal surfaces (mouth, vagina) or tissues.

Fungus Infection—Infection caused by fungus.

Fusiform Bacteria—Bacteria shaped like slender rods.

G

Galactorrhea—1) Continued breast-milk flow after weaning. 2) Excess breast-milk flow during nursing.

Galactosemia—Inherited disease of infants in which milk cannot be digested. Milk should be eliminated from the infant's diet to prevent malnutrition, liver and kidney disease and mental retardation.

Gallbladder—Small organ under the liver that stores bile. For digestion, the gallbladder contracts to empty bile into the intestines.

Gamma Globulin—Protein in the blood manufactured by the immune system to help destroy or neutralize infection-causing germs. Gamma globulin derived and concentrated from blood of other humans is used to help create temporary immunity to some diseases.

Gammaglobulinemia—Extremely low levels in the blood of gamma globulin brought about by a disease of the immune system. The deficiency causes increased susceptibility to many infections by bacteria, viruses and fungi. Also called hypogammaglobulinemia.

Gangrene—Death of tissue, usually due to partial or total loss of blood supply.

Gastrectomy—Removal of part or all of the stomach.

Gastroduodenoscopy—Examination of the stomach and duodenum by means of a gastroscope.

Gastroenterologist—Doctor who specializes in the diagnosis and treatment of diseases of the gastrointestinal system.

Gastrointestinal Series (Upper GI Series)—X-rays of the upper digestive system (esophagus, stomach and duodenum).

Gastrointestinal Tract—See *Digestive System*.

Gastroscope, Gastroscopy—Visual examination of the inside of the stomach by means of a gastroscope, an optical instrument with a lighted tip.

Gene—Basic unit of protein molecules in chromosomes of cells. Genes transmit inherited characteristics such as eye color, blood type, gender or body shape. Defective genes cause many kinds of birth defects and inborn diseases.

Gene, Dominant or Recessive—Dominant gene, if present in either the mother's egg or father's sperm, will transmit its characteristics to the newborn child. Recessive gene must be present in both parents before its characteristic will be transmitted.

General Surgeon—A doctor specially trained to perform operations.

Genetic Counseling—Counseling to help couples decide whether to have children or not when there is a risk of genetic disease being transmitted to the child.

Genetics—Science of determining inherited factors that result in the unique make-up of every human being; also, science that traces the appearance patterns to genetic (inherited) disease.

Genitourinary Tract—Body system that forms, stores and eliminates urine. Also has a role in male and female reproductive functions. Organs include the kidneys, ureters, bladder, urethra, uterus, Fallopian tubes, ovaries, vagina, cervix, penis, scrotum and testicles.

Germs—Organisms that cause infection such as bacteria, viruses or fungi.

Gestation—Time spent in the mother's uterus by the fetus. Average gestation time for the human infant, from conception to delivery, is approximately 39 weeks.

Gigantism—Condition in which the body or a body part grows excessively, sometimes due to an overactive pituitary gland.

Glucagon—Hormone secreted by the pancreas that increases blood sugar. A synthetic form is sometimes used as emergency treatment for patients with diabetes who have temporarily low blood sugar.

Glucose—Major form of sugar in the blood, stored primarily in the liver. It provides energy to most tissues, organs and systems.

Glucose-Tolerance Test—Method of diagnosing diabetes mellitus or functional hypoglycemia. The patient drinks a measured amount of glucose (sugar). The blood and urine are tested at measured intervals for glucose content.

Gluten—Protein found in wheat and other foods that cannot be digested by some persons because of genetic disease. A gluten-free diet allows persons with the disorder to digest food and grow normally.

Glycosuria—Sugar in the urine.

Goiter—An enlargement of the thyroid gland that is visible as a swelling in the neck.

Gonads—Parts of the reproductive system that produce and release female eggs (ovaries) or male sperm (testes).

Growth Disorders—Conditions in children that result in underdevelopment or overdevelopment of the body. Diseases of the endocrine glands, nutritional problems or genetic abnormalities are frequently the causes.

Gynecologist—Doctor specially trained to treat diseases of the female reproductive system.

H

H-2 Blocker Drugs—Class of antihistamines that reduce the production of stomach acid for treatment of peptic ulcers.

Hallucinogens—Substances that produce hallucinations, apparent sights, sounds or other experiences that do not actually exist.

Hand Surgeon—Surgeon specially trained to treat hand diseases, injuries, infections and arthritic conditions.

Hangover—Unpleasant aftereffects of excessive consumption of alcoholic beverages. Symptoms include irritability, headache and nausea. Sometimes, the same feelings result from using certain medications.

Hashimoto's Thyroiditis—One of several kinds of inflammation of the thyroid gland.

Heart Catheterization—Same as *Cardiac Catheterization*.

Heart Tumors—Rare tumors that grow in the heart wall or in the heart chambers, interfering with normal heart function.

Heart-Lung Machine—Complex mechanical device that provides artificial function of a patient's heart and lungs for a short time during open-heart surgery and heart or lung transplantation.

Hematocrit—Blood test used to detect anemia and other blood disorders. It is expressed as the percentage of blood made up of red blood cells (remainder of the blood is made up of serum or plasma). Normal hematocrit range is approximately 35 to 45%, but it varies with age and sex.

Hematologist—Doctor specially trained to diagnose and treat diseases of the blood and blood-forming organs.

Hemochromatosis—Disease in which excessive iron accumulates in the liver, pancreas and skin, resulting in liver disease, diabetes mellitus and a bronzed skin color.

Hemoglobin, Hemoglobin Range—
1) Component that carries oxygen to body tissues.
2) Blood test used to detect anemia and other blood disorders, expressed in grams per 100 cubic centimeters. The normal hemoglobin range is approximately 12 to 18 grams per 100 cubic centimeters and varies according to age and sex.

Hemothorax—blood in the pleural cavity.

Hepatitis—A disease or condition marked by inflammation of the liver.

Hirschsprung's Disease—Congenital defect of infants in which the colon cannot eliminate feces, resulting in severe constipation.

Histamine—Chemical in body tissues that dilates the smallest blood vessels, constricts the muscle around the bronchial tubes, stimulates stomach secretions and produces an allergic response.

HIV—See *Human Immunodeficiency Virus*.

Holter Monitor—Instrument that detects heartbeat-rhythm abnormalities 24 hours or longer. The device is portable for patients to carry wherever they go.

Hormones—Powerful substances manufactured by the endocrine glands and carried by the blood to body tissues and organs. Hormones determine growth and structure of many organs (such as during growth and maturation) and also control many vital body functions.

Host—Person or animal with an infection that has been received from another person, animal or plant, or the environment.

Human Immunodeficiency Virus—Any of a group of retroviruses that infect and destroy helper T cells of the immune system and weaken the body's natural abilities to fight infections and cancer. Also called the AIDS virus.

Hyaline-Membrane Disease—Serious condition of premature infants in which the lungs can't expand normally. Cause is unknown.

Hydatidiform Mole—Disease occurring during early pregnancy resulting in death of the fetus and an overgrowth of tissue within the uterus.

Hydramnios and Polyhydramnios—Condition in which amniotic fluid (fluid in the uterus that surrounds the fetus until birth) becomes excessive.

Hygiene—Personal self-care and cleanliness that reduces the risk of infections and diseases.

Hyoid Bone—V-shaped bone located just above the larynx.

Hyperalimentation—Method of supplying total nutritional needs of patients unable to eat normally. The method (usually intravenous or by tube through the nose into the stomach) provides nutrients containing essential proteins, fats, carbohydrates and vitamins.

Hyperbaric Chamber—Large, sealed room in which air pressure can be raised above normal levels. It is used primarily to treat patients with either decompression sickness or severe burns (sometimes).

Hypercalcemia—Presence of excessive calcium in the blood, occasionally a sign of malignancy.

Hyperlipoproteinemia—Condition in which excessive lipoproteins (cholesterol and other fatty materials) accumulate in the blood.

Hypermetropia—Seeing distant objects clearly while nearby objects appear blurred; also called farsightedness.

Hypersensitivity—Extreme sensitivity to any agent (drugs, pollens, chemicals, etc.) that causes allergic reactions. Some reactions can be life-threatening, but most are less serious.

Hyperthyroidism—Excessive activity of the thyroid gland marked by increased metabolic rate, enlargement of the thyroid gland, rapid heart rate and high blood pressure.

Hypnotics—Medications that produce sleep.

Hypochondriasis—Mental illness in which a person is convinced that serious disease is present, despite examination that proves otherwise. The symptoms of the imagined disease seem real to the patient (often called a hypochondriac).

Hypogammaglobulinemia—An immunologically deficient state characterized by an abnormally low level of all classes of gamma globulin in the blood.

Hypoparathyroidism—Deficiency of parathyroid hormone in the body.

Hypoplastic Anemia (Aplastic Anemia)—Group of anemias that decrease blood-producing bone marrow. This can be life-threatening.

Hypothalamus—Part of the brain that regulates body functions such as temperature, blood pressure, appetite and thirst.

Hypothyroidism—Deficient activity of the thyroid gland, marked by decreased metabolic rate and loss of vigor.

Hysteria—1) Condition in which a person becomes anxious and excitable and experiences impaired sensory and motor abilities. Sometimes, hysterical persons simulate conditions of diseases such as deafness or blindness. 2) Outbreak of uncontrolled emotions, such as fits of laughing or crying.

Hysterogram—An x-ray of the uterus.

Hysterosalpingography—Studying the uterus and Fallopian tubes by injecting material into the uterus that x-rays can detect. It is used primarily to determine if the passageway for the ovum (egg) is open all the way to the uterus. The x-ray image is the hysterosalpingogram.

Hysteroscope—An instrument with lens system and lighted tip used in direct visual examination of the cervix and cavity of the uterus.

Hysterotomy—Incision of the uterus to prepare for cesarean section delivery of a baby.

I

I-131 Uptake—Measuring thyroid activity with radioactive iodine and radiation emission counters.

Idiopathic—Condition caused by unknown factors.

Ileum—Part of the small intestine just above the large intestine (colon).

Ileus—Condition of the small intestine in which either an obstruction or paralysis prevents material from passing through the intestine.

Iliac Arteries—Large arteries in the inner pelvis that supply blood to the legs.

Immune System—Body's system of defense against infection.

Immune, Immunity—Resistance or protection against infection by the body's natural defenses. A person may be immune to one kind of infection but not immune to another. Some infections, such as measles, chickenpox or mumps, cause the body to become immune permanently to that infection.

Immunization—Producing immunity by giving a vaccine (orally or by injection) of germs that have been altered so they cannot produce significant disease. The vaccine causes the body's immune system to produce antibodies that create immunity.

Immunosuppressants—Drugs used in immunosuppression treatment to weaken the immune system and to inhibit immune response.

Immunosuppression—Prevention of the body from forming a normal immune response. It is used to treat diseases (especially when organs must be transplanted) where certain antibodies must be inactivated.

Impotence—Male's inability to achieve or to sustain an erection or to ejaculate sperm during sexual intercourse.

Incise, Incision—To cut open or cut into.

Incomplete Spontaneous Miscarriage—Naturally occurring miscarriage in which the fetus is expelled, but part of the placenta remains in the uterus. Excessive bleeding and infection can result unless the uterus is emptied, usually by dilatation and curettage of the uterus (D & C) or suction curettage.

Incubation Period—The time between exposure to an infecting germ and the appearance of symptoms indicating an infection. Also describes the period of bacterial growth in laboratory cultures.

Infant—Child between the ages of 2 weeks and 1 year.

Infection, Infectious—Disease caused by germs (bacteria, viruses, fungi) that enter the body and cause inflammation or other processes that have an adverse effect on health.

Inflammation, Inflammatory Process—Process by which the body attempts to overcome illness-producing causes such as germs, injuries such as burns, or diseases such as arthritis. The process causes increased body heat (fever or local warmth), swelling, pain and tenderness. If the inflammation is near the skin, redness results.

Inhalation—Breathing air into the lungs.

Inherited—Body characteristic that is transmitted from one generation to the next by chromosomes in the mother's egg and father's sperm. Some inherited characteristics such as brown eyes are normal; others such as Down's syndrome are disorders.

Ingestion—Taking in food, medicine, etc., by mouth.

Inoculation—Injection of infected material such as pus into a nutrient medium where the germs will grow, or incubate. They are then stained and analyzed through a microscope. Also describes any kind of immunization.

Insufflation Test—See *Rubin's Insufflation Test.*

Insulin—Hormone produced by the pancreas that helps regulate sugar in the blood and helps produce energy.

Intensive Care Unit (ICU)—Area of a hospital where patients who are seriously ill or recovering from serious surgery are given more care than is available in other hospital units. As soon as the condition improves, the patient is transferred from the ICU to a regular hospital unit.

Intermittent—Happening only occasionally or under certain conditions.

Internist—Doctor specially trained in nonsurgical diagnosis and treatment of diseases in adults.

Intervertebral Disc—Cartilage that connects adjacent vertebrae in the spinal column.

Intestinal Tract—All parts of the gastrointestinal tract except the mouth, esophagus and stomach. The intestinal tract organs are: duodenum, small bowel, ileum, cecum, appendix, ascending colon, transverse colon, descending colon, sigmoid colon, rectum and anus.

Intestine, Large—Last major portion of the gastrointestinal tract located just under the small intestine. It is also called the colon or large bowel. It processes waste material into feces, which are stored until eliminated from the body.

Intestine, Small—Longest section of the gastrointestinal tract, located just under the stomach and duodenum. It absorbs digested food into the bloodstream and passes waste material into the large intestine.

Intracardiac Pressures—Pressures occurring within the heart.

Intrauterine Death—Death of a fetus while inside the mother's uterus.

Intrauterine Device (IUD)—Birth-control method in which a small device placed permanently in the uterus prevents growth of fertilized eggs.

Intravenous—Within the vein. Fluids, medications and nutrients that cannot be taken orally are given intravenously by a needle placed in a large vein near the surface of the skin.

Intravenous Pyelogram (IVP)—See *Pyelogram, Intravenous.*

Intravenous Urography—Method of studying the kidneys and urinary tract by injecting into the bloodstream a medication that x-rays can detect.

IQ (Intelligence Quotient)—Supposedly a measure of a person's intelligence, rather than what one has learned. Research on intelligence raises questions about the accuracy and meaning of the IQ test.

Iridectomy—Surgery performed to treat some kinds of glaucoma.

Irrigation—Flooding with water or other liquid. It is used frequently to clean wounds or areas of the body that will undergo surgery.

Isolation, Reverse Isolation—Procedures to prevent spread of infection in a hospital. Isolation protects hospital staff and visitors from contracting a contagious disease from a patient. Reverse isolation protects a patient susceptible to infection because of immunosuppression from contracting infection from hospital staff or visitors.

IUD—See *Intrauterine Device*.

IVP— See *Pyelogram, Intravenous*.

J

Jaundice—Yellow skin and whites of the eyes, dark urine and light stools, symptoms of diseases of the liver and blood.

Joint—Structure that enables two or more bones to move easily in relation to each other. A joint consists of ligaments and cartilage that hold bones together.

Joint Capsule—Tough, fibrous tissue that surrounds a joint.

Joint Replacement—Replacement of diseased joints with mechanical joints. The wrist, hip and knee joints are among the most common joints replaced.

K

Ketoacidosis—Serious complication of diabetes mellitus in which the body produces acids that cause fluid and electrolyte disorders, dehydration and sometimes coma.

Klinefelter's Syndrome—Inherited disease of young males in which secondary sex characteristics are underdeveloped. The condition does not become evident until puberty. Mental deficiency and some female characteristics are present.

L

Laceration—Wound with jagged edges.

Lactiferous Ducts—Network of tubes in the female breast that collects milk and delivers it to the nipple.

Laminaria—Freeze-dried seaweed sometimes used to dilate the cervix when performing an abortion.

Laparoscope, Laparoscopy—Exploratory examination of the organs inside the abdominal cavity with a laparoscope, an optical instrument with a lighted tip. The laparoscope is inserted into the abdomen through a small incision. Visual examination can then be made of many abdominal organs.

Laparotomy—Exploratory surgery in the abdomen performed to diagnose and sometimes treat abdominal disease.

Laryngeal Nerve—Nerve located in the neck that controls the vocal cords and enables a person to speak.

Laryngoscopy—Examination of the inside of the larynx with a laryngoscope, an optical instrument.

Larynx—Structure of muscle and cartilage in the upper neck. It contains the vocal cords. Air passes through the larynx into the windpipe and then into the lungs. The "Adam's apple" is part of the larynx.

Laser Therapy—Using a laser beam to treat many diseases. Sharply focused laser light creates intense heat and is valuable in cutting tissue, destroying unwanted tissue and joining tissue together. It is most often used to treat retinal detachment, endometriosis or atherosclerosis.

Latent—Present but inactive; something that exists in an undeveloped form.

Laxatives—Medications used to treat constipation.

Lesion—General term for injury or damage to an organ or tissue.

Lethargy—Fatigue or lack of usual physical or mental energy.

Libido—Sexual desire.

Life Cycle—Growth and development from birth to death.

Ligaments—Strong, flexible cords of tissue near joints that hold bones together and permit bone motion.

Lipoproteins (High Density and Low Density)—Components of the fluid in blood that are measured to help predict the likelihood of atherosclerosis (hardening of the arteries).

Liquid Nitrogen—Nitrogen that has been cooled until it becomes a liquid. It is used most often in cryosurgery.

Local Anesthesia—See *Anesthesia, Local*.

Low-Residue Diet—Diet consisting of foods that are digested almost entirely, leaving minimal material to form feces.

Low-Spinal Anesthesia—Also called "saddle-block" anesthesia. An injection into the lower spinal canal provides anesthesia to the lower body.

Lower GI Series—Same as *Barium-Enema X-Rays*.

Lumbar Puncture (Spinal Tap)—A diagnostic procedure in which a needle is inserted between 2 bones (vertebra) of the lower spine to collect spinal fluid for laboratory examination.

Lumbar Spine—Lower part of the spine, from the lowest ribs to the bottom of the spine.

Lung Function Studies—Tests to determine the effectiveness of a patient's respiration.

Lymph (or Lymphatic) System—Lymph channels and lymph glands considered as a single body system.

Lymph Channels—Tubes of tissue that carry lymph fluid away from tissues and back to the bloodstream. Lymph fluid is composed of proteins and water, varying in composition in different parts of the body.

Lymph Glands—Small collections of tissue (nodes) located along lymph channels in areas such as the elbow, armpit or groin. When infection is present, nearby lymph glands enlarge, become tender and destroy germs that enter lymph channels. Lymph glands also manufacture antibodies to help fight infection.

Lymphangiogram, Lymphangiography—Diagnostic method of studying the lymphatic system by infecting a material into the lymph channels that x-rays can detect. The image on x-ray film is the lymphangiogram.

Lymphatic Leukemia—Class of leukemias, involving primarily lymphatic cells, affecting children and adults.

Lymphedema—Painful swelling of soft tissues, caused by edema due to faulty lymphatic drainage. Swelling is often accompanied by decreased mobility in the affected limb, and by increased risk of infection.

Lymphocytes—One of several types of white blood cells that help fight infection.

Lymphosarcoma—Class of cancers of the lymphatic system.

M

Macular Degeneration of the Eye—Condition of the macula (area on the retina that provides detailed vision) in which impaired blood supply causes gradual vision loss.

Macule—General term for any discolored spot or patch on the skin, such as a freckle.

Malignant—Capable of causing great harm, including death. It usually refers to cancerous growth.

Magnetic Resonance Imaging—See *MRI*.

Mammogram, Mammography—Diagnostic method of studying the female breast by an x-ray technique that detects cancerous growths while they are still treatable. The image on x-ray film is the mammogram.

Manic-Depressive Illness—Mental illness in which behavior alternates between unrealistic enthusiasm and deep depression.

Manometer, Manometry—The measuring of pressure (of either liquid or gas) by means of a manometer.

MAO Inhibitors—See *Monoamine Oxidase Inhibitors*.

Marijuana—Mood-altering substance that is usually taken into the body by smoking. It is derived from Indian hemp or Cannabis leaves, stems and seed pods.

Marrow—Core of many bones, where most of the body's blood cells are produced.

Mastoiditis—Infection of the mastoid (bony area just behind the ear).

Mediators—Substances that: 1) help nerve impulses travel from one cell to the next; 2) participate in the allergic process.

Medic Alert—Nonprofit agency that maintains a medical-record system. Subscribers receive a bracelet or pendant that states their medical condition and provides a toll-free number for more information. The service can save the life of a person with a major medical condition who may not be able to provide medical history. For information write: Medic Alert Foundation, P.O. Box 1009, Turlock, CA 95381, (800) 344-3226.

Medical History—Essential facts about past and present medical conditions. Knowing your medical history enables your doctor to plan the best possible health care. Carry a card stating essential health details in your purse or wallet, and consider joining the Medic-Alert program (see above).

Meibomian Glands—Small glands on the inner eyelid. They secrete a fluid that helps the eyelids move easily over the surface of the eye.

Membrane—Thin tissue lining a body cavity, covering an internal organ or dividing a space.

Meninges—Three-layered membrane covering the brain.

Mental System (Mind)—Functions of the brain that provide the abilities to perceive surroundings, to have emotions, imagination, memory, will, and to process information.

Metastases—Cancerous cells or infectious germs that spread from their original location to other parts of the body.

Metatarsal Bones—Bones in the middle of the foot.

Midwife—Nurse with special training and experience in childbirth.

Mole—Skin lesion, often dark-brown or black.

Monoamine Oxidase (MAO) Inhibitors—Medications used to treat some forms of depression.

Motor Nerve—Nerve that transmits the stimulus that causes muscles to contract.

MRI (Magnetic Resonance Imaging)—A method of studying the body's internal structures that employs a strong magnetic field (rather than x-rays) and a computer to produce detailed pictures.

Mucous Membrane—Thin tissue lining internal cavities (nose, mouth, vagina) and tubular systems (respiratory and gastrointestinal) that produce mucus.

Mucus—Slippery liquid produced by the lining of internal cavities and tubular systems to protect tissue.

Muscle—Tissue that contracts, often with considerable force, when stimulated by the motor-nerve impulses.

Muscle Relaxants—Medications that relieve muscle spasms. They also can have significant side effects.

Muscle Tumors—Benign or cancerous tumors arising from muscle tissue.

Musculoskeletal System—The system of bones, muscles, ligaments, and tendons that enable the body to move.

Myelogram, Myelography—Special x-ray of the spinal canal and spinal cord, requiring a spinal tap and injection of dye that is visible on x-ray film. Myelograms frequently are used to identify the location of ruptured discs.

Myoma—Tumor of the muscle.

Myopia—Disease of the eye in which close objects are clearly visible while distant objects are blurred. Also called nearsightedness.

Myringotomy—A surgical opening made through the eardrum to allow drainage of the middle ear cavity. It is usually performed on children.

N

Narcotics—Medications used to control severe pain. Narcotics should be used only when necessary because of their serious side effects: addiction; reduced breathing; nausea and vomiting; low blood pressure; reduced cough reflex; and constipation.

Nasogastric Tube—Slender tube passed through the nose into the stomach. It is used to drain away stomach secretions or to feed patients unable to eat normally.

Naturopathy—Health-care system relying on diet, sunshine, exercises, herbs and other nonmedicinal treatment.

Nausea—Unpleasant sensation of being about to vomit.

Nearsightedness—Same as *Myopia*.

Nebulizer—Device for administering medications used to treat asthma and similar conditions. It converts medication into a fine mist that is inhaled deeply into the lungs.

Necrosis—Death of living tissue.

Nerve-Block Local Anesthesia—See *Anesthesia, Nerve Block or Local*.

Nerve-Conduction Studies, Nerve Conduction Test—Diagnostic test that measures the rate at which an electrical impulse moves along a nerve. It is used to diagnose disorders of the peripheral nerves and muscle.

Nervous Breakdown—Nontechnical term for mental illness serious enough to interfere with daily activities.

Neuralgia—Severe, sharp pain along a nerve.

Neuritis—Inflammation of a nerve.

Neuromuscular System—Nerves and muscles acting together as a system to control body movements.

Neurological—Relating to the body's nervous system.

Neurologist—Doctor specially trained to diagnose and treat diseases of the nervous system.

Neuroma—Tumor arising from nerve tissue.

Neurosis—Mental illness in which anxiety is controlled by avoidance, blaming others, developing bodily complaints or other mechanisms.

Neurosurgeon—Doctor specially trained to diagnose and surgically treat diseases of the brain, spinal cord and nerves.

Nodes—See *Lymph Glands*.

Nodule—Small, rounded lump or firm swelling underneath the skin.

Nonsteroidal Anti-Inflammatory Drugs—Medications that control inflammation other than that caused by infection. Usually used to treat conditions of the joints and muscles and pain such as menstrual cramps or headache. "Non-steroidal" means they are not steroid hormones such as cortisone, prednisone, dexamethasone and others.

Norwalk Virus—A type of virus that commonly causes epidemics of acute gastroenteritis with diarrhea and vomiting that lasts from 24 to 48 hours.

Nuclear Imaging—See *Radionuclide Scans*.

Nurse Practitioner (NP)—Registered nurse with additional medical training who can diagnose and treat common illness. Nurse practitioners usually work closely with a doctor, although in some states the practitioner can prescribe medicine and work independently of a physician.

Nutrient—Food or material containing elements needed to promote growth and development or to support life.

O

Obsessions—Unpleasant, frightening, senseless thoughts that won't go away despite reasoning.

Obstetrician-Gynecologist—Doctor specially trained to treat diseases of the female reproductive system and provide health care for pregnant mothers.

Occlusion—Closing or obstruction. Usually used to describe blockage in blood vessels. In dentistry, it means the way the teeth come together when the mouth is closed.

Occupational Therapy—Treatment for people disabled by accident or illness to relearn muscular control and coordination to cope with daily living tasks (dressing, eating, bathing, etc.) and if possible, to resume some form of employment.

Omentum—A fold of peritoneum which supports or connects abdominal structures.

Oncologist—Doctor specially trained to diagnose and treat cancer.

Operative Death Rate—Percentage of patients who die as a result of a certain surgery. It provides general measure of the risk of a surgery.

Ophthalmologist—Doctor specially trained to diagnose and treat diseases of the eyes.

Optic Neuritis—Inflammation of the nerve that conducts vision impulses from the eye to the brain.

Oral—Relating to the mouth.

Oral-Fecal—See *Fecal-Oral*.

Organic—Conditions or diseases resulting from change in body organs that can be measured or seen. Organic diseases are distinct from functional diseases in which no change can be observed in an organ that is not functioning normally.

Organic Psychosis—Mental illness that results from disease in the brain.

Orthodontia—Straightening teeth by applying temporary braces.

Orthopedic Surgeon (Orthopedist)—Doctor specially trained to diagnose and treat diseases of the muscles, bones and joints using surgical or mechanical means. A rheumatologist is an internist who diagnoses and treats similar conditions primarily with medications and other nonsurgical means.

Osteogenesis Imperfecta—Inherited condition in which the bones are brittle and easily broken.

Otolaryngologist—See *Ear, Nose and Throat Specialist*.

Ovary—Female sexual gland where eggs mature and ripen for fertilization.

Ovulation—Monthly process in which an egg leaves the ovary for possible fertilization by a sperm cell.

Ovum—Egg produced by the ovary.

P

Pain—Unpleasant sensation arising from stimulation of sensory nerves located in almost every part of the body. Disease, injury and strenuous activity can all cause pain.

Palate—Roof of the mouth, consisting of a bony front portion (hard palate) and a soft back portion (soft palate).

Palpitations—Irregular rapid heartbeat, noticeable to the patient.

Pancreas—Organ located on the back abdominal wall that produces and secretes digestive juices into the small intestine. It also produces and secretes insulin into the bloodstream to regulate the level of sugar and other nutrients.

Pancreatitis—Inflammation of the pancreas.

Pap Smear, Papanicolaou Smear—Test routinely done to screen for cancer of the cervix and uterus in an early and treatable stage.

Papule—Small, raised skin lesion. Papules may be red, brown, yellow, white or skin-colored. They may be flat-topped, pointed or dome-shaped.

Paranoia—Mental illness in which a person believes that he or she is being talked about or plotted against.

Parasite—Organism that lives within, upon or at the expense of another living organism. Human parasites include disease-causing agents such as amoebas or worms that infect the digestive system, or fungi that live on the skin.

Parasympathetic Nervous System—System of nerves that controls digestion, heartbeat, and relaxation or contraction of small muscles.

Parathyroid Glands—Small glands that control calcium levels in the blood and bones. They are located within or next to the thyroid glands at the base of the neck.

Passive Exercises—Exercises in which a therapist moves the arms and legs of a patient while the patient relaxes. These exercises keep the joints limber until the patient is able to move without assistance.

Patency—Blood vessels or any hollow organs that clog or become blocked are said to lose their patency.

Pathogenic—Disease-producing.

Pathological—Relating to an abnormal condition.

Pathological Examination—Laboratory study of abnormal tissue to establish or confirm a diagnosis.

Pediatrician—Doctor specially trained to care for children and adolescents, especially to foster normal growth and development.

Pediculicide—Medication that cures body lice (pediculosis). Usually applied to the skin.

Pelvic Examination—Examination of a woman's reproductive organs to diagnose pregnancy or detect diseases.

Pelvic Ultrasonography—Examination of a woman's reproductive organs that uses high-frequency sound waves to create an image. It is used to determine the age, size and position of a fetus in the uterus or to diagnose disease of the pelvic organs.

Pelvis—Lower part of the trunk of the body.

Penis—Male organ used for urination and sexual intercourse.

Perforation—Abnormal hole or opening.

Perforation, Intestinal—Complication of conditions such as ulcers, cancers, or injury to the digestive system. When this occurs, intestinal contents enter the abdominal cavity, causing severe inflammation.

Perfusionist—Medical professional who controls the heart-lung machine to sustain a patient's life during open-heart and lung-transplant surgery.

Perineum—Area between the vulva and anus in females and between the scrotum and anus in males.

Peripheral Nervous System—Nerves that connect to all parts of the body and carry information via electrical impulses to and from the brain and spinal cord.

Peripheral Vascular System—Network of arteries, veins and lymphatic channels supplying the head, arms and legs.

Perirectal—Skin and underlying tissue around the rectum.

Peristalsis—Rhythmic movements of hollow muscular organs (such as the intestines) that move contents (such as digestive material) in one direction.

Peritoneal Cavity—Space enclosed by the peritoneum.

Peritoneum—Very thin, two-layered tissue. One layer lines the outer surface of all the abdominal organs. The other layer lines the abdominal wall.

Peritonitis—Inflammation of the peritoneum.

Peritonsillar Abscess—Abscess forming in the back of the throat near the tonsils.

Pessary—Small ring-shaped device that is inserted into the vagina to help maintain the uterus in a normal position.

PET Scan—A sectional view of the body constructed by positron-emission tomography, which uses integrated x-ray and computing equipment.

pH Balance—Measure of blood's acidity or alkalinity. The pH is controlled by body fluids and electrolytes. Body tissues cannot function normally if the pH varies from a limited range.

Phallus—Penis.

Phenothiazine Drugs—Medications used to slow and regulate mental-system activity. Usually used to treat anxiety and other mental conditions; also useful in producing sleep.

Phlebitis—Inflammation of a vein.

Phlebotomy—Removing blood from the blood vessels. This was once believed to cure many diseases; today, it is done to remove blood for diagnostic testing.

Phobia—Fear that cannot be overcome by reason.

Photochemotherapy—A treatment for some skin disorders that combines oral medication with exposure to ultraviolet light rays for set periods of time.

Physical Therapy—Treatment of diseases of the bone, muscular and nervous systems to help restore normal function after disease or injury.

Physician's Assistant (PA)—Someone trained to do some of the simpler tasks ordinarily performed by a doctor. The PA works under the direction of the doctor.

Pilocarpine—Medication used principally in eye drops to treat glaucoma.

Pituitary Gland—Small endocrine gland at the base of the brain that controls growth and regulates other endocrine glands.

Placenta—Disk-shaped organ that attaches and grows inside the uterus during pregnancy. It enables the fetus to receive nutrients from and

transfer natural wastes to the mother's bloodstream. The umbilical cord connects the placenta to the fetus.

Placenta previa—An abnormal placement of the placenta in the lower uterine segment, so that it covers or adjoins the internal opening of the uterine cervix.

Plaque—1) Small raised area of abnormal material on a surface such as the skin or lining of a blood vessel. 2) Mixture of bacteria and calcium deposited on the teeth that can cause cavities and gum diseases.

Plasma—Liquid part of blood that remains when blood cells are removed.

Plastic and Reconstructive Surgeon (Plastic Surgeon)—Doctor specially trained to perform plastic and reconstructive surgery.

Plastic and Reconstructive Surgery—Special surgery to repair and change body parts to improve function or appearance. The face, hands, breasts and skin are areas most frequently treated.

Platelet Count—Platelets are blood cells (much smaller than red or white blood cells) that assist in the blood-clotting process. A drop of blood contains about 12.5 million platelets. A platelet count determines if the number of platelets is normal.

Plethysmography—A study that estimates the amount of blood flowing in vessels by measuring changes in the size of a body part.

Pleura—Thin tissue lining the lungs and chest cavity. Inflammation of the pleura (pleurisy) is a painful condition caused by lung diseases.

Pleural Effusion (Pleural Fluid Effusion)—Fluid that collects around the lungs, usually caused by inflammation of the lungs and pleura or congestive-heart failure.

Pneumonia—Infection and inflammation of the lungs.

Pneumothorax—A collection of air or gas in the lung which causes collapse of all or part of a lung.

Podiatrist—Health-care professional trained in the medical and surgical treatment of foot diseases.

Polyp—A growth, often on a stalk arising from dry mucous membranes, such as in the nose, cervix or colon.

Portal-Vein System—Veins that drain blood from the gastrointestinal system. The smaller veins empty into the portal vein, which transports blood into the liver.

Postmature Infant—Infant that spends 3 weeks or more beyond the normal 39 weeks of pregnancy in the womb.

Postoperative—Period of recuperation and return to normal health after surgery.

Postural Drainage—Exercises and body positions that promote drainage of fluid and secretions that collect in the lungs and airways.

Potassium—Electrolyte present in all body cells, blood and body fluids. Potassium is important in maintaining normal heart contractions and the strength and contractions of all muscles. Foods high in potassium include: dried apricots and peaches; whole-grain cereals; plain cocoa, dried lentils and peas; bananas; and molasses.

Precancerous—Characteristic of a growth that has the potential to become cancerous.

Predisposition—Tendency. For example, a person who gets many infections has a predisposition to infection.

Preeclampsia—A toxic condition of late pregnancy characterized by a sudden rise in blood pressure, excessive weight gain, generalized edema, protein in the urine, severe headache and visual disturbances.

Premature Labor—Labor beginning before the usual 39 weeks of pregnancy.

Presbyopia—Form of nearsightedness that normally accompanies aging.

Primary Disorder—Basic disease that may result in complications. Diabetes mellitus, for example, is a primary disorder that often causes secondary complications involving the kidneys, blood vessels and eyes.

Proctoscope, Proctoscopy—Method of examining the rectum and lower part of the colon with a proctoscope, an optical instrument with a lighted tip.

Prolapse—Pushing or falling out of a part or an organ from its normal position.

Prolapsed (Dropped) Uterus—Uterus that has moved from its normal position because of loose pelvic muscles and ligaments. In severe cases, it can protrude completely outside the vagina.

Prophylaxis—Measures taken to prevent an illness.

Prophylaxis, Dental—Regular care (including cleaning) of the teeth and gums that helps prevent tooth decay and gum inflammation.

Prostaglandins—Natural substances found in semen, menstrual fluid and many body tissues. They are involved in basic body functions such as inflammation, immune response and activities of the lungs, heart, kidneys, uterus and digestive system.

Prostate (Prostate Gland)—Male sex gland located at the base of the urinary bladder. It produces a fluid that is added to sperm to produce semen.

Prosthesis—Artificial device used as a substitute for a missing or badly functioning part of the body.

Prothrombin Time—Test to measure one of the components of the body's blood-clotting mechanism. It is used to diagnose clotting diseases and to control blood-thinning (anticoagulation) in treatment of some diseases of the heart and blood vessels.

Protozoa—One-celled organisms, the smallest type of animal life. Amoeba are protozoa. Some protozoa can cause disease.

Psychiatrist—Doctor specially trained to diagnose and treat mental illnesses.

Psychoanalysis—Treatment of some mental illness that involves a detailed understanding of how past events in a person's life may have resulted in mental disturbances.

Psychogenic—A symptom with an emotional origin instead of an organic one.

Psychologist—Health-care professional specially trained to diagnose and treat some kinds of mental illness.

Psychopathy—Psychological or mental illness.

Psychosis—Mental illness characterized by deranged personality, loss of contact with reality, and possible delusions, hallucinations or illusions.

Psychosocial—Influences of society on growth and development.

Psychosomatic Illness—Illness in which thoughts and emotions play an important role.

Psychotherapist—Professional specially trained to diagnose and treat some mental illnesses.

Puberty—Period in early adolescence when hormonal changes bring about full sexual maturity and capacity to reproduce.

Pubic Bone—One of the bones of the pelvis located above the genitals in both sexes.

Pulmonary—Relating to the lungs and breathing.

Pulmonary Angiography—Studies of the arteries and veins in the lungs.

Pulmonary Hypertension—Increased pressure in the blood vessels of the lungs.

Pulse—Heartbeat (contraction of the heart) as felt in an artery. Heart rate is often measured by counting the pulse felt in the artery in the wrist.

Pus—Thick fluid, usually green or yellow, that forms to fight local infection. Pus often collects in an enclosed sac, an abscess, at the site of an infection.

PUVA—A type of phototherapy used to treat some skin conditions. It combines the use of a psoralen drug that sensitizes the skin to sunlight with a controlled dose of ultraviolet light.

Pyelogram, Intravenous—Method of studying the kidneys and urinary tract by injecting into the bloodstream a medication that x-rays can detect.

Pyelogram, Retrograde—Method of studying the kidneys, similar to an intravenous pyelogram, but in which the medication detected by x-rays is placed in the urinary system by a catheter inserted through the bladder into the ureters.

R

Radiation Therapy or Treatment—Use of high-energy waves (generated by special x-ray machines, cobalt machines and other devices) to treat some forms of cancer. Radiation destroys cancerous tissue but does little harm to healthy tissue.

Radioactive Chromium Studies—Diagnostic method used to measure total blood in the body.

Radioactive Iodine Uptake and Scan—Same as *Thyroid Scan*.

Radioactive Studies—Same as *Radioisotope Studies*.

Radioactive Technetium 99 Scan—Radioisotope scan method used to diagnose some disorders of the heart, liver, spleen and other organs.

Radioisotope—Radioactive form of chemicals normally present in the body.

Radioisotope Scan—Scan of radioisotopes given orally or intravenously to a patient that become

concentrated in organs such as the heart, lungs or brain. Instruments measure the radiation given off by the radioisotopes and create a photographic image of the organ being studied.

Radioisotope Studies—Radioisotopes are chemical elements that give off radiation. A radioisotope of a chemical element normally present in the body (such as carbon), if injected into the body, will mix with the non-isotopes. The body doesn't know the difference, but radiation from the isotopes can be detected with special instruments. Determining where radioisotopes go in the body allows diagnosis of diseases that cannot be detected otherwise.

Radioisotope Therapy—Treatment of some cancers with radioisotopes.

Radiologist—Doctor specially trained to use x-rays and other kinds of radiation in diagnosis and treatment.

Radionuclide Scan—Method of studying various body functions by means of photographs or videotape taken by special camera or a scanner after intravenous injection of radioactive chemical.

Rebound Phenomenon—A reversed response to the withdrawal of a stimulus. A common rebound phenomenon occurs when nose drops, which decrease congestion, wear off. The nasal congestion that develops on the rebound is greater than that which existed before the drops were administered.

Recovery Room—Specially equipped and staffed area of a hospital for observing and caring for a patient who has just undergone surgery. Postoperative patients usually remain in the recovery room until they are awake and their vital signs (blood pressure, pulse and respiration) are satisfactory.

Rectum—End of the large intestine, located in the pelvis below the sigmoid colon and above the anus.

Regenerate—Ability of some parts of the body to grow back to normal after being damaged.

Regurgitate—To vomit.

Relapse—Stage of illness in which the patient gets worse after having improved.

Remission—Stage of a chronic illness when the patient's condition improves.

Renal—Having to do with the kidneys.

Renal Dialysis—Mechanical and chemical method of removing normal wastes from the body of a patient whose kidneys cannot function adequately. It is also used to remove harmful poison or a drug overdose from the bloodstream.

Reproductive Organs, Female—Organs of a woman's body that enable her to become pregnant and deliver a baby. The major organs are the vagina, uterus, Fallopian tubes and ovaries.

Reproductive Organs, Male—Organs of a man's body that enable him to produce sperm and impregnate the woman. The major organs are the penis, testicles, seminal vesicles and prostate gland.

Reproductive System—Body system enabling impregnation and delivery of a baby. It also provides characteristic male or female appearance.

Resect—Surgical removal of a part of the body.

Respiratory-Distress Syndrome—A condition of newborn infants (often born prematurely) in which the lungs cannot supply adequate oxygen to the body.

Retained Placenta—Condition occurring immediately after childbirth in which part of the placenta remains attached to the uterus, creating a risk of serious bleeding or infection.

Retina—Light-sensitive part of the eye at the back of the eyeball on which the lens focuses images. The retina converts the image to impulses that go to the brain.

Retinal-Vein Occlusion—Condition in which a clot forms in the vein supplying the retina with blood.

Retinoblastoma—Cancerous tumor that forms in the eye of an infant.

Retrograde Pyelography—See *Pyelogram, Retrograde.*

Retrovirus—Group of viruses that cause HIV (human immunodeficiency virus) and some types of lymphoma and leukemia.

Rh Negative Blood—A subtype of red blood cells. Blood subtypes are inherited. The major subtypes are types A, B, O and Rh negative.

Rheumatologist—A specialist in internal medicine who subspecializes in medical diagnosis and treatment of rheumatic and arthritic disorders.

Rhinitis—Swelling of the nasal passages.

Rinne Test—Test using a tuning fork to diagnose hearing disorders.

Rotavirus—A type of virus that is often responsible for acute gastroenteritis in infants and for diarrhea in young children.

Rubin's Insufflation Test—Test used in diagnosing fertility problems in women. A harmless gas is introduced into the uterus to determine if there is a blockage in the Fallopian tubes.

S

Sacroiliac Region—Area of the lower back where the spine meets the pelvic bone.

Saline—Salt-containing solution similar to normal body fluid that is given intravenously to help correct fluid and electrolyte imbalances.

Salivary Glands—Glands located inside the mouth around the jaw that secrete saliva into the mouth.

Saphenous-Femoral Vein System—Network of large veins in the legs that helps return blood from the leg to the inferior vena cava, then to the heart.

Scale, Scaling—Flakes of dried skin that form as whitish skin lesions.

Schizophrenia—Mental illness characterized by a distorted sense of reality, bizarre behavior and fragmentation of the personality.

Sciatic Nerve—Large nerve that begins at the base of the spine and passes through the buttocks down the back side of the thigh and down the leg.

Sciatica—Painful condition resulting from irritation of the sciatic nerve.

Scleritis—Inflammation of the sclera (the white of the eye).

Scopolamine—Medication used to treat hyperactive or spastic conditions of the digestive system and to prevent motion sickness.

Scrotum—Organ of the male reproductive system that contains the testicles, blood vessels and the vas deferens.

Scurvy—Disease of bones, gums and blood vessels that is caused by a deficiency of vitamin C.

Second Molars—Permanent grinding teeth that appear at about age 11 to 13.

Secondary Infection—Infection that results from some other problem. It may occur after surgery or develop during antibiotic treatment of another infection.

Sedative—Medication used to produce relaxation or sleep.

Sedative-Hypnotics—Class of medications that help relieve anxiety and promote sleep.

Sedimentation Rate—Blood test measuring the rate that blood settles in a test tube. It identifies infection, inflammation or tissue damage.

Self-Care—Treatment that patients can administer for themselves.

Seminal Vesicles—Small sacs next to the prostate that help make and store seminal fluid and contract to eject semen.

Senile Dementia—Permanent loss of mental functions of older persons, resulting from conditions such as Alzheimer's disease and atherosclerosis (hardening of the arteries).

Senile Keratosis—Same as *Seborrheic Keratoses*. (See *Illness section*.)

Sensitivity Studies (Antibiotics)—Laboratory method of determining which antibiotic will most likely be successful in treating infections caused by bacteria.

Sensory—Ability to feel or experience sensations such as sound, light or pain.

Septic—Infected.

Serological Tests—Tests of serum (blood without cells) used to diagnose a variety of diseases, especially infections and autoimmune conditions.

Serum—Liquid portion of blood that remains after blood cells and blood clots have been removed.

Serum Alkaline Phosphatase—Material present in excessive amounts in the blood of patients with some bone and liver diseases.

Serum Electrolytes—Same as *Electrolytes*.

Sesamoid Bones—Small oval-shaped bones in the tendons of the hands and feet.

Sever's Disease—Painful condition of the heel bone of growing children.

Sexual Dysfunction—Inability to participate in sexual relations that are satisfactory for both partners.

Shave Biopsy—Procedure to diagnose skin disorders in which a thin layer of tissue from under a skin lesion is shaved away for laboratory examination.

Shock—Condition in which the blood pressure falls below the level needed to supply blood to the body. Signs and symptoms include weakness, paleness, rapid heartbeat, dry mouth, cold sweat and feelings of doom.

Sick-Sinus Syndrome—Form of heart-rhythm disorder (arrhythmia).

Sigmoid Colon—Lower part of the large colon (intestine) located in the pelvis just above the rectum.

Sigmoidoscope, Sigmoidoscopy—Same as P*roctoscope, Proctoscopy*.

Signs—Evidence of disease that can be observed and measured, in contrast to symptoms, which only patients can experience. For example, blood-pressure measurement or red tonsils are signs; headache or nausea are symptoms.

Silicone—Artificial compound used by plastic and reconstructive surgeons to reshape parts of the body, such as the breast.

Silver Nitrate—Chemical used for cautery.

Sims-Huhner Test—Test used in diagnosis of reasons for infertility in women in which the mucus from the cervix is examined, especially for presence of sperm after sexual intercourse.

Sitz bath—Sitting for a period of time in a bathtub that is filled with several inches of warm water. It provides temporary relief to certain types of infections, pain or swelling in the pelvic or buttocks area.

Skin Clips—Small U-shaped metal strips used instead of stitches to close skin that has been incised during surgery.

Skin Tests for Allergy—Diagnostic method used to determine whether a particular substance is causing allergic reactions. The test is carried out by introducing a small amount of the suspected material, such as pollen or dust, under the skin or on the skin. If inflammation results, the patient is allergic to the material.

Sleep Inducers—Medications used to produce sleep.

Sleep-Study Laboratory—Laboratory where persons are studied with sensitive instruments while asleep. Information from sleep study aids in diagnosis of sleep disorders.

Slow Viruses—Group of viruses that infect the brain but do not cause disease until many years afterward.

Small-Bowel Series—A test used to look for blockage in the small bowel, in which the patient swallows a radiopaque fluid (barium), which allows intermittent x-rays to be taken to follow the flow of the fluid through the esophagus, stomach, duodenum and then through the entire small intestine to the colon.

Soaks—Applying moisture—either plain water or water with dissolved medicines—to an inflamed area of the skin.

Soft Palate—Fleshy part of the roof of the mouth close to the throat.

Sonogram, Sonography—See *Ultrasound.*

Spasmodic—Sudden intermittent symptom, or intermittent muscle spasm.

Spastic, Spasticity—A description of muscles that are continuously contracting and in a state of excessive tension.

Speculum—Instrument used to examine the interior of openings such as the vagina, nose, ear or rectum.

Sperm—Male reproductive cells manufactured in testicles and ejaculated in semen.

Spherocytosis—Abnormally shaped red blood cells caused by some anemias. These cells are sphere-shaped, in contrast to the doughnut shape of normal red blood cells.

Spikes, Temperature—High but brief episodes of fever.

Spina Bifida—Congenital (inherited) disorder in which the base of the spine remains open, sometimes exposing the spinal cord and nerves.

Spinal Anesthesia—Method to provide anesthesia to the lower body by injecting an anesthetic into the fluid in the space that surrounds the lower spinal cord.

Spirometry—Test of lung (pulmonary) function.

Spleen—A large organ in the upper abdomen on the left side, located close to the left side of the stomach. It is the largest structure of the lymph system. The spleen causes disintegration of old red blood cells in adults, manufactures red blood cells in the fetus and newborn, and serves as an important reservoir of blood.

Splenic-Vein Thrombosis—Clot in the major vein that carries blood away from the spleen.

Splints—Rigid supports, made of metal, plastic or plaster, used to immobilize an injured or inflamed part of the body. Splints are used temporarily in the case of injury, following some surgical procedures on joints or ligaments, or occasionally in the case of arthritis.

Spore—Microscopic seed form of fungi. Spores are extremely hardy and survive extremes of temperature. If they enter the body of a susceptible person, they can cause fungal disease.

Sputum—Secretion of the lungs, coughed up in large amounts in some lung diseases.

Staphylococcus—Bacteria which frequently cause boils, abscesses, pneumonias, bone infections and infections in other tissues or organs.

Staples—Small U-shaped metal wires used in place of stitches to close incised skin after some surgeries, especially in the digestive system. Also used to close off some portions of the stomach during operations for extreme obesity.

Stenosis—Constriction or narrowing of a passage or opening.

Sterilized—1) Made completely free of all germs, usually by steam heat, toxic gas or chemicals. All instruments used in surgeries are sterilized, as is most other medical equipment. 2) Made unable to conceive children.

Steroids—Medications that resemble hormones produced by the cortex of the adrenal glands, ovaries and testicles.

Stethoscope—Instrument used to listen to the sounds produced by the heart, lungs, blood vessels and pregnant uterus.

Still's Disease—Form of arthritis in children similar to rheumatoid arthritis in adults.

Stimulant Drugs—Medications that increase the activity of the brain and nervous system.

Stomatitis—Inflammation of the mouth.

Stool—Feces.

Streptococcus—Bacteria that cause illnesses such as laryngitis, cellulitis of the skin, pneumonia, meningitis and others. If not treated, streptococcal infections may also cause serious heart and kidney diseases as complications that appear after the original infection has cleared.

Stricture—An abnormal narrowing of a bodily passage.

Subcutaneous—Under the skin.

Sublingual Salivary Glands—Small glands near the base of the tongue that secrete saliva into the mouth.

Submaxillary Salivary Glands—Small glands near the jaw that secrete saliva into the mouth.

Sulfonamides (Sulfa Drugs)—Class of drugs used to fight infections.

Sulfonylurea Drugs—Medications taken orally to treat some forms of diabetes mellitus.

Surgery—Treatment in which the body is restored to a healthy condition by physical methods (or operations) such as cutting, removing, replacing, straightening, repairing or joining.

Surgical Suite—Group of rooms used to perform surgery. In addition to operating rooms, where surgery takes place, there are supply areas, a recovery room, administrative rooms and a lounge for the staff to rest between surgeries.

Suture—Thread-like material used to hold tissues or skin edges together.

Symmetry, Symmetrical—Refers to the arrangement of the body in pairs, such as two arms, legs, kidneys, lungs, etc.

Sympathomimetics—Medications similar to adrenalin in their actions.

Symptoms—Effects of disease that only the patient can experience, such as pain, nausea, dizziness, anxiety, depression and others.

Synovial Membranes—Delicate tissue that lines the inside of joints.

Systemic—Conditions that affect most or all of the body, in contrast to conditions that affect only a limited area. For example, diabetes mellitus is a systemic condition; an abscess is a local condition.

T

Tartar—Hard deposit that forms on the teeth and causes inflammation of the gums.

Temperature Spike—See *Spikes, Temperature*.

Temporomandibular Joint—Joint that joins the jaw to the other head bones.

Tenderness—Condition that causes pain when pressure is applied.

Tendon—Tough cord of tissue at the end of muscles that attach to bone. Tendons transmit the force of muscle contraction to cause movement.

Testes or Testicles—Male sex glands that produce sex hormones and sperm.

Therapeutic Trial—Form of diagnosis and treatment where medication is used even though the diagnosis is not firmly established. If the patient improves after treatment with a medication known to be useful in treating a specific condition, the improvement suggests that the specific disease was present. Therapeutic trials are somewhat risky and are used only when other forms of diagnosis and treatment have failed.

Therapist—Health-care professional specially trained to provide therapy.

Thermogram, Thermography—Method of diagnosis that measures body heat. The area being studied is scanned by a heat-sensitive instrument capable of producing an image (thermogram) of areas of increased heat. They are useful in studying female breast tumors and some blood-vessel conditions.

Thiazide Diuretics—Class of medications that promote excretion of excess fluids by the kidneys.

Third Molars—Permanent grinding teeth that appear at about age 17 to 25.

Thoracic Duct—The largest channel of the lymphatic system, through which lymph fluid enters the vena cava.

Thoracic Spine—That part of the spinal column below the neck and above the back. Ribs attach to the thoracic spine.

Thoracic Surgeon—A surgeon who specializes in surgical treatment of disorders of the organs in the thorax (chest), including lungs, pericardium, heart, pleura (covering of lungs), bronchial tubes and large blood vessels.

Thyroglossal Duct—Small passageway, normally closed, located in the upper neck. It extends from the back of the tongue to just above the larynx. If an abnormally open duct becomes filled with fluid, a thyroglossal cyst results.

Thyroid Cartilage—Larynx (also called the voice box, or Adam's apple), made of semi-hard cartilage.

Thyroid Gland—Endocrine gland located in the lower neck next to the trachea that produces hormones that regulate the rate at which all body cells function. Thyroid hormones are also essential for normal growth and development.

Thyroid Scan—Method of examination of the thyroid gland in which a small amount of radioactive iodine introduced into the body collects in the thyroid gland. An instrument passed over the thyroid produces an image of the gland based on the concentration of the radioactive iodine.

Thrombocytopenia—A persistent decrease in the number of blood platelets, often associated with hemorrhaging.

TIA—See *Transient Ischemic Attack*.

Ticks—Small biting insects that may cause inflammation of the skin or serious infections such as Rocky Mountain spotted fever.

Tics—Brief, uncontrollable muscle spasms. Tics usually involve the face and the shoulders.

Tissue—Building blocks of body organs; living cells all of one type.

Tonsils—Lymphatic tissues that help fight infection located at the entrance of the throat. They frequently become infected, especially in children.

Topical—Medications applied to the skin, conjunctiva, or mucous membrane of the mouth, nose, vagina or rectum.

Tourette's Syndrome—A rare disorder of movement. It involves repetitive grimaces and tics, usually of the head and neck, sometimes arms, legs and trunk. Involuntary noises and foul language may occur.

Tourniquet—Cord or band wrapped around an arm or leg tightly enough to stop blood circulation temporarily.

Toxic, Toxicity—Harmful; capable of causing body damage.

Toxin—Poison. Usually refers to the chemicals produced by some living organisms that harm the human body.

Tracheostomy Tube—A tube which is connected to an artificial opening into the trachea through the neck, and through which breathing is performed.

Traction—Method of treating some conditions of bones, muscles and ligaments by exerting a steady pull on the affected parts. Some bone fractures and back pain due to a ruptured disc are treated this way.

Tranquilizer—Medication used to help diminish anxiety and to produce calmness.

Tranquilizers, Benzodiazepine—Class of tranquilizers commonly used to treat anxiety, nervousness or tension.

Transfuse—To give a patient blood, necessary in treatment of some conditions.

Transfusion—Process of introducing blood through a needle placed in the patient's vein.

Transfusion Reaction—Undesirable symptom or condition resulting from a blood transfusion.

Transient Ischemic Attack, TIA—A temporary decrease in the blood supply to part of the brain which temporarily interferes with normal brain function.

Transmission, Transmit—Passing a disease to another person.

Transplant, Transplantation—Living organ (such as kidney, cornea, heart, bone marrow or skin), removed from one person (donor), and placed in the body of another (recipient).

Transverse Colon—Middle part of the colon (intestine), lying horizontally in the middle or upper abdomen.

Trauma—Force that injures or damages any part of the body.

Tricyclic Antidepressant Drugs (Tricyclics)—Class of medications used to treat depression.

Trophoblastic Tumors—See *Hydatidiform Mole*.

Tube Feeding—Providing nutrients through a small tube placed in the stomach of patients who are unable to eat. The tube may pass through the nose to the stomach or be inserted through an incision in the stomach.

Tuberous Sclerosis—Rare inherited condition of the skin, nervous system and other organs of the body.

Tumor—Literally, a swelling; usually used to refer to a benign or cancerous growth.

Tympanogram—A test which measures the function of the tympanic membrane in the middle ear.

U

Ulceration—Wearing away of the surface or lining of an organ, exposing underlying tissue. Ulceration of the lining of the stomach exposes blood vessels, which may bleed. Ulceration may erode through the wall of an organ (perforation). Ulceration frequently affects the skin, if rubbed excessively or if diseased.

Ultrasonography, Ultrasound—Diagnostic method in which high-frequency (ultrasound) sound waves are transmitted into the body. Their reflections create images of body organs.

Ultrasound Treatment—Method of treatment in which high-energy sound waves are focused on the affected area, producing mild heat that helps relieve inflammation. It is especially useful in treatment of muscular symptoms.

Underlying—Beneath, below or more basic. Thus, losing weight may result from an underlying condition such as diabetes mellitus or cancer.

Upper Gastrointestinal Series—X-ray examination of the esophagus, stomach and duodenum accomplished by having the patient swallow barium solution that x-rays can detect.

Upper Respiratory System—Upper part of the breathing system, consisting of the nose, throat, larynx, trachea and bronchial tubes.

Uremia—A serious condition associated with kidney failure in which body wastes build up in the blood and body tissues.

Ureters—Slender muscular tubes that carry urine from the kidneys to the urinary bladder, where it is stored until eliminated from the body.

Urethra—Tubular passageway extending from the urinary bladder to the outside of the body.

Uric Acid—Chemical normally produced in the body from metabolism or breakdown of protein and eliminated in the urine. If the level of uric acid rises in the body as a result of disease, gout or kidney stones may result.

Urinalysis—Laboratory test performed on a urine sample that helps diagnose diseases of the kidney and other parts of the body.

Urinary Bladder—Muscular sac in the lower abdomen that stores urine brought to it from the kidneys by the ureters. The bladder stores urine until it can be eliminated through the urethra by contractions of the bladder muscles.

Urinary Studies—Laboratory or x-ray tests of the urinary tract.

Urinary Tract—Organs that produce, store and eliminate urine. The organs are the kidneys, ureters, urinary bladder and urethra.

Urography—See *Intravenous Urography*.

Uterus—Organ of the female reproductive system on the wall of which the fertilized egg (ovum) attaches and develops to form a fetus.

Uveitis—Inflammation of the parts of the eyes that make up the iris (the colored tissue encircling the clear center, the pupil).

Uvula—Soft tissue hanging down from the soft palate at the back of the throat.

V

Vaccination—Method of providing protection against disease (immunity) by giving a patient a small amount of the disease-causing germ that is weakened, killed or otherwise modified so that it cannot itself cause disease. Same as *Immunization*.

Vaccine—Medication used to provide immunity by vaccination. Vaccines are given mostly by injection or by mouth.

Vagus Nerve—Long cranial nerve, arising in the base of the brain and passing to the chest and abdomen. It helps regulate heart rate, breathing, swallowing, digestion and many other body functions.

Varicose—Swollen and twisting; usually used to describe varicose veins.

Vas Deferens—Tube that carries sperm manufactured by the testicles toward the prostate gland and seminal vesicles.

Vasculitis—Inflammation of blood vessels, the basis of many illnesses.

Vasoconstrictor Drugs—Medications that cause blood vessels to contract, tighten or become smaller.

Vasodilator Drugs—Medications that cause small arteries to widen, providing more blood to an area of the body where the blood vessels are constricted by spasm, narrowed or obstructed.

Vector—1) An imaginary line that represents both direction and quantity used to study electrocardiograms (ECG's). 2) An agent that transmits infectious germs from one organism to another.

Veins—Blood vessels that return blood from body organs to the heart and lungs. Veins are much thinner than arteries. Veins carry blood at a much lower pressure than do arteries.

Vena Cava—Largest vein in the body. It collects blood from the venous system and carries it to the heart.

Vena Cavography—Method of studying the vena cava by injecting into the bloodstream a medication that x-rays can detect.

Venereal—Related to sexual intercourse or sexual contact. Venereal diseases such as genital herpes, gonorrhea or syphilis are now usually referred to as sexually transmitted diseases (STDs).

Venography—Method of studying the veins by injecting into the bloodstream a medication that x-rays can detect.

Venous Stasis Ulcer—An open sore on the skin of the lower extremities, caused when normal outflow of blood in the legs is obstructed (as in deep venous thrombosis). The resulting pressure from the back-up of blood causes leaking and weeping of fluid into the surrounding tissues (edema), which then stretches the arteries and deprives the skin of oxygen. The skin then breaks down into open sores which leak serum and are prone to infection.

Venous System—Network of veins that extend from all body organs and transport blood back to the heart.

Ventricles—Chambers containing fluid. The ventricles of the heart pump blood; ventricles of the brain contain cerebrospinal fluid.

Ventricular Aneurysm—Ballooning of the wall of the heart resulting from a weakening of the heart muscle, a complication of scarring from a previous heart attack.

Vertebrae—Bones of the spine that form the vertebral column (backbone).

Vertebral Column—The spine; the bones of the back.

Virulent—Extremely dangerous or harmful. Virulent bacteria are ones capable of causing diseases.

Viruses—Small germs responsible for a variety of infectious illnesses. Viruses are not alive until they enter cells of the body, where they grow and reproduce, causing viral illnesses.

Visual Acuity—Clarity with which objects are seen.

Vitamins—Chemical substances found in food that are necessary for healthy body growth, function and tissue repair.

Vitreous—Clear fluid that fills much of the eye.

Vocal Cords—Two narrow bands of fibrous and muscular tissue in the larynx that vibrate to create the sounds of the voice.

Volvulus—Twisting of loops of intestines, which become closed off (obstructed) and may lose their blood supply.

Vulva—The external genitalia of the female including the clitoris and vaginal lips.

W

Warts—Small, often hard and rough skin growths caused by viruses that infect the skin.

Wasting of Body or Muscles—Severe loss of body tissues (other than surplus fat), especially muscles and vital organs, resulting in weakness, susceptibility to infection, bone fractures and sometimes death.

Weber Test—Hearing test performed with a tuning fork.

Wheezes—High-pitched sounds and whistles produced in the lungs where secretions have partially blocked air passages.

Wheal—A temporary skin elevation usually a result of an allergic reaction.

Whirlpool Treatment—Method of treating minor blood-vessel and musculoskeletal diseases by immersion in a pool where jets of warm water enter and swirl under high pressure.

Wisdom Teeth—Same as *Third Molars*.

X

X-Rays—High energy, invisible waves capable of penetrating the body and creating shadows on photographic film. The shadows provide images of the body tissues through which the x-rays pass.

Xeroradiogram—Method of x-ray diagnosis, usually of the female breast, which uses a process similar to that used to produce photocopies.

Xerosis—Abnormal dryness.

Y

Yellow Fever—An acute disease caused by a virus spread by insect bites. Usually seen in Africa and South America.

Yersinia Infection—A type of foodborne bacteria that can cause gastroenteritis and diarrhea.

Z

Zoster—"Girdle," used to describe a form of virus infection (herpes zoster, shingles) that often produces bands of inflammation across the chest or abdomen.

Zygote—The fertilized egg before division.

EMERGENCY FIRST AID

This section lists basic steps in recognizing and treating immediate effects of emergencies.

If possible, take a course in first aid and learn technique, called cardiopulmonary resuscitation (CPR). This is a lifesaving procedure that is performed when someone's breathing or heartbeat has stopped.

ANAPHYLAXIS (Severe allergic reaction)

Symptoms

Itching, rash, hives, runny nose, wheezing, paleness, cold sweats, dizziness, low blood pressure, coma, cardiac arrest. Symptoms usually occur within 30 minutes after an insect sting or ingestion of certain foods or drugs.

Treatment

If Victim is Unconscious, Not Breathing

1. Yell for help. Don't leave victim.

2. Call or have someone call 911 (emergency) for an ambulance or medical help. The emergency operator may give you first-aid instructions to perform before emergency help arrives.

3. Check to see if the person is carrying special medication to inject to counter the effects of the allergic attack. If so, use it if you know how.

4. Place the heel of your hand in the middle of person's chest. Put your other hand on top of the first with your fingers interlaced. Compress the chest at least 2 inches (4-5 cm). Allow the chest to completely recoil before the next compression. Compress the chest at a rate of at least 100 pushes per minute until emergency help arrives.
(If trained and rescuer is able to perform rescue breaths, compressions and breaths should be provided in a ratio of 30 compressions to 2 breaths.)

5. Don't try to make victim vomit. If vomiting does occur, save vomit to take to emergency room for analysis.

If Victim is Unconscious and Breathing

1. Call or have someone call 911 (emergency) for an ambulance or medical help.

2. Check to see if the person is carrying special medication to inhale, swallow or inject to counter the effects of the allergic attack. If so, use them if you know how.

3. If you can't get help immediately, take patient to nearest emergency room or other facility with adequate equipment and personnel to care for medical emergencies.

BLEEDING (continued on next page)

Symptoms

Bleeding caused by any serious injury should be treated in an emergency facility. There is usually a lot of bright-red blood pumping from an injured artery, or darker blood if a large vein has been injured.

BLEEDING (continued from previous page)

Treatment

1. Call or have someone call 911 (emergency) for an ambulance or medical help. Do not leave the victim. The emergency operator may give you first-aid instructions to perform before emergency help arrives.

2. Lay the person down. If possible, the head should be lower than the trunk of the body or the legs should be elevated. This helps increase blood flow to the brain. If possible, raise a bleeding arm or leg (if not broken) above the level of the victim's heart.

3. Use rubber gloves or plastic bags over your hands or other protection to avoid contact with victim's blood. Apply steady, firm pressure to the wound using a sterile bandage, clean cloth or your hand. Maintain pressure until the bleeding stops (or medical help arrives). Then wrap the wound securely with a bandage or dressing and tape it or tie it in place. Do not tie it so tightly that blood flow to the rest of the body area is cut off. If bleeding seeps through, add more absorbent material. Do not remove the first bandage.

3. If bleeding does not stop with the pressure method, try to stop the bleeding by applying pressure to the artery that that delivers blood to the area of the injury (continue to apply pressure to the bleeding site). Do not apply pressure for longer than 5 minutes to an artery.

BURNS

Symptoms

First- and second-degree burns are not usually life-threatening.
First-degree burns cause only red skin and mild swelling.
Second-degree burns cause blisters, pain and oozing.
Third-degree burns can be life-threatening if extensive. Skin turns white or appears charred.

Treatment for first- and most second- degree burns

1. Place the victim's burned area under cold running water for 15 minutes. If this is not possible, immerse the burn in cool water or cool it with cold compresses. Don't put ice directly on the burn and don't apply butter.

2. For more severe burns, cover the burn area with clean, moist gauze and seek medical help.

3. After cooling minor burns, you can apply an aloe lotion, a triple antibiotic ointment or a moisturizer to prevent drying and to ease some of the discomfort.

Treatment for more extensive burns

1. Keep victim lying flat and lightly covered to prevent shock. Elevate the feet and legs if possible. Wrap or cover the burned area with a clean, moist cloth. Call or have someone call 911 (emergency) for an ambulance or medical help.

2. Remove clothes and jewelry unless they are sticking to burned skin. Do not immerse the victim in a cold bath or apply any type of ointment.

Special instructions

Electrical Burns—Turn off the source of electricity if possible. If not, use a non-conductive material, such as a board or wooden chair, to pull the victim away from the electrical source. Don't use your bare hands. If the victim is not breathing, begin chest compressions.

Chemical Burns of the Eye or Skin—Hold the victim's head or other burned area beneath a faucet. Turn on cool water at medium pressure. Rinse for at least 15 minutes, directing the water away from the unaffected area.

CHOKING

Symptoms

Choking is often caused by food or other foreign body lodged in the throat (airway). Symptoms include clutching at throat and is unable to speak; has trouble breathing or is unable to breathe; skin may turn blue, white or gray; loss of consciousness.

Treatment

1. If the victim can still talk, breathe or cough, don't interfere.

2. If the victim is unable to breathe, cough and talk, perform the Heimlich Maneuver as follows:

Heimlich Maneuver

1. Stand behind person, place both arms around his abdomen and clasp your hands just below the rib cage and above the navel. Make a fist with one hand, thumb side in. Grasp the fist with your other hand.

2. Give 3 or 4 quick forceful squeezes, pushing in and up until the object is coughed up. Keep your elbows away from your body. Be persistent. Continue the maneuver until the obstruction is relieved or medical help is available.

3. In the case of a collapsed person (who is conscious), extreme obesity or late pregnancy, lay the victim on their back and straddle them. Use chest thrusts by placing one hand on top of the other just above the navel and press upward.

4. If victim becomes unconscious, call 911 for emergency help. Lay victim down with head back. Use fingers sweep inside mouth to try and remove the foreign body. Use chest thrust as described above. If necessary, perform chest compressions until help arrives.

5. If the victim is a child under 12 months, turn him or her upside down (such as over your knee). Pat firmly between the shoulder blades with the heel of your hand until the object is dislodged.

Note: If you are alone and are choking, perform thrusts on yourself or thrust your abdomen against back of a chair, sink edge or railing, and push forcefully.

FRACTURES OR DISLOCATIONS

Symptoms

Extreme pain and tenderness in any injured area; change in appearance of injured part, such as swelling, protruding bone or blood under skin. An extremity, such as finger, arm or leg, may be bent out of normal alignment.

Treatment

1. Immobilize any injured area and don't move a broken limb unless absolutely necessary. Keep victim as warm and comfortable as you can. Control any bleeding. Call or have someone call 911 (emergency) for an ambulance or medical help.

2. If you must move a victim, improvise a splint from stiff rolled-up paper, scrap wood or metal. Pad the splint with clothing or blankets. The splint should extend beyond the joint on either end of the injury. Attach splint firmly to injured extremity with strips of cloth, twine or similar material to prevent movement (don't cut off the blood flow).

3. If leg, back or neck is severely injured and possibly fractured or dislocated, keep patient warm and still until ambulance arrives. Don't move the victim.

HEART ATTACK

Symptoms

Chest pain lasting more than 10 minutes that radiates into jaw or arm. Heavy sweating without obvious other cause. Weakness, nausea, pale skin. Irregular pulse.

Treatment

If Victim is Unconscious, Not Breathing

1. Yell for help. Don't leave victim.

2. Call or have someone call 911 (emergency) for an ambulance or medical help. The emergency operator may give you first-aid instructions to perform before emergency help arrives.

3. Place the heel of your hand in the middle of person's chest. Put your other hand on top of the first with your fingers interlaced. Compress the chest at least 2 inches (4-5 cm). Allow the chest to completely recoil before the next compression. Compress the chest at a rate of at least 100 pushes per minute until emergency help arrives.
(If trained and rescuer is able to perform rescue breaths, compressions and breaths should be provided in a ratio of 30 compressions to 2 breaths.)

If Victim is Unconscious and Breathing

1. Call or have someone call 911 (emergency) for an ambulance or medical help.

2. Give the person an aspirin. If possible, get the person into a relaxed sitting position, with the legs up and bent at the knees, to ease the strain on the heart. Loosen tight clothing around the neck and waist.

3. If you can't get help immediately, take patient to nearest emergency room or other facility with adequate equipment and personnel to care for medical emergencies.

Index

Guide to the Index

Alphabetical entries in the index include chart titles and subtitles from the:
Symptoms Section (these titles are shown in *italics*)
Illness & Disorders Section
Surgeries Section
Appendix Section (including Diets)

A

Abdominal Aortic Aneurysm Repair 706
Abdominal Pain, Recurrent Attacks 3
Abdominal Pain, Sudden Attack 4
Abdominal Swelling 6
Abdominoperineal Resection 708
Abdominoplasty 1046
Abortion 710
Abruptio Placenta 126
Abscess Drainage Superficial 712
Acne 127
Acne Rosacea 128
Acne Vulgaris 127
Acquired Immunodeficiency Syndrome 381
Actinic Keratosis 417
Acute Respiratory Syndrome, Severe 597
Addison's Disease 129
Adenoidectomy 1034
Adenomatous Hyperplasia of the Uterus 294
Adhesions, Separation of 714
Adhesive Capsulitis 602
Adjustment Disorders 130
Adrenal Gland Removal 716
Adrenal Insufficiency 129
Adrenalectomy 716
Adult Diet, Standard 1070
Agranulocytosis 131
AIDS & HIV 381
Alcoholism 132
Aldosteronism 384
Allergic Rhinitis 350
Allergic Shock 142
Allergy/Food Sensitivity Diet 1071
Alopecia Areata 133
Altitude Illness 134
Alzheimer's Disease 135
Amebiasis 136
Amebic Dysentery 136
Amenorrhea, Primary 137
Amenorrhea, Secondary 138
Amniocentesis 718

Amputation 720
Amyotrophic Lateral Sclerosis 139
Anal Fissure 140
Anal Fissure Treatment 722
Anal Fistula 141
Anal Fistula Repair 724
Anal Itching 555
Anaphylactoid Purpura 565
Anaphylaxis 142
Anemia, Aplastic 143
Anemia During Pregnancy 144
Anemia, Hemolytic 145
Anemia, Iron-Deficiency 146
Anemia, Pernicious 147
Aneurysm 148
Aneurysm Repair, Ventricular 726
Angina Pectoris 149
Angioplasty, Coronary 728
Angle-Closure Glaucoma 338
Animal Bites 150
Ankle Pain 7
Ankles, Swollen 8
Ankylosing Spondylitis 616
Anorectal Abscess 151
Anorexia Nervosa 152
Anterior Cruciate Ligament Reconstruction 730
Anxiety & Nervousness 9
Anxiety Disorder, Generalized 153
Aortoiliac Bypass Graft 732
Aortoiliofemoral Reconstruction 732
Aphthous Ulcers 199
Aplastic Anemia 143
Appendectomy 734
Appendicitis 154
Appetite Loss 11
Arm or Hand Pain 13
Arrhythmia 360
Arthritis, Infectious 155
Arthritis, Juvenile Idiopathic 156
Arthritis, Psoriatic 561
Arthritis, Reactive 571
Arthritis, Rheumatoid 157